Dermatology Essentials

Content Strategist: Russell Gabbedy
Content Development Specialist: Joanne Scott
Content Coordinator: Humayra Rahman Khan
Project Manager: Caroline Jones, Joanna Souch
Design: Christian J. Bilbow
Illustration Manager: Jennifer Rose
Illustrator: Antbits Ltd.
Marketing Manager(s): Gaynor Jones (UK), Brian McAllister (US)

Dermatology Essentials

Jean L. Bolognia MD
Professor of Dermatology
Yale Medical School
New Haven, CT, USA

Julie V. Schaffer MD
Associate Professor of Dermatology
and Pediatrics
Director of Pediatric Dermatology
New York University School of Medicine
New York, NY, USA

Karynne O. Duncan MD
Clinical Instructor of Dermatology
Yale Medical School
New Haven, CT, USA
Private Practice
St Helena, CA, USA

Christine J. Ko MD
Associate Professor of Dermatology
and Pathology
Yale Medical School
New Haven, CT, USA

For additional online content visit the expertconsult website: www.expertconsult.com

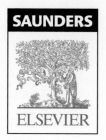

SAUNDERS

ELSEVIER

SAUNDERS

an imprint of Elsevier Inc.

Notices
Knowledge and best practice in this field are constantly changing. As new research and experience broaden our understanding, changes in research methods, professional practices, or medical treatment may become necessary.

Practitioners and researchers must always rely on their own experience and knowledge in evaluating and using any information, methods, compounds, or experiments described herein. In using such information or methods they should be mindful of their own safety and the safety of others, including parties for whom they have a professional responsibility.

With respect to any drug or pharmaceutical products identified, readers are advised to check the most current information provided (i) on procedures featured or (ii) by the manufacturer of each product to be administered, to verify the recommended dose or formula, the method and duration of administration, and contraindications. It is the responsibility of practitioners, relying on their own experience and knowledge of their patients, to make diagnoses, to determine dosages and the best treatment for each individual patient, and to take all appropriate safety precautions.

To the fullest extent of the law, neither the Publisher nor the authors, contributors, or editors, assume any liability for any injury and/or damage to persons or property as a matter of products liability, negligence or otherwise, or from any use or operation of any methods, products, instructions, or ideas contained in the material herein.

ISBN: 978-1-4557-0841-3
E-ISBN: 978-0-7020-5539-3

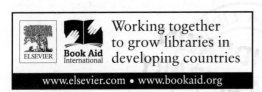

Working together
to grow libraries in
developing countries

www.elsevier.com • www.bookaid.org

Printed in China

Last digit is the print number: 9 8 7 6 5 4 3 2 1

Contents

Contents

Contents

Contents

For further reading and references, a cross-reference is made at the end of each chapter to the corresponding topic in *Dermatology Third Edition*, Bolognia, Jorizzo, & Schaffer, editors. ISBN 9780723435716, published by Elsevier.

Preface

The goal of our *Dermatology Essentials* handbook is to present the broad spectrum of cutaneous diseases in a manner that is straightforward and logical while at the same time maintaining a necessary level of sophistication. The text portion of each section is relatively brief and easy to review, with schematics and tables providing additional and more detailed information. Throughout the handbook are algorithms that present a practical approach to evaluation, differential diagnosis, and treatment of skin disorders. The clinical photographs were chosen with two key objectives in mind – to provide characteristic examples of specific diseases and to offer key teaching points. It is our hope that this handbook will improve the dermatologic care of patients and provide clinicians with greater confidence as they approach patients with cutaneous diseases.

Acknowledgments

We wish to thank all the dermatologists whose clinical photographs are used in this handbook as well as the textbook *Dermatology*. In particular we thank Kalman Watsky, MD, whose photographs appear throughout the book as well as on the front cover. The team at Elsevier has provided enormous support, including Joanne Scott, Humayra Rahman Khan, Dan Hays, Joanna Souch and Caroline Jones. Special thanks goes to Russell Gabbedy who has always delivered on his promises and found humor in our recurring demands.

The following were sourced from the **Yale Residents' Slide Collection**:

1.3c, 1.3f, 1.3h, 1.4aiii, 1.5b, 2.1b, 2.14, 2.17a, 4.15, 5.5b, 6.3b, 6.6a, 6.9a, 6.10, 6.8, 6.11, 6.15, 6.16a, 6.16c, 6.3c, 6.13, 6.14a, 6.14b, 7.2a, 7.2b, 7.3c, 7.3d, 7.3e, 7.5, 7.6a, 7.8, 7.9a, 8.2c, 8.5, 8.8, 9.4a, 9.4d, 9.4e, 9.4g, 9.4h, 9.5a, 9.5b, 9.5c, 9.7c, 9.8a, 9.8b, 10.5, 10.8a, 10.8b, 10.10a (inset), 10.11a, 12.8, 12.10c, 12.10e, 12.10f, 12.14, 12.18, 13.2b, 13.2i, 14.1a, 14.1c, 15.1a, 15.1b, 15.2a, 15.2b, 15.5, 17.3a, 17.3b, 17.3b, 17.8a, 17.9, 17.10b, 17.11a, 17.11b, 18.1d, 18.7, 18.8b, 18.8c, 18.10a, 19.2a, 19.2b, 19.4a, 19.4b, 19.5a, 19.5b, 19.10a,

19.10b, 19.10c, 20.2a, 21.2a, 21.5b, 21.6b, 21.7a, 22.1a, 22.1b, 22.1c, 22.1d, 22.7a, 22.7b, 24.1a, 24.1b, 24.3b, 24.3c, 24.5a, 24.9, 25.2a, 25.2b, 25.4a, 25.4b, 26.2a, 26.3b, 26.4a, 26.7a, 26.7c, 27.1, 28.2a, 28.2b, 28.5c, 28.6a, 28.6b, 28.11, 28.12b, 28.13, 28.14, 29.2c, 29.3b, 29.4b, 30.5b, 31.2a, 31.3a, 31.5, 31.6a, 31.6b, 31.11b, 31.11c, 32.2a, 32.3a, 32.5a, 32.5b, 33.2a, 33.2b, 33.2d, 33.2d, 33.2e, 33.2f, 33.2g, 33.4, 33.5, 33.6c, 33.8b, 33.9, 33.10, 33.3a, 34.2a, 32.10b, 35.5, 35.7, 35.10c, 36.3a, 36.3b, 36.5a, 36.10b, 38.2a, 38.2b, 38.5, 38.7b, 39.3a, 39.8b, 40.1, 41.2a, 41.4, 41.5a, 42.5b, 42.7b, 43.6a, 43.6b, 43.7a, 43.7b, 43.8e, 43.8f, 44.1e, 46.6a, 46.6b, 46.8c, 46.10b, 46.10c, 46.10d, 47.2b, 47.3b, 47.4b, 47.6b, 47.9, 47.10, 48.1b, 48.1d, 48.7, 48.1b, 48.9a, 48.9b, 49.3c, 51.2b, 51.3a, 51.3b, 51.3d, 51.8a, 52.2b, 52.8c, 53.2b, 53.12, 53.15, 54.12, 54.13, 54.15a, 54.15d, 54.15e, 54.15f, 54.15g, 54.16, 54.17, 54.18a, 54.19, 54.22a, 54.23a, 54.23b, 55.6b, 55.8b, 55.17b, 56.4a, 56.4d, 56.11c, 56.11d, 56.11e, 56.11g, 56.11h, 56.11j, 56.11k, 57.5, 58.10a, 58.13, 58.14a, 60.9a, 61.2b, 61.5, 61.8a, 61.8b, 61.11, 61.16, 62.9, 62.10, 62.11b, 62.13, 62.14, 62.15, 62.16a, 62.16b, 62.16c, 63.5, 63.6, 64.5d, 64.7, 64.8a, 64.8c, 64.10, 64.11, 64.13a, 64.13b, 64.13d, 64.13e, 64.15f, 64.19a, 64.25a, 64.25b, 64.25d, 64.25e, 65.2, 65.6, 65.8a, 65.8b, 65.10a, 65.12, 65.13, 65.16, 67.4a, 67.6a, 67.6b, 67.6c, 67.11a, 67.11c, 67.11e, 67.11f, 67.11g, 67.12a, 67.12b, 67.14a, 68.7a, 69.2b, 69.4a, 69.4b, 69.4c, 69.4d, 69.5a, 69.5b, 69.5c, 69.6a, 69.6b, 69.9, 69.12a, 69.12c, 70.1b, 71.2a, 71.2e, 71.10, 71.12a, 72.6, Table 72.1 (insets 1, 2, 3), 73.2c, 73.2h, 73.4a, 73.4c, 74.7b, 76.1a, 76.1c, 76.5, 76.6, 76.10, 76.12, 77.3, 77.4, 77.11, 78.1a, 78.1c, 78.1d, 78.1e, 78.2c, 78.3a, 78.3b, 78.4, 78.9a, 78.18, 79.2, 79.3a, 79.3b, 79.5, 80.1a, 80.1b, 80.1c, 80.2a, 80.2c, 80.3, 81.4b, 81.7, 82.2c, 82.3a, 83.7, 84.4b, 85.3, 85.4c, 85.6b, 85.17a, 85.23, 85.26, 85.27a, 85.27c, 86.2, 86.3a, 86.4a, 86.5e, 86.7, 86.10, 86.11b, 86.13b, 87.7, 87.13, 88.3a, 88.3b, 88.4, 88.6b, 88.6c, 88.7b, 88.9b, 89.1b, 89.7a, 89.7a, 89.10a, 90.1a, 90.2, 90.5b, 90.7, 90.10, 91.2, 91.3, 91.4, 91.5, 91.6, 91.7, 91.8a, 91.10, 91.12, 91.13, 91.14, 92.1, 92.4, 92.6, 92.7, 92.10b, 93.5e, 93.7a, 94.5, 94.9, 94.10, 95.5, 95.11, 95.12, 95.14, 95.16, 96.5a, 96.5b, 96.6, 99.1, 99.3a, 99.5, 100.1, 100.3b, and 100.3c.

The following were sourced from the **NYU Slide Collection**:
7.1b, 7.9b, 8.2a, 8.2b, 8.3, 8.4, 9.7b, 11.2b, 18.11, 19.1b, 20.3, 23.6b, 23.6c, 24.2, 36.2, 36.4b, 40.3a, 46.7b, 53.11a, 55.2a, 55.2b, 55.8a, 56.6b, 57.11, 59.4, 61.9c, 61.9d, 61.12, 63.7a, 63.7b, 65.5, 65.10b, 68.6a, 68.6b, 69.8, 71.12c, 73.2d, 73.3, 73.4b, 78.8a, 78.8b, and 81.6.

The following were sourced from the **USC Residents' Slide Collection**:
4.5, 36.8, 38.1, 51.7c, 54.14, 55.7e, 62.8a, 64.17a, 64.22a, 64.22b, 64.22c, 65.11, 71.2b, 71.2c, 82.2a, 85.29, 91.11, 94.12, and 99.6.

The following were sourced from the **SUNY Stony Brook Residents' Slide Collection**:
Figure 54.15c.

Chapter 58, Nail Disorders—Nail photos are courtesy of Antonella Tosti, the Yale Dermatology Residents' Slide Collection, Julie V. Schaffer, and Jean L. Bolognia.

Acknowledgments

Dedication

To our families, in particular our husbands – Dennis, Andy, David and Peter – who provided the indispensable support required to complete this book, from serving as sounding boards to creating quiet time in busy households.

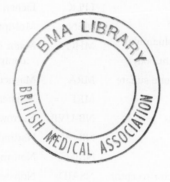

List of Abbreviations

ABI	Ankle-brachial index	EMG	Electromyography
AI-CTD	Autoimmune connective tissue disease	ESR	Erythrocyte sedimentation rate
AK	Actinic keratosis	G6PD	Glucose-6-phosphate dehydrogenase
ANA	Antinuclear antibody	GI	Gastrointestinal
ART	Anti-retroviral therapy	GVHD	Graft-versus-host disease
BB	Broadband	HIV	Human immunodeficiency virus
BCC	Basal cell carcinoma	HPV	Human papillomavirus
BID	Two times daily	HSCT	Hematopoietic stem cell transplant
BSA	Body surface area	HSV	Herpes simplex virus
CBC	Complete blood count	ICU	Intensive care unit
CMV	Cytomegalovirus	IFE	Immunofixation electrophoresis
CNS	Central nervous system	IL	Interleukin
CO	Carbon monoxide	IM	Intramuscularly
COPD	Chronic obstructive pulmonary disease	IV, iv	Intravenous
CRP	C-reactive protein	IVIg	Intravenous immunoglobulin
CS	Corticosteroids	KA	Keratoacanthoma
CSF	Cerebrospinal fluid	KOH	Potassium hydroxide
CT	Computed tomography	LDH	Lactate dehydrogenase
DDT	Dichlorodiphenyltrichloroethane (an insecticide)	LE	Lupus erythematosus
		LFTs	Liver function tests
Dx	Diagnosis	LPLK	Lichen planus-like keratosis
DDx	Differential diagnosis	MEN	Multiple endocrine neoplasia
DEET	N, N-diethyl-meta-toluamide	MHC	Major histocompatibility complex
DFA	Direct fluorescence antibody		
DHEAS	Dehydroepiandrosterone sulfate	MRA	Magnetic resonance angiography
DM	Diabetes mellitus	MRI	Magnetic resonance imaging
DVT	Deep vein thrombosis	NB-UVB	Narrowband UVB
EBV	Epstein-Barr virus	NK	Natural killer
ECG	Electrocardiogram	NMSC	Non-melanoma skin cancer
EGFR	Epidermal growth factor receptor	NSAIDs	Nonsteroidal anti-inflammatory drugs
ELISA	Enzyme-linked immunosorbant assay	OTC	Over-the-counter

PAS	Periodic-acid Schiff	STDs	Sexually transmitted diseases
PCR	Polymerase chain reaction	TB	Tuberculosis
PO, po	Per os (oral administration)	TCAs	Tricyclic antidepressants
PPD	Purified protein derivative	TID	Three times daily
PUVA	Psoralen plus ultraviolet A light	TNF	Tumor necrosis factor
RBC	Red blood cell	TSH	Thyroid stimulating hormone
RPR	Rapid plasma reagin (test for syphilis)	TST	Tuberculin skin test
		UVA	Ultraviolet A
Rx	Treatment	UVB	Ultraviolet B
SC, sc	Subcutaneous	UVA1	Ultraviolet A1 (340-400 nm)
SCC	Squamous cell carcinoma	UVR	Ultraviolet radiation
SLE	Systemic lupus erythematosus	VDRL	Venereal Disease Research Laboratory (test for syphilis)
SPEP	Serum protein electrophoresis		
SSRIs	Selective serotonin reuptake inhibitors	VZV	Varicella zoster virus
		XRT	Radiation therapy

List of Abbreviations

Basic Principles of Dermatology

1

- In the approach to the patient with a dermatologic disease, it is important to think initially of broad categories (Fig. 1.1); this allows for a more complete differential diagnosis and a logical approach.
- Key elements of any clinical description include distribution pattern (Table 1.1; Figs. 1.2 and 1.3), type of primary lesion and its topography (Table 1.2; Fig. 1.4), secondary features (Table 1.3), and its consistency via palpation (Tables 1.4 and 1.5).
- If atrophy is present, it should be categorized as epidermal, dermal, and/or subcutaneous (Fig. 1.5).
- Color is also an important feature, and this can be influenced by the skin phototype

DISTRIBUTION PATTERNS OF CUTANEOUS LESIONS
• Generalized versus localized (see Fig. 1.2) • Unilateral versus bilateral • If bilateral, symmetric or asymmetric pattern • Random versus linear (see Fig. 1.3) or grouped (e.g. herpetiform, clustered) • Special patterns – photodistributed versus photoprotected; along cleavage lines; areas of occlusion; areas of pressure; areas in contact with allergens or irritants

Table 1.1 Distribution patterns of cutaneous lesions.

CLASSIFICATION SCHEME FOR DERMATOLOGIC DISORDERS

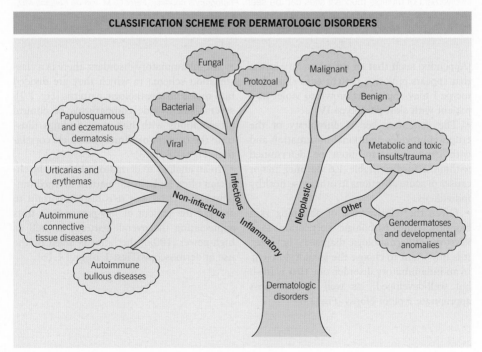

Fig. 1.1 Classification scheme for dermatologic disorders. This scheme is analogous to the structure of a tree with multiple branch points terminating in leaves.

DISTRIBUTION PATTERN – GENERALIZED VERSUS LOCALIZED

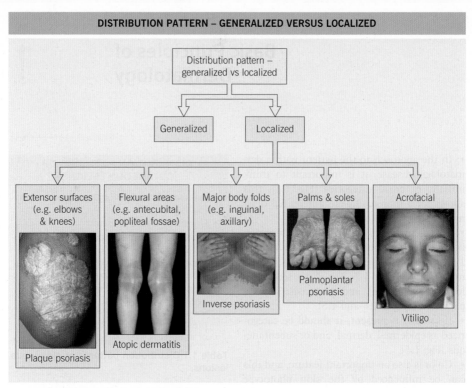

Fig. 1.2 Distribution pattern – generalized versus localized. In addition to these patterns, involvement of multiple mucosal sites can be seen. *Photographs courtesy, Peter C. M. van de Kerkhof, MD, Thomas Bieber, MD, and Julie V. Schaffer, MD.*

(Appendix) such that an inflammatory lesion that appears pink in a patient with skin phototype I may appear red-brown to violet in a patient with skin phototype IV.

• The acuteness versus chronicity of the eruption provides additional information and with experience can often be determined without a history; Table 1.6 outlines major causes of acute eruptions in otherwise healthy individuals.

• Given the relative ease of obtaining skin biopsies, clinicopathologic correlation is a keystone of dermatologic diagnosis; however, it is important to choose the ideal lesion (e.g. in an inflammatory disorder, one that is fresh but well-developed), as well as the most appropriate type of biopsy (Fig. 1.6).

• For inflammatory disorders, there is a classification schema in which they are divided into major histopathologic patterns (Fig. 1.7); several side-by-side comparisons of clinical presentations with histologic findings illustrate the concept of clinicopathologic correlation (Figs. 1.8–1.13).

• In an analogy to dermatopathology, the clinician often looks at the patient at 'medium-power' (i.e. 20×), but it is also important to analyze the patient at low-power (4×), thus appreciating the overall pattern, as well as high-power (100×); the latter is aided by the use of dermoscopy (Figs. 1.14 and 1.15).

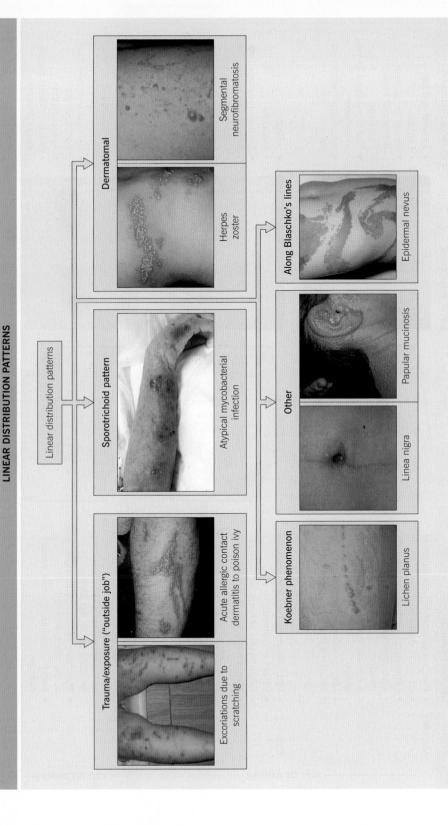

Fig. 1.3 Linear distribution patterns. *Photographs courtesy, Kathryn Schwarzenberger, MD, Jean L. Bolognia, MD, Whitney High, MD, Joyce Rico, MD, and Louis Fragola, MD.*

BASIC PRINCIPLES OF DERMATOLOGY

PRIMARY LESIONS – MORPHOLOGICAL TERMS

Term	Clinical Features		Clinical Example	Clinical Disorders
Macule	• Flat, circumscribed, nonpalpable • <1 cm in diameter • Often hypo- or hyperpigmented • Also other colors (e.g. pink, red, violet) • It can be round, oval, or irregular in shape • May be sharply marginated or blend into the surrounding skin		 Solar lentigines	• Ephelid (freckle) • Lentigo • Idiopathic guttate hypomelanosis • Petechiae • Flat component of viral exanthems • Junctional melanocytic nevus
Patch	• Flat, circumscribed, nonpalpable • >1 cm in diameter • Often hypo- or hyperpigmented • Also other colors (e.g. blue, violet		 Vitiligo	• Vitiligo • Melasma • Dermal melanocytosis (Mongolian spot) • Café-au-lait macule • Nevus depigmentosus • Solar purpura • Port wine stain (early)
Papule	• Elevated, circumscribed • <1 cm in diameter • Elevation due to increased thickness of the epidermis and/or cells or deposits within the dermis • May have secondary changes (e.g. scale, crust, erosion) • Need to distinguish from vesicle or pustule		 Seborrheic keratoses	• Seborrheic keratosis • Cherry hemangioma • Compound or intradermal melanocytic nevus • Verruca or molluscum contagiosum • Acrochordon • Milium, fibrous papule (angiofibroma)

←——— Related by size ———→

←——— Related by size ———→

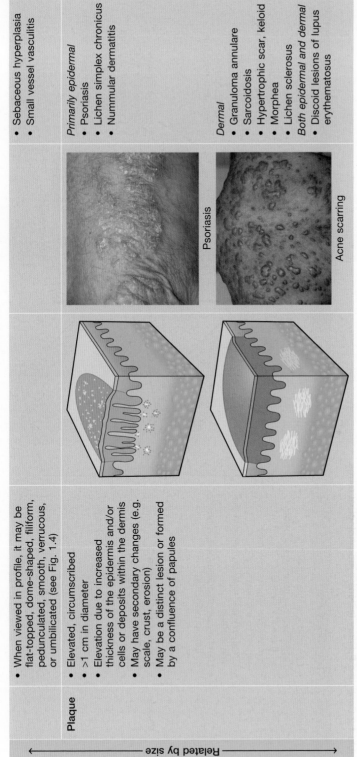

| | Plaque | • When viewed in profile, it may be flat-topped, dome-shaped, filiform, pedunculated, smooth, verrucous, or umbilicated (see Fig. 1.4)

• Elevated, circumscribed

• >1 cm in diameter

• Elevation due to increased thickness of the epidermis and/or cells or deposits within the dermis

• May have secondary changes (e.g. scale, crust, erosion)

• May be a distinct lesion or formed by a confluence of papules | Psoriasis | • Sebaceous hyperplasia
• Small vessel vasculitis

Primarily epidermal
• Psoriasis
• Lichen simplex chronicus
• Nummular dermatitis |
| Related by size | | | Acne scarring | *Dermal*
• Granuloma annulare
• Sarcoidosis
• Hypertrophic scar, keloid
• Morphea
• Lichen sclerosus
Both epidermal and dermal
• Discoid lesions of lupus erythematosus |

Table 1.2 Primary lesions – morphological terms. *Continued*

Table 1.2 *Continued* **Primary lesions – morphological terms.**

Term	Clinical Features		Clinical Example	Clinical Disorders
Nodule	• Elevated, circumscribed • Larger volume than papule, often >1.5 cm in diameter • Involves the dermis and may extend to the subcutis • Greatest mass may be beneath the skin surface • Can be compressible, soft, rubbery, or firm to palpation		 Epidermoid inclusion cysts	• Epidermoid inclusion cyst • Lipoma • Neurofibromas • Nodular melanoma • Metastases • Rheumatoid nodule • Panniculitis, e.g. erythema nodosum
Vesicle	• Elevated, circumscribed • <1 cm in diameter • Fluid-containing, usually clear but may be hemorrhagic • May become pustular, umbilicated, or an erosion		 Herpes zoster	• Herpes simplex • Varicella or zoster • Dyshidrotic eczema • Acute allergic contact dermatitis • Dermatitis herpetiformis

←— Related by size —→

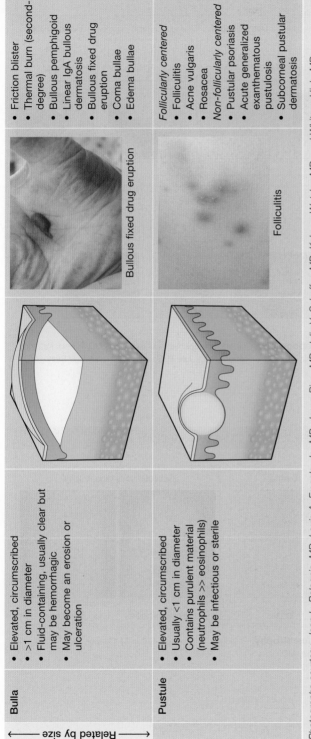

Bulla	• Elevated, circumscribed • >1 cm in diameter • Fluid-containing, usually clear but may be hemorrhagic • May become an erosion or ulceration		Bullous fixed drug eruption	• Friction blister • Thermal burn (second-degree) • Bullous pemphigoid • Linear IgA bullous dermatosis • Bullous fixed drug eruption • Coma bullae • Edema bullae
Pustule	• Elevated, circumscribed • Usually <1 cm in diameter • Contains purulent material (neutrophils >> eosinophils) • May be infectious or sterile		Folliculitis	*Follicularly centered* • Folliculitis • Acne vulgaris • Rosacea *Non-follicularly centered* • Pustular psoriasis • Acute generalized exanthematous pustulosis • Subcorneal pustular dermatosis

← Related by size →

Photographs courtesy, Jean L. Bolognia, MD, Louis A. Fragola, Jr., MD, Joyce Rico, MD, Julie V. Schaffer, MD, Kalman Watsky, MD, and Whitney High, MD.

DESCRIPTIVE TERMS FOR TOPOGRAPHY

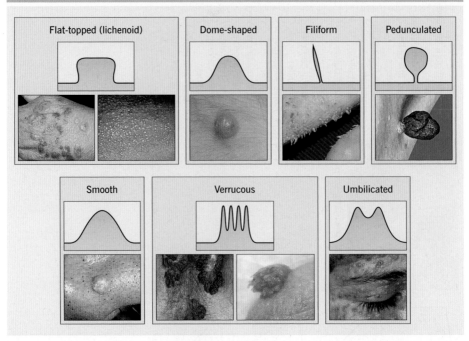

Fig. 1.4 Descriptive terms for topography. *Photographs courtesy, Jennifer Choi, MD, Hideko Kamino, MD, Reinhard Kirnbauer, MD, Petra Lenz, MD, Frank Samarin, MD, Julie V. Schaffer, MD, and Judit Stenn, MD.*

MAJOR TYPES OF CUTANEOUS ATROPHY

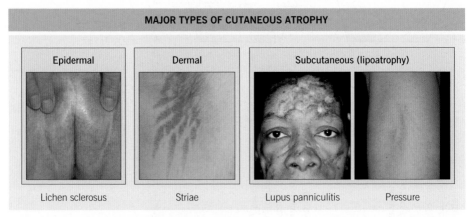

Fig. 1.5 Major types of cutaneous atrophy. *Photographs courtesy, Susan M. Cooper, MD, Fenella Wojnarowska, MD, and Jean L. Bolognia, MD.*

SECONDARY FEATURES – MORPHOLOGICAL TERMS			
Feature	**Description**		**Disorders**
Crust	• Dried serum (serous), blood (hemorrhagic), or pus on the surface • May include bacteria (usually *Staphylococcus*)	Secondarily infected hand dermatitis	• Eczema/dermatitis (multiple types) • Impetigo • Later phase of herpes simplex, varicella or zoster • Erythema multiforme
Scale	• Hyperkeratosis • Accumulation of stratum corneum due to increased proliferation and/or delayed desquamation • Represents a primary rather than a secondary feature in ichthyoses	Psoriasis	• Psoriasis (micaceous [silvery] scale) • Tinea (leading scale) • Erythema annulare centrifugum (trailing scale) • Actinic keratoses (gritty scale) • Pityriasis rosea (peripheral collarette of scale and central scale) • Seborrheic (greasy scale) • Tinea versicolor (powdery [furfuraceous] scale) • Lamellar ichthyosis (plate-like scale)
Fissure	• Linear cleft in skin • Often painful • Results from marked drying, skin thickening, and loss of elasticity	Hand dermatitis	• Angular cheilitis • Hand dermatitis • Sebopsoriasis (intergluteal fold) • Irritant cheilitis
Erosion	• Partial, or sometimes complete, loss of the epidermis (epithelium) • A moist, oozing, and/ or crusted lesion	Pemphigus foliaceus	• Impetigo • Friction • Trauma • Pemphigus, vulgaris and foliaceus • Staphyloccal scalded skin syndrome

Table 1.3 Secondary features – morphological terms. *Continued*

Table 1.3 *Continued* **Secondary features – morphological terms.**

Feature	Description		Disorders
Ulceration	• A deeper defect (compared to an erosion), with loss of at least the entire epidermis plus superficial dermis • May have loss of the entire dermis or even subcutis • Size, shape, and depth of the ulcer should be noted in addition to characteristics of the border, base, and surrounding skin	 Ulcer due to small vessel vasculitis	• Ecthyma gangrenosum • Pyoderma gangrenosum • Venous (stasis) ulcer • Ecthyma • Neuropathic ulcer • Arterial ulcer • Decubitus ulcer • Aphthous ulcer
Excoriation	• Exogenous injury to all or part of the epidermis (epithelium) • Usually due to scratching	 Neurotic excoriations	• A secondary feature of pruritic conditions, including arthropod bites and atopic dermatitis • Neurotic excoriations • Acne excoriée
Atrophy	• Epidermal atrophy – thinning of the epidermis, leading to wrinkling and a shiny appearance • Dermal atrophy – loss of dermal collagen and/or elastin, leading to a depression (see Table 1.4)	 Striae secondary to potent corticosteroids	• Lichen sclerosus • Poikiloderma • Anetoderma • Focal dermal hyoplasia (Goltz syndrome) • Striae
Lichenification	• Thickening (acanthosis) of the epidermis, and accentuation of natural skin lines	 Lichen simplex chronicus	• Lichen simplex chronicus, isolated or superimposed on a pruritic condition, e.g. atopic dermatitis

Photographs courtesy, Louis A. Fragola, Jr., MD, Jeffrey C. Callen, MD, Julie V. Schaffer, MD, and Whitney High, MD.

USE OF PALPATION IN ANALYZING CUTANEOUS LESIONS

Types of Lesion		Examples
Macules and patches (nonpalpable)	Non-palpable	• Solar lentigines • Idiopathic guttate hypomelanosis • Melasma • Vitiligo • Petechiae • Dermal melanocytosis
Papules and plaques (palpable)	Palpable Nests of nevus cells Fibrosis ← Epidermal → ← Dermal →	• Psoriasis • Lichen planus • Dermatitis • Intradermal or compound melanocytic nevus • Hypertrophic scar, keloid • Morphea
Atrophy – dermal and subcutaneous	Soft or depressed ← Dermal atrophy → ← Lipo- → atrophy (A) (B) (C)	(A) • Anetoderma (B) • Focal dermal hypoplasia (Goltz syndrome) (C) • Lipoatrophy due to corticosteroid injections • Lipoatrophy due to panniculitis

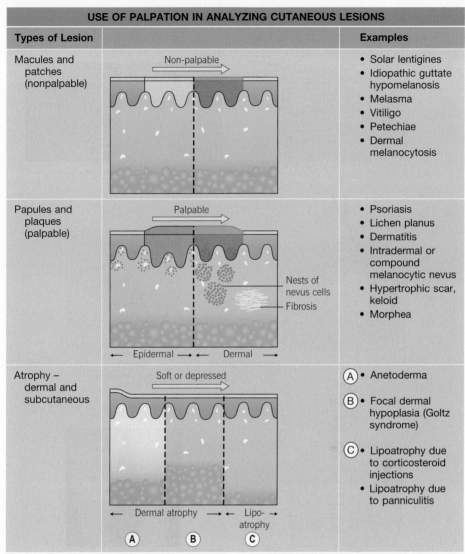

Table 1.4 Use of palpation in analyzing cutaneous lesions. *Courtesy, Whitney High, MD.*

PALPATION OF CUTANEOUS LESIONS

- Soft (e.g. intradermal nevus) versus firm (e.g. dermatofibroma) versus hard (e.g. calcinosis cutis, osteoma cutis)
- Compressible (e.g. venous lake) versus noncompressible (e.g. fibrous papule)
- Tender (e.g. inflamed epidermoid inclusion cyst, angiolipoma, leiomyoma) versus nontender
- Blanchable (e.g. erythema due to vasodilation) versus nonblanchable (e.g. purpura)
- Rough versus smooth
- Mobile versus fixed to underlying structures
- Dermal versus subcutaneous
- Temperature – normal versus elevated
- Other, e.g. thrill, pulsatile

Table 1.5 Palpation of cutaneous lesions.

DIFFERENT CUTANEOUS BIOPSY TECHNIQUES

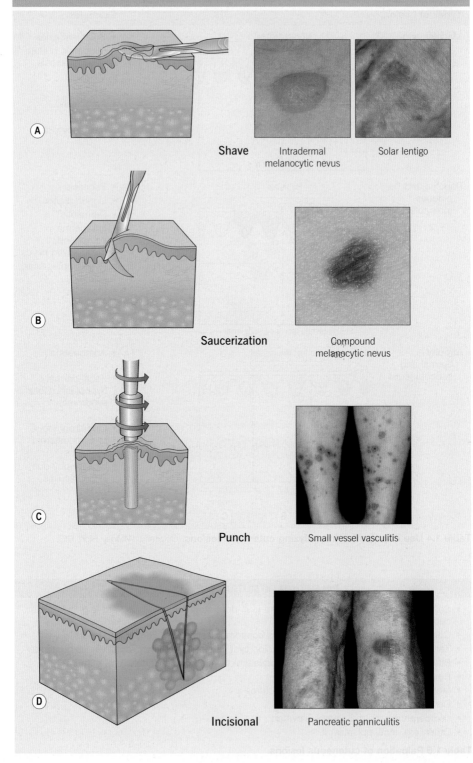

A Shave   Intradermal melanocytic nevus   Solar lentigo

B Saucerization   Compound melanocytic nevus

C Punch   Small vessel vasculitis

D Incisional   Pancreatic panniculitis

Fig. 1.6 Different cutaneous biopsy techniques. A Superficial shave biopsy can be performed to remove the elevated portion of an intradermal nevus or to distinguish a solar lentigo (pictured here) from lentigo maligna. **B** Deep shave biopsy (saucerization); performed to remove a compound melanocytic nevus or atypical melanocytic nevus. **C** Punch biopsy; performed to examine the dermis (as well as the epidermis) and the preferred technique for diagnosing cutaneous small vessel vasculitis. **D** Incisional biopsy; recommended for determining the specific type of panniculitis. *Courtesy, Suzanne Olbricht, MD, Raymond Barnhill, MD, Kenneth Greer, MD, and Frank Samarin, MD.*

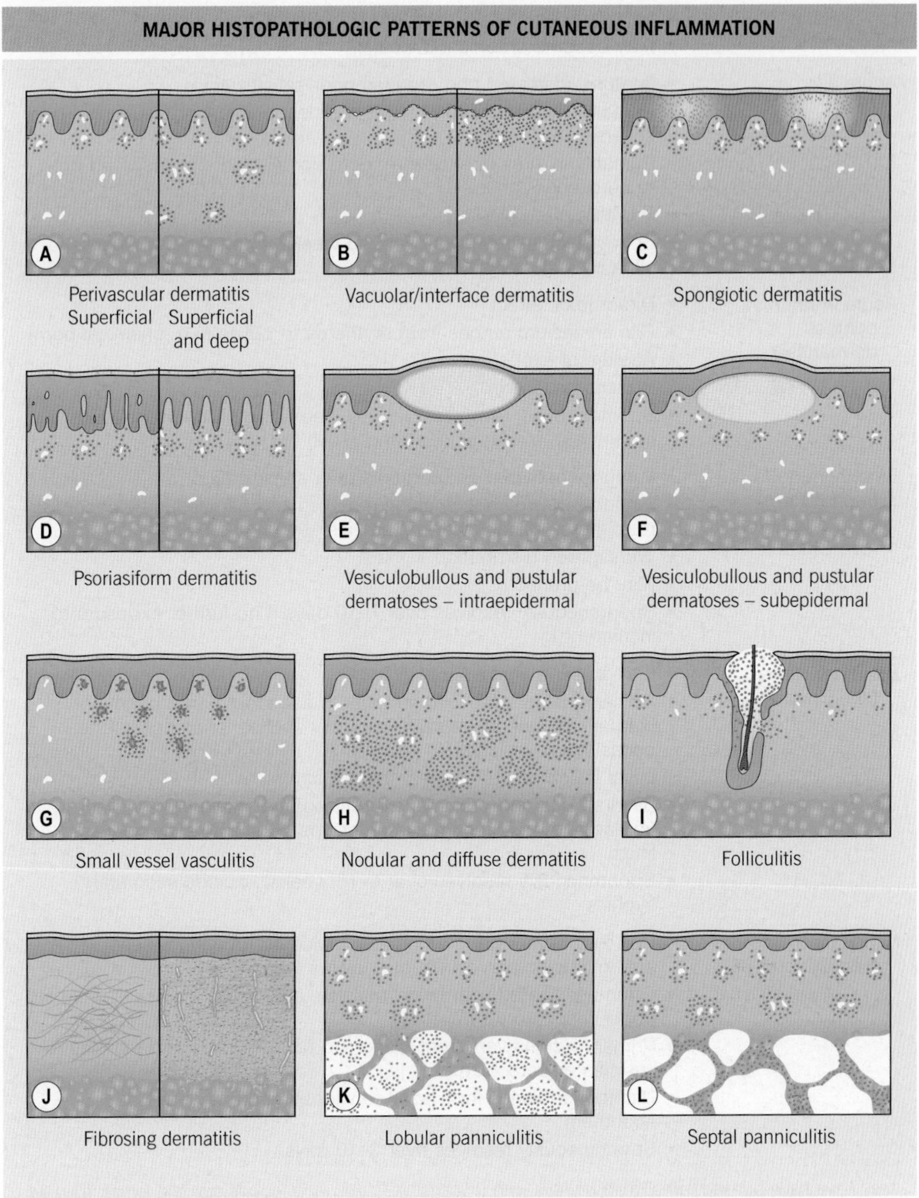

MAJOR HISTOPATHOLOGIC PATTERNS OF CUTANEOUS INFLAMMATION

A Perivascular dermatitis Superficial / Superficial and deep

B Vacuolar/interface dermatitis

C Spongiotic dermatitis

D Psoriasiform dermatitis

E Vesiculobullous and pustular dermatoses – intraepidermal

F Vesiculobullous and pustular dermatoses – subepidermal

G Small vessel vasculitis

H Nodular and diffuse dermatitis

I Folliculitis

J Fibrosing dermatitis

K Lobular panniculitis

L Septal panniculitis

Fig. 1.7 Major histopathologic patterns of cutaneous inflammation (based on Ackerman's classification). Basic patterns of inflammation result primarily from the distribution of the inflammatory cell infiltrate within the dermis and/or the subcutaneous fat (e.g. nodular, perivascular). It also reflects the character of the inflammatory process itself (e.g. pustular), the presence of injury to blood vessels (e.g. vasculitis), involvement of hair follicles (e.g. folliculitis), abnormal fibrous dermal and/or subcutaneous tissue, and formation of vesicles and bullae. *Adapted from Ackerman AB.* Histologic Diagnosis of Inflammatory Skin Diseases: A Method by Pattern Analysis. *Philadelphia: Lea & Febiger, 1978.*

ACUTE CUTANEOUS ERUPTIONS IN OTHERWISE HEALTHY INDIVIDUALS

Disorder	Characteristic Findings
Urticaria (see Chapter 14)	• Pathogenesis involves degranulation of mast cells with release of histamine • Primary lesion: edematous wheal with erythematous flare • Widespread distribution • Very pruritic* • Individual lesions are transient (<24 hours in duration) • May become chronic (>6 weeks)
Acute allergic contact dermatitis (See Chapter 12)	• Immune-mediated and requires prior sensitization • Primary lesion: dermatitis, with vesicles, bullae, and weeping when severe • Primarily in sites of exposure; occasionally more widespread due to autosensitization • Pruritus, often marked • Spontaneously resolves over 2–3 weeks if no further exposure to allergen (e.g. poison ivy, nickel)
Acute irritant contact dermatitis (see Chapter 12)	• Direct toxic effect • Primary lesion: ranges from erythema to bullae (e.g. chemical burn) • At sites of exposure • Burning sensation • Spontaneously resolves over 2–3 weeks if no further exposure to irritant (e.g. strong acid, strong alkali)
Exanthematous (morbilliform) drug eruptions (see Chapter 17)	• Immune-mediated and requires prior sensitization • Pink to red-brown, blanching macules and papules; may become purpuric on distal lower extremities • Widespread distribution • May be pruritic • Spontaneously resolves over 7–10 days if no further exposure to inciting drug
Pityriasis rosea (see Chapter 7)	• May follow a viral illness • Primary lesion: oval-shaped, pink to salmon-colored papule or plaque with fine white scale centrally and peripheral collarette; occasionally vesicular • Initial lesion is often largest (herald patch) • Favors trunk and proximal extremities; may have inverse pattern (axillae and groin); long axis of lesions parallel to skin cleavage lines • Spontaneously resolves over 6–10 weeks; exclude secondary syphilis
Viral exanthems (see Chapter 68)	• Due to a broad range of viruses, including rubeola, rubella, enteroviruses, parvovirus, adenovirus (see Fig. 68.1) • Often associated with fever, malaise, arthralgias, myalgias, nausea, upper respiratory symptoms • Primary lesions vary from blanching pink macules and papules to vesicles or petechiae • Distribution varies from acral to widespread; may have an enanthem • Spontaneously resolves over 3–10 days

*May have have burning rather than pruritus with urticarial vasculitis, and lesions can last longer than 24 hours.

Table 1.6 Acute cutaneous eruptions in otherwise healthy individuals.

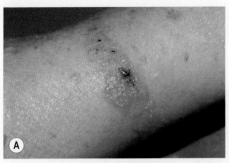

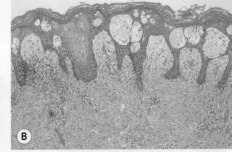

Fig. 1.8 Spongiotic dermatitis. A Acute allergic contact dermatitis to *Toxicodendron radicans* (poison ivy). The central black discoloration is due to the plant's resin. **B** Intercellular edema (spongiosis) and vesicle formation within the epidermis. Lymphocytes are also seen in both the epidermis and dermis. *A, Courtesy, Kalman Watsky, MD; B, Courtesy, James Patterson, MD.*

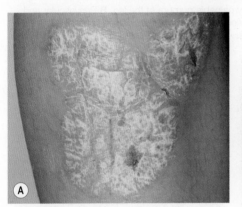

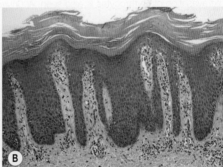

Fig. 1.9 Psoriasiform pattern. A Plaque of psoriasis vulgaris with silvery scale. **B** Regular epidermal hyperplasia and elongated dermal papillae with thin suprapapillary plates and confluent parakeratosis. The parakeratosis represents the histologic correlate of the visible scale. *A, Courtesy, Julie V. Schaffer, MD; B, Courtesy, Carlo F. Tomasini, MD.*

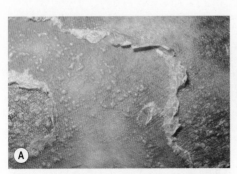

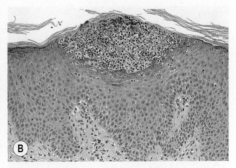

Fig. 1.10 Intraepidermal pustular dermatosis. A Pustular psoriasis. **B** Collection of neutrophils beneath the stratum corneum (subcorneal pustule). Scattered neutrophils are in the upper malpighian layer. *A, Courtesy, Kenneth Greer, MD; B, Courtesy, Lorenzo Cerroni, MD.*

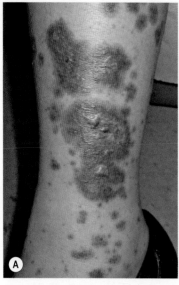

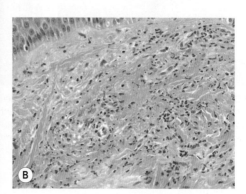

Fig. 1.11 Small vessel vasculitis. A Inflammatory palpable purpura of the leg. **B** Perivascular and interstitial infiltrate of neutrophils with nuclear dust (leukocytoclasia). Fibrin within the vessel wall and extravasation of erythrocytes is also seen. *A, Courtesy, Carlo F. Tomasini, MD; B, Courtesy, Christine Ko, MD.*

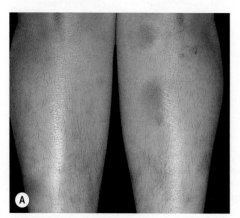

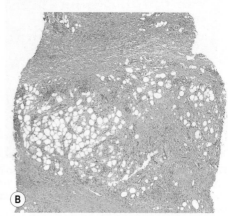

Fig. 1.12 Septal panniculitis. A Multiple red-brown nodules of erythema nodosum on the shins, admixed with healing bruise-like areas. **B** Predominantly septal granulomatous infiltrate with formation of characteristic Miescher's granulomas. *A, Courtesy, Kenneth Greer, MD; B, Courtesy, Christine Ko, MD.*

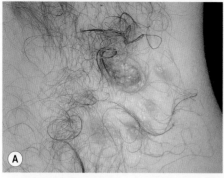

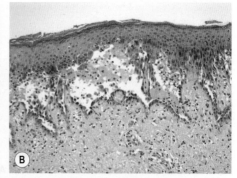

Fig. 1.13 Intraepidermal vesiculobullous dermatosis, acantholytic type. A Pemphigus vulgaris with flaccid bullae and erosions. **B** The keratinocytes within the lower epidermis have lost their intercellular attachments and have separated from one another, resulting in an intraepidermal blister. *A, Courtesy, Louis A. Fragola, Jr., MD; B, Courtesy, Carlo F. Tomasini, MD.*

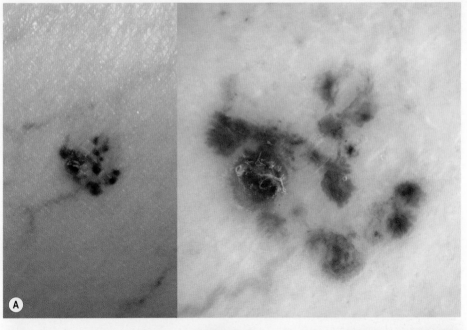

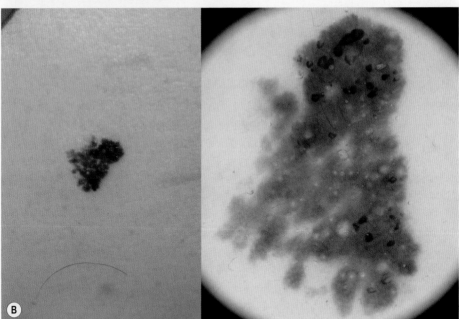

Fig. 1.14 Use of dermoscopy to aid in the diagnosis of four common pigmented (nonmelanocytic) cutaneous lesions. A Pigmented basal cell carcinoma with leaf-like areas (islands of blue-gray color) at the periphery and a small erosion of reddish color at the left side of the lesion. **B** Seborrheic keratosis with typical milia-like cysts (white shining globules) and comedo-like openings (black targetoid globules). *Continued*

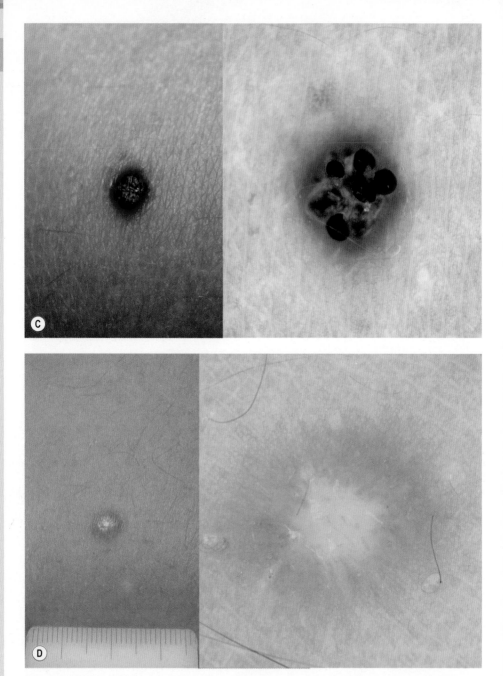

Fig. 1.14 *Continued* **C** Angiokeratoma with red-black lacunas clearly visible as well-demarcated roundish structures. **D** A dermatofibroma with characteristic central white patch and peripheral delicate pseudo-network. Dermoscopic features of melanocytic nevi and melanoma are reviewed in Chapters 92 and 93. *Courtesy, Giuseppe Argenziano, MD, and Iris Zalaudek, MD.*

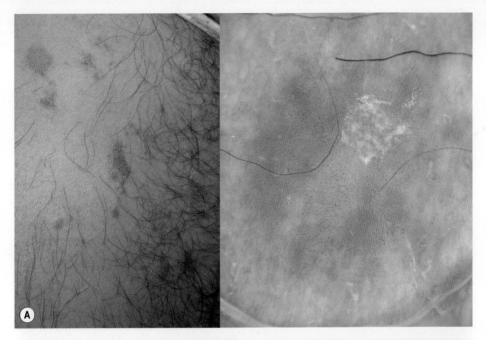

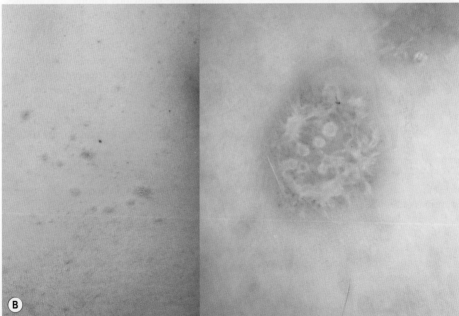

Fig. 1.15 Use of dermoscopy to aid in the diagnosis of inflammatory disorders. A By dermoscopy, classic psoriasis plaques exhibit regular dotted vessels. **B** The dermoscopic pattern of lichen planus is definitely different from the previous one. Here, dotted vessels are seen at the border of typical whitish lines and clods, which closely resemble the Wickham striae found in lichen planus of the oral mucosa. *Courtesy, Giuseppe Argenziano, MD, and Iris Zalaudek, MD.*

For further information see Ch. 0. From *Dermatology, Third Edition.*

2 | Bedside Diagnostics

- A range of bedside diagnostic procedures are performed to assist in the diagnosis of skin disorders.
- The most commonly performed procedures include microscopic examination of skin scrapings mounted in either potassium hydroxide (KOH) or mineral oil and microscopic examination of hair shafts.

Potassium Hydroxide (KOH) Preparation of Scales

- Microscopic examination of scale (stratum corneum), obtained via scraping with a metal blade or glass slide and mounted in KOH, is commonly performed to confirm superficial cutaneous fungal infections (Fig. 2.1).
- These fungal infections include tinea (pityriasis) versicolor, tinea corporis/faciei/manuum/cruris/pedis, and cutaneous candidiasis (see Chapter 64 on fungal diseases).
- Addition of chlorazol black to the KOH can improve detection (see Fig. 2.1B).
- Neither the genus nor the species of a dermatophyte can be determined by the KOH examination of scale.
- For onychomycosis, both nail plates and subungual debris are examined; in addition, nail plates can be fixed in formalin and stained with periodic acid–Schiff (PAS) or Gomori methenamine silver stain (see Chapter 64).

Potassium Hydroxide (KOH) Preparation of Hair Shafts

- Tinea capitis is divided into two major forms: (1) endothrix – conidia occur within the hair shaft; and (2) ectothrix – while the fungus grows inside the hair shaft, conidia form on its surface (Figs. 2.2 and 2.3; see Chapter 64).

- For KOH examination and fungal culture, fragile and broken hairs are preferred and can be obtained by scraping with a metal knife or, in children, a sterile toothbrush or moistened cotton applicator (Q-tip).

Mineral Oil Scraping for Suspected Scabies

- Place 2–3 drops of mineral oil on a glass slide. Dip the metal blade into the oil and then scrape suspicious lesions, e.g. burrows, inflammatory papules. Next place skin scrapings on a glass slide. Several skin lesions should be scraped. Dermoscopy can be used to better identify burrows and an adult female mite at the end of the burrow prior to scraping (see Chapter 71). Sometimes, KOH is used rather than mineral oil. Firm application of transparent adhesive tape to suspicious lesions followed by rapid removal and transfer to a glass slide is another technique that can be used, providing easier transport to a laboratory.
- In addition to adult mites, eggs and feces (scybala) can be seen when scrapings are examined microscopically (Figs. 2.4 and 2.5).

Tzanck Smear

- The advent of direct fluorescent antibody (DFA) and polymerase chain reaction (PCR) assays to detect herpes simplex and varicella–zoster viral infections has led to a decline in the performance of Tzanck smears.
- Nonetheless, it can serve as rapid, easy-to-perform bedside test and is most sensitive when an intact vesicle or bulla is present; in immunocompromised hosts, crusted lesions may also be positive.
- The roof is retracted and scraping of the base and angles of the vesicle should be

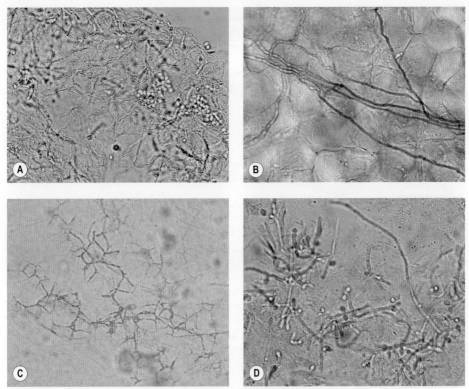

Fig. 2.1 Microscopic examination of potassium hydroxide (KOH) preparations of scale.
A Tinea (pityriasis) versicolor due to *Malassezia* spp. with short mycelial forms and clusters of yeast forms. **B** Tinea corporis due to a dermatophyte with hyphae that cross over more than one cell (squame) and are branching. Chorazol black has been added to the KOH and the stained hyphae are easier to detect. **C** Branching mosaic pattern that represents the junctures of normal epidermal cells; this is a cause of false-positive KOH exams. **D** Cutaneous candidiasis with yeast forms and pseudohyphae. Pseudohyphae can sometimes be difficult to distinguish from hyphae. *A, Courtesy, Ronald Rapini, MD; C, Courtesy, Louis Fragola, MD; D, Courtesy, Frank Samarin, MD.*

performed in order to obtain virally infected keratinocytes, which are thinly spread onto a glass slide, allowed to dry, and then stained with Giemsa stain (Figs. 2.6 and 2.7).

Microscopic Examination of Molluscum Bodies

• In some patients, lesions of molluscum contagiosum may not have a classic appearance – e.g. due to inflammation, previous treatments, large size – and confirmation of the diagnosis without performing a skin biopsy can be helpful.
• The center of the papulonodule, which is often paler in color, is gently curetted to remove a core composed of the viral particles,

and the contents are then thinly spread onto a glass slide; saline or KOH can be added prior to placing the coverslip (Fig. 2.8).

Gram Stain

• Performed when pustular material is available and identifies both gram-positive and gram-negative bacteria (Fig. 2.9).
• In addition, fungal organisms (e.g. *Candida*) can be identified.

Dermal Scrapings and Touch Preps

• When there is suspicion of a septic embolus or a primary infection involving the dermis and/or subcutis (bacterial, fungal, parasitic),

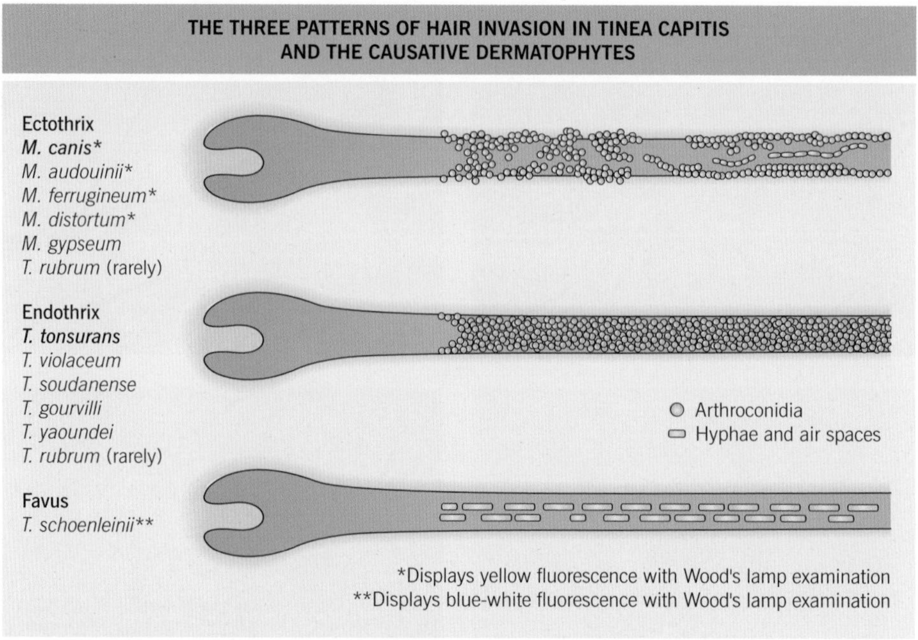

THE THREE PATTERNS OF HAIR INVASION IN TINEA CAPITIS AND THE CAUSATIVE DERMATOPHYTES

Ectothrix
M. canis*
*M. audouinii**
*M. ferrugineum**
*M. distortum**
M. gypseum
T. rubrum (rarely)

Endothrix
T. tonsurans
T. violaceum
T. soudanense
T. gourvilli
T. yaoundei
T. rubrum (rarely)

○ Arthroconidia
▭ Hyphae and air spaces

Favus
*T. schoenleinii***

*Displays yellow fluorescence with Wood's lamp examination
**Displays blue-white fluorescence with Wood's lamp examination

Fig. 2.2 The three patterns of hair invasion in tinea capitis and the causative dermatophytes. See Chapter 64 for additional details.

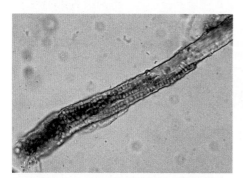

Fig. 2.3 Microscopic examination of a KOH preparation of a hair shaft with an endothrix dermatophyte infection (tinea capitis). The most common species for endothrix infections is *Trichophyton tonsurans*. Chlorazol black has been added to the KOH.

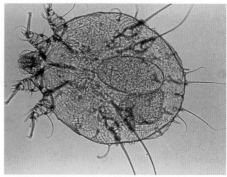

Fig. 2.4 Microscopic examination of scrapings from a patient with scabies. Female *Sarcoptes scabiei* var. *hominus* mite with eggs. There is a flattened, oval body with wrinkle-like corrugations and eight legs. *With permission from Taplin D, Meinking TL. Infestations. In: Schachner LA, Hansen RC (Eds.), Pediatric Dermatology, 4th edn. Edinburgh, UK: Mosby, 2011:1141–1180.*

then in addition to a sterile skin biopsy (Fig. 2.10), a touch prep or a dermal scraping can be performed. Often, the patient is immunocompromised. If there is pustular drainage, then a Gram stain and KOH preparation is performed first.

• In a touch prep, the base of a skin biopsy which includes dermis ± subcutis is tapped multiple times against a glass slide. After

drying for several minutes, the glass slide is stained (e.g. Gram stain, Giemsa stain; Fig. 2.11).

• In a dermal scraping, the epidermis (if present) is reflected back after injection of

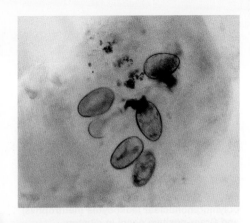

Fig. 2.5 Microscopic examination of scrapings from a patient with scabies. Both oval-shaped eggs and scybala (feces) are seen. *Courtesy, Craig N. Burkhart, MD, and Craig G. Burkhart, MD.*

DEMONSTRATION OF LOCATION OF VIRALLY INFECTED KERATINOCYTES IN VESICULOBULLOUS LESIONS OF HERPES SIMPLEX, VARICELLA AND HERPES ZOSTER

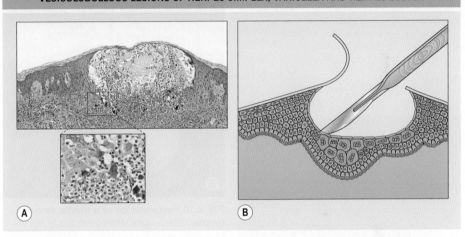

Ⓐ   Ⓑ

Fig. 2.6 Demonstration of location of virally infected keratinocytes in vesiculobullous lesions of herpes simplex, varicella, and herpes zoster. A Histologically, viral changes (e.g. multinucleated giant cells) are seen at the base of the vesicle; note their absence on the roof. **B** Scraping of the base of the vesicle is performed after the roof of the blister is reflected. *A, Courtesy, Lorenzo Cerroni, MD.*

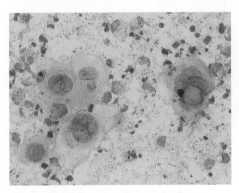

Fig. 2.7 Tzanck smear demonstrating multinucleated giant cells. Such cells are seen in herpes simplex, varicella, and herpes zoster viral infections (Giemsa stain). *Courtesy, Louis Fragola, MD.*

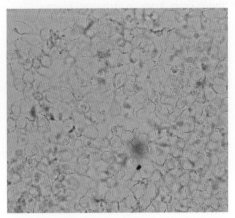

Fig. 2.8 Large, round molluscum bodies are present in a scraping of the center of a papulonodule. The scrapings can be mounted in saline or KOH solution. *Courtesy, Bradley Bloom, MD.*

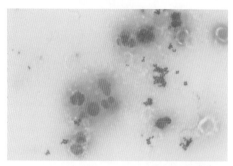

Fig. 2.9 Gram stain of pus demonstrating polymorphonuclear leukocytes (neutrophils) and Gram-positive cocci in clusters (*Staphylococcus aureus*). *From Ekkelenkamp, MB, Rooijakkers, SHM, Bonten, MJM. In: Cohen J, Powderly W, Opal S (Eds.),* Infectious Diseases, *3rd edn. Edinburgh, UK: Mosby, 2010.*

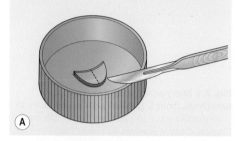

(A)

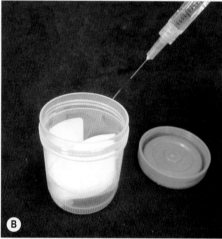

(B)

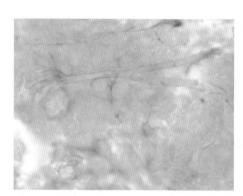

Fig. 2.11 Microscopic examination of a 'touch prep' from an incisional biopsy performed of a necrotic lesion on the chest of an immunocompromised patient. Note the branching, ribbon-like, nonseptate hyphae characteristic of *Rhizopus*. *Courtesy, Jean L. Bolognia, MD.*

Fig. 2.10 Performance of a sterile skin biopsy. This is done when there is a suspicion of a septic embolus or primary skin infection of the dermis and/or subcutis. The equipment required includes a chemical antiseptic (e.g. chlorhexidine), alcohol pads, local anesthetic, punch biopsy instrument or scalpel, sterile scissors and forceps, sterile urine cup containing sterile gauze dampened with nonbacteriostatic saline, and glass slides. Following cleansing of the skin (antiseptic followed by alcohol), the skin is injected with local anesthesia, and a biopsy of dermis plus subcutaneous fat is performed (see Chapter 1). **A** The specimen is cut into two pieces on the sterile side of the urine container lid, while avoiding compression of the tissue. **B** One piece is placed in a sterile urine cup with moistened gauze, and the bottom of the second piece is tapped several times against a glass slide before being placed in formalin. The sealed sterile urine cup is hand carried to the microbiology laboratory.

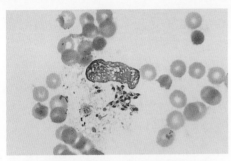

Fig. 2.12 Dermal tissue obtained from a skin slit and scraping of a cutaneous lesion of leishmaniasis shows amastigotes within macrophages. *From Peters W, Pasvol G.* Tropical Medicine and Parasitology, *6th edn. London: Mosby, 2007.*

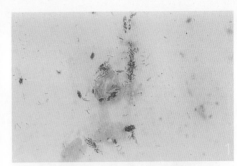

Fig. 2.13 Smear stained with a Ziehl–Neelsen stain demonstrating acid-fast bacilli in a patient with leprosy. *From Peters W, Pasvol G.* Tropical Medicine and Parasitology, *6th edn. London: Mosby, 2007.*

local anesthesia, and a curette is used to scrape dermal tissue onto a slide.

Giemsa Stain for Eosinophils or Amastigotes

• Identification of eosinophils can assist in distinguishing the pustulovesicular lesions of erythema toxicum neonatorum from neonatal pustular melanosis and congenital candidiasis.
• A skin slit and scraping of cutaneous lesions of leishmaniasis demonstrate amastigotes in macrophages when stained with a Giemsa stain (Fig. 2.12).

Acid-Fast Stain for Leprosy

• When leprosy is suspected, a fold of skin is firmly squeezed and a small incision is made with a scalpel, with the liquid expressed smeared onto a slide, allowed to dry, and stained with a Fite or Ziehl–Neelsen stain (Fig. 2.13).
• For bacilloscopy, the skin sites that are examined include the earlobes, forehead, chin, extensor forearms, dorsal fingers, buttocks, and trunk.
• While acid-fast *Mycobacterium leprae* organisms are found in ≤5% of patients with tuberculoid leprosy, they are seen in 100% of patients with lepromatous leprosy (see Chapter 62 on mycobacteria).

Evaluation of Folliculitis

• While the most common forms of folliculitis are associated with normal flora or *Staphylococcus aureus*, there are forms due to gram-negative rods (e.g. *Pseudomonas*), *Pityrosporum* (*Malassezia*) spp., herpes simplex, and *Demodex* spp.
• For bacteria, cultures are the primary means of diagnosis, but for *Pityrosporum* and *Demodex* folliculitis, bedside diagnosis is key (Fig. 2.14).

Dark Field Microscopy for Treponemal Infections

• Dark field microscopy is utilized for the examination of unstained live organisms and in dermatology, primarily for the diagnosis of primary syphilis and less often secondary cutaneous syphilis (see Chapter 69).
• Expressed serous exudate with a minimal number of red blood cells is placed on slide and then a coverslip applied.
• The *Treponema* spirochetes have a characteristic morphology and movement pattern (Fig. 2.15).

Hair Shaft Examination

• Assessment of hair thinning, which may be due to miniaturization, shedding, or breakage, most commonly includes a gentle hair pull and a hair shaft examination of cut,

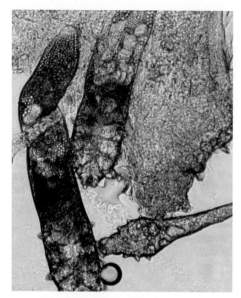

Fig. 2.14 Microscopic examination of follicular contents in a patient with *Demodex* folliculitis.

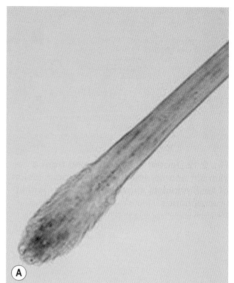

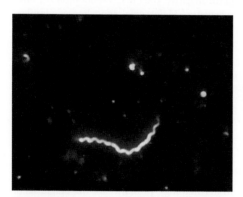

Fig. 2.15 Dark field microscopic examination of a spirochete. Treponemes are recognized by their characteristic corkscrew shape and deliberate forward and backward movement with rotation about the longitudinal axis. *From Morse et al. Atlas of Sexually Transmitted Diseases and AIDS, 3rd edn. London: Mosby; 2003.*

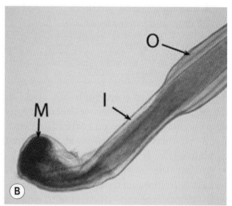

Fig. 2.16 Comparison of a telogen versus anagen hair shaft. A A telogen hair shaft has a club-shaped bulb. **B** An anagen hair has attached root sheaths as well as a pigmented and distorted bulb, sometimes resembling a hockey stick. M, matrix; I, inner root sheath; O, outer root sheath. *B, Courtesy, Leonard Sperling, MD.*

rather than pulled, hairs; some clinicians also do a vigorous hair pluck referred to as a trichogram (20–40 scalp hairs grasped by a hemostat with rubber-covered jaws).

• In general, telogen hairs are observed with a gentle hair pull, but in disorders such as loose anagen syndrome, anagen hairs may be seen (see Chapter 56 on alopecia).

• In a trichogram, the ratio of anagen:telogen hairs is determined by microscopic examination of the hair bulbs (Fig. 2.16). The normal anagen-to-telogen ratio is 9 : 1, but in telogen effluvium, it can be 7 : 3 or less.

• Hair shaft examination can also detect bacterial and fungal infections (e.g. trichomycosis

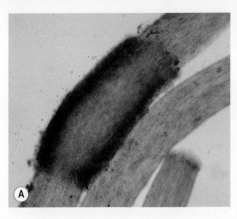

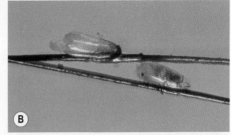

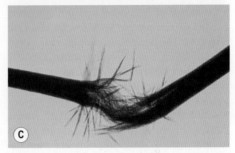

Fig. 2.17 Hair shaft examination as a diagnostic tool. A Nodule composed of numerous conidia of *Trichosporon inkin* in a patient with white piedra. **B** Two head louse egg casings (nits) are seen attached to hair shafts. **C** In trichorrhexis nodosa, the two ends of the hair shaft resemble opposing broomsticks. *B, With permission from Taplin D, Meinking TL. Infestations. In: Schachner LA, Hansen RC (Eds.), Pediatric Dermatology, 4th edn. Edinburgh, UK: Mosby, 2011:1141–1180; C, Courtesy, Christine Ko, MD.*

axillaris, white piedra, black piedra), hair casts, nits due to head lice infestation, and hair shaft abnormalities (e.g. trichorrhexis nodosa) (Fig. 2.17) (see Chapters 56, 64, and 71).

• For optimal detection of hair shaft abnormalities, mounting in Permount (an adhesive composed of polymers dissolved in toluene) is performed.

• Another bedside diagnostic procedure is the identification of lice, insects (e.g. bedbugs), and arachnids (e.g. ticks). Chapters 71 and 72 review their identification via macroscopic and microscopic findings.

3 | Fever and Rash

- A variety of infectious and inflammatory conditions can present with fever and a rash (Fig. 3.1). The cutaneous findings range from a morbilliform eruption or urticaria (Figs. 3.2 and 3.3) to confluent erythema (Fig. 3.4) to petechial, vesiculobullous, and pustular lesions (Figs. 3.5–3.9).
- Clinical features that differentiate among entities in the differential diagnosis of an exanthematous drug eruption are summarized in Fig. 3.10.
- Although the initial skin findings of some potentially life-threatening disorders can mimic a more common benign disorder, the development of other cutaneous and extracutaneous features as the condition evolves points to the correct diagnosis (Table 3.1).

Kawasaki Disease

- Acute febrile multisystem vasculitic syndrome that primarily affects children <5 years of age (rarely adults), with ~3-fold higher incidence in Asians than Caucasians.
- Most common cause of pediatric acquired heart disease in the United States, with greatest morbidity from coronary artery aneurysms.
- Etiology remains unknown; factors include a genetic predisposition to immune activation and possibly an infectious trigger.
- Diagnostic criteria include fever (>39°C/102°F) for ≥5 days plus the presence of ≥4 of the following five criteria.
  - Bilateral nonpurulent bulbar conjunctival injection.
  - Oropharyngeal changes such as 'chapped'/ fissured lips (Fig. 3.11), a 'strawberry' tongue, and diffuse hyperemia.
  - Cervical lymphadenopathy (>1.5 cm; usually unilateral).
  - Erythema, edema, and (eventually) desquamation of the hands and feet (Fig. 3.12A).

- Polymorphous exanthem – morbilliform or urticarial > erythema multiforme-like (Fig. 3.12B), scarlatiniform, or pustular.
- Initial manifestation is often erythema in the perineal area, followed by desquamation (Fig. 3.12B–3.12D).
- 'Incomplete' Kawasaki disease (more common in infants) is diagnosed if fever for ≥5 days and coronary artery abnormalities (via echocardiography or angiography) but <4 other criteria.
- Other cardiac (e.g., myo-/pericarditis, valvular abnormalities), CNS (e.g., irritability, aseptic meningitis), musculoskeletal (e.g., arthritis), gastrointestinal, and genitourinary involvement can occur.
- Laboratory findings of acute disease include leukocytosis with neutrophilia, anemia, elevated ESR/CRP and hepatic transaminase levels, hypoalbuminemia and sterile pyuria; thrombocytosis typically develops by the 2nd or 3rd week (occasionally thrombocytopenia early).
- **DDx:** viral exanthem, scarlet fever, toxic shock syndrome, early staphylococcal scalded skin syndrome, drug reaction, erythema multiforme, Still's disease, periodic fever syndrome.
- **Rx:** IVIg and aspirin are first-line; corticosteroids and infliximab are options for refractory disease.

Periodic Fever Syndromes

- Group of hereditary autoinflammatory disorders that feature recurrent episodes of fever and rash (Table 3.2).
- Cutaneous findings, which range from erysipeloid erythema to urticarial eruptions, represent clues to the underlying diagnosis.
- Acute inflammation in other organ systems can lead to manifestations such as arthritis, serositis, and conjunctivitis; over time, secondary systemic amyloidosis may develop.

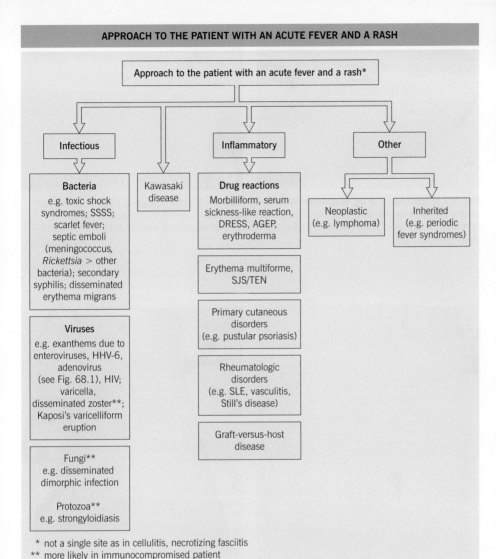

* not a single site as in cellulitis, necrotizing fasciitis
** more likely in immunocompromised patient

Fig. 3.1 Approach to the patient with an acute fever and a rash. AGEP, acute generalized exanthematous pustulosis; DRESS, drug reaction with eosinophilia and systemic symptoms (also referred to as drug-induced hypersensitivity syndrome [DIHS]); HHV, human herpes virus; HIV, human immunodeficiency virus; SJS, Stevens–Johnson syndrome; SLE, systemic lupus erythematosus; SSSS, staphylococcal scalded skin syndrome; TEN, toxic epidermal necrolysis.

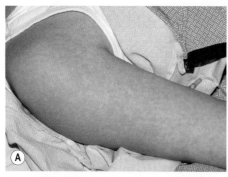
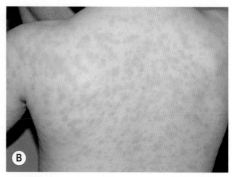

Fig. 3.2 Morbilliform drug eruptions. A Fine pink macules and thin papules, becoming confluent on the posterior upper arm, which is a dependent area in this hospitalized patient. **B** More edematous ('urticarial') pink papules; unlike true urticaria, these lesions are not transient. *Courtesy, Julie V. Schaffer, MD.*

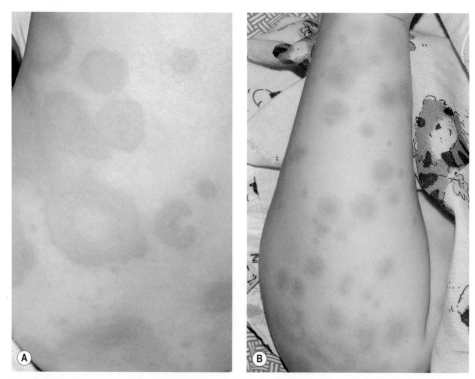

Fig. 3.3 Urticaria and serum sickness-like reaction. A Giant annular urticaria (urticaria 'multiforme') in a young child with a recent viral upper respiratory tract infection. Individual lesions last <24 hours, but they often resolve with a dusky purplish hue that can lead to misdiagnosis as erythema multiforme. **B** Serum sickness-like reaction due to amoxicillin. Some of the urticarial papules and annular plaques have a purpuric component, and the eruption was accompanied by high fevers, lymphadenopathy, arthralgias, and acral edema. *Courtesy, Julie V. Schaffer, MD.*

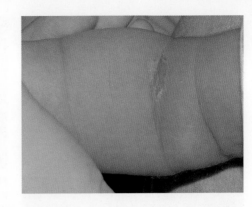

Fig. 3.4 Staphylococcal scalded skin syndrome. Diffuse, tender erythema, with an early superficial erosion in the antecubital fossa. *Courtesy, Julie V. Schaffer, MD.*

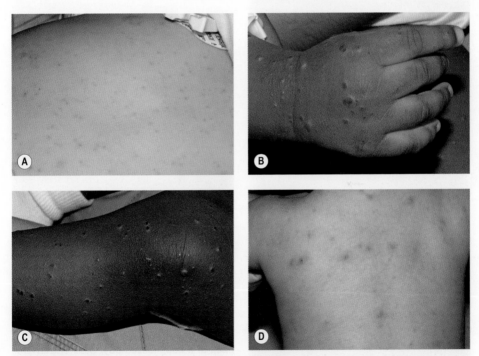

Fig. 3.5 Viral exanthems. A Enteroviral exanthem presenting as widespread small pink papules, many with petechiae centrally. **B, C** Widespread vesicular eruption due to coxsackievirus A6 infection. **D** Scattered vesicles on erythematous bases in varicella, with lesions in different stages of evolution. *Courtesy, Julie V. Schaffer, MD.*

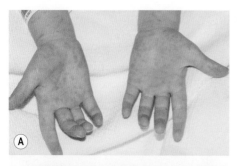

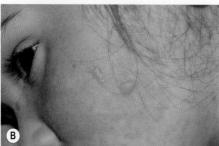

Fig. 3.6 Stevens–Johnson syndrome. The patient initially developed multiple small pink papules mimicking a morbilliform eruption, but with accentuation on the palms **(A).** A day later, confluent erythema and bullae had developed **(B),** and involvement of the vermilion lips and conjunctiva was evident. *Courtesy, Julie V. Schaffer, MD.*

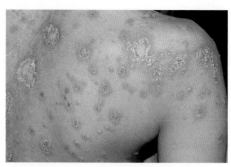

Fig. 3.8 Pustular psoriasis in a pediatric patient. Multiple sterile papulopustules and expanding annular red plaques with pustulation at the advancing edge. This eruption was widespread and associated with fever and malaise. *Courtesy, Julie V. Schaffer, MD.*

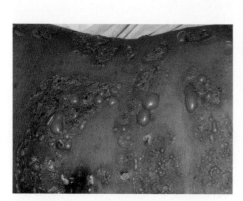

Fig. 3.7 Bullous pemphigoid. Multiple tense bullae and crusted erosions on a background of erythematous skin. *Courtesy, Julie V. Schaffer, MD.*

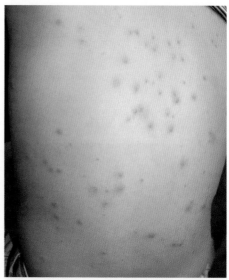

Fig. 3.9 Staphylococcal folliculitis on the back of a hospitalized boy. Other eruptions with a predilection for occluded sites such as the back of a bedridden patient include miliaria rubra (especially if febrile), non-infectious folliculitis, Grover's disease (in the setting of chronic photodamage), and candidiasis. *Courtesy, Julie V. Schaffer, MD.*

APPROACH TO THE PATIENT WITH A SUSPECTED DRUG-INDUCED EXANTHEM

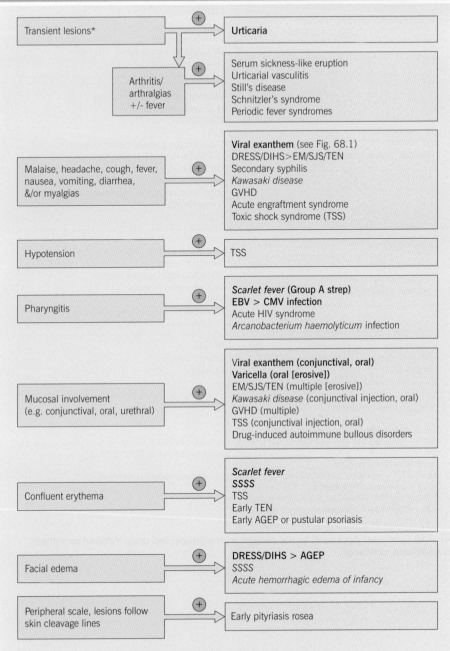

*Individual lesions last <24 hours, which can be documented by outlining them with ink; exceptions include urticarial vasculitis and, occasionally, Schnitzler's or periodic fever syndromes

Fig. 3.10 Approach to the patient with a suspected drug-induced exanthem (morbilliform, urticarial). With a few exceptions (e.g., pityriasis rosea, drug-induced autoimmune bullous disorders), patients with these entities may be febrile. *Entities in italics occur primarily in children.* Toxic shock syndrome can be staphylococcal or streptococcal (see Ch. 61). Acute generalized exanthematous pustulosis (AGEP) is also referred to as a pustular drug eruption. Drug-induced autoimmune bullous disorders: bullous pemphigoid or linear IgA bullous dermatosis > drug-induced pemphigus. *Continued*

APPROACH TO THE PATIENT WITH A SUSPECTED DRUG-INDUCED EXANTHEM

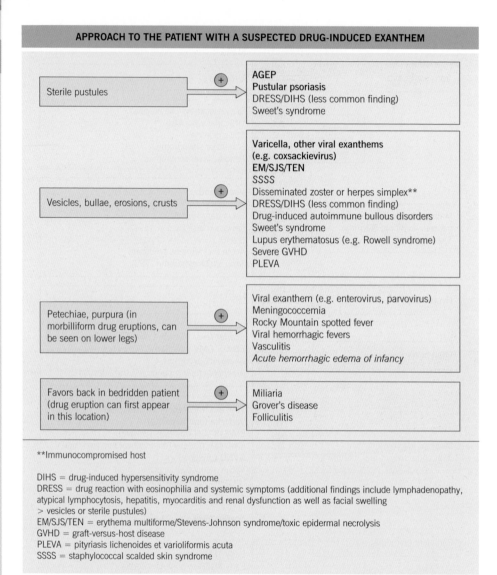

Sterile pustules (+) →
AGEP
Pustular psoriasis
DRESS/DIHS (less common finding)
Sweet's syndrome

Vesicles, bullae, erosions, crusts (+) →
Varicella, other viral exanthems
(e.g. coxsackievirus)
EM/SJS/TEN
SSSS
Disseminated zoster or herpes simplex**
DRESS/DIHS (less common finding)
Drug-induced autoimmune bullous disorders
Sweet's syndrome
Lupus erythematosus (e.g. Rowell syndrome)
Severe GVHD
PLEVA

Petechiae, purpura (in morbilliform drug eruptions, can be seen on lower legs) (+) →
Viral exanthem (e.g. enterovirus, parvovirus)
Meningococcemia
Rocky Mountain spotted fever
Viral hemorrhagic fevers
Vasculitis
Acute hemorrhagic edema of infancy

Favors back in bedridden patient (drug eruption can first appear in this location) (+) →
Miliaria
Grover's disease
Folliculitis

**Immunocompromised host

DIHS = drug-induced hypersensitivity syndrome
DRESS = drug reaction with eosinophilia and systemic symptoms (additional findings include lymphadenopathy, atypical lymphocytosis, hepatitis, myocarditis and renal dysfunction as well as facial swelling
> vesicles or sterile pustules)
EM/SJS/TEN = erythema multiforme/Stevens-Johnson syndrome/toxic epidermal necrolysis
GVHD = graft-versus-host disease
PLEVA = pityriasis lichenoides et varioliformis acuta
SSSS = staphylococcal scalded skin syndrome

Fig. 3.10 *Continued* **Approach to the patient with a suspected drug-induced exanthem (morbilliform, urticarial).**

POTENTIALLY LIFE-THREATENING CONDITIONS WITH INITIAL SKIN FINDINGS THAT CAN MIMIC A MORE COMMON BENIGN DISORDER		
Potentially Life-Threatening Condition	**Benign Disorder That is Mimicked Early in the Course**	**Clues to the Diagnosis as the Condition Evolves**
DRESS/DIHS*	Morbilliform/urticarial drug eruption > viral exanthem	• Facial swelling • High fever • Prominent lymphadenopathy • Marked peripheral blood eosinophilia, atypical lymphocytes • Elevated transaminases, other signs of internal organ involvement
Stevens–Johnson syndrome/toxic epidermal necrolysis	Morbilliform/urticarial drug eruption > viral exanthem	• Early involvement of palms and soles • Duskiness or blistering (often initially in the center of lesions) • Painful/tender skin • Mucosal erosions (oral, nasal, ocular, genital)
Rocky Mountain spotted fever (RMSF)/other rickettsial spotted fevers	Viral exanthem	• Potential exposure to ticks (e.g., season [spring–late summer for RMSF], geographic location) • High fever, myalgias, headache (often for 2–5 days prior to rash) • Rash begins on wrists/ankles → spreads centripetally (± palms/soles) • Petechiae within erythematous macules/papules
Meningococcemia	Viral exanthem	• Petechiae → retiform purpura • Fever with chills, myalgias • Headache, stiff neck
Kawasaki disease	Viral exanthem, morbilliform/urticarial drug eruption, erythema multiforme, 'diaper dermatitis' (for early perineal eruption)	• Early perineal erythema → desquamation • Conjunctival injection • 'Chapped' lips, 'strawberry' tongue • Acral erythema and edema • Continued high-spiking fever • Prominent unilateral lymphadenopathy
Staphylococcal scalded skin syndrome (SSSS)	Seborrheic dermatitis, viral exanthem	• Painful/tender skin • Periorificial (around mouth and eyes) edema and (later) radial scale-crusts • Confluent erythema → superficial erosions/peeling, especially in intertriginous sites
Necrotizing fasciitis	Cellulitis	• Tense, 'woody' induration • Extreme pain or (later) anesthesia • Rapid evolution • Erythema → dusky gray color • Watery, malodorous discharge

*In general, begins ≥2 weeks after drug is initiated and has a relatively limited set of culprit medications (see Chapter 17).
DIHS, drug-induced hypersensitivity syndrome; DRESS, drug reaction with eosinophilia and systemic symptoms.

Table 3.1 Potentially life-threatening conditions with initial skin findings that can mimic a more common benign disorder. The cutaneous manifestations are most likely to resemble those of milder disorder during the first 24 hours. Diffuse erythema, often beginning on the trunk, or a scarlatiniform exanthem can also be early manifestations of toxic shock syndrome.

FACIAL FINDINGS IN KAWASAKI DISEASE, STAPHYLOCOCCAL SCALDED SKIN SYNDROME AND ERYTHEMA MULTIFORME MAJOR/STEVENS-JOHNSON SYNDROME

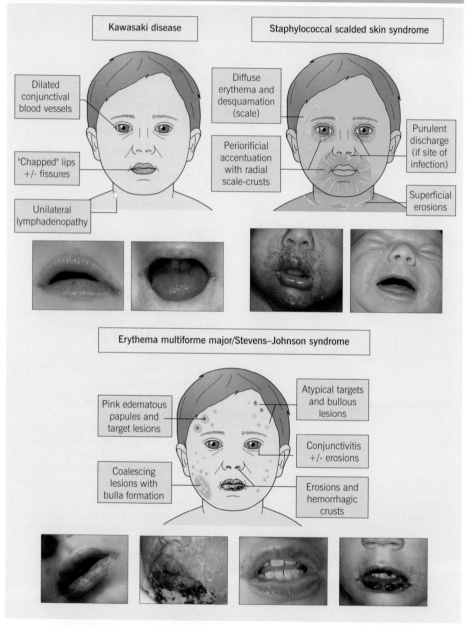

Fig. 3.11 Facial findings in Kawasaki disease, staphylococcal scalded skin syndrome, and erythema multiforme major/Stevens–Johnson syndrome. Hemorrhagic crusting and erosions of the vermilion portion of the lips can also be seen in primary gingivostomatitis due to herpes simplex virus, pemphigus vulgaris, and paraneoplastic pemphigus.

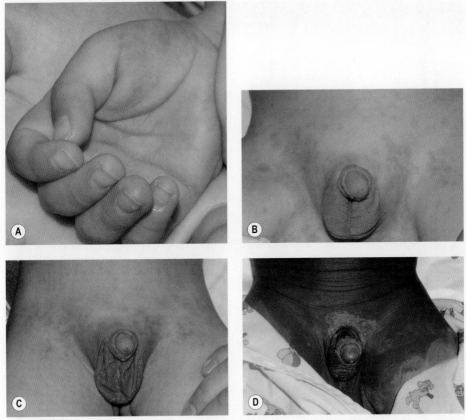

Fig. 3.12 Kawasaki disease. A Erythema and edema of the palm early in the disease course.
B, C Erythema multiforme-like lesions becoming confluent in the perineal region on the second day
of fever **(B)**, followed by desquamation 2 days later **(C)**. **D** Erythema (less evident due to the patient's
darkly pigmented skin) and desquamation in the genital area. Involvement of the skin in this location
is a characteristic early finding in Kawasaki disease. *A–C, Courtesy, Julie V. Schaffer, MD. D, Courtesy,
Anthony Mancini, MD.*

For further information see Chs. 20, 21, 45 and 81. From *Dermatology, Third Edition.*

HEREDITARY PERIODIC FEVER SYNDROMES THAT PRESENT WITH A RASH

	Familial Mediterranean Fever (FMF)	Hyper-IgD with Periodic Fever Syndrome (HIDS)	TNF Receptor-Associated Periodic Syndrome* (TRAPS)	Cryopyrin-Associated Periodic Syndromes** (CAPS)
Ethnic predilection	Armenians, Turks, Jews (especially Sephardic), Arabs, Italians	Dutch, northern Europeans	Variable	Variable
Inheritance	AR	AR	AD	AD
Gene	MEFV	MVK	TNFRSF1A	NLRP3
Protein	Pyrin	Mevalonate kinase	TNF receptor-1	Cryopyrin
Episode length	1–4 days	3–7 days	Often >7 days	<1–3 days
Mucocutaneous and ocular findings	Erysipeloid erythema and edema favoring leg/foot; ± palpable purpura (due to vasculitis)	Erythematous macules/papules; may become purpuric; ± oral or genital ulcers	Annular/serpiginous erythematous patches/plaques; distal migration on extremity (with myalgia); later ecchymotic; periorbital edema, conjunctivitis; ± oral ulcers	Urticarial papules and plaques; may be cold-induced; conjunctivitis > uveitis; ± oral ulcers
Musculoskeletal findings	Monoarthritis, myalgia	Arthralgia, oligoarthritis	Migratory myalgia > arthralgia > monoarthritis	Myalgia (limbs), arthralgia; arthritis and arthropathy in NOMID
Other clinical manifestations	Serositis (e.g., peritonitis mimicking acute abdomen, pleuritis), scrotal swelling, splenomegaly; amyloidosis	Abdominal pain, diarrhea, vomiting, cervical LAN, HSM	Serositis, scrotal pain, splenomegaly > LAN; amyloidosis	Hearing loss in MWS and NOMID; LAN, HSM, chronic aseptic meningitis and dysmorphic facies in NOMID; amyloidosis
Treatment	Colchicine prophylaxis; TNF inhibitors, IL-1 antagonists	TNF inhibitors, IL-1 antagonists, simvastatin	Corticosteroids, TNF inhibitors, IL-1 antagonists	IL-1 antagonists (rilonacept, canakinumab)

*Includes familial Hibernian fever.

**Cryopyrin-associated periodic syndromes (CAPS) include familial cold autoinflammatory syndrome, Muckle–Wells syndrome (MWS), and neonatal-onset multisystem inflammatory disease (NOMID; also known as chronic infantile neurologic, cutaneous and articular syndrome [CINCA]).

AD, autosomal dominant; AR, autosomal recessive; HSM, hepatosplenomegaly; IL-1, interleukin-1; LAN, lymphadenopathy; TNF, tumor necrosis factor.

Table 3.2 Hereditary periodic fever syndromes that present with a rash. In all of these disorders, episodic 'attacks' are characterized by fever and may be associated with headache.

Pruritus and Dysesthesia | 4

Definitions

• **Pruritus:** an unpleasant sensation of the skin that elicits a desire to scratch.
• **Dysesthesia:** an unpleasant, abnormal sensation that can be either spontaneous or evoked; abnormal, unpleasant sensations may include pain, pruritus ('neuropathic itch'), tingling, burning, 'pins and needles'.

Pruritus

• The most common skin-related symptom in dermatology; can have a profound negative impact on a patient's quality of life.
• Results from the activation of the sensory nervous system, involving four sequential levels: the peripheral nervous system → the dorsal root ganglia → the spinal cord → and the brain.
• There are multiple etiologies of pruritus, and it is often a major clinical challenge to diagnose the underlying etiology and to adequately treat.

Etiologies

• May arise **secondary** to a number of conditions:
  – Dermatologic disorders (Table 4.1).
  – Allergic or hypersensitivity syndromes.
  – Systemic diseases (10–25%) and malignancies (Table 4.2; Figs. 4.1 and 4.2).
  – Toxins associated with kidney or liver dysfunction.
  – Medications.
  – Neurologic disorders (see text below).
  – Psychiatric conditions (see Chapter 5).
• May also be **primary** or **idiopathic** – that is, no readily apparent skin disease, underlying etiology, or associated condition.
• Most patients with pruritus due to an underlying dermatologic disorder present with characteristic or diagnostic skin lesions (e.g., dermatitis of the flexures in atopic dermatitis; see Table 4.1).
• In **primary** pruritus and **secondary** pruritus NOT due to an underlying dermatologic disorder, the lesions are usually nonspecific (e.g., linear excoriations [Fig. 4.3], prurigo simplex, prurigo nodularis [Fig. 4.4]).

Diagnostic Pearls

• Patients with chronic, idiopathic pruritus need serial examinations because pruritus can antedate clinical manifestations of the underlying disorder (e.g., lymphoma) or with time, more specific lesions may appear (e.g., bullous pemphigoid).
• Sparing of the mid upper back, an area of patient-hand inaccessibility ('butterfly sign') (Fig. 4.5), is suggestive of pruritus NOT associated with a dermatologic disorder; note, however, this sign is not seen in those who use back scratchers or similar devices.
• Aquagenic pruritus, provoked by cooling of the skin after emergence from a bath, is often idiopathic but may be a sign of polycythemia vera.
• Of note, some patients may have a combination of specific and nonspecific skin lesions and both may be due to an underlying systemic disorder (e.g., eosinophilic folliculitis associated with HIV infection/AIDS).

Approach to the Patient with Pruritus

• Identifying the underlying etiology of a patient's pruritus is important in determining the appropriate management.
• A simplified approach to the patient with pruritus is presented in Fig. 4.6.

Management of Pruritus

• General treatment measures for pruritus are outlined in Table 4.3.

COMMON DERMATOLOGIC DISEASES WITH PRURITUS AS A MAJOR SYMPTOM	
General Category	**Specific Dermatologic Disease**
Infestations/bites and stings	• Scabies • Pediculosis • Arthropod bites
Inflammation	• Atopic dermatitis • Stasis dermatitis • Allergic > irritant contact dermatitis • Seborrheic dermatitis, especially of scalp • Psoriasis • Lichen planus • Urticaria • Papular urticaria • Drug eruptions (e.g., morbilliform) • Bullous diseases (e.g., BP, DH) • Mastocytosis • Eosinophilic folliculitis • Pruritic papular eruption of HIV
Autoimmune connective tissue disease	• Lichen sclerosus, especially of the vulva • Dermatomyositis • Lupus erythematosus (systemic and cutaneous)
Infection	• Bacterial (e.g., folliculitis) • Viral (e.g., varicella) • Fungal (e.g., inflammatory tinea) • Parasitic (e.g., schistosomal cercarial dermatitis)
Neoplastic	• Cutaneous T-cell lymphoma (e.g., mycosis fungoides, Sézary syndrome)
Other	• Xerosis/eczema craquelé • Scar-associated pruritus • Lichen simplex chronicus • Prurigo nodularis • Pregnancy dermatoses • Neuropathic itch (e.g., notalgia paresthetica) • Actinic prurigo

BP, bullous pemphigoid; DH, dermatitis herpetiformis.

Table 4.1 Common dermatologic diseases with pruritus as a major symptom.

Classic Clinical Findings from Chronic Pruritus

LICHEN SIMPLEX CHRONICUS (LSC)

• Skin-colored to pink or hyperpigmented plaques with exaggerated skin lines and a leathery appearance due to repeated, often habitual, scratching or rubbing (Fig. 4.7).

• Favors the posterior neck and occipital scalp (Fig. 4.8), anogenital region (Fig. 4.9), and ankles as well as the extensor surface of the forearms and shins.

• LSC may be superimposed upon a specific cutaneous disorder, most commonly atopic dermatitis.

• In addition to symptomatic relief (e.g., topical anesthetics such as pramoxine), disruption of the itch–scratch cycle requires discussion of possible psychosocial issues (e.g., stress, depression, anxiety).

• **Rx:** potent topical CS, often under occlusion (e.g., hydrocolloid dressings), can be helpful.

APPROACH TO THE PATIENT WITH GENERALIZED PRURITUS AND NO OBVIOUS SPECIFIC SKIN DISEASE

- History and review of systems, including symptoms in household contacts
- Complete skin examination and lymph node examination
- Exclude infestations (e.g., scabies) and confounding factors (e.g., dermographism, xerosis, irritants; Fig. 4.1) and treat accordingly
- Review medications (prescription, OTC, and illicit) as well as supplements for drug-induced pruritus (e.g., calcium channel blockers, proton pump inhibitors, narcotics, amphetamines)
- If no obvious etiology, obtain screening laboratory tests: CBC with differential, plt, ESR, TSH, BUN/Cr, LDH*, and liver function tests to detect eosinophilia or renal (Fig. 4.2), thyroid or liver dysfunction (cholestatic or hepatocellular), followed by appropriate evaluation if abnormalities present (e.g., viral hepatitis screen, stool exam for ova and parasites)
- Consider patch testing, if history or distribution suggestive
- Consider less common causes, including
  - Early manifestation of autoimmune blistering disorder, particularly bullous pemphigoid, dermatitis herpetiformis
  - Lymphoma (Hodgkin and non-Hodgkin disease), myeloproliferative disorders (e.g., polycythemia vera, hypereosinophilic syndrome), chronic lymphocytic leukemia
  - Endocrinopathies (e.g., hyperparathyroidism, diabetes)
  - Metabolic disorders (e.g., iron deficiency [debatable], hemochromatosis)
  - Celiac disease
- Additional evaluation includes: serum fasting glucose, HbA1c, Ca^{2+}, PO_4^{---}, albumin, ferritin, iron studies; chest x-ray; skin biopsies for routine histology and direct immunofluorescence, anti-tissue transglutaminase antibodies
- In concert with primary care physician, age-appropriate cancer screening examinations
- Depending on history and symptoms, further steps: for example, travel – stool for ova and parasites; iron deficiency anemia – stool guaiac, endoscopies; HIV risk factors – HIV testing; psychiatric illness – consult with psychiatrist

*LDH is often used in a manner similar to an ESR, especially in patients with lymphoma.
BUN, blood urea nitrogen; CBC, complete blood count; Cr, creatinine; ESR, erythrocyte sedimentation rate; HIV, human immunodeficiency virus; LDH, lactic dehydrogenase; OTC, over-the-counter; plt, platelets; TSH, thyroid-stimulating hormone.

Table 4.2 Approach to the patient with generalized pruritus and no obvious specific skin disease.

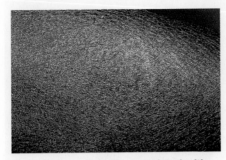

Fig. 4.1 Extreme xerosis associated with pruritus in an HIV-infected patient. *Courtesy, Elke Weisshaar, MD and Jeffrey D. Bernhard, MD.*

- **Other Rx:** intralesional CS or use of an office-applied dressing (e.g., Unna boot) may be required.

PRURIGO NODULARIS

- Multiple, discrete, firm papulonodules with central scale-crust due to chronic and repetitive scratching and picking.
- Degree of pruritus can vary from moderate to intense.
- Lesions usually favor the extensor surfaces of the extremities (see Fig. 4.4), upper back, and buttocks, but they can be widespread in easily reachable areas (Fig. 4.10).
- Disruption of the itch–scratch cycle requires symptomatic relief and discussion of psychosocial issues as in LSC (see above).

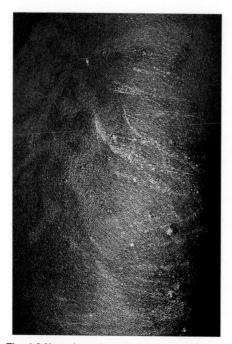

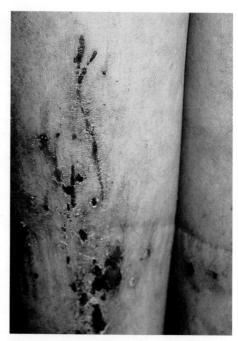

Fig. 4.2 Xerosis and pruritus in a patient with chronic renal failure on hemodialysis. There are a few papules of acquired perforating dermatosis admixed with the scratch marks. *Courtesy, Jean L. Bolognia, MD.*

Fig. 4.3 Linear excoriations on the leg. Although this patient had atopic dermatitis, similar lesions can be seen in patients with 'primary' or 'idiopathic' pruritus. *Courtesy, Elke Weisshaar, MD and Jeffrey D. Bernhard, MD.*

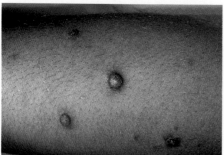

Fig. 4.4 Prurigo nodularis. Firm papulonodules on the extensor forearm due to repeated scratching and picking. *Courtesy, Ronald P. Rapini, MD.*

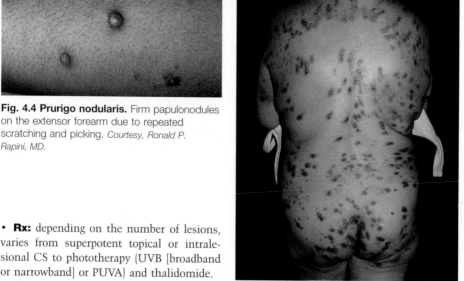

- **Rx:** depending on the number of lesions, varies from superpotent topical or intralesional CS to phototherapy (UVB [broadband or narrowband] or PUVA) and thalidomide.
- If no underlying reversible disorder is detected (see Table 4.2), prurigo nodularis can be difficult to treat.

Fig. 4.5 Multiple lesions of prurigo nodularis. Note the sparing of the mid upper back ('butterfly sign').

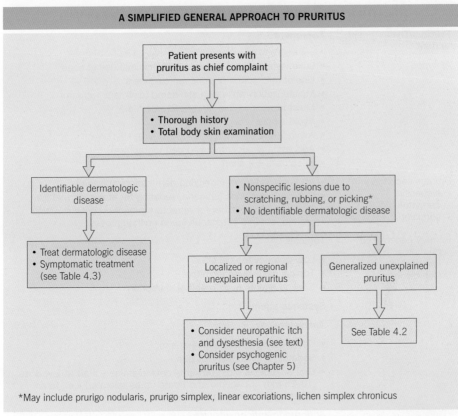

A SIMPLIFIED GENERAL APPROACH TO PRURITUS

Patient presents with pruritus as chief complaint

- Thorough history
- Total body skin examination

Identifiable dermatologic disease

- Nonspecific lesions due to scratching, rubbing, or picking*
- No identifiable dermatologic disease

- Treat dermatologic disease
- Symptomatic treatment (see Table 4.3)

Localized or regional unexplained pruritus

Generalized unexplained pruritus

- Consider neuropathic itch and dysesthesia (see text)
- Consider psychogenic pruritus (see Chapter 5)

See Table 4.2

*May include prurigo nodularis, prurigo simplex, linear excoriations, lichen simplex chronicus

Fig. 4.6 A simplified approach to the patient presenting with a chief complaint of pruritus.

Neurologic Etiologies of Pruritus and Dysesthesia

- The same neurological diseases that can cause neuropathic pain and dysesthesia can also cause neuropathic itch, with some differences (e.g., opioid pain relievers that help treat neuropathic pain may cause or worsen neuropathic itch).

Neuropathic Itch

- Neuropathic itch syndromes are typically due to either peripheral (PNS) or central nervous system (CNS) disorders and can be further categorized into focal or regional presentations.
- CNS-related neuropathic itch syndromes involve abnormalities of the brain.
- PNS-related neuropathic itch syndromes involve abnormalities of the spinal cord, cranial or spinal nerve roots, or peripheral nerves.

- Neuropathic itch is more likely to develop in the head and neck region than on the lower body (e.g., facial zoster is more likely to cause post-herpetic itch [PHI] than zoster on the torso).
- Neuropathic itch differs in quality from other forms of pruritus and often makes afflicted individuals want to 'dig at' or 'gouge out' their skin; it is not responsive to antihistamines, but patients may find relief with application of ice packs.
- Patients with neuropathic itch often present first to a dermatologist.

TRIGEMINAL TROPHIC SYNDROME (TTS)

- A type of intractable facial neuropathic itch characterized by 'painless scratching' to the point of self-harm and cutaneous ulceration.
- Classically involves the nasal ala and typically results from impingement or damage to the sensory portion of the trigeminal nerve (Figs. 4.11 and 4.12).

TREATMENT FOR PRURITUS/DYSESTHESIA – GENERAL MEASURES

Pruritus/Dysesthesia Variant	Treatment
All types	• Lukewarm baths or showers with minimal use of soap • Use of mild soaps or nonsoap cleansers • Moisturization while skin still damp (ointment > cream) • Moisturization in a.m. and before bedtime • Avoid woolens and harsh fabrics • Avoid fabric softeners • Address any superimposed dermographism • Keep nails cut short
Pruritus secondary to a specific dermatologic condition	• Address and treat underlying dermatologic disease • Oral antihistamines (urticaria, sedating for atopic dermatitis) • Thalidomide (consider for refractory prurigo nodularis, actinic prurigo, chronic cutaneous lupus erythematosus)
Primary generalized pruritus with no identifiable specific skin disorder	**Topicals** • Low-potency topical CS • Topical calcineurin inhibitors • Cooling agents (e.g., menthol, camphor) **Systemic agents** *Antihistamines* • Nonsedating antihistamine in a.m. • Sedating antihistamine in p.m. • Oral doxepin is most powerful antihistamine – start at low dose (10–25 mg) at bedtime and titrate up as tolerated (i.e., to an acceptable level of a.m. drowsiness) *Antipruritic anticonvulsants* • Gabapentin (± mirtazapine) • Pregabalin (± mirtazapine) *Antipruritic antidepressants* (consider first-line if underlying depression, associated paraneoplastic condition, or underlying polycythemia vera) • SSRIs and SNRIs (e.g., fluoxetine, paroxetine, sertraline, venlaxafine) • TCAs (e.g., amitriptyline, doxepin) *Opioid antagonists and agonists* (consider first-line if underlying renal or hepatic dysfunction) • Naltrexone • Nalfuraline (renal itch) *Thalidomide* (see above; also consider for cancer-associated pruritus) **Physical treatment modalities** • UV light therapy (UVB [broadband or narrowband] or PUVA) • Acupuncture **Other** • Psychosocial intervention

Table 4.3 Treatment for pruritus/dysesthesia – general measures. *Continued*

Table 4.3 *Continued* **Treatment for pruritus/dysesthesia – general measures.**

Pruritus/Dysesthesia Variant	Treatment
Neuropathic pruritus/ dysesthesia (refer to text for disease-specific therapies)	**Topicals**
	• Antipruritics (CS, calcineurin inhibitors)
	• Anesthetics (pramoxine, lidocaine, prilocaine)
	• Counter-irritants (menthol, capsaicin)
	Systemic neuromodulators
	• Antipruritic anticonvulsants (e.g., gabapentin, pregabalin)
	• TCAs (e.g., amitriptyline, doxepin)
	• Other anticonvulsants (e.g., carbamazepine, phenytoin)
	Other
	• Paravertebral/spinal nerve block (temporary relief)
	• Physical therapy, acupuncture
	• Behavioral therapy
	• Botulinum toxin injections (to weaken impinging muscles)
	• Surgical intervention (last resort)

SNRIs, selective norepinephrine reuptake inhibitors; SSRIs, selective serotonin reuptake inhibitors; TCAs, tricyclic antidepressants.

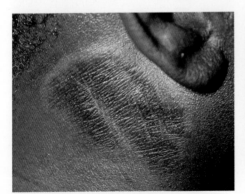

Fig. 4.7 Lichen simplex chronicus of the lateral neck. Note the increased skin markings. Use of topical corticosteroids can lead to a shiny appearance and a rim of hypopigmentation. *Courtesy, Elke Weisshaar, MD and Jeffrey D. Bernhard, MD.*

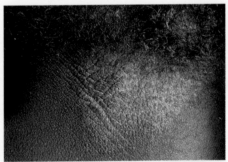

Fig. 4.8 Lichen simplex chronicus of the posterior neck. The increased skin markings have been likened to the bark of a tree. *Courtesy, Ronald P. Rapini, MD.*

• Common inciting factors include iatrogenesis (ablation of the Gasserian ganglion to treat intractable trigeminal neuralgia), infection (varicella zoster virus [VZV], herpes simplex virus), stroke (infarction of the posterior cerebellar artery), CNS tumors or their resultant treatment.

• Clinically may present as a small crust that develops into a crescentic ulcer that may gradually extend to involve the cheek and upper lip.

• The nasal tip is usually spared because its nerve supply is derived from the external branch of the anterior ethmoidal nerve.

• Treatment is difficult and should involve protective barriers, patient education, and surgical consultation; oral pimozide and carbamazepine have been anecdotally reported as helpful.

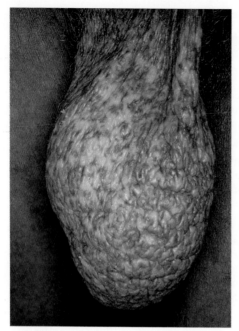

Fig. 4.9 Lichen simplex chronicus of the scrotum. Secondary pigmentary changes are seen more commonly in darkly pigmented skin. *Courtesy, Louis A. Fragola, Jr., MD.*

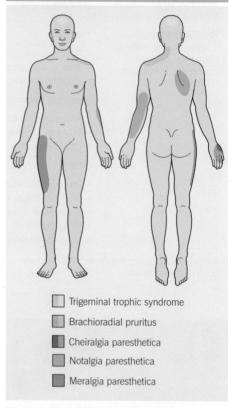

DISTRIBUTIONS OF DYSESTHESIA IN SELECTED NEUROPATHIC CONDITIONS

☐ Trigeminal trophic syndrome

☐ Brachioradial pruritus

☐ Cheiralgia paresthetica

☐ Notalgia paresthetica

☐ Meralgia paresthetica

Fig. 4.11 Distributions of dysesthesia in selected neuropathic conditions. Cheiralgia paresthetica is caused by entrapment of the superficial branch of the radial nerve. Darker shades indicate more common areas of involvement. *Courtesy, Karynne O. Duncan, MD.*

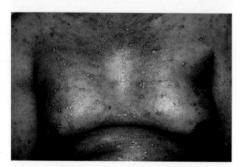

Fig. 4.10 Widespread prurigo nodularis. This patient had underlying atopic dermatitis. *Courtesy, Elke Weisshaar, MD and Jeffrey D. Bernhard, MD.*

RADICULOPATHIES

• Characterized by a pattern of focal or regional neurological dysfunction that is caused by 'injury' to a single sensory nerve root (SNR) or less often to a few adjacent nerve roots, resulting in pruritus or dysesthesia.

• 'Injuries' that can cause damage to these SNRs may include (1) impingement from spinal osteoarthritis; (2) distal impingement or irritation by inflamed muscles or connective tissues; (3) infections (e.g., VZV, Lyme disease, leprosy); and (4) other rare causes, such as tumors (schwannomas, metastases), vascular malformations, and cysts.

• The abnormal sensation (e.g., pruritus or other dysesthesia) is perceived in the skin area that is innervated by the damaged SNR(s), and these areas are known as dermatomes (see Fig. 67.10).

• Clinical presentations are usually unilateral and on the side of the damaged SNR, but occasionally may be bilateral.

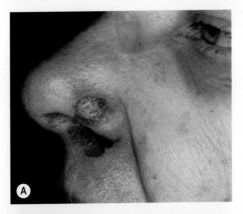

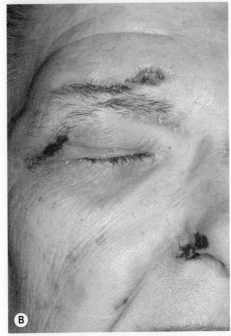

Fig. 4.12 Trigeminal trophic syndrome.
Erosions and ulcerations with hemorrhagic crusts favor the ala nasi **(A, B)**. Obvious linear excoriations are seen in the second patient **(B)**.
Courtesy, Kalman Watsky, MD.

• The evaluation of an unexplained radiculopathy should include a neurologic examination.
• If the symptoms are severe, sudden in onset, or worsen significantly, then radiologic imaging (magnetic resonance imaging is most sensitive) of the appropriate area of the spine can be performed.

• If radiologic imaging is negative, electromyogram and nerve conduction studies can be considered.
• In general, symptomatic treatment may include (1) topical agents (e.g., anesthetics, capsaicin); (2) various oral neuromodulators (e.g., gabapentin, pregabalin, other anticonvulsants); (3) physical therapy and acupuncture (if underlying muscle or connective tissue inflammation); and (4) botulinum toxin injections to weaken impinging muscles, if deemed safe.
• Several classic radiculopathies encountered in dermatology are (1) 'shingles' or postherpetic neuralgia (PHN) or post-herpetic itch (PHI); (2) notalgia paresthetica; (3) brachioradial pruritus, and (4) meralgia paresthetica (Fig. 4.11).

NOTALGIA PARESTHETICA
• Affects roughly 10% of the adult population and thought to be related to SNR impingement at the level of the spinal cord due to osteoarthritis or more distally, due to impingement or irritation from inflamed muscles or other connective tissue.
• Presents with focal, intense pruritus of the upper back, most commonly along the medial scapular borders (see Fig. 4.11); sometimes the pruritus is accompanied by other dysesthesias (e.g., pain, burning).
• Often, a hyperpigmented patch that is a result of chronic rubbing is seen in the area of pruritus (Fig. 4.13).
• **DDx:** macular amyloidosis, which is also due to chronic rubbing and is probably a related entity; both disorders can be a cutaneous marker of Sipple syndrome, especially if the onset is during childhood or adolescence.
• **Rx:** topical capsaicin, a natural plant product that depletes substance P from cutaneous nerve endings, 5 times daily for 1 week followed by 3 times daily for 3–6 weeks may be effective.
• **Other Rx:** topical anesthetics, gabapentin, and acupuncture.

BRACHIORADIAL PRURITUS
• Chronic, intermittent pruritus or burning pain of the dorsolateral aspects of the forearms and elbows; sometimes more extensive area of involvement (e.g., shoulder region) (see Fig. 4.11).

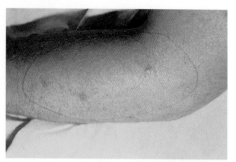

Fig. 4.14 Brachioradial pruritus. The affected area is outlined by ink. *Courtesy, Elke Weisshaar, MD and Jeffrey D. Bernhard, MD.*

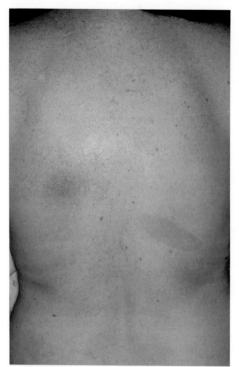

Fig. 4.13 Notalgia paresthetica. A circumscribed area of hyperpigmentation on the left mid back (overlying the medial aspect of the scapula) due to chronic rubbing and scratching. The patient complained of significant pruritus in that area. An incidental café au lait macule is on the right mid back. *Courtesy, Jean L. Bolognia, MD.*

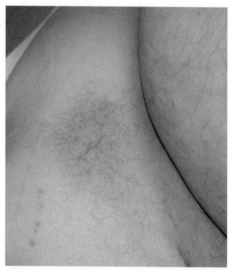

Fig. 4.15 Meralgia paresthetica. A circumscribed area of hyperpigmentation, lichenification, and hypertrichosis due to chronic rubbing and scratching.

• Most patients have photodamaged skin and degenerative cervical spine disease, with UV light exposure and heat serving as triggers.

• The patient can often precisely delineate the affected area with a marking pen, and within this area are excoriations, prurigo simplex lesions, and sometimes even scarring (Fig. 4.14).

• The 'ice-pack sign' is another diagnostic clue, because application of ice is often reported as the only modality that provides relief.

• **Rx:** sun protection, cold packs, topical medications (pramoxine, capsaicin), oral neuromodulating drugs (gabapentin, amitriptyline).

MERALGIA PARESTHETICA

• Due to impingement of the lateral femoral cutaneous nerve as it passes through the inguinal ligament; rarely due to trauma or ischemia.

• Presents with pruritus or dysesthesia of the anterolateral thigh, most often numbness or burning pain (Fig. 4.15; see Fig. 4.11).

• Predisposing factors include obesity, pregnancy, tight clothing, and, rarely, mass effect from tumor or hemorrhage.

• **Rx:** removal of the cause of compression, focal nerve block at the inguinal ligament, and lastly surgical decompression.

• Neuromodulating medications are not typically helpful.

SMALL FIBER POLYNEUROPATHIES (SFPN)

• Perhaps the most common cause of chronic pruritus in the following areas: bilateral feet;

feet and legs; hands and legs; or other widespread bilateral areas of the body.
• Typically presents with pruritus, dysesthesias, paresthesias, and/or neuropathic pain in a 'stocking-glove' distribution; muscle function is usually intact.
• If the diagnosis of SFPN is suspected based on history and neurologic examination, then potentially treatable causes should be identified, including.
  – Fasting blood glucose, HbA1c (diabetes mellitus).
  – Serum B_{12}, RBC folate, methylmalonic acid, homocysteine, and copper levels (B_{12}, folate, or copper deficiencies).
  – Serum (SPEP) and urine (UPEP) protein electrophoreses, immunofixation and serum-free light-chain analysis (monoclonal gammopathy).
  – CBC with differential and platelets (hematologic malignancies).
• For SFPN, there are two diagnostic tests:
  – Immunohistochemical staining (e.g., anti-PGP9.5) of a (nontraumatized) distal leg skin punch biopsy specimen to evaluate the small nerve fibers (requires a special fixative).
  – Autoimmune function testing (e.g., sweat functioning).

Dysesthesia Syndromes

• Typically caused by an underlying neurological disorder (either peripheral or central), but it is not always identifiable.
• Several locoregional dysesthesia syndromes are encountered in dermatology: burning mouth syndrome (orodynia), burning scalp syndrome (scalp dysesthesia), and several dysesthetic anogenital syndromes.
• **DDx:** includes psychogenic pruritus/dysesthesia (see Chapter 5).

Burning Mouth Syndrome (Orodynia)

• Burning mucosal pain without clinically detectable oral lesions; most commonly affects middle-aged to elderly women.
• Typically bilateral, involving the anterior two-thirds of the tongue, palate, and lower lip.
• Diagnosis requires exclusion of secondary causes such as malignancy (e.g., oral SCC),

vitamin deficiencies (e.g., folate, B_{12}), candidiasis, xerostomia (e.g., previous radiation therapy, Sjögren syndrome), contact stomatitis, and ill-fitting dentures.
• Depression and anxiety are more common in patients with burning mouth syndrome.
• **Rx:** oral tricyclic antidepressants and gabapentin in addition to topical anesthetics (e.g., lidocaine, dyclonine) and mouthwashes (various combinations of tetracycline, hydrocortisone, diphenhydramine, nystatin, and Maalox®).

Burning Scalp Syndrome (Scalp Dysesthesia)

• Diffuse scalp burning, pain, pruritus, numbness or tingling without any specific cutaneous lesions.
• Strongly correlated with underlying depression and anxiety.
• Occasionally associated with primary neurologic disorders (e.g., multiple sclerosis).
• Diagnosis requires exclusion and treatment of secondary causes, such as seborrheic dermatitis, folliculitis, lichen planopilaris, allergic or irritant contact dermatitis, dermatomyositis, and discoid lupus erythematosus.
• **Rx:** oral tricyclic antidepressants.

Dysesthetic Anogenital Syndromes

• Various names: pruritus ani, anodynia, pruritus vulvae, vulvodynia, pruritus scroti, scrotodynia, penile pain syndrome.
• Severe, intractable pruritus or dysesthesia despite either a normal clinical examination or the presence of nonspecific cutaneous findings.
• When all typical secondary causes of anogenital pruritus and dysesthesia have been investigated and treated (e.g., candidiasis, fecal incontinence; see Chapter 60), and the patient still has symptoms, consider lumbosacral radiculopathy (imaging studies), dermographism (trial of oral antihistamines), and contact dermatitis (patch testing).
• If no etiology detected, consider both psychiatric counseling and treatment with a neuromodulator medication (e.g., tricyclic antidepressant or gabapentin).

For further information see Ch. 6. From *Dermatology, Third Edition*.

5 | Psychocutaneous Disorders

Introduction

• Psychodermatology refers to any aspect of dermatology in which psychological factors play a significant role.
• Psychodermatologic disorders can be classified in two ways: (1) by the specific psychodermatologic condition or (2) by the underlying psychopathology (Fig. 5.1).
• Treatment is simplified by basing the choice of psychotropic medication or therapy on the underlying psychopathology (Table 5.1).
• The more commonly encountered primary psychiatric disorders in dermatology include body dysmorphic disorder, psychogenic (neurotic) excoriations, acne excoriée, trichotillomania, dermatitis artefacta, and delusions of parasitosis.
• Because many of these patients with primary psychiatric disorders present to the dermatologist and not the psychiatrist, it is important to establish the correct diagnosis and to offer appropriate treatment options.

The More Common Primary Psychiatric Disorders Seen in Dermatology

Body Dysmorphic Disorder

• Characterized by a distressing or impairing preoccupation with a nonexistent or slight defect in appearance.
• On a psychiatric spectrum from obsessional to delusional.
• Mean age of onset is 30–35 years; females = males; present in up to 10–15% of dermatologic patients.
• Patients usually concerned with nose, mouth, hair, breasts, or genitalia.
• Often adopt obsessional (e.g., numerous visits to physician for reassurance), ritualistic (e.g., excessive grooming routines), or delusional (e.g., multiple unnecessary surgeries) behaviors.

• Consider and assess for this diagnosis in patients seeking multiple cosmetic procedures.
• **Rx:** selective serotonin reuptake inhibitors (SSRIs) for obsessive–compulsive disorder (OCD) variant or antipsychotics for delusional variant.

Psychogenic (Neurotic) Excoriations

• A conscious, repetitive, uncontrollable desire to pick, rub, or scratch skin.
• On a psychiatric spectrum most closely related to OCD but may also be an expression of generalized anxiety disorder or depression.
• Most common in middle-age; females > males.
• Favors scalp, face, upper back, extensor forearms, shins, buttocks.
• Lesions usually in all stages of evolution: erosions (prurigo simplex), deep circular or linear ulcerations with hypertrophic borders, hypo- or hyperpigmented scars (Fig. 5.2); admixed well-healed scars point to chronicity.
• **DDx:** (1) underlying causes of primary pruritus (see Chapter 4); (2) underlying primary cutaneous disorder (e.g., folliculitis).
• **Rx:** symptomatic treatment of pruritus (topicals, oral antihistamines); tricyclic antidepressants (TCAs) or SSRIs (if underlying depression); SSRIs (if underlying OCD); consultation with a psychiatrist.

Acne Excoriée

• Considered a subset of psychogenic (neurotic) excoriations, characterized by ritualistic picking of acne lesions (Fig. 5.3).
• Often associated with OCD; most common in young females.
• **Rx:** aggressively treat underlying acne; TCAs or SSRIs (if underlying depression); SSRIs (if underlying OCD); consultation with a psychiatrist.

CLASSIFICATION OF PSYCHODERMATOLOGIC DISORDERS

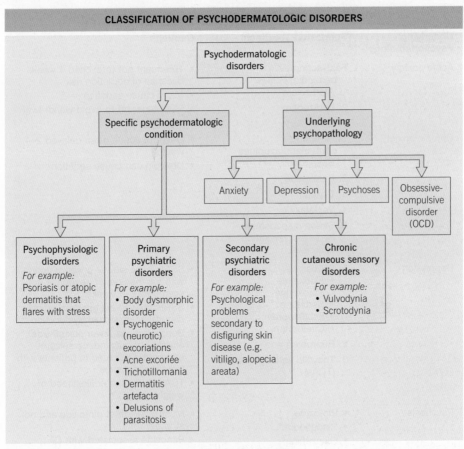

Fig. 5.1 Classification of the psychodermatologic disorders.

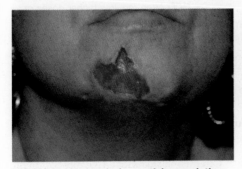

Fig. 5.2 Psychogenic (neurotic) excoriations.
Deep, angulated, unnatural-shaped ulceration on
the chin. *Courtesy, Kalman Watsky, MD.*

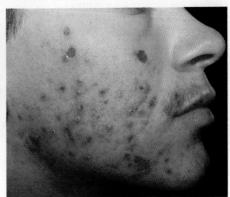

Fig. 5.3 Acne excoriée. This patient
compulsively picked at his acne lesions. *Courtesy,
Richard Odom, MD.*

COMMON PSYCHOTROPIC MEDICATIONS USED IN DERMATOLOGY		
Underlying Psychopathology	Suggested Treatment	Cautions
Acute anxiety	Fast-acting benzodiazepines 1. Alprazolam 2. Lorazepam	• Treatment not to exceed 4 weeks because of addiction risk • Might cause sedation • Must taper off to avoid withdrawal symptoms
Chronic anxiety	Slow-acting nonbenzodiazepines 1. Buspirone 2. Paroxetine 3. Doxepin 4. Venlafaxine 5. Stress management, hypnosis, relaxation exercises	• Onset of action often delayed 2–4 weeks • Doxepin can cause sedation
Depression	1. SSRIs • Fluoxetine • Paroxetine • Sertraline • Escitalopram • Citalopram 2. Bupropion 3. Tricyclic antidepressants (TCAs)	• SSRIs have slower onset of action, with full therapeutic response not seen until 6–8 weeks • SSRIs may cause gastrointestinal disturbances, sexual dysfunction • Bupropion has fewer sexual side effects but may induce seizures and contraindicated in patients with history of seizures • TCAs have greater likelihood of weight gain
Psychosis	• Pimozide • Risperidone* • Olanzapine* • Quetiapine*	• Must taper off of pimozide and not stop abruptly • Pimozide associated with QT prolongation, cardiac toxicity, extrapyramidal side effects, drug interactions (avoid if taking macrolides, protease inhibitors, azole antifungals, grapefruit juice) • Baseline ECG often recommended when starting pimozide
Obsessive– compulsive disorder (OCD)	1. SSRIs • Fluoxetine • Paroxetine • Sertraline • Fluvoxamine 2. Behavioral therapy	• OCD often requires higher doses of SSRIs and may take longer to respond (10–12 weeks)

*Increasing frequency of use because of lower risk of tardive dyskinesia, compared with pimozide.
SSRI, selective serotonin reuptake inhibitors.

Table 5.1 Common psychotropic medications used in dermatology.

Trichotillomania

• Defined as hair loss from a patient's repetitive self-pulling of hair.

• On a psychiatric spectrum from inattentive habitual hair pulling to impulse disorder to OCD to other underlying psychiatric disorder.

• Most helpful to approach the patient by age of onset, in terms of discussing prognosis and treatment.

– *Preschool onset:* typically benign course; most children outgrow the habit; **Rx** involves bringing awareness to parents and patient.

– *Pre-adolescent to young adult onset:* more chronic, relapsing course; on a spectrum from habit/unawareness to underlying psychopathology; **Rx** includes bringing awareness, behavioral modification therapy, psychotropic medications as necessary.

– *Adult onset:* more protracted course; often due to underlying psychopathology; **Rx** most often entails referral to psychiatrist/psychologist and treatment of underlying psychiatric disorder.

• Peak onset ages 8–12 years; females > males.

• Most commonly scalp hair, but also eyebrows, eyelashes, or pubic hair.

• Classically see hairs of varying lengths distributed within the area of alopecia; uninvolved areas are normal (Fig. 5.4).

• Sometimes associated ritualistic behavior or trichophagy.

• **DDx:** other causes of non-scarring alopecia (e.g., alopecia areata, tinea capitis).

• A helpful diagnostic test is the 'clipped hair square,' in which a small section of hair is clipped close to the scalp with scissors; in trichotillomania the hairs (being too short to pull out) display uniform hair regrowth.

• **Rx:** behavioral modification is primary treatment; psychosocial support; SSRIs; case reports of *N*-acetyl cysteine replacement.

Cutting (Self-Injury)

• Cutting is a form of nonsuicidal self-injury that has received increased attention by the medical community and media in recent years.

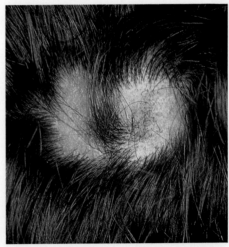

Fig. 5.4 Trichotillomania. Classic findings with small areas of sparing. *Courtesy, John Koo, MD.*

• It is a practice in which the individual makes small cuts on his/her body, most often on the arms and legs, with a sharp instrument such as a razor blade.

• Typically seen in adolescents and young adults (females > males) as a maladaptive response to psychological distress; may also be a symptom of an underlying psychological disorder (e.g., anxiety, depression, borderline personality disorder).

• In contrast to dermatitis artefacta, patients acknowledge that they inflicted the lesions upon themselves.

• Clinically, lesions present as an admixture of linear erosions or well-healed scars, often in an array of parallel lines (likened to 'railroad ties'); some individuals will cut words into their skin; with time, the cutting will typically escalate to more frequent and numerous lesions.

• Unexplained, recurrent 'cuts and scratches' on the forearms and legs of adolescents should arouse suspicion for this behavior.

• **Rx:** familial and psychological support; treatment of underlying psychopathology.

Dermatitis Artefacta

• Characterized by self-inflicted lesions as a means to satisfy a psychological need that is not consciously understood; self-denial.

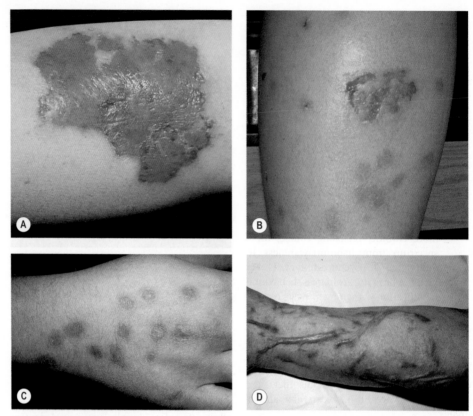

Fig. 5.5 Dermatitis artefacta. A 'Bizarre' and unnatural appearance of the skin with angulated borders, possibly created with a sharp instrument. **B** Lesions in multiple stages of evolution, from circular, crusted erosions to 'bizarre-shaped' erosions on the mid-shin to hyperpigmented scars. This teenage girl denied knowing how the lesions developed or having any role in the process. **C** Scars from cigarette burns. **D** Unusual, linear, hypertrophic scars resulting from self-carving with a sharp instrument. *A, Courtesy, John Koo, MD; C, Courtesy, Ronald P. Rapini, MD; D, Courtesy, M. Joyce Rico, MD.*

- Rare disorder; majority of patients suffer from borderline personality disorder; may have underlying depression and/or anxiety.
- Onset typically in adolescence or young adulthood; females >> males.
- Lesions often appear in easy-to-reach areas and appear in bizarre shapes and configurations; may employ outside instruments (Fig. 5.5).
- **DDx:** (1) primary dermatologic disorder; (2) monosymptomatic hypochondriacal disorder; (3) malingering (conscious gain); (4) OCD; (5) Münchhausen syndrome by proxy.
- **Rx:** symptomatic treatment of wounds; psychosocial support; psychotropic medications tailored to underlying psychopathology.

Delusions of Parasitosis

- A monosymptomatic, hypochondriacal psychosis characterized by a fixed and false (delusional) belief that an individual is infested with parasites, despite any objective evidence.
- This delusion is 'encapsulated' and other mental functions are usually intact.
- Typical onset is in the mid 50s–60s.
- Patients often bring in bits of skin, lint, and other specimens to prove the existence of the supposed parasites (Fig. 5.6).
- Often experience 'formication,' which is a cutaneous sensation of crawling, biting, and/or stinging.
- **DDx:** (1) legitimate primary dermatologic disorder; (2) true formication without

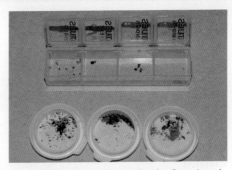

Fig. 5.6 Delusions of parasitosis. Samples of alleged 'parasites' brought in by a patient ('matchbox sign'). *Courtesy, Kalman Watsky, MD.*

delusion; (3) formication plus delusion, related to substance abuse (e.g., methamphetamines); (4) delusional ideation (i.e., mentally fixated but not completely inflexible).

• A recent investigation by the Centers for Disease Control and Prevention supported the categorization of Morgellons disease as a form of delusions of parasitosis.

• **Rx:** establish rapport with patient first; pimozide or atypical antipsychotics.

For further information see Ch. 7. From *Dermatology, Third Edition*.

6 | Psoriasis

Key Points

- Affects up to 2% of the population.
- Chronic disorder in those with a polygenic predisposition combined with triggering factors such as infections (especially streptococcal pharyngitis, but also HIV infection) or medications (e.g. interferon, β-blockers, lithium, or oral CS taper).
- Koebner phenomenon – elicitation of psoriatic lesions by traumatizing the skin.
- Common sites.
  - Scalp.
  - Elbows and knees.
  - Nails, hands, feet, trunk (intergluteal fold).
- Skin lesions.
  - Most commonly – well-demarcated, erythematous plaques with silvery scale (Fig. 6.1).
  - Other lesions include sterile pustules, glistening plaques in intertriginous zones.
- Histopathologic findings.
  - Regular acanthosis, confluent parakeratosis with neutrophils, hypogranulosis, dilated blood vessels (see Chapter 1).
- Major systemic association is psoriatic arthritis (see Table 6.1), most commonly presenting as asymmetric oligoarthritis of hands/feet; the metabolic syndrome is also common.
- Pathogenesis.
  - Regarded as a T-cell-driven disease involving cytokines, including TNF-α and IL-23 (stimulates Th17 cells).
  - Genes that have been associated with psoriasis include those encoding

FIVE TYPES OF PSORIATIC ARTHRITIS
• Mono- and asymmetric oligoarthritis
• Arthritis of distal interphalangeal joints
• Rheumatoid arthritis-like presentation
• Arthritis mutilans
• Spondylitis and sacroiliitis

Table 6.1 Five types of psoriatic arthritis.

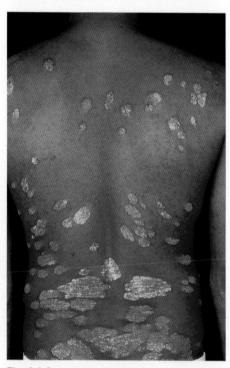

Fig. 6.2 Symmetric distribution of psoriatic plaques. *Courtesy, Peter C. M. van de Kerkhof, MD.*

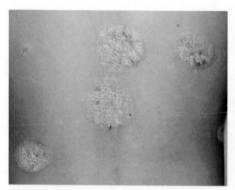

Fig. 6.1 Psoriatic plaques. Note the sharp demarcation and silvery scale. *Courtesy Julie V. Schaffer, MD.*

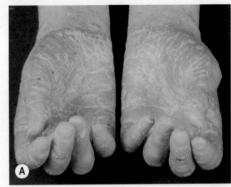

Fig. 6.3 Palmoplantar psoriasis. Erythematous scaling plaques of the palmar **(A)** and plantar surfaces **(B)**. Occasionally, there is well-demarcated hyperkeratosis with minimal erythema **(C)**. *A, Courtesy, Peter C. M. van de Kerkhof, MD.*

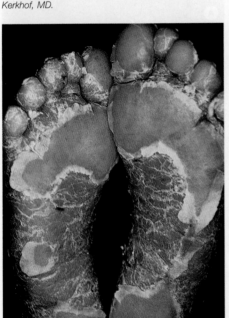

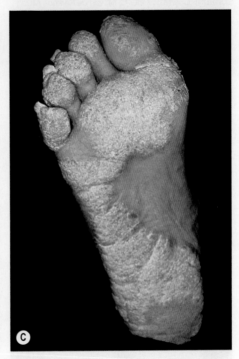

caspase recruitment domain family member 14 (CARD14, a regulator of NF-κB signaling) and, for generalized pustular psoriasis, the IL-36 receptor antagonist (a regulator of IL-8 production and IL-1β responses).

Variants

Chronic Plaque Psoriasis

• Typical lesion – well-demarcated, erythematous plaque with silvery scale.
• Often symmetrical lesions on the elbows and knees; additional sites include the scalp,

presacrum, hands, feet, intergluteal fold, and umbilicus (Figs. 6.2–6.4).
• May be generalized (Fig. 6.5).
• Lesions may be surrounded by a peripheral, blanching ring (Woronoff's ring), especially when patient is receiving phototherapy.

Guttate Psoriasis

• Typical lesion – small papule or plaque (3 mm to 1.5 cm) with adherent scale (Fig. 6.6).
• Generalized distribution.
• Affects children > adults.
• Often preceded by an upper respiratory tract infection.

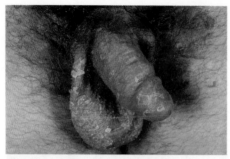

Fig. 6.4 Psoriasis of the genitalia.
Erythematous plaques with scale on the penis and scrotum. *Courtesy, Peter C. M. van de Kerkhof, MD.*

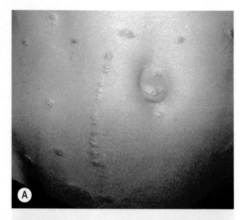

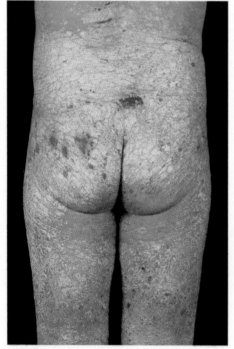

Fig. 6.5 Widespread chronic plaque psoriasis. *Courtesy, Peter CM van de Kerkhof, MD.*

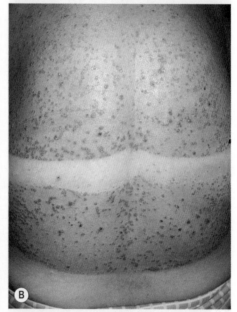

Fig. 6.6 Guttate psoriasis. A Small discrete papules and plaques of guttate psoriasis in an adolescent; note the Koebner phenomenon. **B** Numerous papules due to the Koebner phenomenon after a sunburn. *B, Courtesy Ronald P. Rapini, MD.*

• In children, may have spontaneous remission but often responds well to UVB phototherapy.
• **DDx:** pityriasis rosea, syphilis, id reaction to tinea pedis, and small plaque parapsoriasis.

Linear Psoriasis

• Linear, erythematous, scaly lesions that often follow the lines of Blaschko.
• **DDx:** inflammatory linear verrucous epidermal nevus (ILVEN; follows the lines of Blaschko; resistant to therapy), epidermal nevus with superimposed psoriasis.

Erythrodermic Psoriasis

• Generalized erythema of the skin, with areas of scaling.
• Gradual or acute onset.
• Nail changes, facial sparing, and a history of typical plaque-type psoriasis may be helpful clues.

- May be seen after abrupt tapering of medications, especially CS.
- **DDx:** other causes of erythroderma, e.g., pityriasis rubra pilaris, generalized atopic dermatitis, Sézary syndrome (see Table 8.2).

Pustular Psoriasis

- Generalized pustular psoriasis (von Zumbusch pattern).
  - Erythema and sterile pustules arising within erythematous, painful skin; lakes of pus characteristic (Fig. 6.7).

- Often associated fever.
  - Triggering factors – pregnancy (termed impetigo herpetiformis), rapid tapering of CS, hypocalcemia, infections.
  - **DDx:** acute generalized exanthematous pustulosis (AGEP; pustular drug reaction) (see Chapter 17).
- Palmoplantar (pustulosis).
  - Sterile pustules on palms/soles (Fig. 6.8).
  - May have no evidence of psoriasis elsewhere.
  - Triggering factors – infections, stress.
  - May be aggravated by smoking.
  - Associated with inflammatory bone lesions (see Chapter 21).

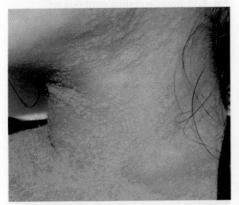

Fig. 6.7 Pustular psoriasis. Large areas of erythema with numerous pustules. Confluence of pustules creates lakes of pus. *Courtesy, Julie V. Schaffer, MD.*

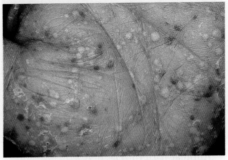

Fig. 6.8 Pustulosis of the palms and soles. Multiple sterile pustules are admixed with yellow-brown macules on the palm.

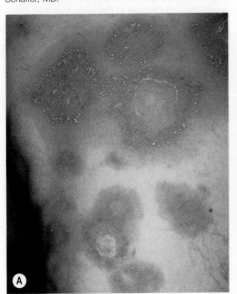

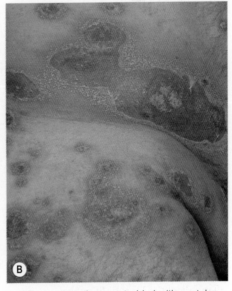

Fig. 6.9 Annular pustular psoriasis. Multiple annular inflammatory plaques studded with pustules. As the lesions enlarge, there can be central clearing, dry desquamation **(A)**, and/or moist desquamation that resembles wet cigarette paper **(B)**. *B, Courtesy, Peter C. M. van de Kerkhof, MD.*

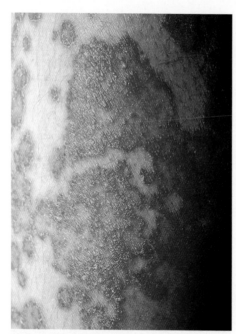

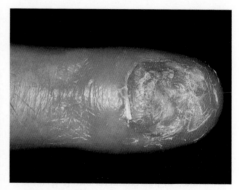

Fig. 6.11 Acrodermatitis continua (of Hallopeau). Erythema and scale of the distal digit, pustules within the nail bed, and partial shedding of the nail plate.

Fig. 6.10 'Localized' pattern of pustular psoriasis. The pustules are limited to preexisting plaques of psoriasis.

- Annular pattern (Fig. 6.9).
  - **DDx:** includes Sneddon–Wilkinson disease (see below).
- Exanthematic type.
  - Significant overlap with AGEP.
- Localized pattern – within plaques, often due to irritants (Fig. 6.10).
- Acrodermatitis continua (of Hallopeau).
  - Erythema and scale of distal digit with pustules (Fig. 6.11).
  - Often associated fever.

Special Sites

Scalp

- Well-demarcated, erythematous plaques with silvery scale.
- Scale may be attached for some distance onto scalp hairs, giving an asbestos-like appearance (pityriasis amiantacea).
- Occasionally alopecia may be seen within lesions.
- **DDx:** seborrheic dermatitis (more diffuse pattern), tinea capitis, dermatomyositis.

Flexural (Inverse Psoriasis)

- Shiny, pink, well-demarcated thin plaques with minimal scale (Fig. 6.12).

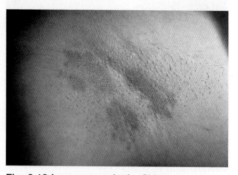

Fig. 6.12 Inverse psoriasis. Shiny erythematous plaques in the axilla that lack scale. *Courtesy, Ronald P. Rapini, MD.*

- Common sites include the axilla, inguinal crease, intergluteal cleft, inframammary area, and retroauricular fold.
- Sebopsoriasis – seborrheic dermatitis and psoriasis are at either ends of a spectrum, with intermediate forms termed sebopsoriasis.
- Additional **DDx:** seborrheic dermatitis, candidiasis, tinea cruris, erythrasma, granular parakeratosis (see Fig. 13.4).

Oral

- Migratory, annular lesions with central denuded areas and white borders.
- Similar to geographic tongue clinically and histopathologically.

Nail (See Chapter 58)

- Fingernails > toenails (Fig. 6.13).
- Associated with psoriatic arthritis.

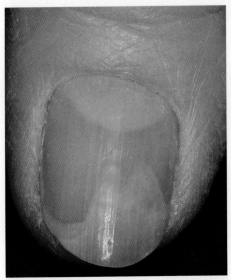

Fig. 6.13 Nail psoriasis. Changes include distal onycholysis, pitting, and 'oil spot' (salmon patch) phenomenon.

• Findings include nail pitting, oil spots (salmon patch), onycholysis with proximal red rim, splinter hemorrhages, subungual debris.

Sneddon–Wilkinson Disease (Subcorneal Pustular Dermatosis)

• Often begins in body folds or major intertriginous zones.
• Lesions are annular with superficial pustules on the border.
• Classic sign is a half and half pustule with clear fluid superiorly and pus inferiorly (dependent portion).
• Two schools of thought – this disease is (1) a variant of psoriasis vs. (2) a separate entity (Fig. 6.14).

Psoriatic Arthritis (See Table 6.1)

• Seen in 5–30% of patients with cutaneous psoriasis.
• Most commonly is an asymmetric oligoarthritis affecting the distal interphalangeal joints (Fig. 6.15).
• More rarely, but classically, is arthritis of all the interphalangeal joints.

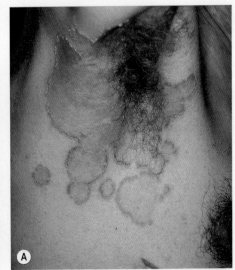

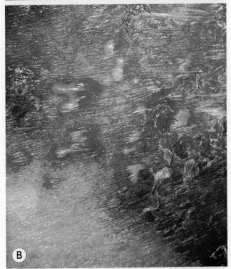

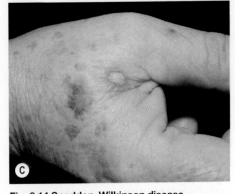

Fig. 6.14 Sneddon–Wilkinson disease.
A Annular and polycyclic plaques in the axilla.
B Subcorneal pustules with scale and crusts as well as background erythema. **C** Discrete pustule with an erythematous rim. *C, Courtesy, Joyce Rico, MD.*

• Occasionally, presentation is rheumatoid arthritis-like, affecting small- and medium-sized joints symmetrically.

• Arthritis mutilans – rare form with acute, rapidly progressive joint inflammation and destruction; softening and telescoping of the digits.

• Spondylitis and sacroiliitis – axial arthritis as well as arthritis of the knees and sacroiliac joints; may be HLA-B27-positive and may have associated inflammatory bowel disease or uveitis.

• **DDx:** reactive arthritis (previously referred to as Reiter's disease).

   – Urethritis, arthritis, ocular findings (e.g., conjunctivitis), and oral ulcers in addition to psoriasiform lesions, especially on the soles (keratoderma blennorrhagicum) or genitalia (balanitis circinata) (Fig. 6.16).

   – More common in men.

   – Strongly associated with HLA-B27.

   – Course is often self-limited.

   – May be severe in HIV-positive individuals.

Treatment

• Topical agents.
   – First-line.
     • CS (Table 6.2).
     • Vitamin D₃ analogues (calcipotriene, calcitriol) (Table 6.3).
   – Second-line.
     • Calcineurin inhibitors (may be first-line for sensitive areas such as the face or flexures).

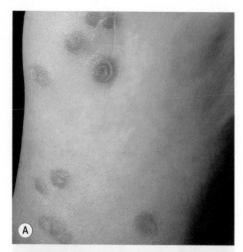

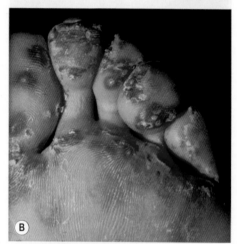

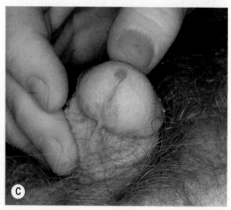

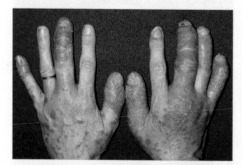

Fig. 6.15 Psoriatic arthritis. Asymmetric involvement of the distal interphalangeal (DIP) and proximal interphalangeal (PIP) joints. A 'sausage' digit (third digit bilaterally) results from involvement of both the DIP and PIP joints.

Fig. 6.16 Reactive arthritis (formerly Reiter's disease). A, B Plantar lesions of keratoderma blennorrhagicum. **C** Papulosquamous lesions of balanitis circinata on the penis. *B, Courtesy, Eugene Mirrer, MD.*

INDICATIONS AND CONTRAINDICATIONS FOR TOPICAL CORTICOSTEROIDS

Indications

- Mild to moderate psoriasis: first-line treatment as monotherapy or in combination
- Severe psoriasis: often in combination with a vitamin D_3 analogue, a topical retinoid, anthralin, or tar
- Monotherapy for flexural and facial psoriasis (usually mild strength)
- Recalcitrant plaques often require occlusion (plastic, hydrocolloid)

Contraindications

- Bacterial, viral, and mycotic infections
- Atrophy of the skin
- Allergic contact dermatitis due to corticosteroids or constituents of the formulation
- Pregnancy or lactation*

Relative; can consider limited use of mild- to moderate-strength corticosteroids.

Table 6.2 Indications and contraindications for topical corticosteroids. Maximal quantities: 50 g/week of a superpotent corticosteroid; 100 g/week of a potent corticosteroid. *Courtesy, Peter C. M. van de Kerkhof, MD.*

INDICATIONS AND CONTRAINDICATIONS FOR VITAMIN D_3 ANALOGUES

Indications

- Mild to moderate psoriasis: first-line treatment as monotherapy or in combination
- Severe psoriasis: combination treatment

Contraindications

- Involvement requiring more than the maximally recommended quantity, e.g. 100 g/week of calcipotriene/calcipotriol
- Abnormality in bone or calcium metabolism*
- Renal insufficiency
- Allergy to the vitamin D_3 analogue or constituents of the preparation
- Pregnancy or lactation

For example, sarcoidosis and bone metastases.

Table 6.3 Indications and contraindications for vitamin D_3 analogues. If used in conjunction with phototherapy, vitamin D_3 preparations need to be applied after UV irradiation or at least several hours prior, because they may reduce UV penetration into the skin. *Courtesy, Peter C. M. van de Kerkhof, MD.*

- Tars (e.g. liquor carbonis detergens [LCD] 5%).
- Anthralin.
- Tazarotene.
- Phototherapy and systemic agents.
  - First-line.
    - Phototherapy – UVB (narrowband or broadband > PUVA) (Table 6.4); if thick keratotic plaques, can combine with oral retinoids.
    - Methotrexate (oral or intramuscular, occasionally subcutaneous) (Table 6.5).
    - Oral retinoids (e.g. acitretin, isotretinoin).
  - Second-line systemic.
    - Targeted immunomodulators ('biologic' agents) (Tables 6.6 and 6.7).
    - Cyclosporine.
- See Table 6.8 for treatment options in patients with comorbidities or special situations.
- See Table 6.9 for the recommended laboratory evaluation for patients receiving targeted immunomodulators.

INDICATIONS AND CONTRAINDICATIONS FOR PHOTOTHERAPY
Indications
• Moderate to severe psoriasis: first-line treatment as monotherapy or in combination
Contraindications (Absolute or Relative)
• Genetic disorders characterized by increased photosensitivity or an increased risk of skin cancer (UVB and PUVA)*
• Skin type I (UVB and PUVA)†
• Photosensitive dermatoses (UVB and PUVA)†
• Unavoidable phototoxic systemic or topical medications (UVB and PUVA)†
• Vitiligo (UVB and PUVA)†
• Previous history of arsenic exposure, ionizing irradiation, or excessive phototherapy (UVB and PUVA)
• High cumulative number of PUVA treatments, i.e. >150–200 individual treatments (PUVA)*
• Treatment with cyclosporine (UVB and PUVA)*
• Immunosuppressive medication (UVB and PUVA)
• Previous history of skin cancers (PUVA > UVB)
• Atypical melanocytic nevi (UVB and PUVA)
• Seizure disorder (risk of fall/injury; UVB and PUVA)
• Poor compliance (UVB and PUVA)
• Men and women in reproductive years without contraception (PUVA)
• Pregnancy or lactation (PUVA)*
• Impaired liver function or hepatotoxic medication (PUVA)
• Cataracts (PUVA)
*Absolute contraindication. †Need to adjust the dose and monitor closely. PUVA, psoralen + ultraviolet A; UVB, ultraviolet B.

Table 6.4 Indications and contraindications for phototherapy. *Courtesy, Peter C. M. van de Kerkhof, MD.*

INDICATIONS AND CONTRAINDICATIONS FOR METHOTREXATE (MTX)
Indications
• Severe psoriasis
• Chronic plaque psoriasis (>10–15% BSA or interference with employment or social functioning)
• Pustular psoriasis (generalized or localized)
• Erythrodermic psoriasis
• Psoriatic arthritis (moderate to severe)
• Severe nail psoriasis
• Psoriasis not responding to topical treatments, phototherapy, and/or systemic retinoids

Table 6.5 Indications and contraindications for methotrexate (MTX). *Courtesy, Peter C. M. van de Kerkhof, MD. Continued*

Table 6.5 *Continued* **Indications and contraindications for methotrexate (MTX).** *Courtesy, Peter C. M. van de Kerkhof, MD.*

Contraindications (Absolute or Relative)

- Impaired kidney function (creatinine clearance <60 ml/min)[†]
- Severe anemia, leukopenia, and/or thrombocytopenia*
- Significant liver function abnormalities, hepatitis (active and/or recent), severe fibrosis, cirrhosis, excessive alcohol intake*
- Concomitant hepatotoxic medications
- Concomitant medications that increase MTX levels, e.g. trimethoprim–sulfamethoxazole*
- Significantly reduced pulmonary function*
- Pregnancy or lactation*
- Currently planning to have children (male and female patients)[‡]
- Immunodeficiency syndromes
- Severe infections*
- Active infections
- Peptic ulcer (active)*
- Gastritis
- Concomitant radiation therapy
- Pleural effusion or ascites[†]
- Hypersensitivity to MTX*
- Unreliable patient*

Absolute contraindication.
[†]*Requires significant reduction in dosage.*
[‡]*Because of possible mutagenic risk and teratogenicity, discontinue MTX 3 months prior to attempts to conceive; continue contraception during these 3 months.*
BSA, body surface area.

COMMERCIALLY AVAILABLE BIOLOGIC AGENTS USED FOR THE TREATMENT OF PSORIASIS			
Biologic Agent	**Target**	**Molecule**	**Approved***
Alefacept**	CD2	Human fusion protein	FDA
Etanercept	TNF-α[†]	Human fusion protein	FDA + EMA
Infliximab	TNF-α[‡]	Chimeric antibody	FDA + EMA
Adalimumab	TNF-α[‡]	Human antibody	FDA + EMA (psoriatic arthritis)
Ustekinumab	p40 subunit of IL-12/23	Human antibody	FDA + EMA

By registration authorities for the treatment of psoriasis.
**Production of alefacept in the United States was discontinued in 2011.*
[†]*Soluble form.*
[‡]*Soluble form and transmembrane TNF receptor.*
EMA, European Medicines Agency; FDA, Food and Drug Administration; IL, interleukin; TNF, tumor necrosis factor.

Table 6.6 Commercially available biologic agents used for the treatment of psoriasis.

INDICATIONS AND CONTRAINDICATIONS FOR COMMERCIALLY AVAILABLE TARGETED IMMUNE MODULATORS ('BIOLOGIC' AGENTS)

Indications

General Indications

- Patients with moderate to severe psoriasis, eligible for a systemic treatment
- Patients with psoriatic arthritis, particularly those who have failed to improve with other disease-modifying antirheumatic drugs (DMARDs)

Restricted Indication

- Patients with moderate to severe psoriasis who are not candidates for topical treatments, phototherapy, or classic systemic treatments because of insufficient efficacy or contraindications

Contraindications

(The exact contraindications vary by agent; some listed below are relative, while others are absolute [*])

- Significant viral, bacterial, or fungal infections*
- Increased risk for developing sepsis*
- Active tuberculosis*
- Immunosuppressed patient
- Past history of hepatitis B
- Pregnancy (TNF-α inhibitors, alefacept[†] and ustekinumab are category B)
- Breast-feeding
- Malignancy within the past 5 years (does not include adequately treated cutaneous squamous or basal cell carcinoma)
- Excessive chronic sun exposure or phototherapy
- Allergic reaction to the biologic agent*
- Selective for alefacept[†]: CD4 counts <250 cells/mcl*; HIV infection*
- Selective for TNF-α inhibitors: ANA+ (especially if high titer) or autoimmune connective tissue disease, lymphoma, congestive heart failure (NYHA grade III or IV), or demyelinization disorders (the latter also in first-degree relatives)*
- Selective for ustekinumab: BCG vaccination within the past 12 months (mode of action expected to increase susceptibility to mycobacterial infections)

[†]*Production of alefacept in the United States was discontinued in 2011.*
BCG, bacillus Calmette–Guérin; NYHA, New York Heart Association.

Table 6.7 Indications and contraindications for commercially available targeted immune modulators ('biologic' agents). Administration of live vaccines is contraindicated in patients receiving biologic agents for psoriasis. *Courtesy, Peter C. M. van de Kerkhof, MD.*

TREATMENT OF THE PSORIATIC PATIENT WITH COMORBIDITIES OR SPECIAL SITUATIONS

Comorbidity or Special Situation	Potential Treatment(s)
History of internal malignancy (e.g. lymphoma and lung cancer)	Topical agents UVB phototherapy Oral retinoids
Liver disease	Topical agents UVB phototherapy Targeted immunomodulators ('biologic' agents) (e.g. etanercept)
Hepatitis B* or C viral infection	Etanercept > adalimumab, ustekinumab

Table 6.8 Treatment of the psoriatic patient with comorbidities or special situations. Targeted immunomodulators ('biologic' agents) are contraindicated in patients with active tuberculosis. *Continued*

Table 6.8 *Continued* **Treatment of the psoriatic patient with comorbidities or special situations.** Targeted immunomodulators ('biologic' agents) are contraindicated in patients with active tuberculosis.

Comorbidity or Special Situation	Potential Treatment(s)
Metabolic syndrome	Topical agents Phototherapy Methotrexate[†] Oral retinoids[†] Targeted immunomodulators ('biologic' agents)
Pregnancy	Topical CS (limited use of mild- to moderate-strength CS) UVB phototherapy Targeted immunomodulators ('biologic' agents) (anti-TNF agents and ustekinumab are category B) Cyclosporine (category C)
Immunosuppression (e.g. HIV infection/AIDS)	Topical agents UVB phototherapy Oral retinoids
Numerous skin cancers	Topical agents Oral retinoids

In hepatitis B surface antigen (HBsAg) carriers, either anti-HBV treatment or prophylaxis is required to prevent hepatitis reactivation; others require careful monitoring.
[†]*Caution with use in patients with fatty liver.*

RECOMMENDED LABORATORY EVALUATION FOR PATIENTS RECEIVING TARGETED IMMUNOMODULATORS FOR PSORIASIS

Drug	Prior to treatment	During treatment
TNF-α inhibitors (e.g. adalimumab, etanercept, infliximab) or ustekinumab	Tuberculin skin test*/interferon-γ release assay** and/or (e.g. if immunosuppression or history of tuberculosis) chest x-ray CBC, CMP Hepatitis B and C virus serologic profiles Consider HIV testing	Annual tuberculin skin test*/interferon-γ release assay** and/or chest x-ray CBC or CMP every 3-12 months (or as clinically indicated)

≥5 mm of induration should be considered as positive.
***e.g. QuantiFERON® TB Gold or T-SPOT®.TB.*
CMP, comprehensive metabolic panel (includes liver function tests); PPD, purified protein derivative.

Table 6.9 Recommended laboratory evaluation for patients receiving targeted immunomodulators for psoriasis. A complete medical history and physical examination should also be performed, with particular attention to history/risk/symptoms/signs of tuberculosis, other chronic infections, malignancy, neurologic disorders and cardiac disease (especially congestive heart failure in patients receiving TNF-α inhibitors).

For further information see Ch. 8. From *Dermatology, Third Edition*.

7 | Other Papulosquamous Disorders

Parapsoriasis

- Chronic, usually asymptomatic patches or thin plaques with fine scale whose color varies from pink to red-brown; may have associated epidermal atrophy and occasionally poikiloderma (large plaque parapsoriasis).
- Two major forms of parapsoriasis are small plaque (lesions usually <5 cm in diameter) and large plaque (usually >5 cm); digitate dermatosis is a form of the former, whereas retiform parapsoriasis is a variant of the latter (Figs. 7.1 and 7.2).
- While the distribution may be limited or more generalized, there is a tendency for an increase in extent over time; large plaque parapsoriasis can favor the sun-protected 'girdle' area; both forms usually occur in adults.
- Controversy exists regarding the percentage of cases of large plaque parapsoriasis that eventually evolve into mycosis fungoides.
- Histologically, parakeratosis and nonspecific spongiotic dermatitis is seen in small and large plaque; large plaque may have a more lichenoid infiltrate.
- Infiltrate of CD4+ T lymphocytes, often clonal, in large plaque > small plaque, leading to the term 'clonal dermatitis'.
- **DDx:** small plaque – pityriasis rosea (PR), PR-like drug eruption, pityriasis lichenoides chronica, guttate psoriasis, secondary syphilis; large plaque parapsoriasis – patch stage mycosis fungoides (MF), MF-like drug eruption; if a few lesions, consider tinea corporis.
- **Rx:** topical CS, sunlight, phototherapy (e.g. NBUVB).

Pityriasis Lichenoides et Varioliformis Acuta (PLEVA) and Pityriasis Lichenoides Chronica (PLC)

- PLEVA, also known as Mucha–Habermann disease, and PLC exist along a clinicopathologic spectrum such that patients can have characteristic lesions of both disorders, either concurrently or in tandem.

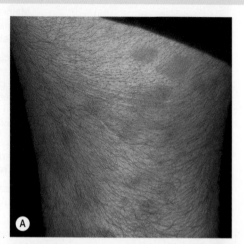

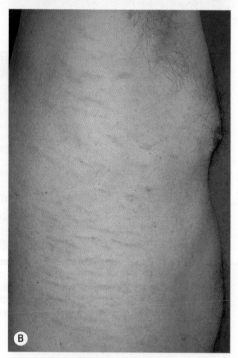

Fig. 7.1 Small plaque parapsoriasis. A Small (<5 cm), pink slight scaly patches. **B** Digitate dermatosis with elongated finger-like lesions on the flank. Digitate dermatosis is the exception to the 5-cm rule as the lesions may measure 10 cm or more along their long axes. *A, Courtesy, Gary Wood, MD, and George Reizner, MD.*

- In both forms, there are recurrent crops of papules with individual lesions spontaneously resolving over weeks (PLEVA) to months (PLC); only occasionally is there an obvious trigger (e.g. viral infection, medication); the entire course of the disorder can last for years.
- PLEVA occurs more commonly in younger age groups; it is characterized by widespread erythematous papules that are often crusted but may be vesicular or pustular (Fig. 7.3A–C).
- The onset of PLEVA can be abrupt, and recurrences typically occur for months to years; there is an unusual ulcerative form that is accompanied by fever, lymphadenopathy, arthritis, and mucosal involvement.
- PLC is characterized by pink to red-brown papules with scale and can resolve with post-inflammatory guttate hypopigmentation (Fig. 7.3D,E).
- Histologically, parakeratosis, an interface dermatitis with necrotic keratinocytes, and extravasation of red blood cells are seen; the infiltrate is composed of T cells that are often monoclonal; in PLEVA, the infiltrate may be wedge-shaped and neutrophils may be seen.
- **DDx:** PLEVA – varicella or other viral exanthem, e.g. Coxsackie, disseminated zoster without a dermatome (more limited duration), lymphomatoid papulosis (often fewer larger lesions), arthropod reactions, small vessel vasculitis; PLC – small plaque parapsoriasis, pityriasis rosea, secondary syphilis, guttate psoriasis, lichen planus.
- **Rx:** topical CS, prolonged courses of antibiotics (e.g. erythromycin, tetracyclines), phototherapy (e.g. NBUVB); severe cases may require MTX in consultation with a dermatologist.

Pityriasis Rosea

- Occurs more commonly in adolescents and young adults; in general, individuals are healthy and have no systemic complaints/symptoms.
- The etiology is unknown, but viral infections may serve as a trigger.
- Lesions increase in number and extent over a few weeks but then spontaneously resolve; classically, the initial lesion, known as the 'herald patch,' is often the largest (Fig. 7.4).

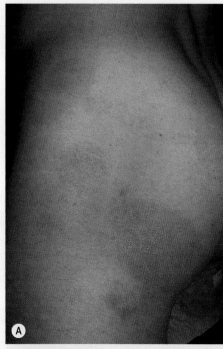

Fig. 7.2 Large plaque parapsoriasis. A Large, red-brown patches in the bathing trunk region – a classic clinical presentation. **B** Retiform parapsoriasis with pink-brown lesions forming a net-like pattern, hence the term retiform; note the associated wrinkling due to epidermal atrophy.

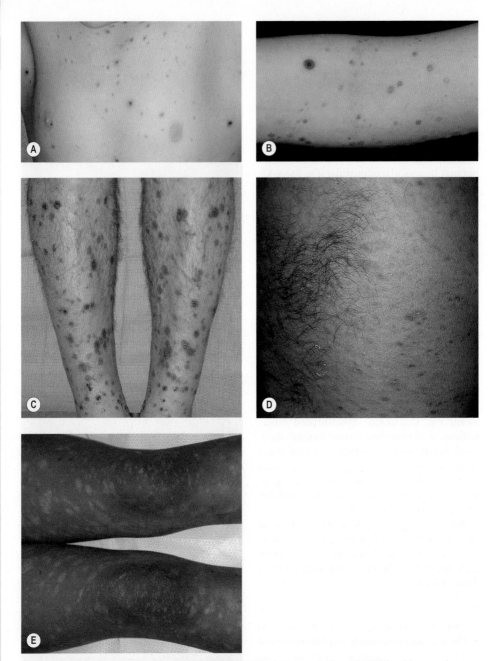

Fig. 7.3 Clinical spectrum of pityriasis lichenoides. In the acute form (PLEVA), widespread erythematous papules and papulovesicles are admixed with crusted lesions **(A, B);** sometimes there can be an ulcerative component **(C).** Lesions can heal with varioliform scars. Individuals with the chronic form (PLC) develop multiple red-brown papules, some of which have scale **(D);** these lesions often heal with hypopigmentation, especially in patients with darkly pigmented skin **(E).** *A, Courtesy, Julie V. Schaffer, MD; B, Courtesy, Thomas Schwarz, MD.*

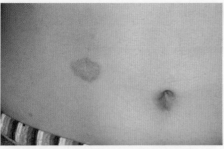

Fig. 7.4 Pityriasis rosea – herald patch. It typically precedes the development of a more widespread eruption. *Courtesy, Kalman Watsky, MD.*

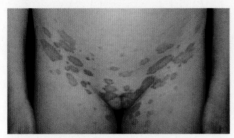

Fig. 7.5 Inverse pityriasis rosea. In this variant, the lesions are limited to the groin and/or axillae. The long axes of the lesions follow the lines of cleavage.

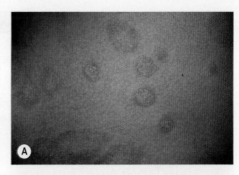

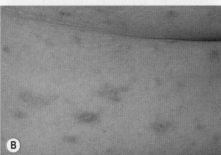

- The distribution is that of a 1920s bathing suit – proximal extremities and trunk; occasionally, an inverse pattern is seen in which the majority of lesions are in the axillae and/ or groin (Fig. 7.5).
- Pink to salmon-colored papules or plaques are round or oval in shape (Fig. 7.6), with their long axes following Langer's lines of cleavage (Fig. 7.7), creating a 'Christmas tree' pattern on the trunk; scale, both fine white centrally and as a collarette at the edge of the lesion, is the most common secondary change, but occasionally crusting, vesicles, purpura, or even pustules may be seen.
- The average duration is 6–8 weeks, with some cases lasting for months.
- Histologically, mounds of parakeratosis are seen, accompanied by spongiosis and a mild perivascular and interstitial lymphocytic infiltrate; extravasation of red blood cells may occur.
- **DDx:** guttate psoriasis, secondary syphilis (preceding chancre, usually genital; accompanied by malaise, lymphadenopathy, other

Fig. 7.6 Pityriasis rosea. A, B Both round and oval-shaped plaques can be seen as well as fine white scale and collarettes of scale. **C** In patients with more darkly pigmented skin, central hyperpigmentation can develop and there may be a more follicular pattern. *B, Courtesy, Julie V. Schaffer, MD; C, Courtesy, Aisha Sethi, MD.*

SECTION 3: Papulosquamous and Eczematous Dermatoses

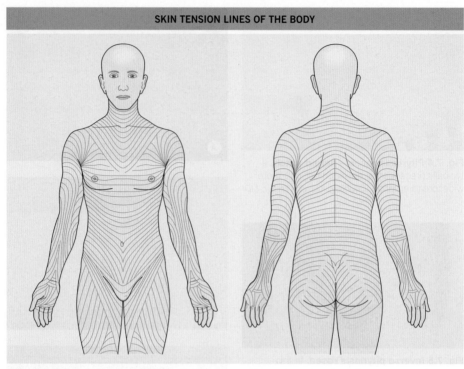

Fig. 7.7 Langer's lines of cleavage. These represent skin tension lines on the body.

mucocutaneous signs such as condyloma latum, palmoplantar lesions; positive Venereal Disease Research Laboratory [VDRL] or rapid plasma reagin [RPR] test), pityriasis lichenoides chronica (especially if persistent), nummular dermatitis (if vesicular), pityriasis rosea-like drug eruptions (e.g. ACE inhibitors, metronidazole).

• **Rx:** topical anti-pruritic lotions or CS (for the minority of patients with associated pruritus), natural sunlight, 14-day course of erythromycin, 10-day course of azithromycin, NBUVB.

Pityriasis Rubra Pilaris

• One of the dermatologic disorders that can lead to an erythroderma (Fig. 7.8), often with an onset in the head and neck region; peaks of incidence – first to second decade of life and sixth decade of life.

• It is characterized by a salmon or orange-red color, islands of sparing, follicular papules (including within the relatively spared areas

and on the dorsal fingers), and a waxy keratoderma (Fig. 7.9).

• May be exacerbated by exposure to UV light; classic forms spontaneously resolve within 3–5 years (Fig. 7.10).

• Five major forms have been described, with distinctions based on age of onset and distribution, with the adult classic form being the most common (Fig. 7.10); occasionally PRP is familial and can be due to *CARD14* mutations.

• Histologically, there is alternating ortho- and parakeratosis, both vertically and horizontally, within the stratum corneum (checkerboard pattern); additional findings are follicular plugging with a shoulder of parakeratosis, acantholysis within the epidermis, and variable inflammation.

• **DDx:** other causes of erythroderma, in particular psoriasis and Sézary syndrome, and an unusual form of dermatomyositis seen more often in Asians (Wong type); in children, also progressive symmetric erythrokeratoderma; early on, seborrheic dermatitis.

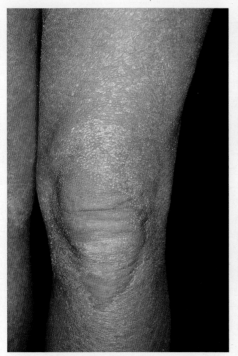

Fig. 7.8 Erythroderma due to pityriasis rubra pilaris. Within areas of erythema, follicular hyperkeratosis (knee) may be more difficult to appreciate than in areas of relative sparing (compare to Fig. 7.9A).

• **Rx:** oral isotretinion, acetretin, methotrexate, tumor necrosis factor-α inhibitors (mixed results); response should be seen within 6 months.

Pityriasis Rotunda

• Seen primarily in the Far East, Mediterranean basin, and Africa; favors individuals with darker skin phototypes.

• Large, asymptomatic, circular and polycyclic patches with scale that are often hyperpigmented; the lesions are also well demarcated and lack inflammation clinically, occurring on the trunk and extremities.

• Associated with malnutrition and secondarily internal malignancies or systemic infections; occasionally, familial, especially in Caucasians.

• Histologically, resembles ichthyosis vulgaris with hyperkeratosis and a reduced granular layer.

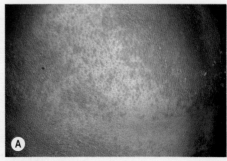

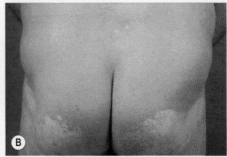

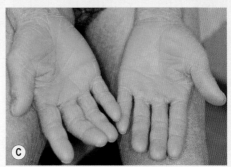

Fig. 7.9 Pityriasis rubra pilaris. A Follicular papules within islands of sparing and confluent orange-red scaly plaques. **B** The islands of sparing may be sharply demarcated; note the salmon color of the plaques. **C** Waxy keratoderma, again with an orange hue.
C, Courtesy, Irwin Braverman, MD.

• **DDx:** leprosy, large plaque parapsoriasis, tinea corporis, tinea versicolor.

Granular Parakeratosis

• Originally described in the axillae of adults (primarily women), but can involve other intertriginous zones and in infants, the diaper area.

• Red-brown plaques with scale, often thick, that may be related to chronic irritation

CLASSIFICATION OF PITYRIASIS RUBRA PILARIS

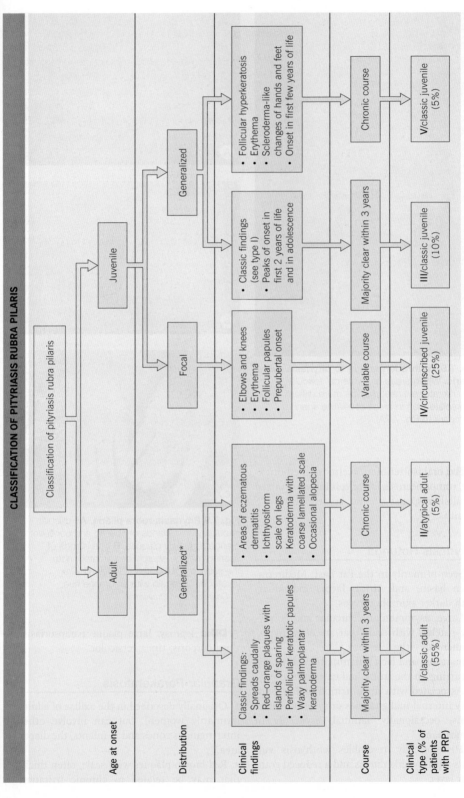

Fig. 7.10 Classification of pityriasis rubra pilaris (PRP). *A generalized distribution of PRP, often with findings similar to type I, may be seen in association with elongated follicular spines, acne conglobata, and hidradenitis suppurativa in HIV-infected individuals; this has been referred to as type VI PRP or the HIV-associated follicular syndrome.

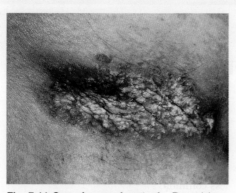

Fig. 7.11 Granular parakeratosis. Brownish-red papules that have coalesced into a keratotic plaque in the axilla. *Courtesy, David Mehregan, MD.*

(Fig. 7.11); there may be secondary maceration and pruritus.

• Diagnostic histologic findings of marked compact parakeratosis with retained keratohyaline granules within the stratum corneum.

• **DDx:** other causes of intertrigo (e.g. seborrheic dermatitis, inverse psoriasis, candidiasis), irritant or allergic contact dermatitis, erythrasma, Hailey–Hailey disease.

• **Rx:** discontinuation of topical irritants (e.g. mineral salt-containing crystals used as 'natural' deodorants, biodegradable diapers), mild topical CS.

For further information see Ch. 9. From *Dermatology, Third Edition.*

8 Erythroderma

Introduction

- Defined as generalized redness and scaling involving more than 90% of the body surface area (BSA); occasionally applied to patients with slightly less BSA involvement, e.g. when diagnosed earlier in the course of their disease.
- A clinical presentation for a variety of diseases, often divided into three major categories: (1) primary skin disorders; (2) drug-related (Table 8.1); and (3) malignancies, particularly Sézary syndrome and erythrodermic mycosis fungoides.
- In adults (Table 8.2), the most common primary skin disorders are psoriasis (Fig. 8.1) and atopic dermatitis, with allergic contact dermatitis or pityriasis rubra pilaris (Fig. 8.2) less common.
- In addition to atopic dermatitis, causes in infants and neonates (Table 8.3) include inherited ichthyoses, immunodeficiencies, staphylococcal scalded skin syndrome (SSSS), and seborrheic dermatitis.
- Despite varied etiologies, patients have a number of clinical features in common: generalized erythema and desquamation (scaling) (Fig. 8.5), pruritus with secondary changes (e.g., lichenification), dyspigmentation, eruptive seborrheic keratoses (Fig. 8.6), secondary cutaneous infections, ectropion and purulent conjunctivitis; additional findings include palmoplantar keratoderma, nail dystrophy (Fig. 8.7), and alopecia.

DRUGS ASSOCIATED WITH ERYTHRODERMA	
Common	**Less Common***
• Allopurinol • Beta-lactam antibiotics • Carbamazepine/oxcarbazepine • Gold • Phenobarbital • Phenytoins • Sulfasalazine • Sulfonamides**	• Captopril • Carboplatin/cisplatin • Cytokines (IL-2/GM-CSF) • Dapsone • Diflunisal • Fluindone • Hydroxychloroquine/chloroquine • Isoniazid • Isotretinoin/acitretin • Lithium • Mercury compounds • Minocycline • Nifedipine/diltiazem • Omeprazole/lansoprazole • Thalidomide • Vancomycin[†]

*Reference for additional drugs: Litt, JZ. 2010. Litt's Drug Eruptions & Reactions Manual, 16th ed. London. Informa Healthcare.
**Includes furosemide.
[†]Not to be confused with red man syndrome due to rapid infusion of vancomycin.

Table 8.1 Drugs associated with erythroderma.

CAUSES OF ERYTHRODERMA IN ADULTS	
Underlying Disease	**Major Features**
Common	
Psoriasis (Chapter 6) (see Fig. 8.1)	• Pre-existing psoriatic plaques • Often spares face • Nail changes (pits, oil drop, onycholysis) • Subcorneal pustules (pustular psoriasis) • Inflammatory arthritis • Personal or family history of psoriasis • Onset after withdrawal of CS or methotrexate
Atopic dermatitis (Chapter 10)	• Pre-existing lesions in flexures • Severe pruritus • Lichenification, including eyelids • Prurigo nodularis • Elevated serum IgE, eosinophilia • Personal or family history of atopy
Drug reactions (Chapter 17) (see Table 8.1)	• Often preceded by morbilliform or scarlatiniform exanthem • Typically more abrupt onset • Facial edema • In dependent areas, may become purpuric • No history of skin diseases • Usually resolves within 2–6 weeks after withdrawal of culprit drug; with the possible exception of DRESS/DIHS (see Chapter 17)
Idiopathic erythroderma (see Fig. 8.3)	• Elderly men • Chronic, relapsing • Severe pruritus • Palmoplantar keratoderma • Dermatopathic lymphadenopathy • Consider less commonly associated drugs (Table 8.1) • Continue to re-evaluate for cutaneous T-cell lymphoma
Less Common	
Cutaneous T-cell lymphoma (CTCL; see Chapter 98)	• Sézary syndrome more common than erythrodermic mycosis fungoides or other forms of CTCL • Intense pruritus • Deep purple-red hue • Painful fissured keratoderma • Alopecia • Leonine facies • Elevated $CD4^+:CD8^+$ ratio (blood) • Detection of clonal T-cell population in skin and blood (flow cytometry)

Table 8.2 Causes of erythroderma in adults. *Continued*

Table 8.2 *Continued* **Causes of erythroderma in adults.**

Underlying Disease	Major Features
Pityriasis rubra pilaris (Chapter 7) (see Fig. 8.2)	• Cephalocaudal progression • Salmon-colored erythema • Islands of sparing (*nappes claires*) • Waxy keratoderma • Perifollicular keratotic papules • Flare after sun exposure
Dermatitis (non-atopic) • Contact (Chapter 12) • Seborrheic (Chapter 11) • Stasis with autosensitization (Chapter 11)	• Pre-existing localized disease • Distribution of initial lesions • Occupation and hobbies • Patch testing • Review oral medications (systemic contact dermatitis)
Chronic actinic dermatitis (Chapter 73)	• Initial lesions in photodistribution • Drug history • UVA, UVB, and visible light phototesting • Photopatch testing
Rare	
Crusted (Norwegian) scabies (Chapter 71)	• Elderly, infants, immunocompromised • Crusted keratoderma
Papuloerythroderma of Ofuji	• Widespread, pruritic, red-brown, flat-topped papules; may become confluent • Sparing of skin folds ('deck chair' sign) • Favors elderly men • May be associated with lymphoma or HIV infection
Other	

- Hypereosinophilic syndrome (Chapter 20)
- Lichen planus
- Autoimmune connective tissue disease (dermatomyositis, lupus)
- Autoimmune bullous dermatoses (e.g., pemphigus foliaceus [Fig. 8.4])
- Dermatophyte infection
- Mastocytosis
- Graft-versus-host disease (GVHD)

DRESS, drug reaction with eosinophilia and systemic symptoms (also referred to as drug-induced hypersensitivity syndrome [DIHS]).

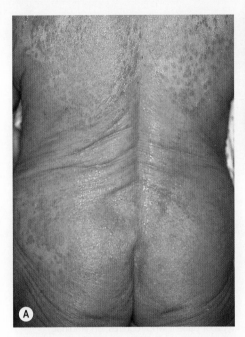

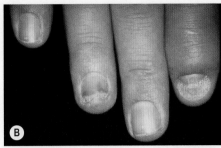

Fig. 8.1 Psoriatic erythroderma. A The disease flare correlated with the administration of lithium. **B** Nail findings (subungual hyperkeratosis, nail plate thickening, and oil-drop changes) point to the diagnosis of psoriasis. There is also soft tissue swelling of the forefinger due to psoriatic arthritis. *A, Courtesy, Jean L. Bolognia, MD; B, Courtesy, Wolfram Sterry, MD.*

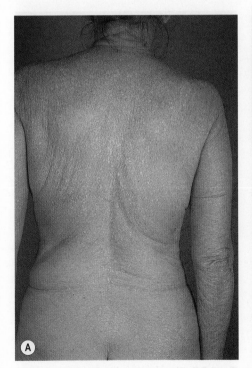

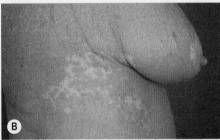

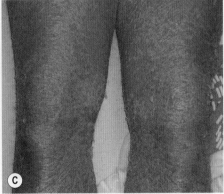

Fig. 8.2 Erythroderma secondary to pityriasis rubra pilaris. A few islands of sparing are noted on the upper back **(A)** but are more noticeable on the flank and breast **(B). C** Large thin scales are seen as well as the distinctive salmon to orange-red color.

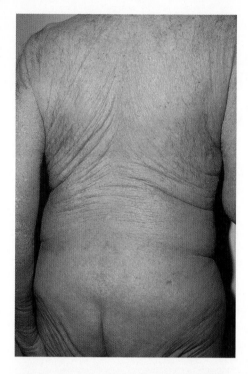

Fig. 8.3 Idiopathic erythroderma. This is the type of patient who requires longitudinal evaluation to exclude the development of cutaneous T-cell lymphoma.

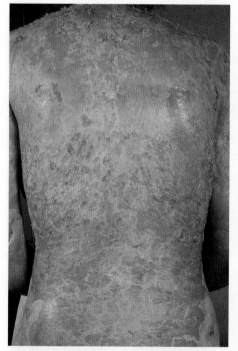

Fig. 8.4 Erythroderma due to pemphigus foliaceus. Generalized erythema with widespread scale-crusts and large areas of erosion.

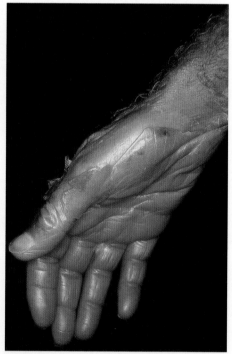

Fig. 8.5 Erythroderma with desquamation. Obvious exfoliation of scale with underlying erythema.

CAUSES OF ERYTHRODERMA IN NEONATES AND INFANTS

Inherited Ichthyoses (Chapter 46)

- Epidermolytic ichthyosis (bullous congenital ichthyosiform erythroderma)
- Nonbullous congenital ichthyosiform erythroderma (NBCIE)
- Netherton syndrome
- Conradi–Hünermann–Happle syndrome (X-linked dominant chondrodysplasia punctata)

Immunodeficiencies (Chapter 49)

- Omenn syndrome and other forms of severe combined immunodeficiency (SCID)
- Agammaglobulinemia, complement disorders (e.g., C3, C5)
- Wiskott–Aldrich syndrome, hyper-IgE syndrome

Primary Dermatoses

- Atopic dermatitis
- Seborrheic dermatitis
- Psoriasis

Drug Reactions (See Table 8.1)

Infections

- Staphylococcal scalded skin syndrome (Chapter 61)
- Neonatal toxic shock-like exanthematous disease
- Congenital cutaneous candidiasis

Other

- Diffuse cutaneous mastocytosis
- Pityriasis rubra pilaris (Chapter 7)
- Graft-versus-host disease (GVHD)
- Rare ichthyoses
- Ankyloblepharon, ectodermal dysplasia, and cleft lip/palate (AEC) syndrome (Chapter 52)
- Nutritional dermatitis

Table 8.3 Causes of erythroderma in neonates and infants.

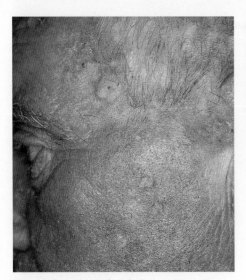

Fig. 8.6 Eruptive seborrheic keratoses in a patient with idiopathic erythroderma.
Courtesy, Jean L. Bolognia, MD.

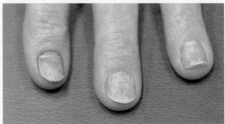

Fig. 8.7 Nail dystrophy in a patient with idiopathic erythroderma. In addition to yellowing and thickening of the nail plate as well as subungual debris, splinter hemorrhages, and onycholysis, there is impending onychomadesis of at least one fingernail. *Courtesy, Karynne O. Duncan, MD.*

GENERAL TREATMENT STRATEGIES FOR ADULT ERYTHRODERMA

General Measures

- Consider hospitalization
- Nutritional assessment
- Correct fluid/electrolyte imbalances
- Prevent hypothermia
- Treat secondary infections (e.g., *Staphylococcus aureus*)
- Oral antihistamines to suppress pruritus (via sedation)

Topical Measures

- Open wet dressings (Appendix)
- Bland emollients
- Low- to mid-potency topical CS (ointments > creams)
- Reserve high-potency topical CS for lichenified areas
- Avoid coal tar ointments and anthralin, may aggravate condition

Additional Measures

- Treat specific underlying disease, if known
- Idiopathic and/or refractory to topical medications and general measures, consider
  - Systemic CS (start dose of prednisone: 1 mg/kg/day with maintenance dose of ≤0.5 mg/kg/day with slow taper)
  - Methotrexate (7.5–10 mg/week)
  - Cyclosporine (initial dose of 4–5 mg/kg/day with reduction to 1–3 mg/kg/day)
  - Azathioprine (as dosed for atopic dermatitis; see Chapter 10)
  - Mycophenolate mofetil
- Psoriasis
  - Avoid systemic CS
  - Consider methotrexate,* acitretin, cyclosporine, targeted immune modulators ('biologics')
- Drug eruptions
  - Stop offending drug
  - In severe cases (e.g., DRESS/DIHS), may need to use systemic CS

May take 4–6 weeks to see any significant improvement.
DRESS, drug reaction with eosinophilia and systemic symptoms (also referred to as drug-induced hypersensitivity syndrome [DIHS]).

Table 8.4 General treatment strategies for adult erythroderma.

- In addition to these shared features, more specific clinical findings and initial sites of involvement may suggest the underlying etiology (see Table 8.2).
- Potential systemic complications: generalized lymphadenopathy, edema, tachycardia, high-output cardiac failure, hepatomegaly, thermoregulatory disturbances, compensatory hypermetabolism, cachexia, hypoalbuminemia, and anemia.
- Dx is often challenging because both clinical and histologic features may be nonspecific; repeat clinical examinations, laboratory evaluations, and skin biopsies are often necessary (Fig. 8.8).

- Despite a thorough evaluation, the cause can remain unknown (idiopathic) in up to a third of patients (see Fig. 8.3).
- Some patients with idiopathic erythroderma eventually develop a cutaneous T-cell lymphoma (CTCL).
- Treatment strategies should address the dermatological symptoms, the underlying etiology, and the associated systemic complications (Table 8.4).
- May represent a serious medical threat to the patient and require hospitalization.

For further information see Ch. 120. From *Dermatology, Third Edition*.

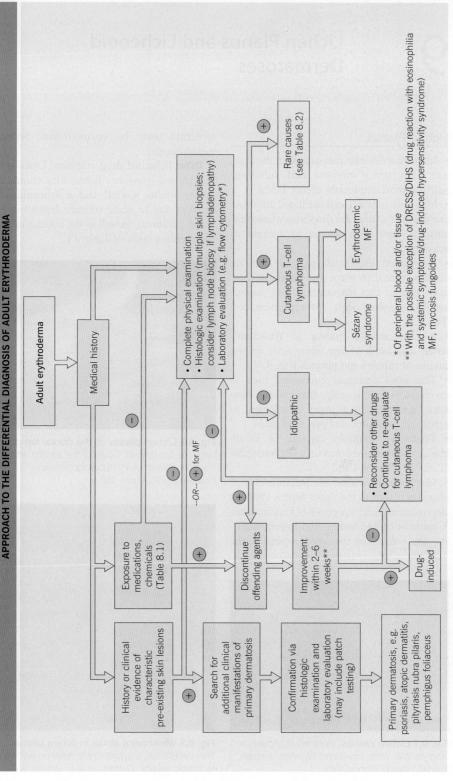

Fig. 8.8 Approach to the differential diagnosis of adult erythroderma.

9

Lichen Planus and Lichenoid Dermatoses

Lichen Planus

- Idiopathic disorder that can affect the skin, hair, nails, and/or mucosae (oral, vulvovaginal) and most commonly affects adults.
- May represent a T cell-mediated autoreactive disorder against keratinocytes whose self-antigens have been altered by trauma or infection.
- Flat-topped (lichenoid) papules that are often polygonal in shape and purple in color may coalesce into plaques (Fig. 9.1); lesions usually resolve with hyperpigmentation (Fig. 9.2).
- A characteristic finding is Wickham's striae, a network of fine white lines on the surface of papules and plaques (Fig. 9.3).
- The most common cutaneous sites of involvement are the scalp, flexor wrists, forearms, genitalia, distal lower extremities, in particular the shins, and presacral areas.
- There are multiple variants of lichen planus, from exanthematous to hypertrophic (Table 9.1; Figs. 9.4 and 9.5).
- Histologically, a band-like infiltrate of lymphocytes is seen in the upper dermis abutting the epidermis, with apoptosis of keratinocytes (Civatte or colloid bodies) and hypergranulosis; the outline of the lower aspect of the epidermis may be sawtooth-like; dermal melanophages.
- **DDx:** lichenoid drug eruption, lupus erythematosus, pityriasis lichenoides chronica, lichen nitidus, GVHD and a lichenoid 'id' reaction due to acute contact dermatitis to nickel (children), as well as the entities in the comments section of Table 9.1.

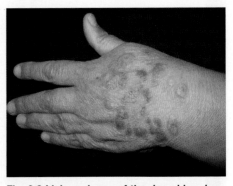

Fig. 9.2 Lichen planus of the dorsal hand. Note the flat-topped nature of the lesions and the post-inflammatory hyperpigmentation. *Courtesy, Frank Samarin, MD.*

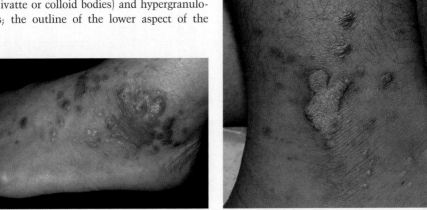

Fig. 9.1 Lichen planus. Violaceous papules and plaques with white scale and Wickham's striae. *Courtesy, Tetsuo Shiohara, MD.*

Fig. 9.3 Wickham's striae in lichen planus. This patient has a hypertrophic lesion in addition to classic lesions. *Courtesy, Julie V. Schaffer, MD.*

VARIANTS OF LICHEN PLANUS		
Type	Clinical Aspects	Comments
Actinic LP	Sun-exposed sites, especially face, neck, dorsal aspect of arms Red-brown annular plaques or melasma-like appearance	Middle East Young adults, children
Acute (exanthematous; eruptive) LP (Fig. 9.4A)	Abrupt onset Widespread distribution	Usually self-limited (3–9 months) Exclude lichenoid drug eruption, pityriasis rosea, secondary syphilis
Annular LP (Fig. 9.4B)	Thin raised border, with hyperpigmented or skin-colored center	Favors axillae, groin/penis, extremities
Atrophic LP (Fig. 9.4C)	Large plaques with epidermal atrophy Later stage of disease	**DDx:** lichen sclerosus Annular variant with loss of elastic fibers centrally
Bullous LP (Fig. 9.4D)	Bullae within pre-existing lesions	Separation of epidermis from dermis with underlying lichenoid lymphocytic infiltrate
Hypertrophic LP (Fig. 9.4E; see Fig. 9.3)	Favors shins and dorsal feet Thick pruritic plaques with scale Can develop SCC	Average duration – 6 years **DDx:** lichen amyloidosis and LSC
Inverse LP (Fig. 9.4F)	Violaceous plaques Axillae > inguinal or other major body folds	Overlap with LP pigmentosus as lesions resolve with hyperpigmentation
LP pemphigoides	Variable distribution of vesicobullae, including previously uninvolved skin	Routine histology and DIF of bullous lesions – similar to BP; IIF: autoAb to BPAG2
LP pigmentosus (Fig. 9.4G)	Brown to gray-brown macules and patches in sun-exposed areas of the face and neck *or* intertriginous zones Inflammatory phase usually absent	Skin phototypes III and IV Coexisting LP lesions in 20% of patients **DDx:** erythema dyschromicum perstans
Lichen planopilaris (see Chapter 56)	Keratotic plugs within hair follicles with narrow surrounding red to violet-colored rim Hair-bearing sites, especially the scalp	A form of scarring alopecia Variant – frontal fibrosing alopecia (see Chapter 56) **DDx** for scalp: discoid LE
Linear LP (Fig. 9.4H)	Need to distinguish Koebner phenomenon from lesions following Blaschko's lines	See Chapters 1 and 51 **DDx:** lichen striatus if along Blaschko's lines
LP/LE overlap	Lesions favor acral sites Overlapping features	Spectrum – from only cutaneous LE to systemic LE
Nail LP (see Chapter 58)	Lateral thinning, longitudinal ridging, fissuring Dorsal pterygium	Variant – twenty-nail dystrophy (more common in children)

Table 9.1 Variants of lichen planus. *Continued*

Table 9.1 *Continued* **Variants of lichen planus.**

Type	Clinical Aspects	Comments
Oral LP	Reticular form – white lacy lines or circle with short radiating spikes (buccal mucosa) Erosive form* – includes chronic desquamative gingivitis	Patients can have both gingival and vulvovaginal involvement May be associated with HCV infection
Ulcerative LP	Plantar surface > palms	
Vulvovaginal LP (see Chapter 60)	Inner aspects of labia minora Glazed erythema that easily bleeds	DDx: lichen sclerosus

*If erosive variant plus lichenoid cutaneous lesions, **DDx** includes paraneoplastic pemphigus.
AutoAb, autoantibody; BP, bullous pemphigoid; BPAG2, bullous pemphigoid antigen 2 (type XVII collagen); DIF, direct immunofluorescence; HCV, hepatitis C virus; IIF, indirect immunofluorescence; LE, lupus erythematosus; LSC, lichen simplex chronicus; SCC, squamous cell carcinoma.

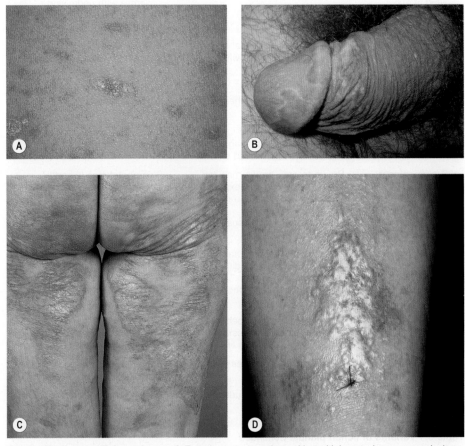

Fig. 9.4 Variants of lichen planus. A Exanthematous variant with multiple papulosquamous lesions. **B** Annular variant with thin elevated rim and central hyperpigmentation. **C** Atrophic variant with large, long-standing lesions. **D** Bullous variant with vesicobullae arising in pre-existing plaque. *B, Courtesy, Frank Samarin, MD; C, Courtesy, Tetsuo Shiohara, MD.* **Continued**

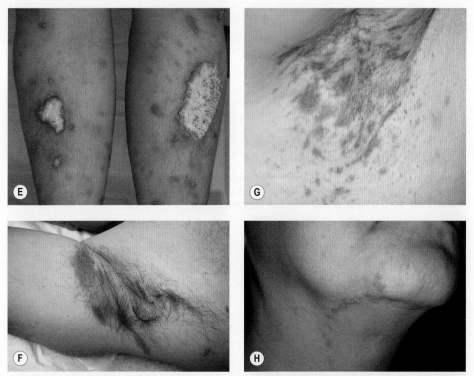

Fig. 9.4 *Continued* **E** Hypertrophic variant with thick plaques on the shins, a common location for this variant. **F** Inverse variant of the axillae; note the purple color. **G** Pigmentosus variant with only hyperpigmented lesions in an intertriginous zone. **H** Linear variant along Blaschko's lines with follicular spines. *F, Courtesy, Jeffrey Callen, MD.*

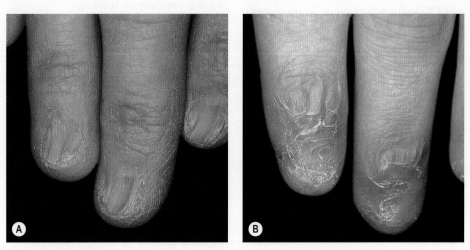

Fig. 9.5 Lichen planus of the nails and oral mucosa. A Thinning of the nail plate with lateral loss. **B** Violaceous discoloration of the periungual area with pterygium formation. *Continued*

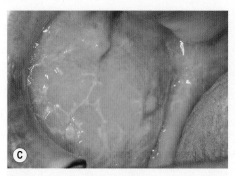 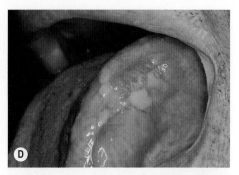

Fig. 9.5 *Continued* **C** Reticular oral form characterized by a white lacy pattern composed of rings with short radiating spikes; there is also an erosion of the buccal mucosa. **D** Erosions, lacy pattern, and scarring of the tongue. *D, Courtesy, Louis Fragola, MD.*

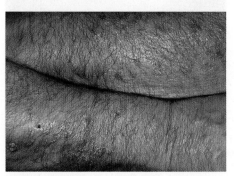

Fig. 9.6 Lichenoid drug eruption in a photodistribution. The patient was taking hydrochlorothiazide (HCTZ).

• **Rx:** topical or intralesional CS, topical calcineurin inhibitors, phototherapy (NBUVB), and if severe, consider systemic therapy (e.g. oral CS, hydroxychloroquine [scalp disease], acitretin).

Lichenoid Drug Eruption

• A drug-induced eruption that has an appearance similar to lichen planus; often more generalized or in a photodistribution (e.g. HCTZ-induced [Fig. 9.6]).
• Often a latent period of months after instituting drug.
• Lesions tend to be more eczematous, psoriasiform, or pityriasis rosea-like.
• Most commonly incriminated drugs are angiotensin-converting enzyme (ACE) inhibitors, thiazide diuretics, antimalarials, β-blockers, TNF-α inhibitors, and quinidine.
• Despite discontinuation of the offending drug, the eruption may be persistent,

requiring treatments employed for lichen planus (e.g. topical corticosteroids).

Lichen Striatus

• Linear array of small, 2–4 mm, flat-topped (lichenoid) papules whose color ranges from skin-colored to pink to tan (i.e., hypopigmented, especially in darkly pigmented patients) (Fig. 9.7).
• Lesions appear over several days to weeks along the lines of Blaschko (see Chapter 51) and are usually asymptomatic.
• Favors children (median age = 2–3 years), with a single streak along one extremity; spontaneously resolves over months to a few years.
• Acral streaks associated with nail dystrophy (e.g. onycholysis, splitting).
• No consistently identified trigger and mosaicism for a particular gene not detected to date.
• **DDx:** linear lichen planus, Blaschkitis (multiple streaks; adults; relapsing course; trunk > extremities), subtle or inflamed epidermal nevus > linear GVHD (specific setting), linear porokeratosis, linear psoriasis.
• **Rx:** no specific effective therapy; observation given spontaneous resolution; can try topical corticosteroids or topical calcineurin inhibitors.

Lichen Nitidus

• Multiple, tiny, discrete, flat-topped papules that are uniform in size and usually skin-colored (Fig. 9.8); may occasionally be pink to

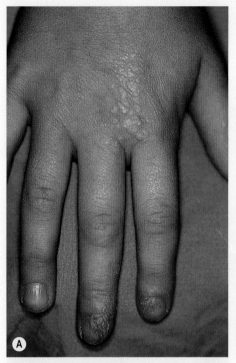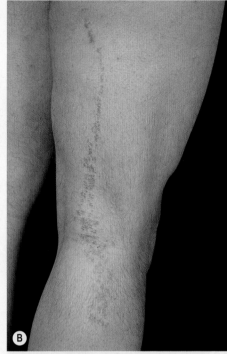

Fig. 9.7 Lichen striatus. A Linear array of pink flat-topped papules on the hand in association with splitting and fraying of the lateral aspect of R2 and the medial aspect of R3. **B** Single streak on the posterior lower extremity composed of multiple pink flat-topped papules. The differential diagnosis would include Blaschkitis and linear lichen planus.

brown in color or hypopigmented (darkly pigmented individuals).

• Lesions favor the anterior trunk, genitalia, and upper extremities and tend to cluster; variants include vesicular, hemorrhagic, linear, and spiny.

• A linear arrangement of papules may be seen, due to Koebner phenomenon (Table 9.2).

• No consistently identified trigger and persists for months to years.

• Histologically, characteristic finding of a 'ball' consisting of a superficial circumscribed infiltrate of lymphocytes and epithelioid cells (2–3 dermal papillae in width) surrounded by a 'claw' of epidermis.

• **DDx:** papular eczema, flat warts, lichen planus, frictional lichenoid dermatitis of the elbows and knees, lichen striatus (when linear), secondary syphilis, lichen spinulosus, lichen scrofulosorum, actinic lichen nitidus (see below).

• **Rx:** no specific effective therapy; can try topical CS or topical calcineurin inhibitors and for extensive disease, phototherapy (e.g. NBUVB).

Erythema Dyschromicum Perstans (EDP; Ashy Dermatosis)

• Symmetric distribution of multiple oval-shaped gray to gray-brown macules and patches (0.5–2.5 cm; Fig. 9.9); occasionally, a transient thin peripheral rim of erythema is present.

• Favors neck, trunk, and proximal upper extremities; as in pityriasis rosea, the long axis of lesions often follows skin cleavage lines, i.e. Langer's lines (see Fig. 7.7).

• Slowly progressive, asymptomatic disorder that favors children and young adults, in particular individuals from Latin America with skin phototypes III and IV.

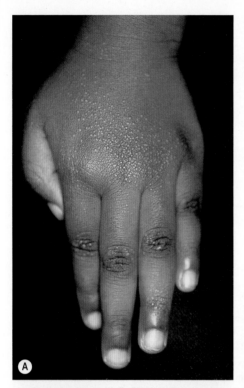

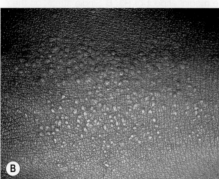

Fig. 9.8 Lichen nitidus. A Numerous tiny flat-topped papules on the hand. **B** A close-up view shows the shiny surface.

Table 9.2 Clinical entities that commonly display Koebner (isomorphic) phenomenon.

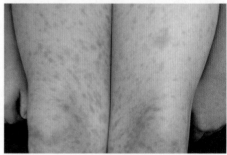

Fig. 9.9 Erythema dyschromicum perstans. Numerous, oval to polygonal, gray-brown (ashy-colored) macules on the lower extremities. *Courtesy, Graham Dermatopathology Library Collection, Wake Forest University.*

- No consistently identified trigger.
- In children, may resolve after a few years (~70% of patients by 2 or 3 years), but often more chronic in adults.
- Histologically, melanin-containing dermal macrophages (melanophages; incontinent pigment) is predominant finding.
- **DDx:** multiple fixed drug eruption (lesions more circular and browner color), post-inflammatory hyperpigmentation (e.g. previous lichenoid drug eruption, pityriasis rosea), lichen planus pigmentosus.
- Idiopathic eruptive macular pigmentation is often considered to be a variant of EDP.
- **Rx:** no specific effective therapy; can try sunscreens and mild topical CS.

Keratosis Lichenoides Chronica

- Violaceous keratotic lichenoid papules are arranged in a linear or reticulated pattern (Fig. 9.10); can resemble Chinese characters.
- Involvement of the limbs and trunk in a symmetric fashion, in addition to facial plaques that may be psoriasiform.

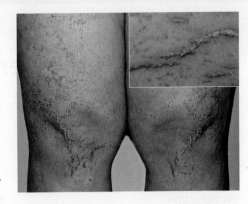

Fig. 9.10 Keratosis lichenoides chronica.
Symmetrical distribution of linear and reticulated keratotic plaques admixed with small violaceous lichenoid papules. *Courtesy, Kathy Schwarzenberger, MD.*

• Tends to be chronic, progressive, and difficult to treat; occasionally responds to phototherapy (NBUVB or PUVA) ± systemic retinoids.

Actinic Lichen Nitidus (Summertime Actinic Lichenoid Eruption)

• Pinhead-sized papules in sun-exposed sites in young adults with darker skin phototypes (IV, V); histologic features similar to lichen nitidus.
• Some clinicians have expanded the clinical spectrum such that it overlaps with actinic lichen planus.

Annular Lichenoid Dermatitis (of Youth)

• Limited number of annular red-brown lesions with central hypopigmentation; they are often 5–15 cm in diameter and favor the groin and flanks.
• More commonly seen in children and young adults.
• **DDx:** inflammatory morphea, mycosis fungoides, inflammatory vitiligo, figurate erythemas.

For further information see Ch. 11. From *Dermatology, Third Edition.*

10 | Atopic Dermatitis

Introduction

• Common inflammatory skin disease that affects 10–25% of children and 2–10% of adults in most high-income and some low-income countries.

• Eczematous dermatitis characterized by intense pruritus and a chronic or chronically relapsing course.

• Sequelae often include sleep disturbances, psychological distress, disrupted family dynamics, and impaired functioning at school or work.

• Onset usually in infancy or early childhood, with development in the first year of life in >50% and before 5 years of age in >85% of affected individuals.

• Often accompanied by other atopic disorders such as asthma and allergic rhinoconjunctivitis (hay fever), which develop in an age-dependent sequence referred to as the atopic march (Fig. 10.1).

• Atopy is linked to the presence of allergen-specific serum IgE antibodies, which exist in ~70% of individuals who meet diagnostic criteria for atopic dermatitis (AD) (Table 10.1).

• The 'hygiene hypothesis' postulates that decreased exposure to infectious agents in early childhood increases susceptibility to atopic diseases.

• Both a genetic predisposition and environmental triggers (e.g., irritation, epicutaneous sensitization, microbial colonization) have pathogenic roles in AD.

• Loss-of-function variants in the filaggrin gene (*FLG*), which encodes a protein important to epidermal barrier function, represent a major predisposing factor for AD that is present in 20–50% of AD patients of European or Asian descent; these *FLG* variants are also implicated in ichthyosis vulgaris.

Clinical Features and Disease Stages of AD

• Pruritic eczematous lesions are often excoriated and exist on a spectrum of acuity:
  – *Acute lesions*: edematous, erythematous papules and plaques that may have vesiculation, oozing, and crusting.
  – *Subacute lesions:* erythematous patches or plaques with scaling and variable crusting.
  – *Chronic lesions:* thickened plaques with lichenification (increased skin markings) as well as scaling.

• Small perifollicular papules (papular eczema) are especially common in patients with darkly pigmented skin.

• Regional variants of AD are depicted in Fig. 10.2.

• Post-inflammatory hyper-, hypo-, or (in severe cases) depigmentation may be seen upon resolution of AD lesions (Fig. 10.3).

• **DDx:** outlined in Table 10.2.

• AD is divided into infantile, childhood, and adolescent/adult stages with characteristic morphologies and distributions (see Fig. 10.2).

Infantile AD (Age < 2 Years)

• Usually develops after 6 weeks of age and often features acute lesions (Fig. 10.4).

• Frequently begins on the cheeks (see Fig. 10.4), forehead, and scalp; also favors the extensor aspects of the extremities and trunk (Fig. 10.5).

• The diaper area and central face tend to be spared.

Childhood AD (Age 2–12 Years)

• Lesions are less acute and typically become lichenified (Fig. 10.6).

THE ATOPIC MARCH

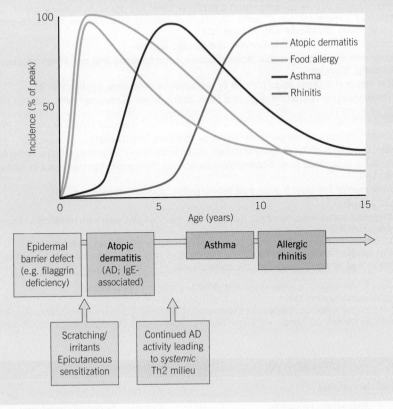

Fig. 10.1 The atopic march.

DIAGNOSTIC FEATURES AND TRIGGERS OF ATOPIC DERMATITIS (AD)

Essential features *(must be present and are sufficient for diagnosis)*

- Pruritus
  - Rubbing or scratching can initiate or exacerbate flares ('the itch that rashes')
  - Often worse in evening and triggered by exogenous factors (e.g., sweating, rough clothing)
- Typical eczematous morphology and age-specific distribution patterns (see text and Fig. 10.2)
- Chronic or relapsing course

Important features *(seen in most cases, support the diagnosis)*

- Onset during infancy or early childhood
- Personal and/or family history of atopy (IgE reactivity)
- Xerosis
  - Dry skin with fine scale in areas *without* clinically apparent inflammation
  - Often leads to pruritus

Table 10.1 Diagnostic features and triggers of atopic dermatitis (AD). *Continued*

SECTION 3: Papulosquamous and Eczematous Dermatoses

Associated features *(helpful in suggesting the diagnosis, but less specific)* (see Figs. 10.2 and 10.10)

- Other filaggrin deficiency-associated conditions: keratosis pilaris, hyperlinear palms, and ichthyosis vulgaris (IV; see Chapter 46; ~15% of patients with AD have moderate–severe IV, and >50% of patients with IV have AD)
- Follicular prominence, lichenification, and prurigo lesions
- Ocular (recurrent conjunctivitis, anterior subcapsular cataract) and periorbital (pleats, darkening) changes
- Other regional findings (e.g., perioral or periauricular dermatitis, pityriasis alba)
- Atypical vascular responses (e.g., mid facial pallor, white dermographism*, delayed blanch)

Triggers

- *Climate:* extremes of temperature (winter or summer), low humidity
- *Irritants:* wool/rough fabrics, perspiration, detergents, solvents, perhaps fabric softeners
- *Infections:* cutaneous (e.g., *Staphylococcus aureus*, molluscum contagiosum) or systemic (e.g., URI)
- *Environmental allergies:* e.g. to dust mites, pollen, contact allergens
- *Food allergies:*
  - Trigger in small minority of AD patients, e.g. 10–30% of those with moderate to severe, refractory AD
  - Common allergens: egg > milk, peanuts/tree nuts, (shell)fish, soy, wheat
  - Detection of allergen-specific IgE (via blood and skin-prick tests) does *not* necessarily mean that allergy is triggering the patient's AD

Stroking the skin leads to a white streak that reflects excessive vasoconstriction.
URI, upper respiratory infection.
Adapted from the American Academy of Dermatology Consensus Conference on Pediatric Atopic Dermatitis (Eichenfield LF, Hanifin JM, Luger TA, et al. J. Am. Acad. Dermatol. 2004;49:1088–1095).

DIFFERENTIAL DIAGNOSIS OF ATOPIC DERMATITIS (AD)		
Chronic dermatoses		
C	Seborrheic dermatitis	Common (especially in infants)
B	Contact dermatitis (allergic* or irritant)	Common
B	Psoriasis (especially palmoplantar)	Common
A>C	Nummular eczema	Uncommon (although nummular lesions can be seen in AD, true nummular eczema is uncommon)
A	Asteatotic eczema	Common
B	Lichen simplex chronicus	Common
Infections and infestations		
B	Scabies	Common
B	Dermatophytosis*	Common
B	Impetigo	Especially for nummular lesions
Primary immunodeficiencies (e.g., hyper-IgE and Wiskott–Aldrich syndromes; C)		
Malignancies (e.g., mycosis fungoides, Sézary syndrome; A > C)		
Genetic/metabolic disorders (e.g., Netherton syndrome, ectodermal dysplasias)		
Autoimmune disorders (e.g., dermatitis herpetiformis, pemphigus foliaceus, dermatomyositis)		
Other (e.g., keratosis pilaris, photoallergic drug eruptions, eczematous drug eruptions**)		

Common causes of autosensitization dermatitis (id reaction).
**Although drug eruptions are common, those resembling AD are uncommon.*
A, adults; B, both; C, children/infants.

Table 10.2 Differential diagnosis of atopic dermatitis (AD).

DISTRIBUTION PATTERNS OF ATOPIC DERMATITIS AND REGIONAL VARIANTS

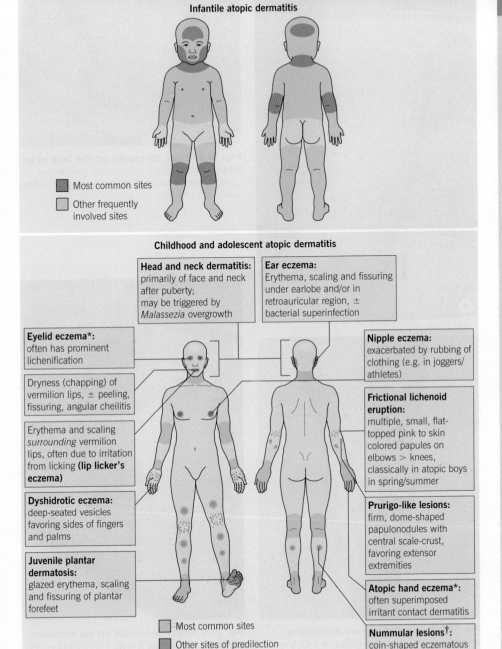

Infantile atopic dermatitis

- Most common sites
- Other frequently involved sites

Childhood and adolescent atopic dermatitis

Head and neck dermatitis: primarily of face and neck after puberty; may be triggered by *Malassezia* overgrowth

Ear eczema: Erythema, scaling and fissuring under earlobe and/or in retroauricular region, ± bacterial superinfection

Eyelid eczema*: often has prominent lichenification

Dryness (chapping) of vermilion lips, ± peeling, fissuring, angular cheilitis

Erythema and scaling *surrounding* vermilion lips, often due to irritation from licking **(lip licker's eczema)**

Dyshidrotic eczema: deep-seated vesicles favoring sides of fingers and palms

Juvenile plantar dermatosis: glazed erythema, scaling and fissuring of plantar forefeet

Nipple eczema: exacerbated by rubbing of clothing (e.g. in joggers/ athletes)

Frictional lichenoid eruption: multiple, small, flat-topped pink to skin colored papules on elbows > knees, classically in atopic boys in spring/summer

Prurigo-like lesions: firm, dome-shaped papulonodules with central scale-crust, favoring extensor extremities

Atopic hand eczema*: often superimposed irritant contact dermatitis

Nummular lesions†: coin-shaped eczematous plaques, often with oozing/crusting, favoring extremities

- Most common sites
- Other sites of predilection
- Specific variants

Fig. 10.2 Distribution patterns of atopic dermatitis (AD) and regional variants. *May be the only manifestation of AD in adults. †Not to be confused with nummular eczema occurring outside the setting of AD (see Chapter 11).

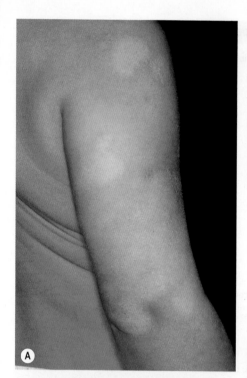

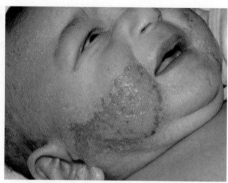

Fig. 10.4 Atopic dermatitis on the face of an infant. Acute lesions with oozing and serous crusting are common in this age group. *Courtesy, Julie V. Schaffer, MD.*

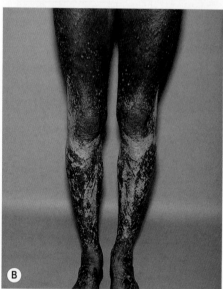

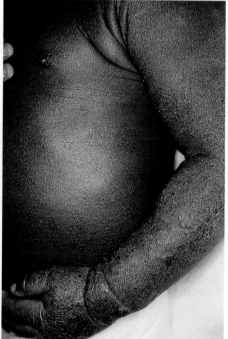

Fig. 10.3 Post-inflammatory pigmentary alteration in atopic dermatitis. A Ill-defined hypopigmented patches with variable residual erythema and scale on the shoulder and upper arm. **B** Post-inflammatory depigmentation in a patient with widespread, severe disease and multiple lesions of prurigo nodularis. *A, Courtesy, Thomas Bieber, MD, and Caroline Bussman, MD; B, Courtesy, Jean L. Bolognia, MD.*

Fig. 10.5 Atopic dermatitis on the extensor surface of an infant's arm. Involvement of the extensor aspects of the extremities is common in this age group. Note the follicular prominence on the trunk.

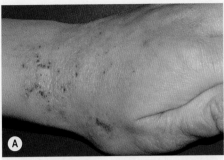
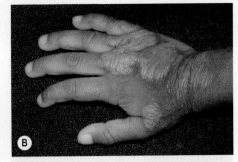

Fig. 10.6 Lichenified atopic dermatitis on the wrists and hands of children. A Pink plaques with excoriation and hemorrhagic crusting as well as lichenification. **B** Thick lichenified plaques. *Courtesy, Julie V. Schaffer, MD.*

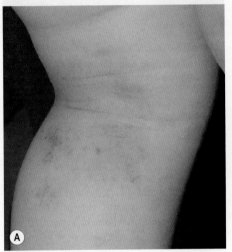
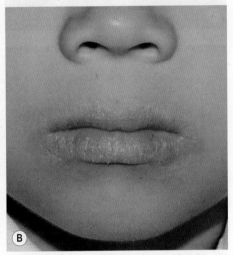

Fig. 10.7 Childhood atopic dermatitis. A Flexural eczema in the popliteal fossa. Note the excoriations and hemorrhagic crusting. **B** Atopic cheilitis involving both the vermilion lip and surrounding skin (lip licker's eczema). *Courtesy, Julie V. Schaffer, MD.*

- Favors the antecubital and popliteal fossae (flexural eczema) (Fig. 10.7), wrists (see Fig. 10.6)/ankles, hands/feet, neck, and periorificial regions of the face.
- Often associated with widespread xerosis.
- ≥50% of children with AD go into remission by 12 years of age.

Adolescent/Adult AD (Age > 12 Years)

- Subacute to chronic, lichenified lesions with distribution similar to childhood AD.
- Some patients have chronic involvement limited to a particular site, e.g. the hands or

face (especially the eyelids) (Fig. 10.8; see Fig. 10.2).
- Chronic papular lesions may develop due to habitual scratching or rubbing (Fig. 10.9).
- More often extensive or even erythrodermic if continuous since childhood.

Associated Features of AD

- Figs. 10.10 and 10.11 present findings that are frequently associated with AD.

Keratosis Pilaris

- Affects >40% of patients with AD and ~15% of the general population.

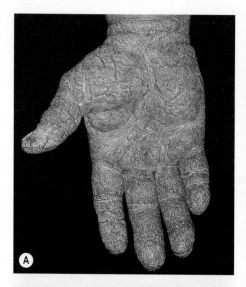

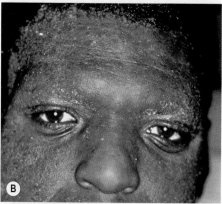

Fig. 10.8 Atopic dermatitis in adolescents and adults. A Severe chronic hand eczema with an irritant as well as atopic component in an adult. **B** Extensive facial involvement in an adult.

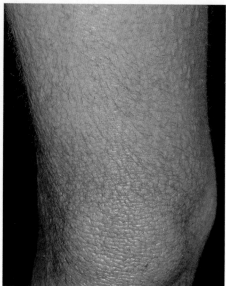

Fig. 10.9 Chronic papular lesions in an adult with atopic dermatitis. This resulted from habitual scratching and rubbing in the setting of long-standing disease. *Courtesy, Thomas Bieber, MD, and Caroline Bussman, MD.*

• Onset typically in childhood; may improve after puberty (especially facial involvement).
• Affects the lateral aspect of the upper arms, thighs, and lateral cheeks (especially in children); the trunk and distal extremities are much less common sites.
• Keratotic follicular papules, often with a rim of erythema (see Fig. 10.11A) or (especially on the cheeks) a background of patchy erythema.
• *Keratosis pilaris rubra* (KPR) has prominent, confluent background erythema (see Fig. 10.11B,C).
• *Keratosis pilaris atrophicans* is a rare atrophic variant that favors the lateral eyebrows.

• Keratolytic agents (e.g., lactic, glycolic, or salicylic acid) and topical retinoids are sometimes used to decrease the hyperkeratotic component, but the benefit is limited and irritation can occur, especially in AD patients.

Pityriasis Alba

• Common in children/adolescents, especially those with AD and tan or darkly pigmented skin.
• Ill-defined hypopigmented macules and patches (usually 0.5–3 cm) with subtle fine scaling.
• Located on face (especially cheeks) (see Fig. 10.11D) > shoulders and arms.
• Represents a low-grade eczematous dermatitis with post-inflammatory hypopigmentation as the primary clinical manifestation.
• **DDx:** post-inflammatory hypopigmentation (e.g., from AD, psoriasis, or pityriasis lichenoides chronica; usually also extrafacial lesions), tinea versicolor (individual lesions more sharply demarcated and smaller), vitiligo (depigmented).
• **Rx:** regular use of sunscreens may make pityriasis alba less noticeable.

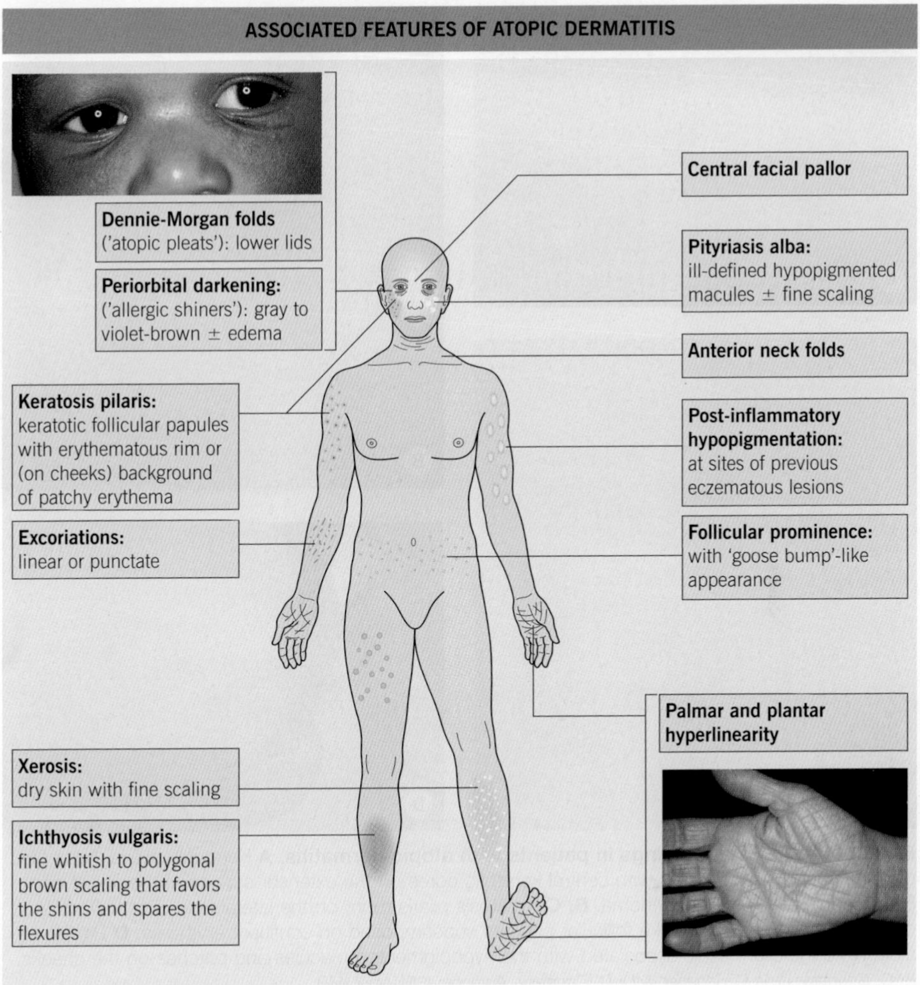

ASSOCIATED FEATURES OF ATOPIC DERMATITIS

Dennie-Morgan folds
('atopic pleats'): lower lids

Periorbital darkening:
('allergic shiners'): gray to
violet-brown ± edema

Keratosis pilaris:
keratotic follicular papules
with erythematous rim or
(on cheeks) background
of patchy erythema

Excoriations:
linear or punctate

Xerosis:
dry skin with fine scaling

Ichthyosis vulgaris:
fine whitish to polygonal
brown scaling that favors
the shins and spares the
flexures

Central facial pallor

Pityriasis alba:
ill-defined hypopigmented
macules ± fine scaling

Anterior neck folds

**Post-inflammatory
hypopigmentation:**
at sites of previous
eczematous lesions

Follicular prominence:
with 'goose bump'-like
appearance

**Palmar and plantar
hyperlinearity**

Fig. 10.10 Associated features of atopic dermatitis. *Inset of hand: Courtesy, Jean L. Bolognia, MD.*

Complications of AD

• An impaired skin barrier and modified immune milieu predispose AD patients to cutaneous infections.
• Affected skin is usually colonized by *Staphylococcus aureus*, and impetiginization (which can also result from *Streptococcus pyogenes*) (Fig. 10.12), folliculitis, and furunculosis frequently occur.
• Eczema herpeticum typically presents with rapid development of numerous monomorphic, punched-out erosions with hemorrhagic crusting (Fig. 10.13); vesicles may or may not be evident.

• Molluscum contagiosum infections result in an increased number of lesions, usually with associated dermatitis (see Chapter 68).
• Potential ocular complications of AD are listed in Table 10.1.

Triggers of AD

• Multiple environmental and psychological factors can trigger or exacerbate AD (see Table 10.1).
• Avoidance of relevant triggers represents an important consideration in AD management.

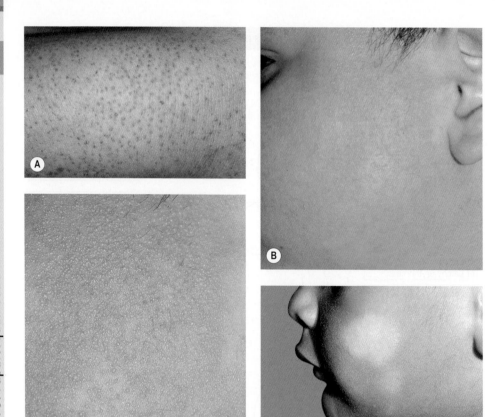

Fig. 10.11 Associated findings in patients with atopic dermatitis. A Keratosis pilaris. Note the discrete perifollicular papules with central keratotic cores on the extensor surface of the upper arm. Each papule has a rim of erythema. **B, C** Keratosis pilaris rubra on the lateral face. This variant is characterized by tiny, grain-like follicular papules superimposed on confluent erythema. **D** Pityriasis alba. Note the slight scale associated with the hypopigmented macules and patches on the cheeks. *B, C, Courtesy, Julie V. Schaffer, MD; D, Courtesy, Anthony J. Mancini, MD.*

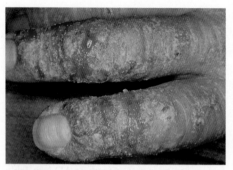

Fig. 10.12 Infected hand dermatitis in a patient with atopic dermatitis. There is impetigo-like crusting as well as pustules. *Courtesy, Louis Fragola, MD.*

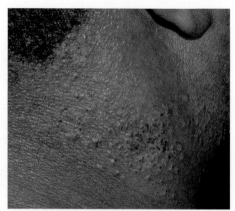

Fig. 10.13 Eczema herpeticum. Note the monomorphic erosions and hemorrhagic crusts. *Courtesy, Julie V. Schaffer, MD.*

Treatment of AD

- There are two major components to management of AD (Fig. 10.14).
  - Treatment of active dermatitis with anti-inflammatory agent(s).
  - Maintenance designed to improve skin barrier function, control subclinical inflammation, and avoid trigger factors.
- Proactive treatment of AD provides better long-term disease control and could potentially interrupt the atopic march.
- Basics of skin care.
  - Daily luke-warm bath (preferred for infants/children) or shower with limited use of a mild cleanser.
  - Within 3 minutes of exit from bath/shower, application of (1) a topical CS (or calcineurin inhibitor) when/where indicated; and then (2) liberal use of an emollient to the entire skin surface.
  - Ointments (minimize stinging) and creams (less greasy) are preferred to lotions as emollients and should be applied twice daily; ceramide-dominant emollients may optimize barrier repair, whereas products containing lactic or glycolic acid can lead to stinging and should be avoided.
- Topical anti-inflammatory agents.
  - First-line: topical CS of appropriate strength – higher potency for thick/lichenified plaques and lesions on hands/feet, lower potency for thinner lesions and body folds – used once or twice daily until eczema is completely clear.
    - CS ointments (minimize stinging) and creams are generally preferred, but CS solutions, foams, and oils are useful for AD on the scalp.
    - Addressing patients'/parents' specific concerns about CS use helps to maximize adherence to the treatment plan.
    - Tap water compresses followed by CS application or wet wraps after CS application can speed improvement of acute flares.
  - Second-line: topical calcineurin inhibitors (TCIs; e.g., tacrolimus) are helpful primarily for thinner lesions on the face and in intertriginous areas.
    - High-level maintenance with intermittent use of a topical CS and/or TCI (see Fig. 10.14) to usual sites of eczema once clear can help to control subclinical inflammation and prevent flares.
- Phototherapy and systemic anti-inflammatory agents.
  - Narrowband UVB (often induces remission) > UVA1 (for acute flares) > UVA-broadband UVB combination.
  - Systemic anti-inflammatory therapy should be restricted for severe, recalcitrant AD.
  - Oral cyclosporine has the most evidence for efficacy, but its use is limited by potential side effects such as nephrotoxicity; other systemic agents (e.g., azathioprine, mycophenolate mofetil, methotrexate) have less dramatic benefit but better long-term safety profiles.
  - Systemic CS therapy should be avoided due to the high likelihood of significant rebound flares (see Fig. 10.14) and the unacceptable side effects of long-term use; uncommon exception: severe acute flare (e.g., with a specific trigger) resistant to aggressive topical management – this short course of systemic CS must be transitioned to a topical regimen, phototherapy, or another systemic agent.
- Adjunctive pharmacologic therapy.
  - Sedating antihistamines (e.g., hydroxyzine, diphenhydramine, doxepin) given at bedtime may help to break the itch–scratch cycle, especially if pruritus disrupts sleep.
  - Controlled trials of nonsedating antihistamines, leukotriene antagonists, antibiotics (oral or topical) aimed at reducing colonization, and probiotics have not consistently demonstrated efficacy as treatments of AD; dilute sodium hypochlorite (bleach) baths may be of benefit (see Fig. 10.14).

MANAGEMENT PLAN FOR ATOPIC DERMATITIS

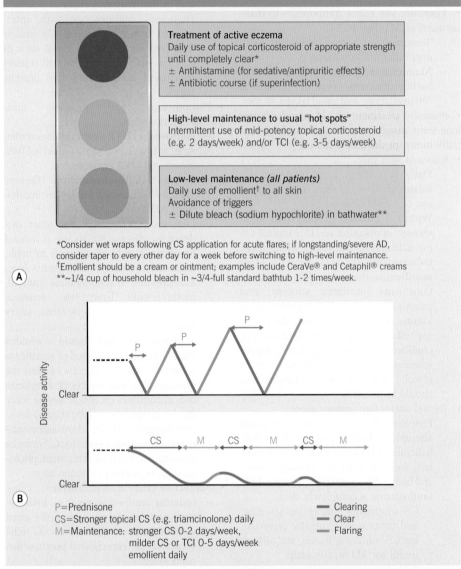

Treatment of active eczema
Daily use of topical corticosteroid of appropriate strength
until completely clear*
± Antihistamine (for sedative/antipruritic effects)
± Antibiotic course (if superinfection)

High-level maintenance to usual "hot spots"
Intermittent use of mid-potency topical corticosteroid
(e.g. 2 days/week) and/or TCI (e.g. 3-5 days/week)

Low-level maintenance *(all patients)*
Daily use of emollient† to all skin
Avoidance of triggers
± Dilute bleach (sodium hypochlorite) in bathwater**

*Consider wet wraps following CS application for acute flares; if longstanding/severe AD,
consider taper to every other day for a week before switching to high-level maintenance.
†Emollient should be a cream or ointment; examples include CeraVe® and Cetaphil® creams
**~1/4 cup of household bleach in ~3/4-full standard bathtub 1-2 times/week.

(A)

(B)

P=Prednisone
CS=Stronger topical CS (e.g. triamcinolone) daily
M=Maintenance: stronger CS 0-2 days/week,
                milder CS or TCI 0-5 days/week
                emollient daily

— Clearing
— Clear
— Flaring

Fig. 10.14 Management plan for atopic dermatitis. A The therapeutic regimen should include
both treatment of active eczema and maintenance (low-level in all and high-level in some patients).
B Intermittent courses of a systemic CS result in rebound flares and worsening of disease over time.
In contrast, a proactive regimen utilizing topical CS leads to longer clear periods and milder disease
over time. TCI, topical calcineurin inhibitor.

For further information see Ch. 12. From *Dermatology, Third Edition.*

Other Eczematous Eruptions | 11

The major forms of dermatitis include atopic (see Chapter 10), contact (see Chapter 12), seborrheic, asteatotic (xerotic), stasis, and nummular. Dermatitis of special sites – i.e. hands, feet, lips, diaper area, and major body folds – is reviewed in Chapter 13, and pityriasis alba is reviewed in Chapters 10 and 54.

Seborrheic Dermatitis

• Common disorder with both an infantile and an adult form (Figs. 11.1 and 11.2); unusual in children.
• Possibly related to components of sebum and *Malassezia* spp.
• Severe or recalcitrant seborrheic dermatitis can be a sign of underlying HIV infection or neurologic disorder.
• In adults, tends to be a chronic relapsing disorder; stress or tapering of systemic CS can lead to a flare.
• Symmetric distribution pattern that includes sites of greater sebum production – scalp, ears (external canal, retroauricular fold), medial eyebrows, upper eyelids, nasolabial folds, central chest – and major body folds.
• Lesions are pink-yellow to red-brown in color, depending on the underlying skin phototype, and they often have greasy scale, especially in the head and neck region; occasionally annular in configuration.
• On the scalp, involvement tends to be more diffuse, with well-circumscribed plaques with thicker silvery scale more characteristic of psoriasis.
• In some patients, the lesions of the scalp, ears, and major body folds have features of both seborrheic dermatitis and psoriasis, leading to the term 'sebopsoriasis'.
• **DDx:** psoriasis, contact dermatitis, other causes of diaper dermatitis (see Fig. 13.4), intertrigo (see Fig. 13.2) or blepharitis, tinea versicolor (presternal), tinea capitis

(especially in children), atopic dermatitis, pityriasis amiantacea and dermatomyositis (scalp); may coexist with rosacea.
• **Rx:** topical anti-fungal creams and daily shampooing (e.g. ketoconazole, ciclopirox, selenium sulfide or zinc-containing shampoo alternating with a gentle shampoo), mild topical CS on the face and in body folds and moderate-strength topical CS for the scalp and ears; topical calcineurin inhibitors (e.g. tacrolimus ointment).

Asteatotic Eczema (Xerotic Eczema, Eczema Craquelé)

• Arises in areas of dry skin, especially during winter months, in dry climates and in older adults.
• The areas of dermatitis resemble a 'dried riverbed' or 'crazy-paving' with superficial cracking of the skin (Fig. 11.3).
• May be associated with pruritus; stinging can occur with application of water-based topical agents, including those that contain lactic or glycolic acid.
• Favors the shins, thighs, lower flanks, and posterior axillary line; may become more widespread but with sparing of the face, palms, and soles.
• Involvement of the posterior axillary line seen in chronic GVHD; when widespread, consider the possibility of an underlying systemic lymphoma.
• **DDx:** stasis dermatitis ± autosensitization, ichthyosis vulgaris, adult atopic dermatitis, allergic or irritant contact dermatitis.
• **Rx:** decrease frequency of bathing and use of soaps, liberal use of water-in-oil emollients, mild topical CS ointments.

Stasis Dermatitis

• Pruritic dermatitis with scale-crust and sometimes oozing that favors the shins and

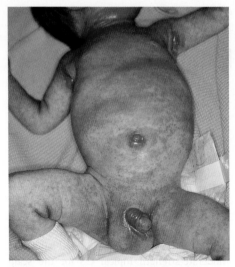

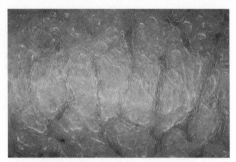

Fig. 11.3 Asteatotic eczema (eczema craquelé). The distal lower extremity has obvious inflammation and xerosis with adherent white scale (pseudo-ichthyosis) as well as a crisscross pattern of superficial cracks and fissures said to resemble a dried riverbed. *Courtesy, Louis A. Fragola, MD.*

Fig. 11.1 Infantile seborrheic dermatitis. Glistening red plaques of the neck, axillary and inguinal folds as well as the penis and umbilicus. Note disseminated lesions on the trunk and extremities. *Courtesy, Robert Hartman, MD.*

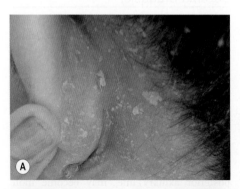

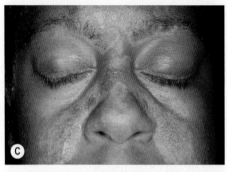

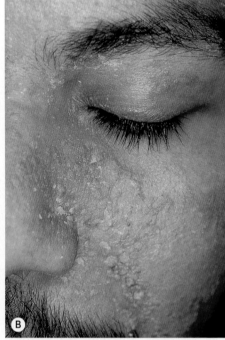

Fig. 11.2 Adult seborrheic dermatitis of the scalp, ear, and face. A Fairly sharply demarcated pink plaque with white and greasy scale. Note the fissure in the retroauricular fold. **B** Thin pink-orange plaques with yellow, greasy scale, especially of the melolabial fold and eyebrows.
C Symmetric red-brown to violet plaques of the central forehead, nasal bridge, and medial cheeks with an associated hypopigmented figurate rim. *A, Courtesy, Norbert Reider, MD, and Peter O Fritsch, MD; C, Courtesy, Jeffrey Callen, MD.*

11

CUTANEOUS SIGNS OF CHRONIC VENOUS HYPERTENSION

- Edema, often tender
- Varicosities
- Stasis dermatitis
- Petechiae superimposed on a yellow-brown discoloration due to hemosiderin deposits (stasis purpura)
- Lipodermatosclerosis, acute and chronic
- Stasis ulcerations, in particular above the medial malleolus
- Acroangiodermatitis (pseudo-Kaposi's sarcoma)
- Livedoid vasculopathy (porcelain-white scars surrounded by punctate telangiectasias and painful ulcerations)*

*Need to exclude causes of hypercoagulability.

Table 11.1 Cutaneous signs of chronic venous hypertension.

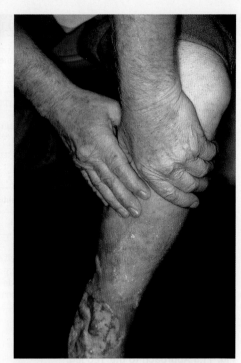

Fig. 11.4 Autosensitization dermatitis. There is dermatitis of the extensor surfaces of the upper extremities in this patient with allergic contact dermatitis to neomycin as well as stasis dermatitis and venous ulceration. *Courtesy, Jean Bolognia, MD.*

calves; historically often begins near the medial malleolus.
• Patients often have a history of chronic lower extremity edema and may have a history of deep vein thromboses and/or recurrent cellulitis.
• Often accompanied by other signs of chronic venous hypertension (Table 11.1).
• One of the more common causes of autosensitization (Fig. 11.4).
• **DDx:** allergic contact dermatitis, irritant contact dermatitis, asteatotic eczema, nummular dermatitis; may accompany other causes of the red leg, especially cellulitis and acute or chronic lipodermatosclerosis (Fig. 11.5), but the latter lack the clinical and histologic findings of dermatitis.
• **Rx:** exclude superimposed allergic contact dermatitis (e.g. neomycin, preservatives in topical creams) or component of infectious eczematous dermatitis if draining ulcer; open wet dressings for a few days, mild topical CS ointments, leg elevation, pressure stockings (after excluding arterial insufficiency via ankle–brachial index), endovascular ablation of large varicosities, water-in-oil emollients for maintenance therapy.

Autosensitization Dermatitis (Id Reaction)

• More widespread distribution of dermatitis that follows by days to weeks the development of localized areas of dermatitis, e.g. allergic contact dermatitis, stasis dermatitis, inflammatory tinea infections.
• Can also represent a rebound phenomenon when there has been too rapid a taper of systemic CS, as in 6-day taper of prednisone or methylprednisolone (Medrol® dose pack) for poison ivy.
• Favored sites of involvement (in addition to primary site): extensor aspects of extremities (see Fig. 11.4), palms and soles, usually in a symmetric pattern.
• In children with tinea capitis, the id reaction often involves the head and neck region.
• Areas of dermatitis, often ill-defined, can be accompanied by excoriated papules (Fig. 11.6).
• **DDx:** atopic dermatitis, widespread contact dermatitis (e.g. textiles), Gianotti–Crosti syndrome, drug eruption to systemic anti-fungal

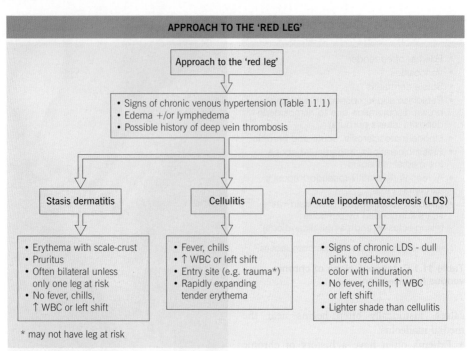

Approach to the 'red leg'

- Signs of chronic venous hypertension (Table 11.1)
- Edema +/or lymphedema
- Possible history of deep vein thrombosis

Stasis dermatitis

- Erythema with scale-crust
- Pruritus
- Often bilateral unless only one leg at risk
- No fever, chills, ↑ WBC or left shift

Cellulitis

- Fever, chills
- ↑ WBC or left shift
- Entry site (e.g. trauma*)
- Rapidly expanding tender erythema

Acute lipodermatosclerosis (LDS)

- Signs of chronic LDS - dull pink to red-brown color with induration
- No fever, chills, ↑ WBC or left shift
- Lighter shade than cellulitis

* may not have leg at risk

Fig. 11.5 Approach to the 'red leg.'

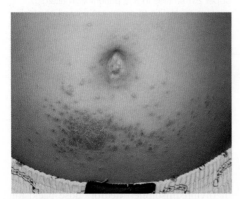

Fig. 11.6 Id reaction in a child due to allergic contact dermatitis (ACD) to nickel. Square-shaped area of ACD due to nickel in a buckle surrounded by multiple crusted edematous papules. *Courtesy, Julie V. Schaffer, MD.*

medication (tinea capitis id), eczematous drug eruptions (e.g. calcium channel blockers [unusual]).

- **Rx:** in addition to aggressively treating the primary dermatitis, topical CS and oral antihistamines usually suffice; occasionally, when severe, systemic CS.

Infectious Eczematous (Eczematoid) Dermatitis

- Dermatitis that initially involves the skin surrounding a site of infection, usually bacterial, which is weeping or has drainage (e.g. otitis externa, infected leg ulcer, toe web infection).
- An id reaction can develop and treatment of both the infection and the dermatitis is recommended.

Nummular Eczema (Nummular Dermatitis)

- Markedly pruritic, coin-shaped lesions of dermatitis, usually measuring 2 or 3 cm in diameter (Fig. 11.7).
- Occurs primarily on the extremities, classically the legs in men and the arms in women.
- Favors adults and can develop in the absence of an atopic diathesis; a chronic relapsing course is common.

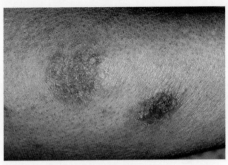

Fig. 11.7 Nummular eczema. Coin-shaped lesions of acute and subacute dermatitis that are fairly well demarcated. There is often marked pruritus. *Courtesy, Kalman Watsky, MD.*

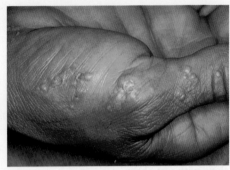

Fig. 11.8 Dyshidrotic eczema. Clusters of firm vesicles along the lateral aspect of the thumb and hypothenar eminence. *Courtesy Louis A. Fragola, MD.*

- **DDx:** atopic dermatitis, autosensitization dermatitis, impetigo, stasis dermatitis, allergic contact dermatitis, tinea corporis, vesicular pityriasis rosea, mycosis fungoides.
- **Rx:** in addition to topical CS and calcineurin inhibitors, often requires phototherapy to clear.

Dyshidrotic Eczema (Acute and Recurrent Vesicular Hand Dermatitis)

- Firm, pruritic vesicles of the palms > soles as well as the lateral and medial aspects of the digits (Fig. 11.8); chronic and recurrent.
- Intact vesicles due to edema within the epidermis are more long-lived because of the thick stratum corneum in acral sites.
- When the vesicles are small and grouped, they are said to have an appearance similar to tapioca pudding.
- When larger vesicles develop, the term pompholyx is sometimes used.
- Can flare with stress, allergic or irritant contact dermatitis and administration of IVIg; seen in patients with atopic dermatitis and hyperhidrosis.
- **DDx:** id reaction (overlap), inflammatory tinea pedis or manuum, allergic contact dermatitis, scabies, dyshidrosiform bullous pemphigoid; if secondarily infected, palmoplantar pustulosis; when localized to a single digit, whitlow (herpes simplex infection) or blistering digital dactylitis (staphylococcal or group A streptococcal infection).

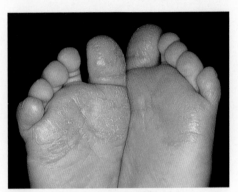

Fig. 11.9 Juvenile plantar dermatosis in a child. Erythema and scaling of the plantar surface of the forefoot, especially the ball of the foot and the great and fifth toes. Note the glazed appearance of the skin of the left foot. *Courtesy, Kalman Watsky, MD.*

- **Rx:** exclude allergic or irritant contact dermatitis; topical CS, topical calcineurin inhibitors, bath PUVA; occasionally, when severe, systemic CS.

Juvenile Plantar Dermatosis

- Favors the plantar surface of the forefeet in prepubertal children, usually with an atopic diathesis.
- The skin is dry and scaly with mild inflammation and a characteristic glazed appearance (Fig. 11.9).

• Thought to be related to hydration of the stratum corneum from wearing shoes made of impermeable materials and subsequent shearing of skin due to friction.
• **DDx:** other causes of foot dermatitis (see Table 13.1), especially psoriasis, allergic contact dermatitis (e.g. rubber, chromates in leather), tinea pedis (interdigital toe webs involved), atopic dermatitis.
• **Rx:** permeable socks and shoes, emollients, CS ointments, removal of wet socks along with wet shoes.

Infective Dermatitis

• Rare disorder of childhood or adolescence associated with human T-cell lymphotropic virus type 1 (HTLV-1) infection.
• Dermatitis of the scalp, ears, eyelid margins, paranasal skin, axillae, and groin that clears with oral antibiotics.

For further information see Ch. 13. From *Dermatology, Third Edition*.

Irritant and Allergic Contact Dermatitis, Occupational Dermatoses, and Dermatoses Due to Plants

12

Key Points

- Irritant contact dermatitis (ICD).
  - Accounts for 80% of all causes of contact dermatitis.
  - Secondary to a local toxic effect caused by a topical substance or physical insult.
- Allergic contact dermatitis (ACD).
  - Accounts for 20% of all causes of contact dermatitis.
  - A delayed-type hypersensitivity reaction to a substance to which the individual has been previously sensitized.
  - Compared to ICD, more commonly presents with pruritus during the acute phase.
- One of the most common occupational dermatoses is ICD.
- Plants can cause a variety of skin reactions, the most common in North America being ACD to poison ivy.

Irritant Contact Dermatitis

- Localized, non-immunologically mediated cutaneous inflammatory reaction (Figs. 12.1–12.4).
- Secondary to a direct toxic effect.
  - Chronic – erythema, lichenification, fissures, and scale.
  - Acute – erythema, edema, and vesiculation followed by erosions and scaling; in severe cases may lead to epidermal necrosis (a 'chemical burn').
- Commonly affects the hands (see Fig. 13.1); Table 12.1 reviews pertinent questions for when environmental exposures are suspected.
- A common cause of cheilitis (lip-licking; see Fig. 13.4).
- May be secondary to an occupational exposure (Table 12.2).
  - Common causes are soaps and wet work, and less often petroleum products, cutting oils, and coolants.

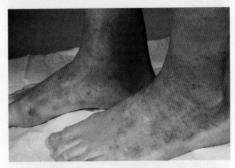

Fig. 12.1 Bilateral irritant contact dermatitis of the feet and ankles due to chronic occlusive footwear. *Courtesy, David Cohen, MD.*

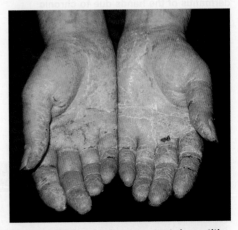

Fig. 12.2 Bilateral irritant contact dermatitis of the palms secondary to repeated contact with paint solvents. Extensive patch testing excluded allergic contact dermatitis in this professional paint and crayon illustrator. *Courtesy, Kalman Watsky, MD.*

- **DDx:** when severe, thermal burn; ACD and other dermatitides; there may be a combination of causes, e.g. ICD and ACD, ICD and atopic dermatitis.
- **Rx:** primarily avoidance of the irritant.

109

Allergic Contact Dermatitis

- In contrast to ICD, more commonly presents with pruritus during the acute phase; the chronic phase has significant overlap with ICD (Fig. 12.5).
- Initially, well demarcated and localized to site of contact with the allergen (Figs. 12.5–12.10).
  - Acute – in addition to erythema and edema, vesicobullae and weeping may develop (Fig. 12.7).

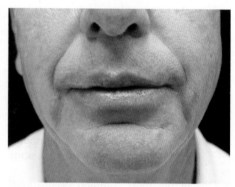

Fig. 12.4 Cheilitis due to irritant contact dermatitis. This patient had the habit of licking his lips and there is involvement of the vermilion and cutaneous lips as well as the perioral region. *Courtesy, Jeffrey P. Callen.*

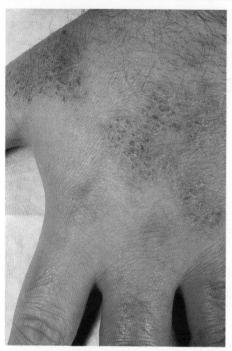

Fig. 12.3 Moderately severe irritant contact dermatitis of the hands due to chronic exposure to disinfecting solutions and antiseptics. The results of patch testing, latex challenge testing, and RAST testing were negative in this practicing dentist. *Courtesy, David Cohen, MD.*

POINTS TO CONSIDER WHEN EVALUATING HAND DERMATITIS AND ENVIRONMENTAL EXPOSURES ARE SUSPECTED	
Occupation	Are findings consistent with work exposure as a cause? Does time off result in improvement?
Materials handled	Do labels and material safety data sheets (MSDS) list potential irritants or allergens? Is there a relationship to handling food? Other persons in workplace affected? Protective equipment (e.g. gloves) used?
Previous skin disease or history of atopy	Is there a history of eczema as a child?
Known allergies	Is there unrecognized exposure?
Treatment	May cause allergic contact dermatitis
Hobbies	Including exposure to plants

Table 12.1 Points to consider when evaluating hand dermatitis and environmental exposures are suspected. *Courtesy, Peter S. Friedmann, MD.*

COMMON IRRITANTS AND EXAMPLES OF MAJOR EXPOSURE(S)

Irritant	Examples of Major Exposure(s)
Inorganic acids	
Hydrofluoric acid	Etching of glass/metal/stone; rust/stain/limescale removers
Sulfuric acid	Manufacturing of fertilizers, textile fibers, explosives, paper
Hydrochloric acid	Production of fertilizers, dyes, paints; used in food processing
Chromic acid	Used in metal treatments
Nitric acid	Production of fertilizers and explosives; in cleaning products
Phosphoric acid	Used in fertilizer, pharmaceuticals, water treatment
Organic acids	
Formic acid	Used as a neutralizer in leather manufacturing
Alkalis	
Sodium hydroxide	Used in the manufacture of bleaches, dyes, vitamins, pulp,
Calcium oxide	paper, plastics, soaps and detergents
Metal salts	
Arsenic trioxide	Aerosolized in the smelting of metals
Beryllium compounds	Used in the production of hard, corrosion-resistant alloys
Solvents	
Stoddard solvent	Used in dry cleaning
Water	Ubiquitous
Alcohols	
Glycols	Commonly used in cosmetic products
Detergents and cleansers	
Sodium lauryl sulfate	Detergents and cleansers
Cocamidopropyl betaine	Detergents, therapeutic formulations, personal care products
Disinfectants	
Ethylene oxide	Medical sterilization
Chloroxylenol	Baby powders and shampoos
Iodines	Surgical scrub, shampoo, skin cleansers
Benzalkonium chloride	Used for instrument cleansing; in ophthalmic solutions
Food	Pineapples, garlic, mustard
Plants	Thistles, prickly pears, grasses
Plastics	
Bodily fluids	
Fabric/man-made vitreous fibers (e.g. fiberglass)	

Table 12.2 Common irritants and examples of major exposure(s). *Courtesy, David Cohen, MD.*

– Chronic – often lichenified with scale (Figs. 12.5B and 12.9).
• Can have autosensitization with extension beyond original site (see Chapter 11).
• Occasionally, there is a diffuse, patchy distribution, depending on the allergen (e.g. body wash or shampoo) and/or concomitant atopic dermatitis.
• Common allergens are metals, fragrances, preservatives, and topical antibiotics, as well as plants, in particular poison ivy/oak (see below) (Fig. 12.10).
• Common causes of occupational ACD are rubber, nickel, epoxy resin, and aromatic amines.
• Suspected allergens should be avoided; an open use test can be tried first but patch testing is required for accurate diagnosis; detailed lists of allergen-containing products are available.

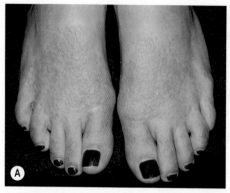
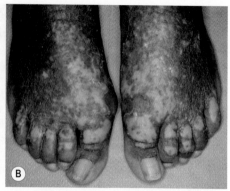

Fig. 12.5 Allergic contact dermatitis to shoes – acute versus chronic. A Extremely pruritic erythematous papules and papulovesicles appeared within days of wearing new sneakers; note the distribution pattern. **B** Pebbled and lichenified plaques with both hypo- and hyperpigmentation. The patient had a positive patch test to potassium dichromate. *Courtesy, Louis A. Fragola, MD.*

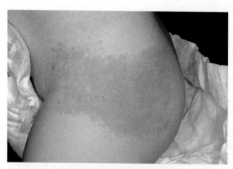

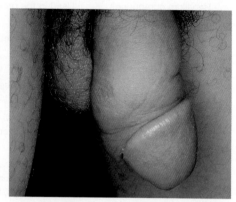

Fig. 12.6 Allergic contact dermatitis. This erythematous plaque with vesiculation developed in a 14-month-old boy following the application of neomycin ointment. *Courtesy, Anthony J. Mancini, MD.*

Fig. 12.7 Acute allergic contact dermatitis with a prominent component of edema. Obvious edema of the shaft of the penis plus subtle crusts of the glans due to application of tiger balm (contains extracts of several plants, including mint, clove, and Chinese cinnamon). *Courtesy, Louis A. Fragola, Jr., MD.*

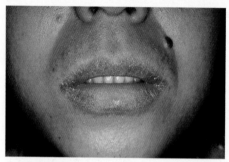

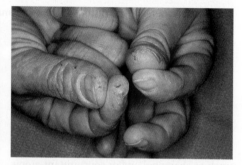

Fig. 12.8 Allergic contact dermatitis due to aloe-containing cream. The degree of involvement on the upper and lower lips is similar, as opposed to actinic cheilitis.

Fig. 12.9 Chronic allergic contact dermatitis due to glutaraldehyde. The patient was an optometrist. *Courtesy, Kalman Watsky, MD.*

112

- In patch testing, specific concentrations of allergens are dissolved in petrolatum or water and placed in wells that are then applied to the patient's back for 48 hours (Figs. 12.11 and 12.12); grading of reactions is performed at two time points (Table 12.3).
- **DDx:** other forms of dermatitis (ICD, atopic dermatitis, stasis dermatitis, seborrheic dermatitis), erythematotelangiectatic rosacea, dermatophyte infection.
- **Rx:** short term: topical and systemic CS depending on severity; long term: avoidance of allergen(s).

Common Allergens

Metals

- Cross-reactivity not uncommon within each broad category.
- Nickel – found in costume jewelry, snaps on jeans, backs of watches, belt buckles; dimethylglyoxime test (Fig. 12.13) identifies objects that release nickel (can purchase dimethylglyoxime at http://www.drrecommended.com).
- Chromate – found in metals, leather, cement.
- Cobalt – used to harden metals; cosmetics, enamel, ceramics, hair dyes, and joint replacements.

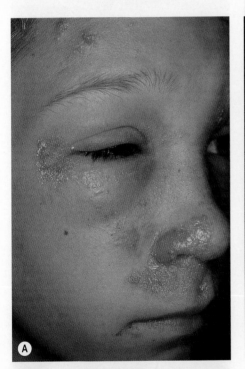

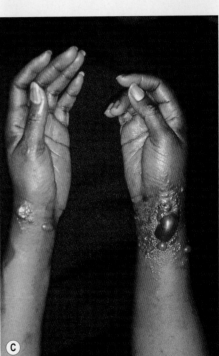

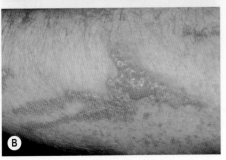

Fig. 12.10 Clinical manifestations of Anacardiaceae dermatitis. *Acute poison ivy dermatitis:* **A** Periorbital edema, in addition to crusted and weeping plaques; **B** Erythematous streaks with linear vesicles; **C** This distribution pattern is seen in patients who wear gloves. *A, Courtesy, Jean L Bolognia, MD; B, Courtesy, Joyce Rico, MD.* **Continued**

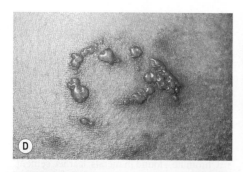

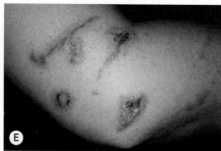

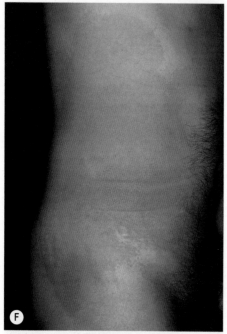

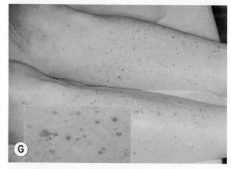

Fig. 12.10 *Continued* **D** Patterned erythema with superimposed vesicles and bullae; **E** 'Black-spot' dermatitis: Note the black discoloration in the central portion of the edematous plaques due to plant resin. *Other:* **F** Widespread erythema and edema associated with intense pruritus after carrying logs of the poisonwood tree *(Metopium toxiferum)* of the family Anacardiaceae. **G** Weed-whacker dermatitis with widespread spotted pattern. *D, Courtesy, Fitzsimons Army Medical Center Dermatology slide teaching library; G, Courtesy Louis A. Fragola, Jr., MD.*

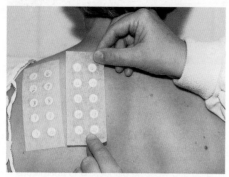

Fig. 12.11 Fixing allergens to patient's back using Scanpor tape. The allergens will remain in place for 48 hours. *Courtesy, Christen M. Mowad, MD, and James G. Marks, Jr., MD.*

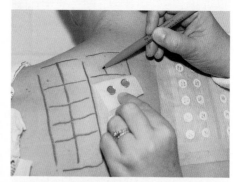

Fig. 12.12 Allergens being marked upon removal of Scanpor tape. *Courtesy, Christen M. Mowad, MD, and James G. Marks, Jr., MD.*

INTERNATIONAL GRADING SYSTEM FOR PATCH TESTS

+/−	Doubtful reaction, faint macular erythema
+	Weak, nonvesicular reaction with erythema, infiltration, and papules
++	Strong, vesicular reaction with infiltration and papules
+++	Spreading bullous reaction
−	Negative reaction
IR	Irritant reaction

Grading is performed at two time points after the patch tests have been in place for 48 hours (then removed; see Fig. 12.12): initially after removal and then 1–7 days later..

Table 12.3 International grading system for patch tests.

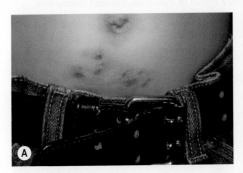

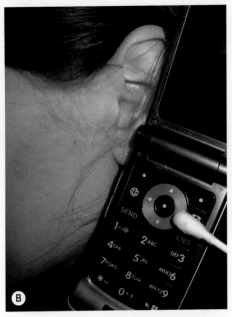

Fig. 12.13 Allergic contact dermatitis to nickel. A Excoriated pink plaques due to nickel within the belt buckle. **B** Facial dermatitis due to nickel within a cellular phone. The latter is demonstrated by a positive dimethylglyoxime test (pink indicator). *A, Courtesy, Julie V. Schaffer, MD; B, Courtesy, Christen M. Mowad, MD, and James G. Marks, Jr., MD.*

• Gold – found in jewelry, dental fillings, and some electronics.

Topical Antibiotics

• Neomycin sulfate – found in many over-the-counter preparations (e.g. hemorrhoid creams).
• Bacitracin – in many products, including some that are labeled 'unscented'.

Fragrances

• Balsam of Peru (*Myroxylon pereirae*) – one of the naturally occurring fragrances; also found in spices (cloves, Jamaican pepper, cinnamon).

Preservatives

• Formaldehyde – cosmetics and textiles (permanent press), medications, paints.
• Thimerosal – found as a preservative in vaccines, contact lens solution, antiseptics, and cosmetics.
• Quaternium-15 – formaldehyde-releasing preservative; found in shampoos, moisturizers, cosmetics, and soaps.

EXAMPLES OF TOPICAL ALLERGENS THAT MAY RESULT IN SYSTEMIC CONTACT DERMATITIS AFTER SYSTEMIC EXPOSURE	
Cutaneous Allergen	**Systemic Exposure**
Ethylenediamine hydrochloride	Aminophylline, hydroxyzine/cetirizine
Poison ivy	Cashews, mango peel
Fragrance (balsam of Peru)	Foods, sodas, mouthwashes, spices
Sorbic acid	Preservative in food
Nickel and other metal salts	Nickel (and other metal salts) in food
Quinolones	Oral antibiotics
Neomycin	Streptomycin, kanamycin
Thiuram	Disulfiram

Table 12.4 Examples of topical allergens that may result in systemic contact dermatitis after systemic exposure.

Other Important Allergens

Topical Corticosteroids

• Can cause ACD in up to 6% of patients.

• Consider CS allergy if an existing dermatitis worsens with CS use or fails to clear; testing with topical tixocortal pivalate (class A) and budesonide (class B) will detect ~90% of CS allergy.

• If CS allergy is suspected/confirmed, use of a CS from a different class can be considered (see Appendix).

Additional allergens include paraphenylenediamine in temporary tattoos and hair dyes, acrylates in artificial nails, thiuram in rubber and makeup applicators, formaldehyde resin in nail polish, components of adhesives, and blue dyes in textiles.

Systemic Contact Dermatitis

• Systemic exposure to a chemical/allergen to which the patient has had prior sensitization (Table 12.4; Fig. 12.14); e.g. administration of oral diphenhydramine to a patient previously sensitized to the topical formulation.

Occupational Dermatoses

• Most commonly an irritant > allergic contact dermatitis.

• Other occupational dermatoses include contact urticaria (see Chapter 14), skin cancer, folliculitis (see Chapter 31), contact leukoderma (see Chapter 54), foreign body reactions, and infections (Table 12.5).

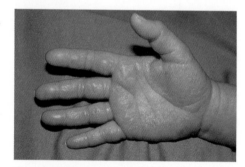

Fig. 12.14 Systemic contact dermatitis. This patient, who was previously sensitized to ethylenediamine, received intravenous aminophylline.

Plant Dermatoses

• Plants can cause a variety of skin reactions, including ACD (Fig. 12.10), ICD, urticaria, and phytophotodermatitis (Table 12.6).

• ACD to plants that contain urushiol.

– Commonly secondary to poison ivy, genus *Toxicodendron* (Fig. 12.16) – compound leaves with three leaflets and flowers/fruits arising from the axillary position; black dots of urushiol often present on leaves.

– Chemicals that cross-react with urushiol are found in the cashew nut tree (nutshell oil and bark), mango tree (leaves, bark, stems, fruit skin), Brazilian pepper tree (sap and crushed berries), Japanese lacquer tree (bark sap), Indian marking tree nut (black juice), and Ginkgo tree (seed coat).

SELECTED OCCUPATIONAL DERMATOSES	
Dermatosis	**Key Features**
Fiberglass dermatitis	Pruritus, tingling Erythematous papules (sometimes with follicular accentuation) Paronychia
Skin cancer	Major hazards are ultraviolet radiation, ionizing radiation, and carcinogenic chemicals Most common tumor is squamous cell carcinoma
Acne	Clinical features similar to non-occupationally related acne In addition, unusual sites may be affected (arms, abdomen) Inciting factors – exposures to oils, halogenated polycyclic hydrocarbons (chloracne), and repeated frictional trauma Chloracne – open comedones predominate; concentration of lesions on malar cheeks and behind ears (Fig. 12.15)
White finger(s)	Workers at risk include operators of chainsaws and pneumatic tools with exposures to vibrations from 30 to 300 Hz and cold Transient loss of sensation with possible permanent neuropathy
Orf	Seen in farmers, slaughterhouse workers, veterinarians Secondary to a parapoxvirus from exposure to sheep, goats, or reindeer
Herpetic whitlow	Exposure to herpes simplex virus, e.g. health care workers
Erysipeloid	Seen in farmers, fishermen, butchers Exposure to *Erysipelothrix rhusiopathiae* in shellfish, fish, birds, and mammals, especially pigs

Table 12.5 Selected occupational dermatoses.

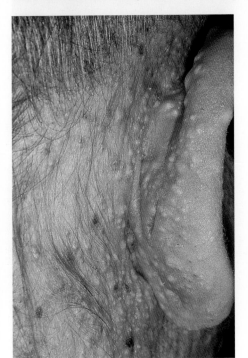

Fig. 12.15 Chloracne. Note involvement of retroauricular skin with numerous comedones (primarily closed) and cysts. The clinical differential diagnosis includes folliculotropic mycosis fungoides.

- Allergen-containing smoke can cause respiratory tract inflammation, systemic contact dermatitis, and temporary blindness.
- After contact with urushiol, a sensitized person develops erythema, vesicles/bullae, and edema within 2 days; the reaction can last 2 or 3 weeks (Fig. 12.10).
- **Rx:** topical, or if severe, systemic CS; treatment should be for at least 2 weeks, otherwise rebound phenomenon common (i.e., avoid the use of a 6-day Medrol® dose pack).
• Phytophotodermatitis.
- Non-immunologic reaction to topical contact with a photosensitizer and subsequent exposure to ultraviolet A light.
- Erythema, vesicles/bullae, and subsequent hyperpigmentation; often in linear streaks or bizarre configurations; however, hyperpigmentation may be the only clinical finding (Figs. 12.17 and 12.18).
- Commonly secondary to furocoumarins (psoralens and angelicins) in plants, e.g. limes, celery, false Bishop's weed, and rue (Fig. 12.18).

MOST COMMON SKIN REACTIONS TO PLANTS

Reaction Type	Plants/Fruit	Inciting Agent
Allergic contact dermatitis	Poison ivy	Alkyl-catechols and resorcinols in urushiol
	Peruvian lily	Tulipalin A > B
	Chrysanthemum	Sesquiterpene lactones*
Irritant contact dermatitis	Dumb cane	Calcium oxalate
	Daffodils	Calcium oxalate
	Prickly pear	Glochids
Urticaria	Stinging nettle	Histamine
Phytophotodermatitis	Persian lime	Furocoumarins (psoralens and angelicins)
	Celery	Same
	Rue	Same
Other – burning/edema	Hot peppers	Capsaicin

*Can cause airborne contact dermatitis and positive in chronic actinic dermatitis.

Table 12.6 Most common skin reactions to plants. Some plants can cause more than one reaction; e.g. garlic can cause ACD (diallyldisulfide), ICD, and urticaria.

IDENTIFICATION OF POISON IVY, OAK AND SUMAC

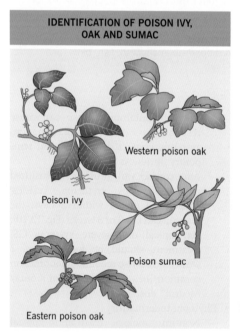

Fig. 12.16 Characteristic features useful for identifying poison ivy, poison oak, and poison sumac. *With permission from the American Journal of Contact Dermatitis.*

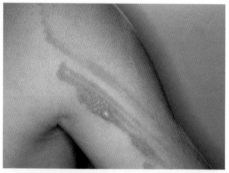

Fig. 12.17 Bullous phase of phytophotodermatitis. There was associated burning but no pruritus, and the linear bullae were replaced by hyperpigmentation. *Courtesy, Jean L. Bolognia, MD.*

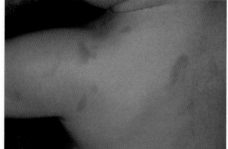

Fig. 12.18 Phytophotodermatitis. Streaky hyperpigmentation due to contact with lime followed by exposure to sunlight. *Courtesy, Anthony J. Mancini, MD.*

For further information see Chs. 14, 15, 16 and 17. From *Dermatology, Third Edition.*

Clinical Approach to Regional Dermatoses

13

- Some inflammatory, infectious, metabolic, neoplastic, and genetic skin conditions have a predilection for particular areas of the body.
- This chapter addresses the diagnosis and treatment of regional dermatoses affecting the hands, feet, intertriginous regions, diaper area, lips, and eyelids.

Dermatitis of the Hands and Feet

- An approach to the classification of hand dermatitis is presented in Fig. 13.1, and the differential diagnosis of foot dermatitis is summarized in Table 13.1.
- Because the hands and feet have a thicker stratum corneum than other areas of the body, percutaneous absorption of topical medications is decreased.
- High-potency topical CS or the use of occlusion may be needed to effectively treat inflammatory dermatoses in these sites.

Intertriginous Dermatitis

- Intertriginous areas include the inguinal creases, gluteal cleft, axillae, inframammary folds, and beneath pannus in obese patients.
- The differential diagnosis of dermatitis in the major skin folds is presented in Fig. 13.2.
- Other conditions with a predilection for intertriginous regions include skin tags, hidradenitis suppurativa, Fox–Fordyce disease, scabies, erythema migrans, variants of lichen planus (e.g. inverse, pigmentosus), inverse pityriasis rosea, vitiligo, lentigines in the setting of neurofibromatosis type 1, Dowling–Degos disease, and pseudoxanthoma elasticum.
- Occlusion and a high level of cutaneous hydration in intertriginous sites increase the absorption of topical medications.
- Low-potency topical CS are often effective for dermatoses in these areas, and prolonged use of more potent agents (including

antifungal combination products; see below) has increased potential to result in side effects such as cutaneous atrophy (Fig. 13.3).

Diaper Dermatitis

- Develops in >50% of infants and has a variety of causes (Fig. 13.4).
- Dampness and exposure to urine and feces represent factors in the etiology of irritant and infectious forms of diaper dermatitis.
- Frequent changing of highly absorbent disposable diapers decreases the incidence and severity of diaper dermatitis.
- Seborrheic dermatitis and psoriasis in the diaper area predispose infants and toddlers to other forms of diaper dermatitis.
- An exuberant, multifactorial diaper dermatitis (e.g. sebopsoriasis with Candida or bacterial superinfection) can trigger the rapid development of numerous small, scaly erythematous papules in a widespread distribution on the trunk and extremities (psoriasiform 'id' reaction).
- Mild topical CS are helpful for the inflammatory component of irritant dermatitis and primary dermatoses in the diaper area, while topical imidazole creams treat candidiasis and have additional anti-inflammatory effects; these agents can be used together for seborrheic dermatitis or psoriasis.
- Combination products containing a potent CS (e.g. Lotrisone® [clotrimazole + betamethasone dipropionate], Mycolog® [nystatin + triamcinolone]) and long-term daily use of any CS in the diaper area should be avoided (see above).
- Barrier ointments containing zinc oxide provide protective and soothing effects; a thick layer should be used (following application of anti-inflammatory/antimicrobial agents if needed) with each diaper change in patients with diaper dermatitis.

CLASSIFICATION OF HAND DERMATITIS

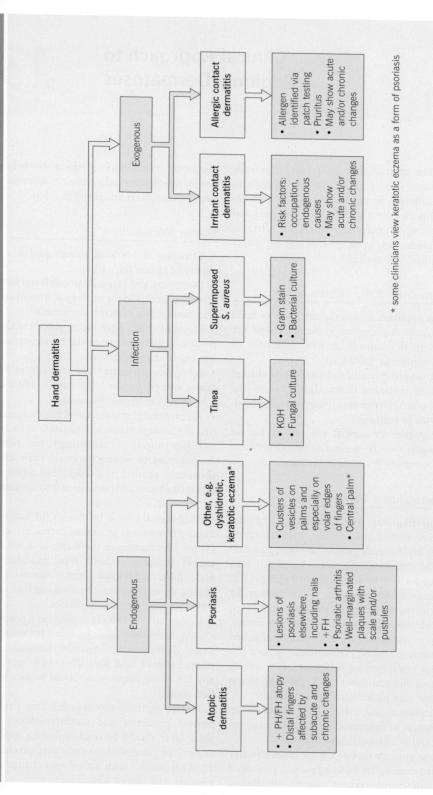

Fig. 13.1 Classification of hand dermatitis. More than one etiology may be present, e.g. atopic dermatitis plus irritant contact dermatitis. FH, family history; PH, personal history. *Courtesy, David E. Cohen, MD.*

DIFFERENTIAL DIAGNOSIS OF FOOT DERMATITIS

Allergic Contact Dermatitis

- Location of the dermatitis on the dorsal surface versus plantar surface (especially weight-bearing areas) of the feet can reflect an allergen in the top portion or sole of the shoe, respectively
- Common shoe allergens include dichromate (used to tan leather), adhesive components (e.g. formaldehyde resins, colophony), rubber accelerators, and dyes; allergens implicated in foot dermatitis also include topical antibiotics (e.g. bacitracin)
- Often associated with atopy and/or hyperhidrosis
- Lesions extend more proximally in sock/stocking dermatitis, where the most common allergen is azo dyes

Dyshidrotic Eczema

- Pruritic, deep-seated vesicles (often pinhead-sized) on the palms/soles and sides of the fingers/toes
- Referred to as 'pompholyx' when larger vesicles/bullae are present
- Frequently associated with atopy or contact dermatitis (allergic and irritant)

Keratolysis Exfoliativa (Recurrent Focal Palmar and Plantar Peeling)

- Circinate pattern of superficial desquamation (collarettes) on the palms and/or soles
- Worsens in warm weather and is associated with low-grade irritation/friction

Juvenile Plantar Dermatosis

- 'Glazed' erythema, scale and fissuring on the balls of the feet and plantar aspect of the toes
- Usually occurs in prepubertal children
- Associated with atopic dermatitis, sweaty feet, and occlusive footwear

Tinea Pedis (Athlete's Foot)

- Dermatophyte infections of the plantar skin are usually accompanied by involvement of the interdigital spaces (e.g. maceration)
- A 'moccasin' distribution of diffuse scaling/erythema and a vesicular inflammatory variant favoring the medial foot can also occur
- Lesions on the lateral and dorsal aspects of the feet tend to have an annular configuration
- Often associated with tinea unguium

Keratoderma Climactericum

- Mechanically induced hyperkeratosis and fissuring on the heels and weight-bearing areas of the soles
- Typically occurs in women >45 years of age
- Predisposing factors include obesity and a cold, dry climate

Psoriasis

- Well-demarcated areas of erythema, adherent scale, and often fissuring
- Psoriasiform plaques elsewhere (e.g. dorsal hands/feet, elbows/knees, scalp) and nail involvement (e.g. pitting, oil spots)

Pustulosis of the Palms and Soles

- 'Sterile' pustules admixed with yellow-brown macules favoring the instep
- Often *not* associated with plaque psoriasis elsewhere

Other

- Atopic dermatitis
- Irritant contact dermatitis (e.g. related to occlusive footwear)
- Crusted scabies
- Pityriasis rubra pilaris
- Keratoderma blennorrhagicum (in setting of reactive arthritis)
- Inherited palmoplantar keratoderma (diffuse or focal)
- Erythrodermic mycosis fungoides, Sézary syndrome
- Acquired keratoderma associated with hypothyroidism or cancer

Table 13.1 Differential diagnosis of foot dermatitis.

DIFFERENTIAL DIAGNOSIS OF INTERTRIGINOUS DERMATITIS IN ADULTS

Common ———— Less common ————▷ Uncommon

Irritant/frictional intertrigo
- Ill-defined erythema/maceration
- Predisposing factors: obesity, heat & humidity, hyperhidrosis, diabetes mellitus, poor hygiene
- Secondary infections common

Seborrheic dermatitis*
- Well-demarcated, pink to red, moist patches/plaques
- Centered along inguinal creases
- Involvement of scalp, face, ears

Inverse psoriasis*
- Well-demarcated, pink to red plaques
- Shiny with little scale in folds
- Centered along inguinal creases
- Psoriasiform plaques elsewhere (e.g. genitals, intergluteal cleft, scalp, elbows/knees, hands/ feet)
- Nail psoriasis (pitting, oil spots)

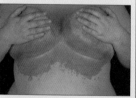

Dermatophytosis (e.g. tinea cruris)
- Less often centered along inguinal creases
- Expanding annular lesions with scaly erythematous border that may contain pustules or vesicles
- Extension to inner thigh, buttock; usually spares scrotum
- Coexisting tinea pedis/unguium

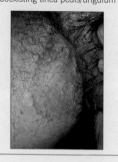

Candidiasis
- Intense erythema with desquamation and satellite papules/pustules
- Often involves scrotum as well as skin folds
- Predisposing factors: occlusion, hyperhidrosis, diabetes mellitus, antibiotic or CS use, immunosuppression

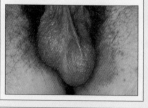

Erythrasma
- Pink-red to brown patches with fine scale
- Coral-red fluorescence with Wood's lamp illumination

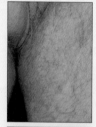

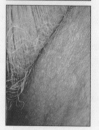

Allergic contact dermatitis
- Consider if fails to respond to usual therapy

Granular parakeratosis
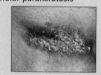

Systemic contact dermatitis, symmetrical drug-related intertriginous flexural exanthema (Table 13.2), toxic erythema of chemotherapy

Hailey-Hailey disease, Darier disease (depicted), pemphigus vegetans
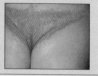

Zinc deficiency, necrolytic migratory erythema, other 'nutritional dermatitis'

'Metastatic' Crohn's disease
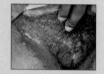

Langerhans cell histiocytosis
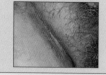

Extramammary Paget's disease
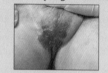

Bowenoid papulosis
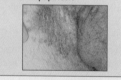

Fig. 13.2 Differential diagnosis of intertriginous dermatitis in adults. *See next page for figure legend.*

Fig. 13.2 Differential diagnosis of intertriginous dermatitis in adults. Individual patients often have multiple disorders superimposed upon one another. Bullous impetigo and streptococcal intertrigo are considerably more common in children than adults (see Fig. 13.4). *The term 'sebopsoriasis' may be used when features of both seborrheic dermatitis and psoriasis are present. *Insets: Courtesy, Eugene Mirrer, MD; Louis Fragola, Jr., MD; David Mehregan, MD and Robert Hartman, MD.*

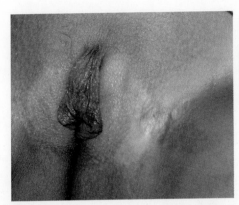

Fig. 13.3 Cutaneous atrophy in the inguinal fold from chronic use of a topical CS. This 10-year-old girl's seborrheic dermatitis had been treated with a mid-potency topical CS on a daily basis for several years, resulting in the development of striae. *Courtesy, Julie V. Schaffer, MD.*

SYMMETRICAL DRUG-RELATED INTERTRIGINOUS AND FLEXURAL EXANTHEMA (SDRIFE): CLINICAL CRITERIA
• Exposure to a systemically administered drug,* occurring with either the initial or a repeated dose (excluding contact allergens)
• Sharply demarcated erythema of the gluteal/perianal area and/or V-shaped erythema of the inguinal/genital area
• Involvement of at least one other intertriginous site/flexural fold
• Symmetric involvement in affected areas
• Absence of systemic symptoms and signs

Not a chemotherapeutic agent, so distinct from toxic erythema of chemotherapy.
Adapted from Häusermann P, Harr TH, Bircher AJ. Baboon syndrome resulting from systemic drugs: Is there strife between SDRIFE and allergic contact dermatitis syndrome? Contact Dermatitis 2004;51:297–310.

Table 13.2 Symmetrical drug-related intertriginous and flexural exanthema (SDRIFE): clinical criteria. This entity is also referred to as drug-induced intertrigo, flexural drug eruption, and baboon syndrome. The latter term is also used for a form of systemic contact dermatitis.

SECTION 3: Papulosquamous and Eczematous Dermatoses

DIFFERENTIAL DIAGNOSIS OF DIAPER DERMATITIS

Common → Less common → Rare

Irritant contact dermatitis
- Glazed erythema ± scale → 'punched out' erosions
- Favors convex surfaces, often spares folds
- Prolonged contact with urine/feces (especially if diarrhea), friction
- Over time pseudoverrucous papules can develop

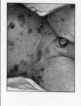

Candidiasis
- Intense erythema with desquamation/superficial erosions & peripheral scale/collarettes
- Satellite pustules
- Favors folds, genitalia
- Yeast/pseudohyphae on KOH preparation
- ±Recent antibiotic use, thrush

Seborrheic dermatitis
- Well-demarcated, salmon-colored to red, moist or scaly patches/plaques
- Favors folds
- Involvement of other flexural sites, scalp

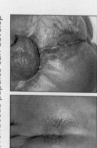

Bacterial infections
Bullous impetigo
- Flaccid bullae, vesiculopustules, superficial shiny red erosions with a collarette of scale
- Gram stain +

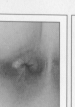 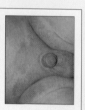

Streptococcal perianal dermatitis & intertrigo
- Sharply demarcated, bright red erythema
- Usually no satellite lesions
- Perianal area, skin folds
- Pain, itch, foul odor
- ± Pharyngitis in patient or family members

Psoriasis
- Well-demarcated erythematous plaques
- Shiny in folds, scaly on convex surfaces
- Psoriasiform lesions elsewhere, ±family history

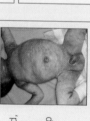

Allergic contact dermatitis*
- Consider if fails to respond to usual therapy
- 'Holster' distribution if reaction to rubber additives in diaper elastics
- May affect folds if reaction to components of baby wipes or topical preparations

Atopic dermatitis (AD)
- Excoriations, lichenification
- Favors skin at diaper margins and convex surfaces
- Often relative sparing of the diaper area
- Marked pruritus
- Other pruritic eczematous lesions in usual sites of AD

Acrodermatitis enteropathica, other forms of 'nutritional dermatitis'

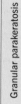

Langerhans cell histiocytosis

Other infections (e.g. congenital syphilis, dermatophytosis)

Granular parakeratosis

Early Kawasaki disease

Fig. 13.4 Differential diagnosis of diaper dermatitis. Patients often have a combination of disorders, one superimposed upon another. Discrete papules or nodules can be seen in scabies, granuloma gluteale infantum, and perianal pseudoverrucous papules, whereas congenital syphilis may present with erosions or even ulcerations. *Potential allergens include sorbitan sesquioleate (an emulsifier in diaper balms), fragrances, disperse dyes, rubber additives (e.g. mercaptobenzothiazole), preservatives in baby wipes, and diaper component. *Insts: Contox, Robert Hartman MD, and Julie V. Schoffer MD.

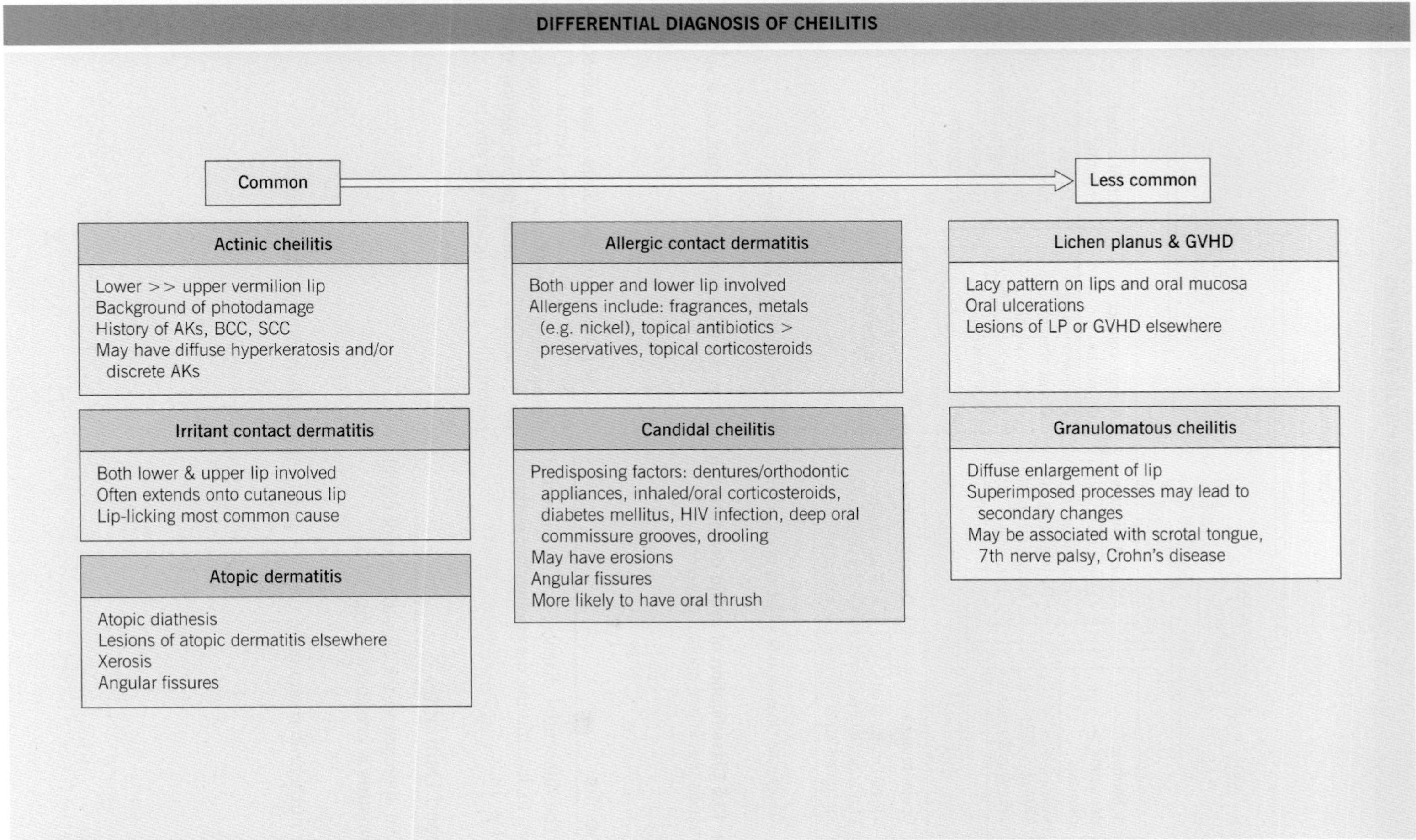

13

DIFFERENTIAL DIAGNOSIS OF CHEILITIS

```
        Common  ──────────────────▶  Less common
```

Actinic cheilitis

Lower >> upper vermilion lip
Background of photodamage
History of AKs, BCC, SCC
May have diffuse hyperkeratosis and/or discrete AKs

Allergic contact dermatitis

Both upper and lower lip involved
Allergens include: fragrances, metals (e.g. nickel), topical antibiotics > preservatives, topical corticosteroids

Lichen planus & GVHD

Lacy pattern on lips and oral mucosa
Oral ulcerations
Lesions of LP or GVHD elsewhere

Irritant contact dermatitis

Both lower & upper lip involved
Often extends onto cutaneous lip
Lip-licking most common cause

Candidal cheilitis

Predisposing factors: dentures/orthodontic appliances, inhaled/oral corticosteroids, diabetes mellitus, HIV infection, deep oral commissure grooves, drooling
May have erosions
Angular fissures
More likely to have oral thrush

Granulomatous cheilitis

Diffuse enlargement of lip
Superimposed processes may lead to secondary changes
May be associated with scrotal tongue, 7th nerve palsy, Crohn's disease

Atopic dermatitis

Atopic diathesis
Lesions of atopic dermatitis elsewhere
Xerosis
Angular fissures

Fig. 13.5 Differential diagnosis of cheilitis. A combination of etiologies is often present, e.g. atopic dermatitis plus irritant contact dermatitis. Other uncommon causes include cheilitis glandularis, actinic prurigo, lichen sclerosus, and nutritional deficiencies. AKs, actinic keratoses; LP, lichen planus; GVHD, graft-versus-host disease. *Courtesy, Jean L. Bolognia, MD.*

CLINICAL APPROACH TO REGIONAL DERMATOSES

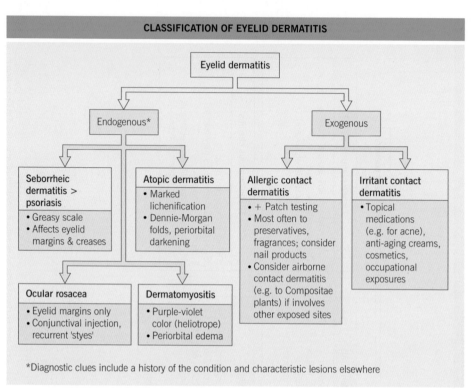

CLASSIFICATION OF EYELID DERMATITIS

Eyelid dermatitis

Endogenous*

Exogenous

Seborrheic dermatitis > psoriasis
• Greasy scale
• Affects eyelid margins & creases

Atopic dermatitis
• Marked lichenification
• Dennie-Morgan folds, periorbital darkening

Allergic contact dermatitis
• + Patch testing
• Most often to preservatives, fragrances; consider nail products
• Consider airborne contact dermatitis (e.g. to Compositae plants) if involves other exposed sites

Irritant contact dermatitis
• Topical medications (e.g. for acne), anti-aging creams, cosmetics, occupational exposures

Ocular rosacea
• Eyelid margins only
• Conjunctival injection, recurrent 'styes'

Dermatomyositis
• Purple-violet color (heliotrope)
• Periorbital edema

*Diagnostic clues include a history of the condition and characteristic lesions elsewhere

Fig. 13.6 Classification of eyelid dermatitis. More than one etiology may be present, e.g. atopic dermatitis plus irritant contact dermatitis.

Cheilitis

• The differential diagnosis of cheilitis and clues to determining the etiology are outlined in Fig. 13.5.

Eyelid Dermatitis

• An approach to the classification of eyelid dermatitis is presented in Fig. 13.6.

• Low-potency topical CS are often effective for dermatitis on the eyelids because of the delicate skin in this site, and prolonged CS use (especially of more potent agents) may potentially lead to ocular side effects.

For further information see Chs. 13 and 15. From *Dermatology, Third Edition.*

Urticaria and Angioedema | 14

- Urticaria and angioedema can occur at any age and are estimated to have an overall lifetime prevalence of 10–25%.
- Urticaria (hives) is characterized by *wheals*: evanescent, pale to pink-red, edematous papules or plaques (Fig. 14.1); lesions often have central clearing, a peripheral erythematous flare, and associated pruritus.
- Individual wheals last <24 hours, which can be documented by outlining them with ink.

- Angioedema represents deeper dermal and subcutaneous or submucosal swelling (Fig. 14.2); affected areas are ill-defined, have minimal or no overlying erythema, and may be painful as well as pruritic.
- In addition to the skin/subcutis, angioedema can affect the mouth and respiratory or gastrointestinal tract; an area of swelling may persist for several days.
- A classification scheme and **DDx** for urticaria and angioedema are presented in

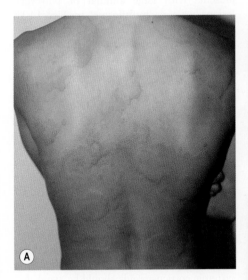

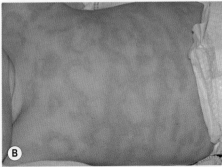

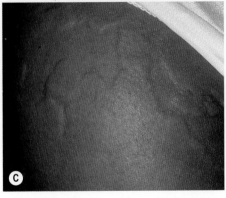

Fig. 14.1 Wheals. Wheals can be small or large in size **(A)** as well as annular or polycyclic **(B)**, but they still retain the classic central pallor and erythematous flare. **C** Occasionally, more uniform edematous plaques are seen. *B, Courtesy, Julie V. Schaffer, MD.*

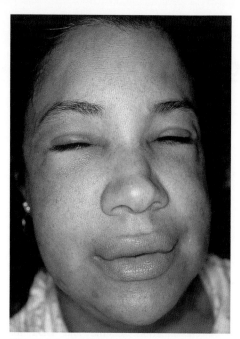

Fig. 14.2 Angioedema. The swelling is deeper than in wheals and may affect mucosal surfaces. Note the swelling of the lips and periorbital region and the lack of erythema. *Courtesy, Clive E. H. Grattan, MD.*

MAST CELL DEGRANULATING STIMULI

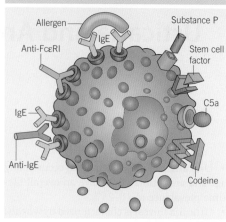

Fig. 14.3 Mast cell degranulating stimuli. Both immunologic and non-immunologic stimuli can lead to release of mediators. Stem cell factor is also known as KIT ligand. Autoantibodies against the high-affinity IgE receptor (FcεRI) and the Fc portion of IgE are implicated in chronic autoimmune urticaria.

Table 14.1; patients with angioedema may have associated urticaria, including physical urticaria.

• Urticaria and urticaria-associated angioedema result from the release of histamine and other proinflammatory and vasoactive substances from mast cells; this leads to extravasation of plasma, vasodilatation, and pruritus.

• Stimuli for mast cell degranulation are shown in Fig. 14.3.

Spontaneous ('Ordinary') Urticaria: Acute and Chronic

• Although both can occur at any age, acute urticaria is most common in children, whereas chronic urticaria has a peak in the fourth decade of life and a female : male ratio of ~2 : 1.

• The most frequent causes of acute and chronic urticaria are listed in Table 14.2.

• Acute urticaria in young children often presents with large annular or polycyclic lesions (urticaria 'multiforme'; see Figs. 14.1B and 3.3A) that tend to resolve with a transient dusky purplish hue, which can lead to misdiagnosis as erythema multiforme.

• Urticaria can result in sleep disturbances and anxiety.

• Chronic autoimmune urticaria is associated with an increased risk of other autoimmune conditions, such as thyroid disorders and celiac disease.

• An approach to the diagnosis of chronic urticaria is outlined in Fig. 14.4; extensive laboratory evaluations (e.g. for food allergies) are extremely low-yield and are not recommended.

• **Rx:** a stepwise therapeutic approach is presented in Fig. 14.5; long-acting antihistamines are the mainstay of treatment, and systemic corticosteroids should be avoided.

Physical (Inducible) Urticaria

• Different forms of physical urticaria may coexist with one another and/or chronic spontaneous urticaria.

• **Rx:** see Fig. 14.5.

14

CLASSIFICATION AND DIFFERENTIAL DIAGNOSIS OF URTICARIA AND ANGIOEDEMA

- Spontaneous ('ordinary') urticaria
  - Acute (duration <6 weeks)
  - Chronic (occurring at least twice weekly for ≥6 weeks*): median duration of ~2–5 years; includes an autoimmune form
- Physical (inducible) urticaria
  - *Due to mechanical stimuli*: dermographism, delayed pressure urticaria[†]
  - *Due to temperature changes*: cold > heat-induced urticaria
  - *Due to sweating/physical exertion*: cholinergic > adrenergic urticaria, exercise-induced anaphylaxis
  - *Other*: solar and aquagenic urticaria
- Contact urticaria (immunologic or non-immunologic)
- Angioedema without wheals (including hereditary angioedema; see Fig. 14.9)
- Related conditions in **DDx****: Schnitzler's syndrome, serum sickness-like reaction (see Chapter 17), urticarial vasculitis[†] (see Chapter 19), hereditary periodic fever syndromes (see Table 3.2)
- Additional **DDx:**
  - *For transient urticarial lesions*: Still's disease, scombroid poisoning, erythema marginatum, cutaneous mastocytosis (also persistent red-brown papules/plaques)
  - *For urticarial lesions lasting >24 hours*: urticarial drug eruption, viral exanthem, erythema multiforme (central duskiness/vesiculation rather than clearing), insect bite reactions, Sweet's syndrome, urticarial bullous pemphigoid, acute hemorrhagic edema of infancy, Kawasaki disease
  - *For angioedema*: early airborne or allergic contact dermatitis, insect bite reaction

*Urticaria occurring less frequently than this over a long period is referred to as episodic or recurrent.
†Individual lesions tend to last >24 hours; urticarial vasculitis features burning/pain, purpura upon resolution, and a subgroup associated with hypocomplementation and autoimmune connective tissue disease (e.g. SLE).
**Consider for chronic urticaria with associated symptoms such as fevers, pain, and arthralgias.
SLE, systemic lupus erythematosus.

Table 14.1 Classification and differential diagnosis of urticaria and angioedema.

CAUSES OF ACUTE AND CHRONIC SPONTANEOUS URTICARIA

Acute Urticaria	Chronic Urticaria
• Infection (e.g. URI) (~40%) • Drug (~10%) • Food (≤1%) • Idiopathic (~50%)	• Autoimmune (histamine-releasing autoantibodies against FcεRI or the Fc portion of IgE; see Fig. 14.3) (40–50%) • Chronic infection (e.g. parasitic) (≤5%) • Idiopathic (~50%)

FcεRI, high-affinity IgE receptor (present on mast cells); IgE, immunoglobulin E; URI, upper respiratory tract infection.

Table 14.2 Causes of acute and chronic spontaneous urticaria.

Dermographism ('Skin Writing')

- Affects at least 10% of the general population; may lead to symptoms such as pruritus.
- Linear or irregularly shaped wheals develop at sites of scratching or friction (Fig. 14.6); lesions typically resolve within an hour.
- Can elicit via stroking the skin, e.g. with a thin wooden stick or tongue depressor.

Delayed Pressure Urticaria

- Pruritic and/or painful erythema and swelling (Fig. 14.7) develop 0.5–12 hours after sustained pressure to the skin (e.g. due to tight clothing or shoes); may last several days, sometimes with associated arthralgias and malaise.

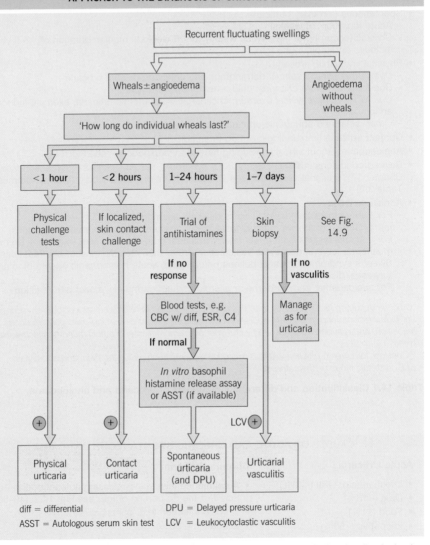

Fig. 14.4 Approach to the diagnosis of chronic urticaria. In a positive ASST, a localized wheal and flare response occurs upon intradermal injection of autologous serum, providing evidence of functional histamine-releasing factors in the blood. Regulations regarding blood products limit the availability of this test. *Courtesy, Clive E. H. Grattan, MD.*

Cold Urticaria

• Wheals ± angioedema develop within minutes of cold exposure, with maximal hiving upon rewarming; systemic reactions (e.g. anaphylaxis) may occur with aquatic activities.

• Can elicit via ice cube test (Fig. 14.8; 1- to 10-minute application within glove, then rewarming).

• Usually primary; <5% of cases are associated with cryoglobulins or cryofibrinogen.

• Rare early-onset variants with autosomal dominant inheritance and a negative ice cube test: cryopyrin-associated periodic syndrome (see Table 3.2), familial atypical cold urticaria (wheals upon evaporative cooling; *PLCG2* mutations).

MANAGEMENT OF SPONTANEOUS AND PHYSICAL URTICARIAS

- Eliminate any modifiable cause
- Avoid physical triggers and drugs that stimulate mast cell degranulation (e.g. aspirin, NSAIDs, codeine, morphine)

↓

Scheduled administration of long-acting, low-sedating H1 antihistamine(s)
- (Levo)cetirizine is especially effective
- Increasing to 2- to 4-times the standard dose of (levo)cetirizine and/or using >1 agent [e.g. adding (des)loratadine] can maximize benefit

↓ If response is not adequate

Add sedating H1 antihistamine at bedtime
- Nightly low-dose doxepin* (10-50 mg in adults) is particularly helpful

↓ If response is not adequate

Add H2 antihistamine (e.g. ranitidine)
- Consider leukotriene antagonist if aspirin/NSAID-sensitive

↓ If response is not adequate

Additional considerations for refractory disease
- Dapsone or colchicine (especially if neutrophilic component)
- Mycophenolate mofetil, methotrexate, cyclosporine
- Omalizumab (anti-IgE monoclonal antibody)

Treatments in specific acute circumstances
- Epinephrine (SC or IM) for anaphylaxis or severe pharyngeal angioedema
- In general, prednisone is not recommended, with the exception of a 2-3 week course for severe acute urticaria with systemic manifestations (e.g. serum sickness-like reactions), with co-administration of antihistamines

*A tricyclic antidepressant with potent H1 and H2 antihistamine effects; contraindications include narrow-angle glaucoma, urinary retention and recent MAOI administration

Fig. 14.5 Management of spontaneous and physical urticarias. IM, intramuscular; IVIg, intravenous immunoglobulin; MAOI, monoamine oxidase inhibitor; SC, subcutaneous.

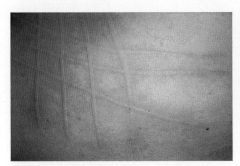

Fig. 14.6 Symptomatic dermographism within minutes of scratching. *Courtesy, Jean L. Bolognia, MD.*

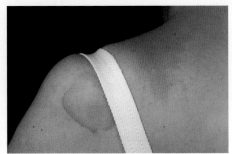

Fig. 14.7 Delayed pressure urticaria. *Courtesy, Clive E. H. Grattan, MD.*

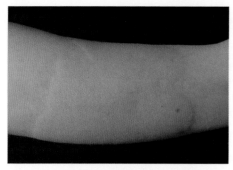

Fig. 14.8 Cold urticaria. Wheals developed on the forearm after placement of an ice cube for 10 minutes, followed by rewarming. *Courtesy, Thomas Schwarz, MD.*

Cholinergic Urticaria

• Multiple small (2–3 mm), monomorphic, pruritic wheals with an erythematous flare develop within 15 minutes of sweat-inducing stimulus (e.g. physical exertion, emotional stress, hot bath); favors the upper body but may be widespread.

• **DDx:** adrenergic urticaria (blanched halo rather than flare), heat urticaria (can occur without sweating), exercise-induced urticaria/anaphylaxis (only with exercise, not a hot bath), aquagenic urticaria (upon contact with water of any temperature).

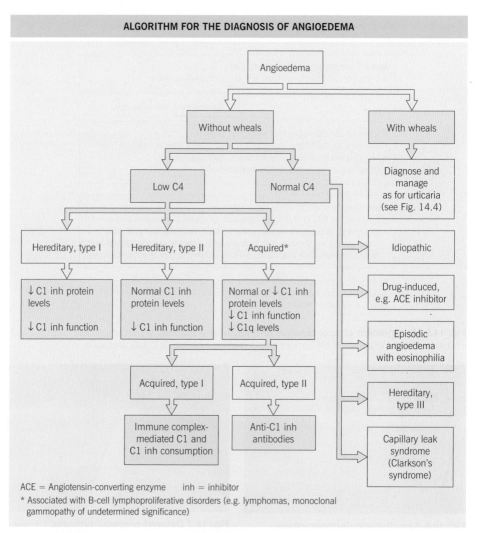

ALGORITHM FOR THE DIAGNOSIS OF ANGIOEDEMA

Angioedema

Without wheals → With wheals

Without wheals → Low C4 / Normal C4

With wheals → Diagnose and manage as for urticaria (see Fig. 14.4)

Low C4 → Hereditary, type I / Hereditary, type II / Acquired*

Hereditary, type I:
↓ C1 inh protein levels
↓ C1 inh function

Hereditary, type II:
Normal C1 inh protein levels
↓ C1 inh function

Acquired*:
Normal or ↓ C1 inh protein levels
↓ C1 inh function
↓ C1q levels

Acquired* → Acquired, type I / Acquired, type II

Acquired, type I → Immune complex-mediated C1 and C1 inh consumption

Acquired, type II → Anti-C1 inh antibodies

Normal C4 / With wheals →
- Idiopathic
- Drug-induced, e.g. ACE inhibitor
- Episodic angioedema with eosinophilia
- Hereditary, type III
- Capillary leak syndrome (Clarkson's syndrome)

ACE = Angiotensin-converting enzyme   inh = inhibitor

* Associated with B-cell lymphoproliferative disorders (e.g. lymphomas, monoclonal gammopathy of undetermined significance)

Fig. 14.9 Algorithm for the diagnosis of angioedema. Episodic angioedema with eosinophilia as well as weight gain and fever is known as Gleich syndrome. Systemic capillary leak syndrome can lead to life-threatening hypotension and is associated with an IgG monoclonal gammopathy.

Solar Urticaria

• Pruritus and wheals within 5–10 minutes of exposure to UVA and/or visible light > UVB (see Chapter 73).

Contact Urticaria

• *Immunologic contact urticaria* presents with localized pruritus and hives within 30 minutes of handling fresh vegetables/fruits or contact with latex in sensitized individuals; occasionally generalizes, and 'protein contact dermatitis' may occur with repeated exposure (especially in atopic patients).

• Evaluation of suspected type 1 latex allergy initially involves a blood test for specific IgE; if negative, a prick test with latex extract can be performed in a controlled setting and, if there is no reaction, confirmed with a usage test (e.g. wearing the suspect glove).

• *'Oral allergy syndrome'* presents with intraoral itching and swelling in individuals with a pollen allergy upon ingestion of cross-reacting fresh fruits or vegetables.

• *Non-immunologic contact urticaria* results from exposure to plants containing toxins (e.g. histamine) within sharp 'hairs' on their leaves (e.g. stinging nettles).

Schnitzler's Syndrome

• Chronic urticaria ± pruritus associated with a monoclonal gammopathy (IgM >> IgG).

• Other features include fevers, arthralgias, bone pain, lymphadenopathy, leukocytosis, and an increased ESR; patients may develop a lymphoproliferative malignancy.

• **Rx:** prednisone, anakinra, and rituximab, as well as treatment of the underlying disorder.

Hereditary Angioedema (HAE)

• HAE due to deficiency (type I) or dysfunction (type II) of the complement C1 esterase inhibitor is an uncommon autosomal dominant disorder that presents with episodic nonpruritic angioedema lasting 2–3 days, often beginning in early childhood and triggered by trauma; although not associated with true urticaria, attacks are occasionally preceded or accompanied by transient, nonpruritic, serpiginous erythematous patches.

• Type I/II HAE favors the extremities and gastrointestinal tract (may mimic an acute abdomen), and airway compromise due to laryngeal edema can occur.

• Type III HAE is a later-onset form with more frequent facial involvement that develops primarily in teenage girls and young women.

• Pathogenesis of HAE is related to excessive generation of bradykinin, which leads to increased vascular permeability.

• Evaluation and **DDx:** outlined in Fig. 14.9.

• **Rx:** *acute attacks or short-term prophylaxis* (e.g. for surgical or dental procedures) – intravenous C1 inhibitor concentrate > subcutaneous ecallantide (kallikrein inhibitor) or icatibant (bradykinin B_2 receptor antagonist); *long-term treatment* – androgens (e.g. oral danazol) > antifibrinolytic agents; antihistamines, epinephrine, and corticosteroids are *not* effective.

For further information see Ch. 18. From *Dermatology, Third Edition*.

15 | Figurate Erythemas

A number of cutaneous diseases can have an annular, arciform, or polycyclic configuration, from urticaria to granuloma annulare and tinea corporis (Table 15.1). Sites of involvement, rate of expansion, and characteristics of the border assist in narrowing the differential diagnosis, along with histologic examination of the active edge. This chapter discusses in more detail the classic figurate erythemas.

Erythema Annulare Centrifugum (EAC)

• Annular, arciform, and polycyclic plaques due to infiltrates of lymphocytes within the dermis; lesions usually last for a few weeks to months and as they migrate centrifugally, there is central clearing; recurrences are common.
• This gyrate erythema is sometimes divided into superficial and deep forms, based on clinicopathologic findings, with the superficial form being minimally elevated with "trailing" white scale (Fig. 15.1A) and the deep form having a more infiltrated border (Fig. 15.1B); some authors reserve the designation EAC for the superficial form.
• Color varies from pink to darker red-violet, with the superficial form favoring the thighs and deeper the trunk; peak incidence is during the fifth decade.
• Often idiopathic, but some cases appear to be a reactive process triggered by fungal infections, in particular tinea pedis, or less often, viral infections or medications.
• **DDx:** Tinea corporis (especially if scale is present); if no surface changes, annular urticaria (Fig. 15.2), benign lymphocytic infiltrate (of Jessner), cutaneous lymphoid hyperplasia, cutaneous lupus erythematosus (tumidus), and lymphoma cutis as well as the other entities covered in this chapter and Table 15.1; in

some patients, the diagnosis of EAC is rendered after exclusion of other disorders.
• **Rx:** if trigger identified, it should be treated; if no trigger is identified, topical CS may be of some benefit.

Erythema Marginatum

• Cutaneous manifestation of rheumatic fever (due to a preceding group A β-hemolytic streptococcal infection) and therefore seen more commonly in children.
• Migratory annular and polycyclic erythematous eruption that represents a major Jones criterion (Fig. 15.3); subcutaneous nodules can also develop, but during a later phase of the disease; both findings are seen in the minority of patients.
• This asymptomatic figurate erythema favors the trunk and proximal extremities, with individual lesions lasting a few hours to days and recurrences occurring over a several-week period.
• Associated systemic manifestations: carditis, migratory polyarthritis, chorea, fever.
• **DDx:** annular urticaria (including urticaria multiforme), annular erythema of infancy, Still's disease, Kawasaki disease, hereditary periodic fever syndromes.
• **Rx:** address the underlying rheumatic fever.

Erythema Gyratum Repens

• Migratory figurate erythema composed of multiple concentric rings that is said to resemble the grain of wood (Fig. 15.4); the lesions can migrate up to 1 cm per day and may have associated scale or pruritus.
• Paraneoplastic dermatosis in the vast majority of patients, with lung cancer and breast cancer representing the most common underlying malignancies; patients may have

ADDITIONAL ENTITIES THAT CAN HAVE AN ANNULAR, ARCIFORM, OR POLYCYCLIC CONFIGURATION

No Epidermal (Surface) Changes

Annular urticaria	Individual lesions are transient, lasting <24 hrs
Urticarial vasculitis	Individual lesions usually last >24 hrs and may resolve with petechiae
Granuloma annulare	Skin-colored to dull pink elevated border, often composed of coalescing papules; favors acral sites, elbows
Sarcoidosis	Skin-colored to red-brown; with pressure (diascopy), has a yellow-brown color; face > trunk, extremities; sometimes has scale
Annular elastolytic giant cell granuloma	Sun-exposed sites; hypopigmented centrally as expands
Leprosy	Primarily tuberculoid and borderline forms, with the former often having central hypopigmentation
Syphilis	Secondary stage, in particular on the face, and tertiary stage (gummas); facial lesions may have central hyperpigmentation
Benign lymphocytic infiltrate (of Jessner)	Favors the head, neck, and upper trunk; erythematous papules and plaques last weeks to months
Lymphoma cutis	Pink to violet papules and plaques; may be primary cutaneous or related to a systemic lymphoma

Scale and/or Crust

Tinea corporis	Scale and pustules in the advancing border; KOH examination is positive
Seborrheic dermatitis	Lesions on the face and central chest; associated scale
Annular psoriasis	Scale is silvery; associated scalp, intergluteal, and nail involvement
Subacute cutaneous LE	Primarily sun-exposed sites, especially upper trunk and upper outer arms; hypopigmented centrally

Wickham's Striae within Border

Annular lichen planus	The elevated border is string-like

Petechiae within Border

Annular capillaritis	Both petechiae and yellow-brown hue due to hemosiderin

Vesicobullae within Border

Linear IgA bullous dermatosis	Border may resemble "string of pearls"; DIF required

More Serpiginous Border

Cutaneous larva migrans	Favor feet, buttocks, and areas in contact with sandy ground

DIF, direct immunofluorescence; KOH, potassium hydroxide; LE, lupus erythematosus.

Table 15.1 Additional entities that can have an annular, arciform, or polycyclic configuration. These disorders are covered in other chapters. See text for discussion of the classic figurate erythemas. Both erythema multiforme and erythema migrans can have a bull's-eye appearance.

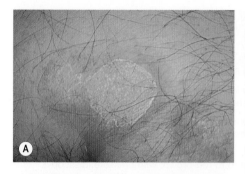

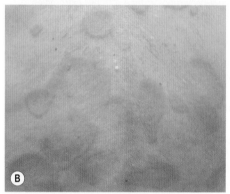

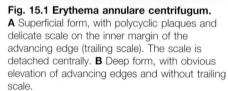

Fig. 15.1 Erythema annulare centrifugum.
A Superficial form, with polyciclic plaques and delicate scale on the inner margin of the advancing edge (trailing scale). The scale is detached centrally. **B** Deep form, with obvious elevation of advancing edges and without trailing scale.

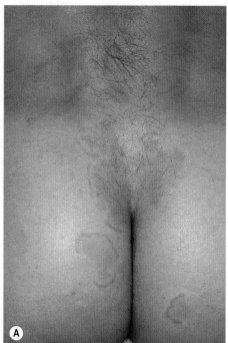

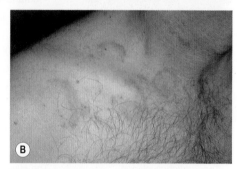

other paraneoplastic phenomena, e.g. acquired ichthyosis, palmoplantar keratoderma.
• Occasionally, patients have no underlying disease or an underlying infection, e.g. pulmonary tuberculosis.
• **DDx:** EAC (slower migration and usually not concentric), tinea imbricata, the resolving phase of pityriasis rubra pilaris, erythrokeratodermia variabilis, mycosis fungoides.
• **Rx:** address the underlying malignancy; if anti-neoplastic treatment is successful, the eruption will resolve.

Erythema Migrans (EM; Erythema Chronicum Migrans [ECM])

• Cutaneous manifestation of the earlier stages of infection with *Borrelia burgdorferi* spirochetes; seen in 60–90% of patients diagnosed with Lyme borreliosis.

Fig. 15.2 A comparison of erythema annulare centrifugum and urticaria. The lesions in **(A)** have no scaling and may be confused with annular urticaria **(B)**. However, individual lesions of urticaria are evanescent.

• Occurs most commonly in the United States (northeast, upper Midwest, west coast), Scandinavia, and central Europe; natural hosts are white-footed mice and white-tailed deer.
• Can be localized to the site of the bite of an infected *Ixodes* tick (Fig. 15.5) or as the disease progresses, become disseminated with multiple secondary lesions (Fig. 15.6); several species of *Ixodes* can transmit disease, including *I. scapularis, I. pacificus, I. ricinus*.

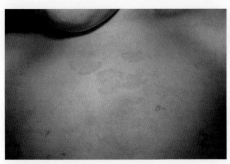

Fig. 15.3 Erythema marginatum (rheumaticum). Polycyclic and evanescent annular lesions are seen on the trunk of this young patient. *Courtesy, Agustin España, MD.*

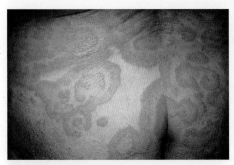

Fig. 15.4 Erythema gyratum repens. Multiple concentric annular plaques, with a wood-grain appearance. *Courtesy, Agustin Alomar, MD.*

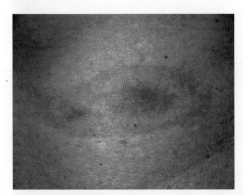

Fig. 15.5 Erythema migrans. Expanding annular plaque that has a bull's-eye appearance.

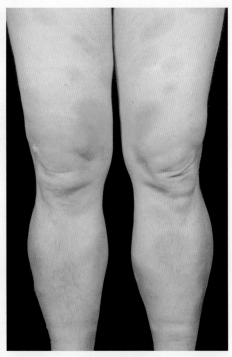

Fig. 15.6 Disseminated erythema migrans. Multiple circular and a few annular plaques are scattered on the lower extremities as well as the trunk (not shown). *Courtesy, Thomas Schwarz, MD.*

result in an annular lesion and sometimes the lesion has a bull's-eye appearance; occasionally, vesicles are seen.

• Primary lesions often favor body folds, are frequently asymptomatic and spontaneously resolve (without treatment) within 6 weeks; primary, and especially disseminated, lesions can be accompanied by flu-like symptoms – headache, malaise, arthralgia, myalgia, and fever.

• Transmission usually requires attachment of the infected *Ixodes* tick for over 24 hours; if untreated, sequelae include arthritis, Bell's palsy, and atrioventricular heart block (Table 15.2); *Ixodes* ticks may also transmit babesiosis and human anaplasmosis.

• Development of additional cutaneous findings (e.g. pseudolymphoma, acrodermatitis chronica atrophicans; Fig. 15.7) is seen in individuals infected outside the United States and reflects the geographic distribution of different genospecies of *Borrelia*, e.g. *B. afzelii* is found in Europe but not the United States.

• At the site of the tick bite, usually after a period of 1 or 2 weeks (range 2–28 days), an erythematous patch or plaque appears that expands over days to weeks to reach a diameter of at least 5 cm; central clearing can

STAGES AND MAJOR ORGAN MANIFESTATIONS OF LYME BORRELIOSIS			
Organ	**Early Localized Disease**	**Early Disseminated Disease**	**Chronic Disease**
Skin	Erythema migrans Disseminated erythema migrans Borrelial lymphocytoma (Europe)		Acrodermatitis chronica atrophicans (Europe)
Nervous system		Meningo- polyradiculoneuritis Cranial neuritis Bell's palsy	Encephalopathy Encephalomyelitis Neuropathy
Musculoskeletal system		Arthralgias, arthritis Myositis	Chronic arthritis
Heart		Atrioventricular block Myopericarditis, pancarditis Tachycardia	
Lymphatic	Regional lymphadenopathy	Regional or generalized lymphadenopathy	
Other		Conjunctivitis, iritis Hepatitis Nonproductive cough Microscopic hematuria or proteinuria	

Adapted from Müllegger RR. Dermatological manifestations of Lyme borreliosis. Eur. J. Dermatol. 2004;14:296–309.

Table 15.2 Stages and major organ manifestations of Lyme borreliosis.

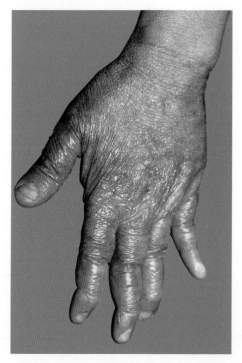

Fig. 15.7 Acrodermatitis chronica atrophicans is another manifestation of Lyme borreliosis. Note the shiny and wrinkled skin plus more visible superficial veins – signs of atrophy.

TREATMENT OPTIONS FOR BORRELIOSIS			
	Antibiotic		
Clinical Features	*First Choice for Adults and Children ≥ 8 Years*,†*	*First Choice for Children < 8 Years and Pregnant Women; Second Choice Otherwise**	*Alternative Choice**
Early localized disease	Doxycycline 100 mg (2 mg/kg) PO q12h, 14–21 days‡	Amoxicillin 500 mg PO q8h (50 mg/kg PO per day divided q8h), 14–21 days§	Cefuroxime axetil 500 mg (15 mg/kg) PO q12h, 14–21 days
Early disseminated disease or chronic disease, **mild** Cranial nerve palsy, 1st or 2nd degree heart block	Doxycycline 100 mg (2 mg/kg) PO q12h, 14–28 days‡	Amoxicillin 500 mg PO q8h (50 mg/kg PO per day divided q8h), 14–28 days	Cefuroxime axetil 500 mg (15 mg/kg) PO q12h, 14–28 days
	First Choice	*Second Choice*	*Third Choice*
Early disseminated disease or chronic disease, **severe** Meningitis, radiculopathy, 3rd degree heart block	Ceftriaxone 2 g (75–100 mg/kg) iv once daily, 14–28 days	Cefotaxime 2 g (50–70 mg/kg) iv q8h, 14–28 days	Penicillin G 18–24 million units (200 000–400 000 units/kg) iv per day divided q4h, 14–28 days

*No comparative trials for early localized disease, so no established superior treatment; doxycycline also treats human anaplasmosis.
†Avoid doxycycline in children <8 years and pregnant women.
‡In a randomized, double-blind, controlled trial, similar outcomes were observed for a 10-day versus 20-day course of doxycycline.
§Recommended for 21 days for pregnant women.

Table 15.3 Treatment options for borreliosis. Doses for children are in parentheses, with adult dose as maximum. A Jarisch–Herxheimer-like reaction with an increase in systemic symptoms and in the size or intensity of the inflammation of the erythema migrans lesion occurs in ~15% of patients within 24 hours after the initiation of antimicrobial therapy.

• **DDx:** exaggerated local reaction to an arthropod bite, cellulitis, allergic contact dermatitis, southern tick-associated rash illness (STARI), nonpigmented fixed drug eruption, and other causes of pseudocellulitis (see Table 61.2); of note, peak specific IgM antibodies usually appear at 3–6 weeks into infection so they may not be detected in patients with early EM (false-negative rate as high as 60%).

• **Rx** is outlined in Table 15.3; for patients who (1) live in an endemic area, (2) had a tick attached for >36 hours, (3) removed the tick within the past 72 hours, and (4) had the tick identified as *I. scapularis*, a single dose of oral doxycycline (200 mg) may reduce the risk of developing Lyme borreliosis from 3.2% to 0.4%.

For further information see Ch. 19. From *Dermatology, Third Edition.*

16 Erythema Multiforme, Stevens–Johnson Syndrome, and Toxic Epidermal Necrolysis

Erythema Multiforme

• Self-limited, but potentially recurrent, disease.
• Two forms: erythema multiforme (EM) major and EM minor (Table 16.1).
• Both forms have an abrupt onset of papular 'target' lesions that favor acrofacial sites.
• Two types of target lesions: (1) typical targets, with at least three different zones; (2) atypical papular targets, with only two different zones and/or a poorly defined border (Fig. 16.1).
• EM minor: typical > atypical *papular* target lesions, little or no mucosal involvement, and no systemic symptoms.
• EM major: typical > atypical *papular* target lesions, moderate to severe mucosal involvement, and some systemic symptoms (fever, asthenia, arthralgia).
• Preceding HSV infection is most common precipitating factor; less often other preceding infections, in particular *Mycoplasma pneumoniae* (Table 16.2; Fig. 16.2); rarely drug exposure.
• Diagnosis based on clinicopathologic correlation and not solely histopathologic findings.
• EM is a distinct disorder from Stevens–Johnson syndrome (SJS) and toxic epidermal necrolysis (TEN) (see Table 16.1).
• EM does not progress to TEN.
• **DDx:** giant urticaria (Fig. 16.3; Table 16.3), morbilliform drug reaction (Fig. 16.4), multiple fixed drug eruption (FDE), acute hemorrhagic edema of infancy, Kawasaki disease, small vessel vasculitis, Rowell's syndrome, GVHD, polymorphic light eruption (PMLE).
• **Rx** *mild* disease: symptomatic and supportive care, treat underlying infection if detected, ophthalmology consultation if ocular involvement.
• **Rx** *recurrent* disease: oral antiviral drug as prophylaxis for HSV infections, administered for at least 6 months (acyclovir 10 mg/kg/day, valacyclovir 500–1000 mg/day, or famciclovir 250 mg BID).
• **Rx** *severe recurrent* disease or *failure to respond* to prophylactic (anti-HSV) treatment: double the antiviral dose and if this fails, then consider referral to a dermatologist for possible immunosuppressive treatment.

Stevens–Johnson Syndrome (SJS) and Toxic Epidermal Necrolysis (TEN)

• SJS and TEN are considered the same disease, but along a clinical spectrum of severity and distinct from EM (see Table 16.1).
• Most likely etiology for both is an adverse reaction to a medication.
• Most common culprit drugs (Table 16.4): NSAIDs, antibiotics (in particular, sulfonamides and penicillins), anticonvulsants, and allopurinol.
• In some patients there may be an underlying genetic predisposition, e.g.
    – Allopurinol-induced SJS/TEN associated with *HLA-B*58:01* allele.
    – Carbamazepine-induced SJS associated with *HLA-B*15:02* in Asian populations.
    – Carbamazepine-induced SJS associated with *HLA-A*31:01* allele in Europeans.
• HLA screening in these at-risk populations prior to beginning these medications has been shown to reduce SJS–TEN risk and has opened the door for the future identification of additional genetic risks.
• Mucocutaneous tenderness, erythema, and varying degrees of epidermal detachment are characteristic features.
• SJS is characterized by <10% body surface area (BSA) epidermal detachment, SJS–TEN overlap by 10–30% BSA epidermal detachment, and TEN by >30% BSA epidermal detachment (Fig. 16.5).

CLINICAL FEATURES THAT DISTINGUISH ERYTHEMA MULTIFORME (EM) FROM STEVENS–JOHNSON SYNDROME (SJS), TOXIC EPIDERMAL NECROLYSIS (TEN), AND SJS–TEN OVERLAP

Clinical Entity	Type of Skin Lesions	Distribution	Mucosal Involvement	Systemic Symptoms	Progression to TEN	Major Precipitating Factors
EM minor (see Fig. 16.1)	• Typical targets (see Fig. 16.1D,E) • ± Papular atypical targets (see Fig. 16.1F)	Acrofacial	Absent or mild	Absent	No	• HSV • Other infectious agents
EM major (see Fig. 16.1)	• Typical targets (see Fig. 16.1D,E) • ± Papular atypical targets (see Fig. 16.1F) • Occasional bullous lesions	Acrofacial	Moderate to severe (see Fig. 16.1H)	Usually present • Fever • Asthenia • Arthralgias	No	• HSV • *Mycoplasma pneumoniae* (see Fig. 16.2) • Other infectious agents • Rarely drugs
SJS (see Fig. 16.6)	• Dusky macules with or without epidermal detachment • Macular atypical targets (see Fig. 16.7) • Bullous lesions • <10% BSA detachment	• Trunk • Face • Neck	Severe (see Fig. 16.6)	Usually present • Fever • Lymphadenopathy • Hepatitis • Cytopenias	Possible	• Drugs • Occasionally *Mycoplasma pneumoniae* • Rarely, immunizations

Table 16.1 Clinical features that distinguish erythema multiforme (EM) from Stevens–Johnson syndrome (SJS), toxic epidermal necrolysis (TEN), and SJS–TEN overlap. *Continued*

ERYTHEMA MULTIFORME, STEVENS–JOHNSON SYNDROME, AND TOXIC EPIDERMAL NECROLYSIS

Table 16.1 *Continued* **Clinical features that distinguish erythema multiforme (EM) from Stevens–Johnson syndrome (SJS), toxic epidermal necrolysis (TEN), and SJS–TEN overlap.**

Clinical Entity	Type of Skin Lesions	Distribution	Mucosal Involvement	Systemic Symptoms	Progression to TEN	Major Precipitating Factors
SJS/TEN overlap (see Fig. 16.8)	• Dusky macules with or without epidermal detachment • Macular atypical targets (see Fig. 16.7) • Bullous lesions • 10–30% BSA detachment	Confluence (++) • Trunk • Face • Neck	Severe	Always present • Fever • Lymphadenopathy • Hepatitis • Cytopenias	More likely	• Drugs
TEN (see Fig. 16.9)	• Dusky macules and macular atypical targets rarely • Poorly delineated erythematous plaques • Bullous lesions • >30% BSA detachment	Confluence (+++) • Trunk • Face • Neck • Elsewhere	Severe (see Fig. 16.9B) • May also involve respiratory and gastrointestinal epithelial linings	Always present • Fever • Lymphadenopathy • Hepatitis • Cytopenias	Already there	• Drugs

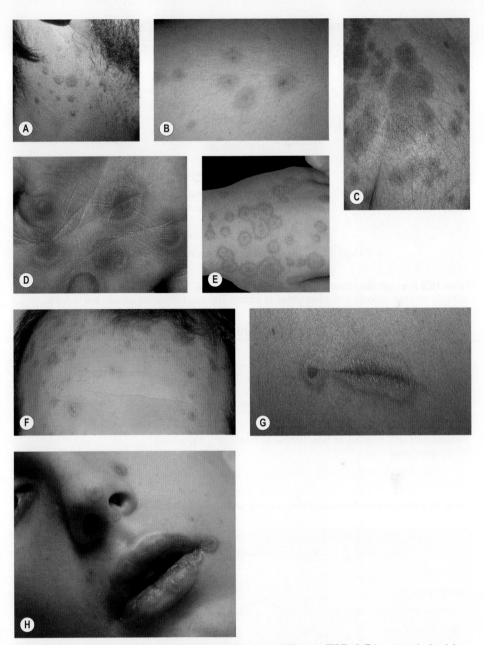

Fig. 16.1 Phenotypic variety in lesions of erythema multiforme (EM). A Edematous/urticarial.
B Urticarial with central crusting. **C** Erythematous plaques with dusky centers; coalescence of the
lesions leads to a well-defined polycyclic outline. **D, E** Typical (classic) target lesions on the palms
and dorsal hand, with three zones of color change ('bull's eye'); note the central vesicles in **(D)**.
F Atypical papular target lesions on the upper forehead mixed with more typical target lesions on the
lower forehead. **G** Isomorphic response. **H** Mucosal involvement in EM major. Typical target lesions
are seen as well as serous crusting of the vermilion lips and eyelid margin. At the margin of the
serous crusting of the lip, there are two zones of color with a polycyclic outline. *A, D, G, Courtesy,
William Weston, MD.*

PRECIPITATING FACTORS IN ERYTHEMA MULTIFORME

Infections (~90% of cases)	Viral	• **Herpes simplex virus (HSV-1, HSV-2)** • Parapoxvirus (orf) • Vaccinia (smallpox vaccine) • Varicella zoster virus (chickenpox) • Adenovirus • Cytomegalovirus • Hepatitis virus • Coxsackievirus • Parvovirus B19 • Human immunodeficiency virus
	Bacterial	• ***Mycoplasma pneumoniae*** (see Fig. 16.2) • *Chlamydophila* (formerly *Chlamydia*) *psittaci* (ornithosis) • *Salmonella* • *Mycobacterium tuberculosis*
	Fungal	• *Histoplasma capsulatum* • Dermatophytes

Table 16.2 Precipitating factors in erythema multiforme. This is a *non-exhaustive* list based primarily on case reports and small series of cases. The most common causes are in bold.

DIFFERENCES BETWEEN URTICARIA AND ERYTHEMA MULTIFORME

Urticaria	Erythema Multiforme
Central zone is normal skin	Central zone is damaged skin (dusky, bullous, or crusted)
Lesions are transient, lasting less than 24 hours*	Lesions 'fixed' for at least 7 days
New lesions appear daily	All lesions appear within first 72 hours
Associated with swelling of face, hands, or feet (angioedema)	No edema

*Confirmed with 'circle test' – circle a given urticarial lesion with pen/marker and re-check to see if still there in 24 hours.

Table 16.3 Differences between urticaria and erythema multiforme.

MEDICATIONS MOST FREQUENTLY ASSOCIATED WITH STEVENS–JOHNSON SYNDROME (SJS) AND TOXIC EPIDERMAL NECROLYSIS (TEN)

Allopurinol	Lamotrigine
Aminopenicillins	Phenylbutazone*,§
Amithiozone (thioacetazone)*,†	Piroxicam
Antiretroviral drugs	Sulfadiazine*,†
Barbiturates	Sulfadoxine†
Carbamazepine	Sulfasalazine
Chlormezanone*,‡	Trimethoprim–sulfamethoxazole
Phenytoin anticonvulsants	

*Not available in the United States.
†Antibacterial.
‡Sedative/hypnotic.
§Nonsteroidal anti-inflammatory drug.

Table 16.4 Medications most frequently associated with Stevens–Johnson syndrome (SJS) and toxic epidermal necrolysis (TEN). For a complete updated list of drugs associated with SJS and TEN, refer to Litt JZ, 2010. *Litt's Drug Eruptions and Reactions Manual*, 16th ed. London: Informa Healthcare.

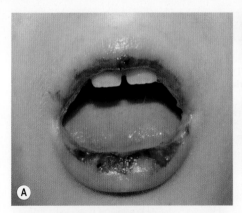

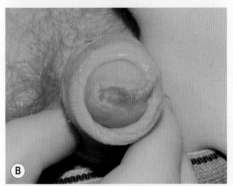

Fig. 16.2 *Mycoplasma pneumoniae*-associated mucositis (MPAM). MPAM is an extrapulmonary manifestation of *M. pneumoniae* infection that falls along the spectrum of EM major or SJS. In MPAM, there may be isolated mucosal lesions (e.g. ocular, oral, and urogenital) or a combination of mucosal and minimal skin lesions. Note the hemorrhagic and serous crusting of the vermilion lips **(A)** in this 12-year-old male with *M. pneumoniae* infection who presented with isolated oral and genital **(B)** lesions. *A, B, Courtesy, Julie V. Schaffer, MD.*

• Onset usually 7–21 days after starting culprit medication.

• Symptoms that typically precede skin findings by 1–3 days: prodromal flu-like syndrome, sore throat, fever, painful skin.

• Tender cutaneous lesions most prominent on trunk, followed by extension to face, neck, proximal extremities.

• Painful erythema and erosions of buccal, ocular, and genital mucosa in >90% of patients (Fig. 16.6).

• Morphologic progression of skin lesions: dusky red or purpuric *macules* (macular atypical targets) of various sizes and shapes that

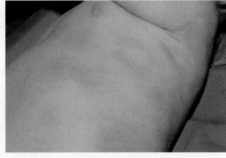

Fig. 16.3 Giant annular urticaria. This form of urticaria is sometimes referred to as urticaria multiforme because lesions can resolve with faint purpura. It does not represent erythema multiforme but is rather a form of urticaria. Refer to Table 16.3 for clinical ways to distinguish urticaria from erythema multiforme. *Courtesy, Julie V. Schaffer, MD.*

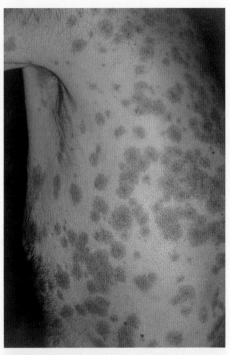

Fig. 16.4 Multiple lesions of erythema multiforme on the trunk. The dusky or crusted centers within the papules help to differentiate it from a morbilliform drug eruption.

begin to coalesce (Fig. 16.7); the gray-colored centers become wrinkled and begin to slough due to the development of flaccid bullae and poor attachment of the necrotic epidermis (likened to wet cigarette paper) (Fig. 16.8);

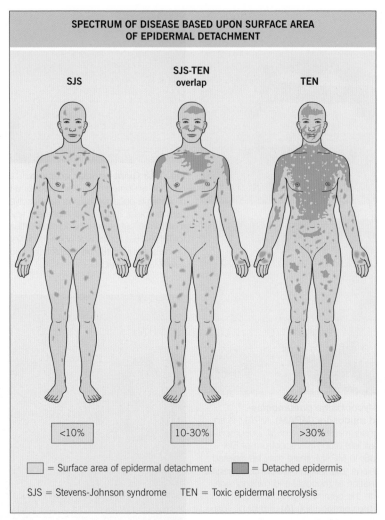

SPECTRUM OF DISEASE BASED UPON SURFACE AREA OF EPIDERMAL DETACHMENT

SJS

SJS-TEN overlap

TEN

<10%

10-30%

>30%

☐ = Surface area of epidermal detachment   ▨ = Detached epidermis

SJS = Stevens-Johnson syndrome   TEN = Toxic epidermal necrolysis

Fig. 16.5 Spectrum of disease based on surface area of epidermal detachment. *Adapted from Bastuji-Garin S, et al. Arch Dermatol. 129:92, 1993.*

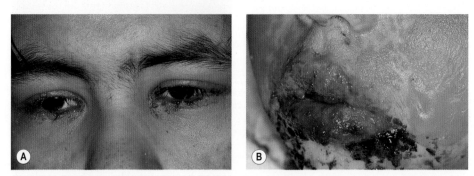

Fig. 16.6 Mucosal involvement in Stevens–Johnson syndrome (SJS). A Conjunctival erosions and exudate. **B** Hemorrhagic crusts and denudation of the lips in a child with SJS secondary to trimethoprim–sulfamethoxazole therapy; note the bullous cutaneous lesions. *A, B, Courtesy, William Weston, MD. Continued*

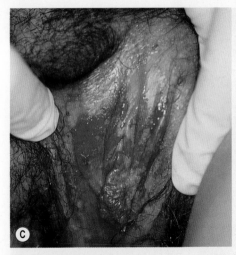

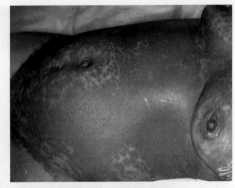

Fig. 16.7 Cutaneous features of toxic epidermal necrolysis (TEN). Characteristic dusky red color of the early macular eruption in TEN. Lesions with this color often progress to full-blown necrolytic lesions with dermal–epidermal detachment. Note the atypical macular target lesions in areas without confluence, e.g. around the umbilicus and left flank.

Fig. 16.6 *Continued* **C** Erosions of the genital mucosa.

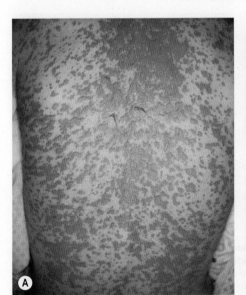

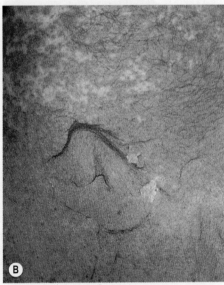

Fig. 16.8 Stevens–Johnson syndrome (SJS) versus SJS–TEN overlap. A In addition to mucosal involvement and numerous dusky lesions with flaccid bullae, there are areas of coalescence and multiple sites of epidermal detachment. Because the latter involved >10% body surface area, the patient was classified as having SJS–TEN overlap. **B** Close-up of epidermal detachment, whose appearance has been likened to wet cigarette paper.

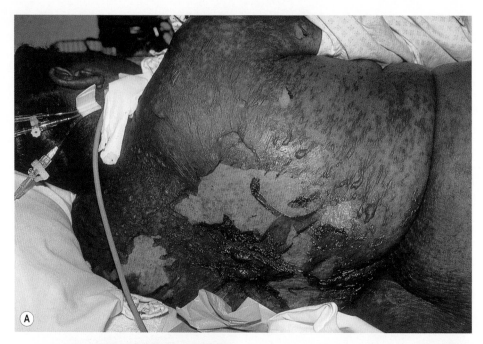

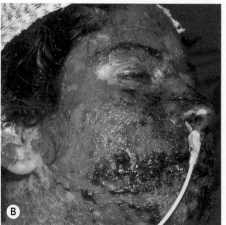

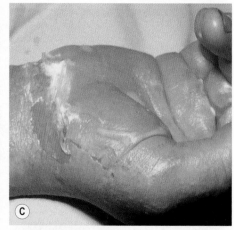

Fig. 16.9 Clinical features of toxic epidermal necrolysis (TEN). A Detachment of large sheets of necrolytic epidermis (>30% body surface area), leading to extensive areas of denuded skin. A few intact bullae are still present. **B** Hemorrhagic crusts with mucosal involvement. **C** Epidermal detachment of palmar skin. *B, C, Courtesy, Lars E. French, MD.*

the result is raw, denuded, bright red dermis (scalding) (Fig. 16.9).
• Additional systemic findings: fever, lymphadenopathy, hepatitis, cytopenias, erosions of epithelium in the gastrointestinal and respiratory tracts.
• Unpredictable course; worse prognosis in the elderly and with increasing BSA involvement (Table 16.5).

• Mortality rate in SJS is 1–5% and in TEN, 25–35%.
• Most important factor in improving outcome is withdrawal of culprit medication.
• Epidermal detachment is due to extensive keratinocyte death via apoptosis, which is mediated by interaction of the death receptor-ligand pair Fas–Fas ligand; perforin, granzyme B, and granulysin also play a role.

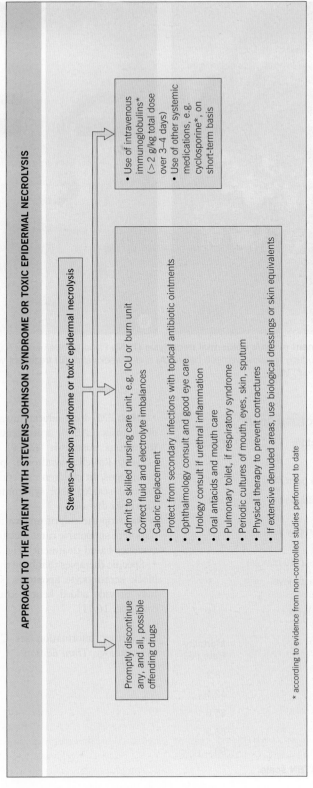

APPROACH TO THE PATIENT WITH STEVENS–JOHNSON SYNDROME OR TOXIC EPIDERMAL NECROLYSIS

Stevens–Johnson syndrome or toxic epidermal necrolysis

Promptly discontinue any, and all, possible offending drugs

- Admit to skilled nursing care unit, e.g. ICU or burn unit
- Correct fluid and electrolyte imbalances
- Caloric replacement
- Protect from secondary infections with topical antibiotic ointments
- Ophthalmology consult and good eye care
- Urology consult if urethral inflammation
- Oral antacids and mouth care
- Pulmonary toilet, if respiratory syndrome
- Periodic cultures of mouth, eyes, skin, sputum
- Physical therapy to prevent contractures
- If extensive denuded areas, use biological dressings or skin equivalents

- Use of intravenous immunoglobulins* (>2 g/kg total dose over 3—4 days)
- Use of other systemic medications, e.g. cyclosporine*, on short-term basis

* according to evidence from non-controlled studies performed to date

Fig. 16.10 Management of the patient with Stevens–Johnson syndrome or toxic epidermal necrolysis. ICU, intensive care unit.

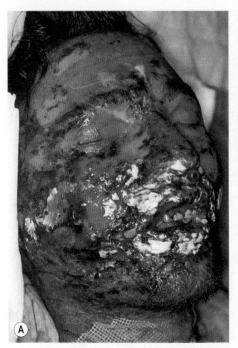
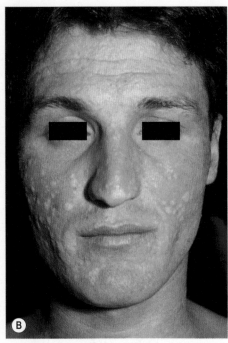

Fig. 16.11 Treatment of toxic epidermal necrolysis (TEN). Facial involvement of a patient with TEN (50% body surface area involvement) before **(A)** and 3 weeks after **(B)** treatment with IVIg. *Courtesy, Lars E. French, MD.*

SCORTEN SCALE	
Prognostic Factors	**Points**
Age >40 years	1
Heart rate >120 bpm	1
Cancer or hematologic malignancy	1
BSA involved on day 1 above 10%	1
Serum urea level (>10 mmol/l)	1
Serum bicarbonate level (<20 mmol/l)	1
Serum glucose level (>14 mmol/l)	1
SCORTEN	**Mortality Rate (%)**
0–1	3.2
2	12.1
3	35.8
4	58.3
≥5	90

Table 16.5 SCORTEN scale.

- **DDx:** EM, drug-induced linear IgA bullous dermatosis (LABD), acute generalized exanthematous pustulosis (AGEP), severe acute GVHD, Rowell's syndrome, paraneoplastic pemphigus; in children can consider staphylococcal scalded skin syndrome (SSSS) and Kawasaki disease.
- **Rx:** stop the culprit medication, rapid initiation of supportive care, specific therapy (no evidence-based treatment) (Fig. 16.10).
- Specific therapies that have the potential to block keratinocyte apoptosis, such as IVIg, may provide added benefit over supportive care (Fig. 16.11).

For further information see Ch. 20. From *Dermatology, Third Edition.*

Drug Reactions

17

- The skin is one of the most common targets for adverse drug reactions.
- Adverse cutaneous drug reactions (ACDR) affect 2–3% of all hospitalized patients.
- Increased risk of ACDR in women (>men), the elderly, and immunocompromised hosts, including those with AIDS (CD4 < 200/mm^3); in individual patients, the risk increases as the number of drugs taken increases.

- Pathogenesis of ACDR not totally understood but can involve immunologic, nonimmunologic, and idiosyncratic mechanisms (Table 17.1).
- Some of the most and least likely culprit drugs are listed in Table 17.2.
- Most common types of ACDR: morbilliform > urticaria > vasculitis (Table 17.3).

MECHANISMS OF CUTANEOUS DRUG-INDUCED REACTIONS	
Immunologic mechanism (unpredictable)	• IgE-dependent drug reactions • Cytotoxic drug-induced reactions • Immune complex-dependent drug reactions • Cell-mediated reactions
Non-immunologic mechanism (sometimes predictable)	• Overdose • Pharmacologic side effects • Cumulative toxicity • Delayed toxicity • Drug–drug interactions • Alterations in metabolism • Exacerbation of disease
Idiosyncratic with a possible immunologic mechanism (unpredictable)	• DRESS (DIHS) • TEN/SJS • Drug reactions in the setting of HIV infection • Drug-induced lupus erythematosus

DRESS, drug reaction with eosinophilia and systemic symptoms (also known as DIHS, drug-induced hypersensitivity syndrome); SJS, Stevens–Johnson syndrome; TEN, toxic epidermal necrolysis.

Table 17.1 Mechanisms of cutaneous drug-induced reactions.

SELECTED MOST AND LEAST LIKELY DRUGS TO CAUSE ADVERSE CUTANEOUS DRUG REACTIONS	
Most Likely Culprit Drugs	Least Likely Culprit Drugs*
Penicillins	Digoxin
Aminopenicillins	Acetaminophen
Sulfonamides	Meperidine
Cephalosporins	Codeine
Packed red blood cells	Morphine
	Multivitamins
NSAIDs	Aspirin
Tetracyclines	Diphenhydramine
Fluoroquinolones	Aminophylline
Anticonvulsants	Spironolactone
Allopurinol	Prednisone
EGFR inhibitors	Ferrous sulfate
	Nitroglycerin
	Insulin, regular
	Thiamine
	Potassium
	Magnesium
	Folic acid
	Lidocaine

With the exception of urticaria with narcotics and aspirin.
NSAIDs, nonsteroidal anti-inflammatory drugs; EGFR, epidermal growth factor receptor.
Adapted from: Arndt KA, Jick H. Rates of cutaneous reactions to drugs. J. Am. Med. Assoc. 1976;235:918–923.

Table 17.2 Selected most and least likely drugs to cause adverse cutaneous drug reactions.

CHARACTERISTICS OF SELECTED ADVERSE CUTANEOUS DRUG REACTIONS (ACDR)

Diagnosis/ % *Drug-Induced*	Selected Responsible Drugs	Time Interval to Onset	Mucocutaneous Features
Severe Cutaneous Adverse Reactions to Drugs (SCARs) (Fig. 17.1)			
SJS *80–90+%* TEN *80–90+%* (Fig. 17.3)	• Sulfonamides • Anticonvulsants* • NSAIDs • Allopurinol	• 7–21 days	• Mucosal erosions • Dusky macular atypical targets • Necrosis and epidermal detachment • SJS <10% BSA • SJS/TEN overlap 10–30% BSA • TEN >30% BSA
Drug reaction with eosinophilia and systemic symptoms (DRESS)/ drug-induced hypersensitivity syndrome (DIHS) *80–90+%* (Fig. 17.4)	• Anticonvulsants*, including lamotrigine (especially in combination with valproic acid) • Sulfonamides • Allopurinol • Antiretroviral medications (e.g. abacavir) • Minocycline • Dapsone	• 15–40 days	• Facial edema • Edematous morbilliform eruption with follicular accentuation • Face, upper trunk, and extremities favored initially • Occasionally other skin findings: vesicles, bullae, pustules, erythroderma, purpura
Cutaneous small vessel vasculitis (CSVV) *~10%*	• Penicillins • NSAIDs • Sulfonamides • Cephalosporins • Diuretics (e.g. furosemide, hydrochlorothiazide) • Allopurinol • Phenytoin	• 7–21 days (initial) • <3 days (rechallenge)	• Purpuric papules, most often on lower extremities • Hemorrhagic blisters • Urticaria-like lesions • Pustules
Cutaneous medium vessel vasculitis (CMVV)	• Hydralazine • Propothiouracil • Methimazole • Minocycline • Penicillamine • Allopurinol • Sulfasalazine	• Hours to years	• Purpuric plaques and nodules (favors face, ears, breasts, and extremities) • Ulcers • Livedo reticularis • Digital necrosis • Occasionally palpable purpura, mimicking a CSSV
'True' serum sickness (due to nonhuman proteins) *>90%* (Fig. 17.5)	• Anti-thymocyte globulin • Tositumomab • Infliximab	• 7–21 days	• Morbilliform eruption • Urticaria • Purpuric papules/plaques

Table 17.3a Characteristics of selected adverse cutaneous drug reactions (ACDR). *Continued*

CHARACTERISTICS OF SELECTED ADVERSE CUTANEOUS DRUG REACTIONS (ACDR)

Systemic Features	Other Helpful Hints	Differential Diagnosis	Treatment (in Addition to Withdrawal of Culprit Drug)
• Prodromal URI symptoms • Fever • Skin pain	• Leukopenia • Skin biopsy • Frozen section to differentiate from SSSS	• EM major • LABD • SSSS • AGEP • Severe acute GVHD • Rowell's syndrome • Kawasaki disease • Generalized FDE • Paraneoplastic pemphigus	Mild disease • Hospitalization • Wound care • Ophthalmology consult Severe disease • ICU/burn care • Consider IVIg
(Always present to some degree) • Fever • Lymphadenopathy • Arthralgias/arthritis • Hepatitis • Myocarditis • Pneumonitis • Nephritis • Thyroiditis • Gastrointestinal bleeding (allopurinol)	• Marked eosinophilia • Lymphocytosis with increased atypical lymphocytes • Increased liver enzymes • Consider skin biopsy • Consider laboratory testing for reactivation of HHV6 in immunocompromised host • Cutaneous and visceral involvement may persist for weeks to months after withdrawal of culprit drug • With rapid taper of CS may see rebound	• Viral exanthem • Other ACDR • Cutaneous lymphoma • Pseudolymphoma • Idiopathic hypereosinophilic syndrome	• Oral CS with a long course (often several months for more severe disease) and slow taper • Topical CS may relieve symptoms • Longitudinal evaluation for up to a year, given delayed manifestations, e.g. thyroiditis, myocarditis
(Not always present) • Fever • Myalgias • Arthralgias/arthritis • Headache • Peripheral edema • Peripheral neuropathy • Glomerulonephritis	• Urinalysis and BUN/Cr to exclude active urine sediment/kidney involvement • Check stools for evidence of GI bleeding • Skin biopsy of early lesion for H&E and DIF	• CSVV that is idiopathic or due to infection, autoimmune connective tissue or disease, malignancy	Mild disease • Observation • High-potency topical CS Severe or systemic disease • Oral CS • Steroid-sparing immunosuppressive agents
(Often present) • Fever • Arthralgias/arthritis • Necrotizing glomerulonephritis • Pulmonary hemorrhage • Peripheral neuropathy	• Skin biopsy may reveal leukocytoclastic vasculitis of superficial and deep vessels • ANCA (+) with propylthiouracil, hydralazine, and minocycline	• Polyarteritis nodosa (classic or cutaneous) • Wegener's granulomatosis (granulomatosis with polyangiitis) • Microscopic polyangiitis • Churg–Strauss syndrome	Mild, early disease • Drug withdrawal is often adequate Severe disease with systemic involvement or late withdrawal of culprit drug • May require immunosuppressive therapy
• Fever • Arthralgias/arthritis • Lymphadenopathy • Renal disease	• Hypocomplementemia • Circulating immune complexes • Vasculitis seen in skin biopsy	• Viral exanthem • Other ACDR	Mild disease • Supportive care Severe disease • Oral CS • Steroid-sparing immunosuppressive agents

SECTION 4: Urticarias, Erythemas, and Purpura

Diagnosis/ % *Drug-Induced*	Selected Responsible Drugs	Time Interval to Onset	Mucocutaneous Features
Serum sickness-like reaction *>90%* (See Fig. 3.3B)	• Cefaclor • Bupropion • Minocycline • Penicillins • Propranolol	• 7–21 days	• Morbilliform eruption • Urticaria, acral edema • Urticarial papules and plaques with a purpuric component
Anticoagulant-induced skin necrosis *100%* (Fig. 17.6)	• Warfarin	• 2–5 days	• Red to violaceous painful plaques evolving into hemorrhagic blisters and necrotic ulcers • Favors areas of greatest subcutaneous fat, e.g. breasts, thighs, buttocks
Heparin-induced thrombocytopenia with thrombosis (HIT) Also referred to as heparin-associated thrombocytopenia and thrombosis (HATT) *100%* (Fig. 17.7; see Fig. 18.2)	• Heparin – all forms (IV, SC, LMWH; and in heparin flushes used for dialysis and IV catheters)	• 5–10 days (initial) • Early-onset, occurs within 24 hours (rechallenge within ~100 days of last exposure) • Delayed-onset, occurs ~9 days after stopping heparin • Anaphylactoid reaction, occurs within 30 minutes of IV bolus	• Skin necrosis at sites of injection and at distant sites (e.g. distal extremities, nose) • Digital ischemia • Petechiae
Angioedema/ anaphylaxis *30%*	• Penicillins • Radiocontrast media • Monoclonal antibodies	• Minutes to hours	• Acute pale or pink subcutaneous swelling • Favors face (eyelids, ears, lips, nose) • Less often extremities and genitalia • Associated with urticaria 50% of the time
	• NSAIDs	• 1–7 days	
	• ACE inhibitors • Angiotensin II receptor blockers	• 1 day to several years	

Aromatic anticonvulsants, e.g. phenytoin, phenobarbital, and carbamazepine, are most often implicated. SJS, Stevens–Johnson syndrome; TEN, toxic epidermal necrolysis; BSA, body surface area; URI, upper respiratory tract infection; LABD, linear IgA bullous dermatosis; SSSS, staphylococcal scalded skin syndrome; AGEP, acute generalized exanthematous pustulosis; GVHD, graft-versus-host disease; FDE, fixed drug eruption; ICU, intensive care unit; IV, intravenous; SC, subcutaneous; BUN/Cr, blood urea nitrogen/creatinine; ANCA, antineutrophil cytoplasmic antibodies; DIC, disseminated intravascular coagulation; GI, gastrointestinal; H&E, hematoxylin and eosin; DIF, direct immunofluorescence; LMWH, low-molecular-weight heparin; FDA, Food and Drug Administration; NSAIDs, nonsteroidal anti-inflammatory drugs; ACE, angiotensin-converting enzyme; 5-FU, 5-fluorouracil.

Table 17.3a *Continued* **Characteristics of selected adverse cutaneous drug reactions (ACDR).**

Systemic Features	Other Helpful Hints	Differential Diagnosis	Treatment (in Addition to Withdrawal of Culprit Drug)
• Fever • Arthralgia/arthritis • Lymphadenopathy	• *No* hypocomplementemia, circulating immune complexes, vasculitis or renal disease	• Viral exanthem • DRESS/DIHS • Early CSVV • EM or early SJS • Kawasaki disease	• Long-acting oral antihistamines, especially if urticaria • Oral CS if significant symptoms
• Extreme pain at affected site	• Protein C deficiency	• DIC • Septicemia	• Vitamin K • IV heparin • IV protein C concentrate

• Venous and arterial systemic thrombosis
• In anaphylactoid reaction, see acute inflammatory (fever, chills) and cardiorespiratory (hypertension, shortness of breath) symptoms
	• Thrombocytopenia or decrease in platelets by >50%
	• Positive functional assay (serotonin release assay or heparin-induced platelet aggregation assay)
	• Positive ELISA immunoassay for antiplatelet factor 4/heparin antibodies
		• DIC
		• Septicemia
		• Anti-phospholipid antibody syndrome
			• Change to another, nonheparin anticoagulant, e.g.
			  • Argatroban (FDA approved for HIT)
			  • Danaparoid currently (available in Canada but not in USA)
			  • Fondaparinux (off-label)
			  • Bivalirudin (FDA approved for patients undergoing percutaneous coronary intervention with or at risk for HIT)
			• Once the thrombocytopenia is resolved, most patients are then transitioned to an oral vitamin K antagonist, e.g. warfarin

• Involvement of oropharynx, larynx, epiglottis, and surrounding tissues may impair breathing and swallowing • Intestinal wall edema can cause nausea, vomiting, diarrhea, pain • Hypotension and circulatory collapse with anaphylaxis		• Severe insect bite reaction • Food allergies • Hereditary angioedema • Acquired angioedema • Estrogen-dependent angioedema	Mild disease • Oral antihistamine Severe disease • Hospitalization • SC epinephrine • IV/oral antihistamines • IV/oral CS

CHARACTERISTICS OF SELECTED ADVERSE CUTANEOUS DRUG REACTIONS (ACDR)

Diagnosis/ % *Drug-Induced*	Selected Responsible Drugs	Time Interval to Onset	Mucocutaneous Features
Less Severe Cutaneous Adverse Reactions to Drugs			
Morbilliform/ exanthematous/ maculopapular drug eruption (Fig. 17.8; see Fig. 3.2)	• Aminopenicillins • Sulfonamides • Cephalosporins • Anticonvulsants • Allopurinol	• 4–14 days (occasionally sooner with rechallenge)	• Erythematous macules and subtle papules that often become confluent • Symmetric distribution favoring trunk, upper extremities • Dependent areas in bed-ridden patients • Purpuric lesions on lower legs and feet • Sometimes annular or targetoid plaques • Typically no mucosal involvement
Urticaria *<10%* (Fig. 17.9; see Fig. 3.3A)	• Penicillins • Cephalosporins • NSAIDs • Monoclonal antibodies • Radiocontrast media	• Minutes to hours	• Transient erythematous, edematous papules and plaques with central pallor • Varied sizes and configurations, including annular; sometimes transient central duskiness in children (urticaria 'multiforme')
Acute generalized exanthematous pustulosis (AGEP) *>90%* (Fig. 17.10)	• Beta-lactam antibiotics • Macrolides • Calcium channel blockers • Antimalarials	• <4 days	• Numerous, small, mostly nonfollicular, sterile pustules that arise within large areas of edematous erythema • Often begins on face and in intertriginous areas, and then becomes widespread • In 50% of patients, additional skin lesions: petechiae, purpura, atypical target-like lesions, vesicles

Table 17.3b Characteristics of selected adverse cutaneous drug reactions (ACDR). *Continued*

CHARACTERISTICS OF SELECTED ADVERSE CUTANEOUS DRUG REACTIONS (ACDR)

Systemic Features	Other Helpful Hints	Differential Diagnosis	Treatment (in Addition to Withdrawal of Culprit Drug)
• Pruritus • Low-grade fever	• Mild eosinophilia • May get a bit worse before getting better upon withdrawal of culprit drug • Eruption resolves in 1–2 weeks after withdrawal of culprit drug	• Viral exanthem	• Supportive care with oral antihistamines and mild topical CS • Can treat through eruption if culprit drug is crucially important to patient and no adequate alternative
• Pruritus	• Individual lesions last <24 hours • Normal skin left behind when lesions resolve	• Other causes of urticaria (e.g. virus, food allergy, idiopathic) • Urticarial vasculitis • Serum sickness-like reaction • EM	• Oral antihistamines with a longer half-life, e.g. cetirizine
• Fever • Pruritus or burning	• Leukocytosis with neutrophilia • Transient renal dysfunction • Hypocalcemia • Skin biopsy helpful • Resolves with superficial desquamation	• Acute pustular psoriasis • DRESS/DIHS • Morbilliform drug eruption • TEN	• Supportive care • Mild topical CS • Antipyretics

Table 17.3b *Continued* **Characteristics of selected adverse cutaneous drug reactions (ACDR).**

Diagnosis/ % *Drug-Induced*	Selected Responsible Drugs	Time Interval to Onset	Mucocutaneous Features

Fixed drug eruption (FDE) *99%* (Fig. 17.11)	• Sulfonamides
	• NSAIDs
	• Tetracyclines
	• Pseudoephedrine (nonpigmenting FDE)
		• 7–14 days (first exposure)
		• Within 24 hours (rechallenge)
			• One or a few round, sharply demarcated erythematous and edematous plaques
			• Sometimes with a dusky violaceous hue, central blister, or detached epidermis
			• Favors lips, face, hands, feet, genitalia
			• Fades over several days; residual post-inflammatory brown pigmentation
			Variants
			  • Generalized FDE (numerous lesions)
			  • Non-pigmenting FDE
			  • Linear FDE

Toxic erythema of chemotherapy (TEC) (Figs. 17.12 and 17.13)	Cytarabine (AraC) Anthracyclines (liposomal doxorubicin > doxorubicin) 5-Fluorouracil Capecitabine Gemcitabine Taxanes Methotrexate Busulfan Multikinase inhibitors (e.g. sorafenib)	• 14–30 days • Delayed onset (2–10 months) with lower-dose, continuous IV infusions (5-FU) and some oral agents	• Erythematous patches and edematous plaques favoring hands, feet and intertriginous zones; less often affects elbows, knees, ears • A dusky hue, petechiae, and/or sterile bullae may develop within areas of intense erythema • Occasionally more generalized distribution (may be confused with TEN) • Resolves spontaneously with desquamation • Recurrence possible with same or higher doses of culprit chemotherapeutic agents

SJS, Stevens–Johnson syndrome; TEN, toxic epidermal necrolysis; EM, erythema multiforme; NSAIDs, nonsteroidal anti-inflammatory drugs; 5-FU, 5-fluorouracil.

• Severe cutaneous adverse drug reactions (SCARs) cause significant morbidity and potential mortality, but fortunately only constitute ~2% of all ACDR.

• SCARs that require immediate attention: Stevens–Johnson syndrome (SJS), toxic epidermal necrolysis (TEN), drug reaction with eosinophilia and systemic symptoms (DRESS)/drug-induced hypersensitivity syndrome (DIHS), vasculitis, serum sickness, serum sickness-like reaction, warfarin-induced skin necrosis, angioedema/anaphylaxis, and heparin-induced thrombocytopenia and thrombosis syndrome (HIT) (see Table 17.3 and Fig. 17.1).

• Features that should alert one to the presence of a SCAR are outlined in Table 17.4.

• A practical approach in determining the cause of an ACDR is outlined in Table 17.5.

Table 17.3b *Continued* **Characteristics of selected adverse cutaneous drug reactions (ACDR).**

Systemic Features	Other Helpful Hints	Differential Diagnosis	Treatment (in Addition to Withdrawal of Culprit Drug)
	• Upon rechallenge lesions recur at exact same sites ± new lesions • Skin biopsy helpful	• Arthropod or spider bite (single lesion) • EM (generalized FDE) • SJS (generalized FDE plus mucosal involvement) • TEN (generalized FDE with blisters/ epidermal detachment) • Cellulitis (nonpigmenting FDE) • Lichen planus (linear FDE)	• Supportive care
• Pain, burning, paresthesias, pruritus, tenderness	• Other chemotherapy-related, self-limited, 'toxic' reactions may coexist, including gastrointestinal 'mucositis' manifesting as diarrhea, ileus, abdominal pain, hematemesis, melena, protein-losing enteropathy; pleuropericarditis	• 'Allergic' drug reactions • Contact dermatitis • GVHD • Cutaneous infection • Vasculitis • Intertrigo	• Supportive care • Cool compresses, bland emollients, topical CS • Oral analgesics • Possibly vitamin B_6 (50–150 mg/day) • Prevention of recurrence with dose reduction, lengthening of interval between chemotherapy cycles, or stopping culprit drug

• Organizing pertinent information into a drug chart (see Fig. 17.2 and Appendix) can be helpful in synthesizing the available information.

• The most important step in the treatment of SCARs is early identification and withdrawal of the culprit drug.

• In non-life-threatening morbilliform drug eruptions, the culprit drug is ideally stopped, but if vitally important to the patient's health and no alternative drug is available, one can consider 'treating through' the eruption with supportive care (topical CS and oral antihistamines).

• An approach to the management of a suspected ACDR is presented in Fig. 17.1.

• Additional reviews of specific types of drug reactions can be found in other chapters (Table 17.6).

• Selected drug-induced eruptions due to chemotherapeutic agents are listed in Table 17.7.

• Localized injection site reactions to selected medications are outlined in Table 17.8.

FEATURES THAT SUGGEST A SEVERE CUTANEOUS ADVERSE REACTION (SCAR) TO A DRUG

Cutaneous Features	Systemic Features	Laboratory Findings
• Skin pain • Confluent erythema • Facial edema • Blisters or epidermal detachment • Mucosal erosions • Necrosis • Palpable purpura • Urticaria • Swelling of lips/tongue	• High fever • Lymphadenopathy • Arthralgia/arthritis • Shortness of breath, wheezing, stridor, hypotension • Other visceral involvement	• Marked eosinophilia • Lymphocytosis with atypical lymphocytes • Leukopenia • Abnormal liver or renal function tests • Thrombocytopenia

Table 17.4 Features that suggest a severe cutaneous adverse reaction (SCAR) to a drug. *Adapted from: Roujeau JC, Stern RS. Severe adverse cutaneous reactions to drugs. N. Engl. J. Med. 1994;331(19):1272–1285.*

LOGICAL APPROACH TO DETERMINE THE CAUSE OF A DRUG ERUPTION

Drug Responsibility Assessment

Clinical characteristics	• Type of primary lesion (e.g. urticaria, erythematous papule, pustule, purpuric papule, vesicle or bulla) • Distribution and number of lesions • Mucous membrane involvement, facial edema • Associated signs and symptoms: fever, pruritus, lymph node enlargement, visceral involvement
Chronological factors	• Document all drugs to which the patient has been exposed (including OTC and complementary) and the dates of administration • Date of eruption • Time interval between drug introduction (or reintroduction) and skin eruption • Response to removal of the suspected agent • Consider excipients (e.g. soybean oil) • Response to rechallenge*
Literature search	• Bibliographic research (e.g. Medline) • Drug Alert Registry or MedWatch • Data collected by pharmaceutical companies • In the case of more recently released medications, extrapolation based on the class of drug and in particular the first drug released in the class

*Often inadvertent.
OTC, over-the-counter.

Table 17.5 Logical approach to determine the cause of a drug eruption. *Courtesy, Jean Revuz MD and Laurence Valeyrie-Allanore MD.*

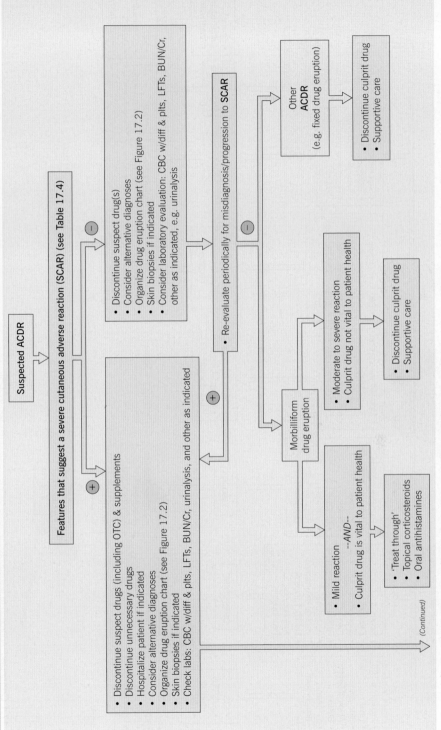

APPROACH TO A SUSPECTED ADVERSE CUTANEOUS DRUG REACTION (ACDR)

Suspected ACDR

Features that suggest a severe cutaneous adverse reaction (SCAR) (see Table 17.4)

(+)

- Discontinue suspect drugs (including OTC) & supplements
- Discontinue unnecessary drugs
- Hospitalize patient if indicated
- Consider alternative diagnoses
- Organize drug eruption chart (see Figure 17.2)
- Skin biopsies if indicated
- Check labs: CBC w/diff & plts, LFTs, BUN/Cr, urinalysis, and other as indicated

(−)

- Discontinue suspect drug(s)
- Consider alternative diagnoses
- Organize drug eruption chart (see Figure 17.2)
- Skin biopsies if indicated
- Consider laboratory evaluation: CBC w/diff & plts, LFTs, BUN/Cr, other as indicated, e.g. urinalysis

- Re-evaluate periodically for misdiagnosis/progression to **SCAR**

(+)

(−)

Other **ACDR**
(e.g. fixed drug eruption)

- Discontinue culprit drug
- Supportive care

Morbilliform drug eruption

- Moderate to severe reaction
- Culprit drug not vital to patient health

- Discontinue culprit drug
- Supportive care

- Mild reaction
  --AND--
- Culprit drug is vital to patient health

- 'Treat through'
- Topical corticosteroids
- Oral antihistamines

(Continued)

Fig. 17.1 Approach to a suspected adverse cutaneous drug reaction (ACDR). SCAR, severe cutaneous adverse reaction to a drug; OTC, over-the-counter; CBC, complete blood count; diff, differential; plts, platelets; LFTs, liver function tests; BUN/Cr, blood urea nitrogen/creatinine; URI, upper respiratory illness (including sore throat); SJS, Stevens–Johnson syndrome; TEN, toxic epidermal necrolysis; ICU, intensive care unit; SC, subcutaneous; IV, intravenous; DRESS, drug reaction with eosinophilia and systemic symptoms; DIHS, drug-induced hypersensitivity syndrome; SLE, systemic lupus erythematosus; RA, rheumatoid arthritis; HIT, heparin-induced thrombocytopenia and thrombosis syndrome. *Continued*

APPROACH TO A SUSPECTED ADVERSE CUTANEOUS DRUG REACTION (ACDR)

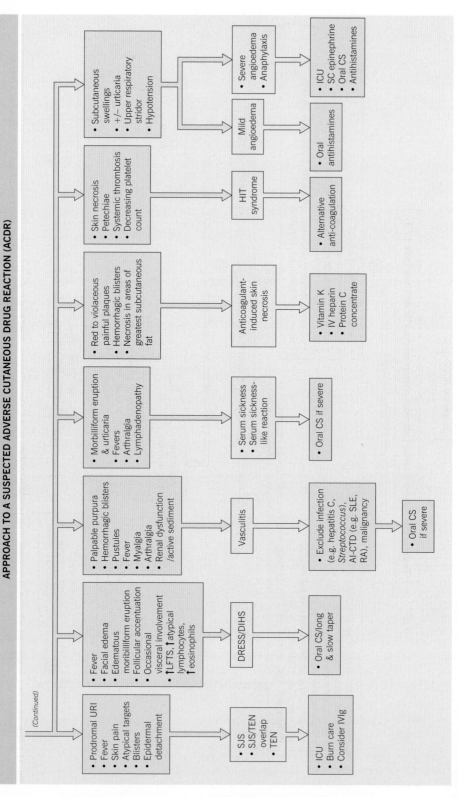

Fig. 17.1 *Continued* Approach to a suspected adverse cutaneous drug reaction (ACDR).

DRUG ERUPTION CHART - SAMPLE

Annotations: Rash onset → 6/21 · Derm consult → 6/22 · Rash worse → 6/24 · Rash better → 6/27

Drugs	Pre-hospital Duration (years)	6/15	6/16	6/17	6/18	6/19	6/20	6/21	6/22	6/23	6/24	6/25	6/26	6/27	6/28	6/29
Aspirin	X/10	X	X	X	X	X	X	X	X	X	X	X	X	X	X	X
Heparin SC			X	X	X	X	X	X	X	X	X	X	X	X	X	X
Famotidine		X	X	X	X	X	X	X								
Insulin	X/5	X	X	X	X	X	X	X	X	X	X	X	X	X	X	X
Digoxin	X/8	X	X	X	X	X	X	X	X	X	X	X	X	X	X	X
Diltiazem	X/6	X	X	X	X	X	X	X	X	X	X	X	X	X	X	X
Multi-vitamin	X/5	X	X	X	X	X	X	X								
Thiamine		X	X	X												
Folate		X	X	X	X	X	X	X	X							
Lorazepam		X	X	X	X	X	X	X	X	X	X	X				
Zolpidem		X	X		X	X		X								
Acetaminophen		X	X													
Ibuprofen				X	X											
Tramadol HC							X	X								
Maalox®			X	X	X							-				
Lactulose						X	X	X								
Diphenhydramine								X	X	X	X	X	X			
Ampicillin/sulbactam		X	X													
Vancomycin				X	X	X	X	X	X							
Ceftazidime				X	X	X	X	X	X							
Levofloxacin											X	X				
Linezolid												X	X	X	X	X
Laboratory																
WBC	20.2	16.5	7.0	7.6	8.1	10.2	11.3	11.5	11.2	11.5	10.5	9.2	7.0	7.0	6.5	
% Eosinophils	0%	0%	<1%	<1%	3%	5%	7%	9%	9%	8%	7%	5%	3%	1%	1%	
% Atypical lymphocytes	0%	→														
Platelets	nl	→														
AST	nl	→														
ALT	nl	→														
BUN/Cr	nl	→														
Temperature (°C)	40			38			38.3		38.5			37.5				
Physical exam*	nl	→														
Type of rash							Morbilliform → Confluence									

* Checking for the presence of lymphadenopathy, arthritis, wheezing, hypotension

Fig. 17.2 Drug eruption chart. This is a helpful working template for organizing all of the available patient information into one document for a patient with a suspected adverse cutaneous drug reaction (ACDR). **Step 1:** Compile all of the recently consumed or administered drugs (including prescription, over-the-counter, and supplements) into the chart. **Step 2:** Review and list the pertinent laboratory information and physical findings at the bottom of the chart. **Step 3:** Referring to Fig. 17.1, exclude a SCAR and categorize the type of ACDR. **Step 4:** Based on time intervals (see Table 17.3) and the most and least likely drugs to cause ACDR (see Table 17.2), begin to formulate the most likely culprit drugs and recommend their discontinuation. In addition, discontinue unnecessary drugs. **Step 5:** Longitudinal evaluation of the patient is necessary to (1) exclude progression to a SCAR, (2) determine the response upon discontinuation of the culprit drug (noting that it might 'get worse before it gets better'), and (3) provide supportive care to the patient. In this sample patient, the most likely culprit drugs are ceftazidime > ampicillin/sulbactam > vancomycin; however, the multi-vitamin, folate, famotidine, zolpidem, acetaminophen, ibuprofen, tramadol, Maalox®, and lorazepam (must taper off and not abruptly stop) were also discontinued. Note that the discontinuation of levofloxacin by the primary physicians was not necessary. Refer to www.expertconsult.com for a blank template of the drug eruption chart. SC, subcutaneous; WBC, white blood cell count; AST, aspartate aminotransferase; ALT, alanine aminotransferase.

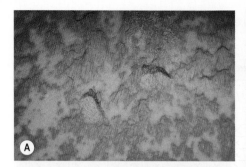

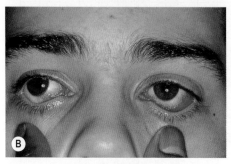

Fig. 17.3 Stevens–Johnson syndrome. Flaccid bullae leading to epidermal detachment (<10% body surface area) **(A)** and involvement of the conjunctivae **(B)** allow distinction from exanthematous drug eruptions.

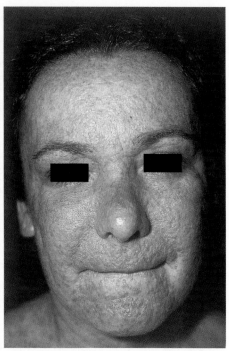

Fig. 17.4 Drug reaction with eosinophilia and systemic symptoms (DRESS). Also known as drug-induced hypersensitivity syndrome (DIHS). Facial edema and multiple edematous papules are present. *Courtesy, Kenneth Greer, MD.*

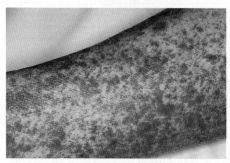

Fig. 17.5 Serum sickness due to antithymocyte globulin. The purpuric lesions are due to small vessel vasculitis in this patient with aplastic anemia. *Courtesy, Jean L. Bolognia, MD.*

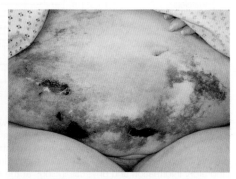

Fig. 17.6 Warfarin-induced skin necrosis. Retiform purpuric plaques with large hemorrhagic crusts and underlying ulcers on the abdominal pannus of a woman who recently initiated warfarin treatment. *Courtesy, Jean L. Bolognia, MD.*

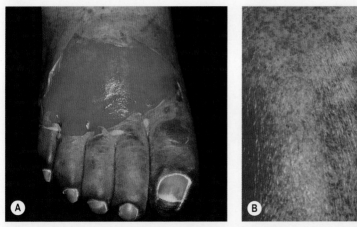

Fig. 17.7 Heparin-induced thrombocytopenia with thrombosis syndrome (HIT). A Ischemia and necrosis of the foot. **B** Petechiae due to thrombocytopenia and an irregular area of cutaneous necrosis. *A, Courtesy, Kalman Watsky, MD. B, Courtesy Jean L. Bolognia, MD.*

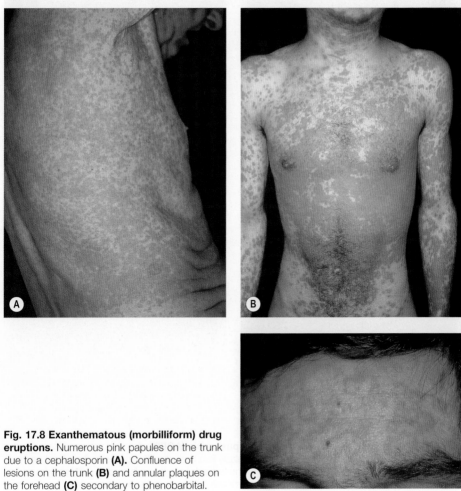

Fig. 17.8 Exanthematous (morbilliform) drug eruptions. Numerous pink papules on the trunk due to a cephalosporin **(A).** Confluence of lesions on the trunk **(B)** and annular plaques on the forehead **(C)** secondary to phenobarbital.

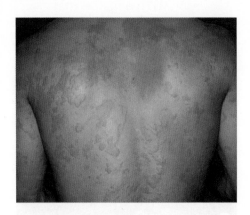

Fig. 17.9 Urticaria secondary to penicillin.
Several of the lesions have a figurate
appearance.

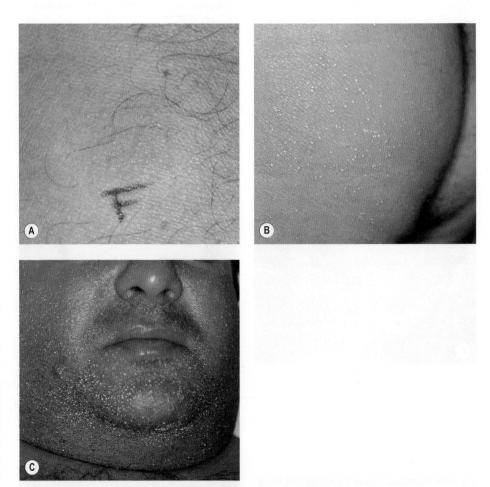

Fig. 17.10 Acute generalized exanthematous pustulosis (AGEP). A A positive patch test result 4 days following the application of 0.75% metronidazole in a patient with a previous pustular drug eruption to that medication. Diffuse erythema of the buttock (due to cephalosporin, **(B)** and face (due to metronidazole, **(C)** studded with sterile pustules. *A and C, Courtesy, Kalman Watsky, MD.*

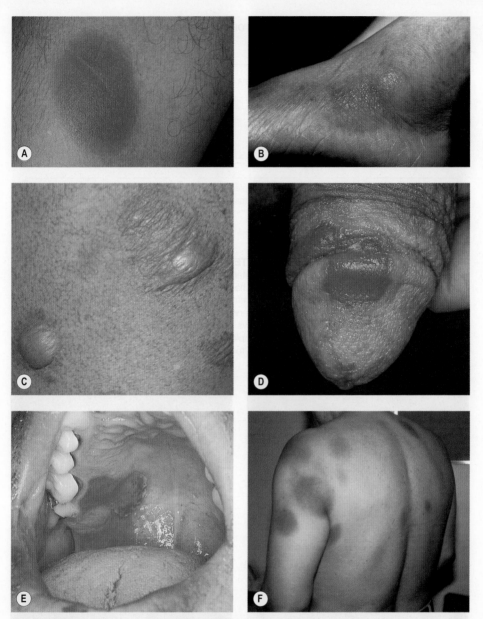

Fig. 17.11 Fixed drug eruptions (FDE). Well-demarcated erythematous **(A)** to violet-brown plaques that can develop a detached epidermis **(B)**, bulla **(C)**, or erosion **(D, E)** centrally. As lesions heal, circular or oval areas of hyperpigmentation are commonly seen **(F)**. Responsible drugs were phenolphthalein **(A)**, naproxen **(B)**, ciprofloxacin **(D)**, allopurinol **(E)**, and trimethoprim–sulfamethoxazole **(F)**. *C, Courtesy, Jean Revuz, MD; D, E, Courtesy, Kalman Watsky, MD; F, Courtesy, Mary Stone, MD.*

TOXIC ERYTHEMA OF CHEMOTHERAPY

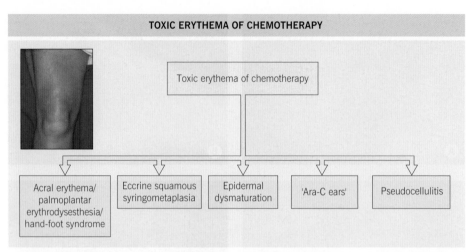

Fig. 17.12 Toxic erythema of chemotherapy (TEC). Use of a number of terms (especially those based on histologic findings), including palmoplantar erythrodysesthesia, eccrine squamous syringometaplasia, and epidermal dysmaturation, has created some confusion for clinicians. There is considerable overlap in the appearance of the symmetric erythematous patches, which can develop edema, erosions, desquamation, or purpura (depending on the patient's platelet count), whether they favor acral sites, intertriginous zones, or the elbows and knees. 'Toxic erythema of chemotherapy' represents an encompassing term that allows simplification. In addition, there is no need to implicate additional diagnoses when lesions are not limited to the hands and feet. *Courtesy, Jean L. Bolognia, MD.*

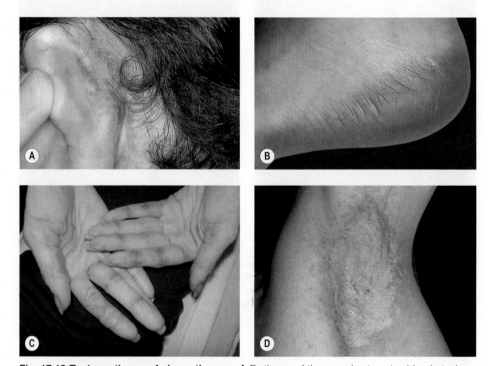

Fig. 17.13 Toxic erythema of chemotherapy. A Erythema of the ears due to cytarabine (cytosine arabinoside), sometimes referred to as 'Ara-C ears'; the petechiae are due to thrombocytopenia. **B** Toxic erythema of chemotherapy due to cytarabine, with obvious erythema of the plantar surface. **C** Acral erythema due to sorafenib. Note the erythema and bullae localizing to the palmar skin folds. **D** Axillary erythema and desquamation in a patient receiving busulfan plus fludarabine. Note that this eruption occurred 1 month after receiving these drugs. *A, B, D, Courtesy, Jean Bolognia, MD, C, Courtesy, Peter W. Heald, MD.*

ADDITIONAL SPECIFIC TYPES OF DRUG-INDUCED ERUPTIONS	
Drug Reaction	**Chapter Text**
Sweet's syndrome	Chapter 21
Psoriasiform (Fig. 17.14)	Chapter 6
Erythroderma	Chapter 8, Table 8.1
Lichenoid	Chapter 9
Urticaria	Chapter 14
Stevens–Johnson syndrome and toxic epidermal necrolysis	Chapter 16
Warfarin and heparin necrosis	Chapter 18
Vasculitis	Chapter 19
Pemphigus and bullous pemphigoid	Chapters 23 and 24
Linear IgA bullous dermatosis (LABD)	Chapter 25, Table 25.1
Acneiform/folliculitis	Chapters 29 and 31
Hyper- and hypohidrosis	Chapter 32
Lupus erythematosus (drug-induced SLE and drug-induced SCLE)	Chapter 33, Table 33.1
Pseudoporphyria	Chapter 41, Table 41.1
Hypopigmentation (skin and hair)	Chapter 54
Hyperpigmentation and dyschromatosis	Chapter 55
Hypertrichosis and hirsutism	Chapter 57
Phototoxic and photoallergic	Chapter 73, Table 73.4

SLE, systemic lupus erythematosus; SCLE, subacute cutaneous lupus erythematosus.

Table 17.6 Additional specific types of drug-induced eruptions.

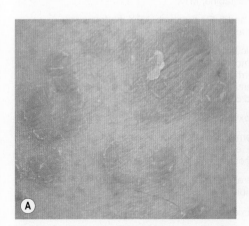
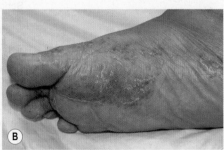

Fig. 17.14 Psoriasiform eruptions due to TNF-α inhibitors. A Widespread papulosquamous lesions in a patient being treated with infliximab for gastrointestinal GVHD. Histopathologically, there was no evidence of cutaneous GVHD. **B** Sterile pustulosis of the plantar surface developed in this patient with rheumatoid arthritis who had received infliximab for the previous 5 years. Neither patient had had a reduction in immunosuppression prior to the onset of the psoriasiform eruption. *A, Courtesy, Dennis Cooper, MD. B, Courtesy, Chris Bunick, MD.*

DRUG-INDUCED ERUPTIONS DUE TO CHEMOTHERAPEUTIC AGENTS

Mucocutaneous Reactions	Responsible Drugs
Alopecia (these alopecias are usually reversible, except for busulfan-induced alopecia, which is often irreversible)	Alkylating agents: cyclophosphamide, ifosfamide, mechlorethamine Anthracyclines: daunorubicin, doxorubicin, idarubicin Taxanes: paclitaxel, docetaxel Topoisomerase 1 inhibitors: topotecan, irinotecan Etoposide, vincristine, vinblastine, actinomycin D, busulfan
Mucositis	Daunorubicin, doxorubicin, high-dose MTX, high-dose melphalan, topotecan, cyclophosphamide, taxanes, continuous infusions of 5-FU and prodrugs of 5-FU
Extravasation reactions (e.g. chemical cellulitis, ulceration)	Anthracyclines, carmustine, 5-FU, vinblastine, vincristine, mitomycin C
Chemotherapy recall (tender sterile inflammatory nodules at sites of previous chemotherapy extravasation or administration)	5-FU, mitomycin C, paclitaxel, doxorubicin, epirubicin
Hyperpigmentation (see Chapter 55)	Alkylating agents: busulfan, cyclophosphamide, cisplatin, mechlorethamine Antimetabolites: 5-FU, 5-FU prodrugs (e.g. capecitabine, tegafur), MTX, hydroxyurea Antibiotics: bleomycin, doxorubicin
Mucosal hyperpigmentation	Busulfan, 5-FU, hydroxyurea, cyclophosphamide
Nail hyperpigmentation	5-FU, cyclophosphamide, daunorubicin, doxorubicin, hydroxyurea, MTX, bleomycin
Onycholysis	Paclitaxel, docetaxel
Radiation recall	MTX, doxorubicin, daunorubicin, taxanes, dacarbazine, melphalan, capecitabine, gemcitabine, cytarabine, pemetrexed
Radiation enhancement	Doxorubicin, hydroxyurea, taxanes, 5-FU, etoposide, gemcitabine, MTX
Photosensitivity	5-FU and 5-FU prodrugs, MTX, hydroxyurea, dacarbazine, mitomycin C, docetaxel
Inflammation of 'keratoses'	Actinic keratosis: 5-FU and 5-FU prodrugs, pentostatin Seborrheic keratosis: cytarabine, taxanes Disseminated superficial actinic porokeratosis: 5-FU and 5-FU prodrugs, taxanes
Ulcerations	Hydroxyurea (lower extremities)
Acneiform eruptions (including folliculitis)	Epidermal growth factor receptor inhibitors (EGFRI): e.g. erlotinib, cetuximab, panitumumab, lapatinib Corticosteroids
Squamous cell carcinoma	Fludarabine, hydroxyurea, topical BCNU, BRAF inhibitors

MTX, methotrexate; 5-FU, 5-fluorouracil; BCNU, carmustine.

Table 17.7 Drug-induced eruptions due to chemotherapeutic agents.

REACTIONS LOCALIZED TO SITES OF INJECTIONS OF MEDICATIONS (IN ADDITION TO EXTRAVASATION OF THOSE ADMINISTERED INTRAVENOUSLY)	
Etanercept	Erythematous plaques, vasculitis, eosinophilic cellulitis
Adalimumab	Erythematous or urticarial plaques
GM-CSF, G-CSF	Pustular reaction, urticarial plaque
Interferon	Vasculopathy with necrosis, development of plaque of psoriasis
Interleukin-2	Lobular panniculitis, granulomas
Vitamin K	Erythematous plaque, often annular; morpheaform plaque (Texier's disease)

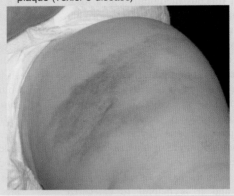

Heparin	Necrosis, ecchymosis
Low-molecular-weight, calcium-containing heparin	Calcinosis cutis
Glatiramer acetate	Fibrosis, panniculitis, lipoatrophy, vasospasm, Nicolau syndrome
Iron	Brown discoloration, hyperpigmentation
Hyaluronic acid, silicone	Swelling, granulomatous reaction
Corticosteroids	Dermal atrophy, lipoatrophy, telangiectasias, deposits, hypopigmentation
Vitamin B₁₂	Pruritus, morpheaform plaque
Enfuvirtide	Erythematous or morpheaform plaque
Aluminum-containing vaccines	Nodules, foreign body reaction

CSF, colony stimulating factor; G, granulocyte; GM, granulocyte–macrophage.

Table 17.8 Reactions localized to sites of injections of medications (in addition to extravasation of those administered intravenously).

For further information see Ch. 21. From *Dermatology, Third Edition.*

18 | Purpura and Disorders of Microvascular Occlusion

- Purpura represents visible hemorrhage into the skin or mucous membranes; as a result and in contrast to erythema due to vasodilation, it is nonblanching upon application of external pressure.
- Purpura can be *primary*, where hemorrhage is an integral part of lesion formation, or *secondary*, where there is hemorrhage into established lesions due to factors such as venous hypertension, gravity, or thrombocytopenia.
- As purpuric lesions fade, their color evolves from red-purple or blue to brown or yellow-green.
- Primary purpura has a broad differential diagnosis, and it is helpful to categorize purpuric lesions based on their size and morphology.

  – *Petechiae*: ≤3 mm and macular (Table 18.1; Fig. 18.1A).
  – *Ecchymoses*: usually >1 cm and macular with round/oval to slightly irregular borders, and typically have an element of trauma in their pathogenesis (see Table 18.1; Fig. 18.1B); a greater volume of hemorrhage leads to a *hematoma*, which is palpable.
  – *Retiform purpura*: reticulated, branching or stellate morphology, which reflects occlusion of the vessels that produce the livedo reticularis pattern (see Chapter 87; Tables 18.2 and 18.3; Figs. 18.1C and 18.2–18.9).

CAUSES OF PETECHIAE AND ECCHYMOSIS WITH MINOR TRAUMA
Petechiae (≤3 mm in diameter)
Significant thrombocytopenia (e.g. <20 000–40 000/mm³)
• Etiologies include ITP, TTP, DIC, drugs, and bone marrow infiltration
Platelet dysfunction
• Hereditary or acquired (e.g. due to aspirin or NSAIDs)
Etiologies unrelated to platelets
• Increased intravenous pressure, e.g. due to the Valsalva maneuver (coughing, childbirth) or use of a blood pressure cuff (Rumple–Leede sign)
• Trauma (often linear configuration)
• Scurvy (perifollicular distribution)
• Inflammatory conditions, especially in dependent sites (e.g. pigmented purpuric dermatoses, hypergammaglobulinemic purpura of Waldenström)
Ecchymosis with Minor Trauma (lesions usually >1 cm in diameter)
Defective coagulation
• Etiologies include anticoagulant use, hepatic insufficiency, and vitamin K deficiency
Poor dermal support of blood vessels
• Etiologies include actinic purpura (Fig. 18.1B), corticosteroid use, scurvy, primary systemic amyloidosis, and Ehlers–Danlos syndrome
Thrombocytopenia or platelet dysfunction (see above)
DIC, disseminated intravascular coagulation; ITP, idiopathic thrombocytopenia purpura; TTP, thrombotic thrombocytopenic purpura.

Table 18.1 Causes of petechiae and ecchymosis with minor trauma.

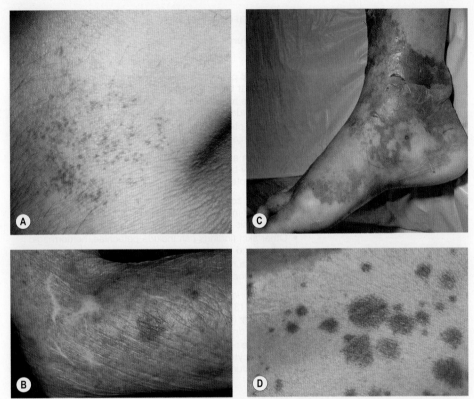

Fig. 18.1 Clinical examples of petechiae and purpura. A Round to oval petechiae, ≤3 mm in diameter. **B** Actinic (solar) purpura and pseudoscars, both in sites of actinic damage plus trauma. **C** Non-inflammatory (bland) retiform purpura as well as hemorrhagic bullae in a patient with disseminated intravascular coagulation (DIC). **D** Palpable purpura due to cutaneous small vessel vasculitis (inflammation plus hemorrhage). *A, Courtesy, Warren Piette, MD; B, Courtesy, Jean L. Bolognia, MD; C, Courtesy, Judit Stenn, MD.*

– *Classic 'palpable purpura'*: round red-purple papules that are occasionally targetoid, with a component of blanching erythema in early lesions; represents the most common presentation of cutaneous small vessel vasculitis (see Chapter 19; Fig. 18.1D).

• A biopsy specimen can be helpful in determining the etiology of a purpuric eruption, e.g. whether there is vascular occlusion with minimal inflammation or vasculitis (inflammation and fibrinoid necrosis of vessel walls); because secondary changes of vasculitis may be seen when an older lesion of microvascular occlusion is sampled, and likewise a late lesion of vasculitis may have minimal residual inflammation, it is preferable to choose a well-developed but relatively early lesion (e.g. 24–48 hours old).

Selected Microvascular Occlusion Syndromes (See Table 18.2)

Antiphospholipid Syndrome (APLS)

• Acquired systemic autoimmune disorder characterized by vascular thrombosis and/or pregnancy complications in the presence of elevated levels of antiphospholipid antibodies (Table 18.4).

CAUSES OF RETIFORM PURPURA

Disorder	Major Features
Microvascular platelet plugs	
Heparin-induced thrombocytopenia (HIT)	• ~1–5% of patients receiving heparin* (IV or SC) develop an Ab that binds to heparin–platelet factor 4 complexes and leads to ↓platelets ± thrombosis, typically with onset on day 5–10 of therapy* • Retiform purpura can be distant from or at sites of heparin injection (Fig. 18.2)
Thrombocytosis due to myeloproliferative disorders	• Occurs in essential thrombocythemia > polycythemia vera; may be associated with secondary erythromelalgia (see Chapter 87)
Paroxysmal nocturnal hemoglobinuria	• Acquired somatic *PIGA* mutation leads to complement-mediated injury of blood cells, resulting in hemolysis, thrombosis (especially venous), and cytopenias • Other skin findings can include petechiae, hemorrhagic bullae, and leg ulcers • **Rx:** eculizumab to inhibit terminal complement cascade (↑meningococcemia risk)
Thrombotic thrombocytopenic purpura (TTP) ± hemolytic uremic syndrome (HUS)	• May be *primary* (Ab against or genetic defect in ADAMTS13 protease → reduced cleavage of vWF) or *secondary* (often with HUS, e.g. due to hemorrhagic colitis or drugs) • Petechiae > retiform purpura; also fever, thrombocytopenia, microangiopathic hemolytic anemia, renal dysfunction, and CNS involvement
Cold-related agglutination	
Cryoglobulinemia type I > cryofibrinogenemia†	• Retiform purpura that favors acral sites (Fig. 18.3); see Table 18.3
Altered coagulation	
Antiphospholipid syndrome	• See text and Table 18.4 (Figs. 18.4 and 18.5)
Protein C or S deficiency/ dysfunction	• *Warfarin necrosis* (protein C – short half-life, so function decreases faster than for procoagulant factors): 2–5 days after starting warfarin without heparin; favors sites of abundant fat in women (Fig. 18.6) • *Sepsis-associated purpura fulminans* (protein C; see Fig. 18.1C) • *Post-infectious purpura fulminans* (Ab blocks protein S): ~2 weeks after streptococcal infection or varicella • *Neonatal purpura fulminans* (homozygous protein C or S defect)
'Vascular coagulopathy'	
Livedoid vasculopathy	• Often associated with hypercoagulability (Table 18.5); see text (Fig. 18.7)

*Less common with low-molecular-weight heparin (≤1%) than unfractionated heparin; a transient decrease in the platelet count can also occur within the first 2 days of heparin therapy due to its direct effects on platelet activation.
†May be an incidental finding in hospitalized patients; cold agglutinins rarely lead to acrocyanosis or purpura.

Table 18.2 Causes of retiform purpura. *Continued*

Table 18.2 *Continued* **Causes of retiform purpura.**

Disorder	Major Features
Degos' disease (malignant atrophic papulosis)	• Vaso-occlusive disorder of skin, GI tract, and CNS; favors young adults • Small erythematous papules on trunk and extremities evolve over 2–4 weeks to porcelain white scars with rim of telangiectasias; similar lesions can be seen in antiphospholipid syndrome
Sneddon syndrome (often associated with antiphospholipid syndrome)	• Triad of widespread livedo reticularis/racemosa ('broken' livedo), labile hypertension, and cerebrovascular disease; favors young women
Embolization and/or crystal deposition	

Cholesterol emboli ('warfarin blue toe syndrome')	• Atherosclerosis (especially in older men) leads to emboli, often triggered by
	  (1) Arterial/coronary catheterization or thrombolytic therapy (hours–days later)
	  (2) Prolonged anticoagulation (after 1–2 months of treatment)
	• Retiform purpura of distal leg(s) + more extensive livedo reticularis (Fig. 18.8)
	• Fever, myalgias, multisystem involvement (e.g. renal, GI, CNS); often peripheral eosinophilia

Other sources of emboli and/or crystal deposition	• Infective endocarditis (acute > subacute**), marantic endocarditis, atrial myxomas, hypereosinophilic syndrome (with intracardiac thrombus‡), systemic oxalosis (e.g. in primary hyperoxaluria), crystalglobulin vasculopathy (associated with monoclonal gammopathy)
Reticulocyte/red blood cell occlusion (e.g. in sickle cell disease or severe malaria)	
Organisms within vessels (usually in immunocompromised patients)	
Ecthyma gangrenosum	• See Chapter 61
Vessel-invasive fungi	• e.g. *Aspergillus*, *Mucor* (see Chapter 64)
Disseminated strongyloidiasis	• 'Thumbprint' purpura in periumbilical region
Lucio phenomenon	• Reactional state in lepromatous leprosy, primarily in Mexico and Central America (see Chapter 62)
Other causes	
Vasculitis (usually involving small and medium-sized vessels)	• e.g. ANCA-associated vasculitides, polyarteritis nodosa (see Chapter 19); early lesions often exhibit prominent erythema and induration
Calciphylaxis	• See Chapter 42
Necrotic spider bite reaction	• See Chapter 72
Intravascular lymphoma	• Most often B cell (Fig. 18.9); see Table 97.3

**Skin lesions associated with subacute endocarditis are more likely to be inflammatory due to immune complex deposition, e.g. Osler's nodes (tender red-purple papules), rather than Janeway lesions (purpuric macules; more common in acute endocarditis) on the hands and feet.*
‡Cutaneous microthrombi and superficial thrombophlebitis have also been described.
Ab, antibody; PIGA, phosphatidylinositol glycan anchor class A; vWF, von Willebrand factor.

CLASSIFICATION OF CRYOGLOBULINS

Type	Composition	Associations	Pathophysiology	Clinical Manifestations
I	Monoclonal IgM or IgG >> IgA	Plasma cell dyscrasias, lymphoproliferative disorders	Vascular occlusion	Retiform purpura (often acral; Fig. 18.3), gangrene, acrocyanosis, Raynaud's phenomenon
II**	Monoclonal IgM* (>IgG*) against polyclonal IgG	HCV, HIV, autoimmune connective tissue diseases, lymphoproliferative disorders	Vasculitis	Palpable purpura, arthralgias, peripheral neuropathy, glomerulonephritis
III**	Polyclonal IgM* against polyclonal IgG			

Typically have rheumatoid factor activity (i.e. are directed against the Fc portion of IgG).
**Referred to as 'mixed' cryoglobulins.*
HCV, hepatitis C virus; HIV, human immunodeficiency virus.

Table 18.3 Classification of cryoglobulins.

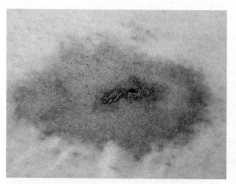

Fig. 18.2 Heparin necrosis at site of subcutaneous heparin injection. Note the branching or retiform pattern of intense hemorrhage and the necrosis in the center of the lesion. *From Robson K, Piette W.* Adv. Dermatol. *1999;15:153–182, used with permission.*

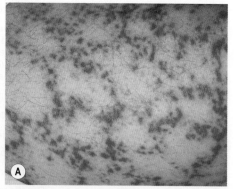

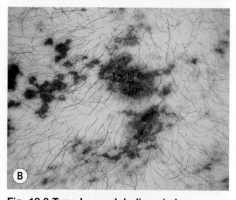

• Predilection for young to middle-aged women (5:1 female:male ratio in adults) and often associated with systemic lupus erythematosus.

• Cutaneous findings can include livedo reticularis, retiform purpura progressing to cutaneous necrosis, leg ulcers, livedoid vasculopathy, Degos-like lesions, nail bed infarcts, superficial thrombophlebitis and anetoderma (see Figs. 18.4 and 18.5).

Fig. 18.3 Type I cryoglobulinemia in a patient with multiple myeloma (IgG type). Note the retiform purpura **(A)** and the areas of necrosis within the purpuric areas **(B)**. Lesions favor the distal extremities, helices of the ears, and nose. *Courtesy, Jean L. Bolognia, MD.*

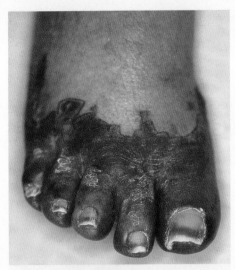

Fig. 18.4 Retiform purpura in antiphospholipid syndrome. Purpura and ischemia of the distal portion of the foot. The purpuric lesions have irregular borders (marked with ink). *Courtesy, Jean L. Bolognia, MD.*

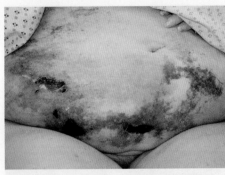

Fig. 18.6 Warfarin (Coumadin®) necrosis. Striking areas of retiform purpura with ischemic necrosis centrally on the pannus. *Courtesy, Jean L. Bolognia, MD.*

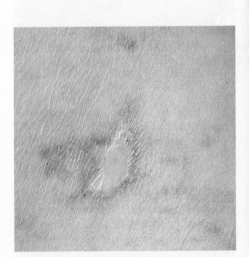

Fig. 18.5 Atrophie blanche-like scarring in antiphospholipid syndrome. This patient had lupus erythematosus. *Courtesy, Warren Piette, MD.*

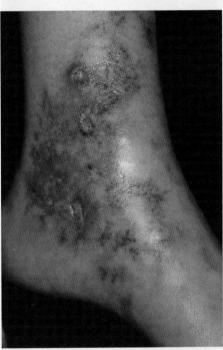

Fig. 18.7 Livedoid vasculopathy. Punched-out ulcers on the ankle as well as multiple stellate purpuric macules.

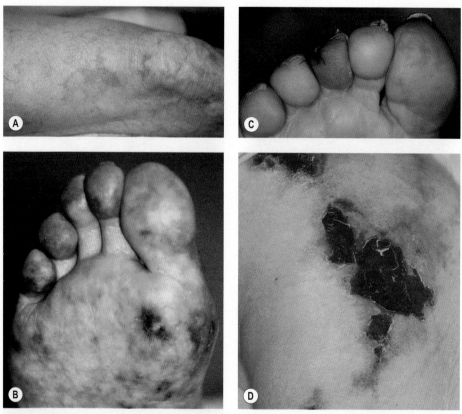

Fig. 18.8 Cholesterol emboli. A Livedo reticularis proximally on the thigh. **B** Both livedo reticularis and retiform purpura distally. **C** Purpura of the digits in 'warfarin blue toe syndrome'. **D** Several irregularly shaped ulcers with eschars surrounded by retiform purpura. *A, B, Courtesy, Norbert Sepp, MD; D, Courtesy, Kalman Watsky, MD.*

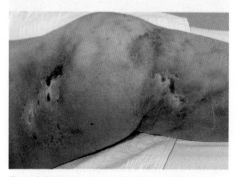

Fig. 18.9 Intravascular B-cell lymphoma. The clinical presentation in this patient was retiform purpura and necrosis with livedo. *Courtesy, Lucinda Buescher, MD.*

• Deep venous thrombosis and CNS disease are the most common extracutaneous manifestations; catastrophic APLS affecting multiple organ systems together with widespread retiform purpura occasionally occurs.

• **Rx:** anticoagulant and antiplatelet agents; also immunomodulatory agents (e.g. systemic CS, rituximab) for catastrophic APLS.

Livedoid Vasculopathy

• Chronic condition that occurs primarily in young to middle-aged women, often with an underlying hypercoagulable state (Table 18.5).

• Recurrent development of hemorrhagic crusts resembling ground pepper and extremely painful, punched-out ulcers on the legs (especially the ankles); frequently arises within a background of retiform purpura ± livedo reticularis (see Fig. 18.7).

• The ulcers heal slowly, forming stellate, ivory-white, atrophic scars bordered by papular telangiectasias and hemosiderin pigmentation; such lesions, referred to as

2006 REVISED CRITERIA FOR THE ANTIPHOSPHOLIPID SYNDROME

Clinical Criteria

1. Vascular thrombosis
   - One or more clinical episodes of arterial, venous, or small vessel thrombosis
2. Complications of pregnancy
   - One or more unexplained deaths of morphologically normal fetuses at or after the 10th week of pregnancy; *or*
   - One or more premature births of morphologically normal neonates at or before the 34th week of gestation; *or*
   - Three or more unexplained consecutive spontaneous abortions before the 10th week of gestation

Laboratory Criteria

1. Anticardiolipin antibodies,* IgG or IgM, present at moderate or high levels[†] on two or more occasions at least 12 weeks apart
2. Lupus anticoagulant antibodies on two or more occasions at least 12 weeks apart
3. Anti-β_2-glycoprotein I antibodies, IgG or IgM (in titer >99th percentile), on two or more occasions at least 12 weeks apart

β_2-glycoprotein I-dependent.
[†]Several thresholds exist for low versus moderate to high: (1) >40 international 'phospholipid' units; (2) 2–2.5× the median level of anticardiolipin antibodies (ACA); and (3) 99th percentile for ACA in the normal population.

Table 18.4 2006 revised criteria for the antiphospholipid syndrome. Definite diagnosis requires at least one clinical and one laboratory criterion.

atrophie blanche, also occur in other settings such as venous hypertension, antiphospholipid syndrome (see Fig. 18.5), and cutaneous vasculitis.
- **Rx:** anticoagulant, antiplatelet, and fibrinolytic agents (especially if hypercoagulability).

Other Purpuric Disorders

Pigmented Purpuric Dermatoses (Capillaritis)

- Group of disorders characterized by clustered petechial hemorrhage due to inflammation affecting capillaries.
- *Schamberg's disease:* most common form, occurring in both children and adults; recurrent crops of discrete yellow-brown patches containing pinpoint petechiae ('cayenne pepper') on the lower legs > thighs, buttocks, trunk, and arms (Fig. 18.10A); the yellow-brown color reflects deposits of hemosiderin, derived from extravasated RBCs, within the dermis.

- *Purpura annularis telangiectodes (of Majocchi):* favors adolescent girls and young women; expanding annular plaques with punctate telangiectasias and petechiae in their borders (Fig. 18.11).
- *Lichen aureus:* solitary golden to rust-colored or purple-brown patch or thin plaque, typically on the leg overlying a perforator vein.
- Other forms include *pigmented purpuric lichenoid dermatitis* presenting as red-brown papules and *eczematid-like purpura* with scaling and pruritus; these variants favor the lower legs of men.
- **DDx:** 'stasis purpura' presenting as petechiae superimposed on diffuse hemosiderin deposition on the legs (see Fig. 18.10B); purpuric forms of allergic contact dermatitis, drug eruptions or mycosis fungoides; suction-induced purpura (e.g. with cupping), hypergammaglobulinemic purpura of Waldenström, angioma serpiginosum; *for lichenoid variant:* primarily small vessel vasculitis.
- **Rx:** difficult; topical CS if pruritic, phototherapy.

EVALUATION FOR HYPERCOAGULABILITY

Disorder	% of Population	Potential Confounding Conditions
Hereditary		
Factor V Leiden (can screen with activated protein C resistance)	5	Warfarin, OCP, pregnancy, ↑ factor VIII levels, lupus anticoagulant
Prothrombin G20210A mutation	3	—
Hyperhomocysteinemia (↑ homocysteine level*)	>5	Deficient folate, B_{12}, or B_6; older age, smoking
Protein C deficiency (↓ activity)	0.3	Warfarin, OCP, pregnancy, liver disease
Protein S deficiency (↓ free antigen level)	≤0.3	Warfarin, OCP, pregnancy, liver disease
Antithrombin III deficiency	0.05	Heparin, liver disease
Excess factor VIII activity	10	Acute-phase response, OCP, pregnancy, old age
Dysfibrinogenemia (↓ fibrinogen activity relative to antigen level; ↑ reptilase time)	—	Liver or renal disease, amyloidosis, malignancy
Excess plasminogen activator inhibitor-1 (PAI-1) activity*	10+	Wide range of normal values
Acquired		
Lupus anticoagulant[†]	—	Warfarin, heparin
Anticardiolipin antibodies (IgG or IgM)[†]	—	Various infectious diseases
Anti-β_2-glycoprotein I antibodies (IgG or IgM)[†]	—	—
Cryoglobulinemia, type I	—	—
Cryofibrinogens	—	Acute-phase response

*May subsequently test for a homozygous MTHFR mutation (e.g. C677T or 1298C; hyperhomocysteinemia can also be due to other genes or acquired) or PAI-1 4G/5G polymorphism.
[†]Antiphospholipid antibodies; additional studies may include anti-phosphatidylserine and/or anti-prothrombin antibodies.
OCP, oral contraceptive pill use.

Table 18.5 Evaluation for hypercoagulability. Evaluation for entities in the rows shaded gray is often considered as second tier. The initial laboratory evaluation should also include a complete blood count with differential and platelet count, examination of a peripheral blood smear, erythrocyte sedimentation rate, activated partial thromboplastin time (PTT), and hepatic and renal function panels. Testing for antineutrophil cytoplasmic antibodies (ANCA) can be considered for patients with retiform purpura, as ANCA-positive vasculitides occasionally present with minimally inflammatory lesions.

Hypergammaglobulinemic Purpura of Waldenström

• Recurrent crops of petechiae, purpuric macules, and/or palpable purpura (Fig. 18.12) on the lower extremities, often in young women with an autoimmune connective tissue disease (especially Sjögren's syndrome).

• Associated with polyclonal hypergammaglobulinemia, an elevated ESR, rheumatoid factor (IgG or IgA), and anti-Ro/La (SS-A/B) antibodies.

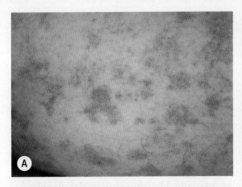

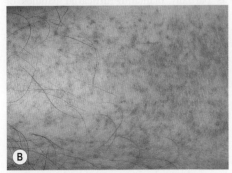

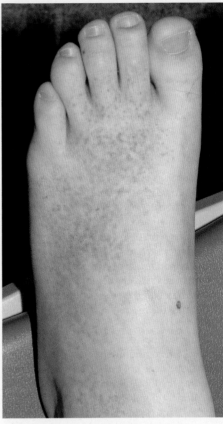

Fig. 18.10 Schamberg's disease versus petechiae and hemosiderin secondary to venous hypertension. A Discrete yellow-pink patches with superimposed petechiae in Schamberg's disease. **B** Petechiae within a background of more diffuse hemosiderin deposition in the setting of venous hypertension, referred to as 'stasis purpura.' *B, Courtesy, Jean L. Bolognia, MD.*

Fig. 18.12 Hypergammaglobulinemic purpura of Waldenström. This young woman with Sjögren's syndrome had recurrent crops of petechiae on her lower legs. Note the hemosiderin deposition at sites of older lesions. *Courtesy, Julie V. Schaffer, MD.*

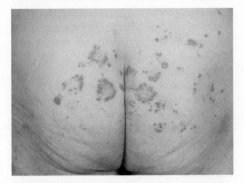

Fig. 18.11 Purpura annularis telangiectodes of Majocchi. Annular plaques with 'cayenne pepper' petechiae in the border.

For further information see Chs. 22 and 23. From *Dermatology, Third Edition.*

19 | Vasculitis

- Vasculitis is characterized by an inflammatory infiltrate that targets blood vessels and leads to destruction of their walls.
- Cutaneous vasculitis can occur in isolation or together with involvement of other organs; in the latter scenario, skin findings may represent important signs of systemic disease.
- Cutaneous vasculitides are classified based on the size of the vessels affected, which determines the morphology of the skin lesions (Table 19.1).
- Other features that assist in categorization include direct immunofluorescence findings (e.g. IgA deposits in Henoch–Schönlein purpura [HSP]), the presence or absence of antineutrophil cytoplasmic antibodies (ANCA), and systemic manifestations (e.g. hematuria, abdominal pain, paresthesias).
- Constitutional symptoms (e.g. fevers, malaise) and arthralgias or arthritis can develop in most forms of vasculitis.
- Favors adults but can occur at any age; HSP accounts for the majority of cases in children.
- The pathogenesis of cutaneous small vessel vasculitis (CSVV) and several other vasculitides (e.g. cryoglobulinemic vasculitis, polyarteritis nodosa) is related to immune complex deposition, which results in complement activation and recruitment of neutrophils; in contrast, neutrophils directly mediate vessel damage in ANCA-associated 'pauci-immune' vasculitis.

Cutaneous Small Vessel Vasculitis (CSVV)

- The clinical hallmark of CSVV is palpable purpura – nonblanching red-purple papules that favor dependent sites and areas of trauma (Koebner phenomenon) or pressure (e.g. from tight clothing); however, lesions often begin as partially blanching urticarial papules or purpuric macules, and occasionally other morphologies may be observed (e.g. vesicles or pustules; see Table 19.1, Figs. 19.1 and 19.2); frequently asymptomatic but can have associated pruritus, burning, or pain.

- Possible underlying conditions are presented in Figs. 19.3 and 19.4.
- Characterized by the histologic finding of *leukocytoclastic vasculitis (LCV)* – transmural infiltration of postcapillary venules by neutrophils that undergo fragmentation (leukocytoclasia), leading to fibrinoid necrosis of the vessel walls (see Fig. 1.11).
- **DDx:** specific CSVV subtypes or systemic vasculitides (see Table 19.1 and below), morbilliform drug eruptions or arthropod bites (with hemorrhage in dependent sites), petechial viral exanthems (see Fig. 68.1), pigmented purpura, erythema multiforme, pityriasis lichenoides, septic emboli.
- Usually resolves within several weeks to months, typically with postinflammatory hyperpigmentation; chronic or recurrent in ~10% of patients, especially if an underlying autoimmune connective tissue disease (AI-CTD) or cryoglobulinemia.
- **Rx:** eliminate possible triggers, evaluate for systemic involvement (see Fig. 19.14), and provide supportive care (e.g. leg elevation, NSAIDs); for more severe or persistent (e.g. >4 weeks) skin disease, oral dapsone ± colchicine; if rapidly progressive or ulcerating, a 4- to 6-week course of prednisone may be considered.

Henoch–Schönlein Purpura (HSP)

- Form of CSVV characterized by prominent vascular IgA deposition, which is evident via DIF of a skin biopsy specimen (see Fig. 23.2); favors children <10 years of age, often

CLASSIFICATION OF CUTANEOUS VASCULITIS

Size of Predominantly Affected Vessels	Types of Vessels Affected in the Skin	Forms of Cutaneous Vasculitis	Cutaneous Morphologies
Small	Arterioles, capillaries and venules in *superficial to mid dermis*	Idiopathic Secondary causes (e.g. drugs, infections, inflammatory disorders; Fig. 19.3) Henoch–Schönlein purpura Urticarial vasculitis Acute hemorrhagic edema of infancy Erythema elevatum diutinum	• Palpable purpura (Fig. 19.1) > macular purpura or petechiae • Urticarial, annular or targetoid papules/plaques (Fig. 19.2A,B) • Vesicles, bullae (Fig. 19.2C), pustules
Small ± medium-sized		Cryoglobulinemic vasculitis ANCA-associated vasculitis • Wegener's granulomatosis • Churg–Strauss syndrome • Microscopic polyangiitis Secondary causes (e.g. drugs, rheumatoid arthritis; Fig. 19.3)	
Medium-sized	Small arteries and veins in *deep dermis to subcutis*	Polyarteritis nodosa (PAN) • Classic (systemic) PAN • Cutaneous PAN	• Livedo racemosa ('broken' livedo reticularis) • Retiform purpura • Subcutaneous nodules • Ulcers, digital necrosis
Large	(*Extracutaneous* named arteries*)	Temporal arteritis Takayasu's arteritis	• Temporal arteritis*: erythema, alopecia, purpura, tender nodules → ulcers on frontotemporal scalp; ulcers on tongue • Takayasu's arteritis*: nodules, ulcers

*Cutaneous involvement is uncommon.
ANCA, antineutrophil cytoplasmic antibodies.

Table 19.1 Classification of cutaneous vasculitis.

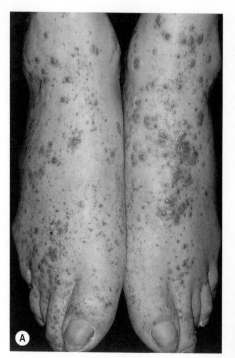

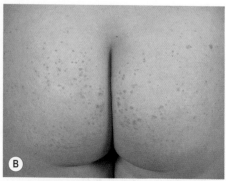

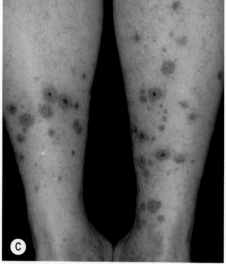

Fig. 19.1 Cutaneous small vessel vasculitis. A Classic presentation of purpuric papules on the distal lower extremities; a few lesions have become vesicular. **B** Early lesions may be pink papules. **C** Central necrosis with formation of hemorrhagic crusts. *A, Courtesy, Kalman Watsky, MD; C, Courtesy, Frank Samarin, MD.*

presenting 1–2 weeks after an upper respiratory tract infection (URI).

• Urticarial papules evolve into palpable purpura, occasionally progressing to bullous or necrotic lesions (Fig. 19.5); typically involves the buttocks and lower extremities, but may be more widespread.

• Other manifestations include acral or scrotal edema, arthralgias/arthritis (especially of the knees and ankles; ~75% of children), colicky abdominal pain (~65%; occasionally intussusception), bloody stools (~30%), and microscopic hematuria ± proteinuria (~30–40%; can be delayed up to 3 months).

• Resolves over several weeks to months, with recurrent purpuric eruptions in ~20%

and long-term renal impairment in ~2% of children with HSP.

• Adults with HSP are more likely to have necrotic skin lesions, renal involvement, and chronic kidney disease; in adults with unexplained persistent or widespread IgA vasculitis, especially if involving medium-sized vessels, an underlying IgA monoclonal gammopathy or malignancy should be considered.

• **Rx:** as for CSVV above, with monitoring for renal disease and systemic CS therapy as needed for arthritis, abdominal pain, and severe nephritis; however, CS administration does not appear to prevent renal disease or its sequelae.

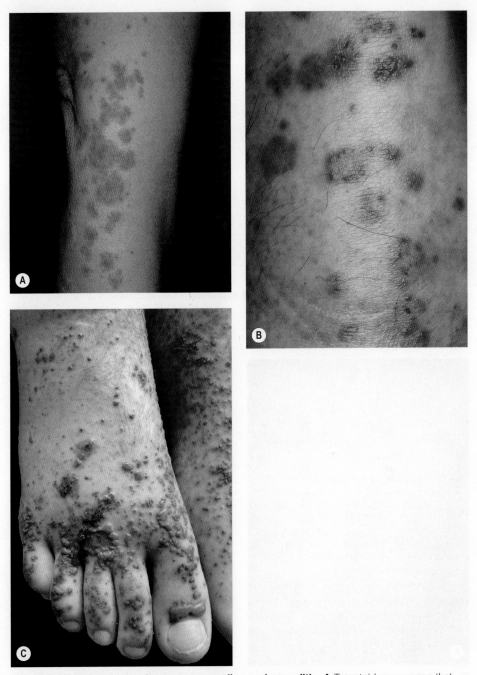

Fig. 19.2 Clinical variants of cutaneous small vessel vasculitis. A Targetoid appearance that can resemble erythema multiforme. **B** Hemorrhagic crusts in annular configuration. **C** Predominantly vesicular lesions on the foot. *C, Courtesy, Karynne O. Duncan, MD.*

ETIOLOGIES OF CUTANEOUS SMALL VESSEL VASCULITIS

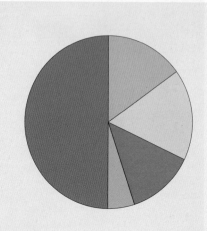

▽ Infection (15–20%)
e.g. streptococcal or upper respiratory tract infections, hepatitis C>B, leprosy, subacute infective endocarditis

▽ Autoimmune connective tissue disease (15–20%)
e.g. rheumatoid arthritis, SLE, Sjögren's syndrome

▼ Drug (10–15%)
e.g. penicillins, quinolones, NSAIDs, propylthiouracil*

▽ Neoplasm (5%)
e.g. plasma cell dyscrasias, myelo- and lymphoproliferative disorders

▼ Idiopathic (45–55%)

Fig. 19.3 Etiologies of cutaneous small vessel vasculitis. *Often associated with antineutrophil cytoplasmic antibodies (ANCA).

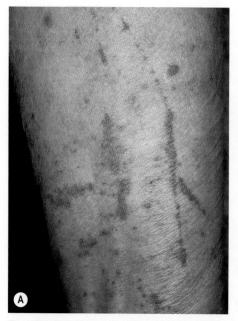

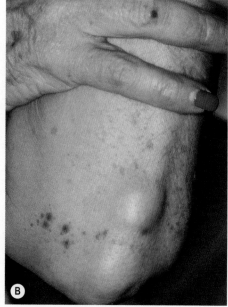

Fig. 19.4 Cutaneous small vessel vasculitis associated with systemic disorders. The underlying diseases were Sjögren's syndrome **(A)** and rheumatoid arthritis **(B).** Note the Koebner phenomenon in **(A)** and the rheumatoid nodules in **(B).**

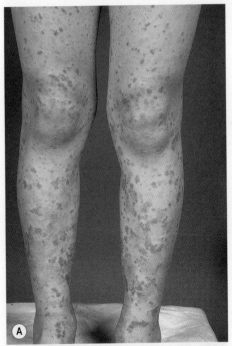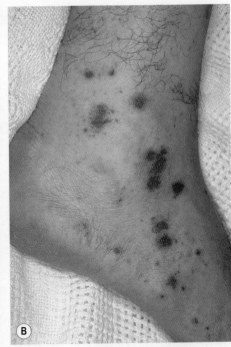

Fig. 19.5 Henoch–Schönlein purpura. A Multiple pink, partially blanching papules on the lower extremities. **B** More developed lesions with central necrosis.

Acute Hemorrhagic Edema of Infancy

• Uncommon CSVV variant that affects children ≤2 years of age, often following a URI.

• Presents with annular or targetoid purpuric plaques and edema favoring the face, ears, and extremities (Fig. 19.6); patients may be febrile, but extracutaneous involvement is rare and spontaneous resolution occurs within 1–3 weeks.

• **DDx:** urticaria 'multiforme' (giant annular urticaria; see Fig. 3.3), serum sickness-like reaction, urticarial vasculitis, Kawasaki disease, erythema multiforme, Sweet's syndrome; findings sometimes overlap with HSP.

Urticarial Vasculitis

• Presents with urticarial plaques that have histologic features of LCV (Fig. 19.7); favors middle-aged women, and a hypocomplementemic subset is associated with AI-CTD (especially SLE and Sjögren's syndrome).

• In contrast to urticaria, individual lesions last >24 hours, resolve with purpura or hyperpigmentation, and produce burning or pain > pruritus.

• Patients with hypocomplementemic urticarial vasculitis may have arthralgias/arthritis, chronic obstructive pulmonary disease, and involvement of the GI tract, kidneys, or eyes.

• **DDx:** see Table 14.1.

Erythema Elevatum Diutinum

• Chronic form of vasculitis that favors middle-aged to older adults; associated disorders include HIV and other infections (e.g. streptococcal), AI-CTD, and IgA monoclonal gammopathy.

• Presents with persistent violaceous to red-brown plaques on extensor surfaces (e.g. elbows, knees) (Fig. 19.8); patients occasionally have arthralgias or ocular disease, and dapsone therapy is usually effective.

Small and Medium-Sized Vessel Vasculitis

Cryoglobulinemic Vasculitis (See Table 18.3)

• 'Mixed' cryoglobulinemia (types II and III) can lead to vasculitis of small ± medium-sized vessels; associated with hepatitis C infection

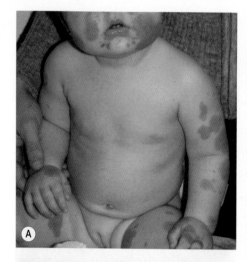

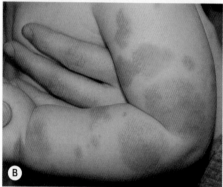

Fig. 19.6 Acute hemorrhagic edema of infancy. Multiple edematous, erythematous plaques on the face and extremities of a toddler. Some of the lesions have begun to become dusky. *Courtesy, Ilona J. Frieden, MD.*

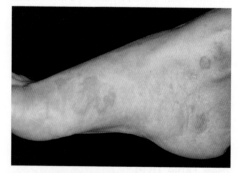

Fig. 19.7 Urticarial vasculitis. Several erythematous urticarial plaques on the foot and ankle. *Courtesy, Cora Whitney Hannon, MD, and Robert Swerlick, MD.*

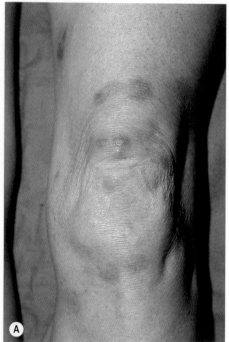

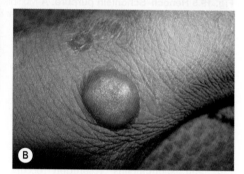

Fig. 19.8 Erythema elevatum diutinum.
A Erythematous papulonodules on the knee (acute lesions) admixed with resolving lesions. **B** Firm nodule on the dorsum of the hand in a patient with HIV infection (late-stage lesion). *A, Courtesy, Kenneth Greer, MD; B, Courtesy, Rachel Moore, MD.*

> other infections (e.g. HIV), AI-CTD, and lymphoproliferative disorders.

• Palpable purpura is the most common cutaneous manifestation (Fig. 19.9); other findings can include arthritis/arthralgias, peripheral neuropathy, glomerulonephritis, and hepatitis.

• **Rx:** treatment of associated hepatitis C with interferon + ribavirin; CS or rituximab for severe or refractory systemic disease.

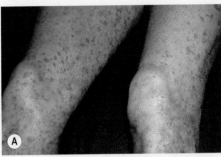

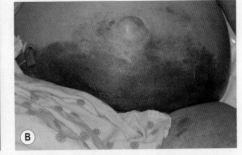

Fig. 19.9 Cutaneous small vessel vasculitis due to mixed cryoglobulinemia. A Palpable purpura represents the most common presentation. B Macular purpura mimicking Cullen's sign in a patient with hepatitis C infection. *B, Courtesy, Kanade Shinkai, MD, and Lindy P. Fox, MD.*

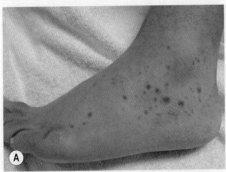

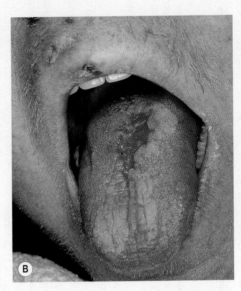

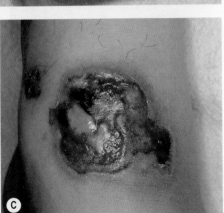

Fig. 19.10 Wegener's granulomatosis. A Palpable purpura on the distal lower extremity due to small vessel (leukocytoclastic) vasculitis. B Ulceration on the tongue. C Sharply demarcated ulcer on the leg. Such lesions may be misdiagnosed as pyoderma gangrenosum. *C, Courtesy, Irwin Braverman, MD.*

ANCA-Associated Vasculitis

• The features of specific ANCA-associated vasculitides are presented in Table 19.2 and Figs. 19.10–19.12.

• Favors middle-aged to older adults, but can occur at any age.

• Requires evaluation for extracutaneous disease (see Fig. 19.14).

• ANCA against various antigens also occur in other diseases (e.g. ulcerative colitis, auto-immune hepatitis); cocaine use can lead to ANCA (typically against myeloperoxidase,

ANTINEUTROPHIL CYTOPLASMIC ANTIBODY (ANCA)-ASSOCIATED VASCULITIDES

Disorder [No. of Diagnostic Criteria Required]	Predominant ANCA Type/ Antigen	Cutaneous and Oral Findings	Extracutaneous Manifestations	Histologic Findings¶
Wegener's granulomatosis (granulomatosis with polyangiitis) [2]	C-/PR3 (90%*) P-/MPO (10%)	• Palpable purpura (Fig. 19.10A) • Friable, micropapular gingivae ('strawberry gums'; see Fig. 59.16), oral ulcers (Fig. 19.10B) • PNGD** • Subcutaneous nodules • Pyoderma gangrenosum-like ulcers (Fig. 19.10C)	• **Upper respiratory:** *nasal ulcers with bloody discharge or nodules; septal perforation/saddle nose* (Table 19.3); *hearing loss; chronic sinusitis, otitis, or mastoiditis*[†] • Pulmonary: *nodules, fixed infiltrates or cavities*[†] • Renal: glomerulonephritis • Ocular: proptosis, scleritis • Less often neurologic, GI, and cardiac involvement	• *Granulomatous inflammation* • Vasculitis of small ± medium-sized vessels
Churg–Strauss syndrome‡ [4]	P-/MPO (60%) C-/PR3 (~10%)	• Palpable purpura (Fig. 19.11A) • PNGD** (Fig. 19.11B) • Subcutaneous nodules • Urticarial plaques • Livedo racemosa, retiform purpura (Fig. 19.11C), ulcers	• **Upper respiratory:** allergic rhinitis§, nasal polyps§, sinusitis[†] • Pulmonary: *asthma*§, *eosinophilic pneumonia*[†] • Hematologic: *peripheral eosinophilia (>10%)*, elevated IgE • Neurologic: *mononeuritis multiplex* • Cardiac: myo- or pericarditis • Less often renal, GI, and ocular involvement	• *Extravascular eosinophils* • Granulomatous inflammation • Vasculitis of small ± medium-sized vessels
Microscopic polyangiitis [4]	P-/MPO (60%) C-/PR3 (30%)	• Palpable purpura (Fig. 19.12A) • Erythematous macules, urticarial or purpuric plaques (Fig. 19.1B) • Livedo racemosa, ulcers, splinter hemorrhages	• Renal: *glomerulonephritis* • Pulmonary: capillaritis/hemorrhage, *no asthma* • Neurologic: mononeuritis multiplex • Less often upper respiratory tract, cardiac, GI, and ocular involvement	• *Vasculitis of small (± medium-sized) vessels* • *No granulomas*

Approximately 60% in patients with limited/localized disease.

**Palisaded neutrophilic and granulomatous dermatitis, which typically presents with umbilicated, crusted papulonodules on extensor surfaces (e.g. elbows) or the face (especially in Wegener's granulomatosis) (see Chapter 37).

[†]Evidence via CT represents a diagnostic criterion.

‡Occasionally triggered by leukotriene inhibitors and/or rapid discontinuation of CS therapy.

§Usually the initial manifestations.

¶May be observed in biopsies of the skin, mucosa, respiratory tract, kidney, or nerve.

C-, cytoplasmic ANCA; MPO, myeloperoxidase; PR3, proteinase-3; P-, perinuclear ANCA.

Table 19.2 Antineutrophil cytoplasmic antibody (ANCA)-associated vasculitides. As in other forms of vasculitis, patients often have constitutional symptoms (e.g. fevers, malaise, weight loss), arthralgias, and arthritis. *Diagnostic criteria for each disorder are in italics.* Alternative criteria that do not specify a lack of granulomatous inflammation have also been proposed for microscopic polyangiitis.

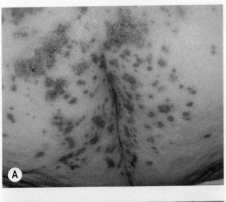

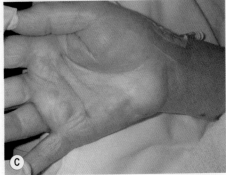

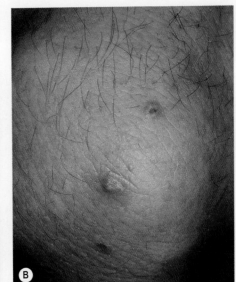

Fig. 19.11 Churg–Strauss syndrome. A Palpable purpura on the buttocks due to small vessel (leukocytoclastic) vasculitis. **B** Palisaded neutrophilic and granulomatous dermatitis presenting with crusted, firm papules on the elbow. **C** Purpuric dermal plaques on the palm due to vasculitis affecting a small artery (representing a medium-sized vessel). *A, C, Courtesy, Kanade Shinkai, MD, and Lindy P. Fox, MD; B, Courtesy, Kalman Watsky, MD.*

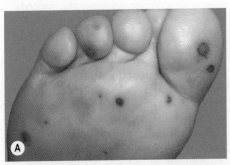

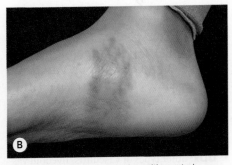

Fig. 19.12 Microscopic polyangiitis. A Petechiae and multiple purpuric papules with central necrosis on the plantar surface. **B** Confluent hemorrhagic plaque on the medial aspect of the foot. *Courtesy, Cora Whitney Hannon, MD, and Robert Swerlick, MD.*

proteinase-3, and neutrophil elastase) together with nasal destruction (Table 19.3) or (with levamisole adulteration) more widespread vasculitis or vasculopathy plus neutropenia (see Fig. 75.3).

- **Rx:** induction of remission with systemic CS ± cyclophosphamide or rituximab; maintenance with CS-sparing agents (e.g. methotrexate, azathioprine), trimethoprim–sulfamethoxazole.

DIFFERENTIAL DIAGNOSIS OF NASAL DESTRUCTION OR DEFORMITY
Inflammatory disorders
• Wegener's granulomatosis • Relapsing polychondritis • Sarcoidosis
Neoplastic disorders
• Nasal natural killer/T-cell lymphoma (lethal midline granuloma) • Squamous cell and basal cell carcinomas • Neuroblastoma, salivary gland tumors, sarcomas (e.g. rhabdomyosarcoma)
Infectious disorders
• *Bacterial*: rhinoscleroma, glanders, noma, syphilis (late congenital or tertiary), yaws • *Mycobacterial*: leprosy, tuberculosis (lupus vulgaris) • *Fungal*: paracoccidioidomycosis, zygomycosis, aspergillosis • *Parasitic*: mucocutaneous leishmaniasis, acanthamoebiasis, rhinosporidiosis
Other
• Cocaine use (cocaine-induced midline destructive lesion) • Nasal myiasis • Factitious or traumatic

Table 19.3 Differential diagnosis of nasal destruction or deformity.

Predominantly Medium-Sized Vessel Vasculitis

Polyarteritis Nodosa (PAN): Classic (Systemic) and Cutaneous Variants

• Segmental vasculitis affecting primarily medium-sized vessels, including small arteries in the deep dermis and subcutis.

• Favors middle-aged adults (men > women), but can occur at any age.

• **DDx:** other types of vasculitis; livedoid vasculopathy, antiphospholipid syndrome, and other microvascular occlusion syndromes (see Chapter 18); superficial thrombophlebitis, panniculitis.

CLASSIC (SYSTEMIC) PAN

• Associated with hepatitis B infection in ~10% of patients.

• Approximately 25% of patients have cutaneous manifestations, including livedo

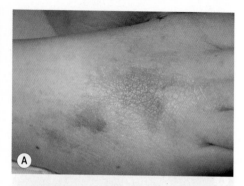

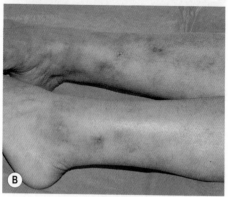

Fig. 19.13 Polyarteritis nodosa (PAN).
A Retiform purpura of the dorsal foot in a patient with systemic PAN. **B** Livedo reticularis of the lower extremities with multiple small 'punched-out' ulcers in an adolescent with cutaneous PAN. This entity can overlap with the PAN-like syndrome with anti-phosphatidylserine–prothrombin complex antibodies that responds to anticoagulation. *A, Courtesy, Kanade Shinkai, MD, and Lindy P. Fox, MD; B, Courtesy, Julie V. Schaffer, MD.*

racemosa, retiform purpura, palpable purpura (when small vessels are affected), and 'punched out' ulcers > subcutaneous nodules and digital infarcts (Fig. 19.13A).

• Extracutaneous manifestations include fevers, weight loss, arthralgias, myalgias, and involvement of arteries supplying the GI tract, kidneys (e.g. renovascular hypertension, *not* glomerulonephritis), nervous system (peripheral > central), heart, and testes.

• **Rx:** systemic CS, treatment of associated hepatitis B; cyclophosphamide for severe or refractory systemic disease.

CUTANEOUS PAN

• Accounts for >30% of childhood PAN and ≤5% of adult PAN.

Patient with suspected cutaneous vasculitis

History and physical examination
- Determine if drug exposure or evidence of an underlying infection; if not, consider an associated inflammatory disorder or malignancy (see Fig. 19.3)

- Evaluate for extracutaneous signs and symptoms
    - Assess for constitutional symptoms: fevers, weight loss, fatigue
    - Review of systems including musculoskeletal, GI, GU, neurologic, respiratory, ENT, eyes & cardiovascular

Biopsy of fresh but well-developed skin lesion(s), 24-48 hours old, to confirm the presence of vasculitis and determine the size of vessels involved:
- If suspect *small vessel* vasculitis (e.g. if palpable purpura): punch biopsies for routine histology and direct immunofluorescence
- If suspect *medium-sized vessel* vasculitis: deep incisional biopsy (including subcutaneous tissue) of a nodule (preferred) or retiform purpura > the edge of an ulcer* (see Fig. 1.6)

Initial basic laboratory evaluation for all patients (repeated with flares of disease activity):
- CBC with differential, platelet count, ESR +/- C-reactive protein
- Hepatic panel, BUN & creatinine, urinalysis, stool guiac

Additional evaluation for associated diseases and specific vasculitides, depending on clinical suspicion:
- Antistreptolysin O and anti-DNase B titers; hepatitis B/C and HIV serologies; throat, urine or blood culture as indicated
- Cryoglobulins; CH50/C3/C4 if suspect urticarial vasculitis (also C1q if low C4)
- Rheumatoid factor, ANA, anti-ENA antibodies (e.g. anti-Ro), ANCA**
- Serum & urine protein electrophoresis, serum immunofixation electrophoresis
- Age-appropriate screening +/- sign/symptom-directed evaluation for malignancies

Additional evaluation for extracutaneous involvement in systemic vasculitides:
ANCA-associated vasculitis
- Chest X-ray, CT of chest & sinuses
- Depending on the specific condition (see Table 19.2) and clinical findings, consider: electromyogram/nerve conduction studies, echocardiogram/electrocardiogram, and biopsy of the respiratory tract (upper or lower), nerve, kidney or muscle
Classic (systemic) polyarteritis nodosa
- Mesenteric/renal/celiac angiogram
- Consider biopsy of muscle, nerve, kidney or testicles

*Include peripheral rim of inflammation if present; vasculitis underlying an ulcer can occur as a secondary phenomenon and is not diagnostic.
**Indirect immunofluorescence (IIF) followed by confirmation with antigen-specific ELISAs for proteinase-3 (PR3) and myeloperoxidase (MPO).

Fig. 19.14 Approach to the patient with suspected cutaneous vasculitis. AI-CTD, autoimmune connective tissue disease; ANCA, antineutrophil cytoplasmic antibodies; BUN, blood urea nitrogen; CBC, complete blood count; ENA, extractable nuclear antigen; ENT, ear, nose, and throat; ESR, erythrocyte sedimentation rate; GU, genitourinary.

• May be associated with infections (e.g. streptococcal) or medications (e.g. minocycline – may be P-ANCA+, unlike most forms of PAN).

• Tender subcutaneous nodules favoring the lower extremities, often in a background of livedo racemosa and sometimes following the course of an artery (see Fig. 19.13B); retiform purpura, ulcers, and annular plaques may also be seen.

• Arthralgias, myalgias, and peripheral neuropathy may occur in areas of skin disease; chronic course without systemic progression.

• **Rx:** intralesional or systemic CS, dapsone, methotrexate.

Diagnostic Approach to Patients with Suspected Cutaneous Vasculitis

• An approach to the evaluation of patients suspected to have vasculitis, including assessment of underlying conditions and systemic manifestations, is presented in Fig. 19.14.

For further information see Ch. 24. From *Dermatology, Third Edition*.

Eosinophilic Dermatoses 20

As with the group of disorders known as neutrophilic dermatoses, there is significant overlap in the cutaneous findings of entities where eosinophils play a role – from papular urticaria triggered by arthropod bites to Wells' syndrome and hypereosinophilic syndrome (Fig. 20.1; Table 20.1). The exception is granuloma faciale, which has a more specific presentation.

Granuloma Faciale

- Idiopathic disorder characterized by a persistent red-brown to violet-brown plaque on the face (Fig. 20.2); prominent follicular openings are often noted and a third of patients have multiple plaques.
- Most commonly occurs in middle-aged adults, and extrafacial involvement is unusual (<10% of patients).
- The clinical diagnosis is confirmed via histopathology where eosinophils, neutrophils, and lymphocytes are seen in the dermis.
- **DDx:** sarcoidosis, foreign body granuloma, granulomatous rosacea, and other entities that lead to persistent red to red-brown plaques of the face (see Fig. 99.2).
- **Rx:** often difficult; intralesional CS, topical calcineurin inhibitors, cryosurgery, vascular lasers.

Exaggerated Insect Bite and Insect Bite-Like Reactions (Eosinophilic Dermatosis Associated with Hematologic Disorders/Malignancies)

- Lesions may occur at sites of known insect bites but a history of bites may be lacking, hence the term insect bite-like reaction; presents as pruritic, erythematous, edematous papulonodules and vesicobullae.

- The most common associated systemic disorder is chronic lymphocytic leukemia, but these reactions can also be seen in patients with myeloproliferative disorders (see Table 99.2) and at sites of mosquito bites in those with Epstein–Barr virus-associated NK/T-cell lymphomas.

Papuloerythroderma of Ofuji

- Widespread red-brown papules that coalesce into an erythroderma with sparing of skin folds ('deck-chair' sign), often with peripheral eosinophilia; primarily elderly men, frequently Japanese.
- Usually idiopathic, but occasionally there is an underlying lymphoma (especially T-cell) or carcinoma (most commonly gastric).
- **DDx:** other causes of erythroderma (see Chapter 8).

Wells' Syndrome (Eosinophilic Cellulitis)

- Recurrent burning, pruritic or painful pink to red plaques that are often edematous, thus resembling infectious cellulitis; over time the lesions may become more infiltrative (Fig. 20.3).
- As the plaques and nodules spontaneously fade over a period of 1–2 months, a residual brown to gray or even green color may be seen.
- Associated symptoms include malaise and occasionally fever; peripheral eosinophilia is common.
- Unknown etiology; the possibility of triggers such as arthropod bites, parasitic infections (e.g. toxocariasis), or an underlying myeloproliferative disorder is a matter of debate.
- Within the dermis, there is a discharge of the granular contents of eosinophils, which then coat collagen fibers and lead to the

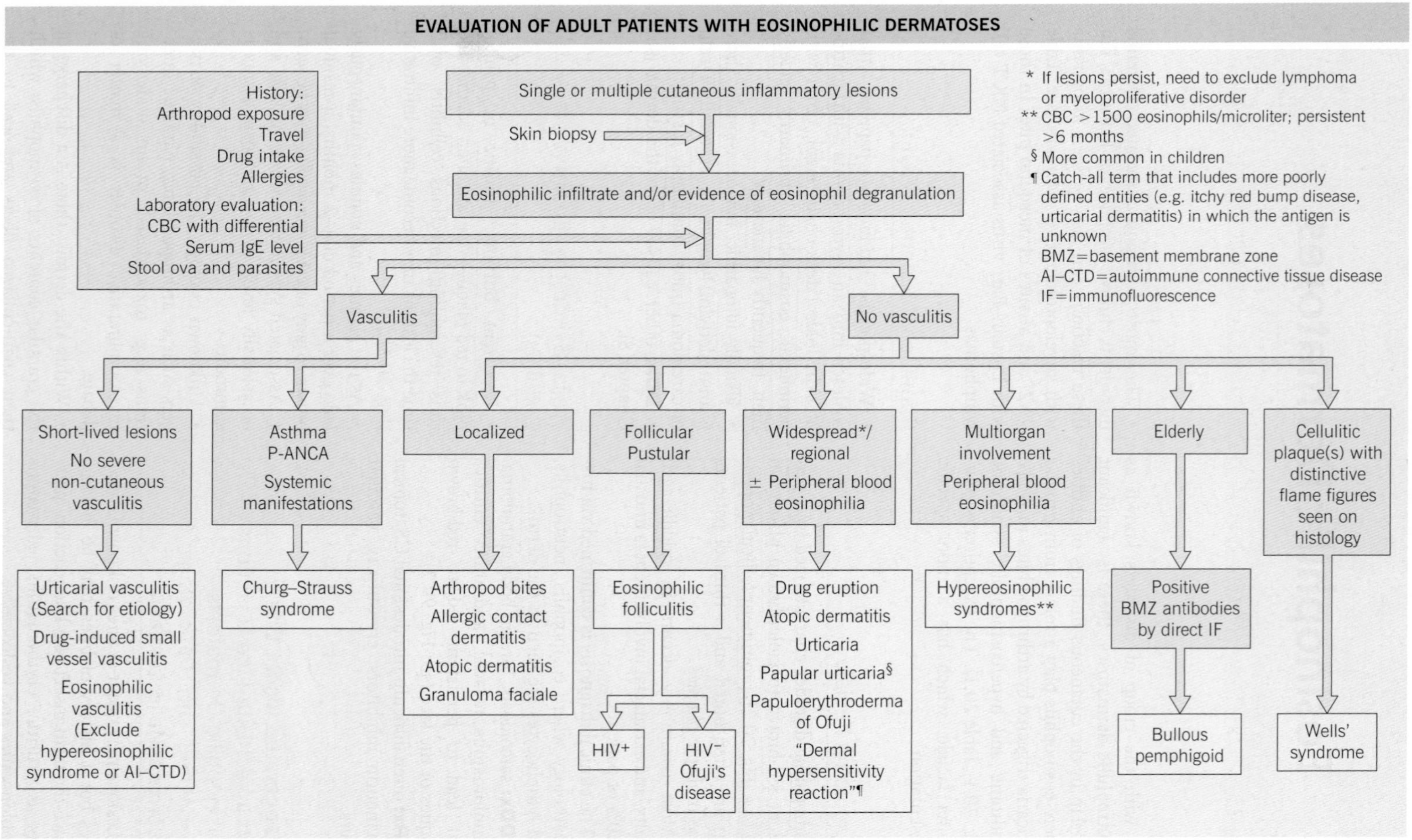

SECTION 4: Urticarias, Erythemas, and Purpura

EVALUATION OF ADULT PATIENTS WITH EOSINOPHILIC DERMATOSES

History:
Arthropod exposure
Travel
Drug intake
Allergies
Laboratory evaluation:
CBC with differential
Serum IgE level
Stool ova and parasites

Single or multiple cutaneous inflammatory lesions

Skin biopsy

Eosinophilic infiltrate and/or evidence of eosinophil degranulation

Vasculitis

Short-lived lesions
No severe non-cutaneous vasculitis

Urticarial vasculitis
(Search for etiology)
Drug-induced small vessel vasculitis
Eosinophilic vasculitis
(Exclude hypereosinophilic syndrome or AI–CTD)

Asthma
P-ANCA
Systemic manifestations

Churg–Strauss syndrome

No vasculitis

Localized

Arthropod bites
Allergic contact dermatitis
Atopic dermatitis
Granuloma faciale

Follicular
Pustular

Eosinophilic folliculitis

HIV+

HIV−
Ofuji's disease

Widespread*/regional
± Peripheral blood eosinophilia

Drug eruption
Atopic dermatitis
Urticaria
Papular urticaria§
Papuloerythroderma of Ofuji
"Dermal hypersensitivity reaction"¶

Multiorgan involvement
Peripheral blood eosinophilia

Hypereosinophilic syndromes**

Elderly

Positive BMZ antibodies by direct IF

Bullous pemphigoid

Cellulitic plaque(s) with distinctive flame figures seen on histology

Wells' syndrome

* If lesions persist, need to exclude lymphoma or myeloproliferative disorder
** CBC >1500 eosinophils/microliter; persistent >6 months
§ More common in children
¶ Catch-all term that includes more poorly defined entities (e.g. itchy red bump disease, urticarial dermatitis) in which the antigen is unknown
BMZ=basement membrane zone
AI–CTD=autoimmune connective tissue disease
IF=immunofluorescence

Fig. 20.1 Evaluation of adult patients with eosinophilic dermatoses. Histologically, these dermatoses are characterized by a prominent eosinophilic infiltrate and/or eosinophil granule protein deposition. Of note, systemic corticosteroids can significantly reduce the peripheral blood eosinophil count.

OTHER DISORDERS WHERE EOSINOPHILS PLAY A ROLE

- Scabies – see Chapter 71
- Parasitic infections (e.g. larva migrans, onchocerciasis, schistosomiasis, strongyloidiasis)
- Seabather's eruption – after ocean swimming, pruritic papules in distribution of swimsuit; due to larvae of either jellyfish (*Linuche unguiculata*) or sea anemones (*Edwardsiella lineata*)
- Pruritic papular eruption of HIV disease – nonfollicular pruritic papules
- Polymorphic eruption of pregnancy (also referred to as PUPPP) – urticarial plaques with involvement of striae and periumbilicial sparing; pregnant women
- Pemphigoid gestationis – urticarial plaques and vesicles similar to bullous pemphigoid; pregnant women
- Angiolymphoid hyperplasia with eosinophilia – nodules of the head and neck; adults

Limited to Neonates or Infants

- Erythema toxicum neonatorum – papules and pustules with erythematous flare; neonates
- Incontinentia pigmenti (stages I and II) – linear streaks of vesicles and keratotic papules along Blaschko's lines
- Infantile eosinophilic folliculitis – recurrent crops of pruritic follicular papules and pustules, primarily of the head and neck

PUPPP, pruritic urticarial papules and plaques of pregnancy.

Table 20.1 Other disorders where eosinophils play a role (in addition to those listed in Fig. 20.1).

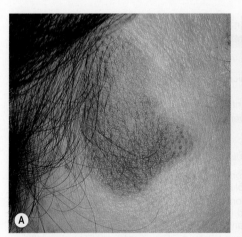 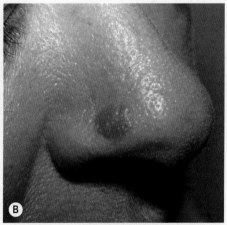

Fig. 20.2 Granuloma faciale. Red-brown plaques on the lateral cheek **(A)** and nose **(B).** Note the prominent follicular openings. *B, Courtesy, Cloyce L. Stetson, MD.*

formation of 'flame figures'; the latter can also be seen in other disorders in which there are numerous eosinophils.
- **DDx:** infectious cellulitis (edematous lesions), exaggerated arthropod reactions (see above), parasitic infections, and other causes of pseudocellulitis (see Table 61.2).
- **Rx:** systemic CS; occasionally steroid-sparing agents are needed.

Hypereosinophilic Syndrome

- Classically defined as peripheral eosinophilia (>1500 eosinophils/microliter) for at least 6 months (or less than 6 months if associated end-organ damage), with multi-organ involvement, but in the absence of an identifiable cause (Table 20.2).
- Divided into major forms: (1) myeloproliferative – characterized by specific mutations, in particular the *FIP1L1-PDGFRA* fusion gene, male predominance, and endomyocardial disease; and (2) lymphocytic – characterized by a clonal proliferation of T cells, as detected by flow cytometry and T-cell receptor gene rearrangement, as well as increased production of Th2 cytokines, e.g. IL-5, which activates eosinophils.

- Mucocutaneous lesions are seen in at least 50% of patients and include nonspecific pruritic erythematous papules and nodules, urticaria, angioedema, dermatitis, erythroderma, and in the myeloproliferative form, mouth or

anogenital ulcers; thromboses can lead to retiform purpura.
- **DDx:** with the exception of granuloma faciale and eosinophilic folliculitis, the entities outlined in Fig. 20.1; several of the entities in Table 20.1, in particular parasitic infections; hereditary and acquired angioedema; for lymphoproliferative form, cutaneous T-cell lymphoma; if oral ulcers, oral aphthae.
- **Rx:** *FIP1L1-PDGFRA*-positive myeloproliferative form – imatinib, other tyrosine kinase inhibitors (e.g. nilotinib); lymphoproliferative form – systemic CS ± mepolizumab (anti-IL-5 monoclonal antibody).

For further information see Ch. 25. From *Dermatology, Third Edition*.

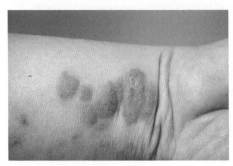

Fig. 20.3 Wells' syndrome. Edematous nodules and plaques.

DIAGNOSTIC CRITERIA AND CLASSIFICATION OF HYPEREOSINOPHILIC SYNDROMES (HES)

Diagnostic Criteria

- Peripheral blood eosinophil counts >1500/microliter for at least 6 months, or less than 6 months with evidence of organ damage
- Lack of evidence for parasitic, allergic, or other recognized causes of eosinophilia
- Symptoms and signs of organ system involvement

Subtypes

Myeloproliferative*	Lymphoproliferative	Other‡
• *FIP1L1-PDGFRA* fusion gene whose product is a constitutively activated tyrosine kinase; other mutations are possible • Includes 'classic HES' with endomyocardial disease, a restrictive cardiomyopathy, and a male predominance • Mucosal ulcers are associated with severe disease • High serum tryptase and vitamin B_{12} levels, tissue fibrosis, splenomegaly, and bone marrow biopsies with increased numbers of CD25⁺ atypical spindle-shaped mast cells	• T-cell clone producing Th2 cytokines, e.g. IL-5 • T-cell clones have occurred in rare cases of EAE and NERDS • High serum levels of IgE • Some patients develop lymphoma	• Eosinophilic vasculitis • Episodic angioedema with eosinophilia (EAE; Gleich syndrome) • Nodules, eosinophilia, rheumatism, dermatitis, and swelling (NERDS) syndrome • A variety of other diseases, including eosinophilic gastroenteritis

*Includes patients with eosinophilic leukemia, who may have other cytogenetic abnormalities; can also screen for other rare fusion genes or rearrangements involving PDGFRB or FGR1, which encode platelet-derived growth factor receptor (beta polypeptide) and fibroblast growth factor receptor-1, respectively.
‡List is not exhaustive.

Table 20.2 Diagnostic criteria and classification of hypereosinophilic syndromes (HES).

Neutrophilic Dermatoses | 21

This group of disorders, in an untreated state, is characterized by infiltrates of neutrophils within the skin. In addition, these dermatoses lack an identifiable infectious etiology, despite the presence of neutrophils (Fig. 21.1). There can be significant overlap in the clinical presentations of the neutrophilic dermatoses; for example, in a patient with acute myelogenous leukemia, bullous pyoderma gangrenosum may be difficult to distinguish from Sweet's syndrome. In addition, infiltrates of neutrophils can occur in other organs, particularly the joints, eyes, lungs, and bones. Bone involvement raises the possibility of SAPHO (synovitis, acne, pustulosis, hyperostosis, osteitis) syndrome.

Sweet's Syndrome (Acute Febrile Neutrophilic Dermatosis)

• Acute onset of erythematous edematous papules and plaques that are tender, but not pruritic; if the edema is intense, the lesions may become bullous and, occasionally, they resemble erysipelas; favored sites are the face, neck, upper trunk, and upper extremities (Fig. 21.2).
• Less commonly, nodules develop due to neutrophilic panniculitis or pustules form within the plaques; a variant occurs on the dorsal aspect of the hands and is referred to as 'neutrophilic dermatosis of the dorsal hands' (Fig. 21.3).
• Associated systemic findings include fever, malaise, and arthralgias, and a peripheral leukocytosis is commonly observed (Table 21.1); some patients also develop systemic manifestations, including ocular, pulmonary, and skeletal involvement (Fig. 21.4, Table 21.2).
• Most often seen in adults, with a female:male ratio of 4:1 (except in the case of malignancy-associated disease); may first appear or flare during pregnancy; idiopathic in up to 50% of patients.
• Underlying disorders include: (1) *infections* – upper respiratory tract (e.g. viral, streptococcal) or gastrointestinal (e.g. yersinosis) > HIV or atypical mycobacteria; (2) *hematologic malignancies* (10–20% of patients), particularly acute myelogenous leukemia (AML) but also myelodysplasia and myeloproliferative disorders; (3) *inflammatory bowel disease*; (4) *autoimmune connective tissue disease*, particularly systemic lupus erythematosus (SLE); (5) *drugs* – G-CSF, all-*trans*-retinoic acid > furosemide, minocycline; and (6) *carcinomas* – genitourinary, breast, colon.
• The vesiculobullous form is more often associated with AML, and in malignancy-associated Sweet's syndrome, the lesions tend to be more widespread, including within the oral cavity.
• Histologically, diffuse infiltrates of neutrophils are seen within the dermis and occasionally the subcutaneous fat; leukocytoclastic vasculitis is absent or minimal.
• **DDx:** bullous pyoderma gangrenosum, neutrophilic eccrine hidradenitis, erysipelas, erythema multiforme, causes of pseudocellulitis (see Table 61.2), infectious cellulitis, vasculitis (urticarial, small vessel, septic), halogenoderma, periodic fever syndromes, as well as additional entities in Fig. 21.1.
• There are differing opinions regarding whether the development of a nonbullous neutrophilic dermatosis in the setting of LE is a distinct entity or is simply Sweet's syndrome associated with LE.
• **Rx:** usually spontaneously resolves over a few months, but may recur in up to 30% to 50% of patients with idiopathic versus malignancy-associated disease, respectively; antimicrobials for any underlying infection

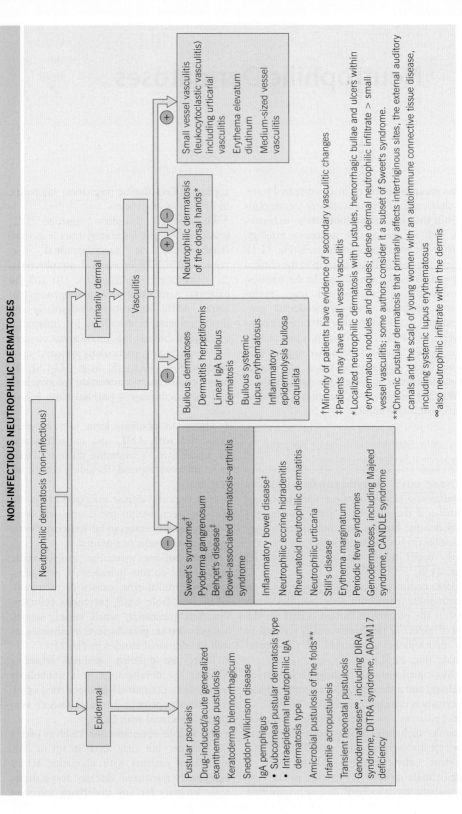

NON-INFECTIOUS NEUTROPHILIC DERMATOSES

Neutrophilic dermatosis (non-infectious)

Epidermal

Pustular psoriasis
Drug-induced/acute generalized exanthematous pustulosis
Keratoderma blennorrhagicum
Sneddon-Wilkinson disease
IgA pemphigus
• Subcorneal pustular dermatosis type
• Intraepidermal neutrophilic IgA dermatosis type
Amicrobial pustulosis of the folds**
Infantile acropustulosis
Transient neonatal pustulosis
Genodermatoses∞, including DIRA syndrome, DITRA syndrome, ADAM17 deficiency

Sweet's syndrome†
Pyoderma gangrenosum‡
Behçet's disease‡
Bowel-associated dermatosis–arthritis syndrome
Inflammatory bowel disease‡
Neutrophilic eccrine hidradenitis
Rheumatoid neutrophilic dermatitis
Neutrophilic urticaria
Still's disease
Erythema marginatum
Periodic fever syndromes
Genodermatoses, including Majeed syndrome, CANDLE syndrome

Primarily dermal

Bullous dermatoses
Dermatitis herpetiformis
Linear IgA bullous dermatosis
Bullous systemic lupus erythematosus
Inflammatory epidermolysis bullosa acquisita

Neutrophilic dermatosis of the dorsal hands*

Vasculitis

Small vessel vasculitis (leukocytoclastic vasculitis) including urticarial vasculitis
Erythema elevatum diutinum
Medium-sized vessel vasculitis

†Minority of patients have evidence of secondary vasculitic changes
‡Patients may have small vessel vasculitis
*Localized neutrophilic dermatosis with pustules, hemorrhagic bullae and ulcers within erythematous nodules and plaques; dense dermal neutrophilic infiltrate > small vessel vasculitis; some authors consider it a subset of Sweet's syndrome.
**Chronic pustular dermatosis that primarily affects intertriginous sites, the external auditory canals and the scalp of young women with an autoimmune connective tissue disease, including systemic lupus erythematosus
∞also neutrophilic infiltrate within the dermis

Fig. 21.1 Non-infectious neutrophilic dermatoses. Entities in the darker box are discussed in this chapter. CANDLE, chronic atypical neutrophilic dermatosis with lipodystrophy and elevated temperature; DIRA, deficiency of interleukin-1 receptor antagonist; DITRA, deficiency of the IL-36R antagonist.

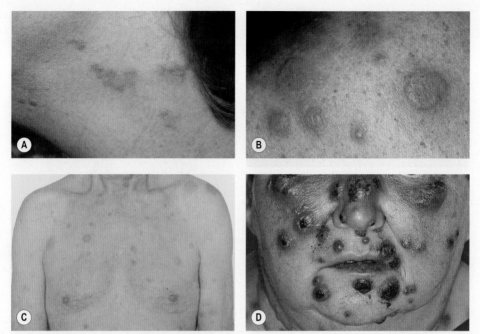

Fig. 21.2 Spectrum of cutaneous findings in Sweet's syndrome. A Edematous erythematous papules and plaques on the neck of a patient with acute myelogenous leukemia. **B** Markedly edematous plaques on the upper back, some of which are pseudovesicular while others are becoming bullous. **C** Some of the edematous lesions have a targetoid appearance. **D** Central hemorrhagic crusts within facial plaques. *B, D, Courtesy, Kalman Watsky, MD; C, Courtesy, Mark Davis, MD.*

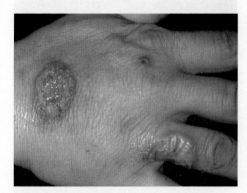

Fig. 21.3 Neutrophilic dermatosis of the dorsal hands. This entity has overlapping clinical and histologic features with both Sweet's syndrome and pyoderma gangrenosum. Some patients have an associated pustular vasculitis. *Courtesy, Jean L. Bolognia, MD.*

CRITERIA FOR THE DIAGNOSIS OF SWEET'S SYNDROME

Major Criteria

1. Abrupt onset of typical cutaneous lesions

2. Histopathology consistent with Sweet's syndrome

Minor Criteria

1. Preceded by one of the associated infections or vaccinations; accompanied by one of the associated malignancies or inflammatory disorders; associated with drug exposure or pregnancy

2. Presence of fever and constitutional signs and symptoms

3. Leukocytosis

4. Excellent response to systemic corticosteroids

Table 21.1 Criteria for the diagnosis of Sweet's syndrome. Both of the major criteria and two of the minor criteria are needed for the diagnosis. *From Su WPD, Liu HNH. Diagnostic criteria for Sweet's syndrome. Cutis 1986;37: 167–174.*

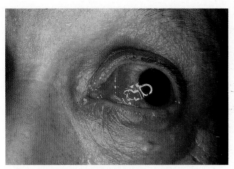

Fig. 21.4 Ocular involvement in Sweet's syndrome. Erythema and hemorrhage of the sclera and conjunctiva. *Courtesy, Kalman Watsky, MD.*

SYSTEMIC MANIFESTATIONS OF SWEET'S SYNDROME

Common (≥50%)
- Fever
- Leukocytosis

Less common (20–50%)
- Arthralgias
- Arthritis: asymmetric, non-erosive, favors knees and wrists
- Myalgias
- Ocular involvement: conjunctivitis, episcleritis, limbal nodules, iridocyclitis

Uncommon
- Neutrophilic alveolitis: cough, dyspnea, and pleurisy; radiographic findings include interstitial infiltrates, nodules, pleural effusions
- Multifocal sterile osteomyelitis (SAPHO syndrome)
- Renal involvement (e.g. mesangial glomerulonephritis): hematuria, proteinuria, renal insufficiency, acute renal failure

Unusual/rare
- Hepatitis
- Acute myositis
- Aseptic meningitis, encephalitis
- Pancreatitis
- Gastrointestinal involvement

SAPHO, synovitis, acne, pustulosis, hyperostosis, osteitis.

Table 21.2 Systemic manifestations of Sweet's syndrome.

such as streptococcal pharyngitis; for moderate to severe disease, systemic CS (e.g. prednisone 0.5–1 mg/kg/day tapered over several months), dapsone, potassium iodide; for milder disease, ultrapotent topical CS and NSAIDs.

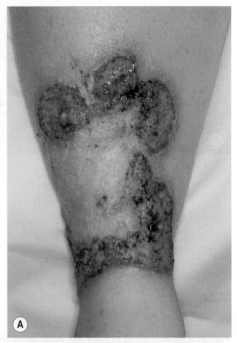

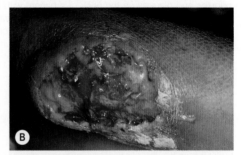

Fig. 21.5 Classic ulcerative pyoderma gangrenosum. A The edge of this ulceration on the shin is undermined with a violet–gray color as well as an inflammatory rim. Note the central scarring. **B** In addition to an overhanging border, this deep ulceration on the elbow has a purulent base. *A, Courtesy, Mark Davis, MD.*

Pyoderma Gangrenosum (PG)

- The most common presentation is a painful, rapidly enlarging ulcer of the lower extremity with a gray-violet, undermined, necrotic border; there is often a peripheral rim of erythema, and the base of the ulcer may be purulent (Fig. 21.5).
- Ulcers can occur at other sites, including the face, upper extremities, and trunk, as well as peristomally (Fig. 21.6); once partially

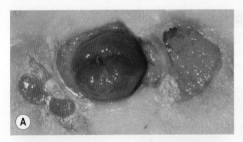

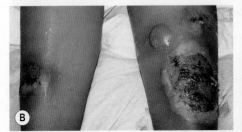

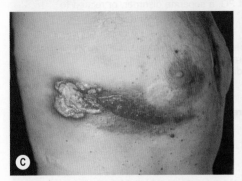

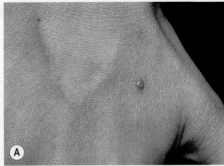

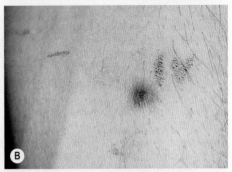

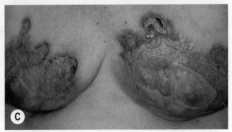

Fig. 21.6 Pyoderma gangrenosum (PG) and underlying disorders – ulcerative colitis and PAPA syndrome. A Multiple ulcers surround an ileostomy (following a total proctocolectomy) in a patient with refractory chronic ulcerative colitis. Although peristomal PG occurs most commonly following intestinal resection of inflammatory bowel disease, it can also follow resection of gastrointestinal or bladder carcinoma. **B** Bullous PG in a patient with ulcerative colitis. **C** PG in a patient with PAPA syndrome (pyogenic arthritis, PG, and acne). *A, Courtesy, Mark Davis, MD; C, Courtesy, Maria Chanco Turner, MD.*

Fig. 21.7 Pyoderma gangrenosum (PG) – early lesion and demonstration of pathergy. A The earliest clinical lesion is a pustule with an inflammatory base; this patient had Crohn's disease. **B** Pathergy with an early lesion at the site of an intravenous catheter. **C** Postsurgical PG following a breast reduction; multiple debridements had been performed and systemic antibiotics administered because the original diagnosis was soft tissue infection. *B, Courtesy, Samuel L. Moschella, MD; C, Courtesy, Mark Davis, MD.*

treated, the ulcer may lose some of its characteristic features.

• Lesions can begin as an inflammatory papulopustule (which may be follicular), as a bulla on a violaceous base, or at the site of trauma (pathergy) (Fig. 21.7); in some patients, especially those with underlying inflammatory bowel disease and/or arthritis, the ulcers may expand more slowly with

significant granulation tissue in their bases; healing of PG ulcers often leads to a distinctive cribriform pattern of scarring.

• There are several clinical variants of PG and they are outlined in Table 21.3; the diagnosis of PG requires clinicopathologic correlation and exclusion of other entities in the **DDx** (Tables 21.4 and 21.5).

CLINICAL VARIANTS OF PYODERMA GANGRENOSUM (PG)

Vesiculobullous (also referred to as atypical or bullous PG)

- Lesions favor the face and upper extremities, especially the dorsal hands
- Clinical appearance overlaps with the superficial bullous variant of Sweet's syndrome (Fig. 21.6B)
- Occurs most commonly in the setting of acute myelogenous leukemia, myelodysplasia, and myeloproliferative disorders such as chronic myelogenous leukemia and when drug-induced (e.g. G-CSF)

Pustular

- Multiple, small, sterile pustules
- Lesions usually regress without scarring, but can evolve into classic PG
- Most commonly observed in patients with inflammatory bowel disease
- Similar eruption may be seen in patients with Behçet's disease or bowel-associated dermatosis–arthritis syndrome

Superficial granulomatous pyoderma

- Localized, superficial vegetative or ulcerative lesion, which favors the trunk and usually follows trauma (e.g. surgery)
- Histologically, a superficial granulomatous response with a less intense neutrophilic infiltrate
- Tends to respond to less aggressive anti-inflammatory therapy
- Controversy as to whether it is a variant of PG, a separate disorder, or related to Wegener's granulomatosis

Pyostomatitis vegetans

- Chronic, vegetative, sterile pyoderma of the labial and buccal mucosa (Fig. 21.8A)
- May be associated with vegetative or ulcerative cutaneous PG (Fig. 21.8B)
- Seen in patients with inflammatory bowel disease

G-CSF, granulocyte colony-stimulating factor.

Table 21.3 Clinical variants of pyoderma gangrenosum (PG).

PROPOSED DIAGNOSTIC CRITERIA FOR CLASSIC ULCERATIVE PYODERMA GANGRENOSUM

Major criteria

1. Rapid[a] progression of a painful,[b] necrolytic cutaneous ulcer[c] with an irregular, violaceous and undermined border
2. Other causes of cutaneous ulceration have been excluded[d]

Minor criteria

1. History suggestive of pathergy[e] or clinical finding of cribriform scarring
2. Systemic diseases associated with pyoderma gangrenosum[f]
3. Histopathologic findings (sterile dermal neutrophilia, ± mixed inflammation, ± lymphocytic vasculitis)
4. Treatment response (rapid response to systemic corticosteroids)[g]

[a]*Characteristic margin expansion of 1–2 cm per day, or a 50% increase in ulcer size within 1 month.*
[b]*Pain is usually out of proportion to the size of the ulceration.*
[c]*Typically preceded by a papule, pustule, or bulla.*
[d]*Usually necessitates skin biopsy and additional evaluation (see Table 21.5) to exclude other causes.*
[e]*Ulcer development at sites of minor cutaneous trauma.*
[f]*Inflammatory bowel disease, arthritis, IgA gammopathy, or underlying malignancy.*
[g]*Generally responds to prednisone (1–2 mg/kg/day) or another corticosteroid at an equivalent dosage, with a 50% decrease in size within 1 month.*

Table 21.4 Proposed diagnostic criteria for classic ulcerative pyoderma gangrenosum.
Diagnosis requires both of the major criteria and at least two minor criteria. *From Su WP, et al. Pyoderma gangrenosum: Clinicopathologic correlation and proposed diagnostic criteria. Int. J. Dermatol. 2004;43:790–800.*

EVALUATION OF A PATIENT WITH PRESUMED PYODERMA GANGRENOSUM

1. Thorough history and physical examination; review medications

2. Sterile skin biopsy of *active* skin lesion with sufficient depth (panniculus) and sufficient tissue for special stains and culture (bacterial, mycobacterial, fungal, and viral). Possibility of future additional biopsies for immunofluorescence or PCR studies

3. Gastrointestinal tract studies – stool for occult blood and parasites, colonoscopy, biopsy, radiography, liver function tests, and, if indicated, hepatitis evaluation

4. Hematologic studies – complete blood and platelet count, peripheral blood smear, and, if indicated, bone marrow examination

5. Serologic studies – serum protein electrophoresis, immunofixation electrophoresis, antinuclear antibodies, antiphospholipid antibodies, ANCA antibodies, VDRL

6. Chest x-ray and urinalysis

ANCA, antineutrophil cytoplasmic antibodies; PCR, polymerase chain reaction.

Table 21.5 Evaluation of a patient with presumed pyoderma gangrenosum.

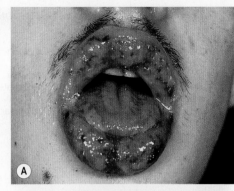

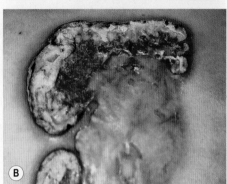

Fig. 21.8 Pyostomatitis vegetans and vegetative pyoderma gangrenosum (PG). **A** Suppurative pyostomatitis vegetans in a patient with ulcerative colitis. **B** Vegetative form of PG following trauma to the skin. *Courtesy, Samuel L. Moschella, MD.*

• Although idiopathic in up to 50% of patients, the age distribution of PG tends to reflect the major underlying disorders, which are: (1) *inflammatory bowel disease*, either ulcerative colitis or Crohn's disease (20–30% of patients); (2) *inflammatory arthritis*, including rheumatoid and seronegative (20%); (3) *plasma cell dyscrasias*, particularly an IgA monoclonal gammopathy (up to 15%); and (4) *other hematologic malignancies*, particularly AML, as well as myelodysplasia, chronic myelogenous leukemia, and hairy cell leukemia; the underlying disorder may be antecedent, coincident, or subsequent.

• PG is included in a few rare syndromes that have various combinations of sterile arthritis, acne, and hidradenitis suppurativa – e.g. PAPA (pyogenic sterile *a*rthritis, *P*G and *a*cne; Fig. 21.6C), PASH (*P*G, *a*cne, *s*uppurative *h*idradenitis), and PAPASH (*p*yogenic

arthritis, *P*G, *a*cne, *s*uppurative *h*idradenitis) syndromes.

• **DDx** for classic ulcerative PG: in the *untreated state*, it consists primarily of infectious etiologies and vasculitis, but in a *partially treated state* (usually with oral CS), it includes a host of other causes of ulcers, from venous ulcers to lymphoma and SCC to drug-induced (see Fig. 86.1).

• **Rx:** treatment of the underlying disorder; systemic CS (e.g. prednisone 1 mg/kg/day), intralesional CS into the edge of the ulcer (e.g. triamcinolone 5–10 mg/cc, but initially only a few test sites to confirm no worsening due to pathergy), pulse CS (1 g IV for 3–5 days), cyclosporine, TNF-α inhibitors; for mild or slowly progressive disease, ultrapotent topical CS, topical tacrolimus, minocycline, dapsone, clofazimine.

SYSTEMIC MANIFESTATIONS OF BEHÇET'S DISEASE

Ocular (leading cause of morbidity)
- Occurs in 90% of patients; favors men, in whom it is more severe
- Can be painful and may lead to blindness
- Retinal vasculitis (more frequently associated with blindness)
- Posterior uveitis (most characteristic ocular finding)
- Anterior uveitis, hypopyon
- Secondary glaucoma, cataracts
- Conjunctivitis, scleritis, keratitis, vitreous hemorrhage, optic neuritis

Joints
- Approximately 50% of patients develop arthritis
- In majority (~80% of patients), duration of attacks is <2 months
- Mono- or polyarthritic and non-erosive
- Most commonly knees, wrists, and ankles

Gastrointestinal
- Abdominal pain and/or hemorrhage may be difficult to distinguish from IBD
- Ulcerations* develop within the small bowel (particularly the ileocecal region) as well as the transverse and ascending colon and esophagus; perforation can occur

Neurologic
- Usually appears later during the evolution of the disease
- Associated with a poor prognosis
- Acute meningoencephalitis that may resolve spontaneously
- Cranial nerve palsies
- Brain stem lesions that can induce swallowing difficulties, laughter, and crying
- Pyramidal or extrapyramidal signs

Vascular
- Aneurysmal or occlusive arterial disease
- Superficial or deep venous thrombosis

Cardiopulmonary
- Coronary arteritis, valvular disease, myocarditis
- Recurrent ventricular arrhythmias
- Pulmonary artery aneurysms

Renal
- Glomerulonephritis

*Resemble anogenital aphthae.
IBD, inflammatory bowel disease.

Table 21.6 Systemic manifestations of Behçet's disease.

Behçet's Disease

- A multisystem disease (Table 21.6) whose mucocutaneous features include aphthous orogenital ulcers (Fig. 21.9), sterile pustules (occasionally follicular), and palpable purpura due to small vessel vasculitis, as well as superficial thrombophlebitis and erythema nodosum-like lesions.
- Because the diagnosis is made clinically, there are several sets of criteria, including the ones outlined in Table 21.7; there are countries in which the disease is more commonly seen, e.g. Turkey, Japan, and those along the ancient Silk Road; the peak incidence is ages 20–35 years.
- **DDx:** recurrent genital and oral HSV (the latter is limited to keratinized mucosa in immunocompetent hosts; see Chapter 59), complex aphthosis, inflammatory bowel disease, SLE, pemphigus vulgaris, Marshall's syndrome (periodic fever, aphthous stomatitis, pharyngitis, cervical adenitis).

- Features of both Behçet's disease and relapsing polychondritis are seen in MAGIC syndrome, which consists of mouth and genital ulcers with inflamed cartilage.

Bowel-Associated Dermatosis–Arthritis Syndrome (Bowel Bypass Syndrome)

- Although initially described following jejunoileal bypass, this syndrome can develop in association with blind loops of bowel due to surgery or inflammatory bowel disease; presumably, there is overgrowth of bacteria and formation of immune complexes containing bacterial antigens that leads to a serum sickness-like picture.
- Cutaneous lesions include erythematous and purpuric papules and vesiculopustules as well as subcutaneous nodules that are accompanied by polyarthritis and tenosynovitis.

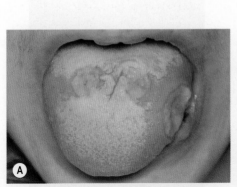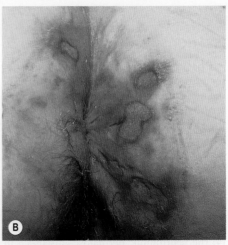

Fig. 21.9 Oral and genital ulcers of Behçet's disease. A Aphthous stomatitis in the form of major aphthae, which are deeper and larger than minor aphthae but share the presence of a pseudomembrane and associated pain. Oral aphthosis is often the initial symptom of Behçet's disease and may flare with the onset of other symptoms. **B** Perianal aphthosis. In men, lesions often occur on the scrotum and penis. *Courtesy, Samuel L. Moschella, MD.*

INTERNATIONAL STUDY GROUP CRITERIA FOR THE DIAGNOSIS OF BEHÇET'S DISEASE	
Criteria	**Required Features**
Major Criterion:	
Recurrent oral ulceration	Aphthous (idiopathic) oral ulceration observed by physician or patient, recurring at least three times in a 12-month period
Plus any two of the following minor criteria:	
Recurrent genital ulceration	Aphthous genital ulceration or scarring, observed by physician or patient
Eye lesions	Anterior or posterior uveitis; cells in the vitreous by slit lamp examination; or retinal vasculitis observed by ophthalmologist
Cutaneous lesions	Erythema nodosum-like lesions observed by physician or patient; papulopustular lesions or pseudofolliculitis; or characteristic acneiform nodules observed by physician in postadolescent patient not on corticosteroids
Pathergy test*	Interpreted at 24–48 hours by physician

Pathergy test is performed on the flexor forearm by obliquely inserting a 20- to 22-gauge sterile hypodermic needle to a depth of 5 mm ± an intradermal injection of 0.1 ml of normal saline. A positive reaction is defined as the development of a papule or pustule.

Table 21.7 International study group criteria for the diagnosis of Behçet's disease. *From International Study Group for Behçet's disease. Criteria for the diagnosis of Behçet's disease. Lancet 1990;335:1078–1080.*

Synovitis, Acne, Pustulosis, Hyperostosis, and Osteitis (SAPHO) Syndrome

• Characterized by aseptic neutrophilic dermatoses plus aseptic osteoarticular involvement, which is also referred to as chronic recurrent multifocal (aseptic) osteomyelitis; the latter favors the anterior chest and axial skeleton (Fig. 21.10).

• Associated skin disorders include: (1) the 'acne family' – acne fulminans, follicular occlusion tetrad; (2) the 'psoriasis family' – palmoplantar pustulosis, pustular psoriasis, psoriasis vulgaris, Sneddon–Wilkinson disease; (3) linear IgA bullous dermatosis; and (4) the neutrophilic dermatoses discussed in this chapter.

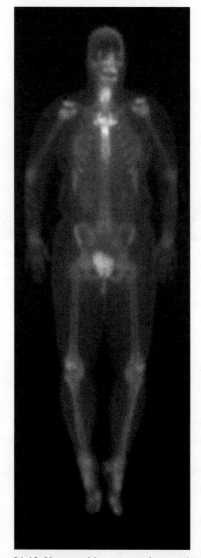

Fig. 21.10 Abnormal bone scan in a patient with SAPHO syndrome. There is abnormal tracer uptake within the mid and lower cervical spine and multiple thoracic vertebral bodies (T3 to T9) in addition to the manubrium and sternoclavicular joints. The pattern and anatomic distribution are indicative of increased osteoblastic activity as in the SAPHO syndrome. *Courtesy, Samuel L. Moschella, MD.*

For further information see Ch. 26. From *Dermatology, Third Edition*.

Pregnancy Dermatoses   22

There are several dermatoses that occur during pregnancy or immediately postpartum, in particular polymorphic eruption of pregnancy, pemphigoid gestationis, and atopic eruption of pregnancy. Pruritus due to intrahepatic cholestasis of pregnancy leads to non-specific skin lesions, including excoriations due to scratching. Impetigo herpetiformis simply represents pustular psoriasis occurring during pregnancy, and this may be related to the relative hypocalcemia of pregnancy. Lastly, there are physiologic changes that occur during pregnancy.

Polymorphic Eruption of Pregnancy (PEP; Pruritic Urticarial Papules and Plaques of Pregnancy [PUPPP])

• Relatively common disorder (~1 in 160 deliveries) that begins late in the third trimester or during the immediate postpartum period; occurs primarily in primiparous women, with an increased frequency in those with multigestational pregnancies.

• Pruritic edematous papules and plaques, whose color varies from pink to red-brown depending on skin phototype, that often involve the abdominal striae but spare the umbilicus (Fig. 22.1); polymorphic presentation includes patches of erythema, targetoid lesions, tiny vesicles, and eczematous plaques (Fig. 22.2).

• Lesions can become widespread, but usually spare the face, palms, and soles; the eruption spontaneously resolves within 4–6 weeks after delivery.

• In general, does not recur with subsequent pregnancies, in contrast to pemphigoid gestationis (PG), and there is no fetal risk.

• **DDx:** PG (may require direct immuno-fluorescence [DIF] of perilesional skin to distinguish), urticarial drug eruption, viral exanthem, allergic contact dermatitis, scabies, erythema multiforme minor.

• **Rx:** topical CS and oral antihistamines usually suffice (see Appendix); occasionally, severe cases require oral CS (prednisolone preferred during pregnancy because of significant inactivation by placenta, leading to a mother : fetus ratio of 10 : 1).

Pemphigoid Gestationis (PG; Gestational Pemphigoid)

• Unusual pruritic vesiculobullous disorder with significant clinical and histologic overlap with bullous pemphigoid (see Chapter 24).

• Usually develops during the later stages of pregnancy or immediately postpartum and is due to circulating autoantibodies against bullous pemphigoid antigen 180 (BP180) present within the hemidesmosome of the basement membrane zone (BMZ).

• In theory, it is related to aberrant expression of MHC class II antigens of paternal origin in the placenta that trigger an autoimmune response to the placental BMZ, followed by cross-reactivity with the BMZ of the skin.

• Lesions often begin on the abdomen, including around and within the umbilicus, but then become more widespread on the trunk as well as the extremities; in addition to vesicles and bullae, edematous urticarial plaques are seen (Fig. 22.3).

• DIF of perilesional skin shows linear deposits of C3 at the BMZ.

• Increased risk of small-for-gestational age and premature neonates and ~10% of

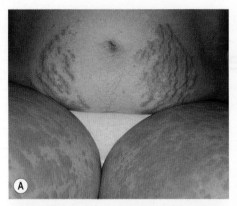

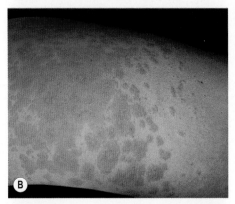

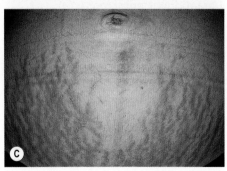

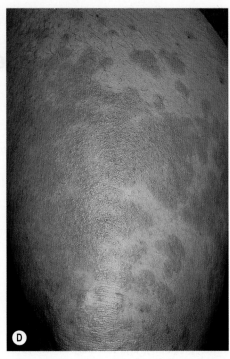

Fig. 22.1 Polymorphic eruption of pregnancy. The edematous urticarial lesions favor the striae **(A, C)** and the upper thighs **(B, D)** and spare the umbilicus. Note the pink color in a woman with skin phototype II versus the red-brown color in a more darkly pigmented patient.

newborns have mild skin involvement; often flares at the time of delivery and recurs during subsequent pregnancies.

• **DDx:** primarily PEP (but in PEP, patients are usually primiparous, large bullae are rare unless there is marked background edema, lesions spare the umbilicus, and DIF of perilesional skin is negative) (Fig. 22.4); urticarial drug eruption, allergic contact dermatitis.

• **Rx:** potent topical or oral CS (prednisolone 0.5 mg/kg/day; see Appendix), depending on severity.

Atopic Eruption of Pregnancy

• Pruritic papules and eczematous plaques that usually develop earlier during pregnancy than other disorders described in this chapter (Fig. 22.5).

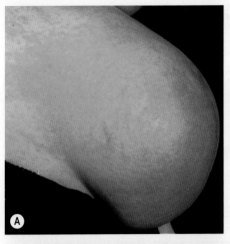

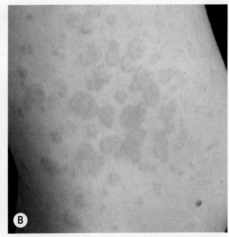

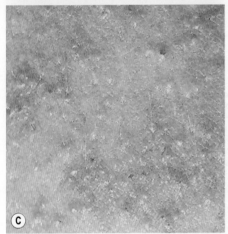

Fig. 22.2 Polymorphic eruption of pregnancy. The clinical spectrum includes: **(A)** macular erythema, which can be widespread; **(B)** targetoid lesions; and **(C)** tiny vesicles due to marked epidermal spongiosis or dermal edema. *Courtesy, Christina M. Ambros-Rudolph, MD.*

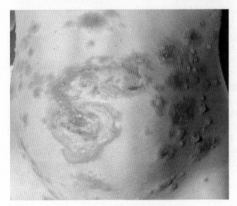

Fig. 22.3 Pemphigoid gestationis. Intact tense bullae arising within areas of edematous erythema as well as erosions due to ruptured bullae. Lesions typically involve the umbilical region. *Courtesy, Christina M. Ambros-Rudolph, MD.*

• Patients have an atopic diathesis, but the eruption is more likely to have its initial presentation during pregnancy and less often it represents a flare of pre-existing atopic dermatitis.
• May be explained by the predominance of a Th2 immune response during pregnancy.
• No maternal or fetal risks, but recurrence during subsequent pregnancies common.
• **DDx:** PEP, intrahepatic cholestasis of pregnancy, scabies, allergic contact dermatitis, drug eruption or viral exanthem (if papular).
• **Rx:** topical CS, oral antihistamines, and other routine therapies for atopic dermatitis (e.g. emollients; oral antibiotics such as cephalexin if secondary bacterial infection; see Chapter 10); NBUVB phototherapy or oral CS for more severe cases.

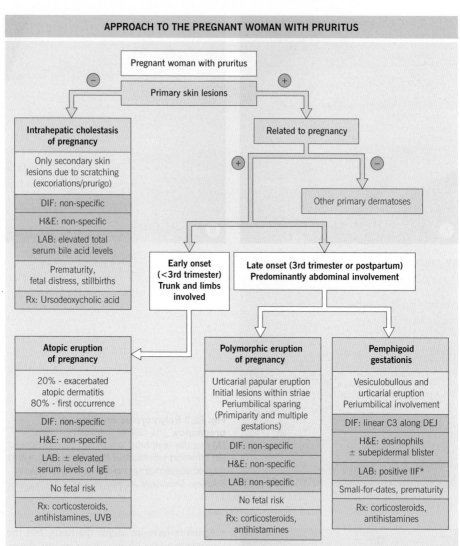

DEJ, dermo-epidermal junction; DIF, direct immunofluorescence; H&E, hematoxylin and eosin-stained histologic sections; IIF, indirect immunofluorescence; LAB, laboratory findings.
*Conventional - 30%; complement-added - nearly all.

Fig. 22.4 Approach to the pregnant woman with pruritus. Patients with refractory pemphigoid gestationis may benefit from plasmapheresis during pregnancy. Prednisolone is the systemic CS of choice for dermatologic indications during pregnancy as it is largely inactivated in the placenta (mother:fetus ratio = 10:1); if use of systemic CS or potent topical CS is long-term during pregnancy, then fetal growth should monitored. During the first trimester, the classic sedating anti-histamines (e.g. chlorpheniramine, clemastine) are preferred and during the second and third trimesters, if a non-sedating agent is requested, loratidine and cetirizine are considered safe. *Courtesy, Christina M. Ambros-Rudolph, MD.*

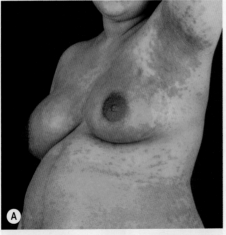
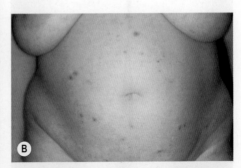

Fig. 22.5 Atopic eruption of pregnancy. A Eczematous lesions involving flexural areas as well as the abdomen and breasts. **B** Excoriated papules (prurigo lesions) that favored the abdomen and extremities. The former presentation is seen in approximately two-thirds of patients, whereas the latter is seen in approximately one-third. *Courtesy, Christina M. Ambros-Rudolph, MD.*

Intrahepatic Cholestasis of Pregnancy

• Onset usually during the third trimester, related in part to peak in estrogen levels; genetic predisposition with higher incidence in native South Americans; hepatitis C viral infection is also a risk factor.

• Cholestasis leads to elevated serum levels of bile acids and this leads to intense pruritus.

• Cutaneous lesions are nonspecific and vary from excoriations to prurigo nodularis (Fig. 22.6); jaundice occurs in a small minority of patients.

• Important to diagnose because cholestasis of pregnancy is associated with intrapartum fetal distress, prematurity, and stillbirths; in severe cases, vitamin K deficiency may occur, with an increased risk of hemorrhage.

• Diagnosis is based on measurement of total serum bile acids, with elevations typically ranging from 3 to 100 times normal.

• **DDx:** other causes of cholestasis (e.g. primary biliary cirrhosis) and hepatitis (e.g. hepatitis B, hepatitis C), especially if pruritus does not resolve within days of delivery; scabies, atopic eruption of pregnancy other causes of primary pruritus (see Fig. 4.1).

• **Rx:** oral ursodeoxycholic acid (15 mg/kg/ daily or 1 g daily); if elevated prothrombin time, vitamin K injections; alert patient that disorder recurs in at least 50% of subsequent pregnancies.

Physiological Changes During Pregnancy

These are outlined in Table 22.1.

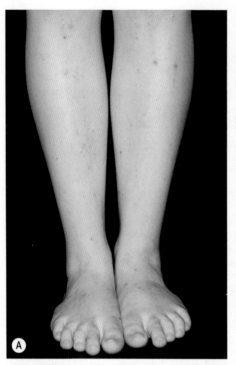
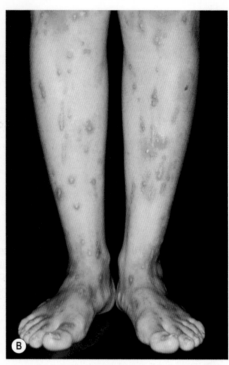

Fig. 22.6 Intrahepatic cholestasis of pregnancy. Marked pruritus leads to secondary skin lesions that vary based on disease duration, from subtle linear excoriations and prurigo simplex early on **(A)** to pronounced prurigo nodularis when the pruritus is longstanding **(B).** *From Ambros-Rudolph CM, Glatz M, Trauner M, Kerl H, Müllegger RR. The importance of serum bile acid level analysis and treatment with ursodeoxycholic acid in intrahepatic cholestasis of pregnancy: A case series from central Europe. Arch. Dermatol. 2007;143:757–762.* © *(2006) American Medical Association. All rights reserved.*

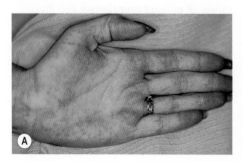

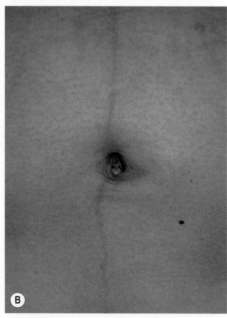

Fig. 22.7 Physiologic changes during pregnancy. Palmar erythema of pregnancy **(A)** and linea nigra **(B).** *B, Courtesy, Jean L. Bolognia, MD.*

PHYSIOLOGIC CHANGES DURING PREGNANCY	
Pigmentary	
Hyperpigmentation (e.g. areolae, linea nigra; Fig. 22.7B) Melasma	Hyperpigmentation (up to 90% of patients) and melasma (up to 70% of patients) are presumably of hormonal etiology. Melasma tends to persist postpartum in those with darkly pigmented skin types
Hair	
Hirsutism Postpartum telogen effluvium Postpartum androgenetic alopecia	Some hirsutism is normal and typically regresses postpartum. Telogen effluvium may last up to 15 months. Postpartum patterned alopecia may or may not revert to normal
Connective Tissue	
Striae	Striae gravidarum develop in up to 90% of patients and often resolve. Both hormonal factors and physical stretching of the skin appear to be relevant in their development
Vascular	
Spider angiomas Palmar erythema (Fig. 22.7A) Nonpitting edema Varicosities Vasomotor instability Purpura Gingival hyperemia or hyperplasia Pyogenic granuloma Hemorrhoids	Vascular changes result from distention, instability, and new vessel formation. Clinically obvious changes are most pronounced during the third trimester, and most changes regress spontaneously following delivery

Adapted from Kroumpouzos G, Cohen LM. Dermatoses of pregnancy. J. Am. Acad. Dermatol. 2001;45:1–19.

Table 22.1 Physiologic changes during pregnancy. Nail changes are nonspecific and include subungual hyperkeratosis, distal onycholysis, transverse grooving, and brittleness.

For further information see Ch. 27. From *Dermatology, Third Edition.*

23 | Pemphigus

Chapters 23–25 review the major autoimmune bullous diseases (Table 23.1). Because of the significant overlap in their clinical presentations, histologic examination of lesional skin (see Fig. 1.12B) as well as direct immunofluorescence (DIF) of perilesional skin (Figs. 23.1–23.3) are usually required in order to establish a specific diagnosis. Indirect immunofluorescence (IIF) and/or ELISA of sera provide additional helpful information; for example, the latter can detect anti-desmoglein 3 (Dsg3) versus anti-Dsg1 antibodies.

Pemphigus is classically divided into three major groups: (1) pemphigus vulgaris, with pemphigus vegetans representing a rare variant; (2) pemphigus foliaceus, with pemphigus erythematosus representing an unusual localized variant, and fogo selvagem, an endemic form; and (3) paraneoplastic pemphigus. Additional subtypes include the two forms of IgA pemphigus and drug-induced pemphigus.

Pemphigus Vulgaris and Pemphigus Vegetans

- Patients have circulating IgG autoantibodies that bind to the cell surface of keratinocytes in the skin and mucous membranes; this binding leads to an inhibition of the function of desmogleins, transmembrane cadherin proteins that are a component of desmosomes and therefore play an important role in cell–cell adhesion.
- In these two disorders, the autoantibodies primarily target Dsg3, which is expressed within the lower portion of the epidermis and is the predominant isoform in mucous membranes; patients with mucosal-dominant disease as well as those with mucocutaneous disease have anti-Dsg3 autoantibodies (the latter group can also have anti-Dsg1 autoantibodies).

- The decrease in cell–cell adhesion leads to the separation of individual keratinocytes from one another (referred to as acantholysis) and the formation of a split within the epidermis or mucosal epithelium, primarily in its lower portion, just above the basal layer (see Fig. 1.12B).
- Clinically, almost all patients with pemphigus vulgaris have painful erosions of the oral mucosa and at least half will have flaccid bullae of the skin plus erosions due to their rupture; lesions can be localized or widespread (Fig. 23.4), and there may be involvement of other mucosal surfaces, e.g. conjunctival, nasal, vaginal.
- Additional clinical clues include the development of hemorrhagic crusts of the vermilion lips (Table 23.2) and a positive Nikolsky sign in areas of active disease – the epidermis can be easily moved laterally with rubbing (due to reduction in intercellular adhesion).
- In pemphigus vegetans, vegetative and papillomatous plaques and nodules develop at sites of erosions (Fig. 23.5); lesions favor major body folds and pustules can also be seen.
- DIF of perilesional skin demonstrates immunostaining of the cell surface of keratinocytes within the epidermis or mucosa in almost all patients, and the staining may be more predominant in the lower portion of the epithelium (see Fig. 23.3A); IIF and ELISA of sera is positive in more than 90% of patients (see Fig. 23.2).
- **DDx:** other forms of pemphigus, bullous pemphigoid, linear IgA bullous dermatosis (LABD), Hailey–Hailey disease; if there is only oral disease, lichen planus, mucous membrane pemphigoid, aphthous stomatitis.
- **Rx:** oral CS, steroid-sparing agents (e.g. mycophenolate mofetil, azathioprine, cyclophosphamide), IVIg, plasmapheresis (plus immunosuppression), and rituximab.

CHARACTERISTICS OF MAJOR AUTOIMMUNE BULLOUS DISEASES

	PV	BP	DH	LABD
Cutaneous lesion	Flaccid vesicles and erosions	Large tense bullae	Grouped papules and small vesicles, often excoriated	Small vesicles and/or large bullae
Distribution	Mucosae; can be widespread	Trunk, extremities, occasionally mucosal surfaces	Extensor surfaces, symmetrical	Similar to DH or BP
Histology	Intraepidermal vesicle with acantholysis	Subepidermal bullae with eosinophilic infiltrate	Subepidermal bullae with neutrophilic infiltrate	Subepidermal bullae with neutrophilic infiltrate
Direct IF	Intracellular C3, IgG; occasionally IgA* ('chickenwire' pattern)	Linear IgG and C3 at BMZ	Granular IgA in dermal papillae	Linear IgA at BMZ, possibly also IgG
Site to biopsy for direct IF	Perilesional	Perilesional	Adjacent normal-appearing skin	Perilesional
Indirect IF	Intracellular IgG (90%)	Linear IgG at BMZ (70%)	Negative	Linear IgA at BMZ (70%)
ELISA	Distinguishes anti-Dsg1 vs. anti-Dsg3 Ab	Detects anti-BP180 and -BP230 IgG antibodies	Anti-tissue transglutaminase (TG2) & anti-epidermal transglutaminase (TG3) antibodies	n/a
Enteropathy	None	None	>90%	Rare
Dapsone responsiveness	Mild**	Minimal to moderate	Excellent	Good, may also require systemic corticosteroids

*Referred to as IgA pemphigus.
**Greater response if IgA +/or neutrophils.
Ab, antibody; BP, bullous pemphigoid; DH, dermatitis herpetiformis; ELISA, enzyme-linked immunosorbent assay; LABD, linear IgA bullous disease; n/a, not commercially available; PV, pemphigus vulgaris.

Table 23.1 Characteristics of major autoimmune bullous diseases.

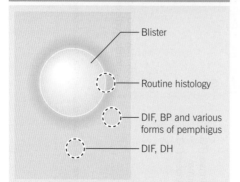

- Blister
- Routine histology
- DIF, BP and various forms of pemphigus
- DIF, DH

Fig. 23.1 Preferred sites for obtaining biopsy specimens in autoimmune bullous diseases. If the edematous papule or vesicle is small enough, it can be removed in its entirety for routine histology. Otherwise, a biopsy specimen that includes the inflammatory rim as well as the edge of a fresh vesicle or bulla is appropriate. In bullous pemphigoid (BP) and pemphigus vulgaris, a perilesional biopsy is done for direct immunofluorescence (DIF), whereas in dermatitis herpetiformis (DH), nearby normal skin is preferred for DIF.

Pemphigus Foliaceus, Pemphigus Erythematosus, and Fogo Selvagem

- In pemphigus foliaceus, the circulating autoantibodies are directed solely against Dsg1 (see above) and can be detected in the vast majority of patients by IIF (~85%) or ELISA (~95%); of note, the expression of Dsg1 is greater in the upper epidermis and minimal in the mucosa.
- As a result, acantholysis and *intra*epidermal blister formation occurs within the upper layers of the epidermis, usually at the granular layer; by DIF, immunostaining of the cell surface of the keratinocytes is seen in >90% of patients and may be more marked in these upper layers.
- Clinically, the more superficial and fragile nature of the blisters leads to a predominance of erosions with scale-crust rather than bullae (Fig. 23.6); the scale is said to resemble cornflakes cereal; mucosal involvement is absent.
- While lesions favor the scalp, face, and upper trunk, they can become widespread, even leading to an exfoliative erythroderma, or they can be localized to the face (pemphigus erythematosus; Fig. 23.7).

**BASIC TECHNIQUES OF DIRECT IMMUNOFLUORESCENCE (DIF)
AND INDIRECT IMMUNOFLUORESCENCE (IIF)**

Direct immunofluorescence (DIF)

Addition of antibody with fluorescent probe

Patient's skin

Pemphigus | Bullous pemphigoid

Indirect immunofluorescence (IIF)

② Addition of secondary antibody with fluorescent probe

① Addition of patient's serum

Normal skin*

Pemphigus | Bullous pemphigoid

*or monkey esophagus, guinea pig esophagus or rat bladder

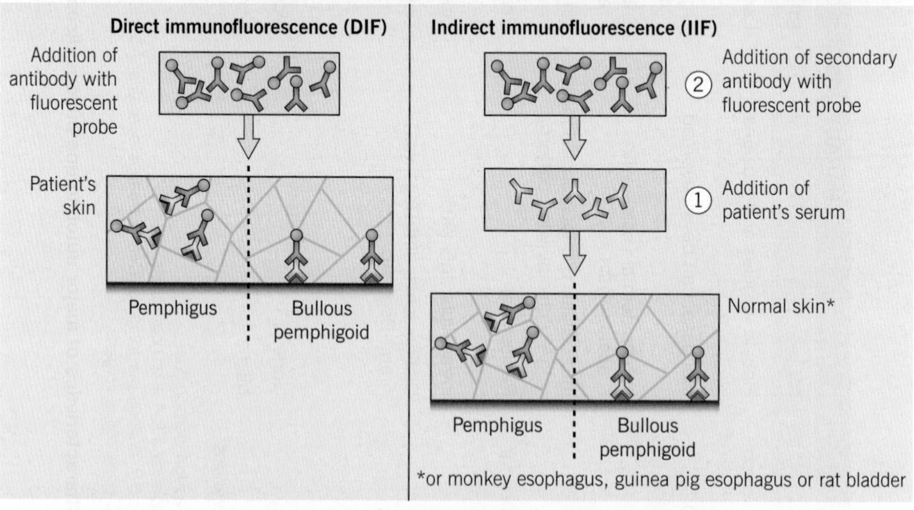

Fig. 23.2 Basic techniques of direct immunofluorescence (DIF) and indirect immunofluorescence (IIF). DIF is performed on skin biopsies to detect tissue-bound immunodeposits (see Fig. 23.1). IIF is performed utilizing patients' sera to detect circulating autoantibodies that bind epithelial antigens. The preferred substrate for IIF is monkey esophagus for pemphigus vulgaris, guinea pig esophagus for pemphigus foliaceus, and human skin for the pemphigoid group and LABD.

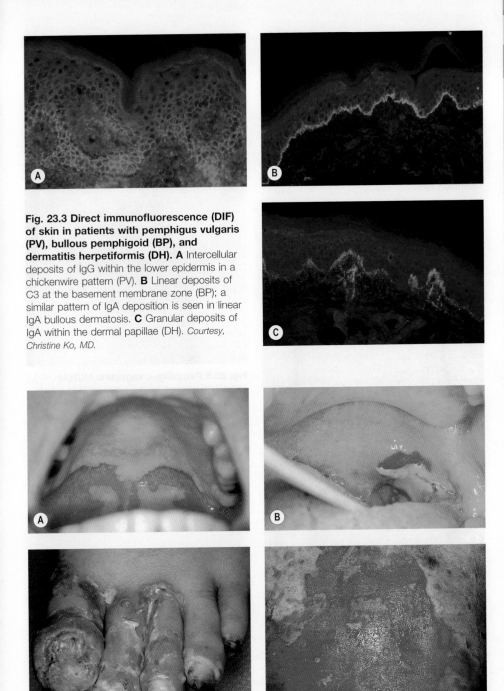

Fig. 23.3 Direct immunofluorescence (DIF) of skin in patients with pemphigus vulgaris (PV), bullous pemphigoid (BP), and dermatitis herpetiformis (DH). A Intercellular deposits of IgG within the lower epidermis in a chickenwire pattern (PV). **B** Linear deposits of C3 at the basement membrane zone (BP); a similar pattern of IgA deposition is seen in linear IgA bullous dermatosis. **C** Granular deposits of IgA within the dermal papillae (DH). *Courtesy, Christine Ko, MD.*

Fig. 23.4 Pemphigus vulgaris. A, B Almost all patients develop painful erosions of the oral mucosa, with the most common locations being the buccal and palatine mucosae; note the sloughing of the mucosa in **(B). C** The flaccid vesicles are fragile and rupture easily, leading to erosions. **D** Extensive involvement is associated with significant fluid loss and risk of secondary infection and bacteremia. *A, Courtesy, Masayuki Amagai, MD; B, C, Courtesy, Louis Fragola, Jr., MD; D, Courtesy, Department of Dermatology, Hamamatsu University School of Medicine.*

HEMORRHAGIC CRUSTS OF THE VERMILION LIPS

- Herpes simplex
- Herpes zoster
- Pemphigus vulgaris
- Paraneoplastic pemphigus (see Fig. 23.8)
- Stevens–Johnson syndrome/TEN spectrum
- Erythema multiforme major (see Fig. 3.11)

Table 23.2 Hemorrhagic crusts of the vermilion lips.

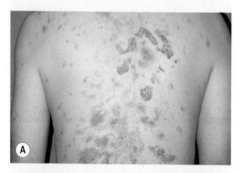

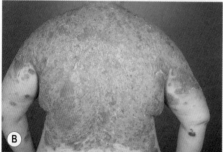

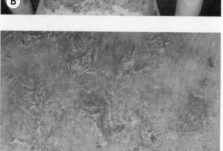

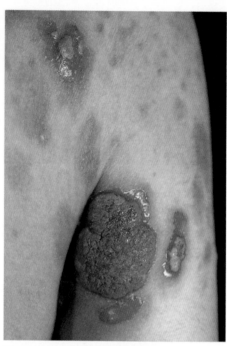

Fig. 23.5 Pemphigus vegetans. Multiple vegetating masses arising within eroded areas. Post-inflammatory hyperpigmentation is seen at previous sites of involvement. *Courtesy, Masayuki Amagai, MD.*

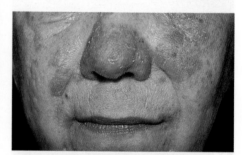

Fig. 23.6 Pemphigus foliaceus. A Scale-crusts overlying widespread erosions. **B** When the disease becomes severe, there is coalescence of lesions; note the large erosions. **C** The scales have been likened to cornflakes cereal. *A, Courtesy, Masayuki Amagai, MD.*

Fig. 23.7 Pemphigus erythematosus. Erythematous plaques with scale-crust on the nose and cheeks. Initially this disorder was thought to be a combination of pemphigus vulgaris plus lupus erythematosus, but now it is classified as a localized variant of pemphigus foliaceus. *Courtesy, Ronald P. Rapini, MD.*

• Fogo selvagem is an endemic form of pemphigus foliaceus seen primarily in rural areas of Brazil and is thought to be related to an immune reaction to antigens introduced by insect bites.

• **DDx:** other forms of pemphigus, impetigo (early limited disease), subacute cutaneous LE, and occasionally psoriasis.

• **Rx:** topical or oral CS, occasionally dapsone; if severe, steroid-sparing agents.

Paraneoplastic Pemphigus

• Develops in patients with an underlying neoplasm, often malignant, and improves slowly following successful treatment of the neoplasm; the most common tumor in children and adolescents is Castleman's disease, whereas the most common ones in adults are non-Hodgkin's lymphoma and chronic lymphocytic leukemia > Castleman's disease and thymomas.

• Cutaneous lesions are variable and they can resemble lichen planus, erythema multiforme, or bullous pemphigoid as well as pemphigus; severe, recalcitrant oral stomatitis is a characteristic feature and conjunctival involvement is common (Fig. 23.8).

• Bronchiolitis obliterans is a serious internal manifestation.

• IgG autoantibodies are directed against at least eight antigens, including desmogleins and plakins; by DIF, there are immunodeposits on the surface of keratinocytes as well as along the basement membrane zone.

• In this disorder, the anti-plakin antibodies also bind to simple epithelia such as rat urinary bladder epithelium and this allows distinction from pemphigus vulgaris.

• **DDx:** other forms of pemphigus, mucous membrane pemphigoid, erythema multiforme major, Stevens–Johnson syndrome, lichen planus, GVHD.

• **Rx:** treatment of the underlying neoplasm, but the stomatitis may prove recalcitrant despite successful eradication of the associated neoplasm.

IgA Pemphigus

• Two forms of this vesiculopustular eruption exist – subcorneal pustular dermatosis type and intraepidermal neutrophilic type, with the intraepidermal pustules histologically involving the upper versus entire epidermis, respectively.

• Clinically, lesions arise within inflamed or normal skin and assume a figurate arrangement (Fig. 23.9); the most common sites are the axillae and groin.

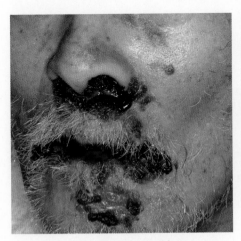

Fig. 23.8 Paraneoplastic pemphigus. Hemorrhagic crusts extend from the nasal and oral mucosae onto the cutaneous and vermilion lips. The chin lesion resembles pemphigus vulgaris. *Courtesy, Masayuki Amagai, MD.*

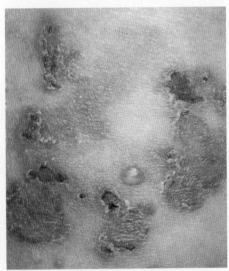

Fig. 23.9 IgA pemphigus – subcorneal pustular dermatosis type. Annular configuration of pink-brown patches and thin plaques with erosions and scale-crust; in the vesiculopustule, the pustular contents have settled into a dependent location (half pustular/ half clear). *Courtesy, Masayuki Amagai, MD.*

- By DIF, there is immunostaining of the cell surface of keratinocytes within the epidermis, as in pemphigus vulgaris, but the immunodeposits are IgA rather than IgG.
- **DDx:** Sneddon–Wilkinson disease (negative DIF), pemphigus foliaceus, impetigo (when more limited), LABD, pustular psoriasis.
- **Rx:** dapsone or sulfapyridine and sometimes oral CS.

Drug-Induced Pemphigus

- Occasionally, medications can induce pemphigus vulgaris or pemphigus foliaceus and discontinuation of those drugs can lead to clinical resolution.
- The most common medications are captopril and penicillamine, both of which contain sulfhydryl groups.

For further information see Ch. 31. From *Dermatology, Third Edition.*

Bullous Pemphigoid, Mucous Membrane Pemphigoid, and Epidermolysis Bullosa Acquisita

24

This chapter, in addition to Chapters 23 and 25, cover the autoimmune bullous diseases. The concepts of direct immunofluorescence (DIF) and indirect immunofluorescence (IIF) are reviewed in Chapter 23 (see Fig. 23.2), as are the recommended sites for performing skin biopsies for DIF (see Fig. 23.1).

Bullous Pemphigoid (BP)

• Immunobullous disease due to circulating autoantibodies that bind two components of hemidesmosomes, i.e. structures that provide adhesion between the epidermis and the dermis; the two antigens are collagen XVII (also referred to BP antigen 2 [BPA2] or BP180) and BPA1/BP230.

• Occurs more commonly in the elderly and can be drug-induced (e.g. furosemide); rarely, lesions are induced by ultraviolet light or radiation therapy.

• Both pruritic fixed urticarial plaques and tense bullae are seen (Figs. 24.1 and 24.2); the latter can develop within normal skin or areas of erythematous skin and produce erosions when they rupture; oral lesions are much less common than in pemphigus vulgaris (10–30% of patients).

• Pruritus and nonspecific eczematous (see Fig. 24.1D) or papular lesions can precede the more characteristic cutaneous lesions and may be the predominant finding; unusual variants include dyshidrosiform (palms and soles), vegetans (major body folds), and localized (e.g. pretibial in adults; vulvar in children, acral in infants), as well as those that mimic prurigo nodularis and toxic epidermal necrolysis (Fig. 24.3).

• Histologically, a subepidermal bulla plus an infiltrate of eosinophils is seen when the lesions are bullous; DIF demonstrates immunodeposits of IgG and/or C3 in a linear array along the basement membrane zone (see Fig. 23.3B); in general, by salt-split skin immunofluorescence studies, the immunodeposits are in the roof (epidermal side) of the blister (Fig. 24.4).

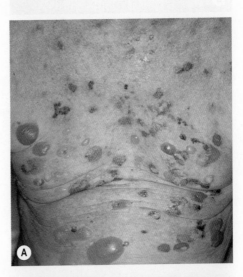

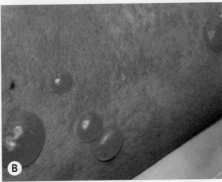

Fig. 24.1 Bullous pemphigoid. A Classic presentation with multiple tense bullae arising on normal and erythematous skin; several of the bullae have ruptured, leaving circular erosions. **B** Urticarial papules and plaques, along with bullae containing serous fluid. *Continued*

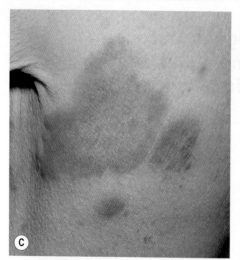

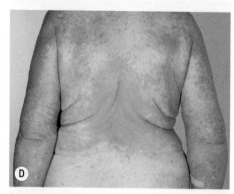

Fig. 24.1 *Continued* **C** Firm annular urticarial plaques. **D** Eczematous presentation with large dermatitic plaques. *C, D, Courtesy, Philippe Bernard, MD, and Luca Borradori, MD.*

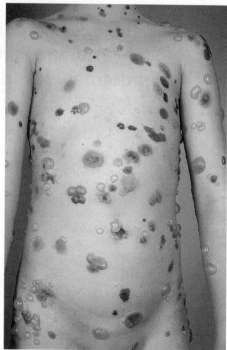

Fig. 24.2 Childhood bullous pemphigoid. Generalized bullae, both tense (fresh) and flaccid (old with re-epithelialization), as well as erosions with hemorrhagic crusts.

- Both enzyme-linked immunosorbant assay and IIF can detect circulating autoantibodies in the sera in at least 70–80% of patients (see Table 23.1).
- At least 50% of patients have a peripheral eosinophilia.
- **DDx:** linear IgA bullous dermatosis (LABD), epidermolysis bullosa acquisita (EBA), mucous membrane pemphigoid, various forms of pemphigus, hypersensitivity reactions (including to drugs), primary pruritus, allergic contact dermatitis, scabies, urticaria (but individual lesions transient).
- **Rx:** see Table 24.1.

Mucous Membrane (Cicatricial) Pemphigoid

- Chronic immunobullous disease due to autoantibodies that bind several components of the BMZ of the skin and mucosae, most often BP180 and laminin 332 (laminin 5); although heterogenous in its presentation, a tendency to scarring is typically seen.
- The mucous membranes represent the major site of involvement, in particular conjunctival (erosions, scarring with symblepharon formation, blindness) and oral mucosae (persistent erosions of the buccal and palatal mucosae, desquamative gingivitis) (Figs. 24.5 and 24.6).
- Additional sites of involvement are the nasopharynx, larynx, and esophagus; a few authors have suggested that patients with anti-laminin 332 immunodeposits have an increased risk of internal malignancy.
- Cutaneous lesions are seen in a quarter of patients and favor the head and neck region and upper trunk; erythematous plaques that

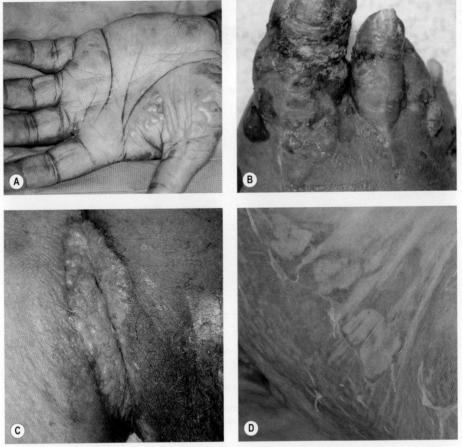

Fig. 24.3 Bullous pemphigoid – unusual clinical variants. Grouped vesicles and bullae on the palms **(A)** and toes **(B)** that can resemble pompholyx (dyshidrosiform pemphigoid). **C** Vegetating plaque in the inguinal crease (pemphigoid vegetans). **D** Toxic epidermal necrolysis-like lesions with large erosions. *A, D, Courtesy, Philippe Bernard, MD, and Luca Borradori, MD.*

CLEAVAGE PLANE IN SALT-SPLIT SKIN AND USUAL SITES BOUND BY AUTOANTIBODIES IN INDIRECT IMMUNOFLUORESCENCE STUDIES

Basal keratinocytes

Lamina lucida

Lamina densa

Sublamina densa

BPAG1
BPAG2

Laminin 332
Type IV collagen
Type VII collagen

Bullous pemphigoid
Pemphigoid gestationis
Linear IgA bullous dermatosis
Mucous membrane pemphigoid*

Mucous membrane pemphigoid**
Epidermolysis bullosa acquisita
The bullous eruption of systemic lupus erythematosus

* Anti-BP180 antibodies
** Anti-laminin 332 (5) antibodies

Fig. 24.4 Cleavage plane in salt-split skin and usual sites bound by autoantibodies in indirect immunofluorescence studies. The cleavage plane in 1 M NaCl salt-split skin is in the lower portion of the lamina lucida. Circulating autoantibodies from patients with various subepidermal immunobullous diseases bind to different sites, e.g. the epidermal versus dermal side of the split. *Courtesy, Kim Yancey, MD.*

THERAPEUTIC LADDER FOR BULLOUS PEMPHIGOID

Mild and/or localized disease

- Superpotent topical corticosteroids (1*)
- Nicotinamide in association with minocycline, doxycycline, or tetracycline (3)
- Erythromycin, penicillins (3)
- Dapsone, sulfonamides (3)
- Topical immunomodulators (e.g. tacrolimus) (3)

Extensive/persistent cutaneous disease

- Superpotent topical corticosteroids (1*)
- Oral corticosteroids[†] (1[‡])
- Azathioprine (2)
- Mycophenolate mofetil (2)
- Methotrexate[§] (2)
- Chlorambucil (3)
- Cyclophosphamide (3)
- IVIg (3)
- Plasma exchange (2)
- Rituximab (3)

Note: Superpotent topical corticosteroids should be considered in any patient and may be combined with a systemic therapy.
*Validated.
[†]Prednisone doses of at least 0.5–0.75 mg/kg/day seem to be necessary to control extensive disease but increase serious side effects, including mortality.
[‡]Validated for prednisone.
[§]In elderly patients, low-dose regimen (2.5–10 mg/week) can be effective.

Table 24.1 Therapeutic ladder for bullous pemphigoid. Key to evidence-based support: (1) prospective controlled trial; (2) retrospective study or large case series; (3) small case series or individual case reports.

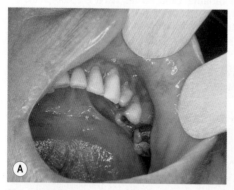 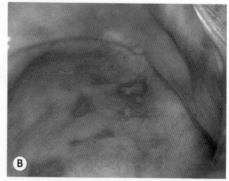

Fig. 24.5 Mucous membrane (cicatricial) pemphigoid – mucosal involvement. A Erythema and erosions of the gingival margins (desquamative or erosive gingivitis). **B** Chronic erosions on the hard palate. *B, Courtesy, C. Prost, MD.*

develop vesicles, erosions, and scarring are characteristic (Fig. 24.7).

• Histologic and DIF features are similar to BP, but there is usually a sparser infiltrate and less eosinophils but fibrosis may be present; DIF positivity (IgG and/or C3 >> IgA) is greater for mucosa (50–90%) than for skin; circulating autoantibodies are detected by IIF in a minority of patients (20–30%).

• **DDx:** pemphigus vulgaris, occasionally BP, EBA, and LABD; if limited to oral mucosa, lichen planus or pemphigus vulgaris (see Fig. 59.5); if limited to scalp, consider other causes of scarring alopecia.

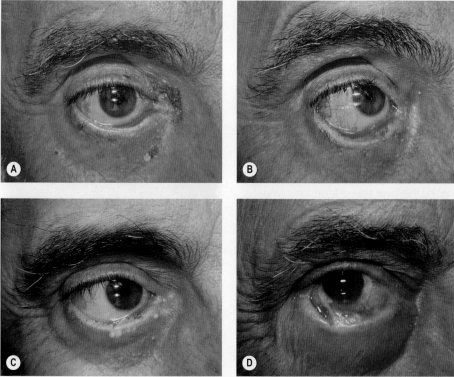

Fig. 24.6 Progression of mucous membrane (cicatricial) pemphigoid. A Erosion of the lower eyelid margin and erythema plus scale-crust of the inner canthus and lower eyelid. **B** Three months later, ectropion and thickening of the lower eyelid in addition to erosions. **C** Six months later, smaller erosions but scarring and milia formation. **D** Seven years later, further scarring with significant shortening of the inferior fornix due to symblepharon. *Courtesy, Louis Fragola, Jr., MD.*

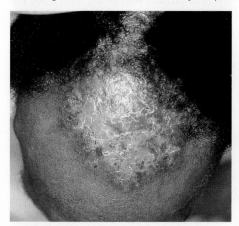

Fig. 24.7 Mucous membrane (cicatricial) pemphigoid – cutaneous involvement. An erythematous plaque with atrophy and crusting; note the scarring alopecia. In the Brunsting–Perry variant, there are cutaneous lesions in the head and neck region but minimal or no mucosal involvement. *Courtesy, Philippe Bernard, MD, and Luca Borradori, MD.*

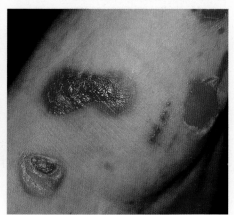

Fig. 24.8 Epidermolysis bullosa acquisita – inflammatory presentation. Bullous and erosive lesions in a patient with multiple myeloma. This form resembles bullous pemphigoid. *Courtesy, Philippe Bernard, MD, and Luca Borradori, MD.*

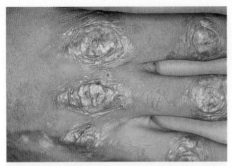

Fig. 24.9 Epidermolysis bullosa acquisita – mechanobullous presentation. Milia and scarring that favor sites of trauma overlying joints, in association with skin fragility.

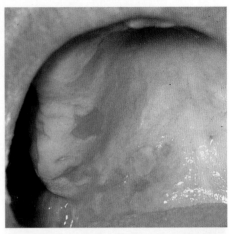

Fig. 24.10 Epidermolysis bullosa acquisita – oral lesions. Multiple erosions of the palate reminiscent of mucous membrane pemphigoid. *Courtesy, C. Prost, MD.*

• **Rx:** potent topical or intralesional CS, dapsone, cyclophosphamide (severe or progressive ocular disease), alone or in combination with systemic CS, and rituximab.

Epidermolysis Bullosa Acquisita (EBA)

• Autoimmune bullous disease due to autoantibodies that bind to collagen VII; the latter forms anchoring fibrils within the upper dermis and they play an important role in adhesion of the epidermis to the dermis.

• Two major clinical forms: (1) mechanobullous which resembles the genetic disorder epidermolysis bullosa; and (2) inflammatory which resembles bullous pemphigoid (Fig. 24.8).

• In the more common mechanobullous form, bullae arise in sites of friction and are followed by erosions, scarring, and milia formation (Fig. 24.9); oral lesions can also be seen (Fig. 24.10).

• Associated systemic disorders include inflammatory bowel disease, in particular Crohn's disease, and plasma cell dyscrasias.

• Histological and DIF features are similar to BP, but there is usually a sparser infiltrate and few eosinophils in the mechanobullous form; DIF studies demonstrate linear IgG > C3 or IgA at the basement membrane zone; circulating autoantibodies are detected in ~50% of patients and by salt-split skin immunofluorescence studies, the immunodeposits are in the floor (dermal side) of the blister (see Fig. 24.4).

• **DDx:** inherited forms of epidermolysis bullosa, porphyria cutanea tarda (and other rare variants of porphyria), pseudoporphyria, bullous pemphigoid, LABD, mucous membrane pemphigoid, bullous systemic lupus erythematosus (also autoantibodies against collagen VII).

• **Rx:** difficult to treat; potent topical CS, oral CS, steroid-sparing agents (e.g. mycophenolate mofetil), dapsone, rituximab.

For further information see Chs. 28 and 30. From *Dermatology, Third Edition.*

Dermatitis Herpetiformis and Linear IgA Bullous Dermatosis

25

This is the third chapter, along with Chapters 23 and 24, that deals with autoimmune bullous diseases (see Table 23.1).

Dermatitis Herpetiformis (DH)

• Autoimmune bullous disease that is a cutaneous manifestation of celiac disease, with >90% of patients having histologic evidence of some degree of gluten-sensitive enteropathy; ~20% of patients with DH have symptomatic celiac disease.
• In predisposed individuals (e.g. those with HLA-DQ2), IgA antibodies form against gliadin cross-linked to *tissue* tranglutaminase; the presumed autoantigen in the skin is *epidermal* transglutaminase (Fig. 25.1).
• Primary lesions consist of pruritic vesicles on an erythematous base and edematous erythematous papules that are often grouped (i.e. herpetiform); however, due to scratching, only excoriated papules and hemorrhagic crusts may be present (Fig. 25.2).
• Favored sites of involvement are the elbows, extensor forearms, knees, posterior neck, and presacral/buttock region, with lesions in a symmetric distribution pattern.
• Histologically, collections of neutrophils are seen within the dermal papillae of involved skin; by direct immunofluorescence (DIF), *granular* deposits of IgA are detected within dermal papillae of adjacent, normal-appearing skin in at least 90% of patients (see Figs. 23.1 and 23.3).
• Patients have circulating anti-tissue transglutaminase and anti-endomysial antibodies, with the level of the latter correlating with degree of enteropathy; they can also develop other autoimmune disorders, in particular Hashimoto's thyroiditis.
• **DDx:** linear IgA bullous dermatosis, bullous pemphigoid, prurigo simplex, and bullous systemic lupus erythematosus; crusted lesions of the elbows are also seen in patients with

Wegener's granulomatosis and Churg–Strauss syndrome.
• **Rx:** gluten-free diet (also reduces risk of enteropathy-associated T-cell lymphoma), dapsone (initially 25–50 mg per day after screening for glucose-6-phosphate dehydrogenase [G6PD] deficiency; average dose on a normal diet is 100 mg), and sulfapyridine; improvement of pruritus within a few days of instituting dapsone supports the diagnosis of DH.

Linear IgA Bullous Dermatosis (LABD)

• Autoimmune bullous disease that occurs in both children and adults and can be drug-induced (Table 25.1); in children, it is sometimes referred to as 'chronic bullous disease of childhood'.
• Vesicles and bullae arise on the trunk and extremities and in children often favor the lower trunk and groin; lesions can assume a figurate arrangement and have been likened to a crown of jewels (Figs. 25.3–25.5).
• Spontaneous remission in children, usually after 2–4 years; ~50% of adults have a spontaneous remission.
• Histologically, a subepidermal bulla is accompanied by an infiltrate of neutrophils; by DIF, *linear* deposits of IgA are detected at the basement membrane zone of perilesional skin (see Figs. 23.1 and 23.3).
• By indirect immunofluorescence (IIF), circulating IgA autoantibodies are detected in ~70% of patients with LABD (see Fig. 23.2); the autoantigen in LABD is a cleavage product of one of the two autoantigens of bullous pemphigoid (BP180; see Chapter 24).
• **DDx:** bullous pemphigoid (linear deposits of IgG), DH (granular deposits of IgA), and mucous membrane (cicatricial) pemphigoid; for vancomycin-induced LABD, toxic epidermal necrolysis.

229

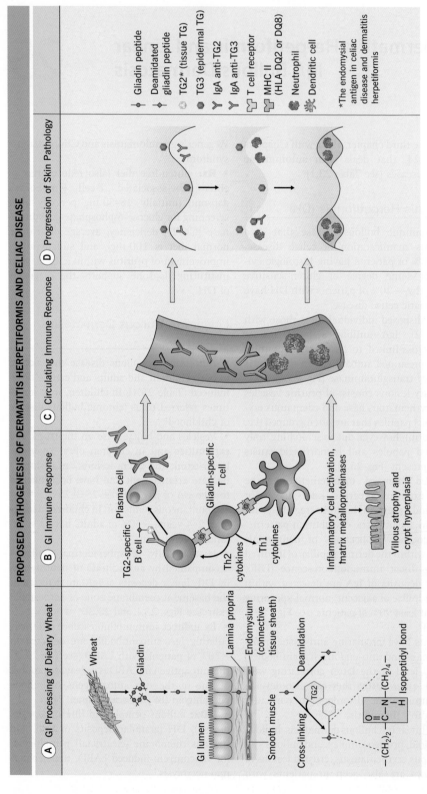

Fig. 25.1 Proposed pathogenesis of dermatitis herpetiformis and celiac disease. *See next page for figure legend.*

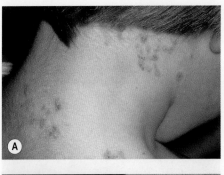

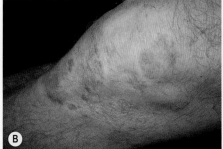

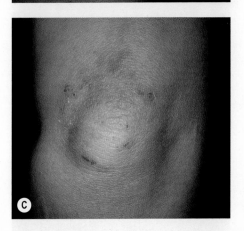

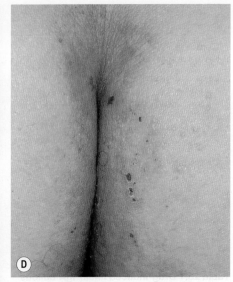

Fig. 25.2 Dermatitis herpetiformis. A Grouped vesicles and pink papulovesicles on the upper back, neck, and scalp of a child. **B** Pink plaques on the knee composed of grouped papules and papulovesicles. **C** Pink papulovesicles admixed with erosions and hemorrhagic crusts on the elbow. **D** Pruritic pink papules of the buttocks, some of which have central hemorrhagic crusts. *C, Courtesy, Thomas Horn, MD; D, Courtesy, Louis A. Fragola, Jr., MD.*

Fig. 25.1 Proposed pathogenesis of dermatitis herpetiformis and celiac disease. A Dietary wheat, barley, or rye is processed by digestive enzymes into antigenic gliadin peptides, which are transported intact across the mucosal epithelium. Within the lamina propria, tissue transglutaminase (TG2) (1) deamidates glutamine residues within gliadin peptides to glutamic acid and (2) becomes covalently cross-linked to gliadin peptides via isopeptidyl bonds (formed between gliadin glutamine and TG2 lysine residues). **B** CD4$^+$ T cells in the lamina propria recognize deamidated gliadin peptides presented by HLA-DQ2 or -DQ8 molecules on antigen-presenting cells, resulting in the production of Th1 cytokines and matrix metalloproteinases that cause mucosal epithelial cell damage and tissue remodeling. In addition, TG2-specific B cells take up TG2–gliadin complexes and present gliadin peptides to gliadin-specific helper T cells, which stimulate the B cells to produce IgA anti-TG2. **C** Over time, IgA directed against TG3 (IgA anti-TG3) forms as a result of epitope spreading and both IgA anti-TG2 and IgA anti-TG3 circulate in the bloodstream. **D** When IgA anti-TG3 antibodies reach the dermis, they complex with TG3 antigens which have been produced by keratinocytes (epidermal TG) and then have diffused into the dermis. That is, IgA/TG3 immune complexes are formed *locally* within the papillary dermis. This leads to neutrophil chemotaxis (with formation of neutrophilic abscesses), proteolytic cleavage of the lamina lucida, and subepidermal blister formation.

DRUG-INDUCED LINEAR IgA BULLOUS DERMATOSIS

Common
- Vancomycin*

Less common
- Penicillins
- Cephalosporins
- Captopril > other ACE inhibitors
- NSAIDs: diclofenac, naproxen, oxaprozin, piroxicam

Uncommon
- Phenytoin
- Sulfonamide antibiotics: sulfamethoxazole, sulfisoxazole

Unusual variants include toxic epidermal necrolysis-like and morbilliform.
ACE, angiotensin-converting enzyme; NSAIDs, nonsteroidal anti-inflammatory drugs.

Table 25.1 Drug-induced linear IgA bullous dermatosis. Based on case reports, additional drugs have been implicated and they are listed in Table 31.5 of *Dermatology, Third Edition*.

- Important to review medications and withdraw possible culprits before instituting systemic therapy.
- **Rx:** dapsone (often higher doses than for DH) or sulfapyridine, occasionally requiring the addition of prednisone; antibiotics (e.g. dicloxacillin, erythromycin, tetracycline) can be tried initially.

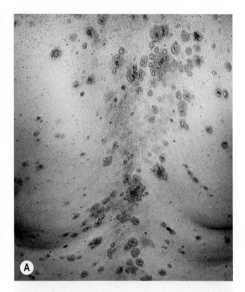

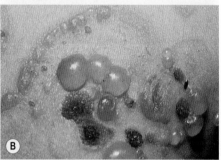

Fig. 25.3 Linear IgA bullous dermatosis.
A Grouped and annular bullae on an erythematous base. **B** The figurate array of the bullae is characteristic of this disorder. *A, B, Courtesy, John J. Zone, MD.*

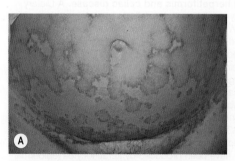

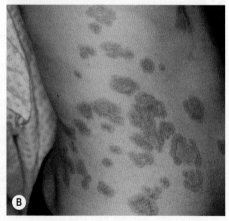

Fig. 25.4 Linear IgA bullous dermatosis. A, B In two women with the disorder, annular and polycyclic plaques of the trunk, with varying degrees of edema. *A, B, Courtesy, John J. Zone, MD.*

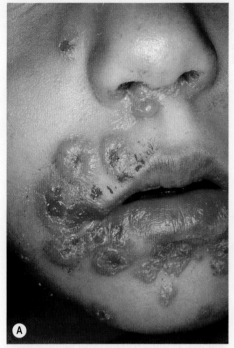

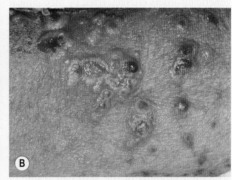

Fig. 25.5 Linear IgA bullous dermatosis. A Annular and herpetiform vesiculobullae on the face of a child. **B** Vancomycin-induced variant with a similar arrangement of vesiculopustules. Note the central hemorrhagic crusts in both patients.

For further information see Ch. 31. From *Dermatology, Third Edition*.

26 | Epidermolysis Bullosa

• Epidermolysis bullosa (EB) is a group of genetic disorders characterized by mechanical fragility of the skin that leads to blister formation with minor trauma or friction.

• Inherited EB is traditionally divided into three major categories – EB simplex (EBS), junctional EB (JEB), and dystrophic EB (DEB) – that differ in the ultrastructural site of blister formation (Fig. 26.1).

• The overall incidence is approximately 1 in 50 000 births, with EBS representing the most common form.

• Mutations in the genes encoding at least 15 structural proteins of the skin can result in EB, with variable clinical phenotypes, ultrastructural findings, and inheritance patterns.

• The major subtypes of EB and Kindler syndrome (now classified as a fourth form of EB) are summarized in Table 26.1.

• The subtype of EB can be determined by immunofluorescence antigenic mapping and/ or transmission electron microscopy on a punch biopsy specimen obtained after inducing a blister on intact skin (e.g. via twisting a pencil eraser on the inner upper arm); blister induction may be difficult for localized EBS and dominant DEB.

Clinical Features of EB

• The severity and distribution of blistering vary depending on the EB subtype (see Table 26.1), the patient's age (e.g. improving over time, especially for EBS), and environmental factors (e.g. sweating, friction).

• Scarring (usually atrophic), milia and nail dystrophy may develop in any subtype of EB, but they are most common in DEB (Fig. 26.8; see Figs. 26.5 and 26.6).

• The molecular defects in EB can also affect other organs/tissues with an epithelial surface, such as the oral mucosa (most common), eye,

and gastrointestinal and genitourinary tracts (see Table 26.1).

• **DDx:** sucking blisters and other genetic (e.g. epidermolytic ichthyosis), infectious (e.g. bullous impetigo, staphylococcal scalded skin syndrome) or autoimmune blistering disorders of infancy (see Chapter 28).

Management of EB

• Management focuses on avoidance of mechanical trauma (e.g. padding, soft clothing, no adhesive use) and prevention of infection (e.g. bathing/soaking with dilute sodium hypochlorite [0.5 cup household bleach in full standard bathtub] or 0.25% acetic acid [1 : 20 white vinegar : water]).

• Only nonadherent/'low-tack' dressing materials should be applied to EB skin, e.g. petrolatum-impregnated gauze (adding extra petrolatum to prevent sticking) and soft silicone dressings (e.g. Mepitel®, Mepilex®), followed by rolled gauze.

• Lancing and draining blisters (with placement of a small window) can relieve pressure and promote healing; antibiotics should be used judiciously, avoiding chronic treatment with topical mupirocin or oral antibiotics.

• A multidisciplinary approach is helpful, especially for more severe forms of EB, with attention to oral/dental care, growth, nutritional status, and potential complications.

• Older children and adults with recessive DEB require periodic total-body skin examinations, with biopsy of nonhealing ulcers to exclude SCC.

• Cell-based (including hematopoietic stem cell transplantation) and gene therapies for EB are currently under investigation.

• Physicians and families can obtain helpful information from websites such as www.debra.org and www.debra-international.org.

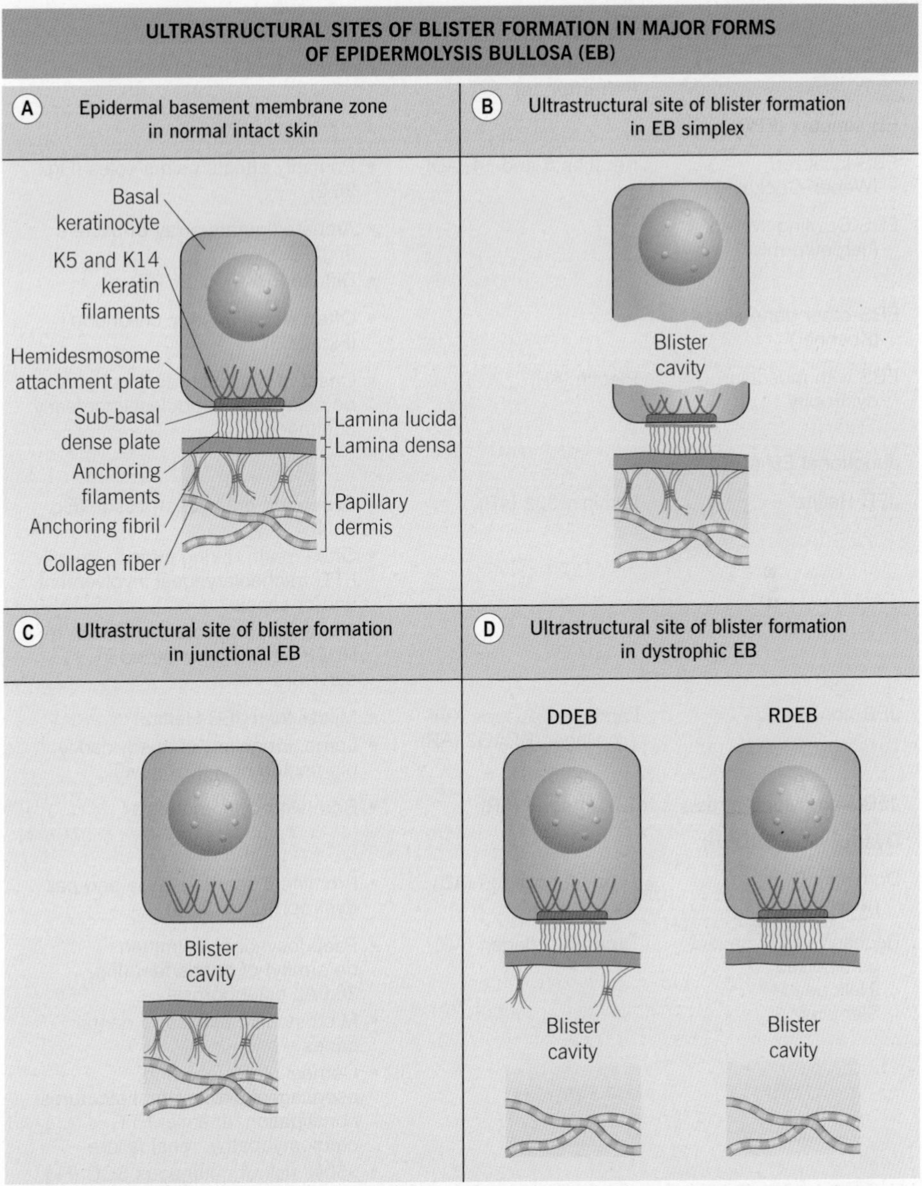

ULTRASTRUCTURAL SITES OF BLISTER FORMATION IN MAJOR FORMS OF EPIDERMOLYSIS BULLOSA (EB)

Fig. 26.1 Ultrastructural sites of blister formation in major forms of epidermolysis bullosa (EB). **A** In intact skin, the ultrastructural regions of the epidermal basement membrane zone consist of (1) basal keratinocytes and the hemidesmosomal plaque; (2) the lamina lucida; (3) the lamina densa; (4) the upper papillary dermis. **B** In EB simplex (EBS), blisters arise within the lower portion of basal keratinocytes. **C** In junctional EB (JEB), blisters form within the lamina lucida. **D** In dystrophic EB (DEB), blisters develop below the lamina densa. Anchoring fibrils are reduced in number in dominant DEB (DDEB) and absent or rudimentary in recessive DEB (RDEB). K5 and K14, keratin 5 and keratin 14, respectively.

EPIDERMOLYSIS BULLOSA (EB) SUBTYPES		
Subtype	**Defective Proteins (Inheritance)**	**Features and Complications**
EB simplex (EBS)		
EBS-localized (Weber–Cockayne)	Keratins 5 and 14 (AD)	• Primarily affects palms/soles (Fig. 26.2)
EBS-Dowling–Meara (herpetiformis)*		• Arcuate/figurate array of blisters (Fig. 26.3A) • Diffuse PPK (Fig. 26.3B)
EBS-other generalized (Koebner)		• Often worse in early childhood (Fig. 26.3C)
EBS with muscular dystrophy	Plectin (AR)	• Onset of muscular dystrophy may be delayed until adolescence/early adulthood
Junctional EB (JEB)**		
JEB-Herlitz*	Laminin-332 (AR)	• Exuberant granulation tissue (Fig. 26.4) • Often death during infancy from FTT, tracheolaryngeal involvement, and/or sepsis • Systemic complications similar to RDEB-severe generalized in survivors
JEB-non-Herlitz	Laminin-332, type XVII collagen/BPAG2 (AR)	• Milder than JEB-Herlitz • Large, irregularly shaped, darkly pigmented nevi ('EB nevi')[†]
JEB with pyloric atresia	$\alpha_6\beta_4$ integrin (AR)	• Born with pyloric atresia
Dystrophic EB (DEB)		
Dominant DEB, generalized	Type VII collagen (AD)	• Prominent scarring, milia and nail dystrophy (Fig. 26.5)
Recessive DEB-severe generalized (Hallopeau–Siemens)*	Type VII collagen (AR)	• Pseudosyndactyly (mitten deformity) of hands/feet (Fig. 26.6A), osteoporosis • Microstomia, excessive dental caries • Corneal ulcers/scarring, esophageal and urethral strictures, constipation, anemia, FTT, cardiomyopathy, renal failure • >50% risk of cutaneous SCC (Fig. 26.6B) by age 30 years[†]; represents leading cause of death
Recessive DEB-other		• Milder generalized and localized forms

Table 26.1 Epidermolysis bullosa (EB) subtypes. Former names are in parentheses. *Suprabasal* forms of EB simplex due to desmosomal defects (e.g. plakophilin deficiency) are also included in the EB spectrum; these rare disorders feature blistering (with acantholysis in skin biopsy specimens), PPK, nail dystrophy, and hypotrichosis. *Continued*

Table 26.1 *Continued* **Epidermolysis bullosa (EB) subtypes.** Former names are in parentheses. *Suprabasal* forms of EB simplex due to desmosomal defects (e.g. plakophilin deficiency) are also included in the EB spectrum; these rare disorders feature blistering (with acantholysis in skin biopsy specimens), PPK, nail dystrophy, and hypotrichosis.

Subtype	Defective Proteins (Inheritance)	Features and Complications
Other		
Kindler syndrome	Kindlin-1‡ (AR)	• Acral blistering, primarily during infancy; ± webbing of fingers/toes (Fig. 26.7A,B), PPK • Photosensitivity that decreases with age • Progressive poikiloderma (Fig. 26.7C), 'cigarette paper' atrophy (Fig. 26.7B) • Gingivitis, colitis, stenoses, ectropion

*Most severe subtype in EBS, JEB, and DEB groups, respectively.
**Dental enamel hypoplasia occurs in all forms of JEB.
†'EB nevi' occasionally occur in other EB subtypes, and patients with RDEB–severe generalized have an increased risk of melanoma.
‡Mediates anchorage between the actin cytoskeleton and the extracellular matrix via focal adhesions.
AD, autosomal dominant; AR, autosomal recessive; BPAG, bullous pemphigoid antigen; FTT, failure to thrive; PPK, palmoplantar keratoderma.

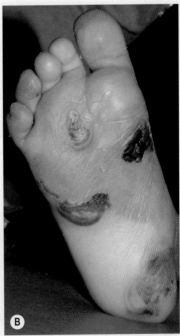
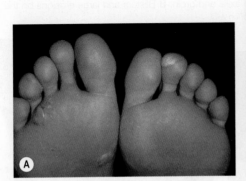

Fig. 26.2 Localized epidermolysis bullosa simplex. A, B Bullae arising on the toes and plantar surfaces at sites of lateral or rotary traction. The majority of blisters occur in acral sites. *B, Courtesy, Julie V. Schaffer, MD.*

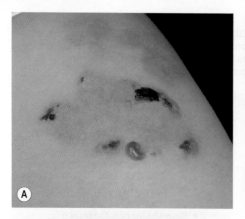

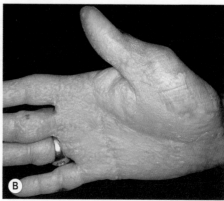

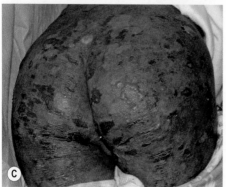

Fig. 26.3 Generalized forms of epidermolysis bullosa simplex (EBS). A Arcuate array of vesicles in a child with EBS, Dowling–Meara. **B** Diffuse palmar keratoderma in an adult with EBS, Dowling–Meara. **C** Widespread blistering in a toddler with EBS, other generalized. *A, C, Courtesy, Julie V. Schaffer, MD.*

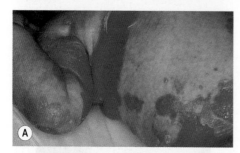

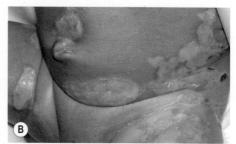

Fig. 26.4 Junctional epidermolysis bullosa, Herlitz. A Blisters on the elbow and large areas of denuded skin; note the bright red color in the axilla and groin. **B** Blisters and large erosions on the abdomen of an infant. *B, Courtesy, Julie V. Schaffer, MD.*

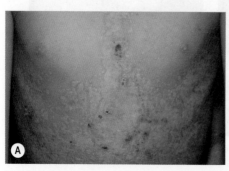

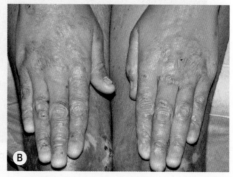

Fig. 26.5 Dominant dystrophic epidermolysis bullosa. Note the prominent scarring on the chest **(A)** and hands **(B)** as well as milia and loss of the fingernails **(B)** in this teenage boy. *Courtesy, Julie V. Schaffer, MD.*

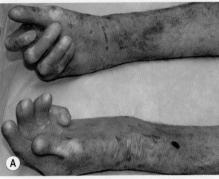
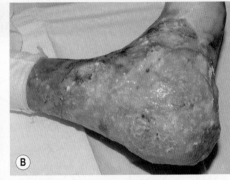

Fig. 26.6 Severe generalized recessive dystrophic epidermolysis bullosa. A Partial pseudosyndactyly (mitten deformities) in a child. **B** Large squamous cell carcinoma in a 21-year-old man. *A, Courtesy, Jo-David Fine, MD; B, Courtesy, Julie V. Schaffer, MD.*

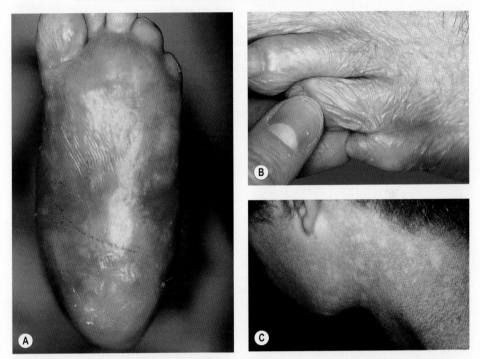

Fig. 26.7 Kindler syndrome. A Atrophy, erosions, and fusion of the toes in an infant. **B** Wrinkling due to atrophy and fusion between the fourth and fifth toes. **C** Poikiloderma of the face and neck with 'skip' areas. *B, Courtesy, Jean L. Bolognia, MD.*

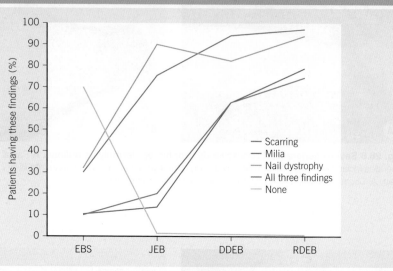

FREQUENCY OF SELECTED CUTANEOUS FINDINGS WITHIN EACH MAJOR SUBTYPE OF INHERITED EB

Fig. 26.8 Frequency of selected cutaneous findings within each major subtype of inherited epidermolysis bullosa (EB). Note the increasing frequency from localized EB simplex (EBS) to recessive dystrophic EB (RDEB). JEB, junctional EB; DDEB, dominant dystrophic EB.

For further information see Ch. 32. From *Dermatology, Third Edition*.

Other Vesiculobullous Diseases

27

There are a number of disorders that can present with vesicles and bullae, including exaggerated insect bite reactions (see Chapter 20), autoimmune and inherited blistering diseases (see Chapters 23–26), porphyrias (see Chapter 41), the Stevens–Johnson syndrome–toxic epidermal necrolysis spectrum (see Chapter 16), and phototoxicity, from sunburn to phototoxic drug reactions (e.g. due to doxycycline). This chapter examines a miscellaneous group of disorders, several of which favor the lower extremities, whereas Chapter 28 reviews vesiculobullous diseases in newborns and infants.

Friction Blisters

• Most commonly develop on the heels, soles, and palms; the blister develops within the epidermis, contains clear or hemorrhagic fluid ('blood blister'), and heals spontaneously without scarring.
• Due to repeated friction (e.g. prolonged walking in ill-fitting shoes) and repetitive actions (e.g. raking leaves).
• **DDx:** if exaggerated response, can consider inherited blistering disease, in particular the localized form of epidermolysis bullosa simplex (see Chapter 26).
• **Rx:** if significant fluid accumulation, drainage of fluid can relieve pressure; the roof of the blister should be left in place to act as a 'natural Band-Aid'; secondary soft tissue infection is unusual in immunocompetent individuals.

Edema Bullae (Edema Blisters)

• The bullae are bland (i.e. non-inflammatory), initially tense, and may reach several centimeters in diameter; they arise within areas of significant edema and contain sterile, usually clear but occasionally blood-tinged, fluid.
• The most common location is the distal lower extremities, often in the setting of an acute exacerbation of chronic edema in an elderly patient; in patients with anasarca and those who are bedridden, the distribution can be more widespread (Fig. 27.1).
• **DDx:** bullosis diabeticorum and bullous pemphigoid, including the variant localized to the lower extremities; if there is surrounding erythema, warmth and tenderness, then bullous cellulitis needs to be excluded.
• **Rx:** as bullae resolve in concert with the edema, only drainage of larger bullae needs to be considered (see below).

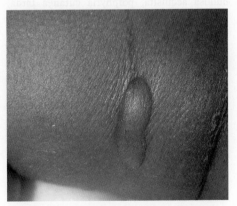

Fig. 27.1 Edema bullae on the thigh of an infant. The bullae are tense and are surrounded by edema. Desquamation from a ruptured bulla is also seen.

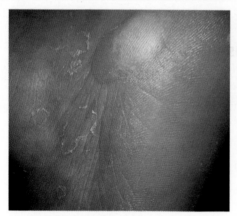

Fig. 27.2 Bullosis diabeticorum. A tense blister on the palm as well as desquamation at sites of previous bullae. *Courtesy, José M. Mascaró Jr., MD.*

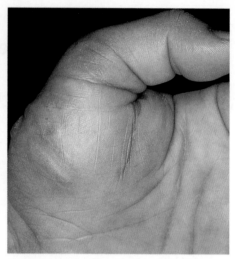

Fig. 27.3 Coma bullae. Blisters developed in an area of pressure in a previously comatose patient. *Courtesy, José M. Mascaró Jr., MD.*

Bullosis Diabeticorum (Diabetic Bullae)

- In patients with diabetes mellitus, tense bland bullae arise rather suddenly within normal-appearing skin (Fig. 27.2); the diameter varies from 0.5 to several centimeters; the blister fluid is sterile and clear, but may be more viscous than that of friction or edema blisters.
- Most commonly develops on the distal extremities (lower > upper) of adults and may be accompanied by peripheral neuropathy.
- **DDx:** bullous pemphigoid, epidermolysis bullosa acquisita, porphyria cutanea tarda, pseudoporphyria, bullous impetigo, and if significant edema, edema bullae; given the increased risk of soft tissue infections in diabetics, the possibility of bullous cellulitis needs to be excluded if there is surrounding erythema.
- **Rx:** placing a small window in a dependent location in the roof of the blister allows for both drainage and preservation of the blister roof; no further treatment is required for uncomplicated lesions, as they spontaneously heal over 3–6 weeks.

Delayed Postburn/Postgraft Blisters

- Tense vesicles or bullae may develop within areas of previous thermal burns as well as within recipient or donor skin graft sites; occur weeks to months after initial injury has healed.
- Possible explanation is enhanced fragility due to a less mature basement membrane zone within the healing wound.
- **DDx:** limited given specific distribution, but includes ischemia within graft recipient sites, herpetic infections, bullous impetigo, and occasionally autoimmune bullous diseases (locus minoris resistentiae phenomenon).
- **Rx:** supportive as lesions heal spontaneously, but can recur.

Coma Bullae (Coma Blisters)

- Tense cutaneous vesicles and bullae can appear within 2 or 3 days of prolonged pressure secondary to immobilization (Figs. 27.3 and 27.4); there is often preceding blanchable erythema.
- The bullae develop at sites of maximum pressure and therefore often develop in the skin overlying joints or bony prominences.
- The prolonged pressure may occur in the setting of a coma, whose cause can vary from drug-induced to metabolic (e.g. hepatic encephalopathy); immobility can also result

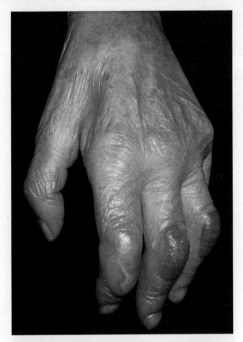

Fig. 27.4 Neurologic blisters. Tense blisters on the dorsal aspect of the fingers on the hemiplegic side of a patient with a previous cerebrovascular accident. *Courtesy, José M. Mascaró Jr., MD.*

from neurologic disorders, especially cerebral vascular accidents.

• Characteristic histologic finding of necrosis of eccrine sweat glands, presumably secondary to local hypoxia.

• **DDx:** usually limited if history of immobilization obtained and distribution pattern limited to pressure points appreciated.

• **Rx:** supportive as lesions heal over 1 or 2 weeks; prevention requires frequent repositioning of the patient.

For further information see Ch. 33. From *Dermatology, Third Edition.*

28 Vesiculopustular and Erosive Disorders in Newborns and Infants

This chapter covers classic transient neonatal eruptions as well as several infectious diseases and other disorders that present with vesiculopustules in the neonatal period or early infancy. Table 28.1 provides a more complete differential diagnosis of vesiculopustules, bullae, erosions, and ulcerations in neonates.

Common Transient Conditions

Erythema Toxicum Neonatorum ('e tox')

• Affects approximately half of full-term neonates; less common in premature infants.
• Typically appears 1–2 days after delivery and lasts up to 1 week, with individual lesions resolving within 1 day; occasionally present at birth, and rarely develops as late as 1 to 2 weeks of age.
• Various combinations of erythematous macules, wheals, and small (≤2 mm) papules, pustules, and vesicles surrounded by a larger erythematous flare (Fig. 28.1); lesions may be grouped at sites of mechanical irritation.
• Often begins on the face and progresses to the trunk, buttocks, and proximal extremities; usually spares the palms and soles.
• Wright's stain of pustular contents shows numerous eosinophils.
• **Rx:** none.

Transient Neonatal Pustular Melanosis

• Affects up to 5% of full-term neonates with darkly pigmented skin; less common in Caucasian newborns.
• Lesions are almost always present at birth.
• Three stages, any of which may be present at a given time (Fig. 28.2).

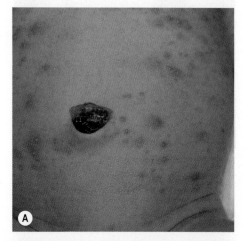

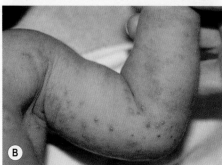

Fig. 28.1 Erythema toxicum neonatorum. Scattered papulovesicles and pustules with an erythematous flare on the abdomen **(A)** and upper extremity **(B)**. *Courtesy, Deborah S. Goddard, MD, Amy E. Gilliam, MD, and Ilona J. Frieden, MD.*

– 2- to 10-mm superficial vesiculopustules with little or no surrounding erythema.
– Collarettes of scale at sites of ruptured vesiculopustules.

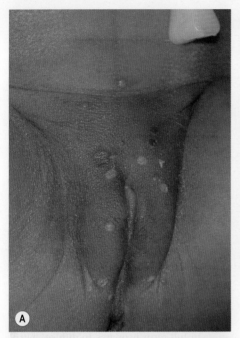

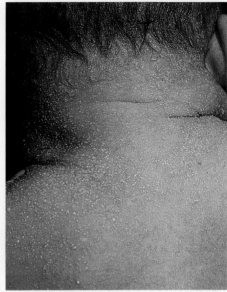

Fig. 28.3 Miliaria crystallina. Tiny, superficial vesicles, seen on the back and neck of this newborn, are characteristic of miliaria crystallina. *From Eichenfield L.F., Frieden I.J., Esterly N.B., et al. (Eds.).* Textbook of Neonatal Dermatology. © 2001 Saunders.

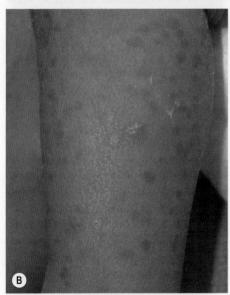

Fig. 28.2 Transient neonatal pustular melanosis in an African-American neonate.
A One hour after birth, flaccid vesiculopustules and superficial erosions with minimal surrounding erythema are present in the groin. **B** On the 8th day of life, hyperpigmented macules and a few collarettes of scale are evident on the lower leg.

- – Residual brown macules representing post-inflammatory hyperpigmentation, which may persist for several months.
- • Any region can be affected, but favors the forehead, chin, neck, lower back, and shins.
- • Wright's stain of pustular contents shows neutrophils > eosinophils.
- • **Rx:** none.

Miliaria (Heat Rash)

- • Common condition in newborns, especially with overheating related to excessive swaddling, warming in an incubator, fever, occlusive dressings, and hot climates.
- • Caused by blockage of eccrine sweat ducts.
- • **Miliaria crystallina**.
  - – Small clear vesicles (likened to 'dew drops') without surrounding erythema (Fig. 28.3); they are fragile and therefore short-lived.
  - – Most often on the forehead, upper trunk, and arms.

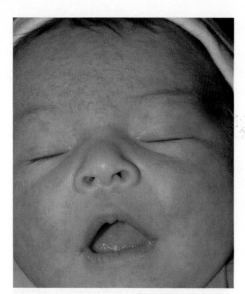

Fig. 28.4 Neonatal cephalic pustulosis.
Papulopustules on the forehead and cheeks of a
3-week-old infant. *Courtesy, Julie V. Schaffer, MD.*

- **Miliaria rubra**.
  – Usually develops at ≥1 week of age.
  – Small erythematous papules, some-times with a tiny central pustule or vesicle.
  – Favors the neck, upper trunk, and occluded areas.
- **Rx:** avoid overheating and occlusion; bathing with lukewarm water.

Neonatal Cephalic Pustulosis (Neonatal Acne)

- Affects ~20% of newborns.
- Onset usually at 2–3 weeks of life, with spontaneous resolution by 2–3 months of age.
- Papulopustular eruption on the face (cheeks > forehead, chin, eyelids) (Fig. 28.4) > neck, upper chest, and scalp.
- An absence of comedones in neonatal cephalic pustulosis distinguishes it from infantile acne, which typically develops at 3–12 months of age and is more persistent (see Chapter 29).
- May represent an inflammatory response to *Malassezia* spp., a normal component of the skin microbiome that may also trigger seborrheic dermatitis.
- **Rx:** usually not required; topical imidazoles (e.g. ketoconazole cream) may be helpful.

Sucking Blister

- Caused by habitual sucking of the affected area *in utero*, and resolves spontaneously within days to weeks of birth.
- Intact bulla, erosion, callus, or ulceration on a non-inflamed base.
- Common sites include the radial forearm, wrist, hand, and fingers.

Infectious Diseases

Cutaneous Candidiasis

- Congenital candidiasis.
  – Uncommon condition that is acquired *in utero*; risk factors include maternal vaginal candidiasis, a foreign body in the uterus or cervix, and prematurity.
  – Evident at birth or during the first few days of life.
  – Findings range from erythematous papules and pustules with fine scaling in full-term neonates to diffuse, 'burn-like' erythema and erosions in premature infants (Fig. 28.5A,B).
  – Often widespread involvement on the face, trunk, and extremities; the palms, soles, and nails (yellow discoloration, transverse ridging) are frequently affected, but the diaper area and oral mucosa are typically spared.
  – **DDx:** budding yeast and pseudohyphae are seen in a potassium hydroxide preparation of skin scrapings, and culture grows *Candida* spp. (usually *C. albicans*).
  – **Rx:** premature infants (especially if <1500 g) are at high risk for disseminated candidiasis and require systemic antifungal agents, as do full-term neonates with extracutaneous involvement (e.g. pneumonia); most full-term neonates have skin-limited disease that can be treated with topical antifungals (e.g. an imidazole cream).
- Neonatal candidiasis (see Chapter 64).
  – Common condition that presents at ≥1 week of age as intense erythema with desquamation and satellite papulopustules, favoring the diaper area > other intertriginous sites (see Fig. 13.4); patients may also have oral thrush.
  – **Rx:** topical imidazole or nystatin.

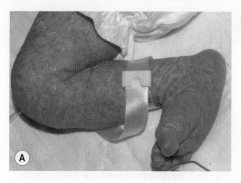

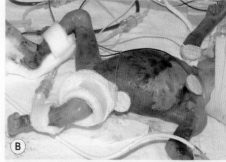

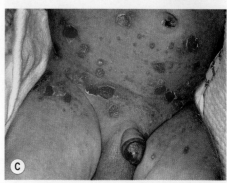

Fig. 28.5 Congenital candidiasis and bullous impetigo. A Numerous pink papules admixed with small superficial pustules and desquamation due to congenital candidiasis in a full-term neonate. Note the plantar involvement. **B** Widespread 'burn-like' erosions due to congenital candidiasis in a premature neonate born at 24 weeks' gestation. **C** Multiple superficial erosions with collarettes of scale in the diaper area of an infant with bullous impetigo. Note the scattered vesiculopustules. *A, B, Courtesy, Julie V. Schaffer, MD.*

Bullous Impetigo (See Chapter 61)

• Presents as early as a few days of age with flaccid bullae, vesiculopustules, and superficial shiny red erosions with collarettes of scale (Fig. 28.5C).

• Favors the diaper area and other intertriginous sites (see Fig. 13.4).

• **DDx:** Gram stain shows gram-positive cocci in clusters, and culture grows *Staphylococcus aureus*.

• **Rx:** topical antibiotic (e.g. mupirocin) for uncomplicated localized disease; systemic anti-staphylococcal antibiotic if more extensive (using an intravenous agent, e.g. vancomycin, if the patient is toxic appearing).

Neonatal Herpes Simplex Virus (HSV) Infection (See Chapter 67)

• Affects ~1 : 10 000 newborns in the United States; risk of transmission is highest (30–50%) for a mother with her first episode of genital HSV infection (which may be asymptomatic) near the time of delivery and low (<1–3%) for recurrent genital herpes.

• Onset from birth to 2 weeks, but usually ≥5 days of age.

• Localized (favoring the scalp and trunk) or disseminated vesicles (Fig. 28.6), pustules, and crusts; lesions are often grouped and may progress to bullae and erosions with scalloped borders.

• Involvement of the oral mucosa, eye, CNS, and other internal organs can occur.

• **Rx:** intravenous acyclovir.

Uncommon Conditions

Eosinophilic Pustular Folliculitis in Infancy

• Onset often in the first few months of life, with cyclical recurrences for several months to years.

• Pruritic perifollicular pustules and crusts favoring the scalp (Fig. 28.7) and forehead.

• **DDx:** Erythema toxicum neonatorum (in neonates), bacterial folliculitis, tinea capitis, scabies, arthropod bite reactions.

• **Rx:** potent topical CS (intermittently for flares), oral antihistamines.

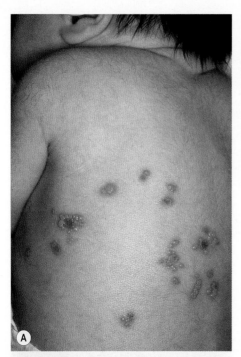

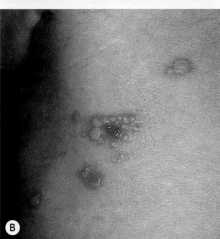

Fig. 28.6 Neonatal HSV infection. Note the clustering of the vesicles on an erythematous base.

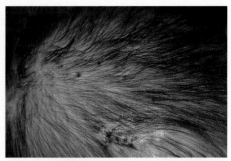

Fig. 28.7 Eosinophilic pustular folliculitis in infancy. Crusted papules and pustules on the scalp of a 1-year-old boy. *Courtesy, Deborah S. Goddard, MD, Amy E. Gilliam, MD, and Ilona J. Frieden, MD.*

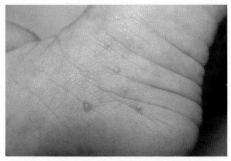

Fig. 28.8 Infantile acropustulosis. Multiple vesiculopustules with an erythematous base on the medial ankle of an infant. *Courtesy, Deborah S. Goddard, MD, Amy E. Gilliam, MD, and Ilona J. Frieden, MD.*

- Onset usually between 3 and 6 months of age; occasionally develops in newborns.
- Pruritic vesicles and pustules on the hands and feet (including palms/soles) (Fig. 28.8) > wrists and ankles.
- Outbreaks last 1–2 weeks, with cyclical recurrences until 2–3 years of age.
- **DDx:** scabies.
- **Rx:** potent topical CS (intermittently for flares), oral antihistamines.

Infantile Acropustulosis (Acropustulosis of Infancy)

- Favors darkly pigmented male infants, sometimes representing a persistent hypersensitivity reaction following successful scabies treatment.

Incontinentia Pigmenti (IP) (See Chapter 51)

- Multisystem X-linked disorder caused by mutations in the *NEMO* gene (NF-κB essential modulator); usually lethal in male fetuses.

DIFFERENTIAL DIAGNOSIS OF NEONATAL VESICULOPUSTULES, BULLAE, EROSIONS, AND ULCERS

Vesiculopustular Eruptions

Infectious Diseases and Infestations
- Bacterial (see Chapter 61): bullous impetigo; group A>B streptococcal or *Listeria* infection
- Candidiasis (congenital or neonatal)
- Viral (see Chapter 67): HSV infection, neonatal varicella, herpes zoster (age ≥2 weeks)
- Scabies (age ≥3–4 weeks) (see Chapter 71)

Common Transient Conditions
- Erythema toxicum neonatorum, transient neonatal pustular melanosis
- Miliaria crystallina and rubra
- Neonatal cephalic pustulosis

Uncommon and Rare Non-Infectious Diseases
- Infantile acropustulosis, eosinophilic pustular folliculitis in infancy
- Incontinentia pigmenti
- Congenital Langerhans cell histiocytosis (Fig. 28.10) (see Chapter 76)
- Neonatal papulopustular eruption of hyper-IgE syndrome (see Chapter 49)
- Vesiculopustular eruption* of transient myeloproliferative disorder in Down syndrome
- Pustular psoriasis (see Chapter 6)

Bullae, Erosions, and Ulcers

Infectious Diseases
- Bacterial (see Chapters 61 and 69): staphylococcal scalded skin syndrome (Fig. 28.11), *Pseudomonas* infection (including noma neonatorum),† congenital syphilis
- Fungal** (see Chapter 64): aspergillosis, zygomycosis
- Intrauterine HSV infection, congenital varicella (see Chapter 67)

Conditions with Exogenous Causes
- Sucking blister, perinatal/iatrogenic injury, irritant contact dermatitis (see Chapter 12)

Uncommon and Rare Non-Infectious Diseases
- Mastocytosis (Fig. 28.12; see Chapter 96), ulcerated infantile hemangioma (see Chapter 85)
- Aplasia cutis congenita (Fig. 28.13; see Chapter 53)
- Genodermatoses, especially epidermolysis bullosa (see Chapter 26) and epidermolytic ichthyosis (Fig. 28.14; see Chapter 46)
- Autoimmune bullous diseases (often due to maternal antibodies; see Chapters 22–25)
- Maternofetal or transfusion-associated GVHD in infants with SCID (see Chapter 49)
- Congenital erosive and vesicular dermatosis (Fig. 28.15)
- Nutritional dermatitis (see Fig. 43.4A)

*Favors the cheeks.
**Evolves into necrotic ulcers; risk factors include prematurity and occlusion.
†Evolves into necrotic ulcers that favor the groin; risk factors include prematurity, immunodeficiency, and (especially for noma) malnutrition.
SCID, severe combined immunodeficiency.

Table 28.1 Differential diagnosis of neonatal vesiculopustules, bullae, erosions, and ulcers. This list is not exhaustive, as other rare diseases such as deficiency of the interleukin-1 receptor antagonist (DIRA), ankyloblepharon–ectodermal dysplasia–clefting (AEC) syndrome, and congenital Behçet's disease can have vesiculopustular and erosive presentations.

• Typically presents in the first 2 weeks of life with vesicles on an inflammatory base in linear streaks that favor the extremities (Fig. 28.9); in subsequent weeks, verrucous streaks may develop, followed by more widespread linear and whorled grayish-brown hyperpigmentation.

• Extracutaneous findings in neonates with IP can include peripheral eosinophilia, leukocytosis, seizures, and retinal vascular abnormalities.

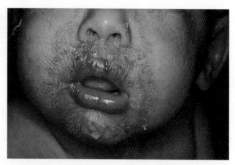

Fig. 28.11 Staphylococcal scalded skin syndrome. Radiating perioral scale-crusts due to exfoliative toxins.

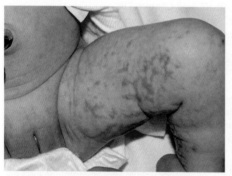

Fig. 28.9 Incontinentia pigmenti stages 1 and 2. Admixture of erythematous streaks containing vesicles and yellow-brown streaks with scale on the lower extremity of a female neonate. *Courtesy, Julie V. Schaffer, MD.*

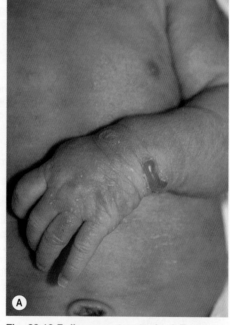

Ⓐ

Fig. 28.12 Bullous mastocytosis. A Tense bulla on the wrist and flaccid bullae on the dorsal hand as well as pink plaques on the trunk in a 1-month-old infant. *A, Courtesy, Deborah S. Goddard, MD, Amy E. Gilliam, MD, and Ilona J. Frieden, MD. **Continued***

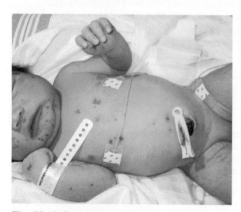

Fig. 28.10 Congenital Langerhans cell histiocytosis. Numerous erosions with crusting on the face and trunk of a newborn. *Courtesy, Deborah S. Goddard, MD, Amy E. Gilliam, MD, and Ilona J. Frieden, MD.*

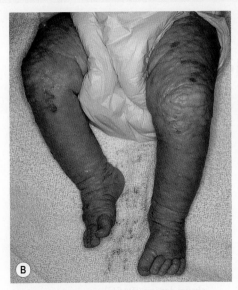

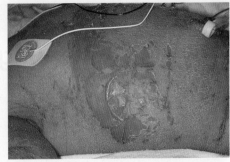

Fig. 28.14 Epidermolytic ichthyosis (bullous congenital ichthyosiform erythroderma). Diffuse scaling and a large erosion with scale-crust in a neonate.

Fig. 28.12 *Continued* **B** Second infant with erosions and diffuse infiltration of the skin with mast cells, leading to a thickened leathery appearance.

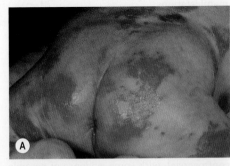

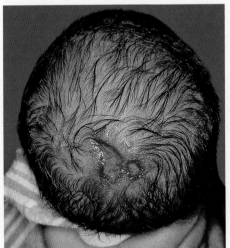

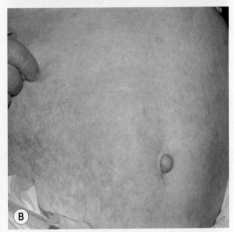

Fig. 28.13 Aplasia cutis congenita. Ulcerations on the vertex of the scalp may be misdiagnosed as an HSV infection. The angulated appearance of the larger ulceration would not be characteristic of HSV infection.

Fig. 28.15 Congenital erosive and vesicular dermatosis. A Bright red, irregularly shaped erosions on the buttocks of a 2-week-old infant. **B** Residual supple and reticulate scarring in a 9-month-old child. *A, Courtesy, Anthony J. Mancini, MD; B, Courtesy, Julie V. Schaffer, MD.*

For further information see Ch. 34. From *Dermatology, Third Edition.*

29 | Acne Vulgaris

- Common pilosebaceous disorder that occurs in ~85% of individuals 12–24 years of age and 15–35% of adults (especially women) in their 30s–40s.
- Clinical presentations range from mild comedones to severe, explosive eruptions of suppurative nodules associated with systemic manifestations.
- May result in scarring and psychosocial repercussions such as anxiety, depression, and social withdrawal.
- A tendency to develop moderate to severe acne can run in families.
- Multiple factors affecting the pilosebaceous unit contribute to acne pathogenesis (Fig. 29.1), a process that typically begins when androgen production increases at adrenarche.
- The relationship between diet and acne is controversial, with some evidence of possible associations with milk intake (especially skim milk) and a high glycemic index diet.

Clinical Features and Variants of Acne

- Favors the face and upper trunk, sites with well-developed sebaceous glands.
- Non-inflammatory acne.
  - *Closed comedones (whiteheads)* are small (~1 mm), skin-colored papules without an obvious follicular opening (Fig. 29.2A,B).
  - *Open comedones (blackheads)* have a dilated follicular opening filled with a keratin plug, which has a black color due to oxidized lipids and melanin (Fig. 29.2B,C).
- Inflammatory acne.
  - Erythematous papules and pustules (Fig. 29.3A).
  - Nodules and cysts filled with pus or serosanguinous fluid; may coalesce and form sinus tracts (Fig. 29.3B).

- *Acne conglobata* (severe nodulocystic acne) is classified in the follicular occlusion tetrad along with dissecting cellulitis of the scalp, hidradenitis suppurativa, and pilonidal cysts (see Chapter 31); it is also a part of *p*yogenic *a*rthritis, *p*yoderma gangrenosum, and *a*cne conglobata (PAPA) and *p*yoderma gangrenosum, *a*cne, and *s*uppurative *h*idradenitis (PASH) syndromes.
- Inflammatory acne commonly results in post-inflammatory hyperpigmentation, especially in patients with darker skin, which fades slowly over time (Fig. 29.4A); nodulocystic acne (and less frequently other inflammatory > comedonal forms) often leads to pitted (Fig. 29.4B) or hypertrophic scars (the latter especially on the trunk; see Fig. 81.4).

Post-Adolescent Acne

- Age >25 years; favors women.
- Tends to flare in the week prior to menstruation; up to one-third of these women have hyperandrogenism.
- Typically features papulonodules on the lower face, jawline, and neck.

Acne Excoriée

- Favors teenage girls and young women.
- Habitual picking at comedones and inflammatory papules, resulting in crusted erosions (often linear/angular) and potential scarring (see Fig. 5.3).
- Some patients have an underlying obsessive–compulsive or anxiety disorder.

Acne Fulminans

- Favors boys 13 to 16 years of age.
- Sudden development of numerous, markedly inflamed nodular lesions on the face, trunk, and upper arms.

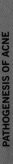

PATHOGENESIS OF ACNE

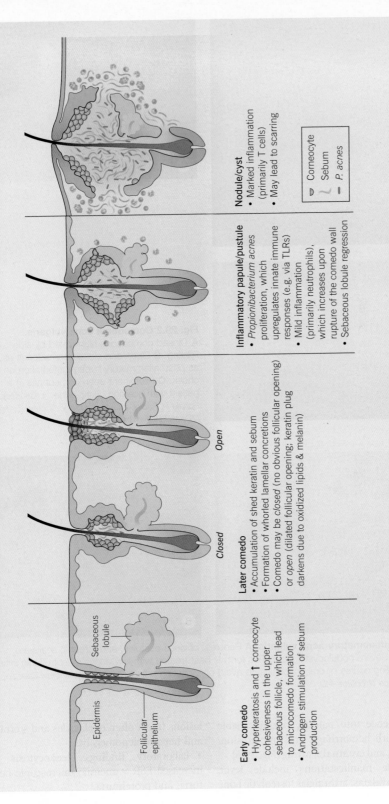

Early comedo
- Hyperkeratosis and ↑ corneocyte cohesiveness in the upper sebaceous follicle, which lead to microcomedo formation
- Androgen stimulation of sebum production

Closed   *Open*

Later comedo
- Accumulation of shed keratin and sebum
- Formation of whorled lamellar concretions
- Comedo may be *closed* (no obvious follicular opening) or *open* (dilated follicular opening; keratin plug darkens due to oxidized lipids & melanin)

Inflammatory papule/pustule
- *Propionibacterium acnes* proliferation, which upregulates innate immune responses (e.g. via TLRs)
- Mild inflammation (primarily neutrophils), which increases upon rupture of the comedo wall
- Sebaceous lobule regression

Nodule/cyst
- Marked inflammation (primarily T cells)
- May lead to scarring

Epidermis

Follicular epithelium

Sebaceous lobule

▽	Corneocyte
∿	Sebum
—	*P. acnes*

Fig. 29.1 Pathogenesis of acne. TLRs, Toll-like receptors.

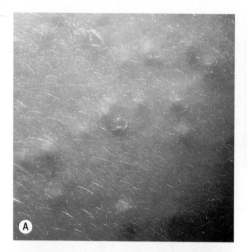

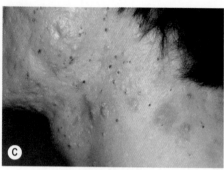

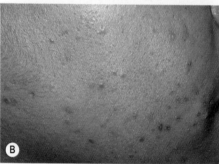

Fig. 29.2 Comedonal acne vulgaris.
A Closed comedones highlighted by side lighting. **B** Open and closed comedones as well as post-inflammatory hyperpigmentation on the cheek. **C** Prominent open comedones in a patient with scarring cystic acne. *A, Courtesy, Ronald P. Rapini, MD; B, Courtesy, Andrew Zaenglein, MD, and Diane Thiboutot, MD.*

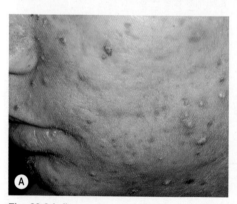

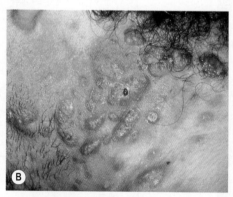

Fig. 29.3 Inflammatory acne vulgaris. A Papules, obvious pustules, and atrophic scars are present. **B** Severe nodulocystic acne. This form is best treated with low doses of isotretinoin initially (± a preceding course of oral antibiotics) to avoid precipitating a flare. *A, Courtesy, Andrew Zaenglein, MD, and Diane Thiboutot, MD.*

- Coalescence into painful, oozing, friable plaques with hemorrhagic crusting, erosion/ulceration, and eventual scarring (Fig. 29.5).
- Systemic manifestations include fever, malaise, myalgias, arthralgias, osteolytic bone lesions (most often of clavicles and sternum), and hepatosplenomegaly.
- Laboratory findings: leukocytosis and increased ESR > anemia, microscopic hematuria, and proteinuria.

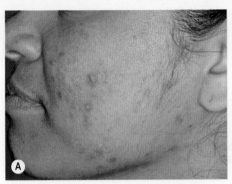
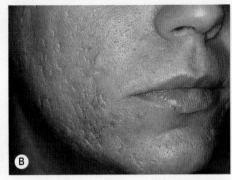

Fig. 29.4 Sequelae of acne. A Post-inflammatory hyperpigmentation. Such pigmentary changes are most common in patients with darker skin colors. **B** 'Ice-pick' scarring secondary to nodulocystic acne. *A, Courtesy, Andrew Zaenglein, MD, and Diane Thiboutot, MD.*

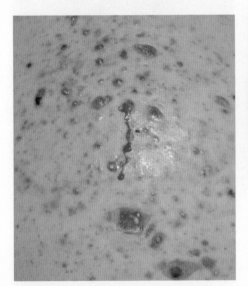

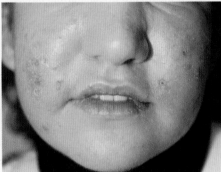

Fig. 29.6 Solid facial edema due to acne vulgaris. There is soft tissue swelling in the central portion of the face. *Courtesy, Andrew Zaenglein, MD, and Diane Thiboutot, MD.*

Fig. 29.5 Acne fulminans. Inflamed, friable papulopustules and plaques with erosions, oozing, and formation of granulation tissue. *Courtesy, Julie V. Schaffer, MD.*

Solid Facial Edema (Morbihan's Disease)

• Woody induration ± erythema of the central face in the setting of chronic inflammation due to acne vulgaris or rosacea (Fig. 29.6).

• **Rx:** isotretinoin (may require an extended course).

• **DDx:** an acne fulminans-like flare occasionally develops upon initiation of isotretinoin therapy for acne, and acne fulminans can be associated with *s*ynovitis, *a*cne, *p*ustulosis, *h*yperostosis, and *o*steitis (SAPHO) syndrome (see Chapter 21).

• **Rx:** isotretinoin (low dose initially with slow escalation) plus prednisone.

Neonatal Acne (Neonatal Cephalic Pustulosis) (See Chapter 28)

• Ages 2 weeks to 3 months.

• Facial papulopustular eruption thought to be triggered by *Malassezia* spp.; comedones are *not* present.

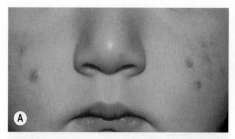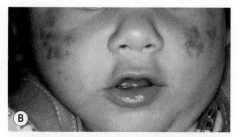

Fig. 29.7 Infantile acne. Presentations can range from scattered papulopustules **(A)** to multiple coalescing papulonodules and inflammatory cysts **(B).** If the latter child failed to improve with a topical retinoid plus an oral antibiotic, consideration would be given to oral isotretinoin. *Courtesy, Kalman Watsky, MD.*

Infantile Acne

• Ages 3 months to 2 years; favors boys.
• Facial comedones, papulopustules, and cysts as in classic acne (Fig. 29.7); may result in scarring.
• Reflects physiologic elevation of androgen levels in infants 6–12 months of age (especially boys); patients often have a family history of severe acne.
• **Rx:** similar to adolescent acne; typically resolves within 1–2 years, becoming quiescent until puberty.

Contact Acne

• *Acne mechanica*: comedogenesis due to chronic friction/occlusion from objects such as chin straps, helmets, collars, and musical instruments (e.g. 'fiddler's neck' in a violinist).
• *Acne cosmetica*, *pomade acne*, and *occupational acne*: comedogenesis caused by exposure to follicle-occluding substances in cosmetics, hair products (favoring forehead and temples), and materials used in the workplace (e.g. cutting oils, coal tar derivatives).

Chloracne

• Results from exposure (usually occupational) to halogenated aromatic hydrocarbons (e.g. polychlorinated dibenzodioxins and dibenzofurans) in agents such as herbicides and insecticides.
• Comedones and cystic papulonodules develop within 2 months of exposure, favoring malar and retroauricular areas of the face

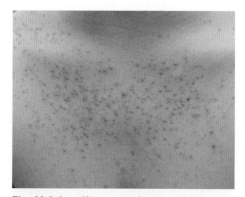

Fig. 29.8 Acneiform eruption secondary to systemic corticosteroid therapy. Abrupt eruption of monomorphous follicular papulopustules on the trunk. *Courtesy, Scott Jackson, MD, and Lee T. Nesbitt, Jr., MD.*

(see Fig. 12.18) as well as the axillae and scrotum; often persists for years.

Drug-Induced Acne and Acneiform Eruptions

• Systemic CS can trigger an eruption of monomorphous follicular papulopustules favoring the upper trunk (Fig. 29.8).
• Acneiform eruptions represent a frequent side effect of epidermal growth factor receptor (EGFR) inhibitors (e.g. cetuximab, erlotinib) used to treat solid tumors; patients present with follicular pustules and papules on the face (Fig. 29.9), scalp, and upper trunk, usually 1–3 weeks after beginning treatment,

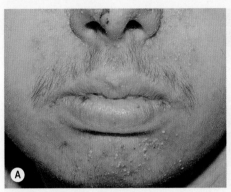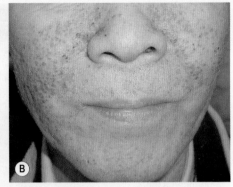

Fig. 29.9 Acneiform eruptions due to epidermal growth factor receptor inhibitors. A, B Numerous monomorphous follicular pustules and crusted papules on the face of two patients treated with erlotinib. *A, Courtesy, Julie V. Schaffer, MD; B, Courtesy, Andrew Zaenglein, MD, and Diane Thiboutot, MD.*

which may correlate with a therapeutic response.

• Other common causes of drug-induced acne include anabolic steroids, bromides (found in sedatives and cold remedies), iodides (found in contrast dyes and supplements), isoniazid (Fig. 29.10), lithium, phenytoin, and progestins.

Acne Associated with a Syndrome

• Examples include Apert, PAPA, PASH, and SAPHO (see Ch. 21) syndromes.

Evaluation and Treatment of Acne

• Table 29.1 lists key components in the history and physical examination of an acne patient.
• **DDx:** presented in Table 29.2.
• **Rx:** outlined in Table 29.3.
• Once active acne has been successfully treated, intralesional CS (for hypertrophic scars) or surgical modalities (e.g. fractional or traditional laser resurfacing, dermabrasion, fillers) can be used for residual scarring if needed.

Tips for Topical Therapy

• Lack of compliance is often an issue, with common reasons including irritated skin, busy schedules, and giving up when the response is not rapid; substantial benefit typically requires 6–8 weeks of treatment.

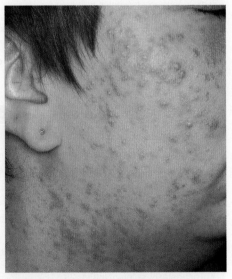

Fig. 29.10 Drug-induced acne due to isoniazid. *Courtesy, Kalman Watsky, MD.*

• The main side effect of topical medications is irritation, which is most problematic in adolescents with atopic dermatitis and adults.
• Patients should be advised to avoid harsh scrubs, other irritating agents (e.g. toners, acne products that are not part of the regimen), and manipulation of lesions, especially inflammatory papulonodules and closed comedones.
• Even if planning combination therapy, a gradual initial approach can improve

HISTORY AND PHYSICAL EXAMINATION OF THE ACNE PATIENT	
History	**Physical Examination**

• Sex
• Age*
• Degree of motivation for treatment
• Lifestyle/hobbies, occupation
• Current and previous acne treatments
• Use of cosmetics, sunscreens, cleansers, moisturizers
• Menstrual history* and oral contraceptive use
• Medications (see text on drug-induced acne)
• Other medical conditions
• Family history of acne
	• Skin type (e.g. oily vs. dry)
	• Skin color/phototype
	• Distribution of acne
	  – Face (e.g. 'T-zone,' cheeks, jawline)
	  – Neck, chest, back, upper arms
	• Overall degree of involvement (mild, moderate, or severe)
	• Lesion morphology
	  – Comedones
	  – Inflammatory papules and pustules
	  – Nodules and cysts, sinus tracts
	• Post-inflammatory pigmentary changes
	• Scarring (e.g. pitted, hypertrophic, atrophic)
	• Signs of virilization* (in female patients)
	  – Hirsutism, androgenetic alopecia
	  – Deep voice, muscular habitus, clitoromegaly

Hyperandrogenism should be suspected in children who develop acne between 2 and 7 years of age, in older adolescents/women with irregular menses, and in female patients with signs of virilization; evaluation often includes serum levels of testosterone (total and free), DHEAS, and 17-hydroxyprogesterone (see Fig. 57.10) as well as hand/wrist x-rays to evaluate bone age in prepubertal children.

Table 29.1 History and physical examination of the acne patient.

DIFFERENTIAL DIAGNOSIS OF ACNE VULGARIS
Comedonal Acne
• Contact acne, chloracne, drug-induced acne • 'Pseudoacne' of the transverse nasal crease (in prepubertal children; Fig. 29.11A)
Closed Comedones • Milia, sebaceous hyperplasia, adnexal neoplasms (e.g. syringomas, fibrofolliculomas) • Eruptive vellus hair cysts or steatocystomas (for truncal lesions)
Open Comedones • Childhood flexural comedones (double-orifice; axilla > groin), dilated pore of Winer (solitary lesion) • Trichostasis spinulosa (Fig. 29.11B) • Favre–Racouchot disease (in photoaged skin), radiation-induced comedones • Nevus comedonicus • Follicular spines (e.g. in viral-associated trichodysplasia spinulosa, multiple myeloma, and HIV-associated follicular syndrome)
Inflammatory Acne
• Rosacea, periorificial dermatitis, idiopathic facial aseptic granuloma (solitary nodule in young children) • Folliculitis: normal flora, staphylococcal, *Pityrosporum*, gram-negative, eosinophilic, *Demodex* • Drug-induced acne/acneiform eruptions, neutrophilic dermatoses • Pseudofolliculitis barbae, acne keloidalis nuchae • Keratosis pilaris, angiofibromas, follicular mucinosis • Tinea faciei, molluscum contagiosum (inflamed lesions), viral-associated trichodysplasia spinulosa

Table 29.2 Differential diagnosis of acne vulgaris. Folliculotropic mycosis fungoides can mimic comedonal or inflammatory acne.

TREATMENT OF ACNE VULGARIS

Topical retinoids (comedolytic > anti-inflammatory effects): tretinoin,* adapalene, tazarotene*
- Response requires 3–4 weeks (sometimes preceded by pustular flare); use a small amount and treat all acne-prone areas
- Initial use of lower concentration and/or alternate-night application can minimize irritation

Topical antimicrobials: benzoyl peroxide (BPO)** and/or antibiotic (e.g. clindamycin,[†] erythromycin,[†] sodium sulfacetamide/sulfur)

Oral antibiotics: *first-line* – tetracycline derivatives (doxycycline, minocycline); *alt.* – azithromycin, trimethoprim–sulfamethoxazole
- Often used for 3–6+ months; tetracyclines are avoided in children <8 years of age and pregnant women

OCPs: FDA-approved for acne – Ortho Tri-Cyclen® (EE 35 microg, norgestimate 180/215/250 microg), Yaz®/Loryna® (EE 20 microg, drospirenone 3000 microg), Estrostep® (EE 20/30/35 microg, norethindrone 1000 microg)

Antiandrogens: spironolactone (50–200 mg/day)

Oral isotretinoin[§]: typically 0.5–1 mg/kg/day (lower initially, especially if acne fulminans) × 4–6 months (cumulative dose 120–150 mg/kg)

	Mild Acne		Moderate Acne	Severe Acne (e.g. Conglobata, Fulminans)
	Comedonal	*Mostly Inflammatory*		
First-line	• Topical retinoid	• Topical antimicrobial[‡] + topical retinoid	• Oral antibiotic + topical retinoid ± BPO	• Oral isotretinoin (+ oral CS for acne fulminans)
Second-line	• Alt. topical retinoid • Azelaic acid • Salicylic acid	• Alt. topical retinoid + alt. topical antimicrobial • Azelaic acid • Topical dapsone	• Alt. oral antibiotic + alt. topical retinoid ± BPO/azelaic acid • Oral isotretinoin (if nodular, scarring or recalcitrant)	• Oral dapsone • High-dose oral antibiotic + topical retinoid + BPO
Options for female patients			• OCP/antiandrogen	• OCP/antiandrogen
Procedural options	• Comedo extraction		• Comedo extraction • Intralesional CS (2–5 mg/ml triamcinolone)	• Intralesional CS (2–5 mg/ml triamcinolone)
Refractory to treatment	Exclude gram-negative folliculitis (see Chapter 31)			
			• Female patient: exclude adrenal or ovarian dysfunction • Exclude use of anabolic steroid or other acne-exacerbating drugs	
Maintenance	• Topical retinoid	• Topical retinoid ± BPO	• Topical retinoid ± BPO	

*Tretinoin is photolabile and inactivated by BPO (so generally applied at night, separately from BPO); tazarotene is the most irritating of the topical retinoids (see text) and is pregnancy category X.

**Can bleach clothing/bedding and cause contact dermatitis (irritant > allergic); unlike topical antibiotics, bacterial resistance does not occur.

[†]Increased effectiveness when used in conjunction with BPO or a retinoid.

[§]Severe teratogenicity; in the United States, prescribers and patients must register in a risk management program (iPLEDGE™) that requires monthly visits. The most common side effects are cheilitis > mucosal dryness (ocular, nasal) and xerosis (Fig. 29.12).

[‡]BPO ± a topical antibiotic may also be used as monotherapy, especially as an initial treatment in a younger patient.

Alt, alternative; EE, ethinyl estradiol; OCP, oral contraceptive pill.

Table 29.3 Treatment of acne vulgaris. Lack of response should prompt consideration of noncompliance and alternative diagnoses. In general, monotherapy with a topical or oral antibiotic should be avoided. Laser (e.g. 1450-nm diode), light (e.g. blue, intense pulsed), or photodynamic therapies may be of benefit to some patients but are not first-line, and superficial chemical peels (e.g. 20–30% salicylic acid, 30–50% glycolic acid) are occasionally useful to reduce comedones.

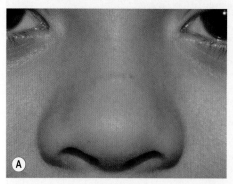

Fig. 29.11 Disorders in the differential diagnosis of comedonal acne vulgaris. A 'Pseudoacne' of the transverse nasal crease in a young child. Note the milia and comedones located along this anatomical demarcation line. **B** Trichostasis spinulosa. Multiple vellus hairs and keratinous debris are found within the dilated follicular orifices. *A, Courtesy, Julie V. Schaffer, MD; B, Courtesy, Judit Stenn, MD.*

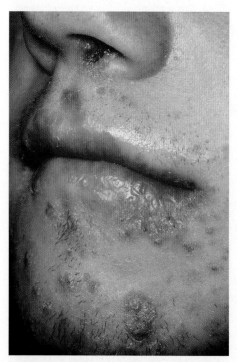

Fig. 29.12 Impetigo in a patient receiving isotretinoin. Multiple serous crusts are evident. Dryness and fragility of the skin, lips, and nasal mucosa in patients treated with isotretinoin increase susceptibility to staphylococcal infections.

tolerance in patients with sensitive skin; for example, a single agent may be used for the first 2–3 weeks (starting every other day for retinoids), followed by slow introduction of a second medication (e.g. transitioning from alternate days to daily).

• Simplifying the regimen and considering combination products (e.g. benzoyl peroxide + adapalene or clindamycin; tretinoin + clindamycin) may improve compliance, especially in less-motivated adolescents.

• In general, topical medications (especially retinoids) should be used to the entire acne-prone region rather than as 'spot treatment' of individual lesions.

• Patients should be instructed to select non-comedogenic products (e.g. moisturizers, sunscreens, make-up) and to avoid having oily hair or using pomades that may contribute to acne.

• Having patients bring everything that they apply to their face to a visit may help to determine the source of problems.

For further information see Ch. 36. From *Dermatology, Third Edition.*

Rosacea and Periorificial Dermatitis

30

Epidemiology

• Seen in all skin types, but considerably more common in patients with skin phototypes I–II.
• Onset generally in the 4th decade of life.

Clinical Features

• Highly variable degree of severity, from a few papulopustules to extreme distortion of the nose.
• Lesions typically develop on the face, especially its central portion; uncommonly other sites such as the scalp and chest are involved.
• Etiology is multifactorial, including vascular hyperreactivity, alterations in innate immunity, e.g. cathelicidins, and *Demodex* plus its commensal bacteria.
• Table 30.1 lists the four major types of rosacea (Figs. 30.1–30.5) and their characteristics.

• Variants include granulomatous rosacea and periorificial dermatitis.
   – Granulomatous rosacea.
      • Red to red-brown papules secondary to granulomatous inflammation (Fig. 30.6).
   – Periorificial dermatitis.
      • Originally referred to as perioral dermatitis but lesions can surround other orifices, hence the term periorificial.
      • Affects children and adults.
      • Lesions around the mouth and nose > eyes.
      • Monomorphic pink papules and fine pustules (Figs. 30.7 and 30.8) admixed with eczematous patches and thin plaques, sometimes with fine scale.

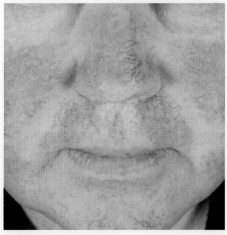

Fig. 30.2 Dermatoheliosis in a skin phototype I patient. Telangiectasias and erythema due to chronic actinic damage are particularly marked on the facial prominences. Features of dermatoheliosis overlap with those of erythematotelangiectatic rosacea. *Courtesy, Frank C. Powell, MD.*

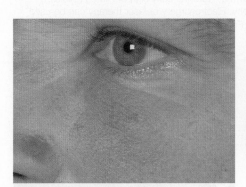

Fig. 30.1 Erythematotelangiectatic rosacea. Persistent erythema of the medial and lateral cheeks is seen. In this patient, there are no telangiectasias, indicating mild disease. *Courtesy, Frank C. Powell, MD.*

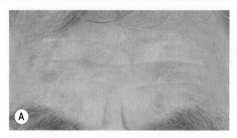
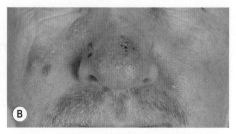

Fig. 30.3 Rosacea. A Moderate papulopustular rosacea of the forehead. Note the superficial nature of the inflammatory lesions. **B** Moderate to severe papulopustular rosacea. There is a typical centrofacial distribution of erythema, telangiectasias, papules, and pustules. In addition, the skin has a scaly, crusty surface, and this is often a sign of more severe disease. *Courtesy, Frank C. Powell, MD.*

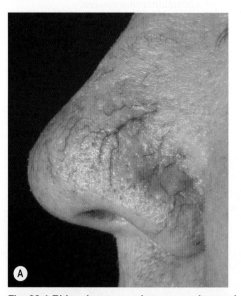
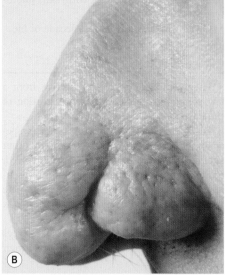

Fig. 30.4 Rhinophyma – early versus advanced disease. A Tortuous, telangiectatic vessels on the distal aspect of the nose contribute to its hyperemic appearance; this hyperemia may predispose to the subsequent hypertrophic changes of rhinophyma. Note the early sign of dilated follicles. **B** Distortion of nasal tissue due to tissue hypertrophy. Electrosurgery or laser therapy can be used to debulk and resculpt this nose. *Courtesy, Frank C. Powell, MD.*

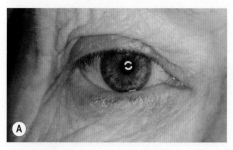
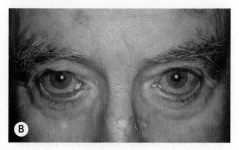

Fig. 30.5 Ocular rosacea. A Tiny concretions of keratin (conical dandruff) are visible at the bases of some of the eyelashes of the lower eyelid. There is also evidence of blepharitis predominantly of the eyelid margin and conjunctival injection. **B** Marked injection of the conjunctivae, leading to the appearance of red eyes. Ectropion is also present. *A, Courtesy, Frank C. Powell, MD.*

FOUR MAJOR TYPES OF ROSACEA		
Type		**Characteristics**
Erythematotelangiectatic (vascular)		Recurrent flushing/blushing, may eventuate in fixed central facial erythema (Figs. 30.1 and 30.2) Telangiectasias
Papulopustular (inflammatory)		Intermittent pink to red papules and inflammatory pustules (Fig. 30.3)
Phymatous		Hypertrophy and irregular (lumpy) thickening of nose (Fig. 30.4) >> forehead, cheeks, chin, or ears
Ocular		Symptoms Burning, stinging, pruritus, foreign-body sensation in the eye, photophobia, dryness, blurry vision Signs Telangiectasias of the sclera, periorbital edema, blepharitis (Fig. 30.5A), conjunctivitis (Fig. 30.5B), recurrent 'styes' (chalazia or hordeola), chronic edema, keratitis

Table 30.1 Four major types of rosacea. An individual patient may have more than one form. Some patients also have seborrheic dermatitis and/or actinic damage.

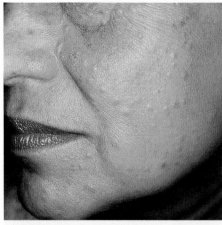

Fig. 30.6 Granulomatous rosacea. Discrete skin-colored to brown papules scattered on the face. *Courtesy, Frank C. Powell, MD.*

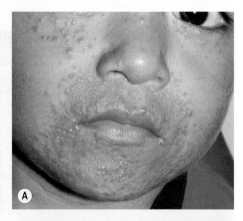

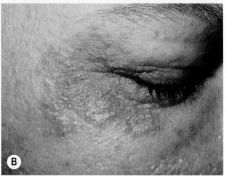

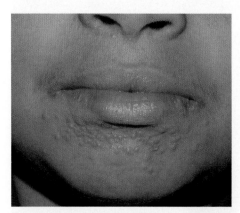

Fig. 30.7 Periorificial dermatitis. Discrete dull pink-red papules around the mouth and nose. While periorificial dermatitis is often misdiagnosed as eczema, this more granulomatous form may be misdiagnosed as sarcoidosis if a biopsy has been performed. *Courtesy, Julie V. Schaffer, MD.*

Fig. 30.8 Periorificial dermatitis.
A Granulomatous periorificial dermatitis in a child with monomorphous pink papules that have become confluent around the mouth. The eruption, which had previously worsened upon treatment with topical and oral corticosteroids, resolved with a 6-week course of azithromycin. **B** Periocular dermatitis with multiple fine papules and pustules superimposed on a pink plaque. The lesions can be misdiagnosed as an irritant or allergic contact dermatitis or atopic dermatitis. Although topical CS will initially improve the lesions, ultimately, there is exacerbation. *A, Courtesy, Julie V. Schaffer, MD; B, Courtesy, Ronald P. Rapini, MD.*

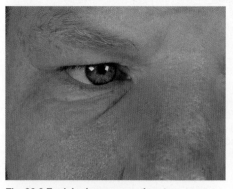

Fig. 30.9 Facial edema secondary to rosacea (Morbihan's disease). Erythematous, firm, nonpitting, nonpainful swelling of the upper face. Areas of greatest involvement have acquired a 'peau d'orange' appearance. *Courtesy, Frank C. Powell, MD.*

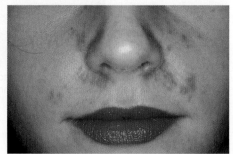

Fig. 30.10 Steroid rosacea. Mild disease in an adult with scattered erythematous papules and papulopustules. *Courtesy, Kalman Watsky, MD.*

DIFFERENTIAL DIAGNOSIS OF ROSACEA	
Disease	Distinguishing Feature(s) from Rosacea
Erythematotelangiectatic Rosacea	
Actinic damage	May be difficult to distinguish because this also leads to telangiectasias and erythema, and some patients have both disorders
Seborrheic dermatitis	Erythema with greasy scale in nasolabial folds, ear canals, eyebrows, and scalp
Keratosis pilaris rubra	• Usually presents during adolescence • Background erythema of the lateral cheeks with superimposed tiny follicular papules
Acute cutaneous lupus erythematosus	• Absence of inflammatory papulopustules and ocular changes • At least 75–80% of patients have systemic signs/symptoms • Often more well-demarcated edematous plaques
Flushing (idiopathic or secondary)	• Intermittent erythema and warmth • Flushing in patients with rosacea is usually limited to the face • Consider other common etiologies (e.g. menopause, anxiety disorder) or a tumor-related phenomenon (carcinoid syndrome, occult pheochromocytoma, mastocytosis) when additional anatomic sites are involved or there are associated symptoms such as tachycardia and sweating
Papulopustular Rosacea	
Acne (vulgaris)	Onset at a younger age Comedones, both open and closed Cysts Greater involvement of the upper trunk
Demodicosis (*Demodex* folliculitis)	Patients often immunosuppressed (HIV infection, leukemia) Responds to topical permethrin ± oral ivermectin
Steroid-induced rosacea	Clinical overlap with periorificial dermatitis (see above) (Fig. 30.10)
Ocular Rosacea	
Seborrheic dermatitis	Involvement beyond the eyelid margin; may be accentuated in the eyelid creases
Drug-induced ocular rosacea	Eyedrops used to treat other ocular disorders, e.g. glaucoma

Table 30.2 Differential diagnosis of rosacea.

- Lesions recur over weeks to months.
- May initially improve with topical CS but ultimately this treatment leads to exacerbation and should not be used.
- If topical CS are an exacerbating factor, taper strength of CS over a period of weeks or substitute topical calcineurin inhibitors in order to reduce rebound.

– Mid-facial edema:
  - Erythematous, firm, nonpitting, painless swelling of the mid-face (Fig. 30.9).
– Rosacea fulminans:
  - Acute facial plaque studded with pustules.
- **DDx:** Table 30.2.
- **Rx:** Tables 30.3 and 30.4.

MEDICAL AND SURGICAL THERAPIES FOR ROSACEA AND PERIORIFICIAL DERMATITIS

Papulopustular Rosacea

Topical Agents – Mild Disease, Adjunct to Oral Therapy or Maintenance after Oral Therapy (Daily to BID)

- Metronidazole (0.75–1%)
- Sodium sulfacetamide (10% ± sulfur 5%; available as a wash)
- Azelaic acid (15%)
- Benzoyl peroxide (5%)/clindamycin (1%)
- Clindamycin (1%)
- Erythromycin (2%)

Oral Medications (Discontinue or Taper to Lowest Effective Dose)

- Initially
  Tetracycline 500 mg orally BID -or-
  Doxycycline 100 mg orally BID -or-
  Minocycline 100 mg orally BID -or-
  Doxycycline 20 mg orally BID or 40 mg orally daily*
- After 4–8 weeks
  Decrease dose by ½ or to once daily
- Long term
  Topicals ± doxycycline 20–50 mg TIW
- If very severe
  Isotretinoin 10–40 mg orally daily for several months

Periorificial Dermatitis

Adults

Similar to papulopustular rosacea, but often unresponsive to topicals and a 4- to 8-week course of oral antibiotics is required

Children

- Topical metronidazole (0.75–1%)
- Oral antibiotic for 4–8 weeks
  Azithromycin 5–10 mg/kg TIW -or-
  Erythromycin 15–25 mg/kg BID -or-
  Doxycycline/minocycline (see below) if age >8 years

Erythematotelangiectatic Rosacea

- Laser (e.g. PDL, KTP) or intense pulsed light therapy
- Use of topical vasoconstrictors (e.g. brimonidine)

Phymatous Rosacea

- Surgical excision
- Electrosurgery (Fig. 30.11)

*Sub-antimicrobial dose.
BID, twice a day; KTP, potassium titanyl phosphate laser; PDL, pulsed dye laser; TIW, three times per week.*

Table 30.3 Medical and surgical therapies for rosacea and periorificial dermatitis.

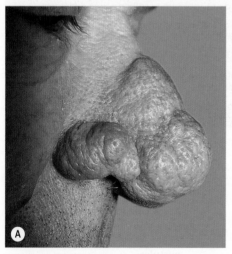
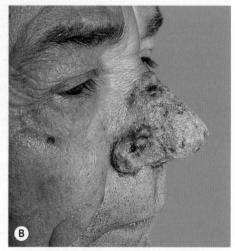

Fig. 30.11 Rhinophyma. A Moderately severe rhinophyma in a middle-aged man. **B** Immediately after electrosurgical planing of excess sebaceous glands. Care is taken to perform subtotal removal as very aggressive therapy can result in significant scarring and possible deformity caused by scar contracture. *Continued*

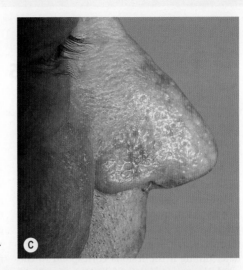

Fig. 30.11 *Continued* **C** Four weeks later, healing with good cosmetic outcome is noted. During healing, the wound is kept moist with an antibiotic ointment and semi-occlusive dressings. *Courtesy, Sheldon V. Pollack, MD.*

GENERAL RECOMMENDATIONS FOR FACIAL SKIN CARE AND EDUCATION IN PATIENTS WITH ROSACEA

Facial Skin Care

- Wash with lukewarm water and use soap-free cleansers that are pH balanced
- Cleansers are applied gently with fingertips
- Use sunscreens with both UVA and UVB protection and an SPF ≥15
- Sun-blocking creams containing the physical barriers titanium dioxide and/or zinc oxide are usually well tolerated
- Use cosmetics and sunscreens that contain protective silicones
- Water-soluble facial powder containing inert green pigment helps to neutralize the perception of erythema
- Moisturizers containing humectants (e.g. glycerin) and occlusives (e.g. petrolatum) help to repair the epidermal barrier
- Avoid astringents, toners, and abrasive exfoliators
- Avoid cosmetics that contain alcohol, menthols, camphor, witch hazel, fragrance, peppermint, and eucalyptus oil
- Avoid waterproof cosmetics and heavy foundations that are difficult to remove without irritating solvents or physical scrubbing
- Avoid procedures such as glycolic peels or dermabrasion

Patient Education

- Reassure the patient about the benign nature of the disorder and the rarity of rhinophyma, particularly in women
- Emphasize the chronicity of the disease and the likelihood of exacerbations
- Direct patients to information websites such as those of the National Rosacea Society (http://www.rosacea.org) or the American Academy of Dermatology (http://www.aad.org)
- Advise to avoid recognized triggers
- Explain the importance of compliance with topical regimens
- Educate on the importance of sun avoidance

Adapted from Powell FC. Rosacea. N. Engl. J. Med. 2005;352:793–803; Pelle MT, Crawford GH, James WD. Rosacea: II. Therapy. J. Am. Acad. Dermatol. 2004;51:499–512; and Del Rosso JQ, Baum EW. Comprehensive medical management of rosacea: An interim study report and literature review. J. Clin. Aesthet. Dermatol. 2008;1:20–25.

Table 30.4 General recommendations for facial skin care and education in patients with rosacea.

For further information see Ch. 37. From *Dermatology, Third Edition.*

31 | Folliculitis

- The folliculitides are divided into superficial and deep forms (Table 31.1).
- Follicular papules and pustules can be distinguished from nonfollicular lesions by the presence of a hair piercing the lesion in the former; if hair shafts are not apparent, then determining if the lesions correspond to the spatial pattern of hair follicles can aid in diagnosis.

Superficial Folliculitis

- Common; characterized by follicular papules or pustules that are often on an erythematous base.

- Often pruritic, sometimes painful.
- Favors areas with terminal hairs, such as the scalp and beard; also common on the trunk, buttocks, and thighs > axillae and groin.
- The most common type is culture-negative/normal flora, followed by bacterial folliculitis caused by *Staphylococcus aureus*.
- Multiple, less common etiologies (Table 31.1), requiring a systematic approach for adequate diagnosis and treatment (Fig. 31.1; Table 31.2).
- **DDx:** acne vulgaris, pseudofolliculitis barbae, rosacea; Grover's disease in adults; pustular miliaria in children.

CLASSIFICATION OF THE FOLLICULITIDES	
Superficial Folliculitides	**Deep Folliculitides**
Infectious	• Furuncles

• Bacterial
  1. *Staphylococcal aureus* (Fig. 31.2)
  2. Gram-negative bacilli
  3. Hot tub folliculitis (Fig. 31.3)
	• Sycosis (Table 31.3)
	  1. Barbae (Fig. 31.2A)
	  2. Lupoid
	  3. Mycotic (Fig. 31.7)
	  4. Herpetic

• Fungal
  1. Dermatophyte (Fig. 31.4A)
  2. *Malassezia* spp. (*Pityrosporum*)
  3. *Candida* spp.
	• Pseudofollicultis barbae
	• Acne keloidalis
	• Follicular occlusion tetrad

• Viral
  1. Herpes simplex (Fig. 31.4B)
  2. Varicella zoster
	1. Acne conglobata (see Chapter 29)
	  2. Hidradenitis suppurativa
	  3. Dissecting cellulitis of the scalp
	    (see Chapter 56)

• Other 1. *Demodex* (Fig. 31.4C,D)	4. Pilonidal sinus/cyst
Non-Infectious	

• Culture-negative/normal flora (Fig. 31.5)
• Irritant
• Drug-induced
• Eosinophilic (Fig. 31.6)
  1. Eosinophilic pustular folliculitis
  2. AIDS-associated eosinophilic folliculitis
  3. Eosinophilic pustular folliculitis of infancy
• Disseminate and recurrent infundibulofolliculitis	

Table 31.1 Classification of the folliculitides.

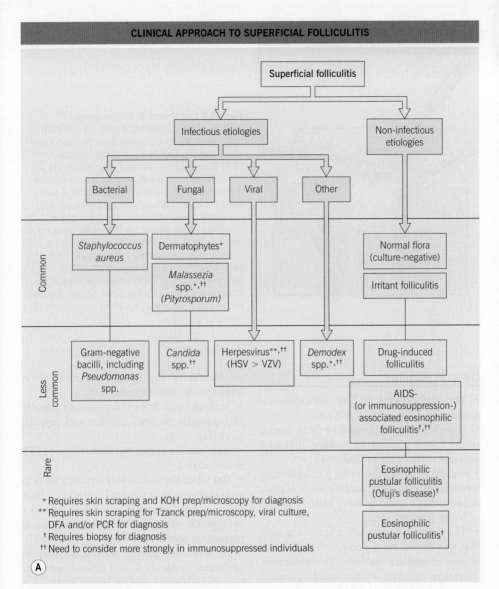

Superficial folliculitis

Infectious etiologies

Non-infectious etiologies

Bacterial

Fungal

Viral

Other

Common

Staphylococcus aureus

Dermatophytes*

Malassezia spp.*,†† (Pityrosporum)

Normal flora (culture-negative)

Irritant folliculitis

Less common

Gram-negative bacilli, including *Pseudomonas* spp.

Candida spp.††

Herpesvirus**,†† (HSV > VZV)

Demodex spp.*,††

Drug-induced folliculitis

AIDS- (or immunosuppression-) associated eosinophilic folliculitis†,††

Rare

Eosinophilic pustular folliculitis (Ofuji's disease)†

Eosinophilic pustular folliculitis†

* Requires skin scraping and KOH prep/microscopy for diagnosis
** Requires skin scraping for Tzanck prep/microscopy, viral culture, DFA and/or PCR for diagnosis
† Requires biopsy for diagnosis
†† Need to consider more strongly in immunosuppressed individuals

A

Fig. 31.1 Superficial folliculitis – clinical approach and initial evaluation. A Clinically, edematous lesions of folliculitis are most suggestive of eosinophilic folliculitis, *Demodex* folliculitis, and *Pseudomonas* 'hot tub' folliculitis. *Continued*

METHOD FOR INITIAL EVALUATION OF SUPERFICIAL FOLLICULITIS

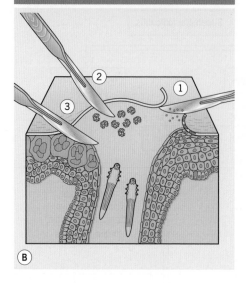

Fig. 31.1 *Continued* **B** If considering dermatophytes, *Malassezia* spp., or *Candida* spp., then obtain scrapings from the peripheral scale and the roof of the follicular pustule for KOH (potassium hydroxide) microscopy (1). If considering bacterial etiologies, and depending on the host, the pustular fluid should be sent for gram stain, culture, and sensitivity (2). If considering viral etiologies, the base of the unroofed lesion should be vigorously scraped in order to collect the viral-laden keratinocytes for Tzanck prep/microscopy, viral culture, DFA (direct fluorescent antibody), and/or PCR (polymerase chain reaction) (3). Likewise, if considering *Demodex* folliculitis, scrape the base of the lesion vigorously for KOH microscopy (3) (see Fig. 31.4D).

Deep Folliculitis

• The major forms of deep folliculitis are outlined in Tables 31.1 and 31.3.
• Lesions are characterized by firm, tender, erythematous papules or nodules that may measure up to 2 cm in diameter.
• Should avoid manipulating (i.e. squeezing) furuncles as may cause bacteremia or seeding of heart valves (endocarditis), brain (abscess), or bones (osteomyelitis).
• The 'follicular occlusion tetrad' is a term that was coined for the common association of acne conglobata, hidradenitis suppurativa, dissecting cellulitis of the scalp, pilonidal sinus; also called 'acne inversa'.

Pseudofolliculitis Barbae (PFB)

• A common, chronic inflammatory disorder occurring most often in the beard area of men who shave.
• Favors males > females; African-Americans and others with darkly pigmented skin and tightly curled hair.
• The proposed etiology is tightly curled hairs that curve back into the skin when shaved (Fig. 31.8).
• Also, there is a genetic predisposition if carrying a mutation in the 1A α-helical subdomain of the hair follicle companion layer-specific keratin K6hf (K75).
• Lesions range from inflammatory papules and pustules to firm papules and keloidal scars (Fig. 31.9).
• Intervention during the acute phase of PFB is essential.
• **Rx:** while the easiest way to cure PFB is to stop shaving, this may not be practical; laser hair removal systems that are skin-color appropriate offer the best option for a more permanent solution.
• In addition, shaving techniques can be optimized (Table 31.4) and other treatments may provide some control (Table 31.5).

Acne Keloidalis

• Begins as a chronic folliculitis of the posterior neck and occipital scalp; with time, keloidal papules and plaques develop (Fig. 31.10).
• Seen almost exclusively in males of African descent.
• Lesions are usually pruritic and sometimes painful and disfiguring.
• Often there is patchy alopecia or complete hair loss; occasionally there are subcutaneous abscesses with malodorous draining sinuses.

CLINICAL FEATURES AND TREATMENT OF SELECTED SUPERFICIAL FOLLICULITIDES

Type	Clinical Features	Therapy
Infectious Folliculitides		
Bacterial		
Staphylococcus aureus folliculitis	• Follicular pustules or papules on erythematous base (Fig. 31.2) • Favors face, trunk, axillae, buttocks • If no pustules present, clue to diagnosis may be a superimposed collarette of scale	**Localized** • Topical mupirocin 2% ointment TID for 7–10 days **Widespread or recurrent** • Culture-guided oral antibiotics • Bleach baths twice weekly* • Weekly use of chlorhexidine cleanser in shower • Treat chronic *S. aureus* nasal carriage
Gram-negative folliculitis	• Due to *Klebsiella*, *Enterobacter*, and *Proteus* spp. • Typically seen in acne patients receiving long-term antibiotics • Also seen in adult men with oily skin	• Pustules in the T-zone and perinasal regions of face • Topical gentamicin or benzoyl peroxide • Systemic quinolones **Severe or recurrent** • Isotretinoin 1 mg/kg/day for 16 weeks
Hot tub folliculitis	• Due to *Pseudomonas aeruginosa* in the setting of hot tub/whirlpool use 12–48 hours prior to onset	• Edematous pink-red follicular papules and pustules • Favors trunk (Fig. 31.3); often pruritic • Usually self-limited in immunocompetent host • More serious in immunocompromised • Antibacterial soap • Maintenance of hot tub/whirlpool to ensure adequate chlorine levels **Severe or immunocompromised host** • Oral quinolones for 1–2 weeks
Fungal		
Dermatophyte folliculitis	• Tinea barbae in beard area • Majocchi's granuloma, often on legs of women who shave	• Inflammatory follicular papules and pustules in beard area; crusts; loosened hairs • Follicular pustules, papules, or nodules, most often on lower legs (Fig. 31.4A) • Topical antifungals often ineffective • Micronized or ultramicronized griseofulvin, 500–1000 mg/day or 500–700 mg/day PO, respectively, for 4–6 weeks • Terbinafine, 250 mg/day PO for 2–3 weeks • Itraconazole, 200 mg PO BID for 1 week per month, for 2 pulses

Table 31.2 Clinical features and treatment of selected superficial folliculitides. *Continued*

Table 31.2 Continued Clinical features and treatment of selected superficial folliculitides.

Type	Clinical Features	Therapy
Pityrosporum folliculitis • Caused by *Malassezia* spp. • Typically young adults • Inciting factors include warm weather, occlusion, excessive sebum production, antibiotic therapy, iatrogenic immunosuppression	• Pruritic follicular pustules and papules • Favors chest, back, shoulders • Abundant yeast forms on KOH microscopy	**Topicals** • Antifungals (e.g. ketoconazole cream) • Selenium sulfide or antifungal shampoos **Systemic** • Fluconazole 100–200 mg/day PO for 3 weeks • Itraconazole 200 mg/day PO for 1–3 weeks
Candida folliculitis • Seen primarily in diabetics • Also in immunocompromised hosts and patients on antibiotic or CS therapy • Common in hospitalized or bedridden, febrile patients on the back	• Pruritic follicular pustules on erythematous base • Favors warm, moist and occluded environments, such as intertriginous areas • Often present as satellite pustules surrounding areas of intertriginous candidiasis • Facial lesions may mimic tinea barbae	• Prevent skin-to-skin contact in intertriginous areas • If possible, discontinue antibiotics or CS therapy **Mild** • Topical antifungals **Severe or recalcitrant** • Fluconazole 100 mg/day PO × 1 week, then qOD × 1 month
Viral *Herpetic folliculitis* • **Immunocompetent host:** most common scenarios are occurrence on the face of men or pubic area of women (with histories of recurrent HSV infections) who shave with blade razors • **Immunocompromised host:** widespread or unusual presentations seen; consider VZV when submitting specimens for culture, DFA, and/or PCR	• Rapid development of individual and grouped follicular pustules and vesicles on an erythematous base (Fig. 31.4B) • Multinucleated giant cells seen on Tzanck smear	• Famciclovir 500 mg PO TID for 5–10 days • Valacyclovir 500 mg PO TID for 5–10 days • Acyclovir 200 mg PO 5 times per day for 5–10 days

Other

Demodex folliculitis

• May be associated with immune suppression • Sometimes associated with flares of rosacea	• Topical 5% permethrin cream • Systemic single dose of ivermectin 200 microg PO • Prevention with daily cleansing using a medicated wash, e.g. sulfacetamide
• Erythematous follicular papules and pustules on the face, often within a background of diffuse erythema (Fig. 31.4C) • Skin scrapings under microscopy reveal numerous *Demodex* mites (Fig. 31.4D)	

Non-Infectious Folliculitides

Culture-negative/normal flora folliculitis

• The most common of all the folliculitides • May look like *S. aureus* folliculitis clinically but cultures reveal no growth or only normal flora • Favors trunk and scalp (Fig. 31.5) • Often pruritic	• Topical benzoyl peroxide • Topical antibiotics (e.g. clindamycin) • Oral antibiotics (e.g. doxycycline, tetracycline) used primarily for their anti-inflammatory effects

Irritant folliculitis

• Usually occurs following the application of a topical medication or ointment (e.g. tar preparations) • May be seen on thighs from rubbing of denim jeans • Follicular pustules in the sites of application or rubbing	• Stop inciting agent • Apply topical medications in the same direction as hair growth • Topical mid-potency CS lotion or cream

Drug-induced folliculitis

• Most common in acne-prone patients and age groups • Can develop within 2 weeks of starting the culprit agent • Risk is proportional to the dose and duration of therapy • Common culprits: CS, androgenic hormones, EGFR inhibitors, iodides, bromides, lithium, isoniazid, anticonvulsants • Acute eruption of monomorphic erythematous follicular papules and pustules • Favors trunk, shoulders, and upper arms • No comedones	• Stop culprit medication, if possible **Topicals** • Benzoyl peroxide, clindamycin, erythromycin, or retinoids **Systemic** • Tetracycline, doxycycline, minocycline

Table 31.2 Continued **Clinical features and treatment of selected superficial folliculitides.**

Type	Clinical Features	Therapy
Eosinophilic Folliculitis		
Eosinophilic pustular folliculitis (Ofuji's disease)		
• Most reported cases from Japan • Not associated with systemic disease	• Recurrent episodes of follicular papulopustules; erythematous patches and plaques with superimposed coalescent pustules; and later central clearing which leads to figurate lesions • Favors face, upper extremities, and trunk; occasionally palms and soles • Pruritus often severe • Lesions last 7–10 days • Spontaneous resolution with relapse is the norm	• Topical antipruritics, oral antihistamines, and topical CS for relief of pruritus **First-line** • Oral indomethacin 50 mg/day PO **Second-line** • UVB phototherapy • Oral minocycline, dapsone, CS, or colchicine
AIDS- (or immunosuppression)-associated eosinophilic folliculitis		
• Correlates with a low CD4 count (<300/mm³) • Also reported in other immunosuppressed individuals, such as those with lymphoma, leukemias, and stem cell transplant recipients • Can be part of the immune reconstitution inflammatory syndrome (IRIS)	• Chronic, persistent pruritic follicular papules; perhaps no pustules (Fig. 31.6A) • Favors the face (Fig. 31.6B), scalp, and upper trunk • Intense pruritus	• Clinical improvement occurs with elevation of CD4 count via ART • Topical and oral antipruritics and CS often inadequate • UVB phototherapy can be helpful for pruritus • Additional: topical tacrolimus, permethrin; oral antibiotics, itraconazole, isotretinoin

*Bleach bath involves mixing ¼ cup of household bleach into a half-filled, regular-sized bathtub.
PO, orally; BID, twice daily; KOH, potassium hydroxide; qOD, every other day; VZV, varicella zoster virus; DFA, direct fluorescence antibody; PCR, polymerase chain reaction; TID, three times a day; ART, antiretroviral treatment.

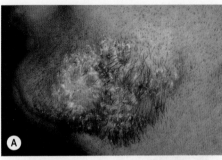
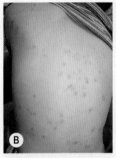
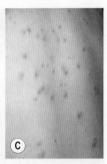

Fig. 31.2 Folliculitis due to _Staphylococcus aureus_. A Folliculitis of the beard area with discrete papulopustules seen posteriorly. Centrally, there is deeper involvement with plaque formation (sycosis barbae). **B** Widespread follicular pustules limited to the back of a sedated psychiatric patient. On closer examination **(C)**, the characteristic follicular papulopustules on an erythematous base are seen, along with a collarette of scale on an older lesion, located centrally in the photo. _B, C, Courtesy, Julie V. Schaffer, MD._

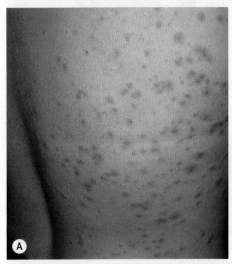
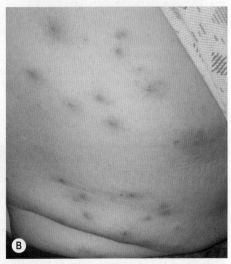

Fig. 31.3 _Pseudomonas_ 'hot tub' folliculitis. A, B Edematous follicular papules on the flank that begin to develop 2–3 days following the use of a hot tub. The number and size can vary. _B, Courtesy, Kalman Watsky, MD._

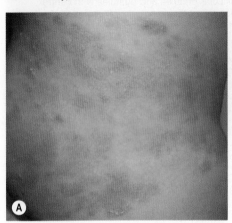
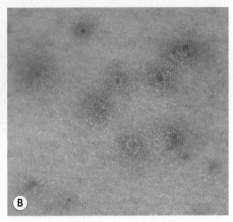

Fig. 31.4 Folliculitis – fungal, viral, and ectoparasitic. A Firm follicular papules of dermatophyte folliculitis (Majocchi's granuloma) in the setting of extensive tinea corporis. **B** Follicular herpes simplex viral infection in an immunocompromised host. _B, Courtesy, Karynne O. Duncan, MD._ **Continued**

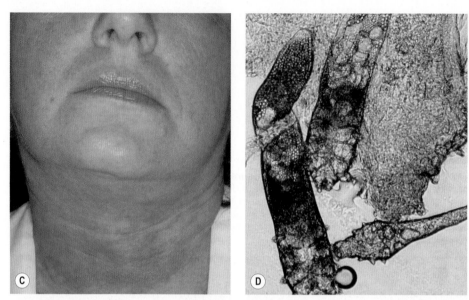

Fig. 31.4 *Continued* **C** Edematous papules of *Demodex* folliculitis superimposed on the characteristic background erythema. **D** Microscopic findings of follicular contents obtained via scraping of *Demodex* folliculitis. *C, Courtesy, Kalman Watsky, MD.*

FORMS OF SYCOSIS	
Type	**Characteristics**
Barbae	• Bacterial folliculitis of the beard and/or mustache areas, usually caused by *Staphylococcus aureus* (see Fig. 31.2A) • Deep-seated, edematous, perifollicular papules and pustules that may coalesce to form plaques studded with pustules and crusts • Subacute to chronic course with frequent relapses
Lupoid	• Scarring form of deep folliculitis, typically affecting the beard area; may be caused by *S. aureus* (although cultures often fail to reveal pathogenic organisms) • Peripheral extension of perifollicular papules and pustules with central atrophic scarring/cicatricial alopecia; granulomatous inflammation can lead to an appearance reminiscent of lupus vulgaris • Chronic course, refractory to treatment
Mycotic	• Dermatophyte folliculitis of the beard area (most often the chin), usually caused by zoophilic organisms • Inflammatory perifollicular papules and pustules coalesce to form nodules and plaques with purulent discharge from patulous follicles, crusting, and loose hairs that can be painlessly removed (Fig. 31.7)
Herpetic	• See Table 31.2

Table 31.3 Forms of sycosis.

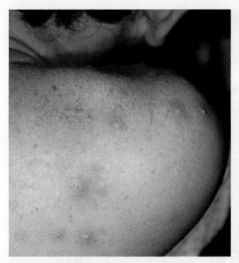

Fig. 31.5 Culture-negative folliculitis.
Follicular pustules with an erythematous rim are
present on the upper back. The differential
diagnosis is primarily folliculitis due to
Staphylococcus aureus and acne.

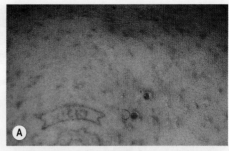

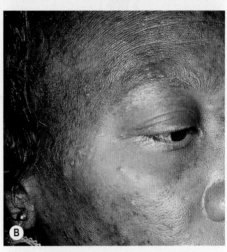

• The sooner this condition is treated, the
less likely it will become disfiguring.
• **Rx:** outlined in Table 31.6.
• Prevention is important, and patients should
avoid mechanical irritation of the posterior
hairline.

Hidradenitis Suppurativa

• A cutaneous disorder that targets the apocrine gland-bearing skin sites, particularly the
axillae and groin.
• A chronic condition characterized by recurrent 'boils' and draining sinus tracts with
subsequent scarring.
• Favors females > males and persons of
African descent; onset at or soon after puberty.
• **Initially** inflammatory nodules and sterile
abscesses arise in the axillae, groin, perianal,
and/or inframammary areas; often very
painful (Fig. 31.11A).
• **With time** sinus tracts (Fig. 31.11B) and
hypertrophic scars develop (Fig. 31.11C);
chronic, malodorous drainage also occurs.
• **Complications** may include anemia of
chronic disease, secondary amyloidosis,
lymphedema, fistulas, arthropathy, and the
rare development of SCCs within the chronic
scars.

**Fig. 31.6 AIDS-associated eosinophilic
folliculitis. A** Multiple follicular papules on the
chest in the setting of AIDS. There are two
punch biopsy sites. Note the edematous nature
of some of the lesions. **B** Multiple pruritic
follicular papules on the face of an HIV-infected
woman. There is also post-inflammatory
hyperpigmentation.

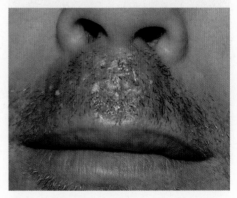

Fig. 31.7 Mycotic sycosis. Firm plaque of the
upper cutaneous lip studded with multiple
pustules due to a zoophilic dermatophye.
Courtesy, Kalman Watsky, MD.

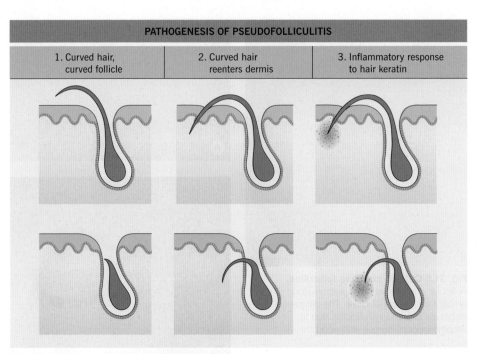

PATHOGENESIS OF PSEUDOFOLLICULITIS

1. Curved hair, curved follicle	2. Curved hair reenters dermis	3. Inflammatory response to hair keratin

Fig. 31.8 Pathogenesis of pseudofolliculitis. *Courtesy, M.A. Abdallah, MD.*

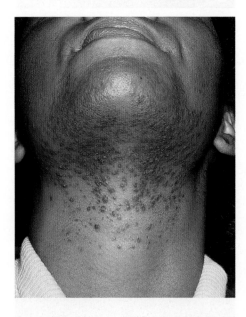

Fig. 31.9 Pseudofolliculitis barbae. Multiple firm hyperpigmented papules on the lower face and neck (beard distribution). *Courtesy, A. Paul Kelly, MD.*

ADVICE ON SHAVING METHODS FOR PATIENTS WITH PSEUDOFOLLICULITIS BARBAE

Important Points

- Do not pull the skin taut
- Do not shave against the grain/direction of hair growth
- Use a sharp razor each time, preferably multiblade
- Take short strokes (with the grain of the hair) and do not shave over the same areas more than twice

Method

1. Remove pre-existing hairs with electric clippers, leaving approximately 1–2 mm of stubble
2. Wash area with nonabrasive acne soap and rough wash cloth; in areas with 'ingrown hairs,' gentle massaging with a soft toothbrush may help
3. Rinse area with water, then compress face with warm tap water for several minutes
4. Using shaving cream of your choice, massage moderate amount of lather on area to be shaved (do not allow lather to dry; if it does, reapply it)
5. Use a sharp blade (whichever type seems to cut best but not too close) and shave with the grain of the hair using short even strokes with minimal tension (and no more than twice over one area); in hard-to-shave areas, you may need to shave against the grain
6. After shaving, rinse with tap water and then apply the most soothing aftershave preparation of your choice. If significant burning or itching ensues, a topical CS cream or lotion (1–2.5% hydrocortisone) can be used as an alternative aftershave preparation

Table 31.4 Advice on shaving methods for patients with pseudofolliculitis barbae. *Courtesy, A. Paul Kelly, MD.*

THERAPEUTIC APPROACH TO PSEUDOFOLLICULITIS BARBAE

Shaving	• Mild to moderate cases: continue shaving daily, but follow guidelines in Table 31.4 • Severe cases: consider discontinuing shaving, with no resumption of shaving until all inflammatory lesions have cleared and all 'ingrown hairs' are released; during this period, the patient can trim beard to a minimum length of 0.5 cm using scissors or electric clippers
Compresses and release of ingrowing hairs	• Warm tap water, saline, or Burow's solution (aluminum acetate) compresses for 10 minutes three times daily to soothe lesions, remove any crusts, reduce drainage secondary to inflammation and/or excoriations, and soften the epidermis to allow easier release of 'ingrown hairs'
Topical therapy	• Low-potency topical CS lotion and/or topical clindamycin should be applied after compresses and freeing of embedded hairs
Secondary bacterial infection	• Appropriate systemic antibiotic should be prescribed, based on bacterial cultures
Recalcitrant disease	• Prednisone (45–60 mg) or its equivalent every morning for 7–10 days may be necessary • Topical eflornithine cream twice daily may be helpful* • Laser hair removal (utilizing appropriate laser for skin color) with goal of permanent hair reduction

Based on case series.

Table 31.5 Therapeutic approach to pseudofolliculitis barbae. *Courtesy, A. Paul Kelly, MD.*

- **DDx:** staphylococcal furunculosis, Crohn's disease, granuloma inguinale, mycetoma, and scrofuloderma (a form of tuberculous lymphadenitis with cutaneous extension).
- **Rx:** difficult to treat and no one perfect treatment exists; surgical excision the closest thing to a 'cure' (Table 31.7).

- Avoid incision and drainage, as may lead to further scarring and sinus tract formation
- In general, medical treatment is recommended in early stages; surgical treatment should be performed as early as possible once abscesses, fistulas, sinus tracts, and scars develop.

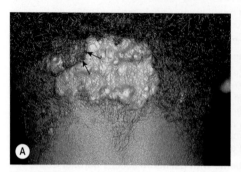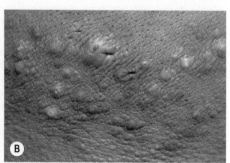

Fig. 31.10 Acne keloidalis. A Keloidal papulonodules and a large plaque of the occipital scalp, associated with scarring alopecia. Note the tufts of hair at the superior border of the scar (arrows). **B** A close-up view, showing an admixture of follicular papules, crusted papules, and firm fibrotic hyperpigmented papules on the posterior neck and occipital scalp. There is associated alopecia. *A, Courtesy, A. Paul Kelly, MD; B, Courtesy, A. Paul Kelly, MD, and Amy McMichael, MD.*

THERAPEUTIC OPTIONS FOR ACNE KELOIDALIS	
Non-inflamed papules and plaques	Mixture of tretinoin gel and potent CS gel twice daily
Inflamed lesions with pustules	Bacterial culture and appropriate systemic antibiotic or a course of oral isotretinoin
Small papules	Punch excision to below level of hair follicles Close primarily or allow to heal secondarily Laser hair removal for permanent hair reduction
Plaques ≤1.5 cm in vertical diameter	Excise and close primarily
Larger plaques and nodules (>1.5 cm in vertical diameter)	Excise with horizontal ellipse Extend excision below posterior hairline and include fascia or deep subcutaneous tissue Allow to heal by second intention Do not inject CS into postoperative site Laser excision and cryosurgery are sometimes successful
Postoperative care	Topical imiquimod daily for 6 weeks (8 weeks every other day if irritation)
Maintenance	Tretinoin–CS gel mixture, intermittent intralesional CS and/or oral or topical antibiotics (when needed)

Table 31.6 Therapeutic options for acne keloidalis. *Courtesy, A. Paul Kelly, MD.*

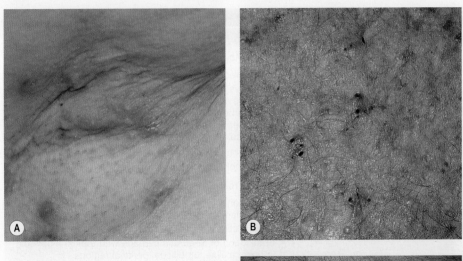

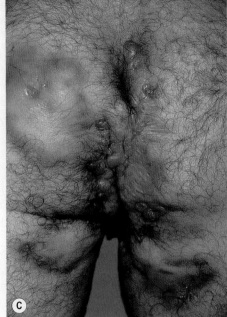

Fig. 31.11 Hidradenitis suppurativa.
A Papulopustules, nodules, sinus tracts, and scarring in the axilla (Hurley stage II). **B** Superficial sinus tracts that serve as a clue to the diagnosis, even in the absence of active disease. **C** Severe disease (Hurley stage III) with inflammatory nodules, hypertrophic scarring, draining fistulae. and sinus tract formation of the perianal region, buttocks, and upper thighs. This is the type of patient who is at risk for the development of squamous cell carcinoma and secondary amyloidosis. *A, Courtesy, Kalman Watsky, MD.*

| THERAPEUTIC OPTIONS FOR HIDRADENITIS SUPPURATIVA ||
Indication	Treatment

All Patients	**General Measures**
	
	• Weight reduction if obese or overweight
	• Measures to reduce friction and moisture
	  1. Loose undergarments
	  2. Absorbent powders
	  3. Antiseptic soaps
	  4. Topical aluminum chloride
	• Warm compresses
	• Stop smoking

Hurley Stage I Disease • Solitary or multiple isolated abscesses • No scarring or sinus tracts	**Medical Treatment** • Intralesional triamcinolone (5 mg/ml) injections into early inflammatory lesions • Topical clindamycin • Eradication of *S. aureus* carriage with topical mupirocin in nose, axillae, umbilicus, perianal regions • Oral antibiotics tailored to results of bacterial cultures from drainage discharge or abscess contents • Oral antibiotic therapy (alone or in combination) for its anti-inflammatory effect (tetracycline, doxycycline, minocycline, clindamycin, rifampin + clindamycin, dapsone, trimethoprim–sulfamethoxazole) • Oral anti-androgen therapy (e.g. finasteride)
Flares	• Short courses of systemic CS

Hurley Stage II Disease (see Fig. 31.11A)
 	
• Recurrent abscesses
• Sinus tract formations
• Early scarring
	Medical Treatment
	
	• Systemic adjuvant or maintenance therapy (may be helpful in selected cases)
	  1. Acitretin
	  2. Infliximab
	  3. Cyclosporine
	
	Surgical Treatment
	
	• Limited local excisions with secondary intention healing
	• CO_2 laser ablation with secondary intention healing

Hurley Stage III Disease (see Fig. 31.11C) • Diffuse or broad involvement with multiple interconnected abscesses and sinus tracts • More extensive scarring	**Surgical Treatment** • Early wide surgical excision of involved areas • CO_2 laser ablation with secondary intention healing

Table 31.7 Therapeutic options for hidradenitis suppurativa.

For further information see Ch. 38. From *Dermatology, Third Edition*.

Disorders of Eccrine and Apocrine Glands

32

Eccrine and apocrine glands represent the two major types of sweat glands (see Fig. 91.1).

Eccrine Glands

• Functional from birth and activated by thermal stimuli via the hypothalamic sweat center; while their major function is thermoregulation by evaporative heat loss, they are also activated by emotional stimuli.
• Innervated by sympathetic fibers that have acetylcholine as their major neurotransmitter.
• Generalized distribution, with greatest concentration on the palms and soles.
• The eccrine duct opens directly onto the skin surface, and the excretory product is a clear hypotonic fluid that is mostly water but also contains NaCl.

Apocrine Glands

• Unclear function in humans; functional development requires androgens.
• More limited distribution – primarily axillae, nipples/areolae, and umbilical and anogenital regions; modified apocrine glands are found in the external auditory canals and eyelid margins.
• The apocrine duct drains into the superficial portion of the hair follicle (see Fig. 91.1).
• 'Decapitation' of apocrine gland cells produces an odorless and viscous fluid; however, its degradation by flora on the skin surface can lead to an odor.

Hyperhidrosis

• Excessive production of eccrine sweat is usually due to *primary cortical* (emotional) hyperhidrosis and the favored sites are the axillae or palms and soles (Fig. 32.1) > the face (Fig. 32.2); involvement is bilateral and symmetric.

• *Secondary cortical* hyperhidrosis is associated with genodermatoses, including palmoplantar keratodermas and epidermolysis bullosa simplex; associated odor reflects maceration and degradation of keratin by bacteria.

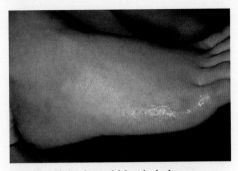

Fig. 32.1 Volar hyperhidrosis (primary cortical). The palmoplantar skin displays excessive eccrine sweat production, including the portions that extend onto the sides of the hands, feet, and digits. Its onset is during childhood as opposed to axillary hyperhidrosis, which has its onset around puberty.

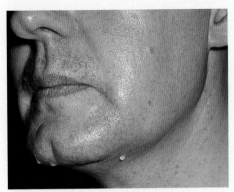

Fig. 32.2 Primary cortical (emotional) hyperhidrosis involving the face. Sweat droplets are evident on the upper cutaneous lip, jawline, and chin. *Reproduced from Hurley HJ. Hyperhidrosis.* Curr. Opin. Dermatol. *1997;4:105–114. Philadelphia: Rapid Science Publishers.*

283

CAUSES OF SECONDARY HYPOTHALAMIC HYPERHIDROSIS
• **Infections**, e.g. acute febrile bacterial and viral infections (defervescence), malaria
• **Neoplasms**, e.g. lymphoma (B symptom), pheochromocytoma
• **Endocrinologic disorders**, e.g. hypoestrogenemia of menopause, hyperthyroidism
• **Vasomotor disorders**, e.g. cold injury, Raynaud's phenomenon, RSD
• **Neurologic diseases**, e.g. CNS tumors, CVAs (contralateral)
• **Drugs and toxins**, e.g. opioid withdrawal, alcohol withdrawal, combination of drugs that result in the serotonin syndrome (MAOI plus tricyclic or SSRI antidepressant)
• **Miscellaneous**, e.g. compensatory in the setting of a sympathectomy, extensive miliaria or diabetes mellitus

CNS, central nervous system; CVA, cerebrovascular accident; MAOI, monoamine oxidase inhibitor; RSD, reflex sympathetic dystrophy, also referred to as complex regional pain syndrome; SSRI, selective serotonin reuptake inhibitor. Linezolid is an MAOI.

Table 32.1 Causes of secondary hypothalamic hyperhidrosis.

• *Secondary hypothalamic* (thermoregulatory) hyperhidrosis can be due to a number of systemic diseases, from infections to neoplasms (Table 32.1).

• *Secondary medullary* (gustatory) hyperhidrosis can be physiologic as exemplified by the facial sweating that occurs with spicy foods or pathologic as occurs in Frey's syndrome (Fig. 32.3); in the former, taste receptors send afferent impulses, whereas in the latter, disrupted nerves for sweat aberrantly connect with nerves for salivation.

• Injuries or diseases affecting the spinal cord can result in segmental hyperhidrosis.

• In addition to embarrassment, hyperhidrosis can lead to overhydration of the skin and a higher risk of bacterial and fungal infections.

• Sweating only during waking hours points to primary cortical (emotional) hyperhidrosis; after consideration of possible underlying etiologies, topical antiperspirants containing aluminum chloride (e.g. Certain-Dri®) or aluminum chloride hexahydrate (e.g. Xerac-AC® [6.25%], Drysol® [20%]) can be applied, and if necessary, initially preceded by oral glycopyrrolate or oxybutynin.

• Injection of botulinum toxin type A every ~6 months is very effective for primary cortical (emotional) hyperhidrosis (Fig. 32.4); tap water iontophoresis is less effective.

Hypohidrosis (and Anhidrosis)

• There are multiple etiologies of hypohidrosis and anhidrosis including the following:

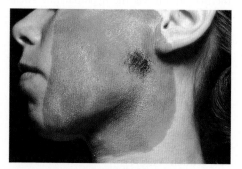

Fig. 32.3 Gustatory sweating in the auriculotemporal (Frey's) syndrome, as a consequence of parotid surgery. The blue-black area represents sweating (starch–iodine technique). Salivary stimulation induced this sweating response. *Reproduced from Hurley HJ. Hyperhidrosis. Curr. Opin. Dermatol. 1997;4:105–114. Philadelphia: Rapid Science Publishers.*

– A side effect of medications with anticholinergic properties (e.g. atropine, tricyclic antidepressants, glycopyrrolate).

– Manifestation of inherited disorders, in particular ectodermal dysplasias (see Chapter 52), as well as acquired disorders such as Sjögren's syndrome.

– Neurologic disorders, from tumors or infarcts of the hypothalamus, pons, or medulla to peripheral neuropathies.

• Increased risk of developing hyperthermia.

• Evaluation includes colorimetric testing (see Fig. 32.4) and biopsy of affected skin.

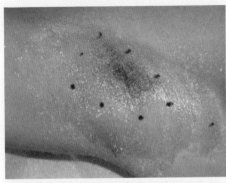

Fig. 32.4 Delineation of area for injections of botulinum toxin A for axillary hyperhidrosis (starch–iodine technique). Blue-black areas represent foci of sweating. In the case of onabotulinumtoxin A, a total of 50–100 U is injected, utilizing 10–15 injection sites. *Courtesy, Alastair Carruthers, MD, and Jean Carruthers, MD.*

Bromhidrosis (Foul-Smelling Sweat)

- *Eccrine* variant associated with degradation of sweat by resident microflora; most commonly involves the feet.
- *Apocrine* variant associated with degradation of odiferous substances (e.g. triglycerides) by skin flora.
- The smell can be rancid (*Corynebacterium*) or sweaty (*Micrococcus*).
- Rarely, it is a sign of an inherited metabolic disorder.

Chromhidrosis

- Colored sweat can be *intrinsic* and due to the lipofuscin content of apocrine sweat (yellow, green, black) or *extrinsic* and due to staining of sweat by clothing or chromogenic bacteria (e.g. *Corynebacterium*) or fungi.

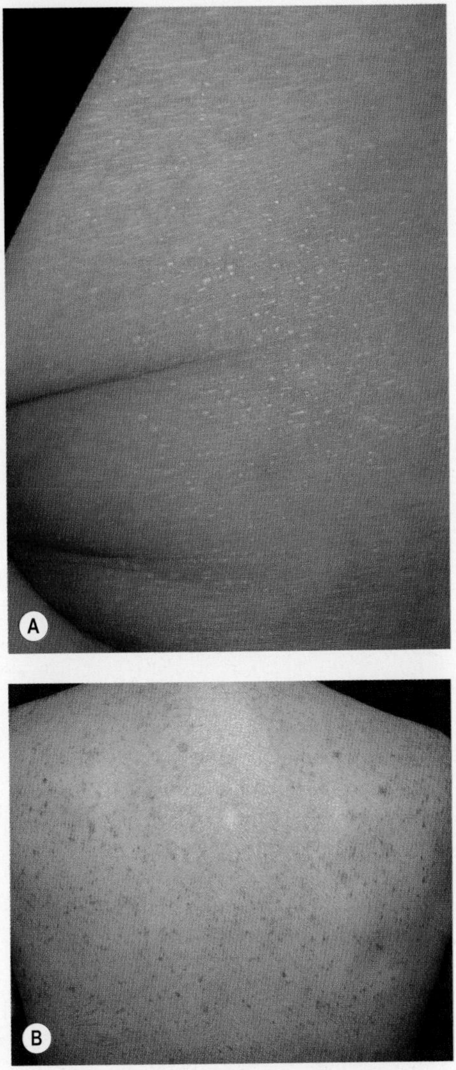

Sweat Retention Disorders

Miliaria

- Excessive sweating leads to maceration and blockage of eccrine ducts; can be exacerbated by occlusion, e.g. clothing, athletic equipment, prolonged bed rest.
- Classically divided into three major types: (1) *crystallina* – tiny, superficial, short-lived, clear vesicles (Fig. 32.5A; see Fig. 28.3); (2) *rubra* (prickly heat) – pruritic erythematous

Fig. 32.5 A Miliaria crystallina. Multiple small superficial vesicles with clear fluid. **B** Miliaria rubra. Multiple erythematous nonfollicular papules and papulovesicles on the back.

papulovesicles and occasionally pustules that favor the upper trunk (Fig. 32.5B); and (3) *profunda* – white papules due to excessive sweating in a hot climate (rare); these three forms reflect ductal occlusion within the stratum corneum, mid-epidermis, and dermal–epidermal junction, respectively.
- If extensive, decrease in eccrine function can give rise to hyperpyrexia.

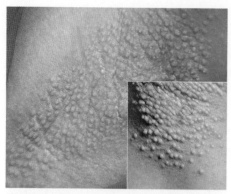

Fig. 32.6 Fox–Fordyce disease. Monomorphic skin-colored papules in the axillary vault. The dome shape is appreciated in the insert.

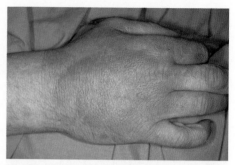

Fig. 32.7 Neutrophilic eccrine hidradenitis. Pink annular plaque on the dorsal hand. *Courtesy, Jami L. Miller, MD.*

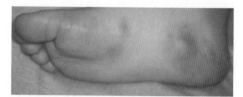

Fig. 32.8 Idiopathic palmoplantar hidradenitits. Tender erythematous papules and nodules on the plantar surface. *Courtesy, Michael L. Smith, MD.*

• **DDx:** miliaria rubra needs to be distinguished from folliculitis, Grover's disease, neutrophilic eccrine hidradenitis, and cutaneous candidiasis.
• **Rx:** cool environment.

Fox–Fordyce Disease (Apocrine Miliaria)

• Occlusion then rupture of apocrine sweat gland ducts in the axillae > anogenital or peri-areolar region > periumbilical or presternal area; seen primarily in women ages 15–35 years.
• Multiple skin-colored papules that are follicular, dome-shaped, and often pruritic (Fig. 32.6).
• May improve with oral contraceptive pills (OCPs) or pregnancy.
• **Rx:** topical CS or calcineurin inhibitors and OCPs.

Grover's Disease

• Grover's disease (transient acantholytic dermatosis) is covered in Chapter 73.

Hidradenitis

Neutrophilic Eccrine Hidradenitis

• Most commonly related to administration of chemotherapy (e.g. cytarabine) and is thought to result from excretion of the drug(s) into the eccrine sweat, leading to a toxic insult.
• Erythematous papules and plaques that may have clinical overlap with Sweet's syndrome (Fig. 32.7).

• **Rx:** spontaneously resolves but sometimes a short course of systemic CS is prescribed once an infectious process such as cellulitis or septic emboli is excluded.

Idiopathic Palmoplantar Hidradenitis

• Occurs following vigorous physical activity, primarily in healthy children.
• Thought to be precipitated by rupture of eccrine glands.
• Erythematous, tender nodules appear suddenly, most often on the soles (Fig. 32.8), and then spontaneously resolve over days to weeks.
• **DDx:** *Pseudomonas* hot-foot syndrome, pernio, symmetric lividity of the soles, delayed pressure urticaria.

Other

Keratolysis Exfoliativa

• Common disorder in healthy individuals; affects the palms >> soles.
• Multiple annular and semi-annular collarettes of white scale that usually measure

<5 mm, but may be larger (Fig. 32.9); no preceding vesicles or inflammation clinically.
• Recurrent and sometimes associated with hyperhidrosis.
• **Rx:** nonspecific; effectiveness of topical agents, e.g. 12% ammonium lactate, 20% urea, is limited.

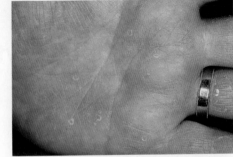

Fig. 32.9 Keratolyis exfoliativa. Small annular collarettes of scale on the palm. *Courtesy, Jean L. Bolognia, MD.*

For further information see Chs. 35 and 39. From *Dermatology, Third Edition.*

33 | Lupus Erythematosus

General

• A multisystem AI-CTD disorder that prominently affects the skin.

• Broadly divided into systemic lupus erythematosus (SLE), cutaneous lupus erythematosus (CLE), and drug-induced lupus erythematosus (DI-LE) (Fig. 33.1).

• CLE is further classified into *specific* and *nonspecific* skin lesions, based on the histopathologic presence (*specific*) or absence (*nonspecific*, Table 33.1) of an 'interface dermatitis'; however, this is not a perfect classification scheme because some specific entities (e.g. LE tumidus, lupus panniculitis) do not demonstrate an 'interface dermatitis' and other, non-lupus entities may display an 'interface dermatitis' on histopathology (e.g. dermatomyositis).

• Classically, the three major forms of *specific* skin lesions are chronic cutaneous LE (CCLE), subacute cutaneous LE (SCLE), and acute cutaneous LE (ACLE), with CCLE being subdivided into four different entities (see Fig. 33.1).

• Cutaneous lesions may be the sole manifestation of LE or they may be associated with systemic disease (SLE), either concurrently or sequentially.

• For all types of LE: women > men; African Americans or black Africans > other populations; onset typically post-puberty to middle age.

• Histopathologic examination of cutaneous lesions often plays an important role in establishing the diagnosis of CLE; direct immunofluorescence of lesional skin can be helpful in distinguishing CLE from other disorders, in particular lichen planus; accurate subtyping requires clinicopathologic correlation.

• Once a diagnosis of CLE is made, initial and longitudinal evaluation for systemic manifestations of SLE is recommended (Tables 33.2–33.4).

• Before making a definitive diagnosis of cutaneous lupus, it is necessary to exclude a drug-induced etiology (Table 33.5).

• Treatment options for the various subtypes of CLE are fairly similar (Table 33.6).

Drug-Induced Lupus Erythematosus

• There are two major forms: *drug-induced SLE (DI-SLE)* and *drug-induced SCLE (DI-SCLE)*; skin lesions are indistinguishable from classic, non-drug-related LE (see Table 33.5).

• Attention should be given to those medications that were initiated within weeks to 9 months prior to the onset of the eruption.

• Usually resolves upon discontinuation of the responsible medication along with sun protection and topical therapy; occasionally a patient will require systemic therapy for persistent disease.

Cutaneous Lupus Erythematosus: Specific Lesions

Chronic Cutaneous Lupus Erythematosus (CCLE)

DISCOID LUPUS ERYTHEMATOSUS (DLE)

• Most common skin manifestation of LE; the terms CCLE and DLE are often used interchangeably, but CCLE encompasses four entities (see Fig. 33.1).

• Overall, ~5–10% of patients will go on to develop SLE (see Table 33.4), but DLE can be a presenting manifestation of SLE.

• Three clinical variants of DLE are recognized.

  – *Localized:* Most common; involves the head and neck region; ≤5% risk of progression to SLE.

  – *Widespread:* Lesions extend beyond the head and neck region to involve the extremities and/or trunk; up to 20% of patients can progress to SLE.

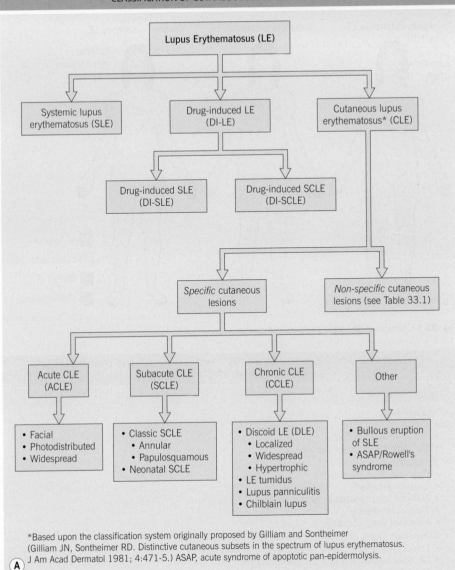

*Based upon the classification system originally proposed by Gilliam and Sontheimer
(Gilliam JN, Sontheimer RD. Distinctive cutaneous subsets in the spectrum of lupus erythematosus.
J Am Acad Dermatol 1981; 4:471-5.) ASAP, acute syndrome of apoptotic pan-epidermolysis.

Fig. 33.1 Classification of cutaneous lupus erythematosus (LE). A Spectrum of LE. *Continued*

CLASSIFICATION OF CUTANEOUS LUPUS ERYTHEMATOSUS

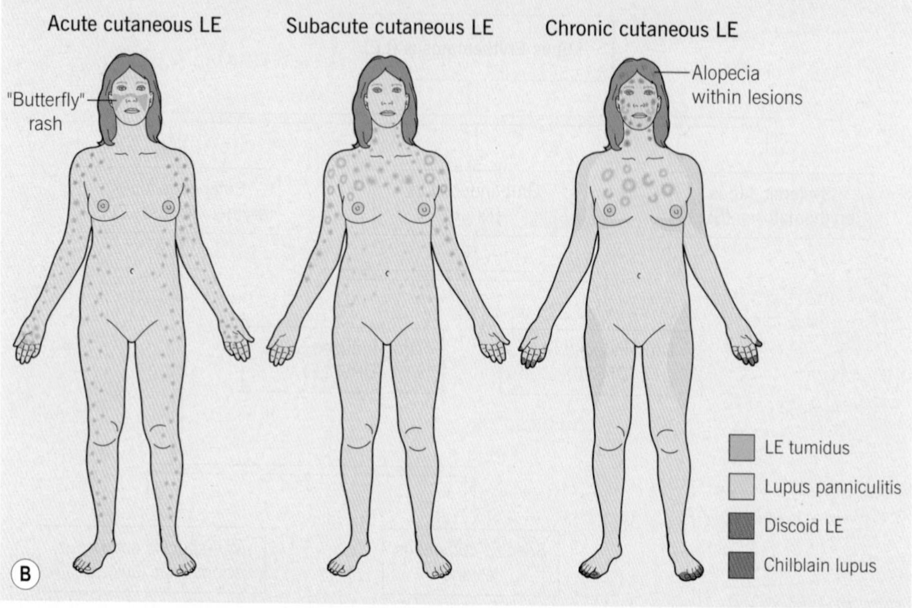

Fig. 33.1 *Continued* **B** Major forms of cutaneous LE.

CUTANEOUS FINDINGS (NONSPECIFIC) THAT SUGGEST THE DIAGNOSIS OF SYSTEMIC LUPUS ERYTHEMATOSUS

Vascular Lesions

- Vasculitis
  - Urticarial vasculitis
  - Small vessel vasculitis
  - Polyarteritis nodosa-like lesions
- Vasculopathy
  - Raynaud's phenomenon
  - Livedo reticularis
  - Nailfold telangiectasias and erythema
  - Palmar erythema
  - Livedoid vasculopathy
- Cutaneous signs of antiphospholipid antibody syndrome
  - Livedo reticularis (more widespread and persistent)
  - Multiple subungual splinter hemorrhages
  - Digital gangrene and cutaneous necrosis
  - Superficial thrombophlebitis
  - Degos'-like lesions
  - Atrophie blanche-like lesions
  - Anetoderma

Other

- Alopecia
  - 'Lupus hair,' diffuse and nonscarring
  - Telogen effluvium
- Papulonodular mucinosis

Table 33.1 Cutaneous findings (nonspecific) that suggest the diagnosis of systemic lupus erythematosus. These cutaneous lesions are associated with LE but are not specific to LE itself. The presence of *nonspecific* LE skin lesions raises the possibility of SLE and may signify more significant internal disease. The presence of these nonspecific lesions should prompt an evaluation for SLE (see Tables 33.2 and 33.3).

THE AMERICAN COLLEGE OF RHEUMATOLOGY 1982 REVISED CRITERIA FOR CLASSIFICATION OF SYSTEMIC LUPUS ERYTHEMATOSUS.*	
Criterion	**Basic Definition**
1. Malar rash	Fixed erythema, flat or raised over malar eminences
2. Discoid rash	Typical DLE lesions
3. Photosensitivity	Skin rash due to an unusual reaction to sunlight
4. Oral ulcers	Oral or nasal ulceration, observed by a physician
5. Arthritis	Non-erosive, involving ≥2 peripheral joints
6. Serositis	Pleuritis *or* pericarditis
7. Renal disorder	Persistent proteinuria *or* cellular casts
8. Neurologic disorder	Seizures *or* psychosis
9. Hematologic disorder	Hemolytic anemia *or* leukopenia *or* thrombocytopenia
10. Immunologic disorder	Anti-dsDNA *or* anti-Sm *or* antiphospholipid antibodies
11. Antinuclear antibody	Abnormal ANA titer, in the absence of drug-induced SLE

*The proposed classification is based on 11 criteria. For the purpose of identifying patients in clinical studies, a person shall be said to have SLE if any 4 or more of the 11 criteria are present, serially or simultaneously, during any interval of observation.
DLE, discoid lupus erythematosus.*

Table 33.2 The American College of Rheumatology 1982 revised criteria for classification of systemic lupus erythematosus. Although these criteria are very helpful in distinguishing SLE from other rheumatologic conditions, they are not very helpful in distinguishing other skin diseases from LE. See Appendix for 2012 Systemic Lupus International Collaborating Clinics classification criteria for SLE.

EVALUATION FOR SYSTEMIC LUPUS ERYTHEMATOSUS
History and Physical Examination
• Specific cutaneous lesions (see Fig. 33.1)   • Nonspecific cutaneous lesions (see Table 33.1)   • Lymphadenopathy, arthritis, friction rubs
Laboratory Tests
• ANA with profile (anti-dsDNA, Sm)   • Urinalysis   • CBC with differential, platelet count   • Chemistries (BUN, creatinine) and LFTs   • Erythrocyte sedimentation rate   • Complement levels (C3, C4)

ANA, antinuclear antibodies; BUN, blood urea nitrogen; CBC, complete blood count; ds, double-stranded; LFTs, liver function tests; Sm, Smith.

Table 33.3 Evaluation for systemic lupus erythematosus.

DIFFERENT FORMS OF CUTANEOUS LUPUS AND THEIR ASSOCIATIONS WITH SYSTEMIC LUPUS ERYTHEMATOSUS (SLE)	
Type of Cutaneous Lupus	**Association with SLE**
• Acute cutaneous lupus erythematosus (ACLE)	++++
• Subacute cutaneous lupus erythematosus (SCLE)	++
• Chronic cutaneous lupus erythematosus (CCLE)	
• Discoid lupus erythematosus (DLE*)	
– Localized (head and neck)	+
– Widespread/disseminated	++
– Hypertrophic	+
• Lupus erythematosus tumidus (LET)	+/–
• Lupus panniculitis	+
• Chilblain lupus	++
• Other variants	
• Bullous eruption of SLE	++++
• Rowell's syndrome	++ to ++++

Risk factors for the development of SLE include widespread DLE, arthralgias/arthritis, anemia, leukopenia, increased ESR, and higher ANA titers.

Table 33.4 Different forms of cutaneous lupus and their associations with systemic lupus erythematosus (SLE).

CLASSIC DISTINCTIONS BETWEEN DRUG-INDUCED SCLE AND DRUG-INDUCED SLE				
Disease	**Most Common Culprit Medications**	**Cutaneous Findings**	**Systemic Findings**	**Serologies**
Drug-induced SCLE	• HCTZ, terbinafine, calcium channel blockers (e.g. diltiazem), ACE inhibitors (e.g. enalapril), TNF-α inhibitors (e.g. infliximab), proton pump inhibitors (e.g. lansoprazole), interferons	• Identical to SCLE, i.e. both annular and papulosquamous presentations in typical photodistributed locations	• Typically no systemic symptoms • Occasional arthralgia	• (+) anti-Ro/SSA antibodies
Drug-induced SLE	• Hydralazine, procainamide, isoniazid, minocycline, TNF-α inhibitors	• **Typically no skin findings** • Occasionally malar or photodistributed erythema (especially with TNF-α inhibitors)	• Constitutional symptoms such as fever, weight loss • Serositis (e.g. arthritis, pericarditis, pleuritis)	• (+) anti-histone antibodies; can also be seen in patients with classic SLE

Table 33.5 Classic distinctions between drug-induced SCLE and drug-induced SLE. Note that *TNF-α inhibitors* can cause both DI-SCLE and DI-SLE.

SUGGESTED THERAPIES FOR CUTANEOUS LUPUS ERYTHEMATOSUS (CLE)

General Measures for All Patients

- Sun protective measures*
- Avoid potentially photosensitizing medications
- Stop smoking
- Oral vitamin D_3 supplementation, guided by serum vitamin D_3 levels

Localized Treatment Options

- Topical and intralesional CS
- Topical calcineurin inhibitors (facial lesions)
- Topical retinoids (perhaps helpful in hypertrophic DLE)
- Topical imiquimod 5% (anecdotal)

Systemic Treatment Options

First-line (antimalarials**)
- Hydroxychloroquine (*Adult*: 6.0–6.5 mg/kg ideal body weight/day; *Children*: ≤5.0 mg/kg ideal body weight/day)
- Chloroquine (*Adult*: 3.5–4.0 mg/kg ideal body weight/day; *Children*: ≤3.5 mg/kg ideal body weight/day)
- Quinacrine*** (in case of retinopathy) (*Adult* and *Children*: 100 mg/day)

Second-line (these agents may be combined with antimalarials or used alone)
- Methotrexate (7.5–25 mg/week, orally, IM, SC)
- Mycophenolate mofetil (1000–2000 mg/day)
- Thalidomide$ (25–100 mg/day)
- Oral retinoids$ (e.g. acitretin, isotretinoin)
- Dapsone$$ (50–150 mg/day)

Third-line (refractory cases)
- IVIg (costly)
- Belimumab (not as effective in African-Americans)

Life-threatening or severe inflammatory cutaneous disease (e.g. ASAP/Rowell's syndrome)
- Systemic CS

Broad-spectrum sunscreen, sun avoidance, sun-protective clothing.
**Delayed onset of action (4–8 weeks); earlier institution may stave off progression of CLE to SLE; recommended monitoring includes baseline and every 3–4 month CBC, LFTs, BUN/Cr, and yearly eye examinations.*
***Quinacrine can be added, as combination therapy, to either hydroxychloroquine or chloroquine.*
$Risk of teratogenicity.*
$$Exclude glucose-6-phosphate dehydrogenase deficiency.*
DLE, discoid lupus erythematosus; IV, intravenous; CBC, complete blood count; LFTs, liver function tests; BUN, blood urea nitrogen; Cr, creatinine; ASAP, acute syndrome of apoptotic pan-epidermolysis.

Table 33.6 Suggested therapies for cutaneous lupus erythematosus (CLE). All patients should be counseled about daily sun protection, as both UVA and UVB can trigger flares of CLE and may even lead to exacerbations of systemic symptoms. Topical therapy is indicated in local disease and as an adjunct to systemic therapy in severe and widespread CLE. Systemic therapy is indicated when skin lesions are widespread, disfiguring, scarring, or refractory to topical agents, or when extracutaneous manifestations are present, e.g. arthritis.

– *Hypertrophic:* Unusual variant; favors extensor arms > face, upper trunk (Fig. 33.2H); thick scale overlying or at periphery of DLE lesions; may resemble hypertrophic actinic keratoses, SCC, hypertrophic lichen planus, or prurigo nodularis.
- Occasionally can involve mucosal surfaces, palms and soles (see Fig. 33.2F,G).

- May occur in sun-exposed or sun-protected sites (e.g. scalp).
- **Early lesions:** inflamed, indurated plaques with erythema and scale.
- **Well-established lesions:** typically display follicular plugging, atrophy, scarring (and alopecia), and dyspigmentation (see Fig. 33.2A–E); the follicular plugging is often best appreciated in the conchal bowl of the ear.

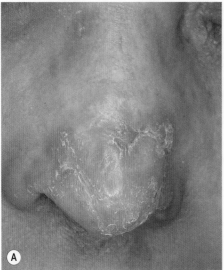

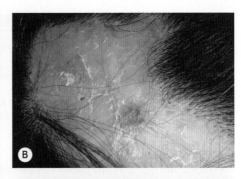

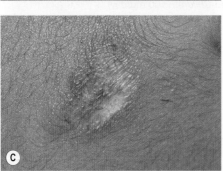

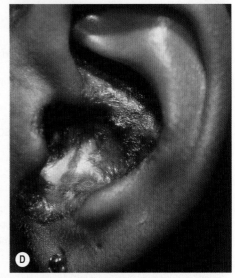

Fig. 33.2 Various presentations of discoid lesions of lupus erythematosus (DLE). Lesions, which favor the head and neck region, may show erythema, scaling, atrophy, and dyspigmentation in addition to scarring (and alopecia) **(A–D).** *C, Courtesy, Kalman Watsky, MD. Continued*

- **DDx: Early lesions:** Jessner's lymphocytic infiltrate, polymorphic light eruption (PMLE), lymphocytoma cutis, lymphoma cutis, granuloma faciale, sarcoidosis; **Late lesions:** lichen planus (hypertrophic, palmoplantar and mucosal variants), sarcoidosis.
- **Typical Rx:** high-potency topical CS, intralesional CS (5 mg/cc), and/or antimalarials (see Table 33.6).

LUPUS ERYTHEMATOSUS (LE) TUMIDUS

- LE tumidus is an entity that overlaps with Jessner's lymphocytic infiltrate and reticular erythematous mucinosis (REM); there is debate as to whether it is a distinct entity or whether it should be considered a specific type of lupus.
- Photo-induced, but often this is not appreciated because of the delay of 1–2 weeks

between UVR exposure and onset of the eruption.
- Most common on the face and upper trunk; reportedly <1% of patients eventually develop SLE.
- Lesions characterized by erythema, induration, and often central clearing (Fig. 33.3); scale, follicular plugging, scarring, and atrophy are absent.
- **DDx:** Jessner's lymphocytic infiltrate, PMLE, REM (chest lesions), papulonodular mucinosis.

LUPUS PANNICULITIS (See Chapter 83)

- Initially characterized by intense inflammation in the subcutaneous fat; eventuates into lipoatrophy.
- The most common sites of involvement are the face, upper outer arms, upper trunk,

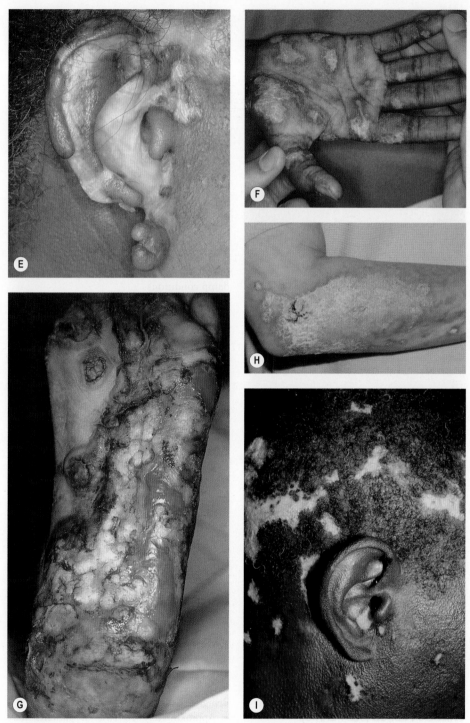

Fig. 33.2 *Continued* The scarring process may be destructive **(E).** Less common sites include the palms and soles, where lesions can be keratotic or ulcerative **(F, G),** as seen in lichen planus. The latter patient had systemic lupus erythematosus and responded well to isotretinoin. **H** Occasionally, hypertrophic lesions develop within significant hyperkeratosis. **I** Discoid lupus lesions with vitiligo-like depigmentation. *H, Courtesy, Julie V. Schaffer, MD; I, Courtesy, Joyce Rico, MD.*

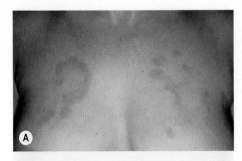

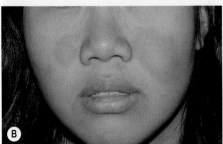

Fig. 33.3 Lupus erythematosus tumidus.
Annular pink plaques on the chest **(A)** and
pink-violet plaques on the face **(B).** None of the
lesions have epidermal change. *B, Courtesy, Julie
V. Schaffer, MD.*

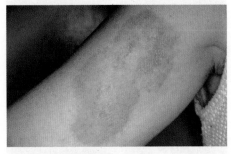

Fig. 33.4 Lupus panniculitis. Erythematous
plaque on the upper arm. The lesions may
resolve with lipoatrophy.

breasts, buttocks, and thighs, with the majority representing sites of abundant fat (Fig.
33.4).

• Sometimes overlying DLE lesions are seen
(termed 'lupus profundus').

CHILBLAIN LUPUS (SLE PERNIO)

• Typically presents with erythematous to
dusky purple papulonodules and plaques on
the toes, fingers > nose, elbows, knees, and
lower legs (Fig. 33.5).

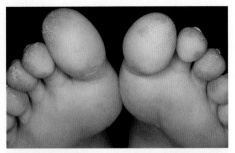

Fig. 33.5 Chilblain lupus. Violaceous plaques,
some with scale, on toes. If there is a family
history of this disorder, the possibility of
mutations in *TREX1*, which encodes a DNA
exonuclease, can be considered.

• Lesions are triggered or exacerbated by cold
temperatures, often in combination with
damp conditions.

• With time, some lesions may progress
to resemble DLE both clinically and
histopathologically.

• **DDx:** idiopathic chilblains (following
exclusion of SLE), familial chilblain lupus
(*TREX1* mutation), other cold-induced syndromes (see Chapter 74).

• Up to 20% of patients may go on to develop
SLE.

Subacute Cutaneous Lupus Erythematosus (SCLE)

• Characterized by non-scarring, annular, or
papulosquamous eruptions in photodistributed sites (Fig. 33.6).

• Favors the upper trunk and upper outer
arms > lateral neck, forearms, hands (see Fig.
33.6).

• Interestingly, often spares the mid-face.

• Two common clinical presentations are
recognized.
  – *Annular*: raised erythematous borders
    with central clearing (see Fig. 33.6B, C).
  – *Papulosquamous*: psoriasiform or
    eczematous appearance (see Fig. 33.6A).

• Long-term residual changes include
dyspigmentation (most often hypo- to
depigmentation).

• Approximately 10–15% of patients may
over time develop SLE (see Table 33.4).

• Depending on the laboratory, ~70%
of patients have associated anti-Ro/SSA
antibodies.

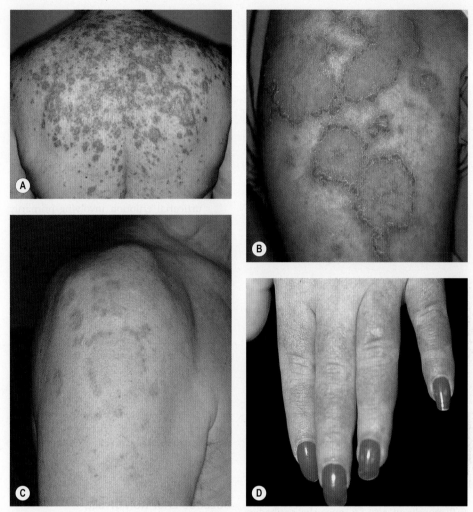

Fig. 33.6 Subacute cutaneous lupus erythematosus (SCLE). A Papulosquamous and annular lesions on the upper back; this site along with the upper, outer arms are the most common distribution patterns. **B, C** The margins of the annular lesions may have scale-crust **(B)** or be composed of multiple papules **(C). D** The lesions on the hands conform to the typical distribution of lupus lesions, sparing the knuckles. *A, Courtesy, Kathryn Schwarzenberger, MD; B, Courtesy, Jean L. Bolognia, MD; D, Courtesy, Lela Lee, MD.*

- Roughly 50% of patients fulfill ≥4 American College of Rheumatology (ACR) criteria for SLE (see Table 33.2), but they rarely develop serious systemic involvement; arthralgias most common.
- **DDx: Annular variant:** dermatophytosis, granuloma annulare, erythema annulare centrifugum, or other annular erythemas (see Chapter 15); **Papulosquamous variant:** photo-lichenoid drug reaction (e.g. HCTZ, antimalarials), psoriasis, photoexacerbated eczema, graft-versus-host disease (GVHD), lichen planus, PMLE.
- Before a diagnosis of classic SCLE can be made, exclude the possibility of DI-SCLE (see Table 33.5).

NEONATAL SCLE (NLE)

- Occurs in infants whose mothers have anti-Ro/SSA autoantibodies that are passively transferred to the fetus.

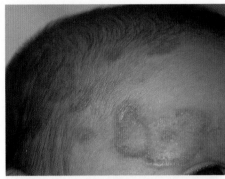

Fig. 33.7 Neonatal lupus erythematosus (NLE). Annular erythematous plaques on the forehead and scalp. Note the resemblance to the annular form of subacute cutaneous lupus erythematosus. *Courtesy, Julie V. Schaffer, MD.*

• These infants primarily have anti-Ro/SSA antibodies (>98%), but may also have anti-La/SSB or anti-U1RNP antibodies.

• Approximately 1–5% of mothers with anti-Ro/SSA antibodies will have infants with NLE, with risk increasing to 10–25% with subsequent pregnancies.

• Cutaneous lesions are similar to adult SCLE but favor the face and periorbital areas and may be atrophic (Fig. 33.7).

• Photosensitivity is common but sun exposure is not necessary for lesion formation.

• New lesions typically cease to develop by 6–9 months of age, i.e. once the antibodies are cleared; however, there may be residual changes such as dyspigmentation and telangiectasias.

• The most common internal manifestations are (1) congenital heart block (± associated cardiomyopathy); (2) hepatobiliary disease; (3) thrombocytopenia > neutropenia or anemia; (4) macrocephaly or skeletal dysplasia.

• Heart block, if it is going to occur, is almost always present at birth and a pacemaker is often required.

• If skin signs of NLE are present, an evaluation, including physical examination, ECG ± echocardiogram, CBC, and liver function tests, is indicated; the latter laboratory tests should be repeated periodically over the first 6 months of life.

Acute Cutaneous Lupus Erythematosus (ACLE)

• The CLE variant most closely associated with SLE and if diagnosed the patient should be evaluated for internal disease.

• Three clinical presentations are recognized:
  – *Facial (malar)*: the classic 'butterfly' eruption, presenting with symmetric erythematous patches or more infiltrated plaques over the nasal bridge and cheeks; spares nasolabial folds (Fig. 33.8A–C).
  – *Photodistributed*: exanthematous to urticarial eruption involving primarily UV-exposed skin, e.g. upper chest, extensor arms (Fig. 33.8D), dorsal hands (with sparing of the knuckles).
  – *Widespread*: extends beyond photodistributed sites.

• A particular patient's ACLE clinical presentation will often repeat itself with subsequent flares, representing a 'signature' pattern.

• Lesions typically respond to systemic CS and resolve without scarring; may leave residual dyspigmentation.

• **DDx: Facial**: seborrheic dermatitis, rosacea, sunburn, perioral dermatitis, tinea faciei, cellulitis, contact dermatitis; **Photodistributed**: drug-induced photosensitivity, dermatomyositis; **Widespread**: exanthem (viral or drug-induced).

Other

BULLOUS ERUPTION OF SLE

• Clinically presents as blisters (ranging from tiny vesicles to large tense bullae) on an erythematous base, typically involving the face, neck, upper trunk, proximal extremities, and mucosal surfaces; seen in patients with underlying SLE (Fig. 33.9).

• Autoantibodies against type VII collagen are present.

• **DDx: Clinical**: autoimmune blistering diseases, contact dermatitis, acute syndrome of apoptotic pan-epidermolysis (ASAP); **Histopathological**: dermatitis herpetiformis.

ACUTE SYNDROME OF APOPTOTIC PAN-EPIDERMOLYSIS (ASAP)/ ROWELL'S SYNDROME

• The term *ASAP* embraces various entities in which there is acute and widespread epidermal cleavage resulting from hyperacute

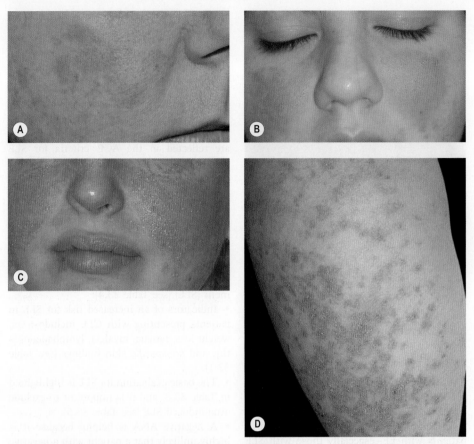

Fig. 33.8 Acute cutaneous lupus erythematosus (ACLE). The facial erythema, often referred to as a 'butterfly rash,' may be variable **(A)**, edematous **(B)**, or have associated scale **(C)**. The presence of small erosions can aid in the clinical differential diagnosis. This patient **(D)** had ACLE lesions on the arms as well as the face. *A, Courtesy, Kalman Watsky, MD; B–D, Courtesy, Lela Lee, MD.*

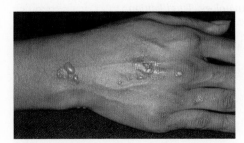

Fig. 33.9 Bullous eruption of systemic lupus erythematosus. Vesicles and bullae due to autoantibodies against type VII collagen can develop in patients with systemic disease.

apoptotic injury of the epidermis from various causes (e.g. drug-induced toxic epidermal necrolysis [TEN], TEN-like GVHD, and TEN-like ACLE).

• Rowell's syndrome and TEN-like ACLE are thought to occur along a spectrum of ASAP, with the former representing a less severe erythema multiforme major-like presentation in the setting of lupus and the latter a potentially life-threatening TEN-like presentation in the setting of ACLE (Fig. 33.10).

• This spectrum of cutaneous findings may occur *de novo* or in the setting of rebound ACLE or SCLE; significant internal organ involvement (e.g. kidney and CNS) is common.

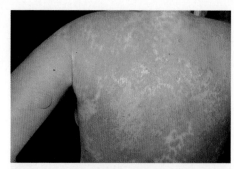

Fig. 33.10 Acute syndrome of apoptotic pan-epidermolysis (ASAP). One form of ASAP is a potentially life-threatening TEN-like presentation in the setting of ACLE.

Cutaneous Lupus Erythematosus: Nonspecific Lesions

• A variety of cutaneous lesions not entirely specific to LE may be seen, signaling not only internal organ involvement (SLE) but also increased systemic disease activity (see Table 33.1).

VASCULAR LESIONS AND THE ANTIPHOSPHOLIPID ANTIBODY SYNDROME (APL)

• Vascular lesions and APL are common in patients with LE, especially those with SLE (see Table 33.1).

• Approximately one-third of APL cases occur in the setting of lupus (see Chapter 18); compared to primary APL, these patients are more likely to have arthritis, livedo reticularis (LR), and cytopenias.

• Patients with LE and APL may benefit from antimalarial therapy.

Systemic Lupus Erythematosus (SLE)

• The organ systems most commonly involved are the joints, skin, hematologic, lungs, kidneys, and CNS, which in large part are reflected in the ACR criteria for SLE diagnosis (see Table 33.2); however, this list is not exhaustive and clinical judgment is required.

• In individual patients it is often only one or a few organs that are significantly affected.

• ACLE is the specific CLE variant most closely associated with SLE, but patients with any type of CLE may develop internal involvement (SLE) (see Table 33.4).

• Indicators of an increased risk for SLE in patients presenting with CLE include fever, weight loss, fatigue, myalgia, lymphadenopathy, and *nonspecific* skin findings (see Table 33.1).

• The basic evaluation for SLE is highlighted in Table 33.3, and it is important to exclude drug-induced SLE (see Table 33.5).

• A negative ANA is helpful because it is highly unlikely that a patient with a negative ANA has SLE.

• A positive ANA is less helpful, as it may occur in normal individuals (usually at low titers) and in patients with CLE.

• Specific antibodies to SLE include dsDNA and Sm.

For further information see Ch. 41. From *Dermatology, Third Edition*.

Dermatomyositis 34

Dermatomyositis is an autoimmune connective tissue disease (AI-CTD) that may overlap with other AI-CTDs, in particular systemic sclerosis. It may be triggered by outside factors, most commonly malignancy (e.g. breast cancer, ovarian cancer) and occasionally drugs (e.g. 'statins') or rarely infectious agents (e.g. picornavirus).

• Bimodal age distribution (juvenile – mean 8 years of age; adult – mean 52 years of age); female predominance.

• Often clinical and laboratory evidence of proximal inflammatory myopathy (the term polymyositis is used when the disease affects muscle only; Table 34.1); patients may report difficulty combing hair or rising from a sitting position.

• Pathogeneses of dermatomyositis and polymyositis are different (humoral immunity versus cell-mediated immunity, respectively).

• May affect the skin only (amyopathic dermatomyositis, formerly termed dermatomyositis sine myositis; see Table 34.1); Fig. 34.1 outlines an approach to the diagnosis of this form of dermatomyositis.

• Characteristic cutaneous findings include a violaceous hue of the upper eyelids with periorbital edema (Fig. 34.2) and nailfold telangiectasias (Fig. 34.3), as well as the cutaneous findings outlined in Table 34.2 and

---

REVISED CLASSIFICATION SYSTEM FOR THE IDIOPATHIC INFLAMMATORY DERMATOMYOPATHIES

This classification scheme recognizes, with equal weighting, the cutaneous and muscle manifestations of this group of disorders.

Dermatomyositis (DM)
  Adult-onset
    Classic DM
    Classic DM with malignancy*
    Classic DM as part of an overlapping connective tissue disorder**
    Clinically amyopathic DM†
      Amyopathic DM
      Hypomyopathic DM
  Juvenile-onset
    Classic DM
    Clinically amyopathic DM†
      Amyopathic DM
      Hypomyopathic DM

Polymyositis
  Isolated polymyositis
  Polymyositis as part of an overlapping connective tissue disorder

Inclusion body myositis

*In up to 25% of adults; ovarian, colon, breast, lung, gastric, pancreatic carcinomas (nasopharyngeal in Southeast Asian populations), and lymphoma; risk decreases to normal after 2–5 years.
**Systemic sclerosis > SLE, Sjögren's syndrome, rheumatoid arthritis.
†Provisional = cutaneous findings without muscle weakness and with normal muscle enzymes for >6 months; confirmed = for 24 months.

Table 34.1 Revised classification system for the idiopathic inflammatory dermatomyopathies.

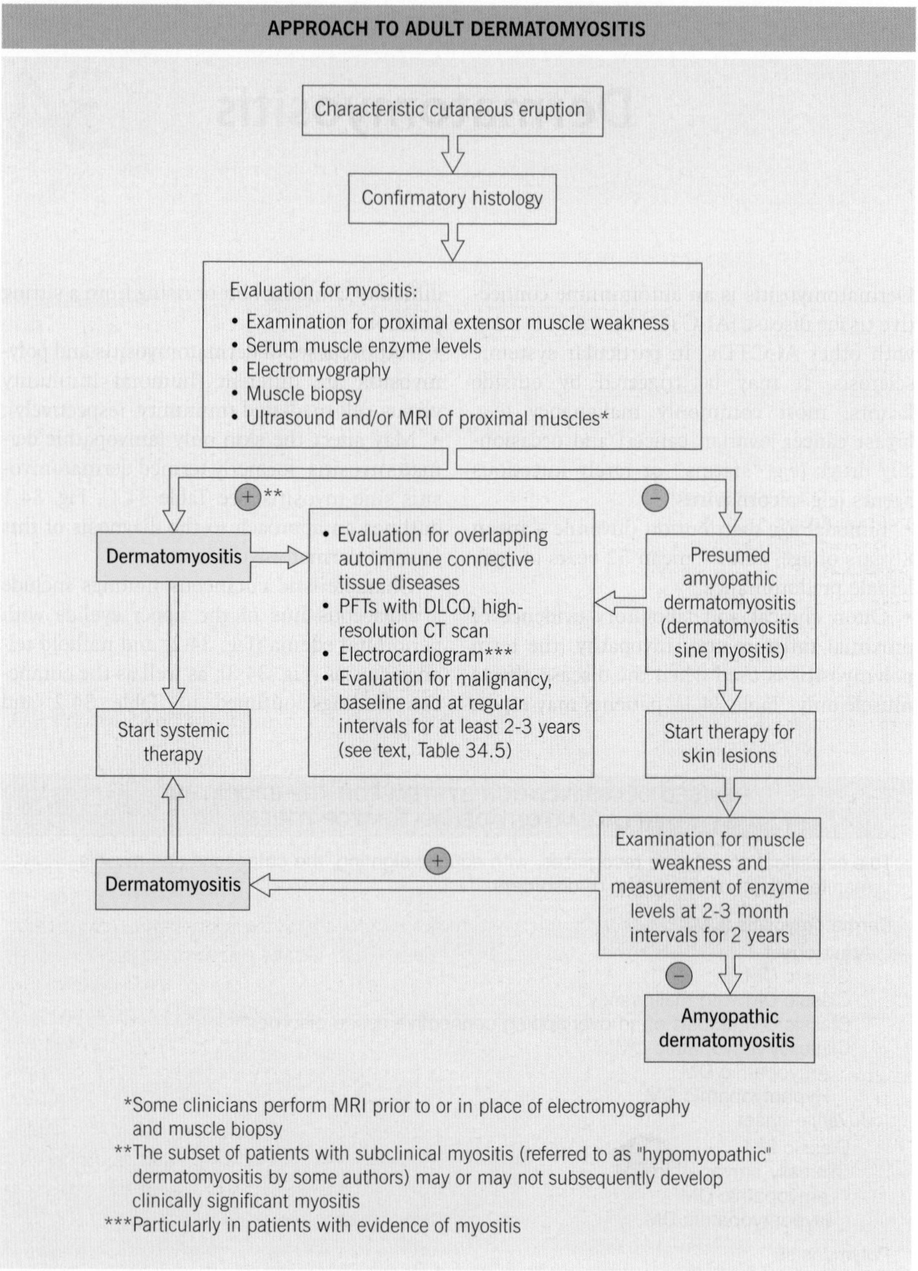

Fig. 34.1 Approach to adult dermatomyositis. The approach for children is similar but without the malignancy evaluation. Some authors classify patients with no evidence of myositis for 6 months after the onset of skin disease as having amyopathic dermatomyositis, but such individuals may go on to develop muscle disease. If planning administration of chronic systemic CS, a baseline DEXA bone density scan is recommended. CT, computed tomography; DLCO, diffusing capacity of the lung for carbon monoxide; PFTs, pulmonary function tests.

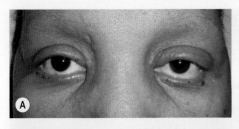

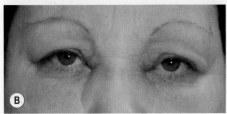

Fig. 34.2 Dermatomyositis – eyelid edema and heliotrope sign. A Inflammation of the upper eyelids can be more subtle in darkly pigmented skin; note involvement of the lateral nasal root and the cheeks. **B** The characteristic pink-violet color is seen with involvement of the hairline, lower forehead, upper eyelids, and cheeks; the edema is striking and involves the nasal root as well as the eyelids. *B, Courtesy, Jean L. Bolognia, MD.*

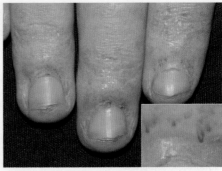

Fig. 34.3 Dermatomyositis – cuticular dystrophy and nailfold telangiectasias. The cuticles are 'ragged' and within the proximal nail fold, dilated capillary loops alternate with vessel dropout (insert). Atrophy, telangiectasias, and hypopigmentation are present on the fingers. *Courtesy, Julie V. Schaffer, MD.*

represented in Fig. 34.4A; these may precede systemic manifestations (Fig. 34.4B).

• Interstitial lung disease affects 15–30% of patients, and baseline pulmonary function tests that include the CO diffusion coefficient are recommended; high-resolution CT may be required to detect involvement.

• May overlap with other AI-CTDs (1 in 5 adult cases) (Table 34.1).

• Histopathologic changes – interface dermatitis of the skin with mucin; lymphocytic myositis in affected muscle.

• Various associated autoantibodies with clinical implications (Table 34.3); antinuclear antibodies may be negative as many autoantibodies are directed against cytoplasmic antigens.

• **DDx** can be broad (Table 34.4).

• **Rx** of cutaneous disease: topical CS, topical tacrolimus, antimalarials, immunosuppressives (e.g. methotrexate); pruritus and scalp involvement often refractory to treatment; skin disease may be less responsive to treatment than muscle inflammation.

• **Rx** of muscle/systemic involvement: systemic CS (e.g. prednisone 1 mg/kg/day with slow taper) ± other immunosuppressive drugs (e.g. methotrexate); for severe cases, consider IVIg.

• In classic dermatomyositis with malignancy (Table 34.5), cutaneous findings may improve gradually over time in the setting of a treatment-responsive tumor.

CUTANEOUS MANIFESTATIONS OF DERMATOMYOSITIS

Distribution of Common Cutaneous Features

Periocular
May resemble an airborne contact dermatitis
Pink-violet discoloration of the upper eyelids (heliotrope rash) (Fig. 34.2)
Periocular edema that may be severe
These findings can be subtle and wax and wane

Nailfolds
Dilated capillary loops alternating with dropout of capillaries (Fig. 34.3)
Ragged cuticles

Sun-exposed sites
May resemble a photodrug eruption
Pink-violet color and/or telangiectasias [e.g. face (Fig. 34.5); V of the chest/upper back, referred to as the 'shawl sign' (Fig. 34.6)]
Poikiloderma with hyperpigmentation, hypopigmentation, and atrophy in addition to telangiectasias

Extensor surfaces of hands (knuckles), elbows, and knees
May resemble psoriasis
Violaceous discoloration over joints (knuckles, knees, elbows), referred to as Gottron's sign (Fig. 34.7)
Over time, flat-topped papules develop on the knuckles (Gottron's papules; Fig. 34.8), and they may become atrophic

Scalp
May resemble seborrheic dermatitis
Scaly, pink patches (Fig. 34.9)
Very pruritic
Posterior > anterior scalp

Additional Cutaneous Features

Calcinosis cutis
More common in juvenile-onset dermatomyositis
Associated with delay in Rx or Rx-resistant disease
Hard, irregular nodules or plaques that can become extensive; may discharge chalky material

Pruritus

Raynaud's phenomenon

Less Common Mucocutaneous Features

When disease is severe, there may be erosions or ulcerations (Fig. 34.10), as well as anasarca
Pink-violet patches of the lateral thighs (holster sign)
Flagellate erythema (Fig. 34.10)
Panniculitis/lipoatrophy (more common in children)
Gingival telangiectasias

Table 34.2 Cutaneous manifestations of dermatomyositis. For a schematic representation of the cutaneous features, see Fig. 34.4A.

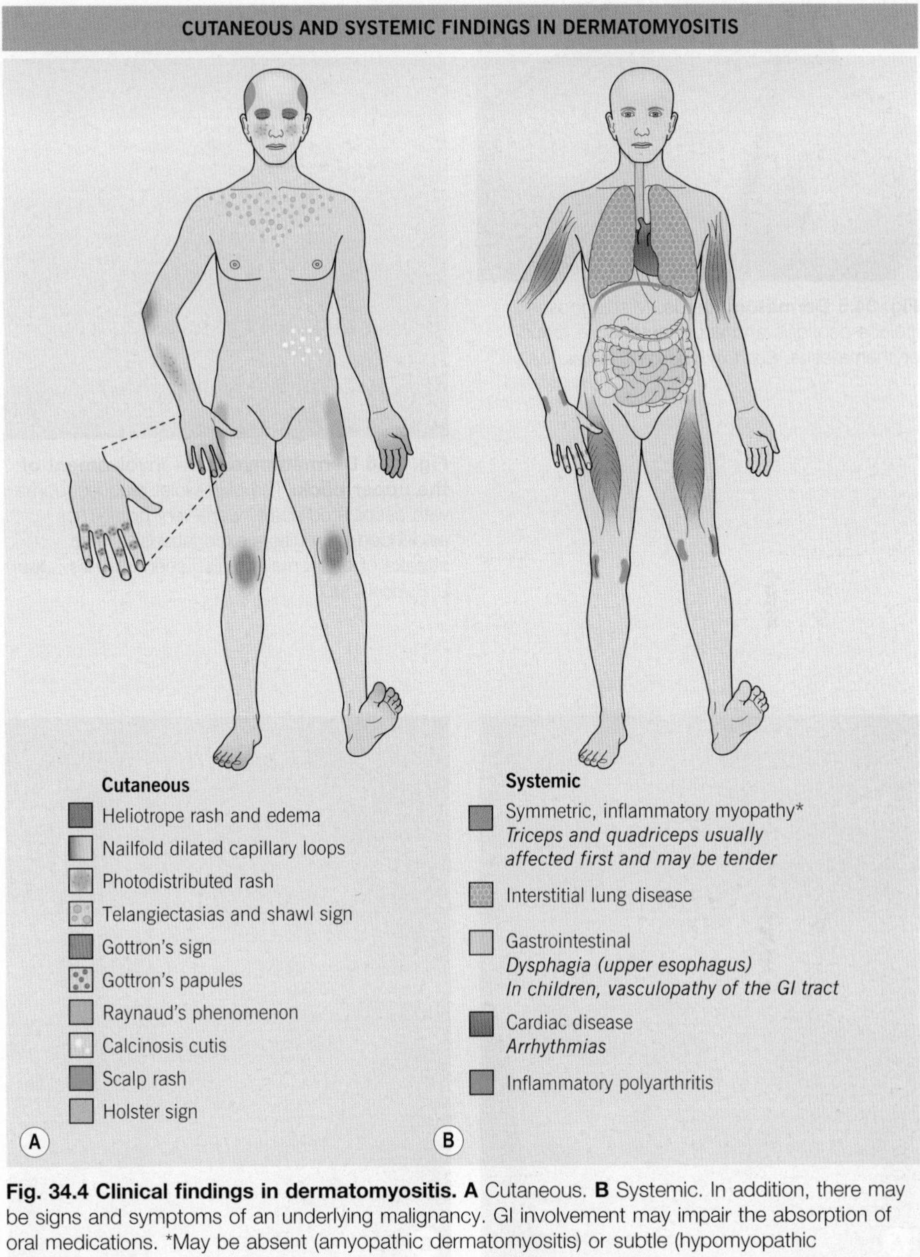
CUTANEOUS AND SYSTEMIC FINDINGS IN DERMATOMYOSITIS
Cutaneous
Heliotrope rash and edema
Nailfold dilated capillary loops
Photodistributed rash
Telangiectasias and shawl sign
Gottron's sign
Gottron's papules
Raynaud's phenomenon
Calcinosis cutis
Scalp rash
Holster sign
A
Systemic
Symmetric, inflammatory myopathy*
Triceps and quadriceps usually affected first and may be tender
Interstitial lung disease
Gastrointestinal
Dysphagia (upper esophagus)
In children, vasculopathy of the GI tract
Cardiac disease
Arrhythmias
Inflammatory polyarthritis
B

Fig. 34.4 Clinical findings in dermatomyositis. A Cutaneous. **B** Systemic. In addition, there may be signs and symptoms of an underlying malignancy. GI involvement may impair the absorption of oral medications. *May be absent (amyopathic dermatomyositis) or subtle (hypomyopathic dermatomyositis).

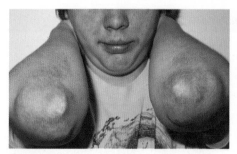

Fig. 34.5 Dermatomyositis. Misdiagnoses include psoriasis and acute cutaneous lupus erythematosus. *Courtesy, Joseph L. Jorizzo, MD.*

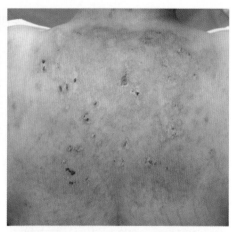

Fig. 34.6 Dermatomyositis – involvement of the upper back. The pink-violet plaques, some with associated scale, were very pruritic, as evidenced by multiple excoriations. Linear streaks of erythema are also seen. *Courtesy, Jean L. Bolognia, MD.*

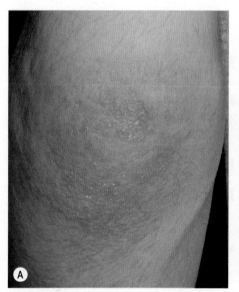

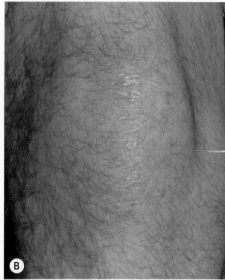

Fig. 34.7 Dermatomyositis – Gottron's sign. Thin pink papules and plaques of the elbow **(A)** and knee **(B)**. Some of the papules on the elbow are flat-topped. *Courtesy, Julie V. Schaffer, MD.*

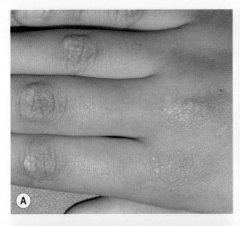

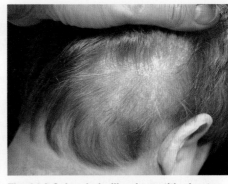

Fig. 34.9 Seborrheic-like dermatitis due to dermatomyositis. This patient presented with severe pruritus of the scalp. In addition to the scalp involvement, she had Gottron's papules and a photodistributed poikiloderma. *Courtesy, Jeffrey P. Callen, MD.*

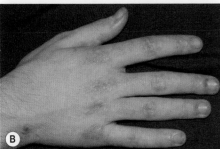

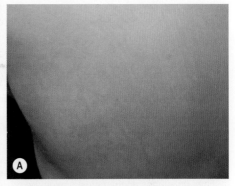

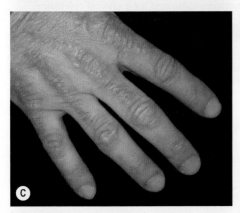

Fig. 34.8 Dermatomyositis – Gottron's papules. A The flat-topped papules overlying the proximal interphalangeal (IP) and metacarpophalangeal (MCP) joints are subtle and were misdiagnosed as verrucae vulgaris in this child. **B** Obvious accentuation of skin lesions over the MCP joints, with coalescence of pink-violet flat-topped papules. **C** Papulosquamous plaques with a somewhat linear configuration proximally; clues against psoriasis are the Gottron's papules of the distal IP joints, cuticular dystrophy, and nailfold telangiectasias. *A, B, Courtesy, Julie V. Schaffer, MD; C, Courtesy, Ruth Ann Vleugels, MD.*

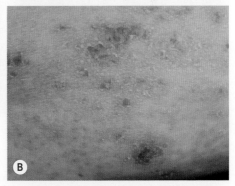

Fig. 34.10 Dermatomyositis – less common presentations. A Flagellate erythema of the posterior trunk. **B** Secondary changes include scale, erosions, and serous as well as hemorrhagic crusts. *A, Courtesy, Ruth Ann Vleugels.*

AUTOANTIBODIES ASSOCIATED WITH DERMATOMYOSITIS AND THEIR CLINICAL RELEVANCE

Autoantibody	Clinical Relevance
Anti-aminoacyl-tRNA synthetases (e.g. anti-Jo-1 [histidyl], anti-PL-7 [threonyl])	• Associated with antisynthetase syndrome (fever, polyarthritis, 'mechanic's hands,' Raynaud's phenomenon, interstitial lung disease) • Present in up to 20% of adult patients
Anti-Mi-2	• Most specific for classic DM • Milder muscle disease • Good response to treatment • Present in up to 10–15% of patients
Anti-TIF1-γ (anti-155/140)	• Severe cutaneous; malignancy-associated; amyopathic
Anti-MDA5 (CADM-140)	• Clinically amyopathic DM (CADM) • Characteristic mucocutaneous findings, including tender palmar papules, ulcerations on the knuckles/elbows, oral/gum pain, diffuse alopecia • Rapidly progressive interstitial lung disease (ILD)
Anti-NXP-2 (anti-p140)	• Juvenile-onset classic DM (calcinosis cutis)
Anti-SAE	• CADM that may progress to myositis and dysphagia • ILD uncommon

DM, dermatomyositis; Mi-2 is a DNA helicase; TIF1, transcriptional intermediary factor 1; MDA5, melanoma differentiation-associated protein 5; NXP-2, nuclear matrix protein; SAE, small ubiquitin-like modifier-activating enzyme. Patients with anti-SRP (signal recognition particle) antibodies have severe myositis and an increased risk of cardiac involvement.

Table 34.3 Autoantibodies associated with dermatomyositis and their clinical relevance.

DIFFERENTIAL DIAGNOSIS OF DERMATOMYOSITIS

Systemic lupus erythematosus
Physician might notice the nail fold telangiectasias and photodistributed poikiloderma but miss the muscle weakness, heliotrope rash, extensor distribution, pruritus, and the violaceous hue (true lupus erythematosus might be present in the setting of an overlap syndrome)

Psoriasis
Involvement of elbows and knees with papulosquamous lesions can lead to misdiagnosis

Airborne or allergic contact dermatitis
Eyelid edema can be marked in dermatomyositis; look for additional sites of dermatitis

Photodrug eruption
Photodistribution

Cutaneous T-cell lymphoma
The poikiloderma often begins in intertriginous zones rather than on the scalp, face, and extensor surfaces

Atopic dermatitis
Usually in children, where the physician focuses on the pruritus and secondary lichenification

Systemic sclerosis (scleroderma)
The nail fold telangiectasias are similar in appearance, but the dyspigmentation is quite different; edema of the hands is an early sign (true systemic sclerosis may be present in the setting of an overlap syndrome)

Trichinosis
Patients have painful muscles and periorbital edema, but not other features

Photodistributed form of multicentric reticulohistiocytosis (rare)
Firm papules have distinct histologic features

Table 34.4 Differential diagnosis of dermatomyositis.

SUGGESTED MALIGNANCY SCREENING TESTS FOR ADULTS WITH DERMATOMYOSITIS

- Urinalysis
- Stool occult blood testing
- Serum prostate-specific antigen (PSA) in men
- Serum CA125 (women)
- Mammogram and transvaginal pelvic ultrasound (women)
- CT of chest, abdomen, and pelvis
- Colonoscopy (if age-appropriate, iron deficiency anemia, occult blood in stool, or symptoms)
- Upper endoscopy (if colonoscopy negative in the setting of iron deficiency anemia, occult blood in stool, or symptoms)
- Serum protein and immunofixation electrophoresis

CT, computed tomography.

Table 34.5 Suggested malignancy screening tests for adults with dermatomyositis.
Screening should be performed at the time of diagnosis and annually for a minimum of 3 years thereafter; history and physical examination can be performed more frequently.

For further information see Ch. 42. From *Dermatology, Third Edition.*

35 | Systemic Sclerosis and Sclerodermoid Disorders

- The spectrum of sclerosing skin disorders is outlined in Fig. 35.1.

Systemic Sclerosis (SSc)

- An uncommon autoimmune connective tissue disease (AI-CTD) that affects the skin, blood vessels, and several other organs (e.g. kidney, lung).

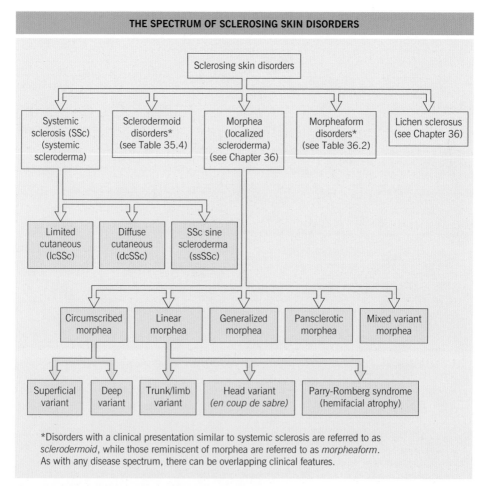

THE SPECTRUM OF SCLEROSING SKIN DISORDERS

*Disorders with a clinical presentation similar to systemic sclerosis are referred to as *sclerodermoid*, while those reminiscent of morphea are referred to as *morpheaform*. As with any disease spectrum, there can be overlapping clinical features.

Fig. 35.1 The spectrum of sclerosing skin disorders.

SYSTEMIC SCLEROSIS AND SCLERODERMOID DISORDERS

Limited cutaneous SSc (lcSSc)
(Anti-centromere antibody)

Diffuse cutaneous SSc (dcSSc)
(Anti-topoisomerase-1 antibody)

SSc sine scleroderma (ssSSc)

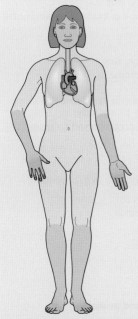
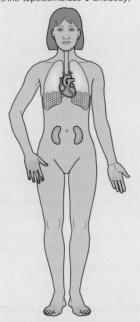
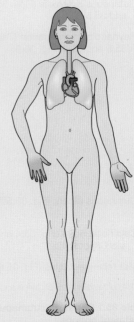

- Formerly called CREST syndrome
- Long preceding history of Raynaud's phenomenon
- Slower development of limited cutaneous sclerosis involving the distal extremities and face
- Later onset of internal organ involvement (after 10-15 years)
- Pulmonary arterial hypertension
- More favorable long-term prognosis

- Sudden onset of Raynaud's phenomenon
- Rapidly progressive, more widespread cutaneous sclerosis (usually peaks within 12-18 months)
- >90% demonstrate internal organ involvement within the first 5 years
- Interstitial lung disease (ILD)
- Kidney disease

- No cutaneous sclerosis
- Otherwise similar to lcSSc

	Cutaneous sclerosis
	Raynaud's phenomenon
	Nail fold capillary abnormalities

Fig. 35.2 Clinical classification of systemic sclerosis (SSc). In addition to the three major clinical subsets shown here, two others are recognized: pre-SSc, in which the full extent of the patient's skin sclerosis has not been reached; and overlap syndrome, in which either lcSSc or dcSSc coexists with another AI-CTD, e.g. polymyositis or SLE. CREST, calcinosis, *R*aynaud's phenomenon, *e*sophageal dysmotility, *s*clerodactyly, *t*elangiectasias.

| Esophageal dysmotility | Cardiomyopathy, heart failure | Hypertension, renal crisis |
| Interstitial lung disease (ILD) | Pulmonary arterial hypertension (PAH) | |

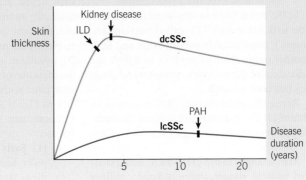

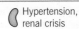

COMMON CUTANEOUS FEATURES OF SYSTEMIC SCLEROSIS AND AVAILABLE TREATMENT OPTIONS	
Cutaneous Feature	**Available Treatment Options**
Cutaneous sclerosis (Figs. 35.3 and 35.5)	• UVA1 therapy for localized disease • Tyrosine kinase inhibitors, e.g. imatinib (experimental)
Raynaud's phenomenon (Tables 35.5 and 35.6; Fig. 35.8)	**First-line** • Cold avoidance • Hand and feet warming packets • Discontinue all tobacco products **Second-line** • Calcium channel blockers (e.g. nifedipine SR 30 mg daily-BID, amlodipine 2.5-10 mg daily) **Third-line** (especially when accompanied by ulceration) • Sildenafil, tadalafil • Prazosin • Angiotensin II receptor blockers • Endothelin receptor antagonists (e.g. bosentan)
Cutaneous ulcers (Fig. 35.5B)	• Avoid excessive debridement • Moist, nonadherent dressings
Calcinosis cutis (Fig. 35.4 and see Chapter 42)	• Low-dose warfarin • Calcium channel blockers
Mat telangiectasias (Fig. 35.6)	• Various lasers

UVA, ultraviolet A; BID, twice a day; SR, slow release.

Table 35.1 Common cutaneous features of systemic sclerosis and available treatment options.

• Etiology unknown but pathogenesis involves vasculopathy, endothelial dysfunction, tissue fibrosis, and immune system activation.

• Seen more frequently in women; onset typically in the 3rd to 4th decades of life; diffuse cutaneous SSc more frequently seen in African-Americans.

• There are three *major* clinical subtypes of SSc, based on the amount of skin sclerosis (Fig. 35.2):
   – Limited cutaneous SSc (lcSSc).
   – Diffuse cutaneous SSc (dcSSc).
   – SSc sine scleroderma (ssSSc).

• LcSSc and dcSSc can also occur in conjunction with other AI-CTD (called 'overlap syndrome'), most notably polymyositis and SLE; another *minor* form is pre-SSc, in which the full extent of the patient's cutaneous sclerosis has not been reached.

• Raynaud's phenomenon (RP) is present in almost all SSc patients and is often the earliest presenting feature (Table 35.1; Figs. 35.3–35.5).

• Mat telangiectasias (Fig. 35.6) and proximal nailfold abnormalities (dilated capillary loops) are present in both lcSSc and dcSSc subtypes and are important clues to the Dx; additional common cutaneous findings are outlined in Table 35.1.

• Patients often have a characteristic facies with microstomia, retraction of the lips, perioral furrows, and a beaked nose; three types of dyspigmentation can also be seen, including diffuse hyperpigmentation and leukoderma of SSc (Fig. 35.7).

• In all three subtypes there can be internal organ involvement (Table 35.2), but patients with dcSSc are at increased risk for more clinically severe extracutaneous disease and overall worse outcomes.

• Most patients (~98%) with SSc are ANA (+), usually in a speckled or nucleolar pattern; the presence of certain nucleolar antibodies is associated with characteristic clinical presentations (Table 35.3).

• There are three phases of cutaneous disease:
   – **(1) Early edematous phase**, featuring puffy hands and pitting edema of the digits (see Fig. 35.5A).

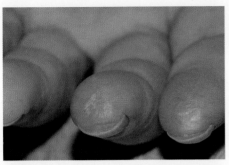

Fig. 35.3 Pitted scars of the digital pulp in a patient with systemic sclerosis. *Courtesy, Kalman Watsky, MD.*

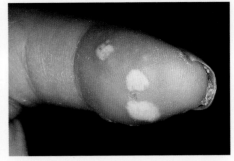

Fig. 35.4 Calcinosis cutis of the finger in a patient with systemic sclerosis.

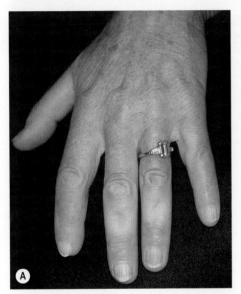

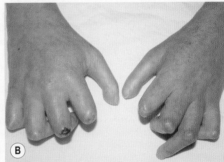

Fig. 35.5 Early versus late stages of systemic sclerosis (SSc) involving the hands. A Early edematous phase of SSc (note the demonstration of pitting edema on two of the digits). **B** Late stage of SSc with fixed flexion contractures, sclerodactyly, and digital ulceration overlying the third proximal interphalangeal joint. *A, Courtesy, Jean L. Bolognia, MD; B, Courtesy, M. Kari Connolly, MD.*

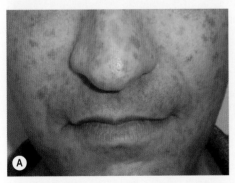

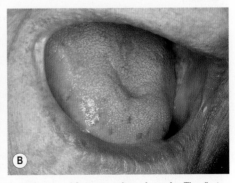

Fig. 35.6 Mat (squared-off) telangiectasias in two patients with systemic sclerosis. The first patient **(A)** had limited cutaneous systemic sclerosis (lcSSc, formerly called CREST syndrome) while the second patient **(B)** presented with diffuse hyperpigmentation and had interstitial lung disease. *A, Courtesy, M. Kari Connolly, MD; B, Courtesy, Jean L. Bolognia, MD.*

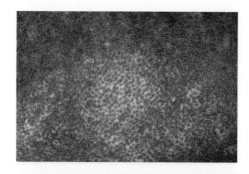

Fig. 35.7 The 'salt and pepper' sign.
Leukoderma with retention of perifollicular
pigmentation in a patient with systemic sclerosis.

EXTRACUTANEOUS FEATURES OF SYSTEMIC SCLEROSIS AND AVAILABLE SCREENING AND TREATMENT OPTIONS		
Extracutaneous Features	**Screening Tools***	**Treatment Options**
Pulmonary*		
• Interstitial lung disease (ILD) *(more common in dcSSc than lcSSc)*	• PFTs (DLCO, spirometry, and lung volumes) • High-resolution CT • Bronchoalveolar lavage and lung biopsy	• Early detection and intervention with immunosuppression (e.g. cyclophosphamide vs. mycophenolate mofetil plus prednisone for 1 year) • Lung transplantation
• Pulmonary arterial hypertension (PAH) *(more common in lcSSc than dcSSc)*	• **Transthoracic echocardiography** • **Serum *N*-Tpro-BNP level** • Right heart catheterization	• Oxygen • Anticoagulation • Endothelin receptor antagonists (e.g. bosentan) • Phosphodiesterase inhibitors (e.g. sildenafil) • Prostaglandins (e.g. epoprostenol) • Lung transplantation
Renal		
• Renal crisis • Hypertension	• **Close monitoring of blood pressure** • **BUN/Cr** • **Urinalysis**	• ACE inhibitors instituted early for treatment but not helpful for prevention
Cardiac		
• Fibrosis/restrictive cardiomyopathy • Heart failure secondary to PAH	• Echocardiography	• ACE inhibitors
Gastrointestinal		
• Esophageal dysmotility • Small bowel involvement	• Barium swallow with small bowel follow through • Manometry • Endoscopy	• Proton pump inhibitors • Promotility agents (e.g. ondansetron)

Patients are typically asymptomatic in the early stages of ILD and PAH, which is when the diagnosis should be made and treatment instituted; cough, dyspnea on exertion, and shortness of breath are typical later-onset symptoms.
PFTs, pulmonary function tests; CT, computed tomography scan; DLCO, diffusing capacity of the lung for carbon monoxide; N-Tpro-BNP, N-terminal pro b-type natriuretic peptide; BUN, blood urea nitrogen; Cr, creatinine; ACE, angiotensin converting enzyme.

Table 35.2 Extracutaneous features of systemic sclerosis and available screening and treatment options. Items in bold signify those screening tests that are recommended at baseline in all newly diagnosed patients.

- (2) **Indurated phase**, characterized by hardening of the skin with taut and shiny appearance (see Fig. 35.5B).
- (3) **Atrophic phase**, with potential/ gradual softening of the skin.

• The degree of skin sclerosis does not predict the degree of internal organ involvement, and survival is dependent on the type and degree of internal organ involvement.

• Pulmonary disease (interstitial lung disease (ILD) > pulmonary arterial hypertension (PAH)) is the most common cause of mortality.

• All SSc patients should be screened and periodically monitored for internal organ involvement, especially lung and renal disease (Table 35.2).

• **DDx** includes other sclerodermoid conditions (Table 35.4) and other AI-CTD (e.g. mixed connective tissue disease; see Chapter 37).

• Recommendations for the initial evaluation of all patients with suspected SSc are presented in Table 35.2.

• **Rx** options for various cutaneous and extracutaneous features of SSc are outlined in Tables 35.1 and 35.2.

Raynaud's Phenomenon

• Characterized by episodic vasospasm of the digital arteries, resulting in white, blue, and red discoloration of the fingers and toes secondary to cold stimuli.

• Occurs in two settings: *primary* Raynaud's phenomenon (Raynaud's disease) and *secondary* Raynaud's phenomenon (Table 35.5).

• *Primary* Raynaud's phenomenon is common, affecting 3–5% of the population and typically develops in adolescent girls and young women (median age at onset, ~14 years) and is not associated with any underlying medical issues.

• *Secondary* Raynaud's phenomenon is uncommon and is associated with an underlying medical problem (Table 35.6).

• SSc is one of the leading causes of secondary Raynaud's phenomenon.

• An approach to differentiating primary from secondary Raynaud's phenomenon is presented in Fig. 35.8.

• **Rx:** Table 35.1.

Sclerodermoid Disorders

• Disorders with a clinical presentation similar to SSc are referred to as 'sclerodermoid disorders' (Table 35.4).

Eosinophilic Fasciitis (Shulman's Syndrome)

• May be one of the presentations of chronic GVHD; Dx by MRI or biopsy of involved fascia.

• Characterized initially by the rapid onset of edema and pain of the extremities, followed by symmetric, woody induration (spares hands, feet, face) (Fig. 35.9); associated with peripheral eosinophilia.

• About 30% preceded by strenuous physical activity.

• Prompt treatment with oral CS necessary to preserve mobility and function; slow taper over 6–24 months.

Nephrogenic Systemic Fibrosis (NSF)

• Occurs in individuals with impaired renal function, most commonly (~90%) dialysis-dependent chronic kidney disease.

• Associated with exposure to gadolinium-based contrast medium.

• Presents on the extremities with symmetrically distributed, ill-defined, thick, indurated, erythematous to hyperpigmented plaques (Fig. 35.10).

• Confluence of lesions can result in joint contracture, pain, and loss of mobility.

• Systemic fibrosis affecting the heart, lungs, and skeletal muscles can also occur.

• No effective treatment; most helpful intervention is to restore renal function (e.g. via renal transplantation).

Stiff Skin Syndrome

• Congenital or onset in early childhood; pathogenesis unknown, but a subset with fibrillin gene mutations; chronic course with no effective treatment, other than physical therapy to prevent contractures.

• Characterized by 'rock hard' induration of the skin and subcutaneous tissues of thighs and buttocks, usually bilateral; noticeable sparing of inguinal folds; joint contractures.

• No internal organ involvement.

SYSTEMIC SCLEROSIS (SSc) AUTOANTIBODY PROFILE AND ITS MORE FREQUENTLY ASSOCIATED CLINICAL PRESENTATION	
SSc Autoantibody	**Clinical Features**
Limited Skin Sclerosis	
Anti-centromere*	• Increased risk isolated PAH
Anti-Th/To	• Frequent in patients with ssSSc • More severe internal organ involvement (PAH, ILD)
Anti-U11/U12 RNP**	• Greatest risk for developing ILD, which is often severe and rapidly progressive
Diffuse Skin Sclerosis	
Anti-topoisomerase-I* (*formerly Scl-70*)	• Increased risk ILD • Poor prognosis
Anti-RNA polymerase III*	• Most severe diffuse skin sclerosis • Increased risk renal crisis • Usually better prognosis
Anti-U3 RNP	• More frequent in African-Americans • Myopathy and cardiomyopathy • Increased risk PAH
Overlap Syndromes	
Anti-PM/Scl	• Polymyositis – SSc overlap • Acute onset inflammatory myositis • Less serious internal organ involvement • Usually better prognosis because responsive to oral CS
Anti-U1RNP†	• MCTD • Increased risk ILD and PAH • Usually better prognosis because responsive to oral CS
Anti-Ku	• Myositis

The most frequently identified autoantibodies in systemic sclerosis patients.
**Currently not commercially available.*
†*The U1RNP antibody is specific for MCTD, which is often considered a distinct clinical entity (see Chapter 37).*
PAH, pulmonary arterial hypertension; ILD, interstitial lung disease or pulmonary fibrosis; ssSSc, systemic sclerosis sine scleroderma; MCTD, mixed connective tissue disease.

Table 35.3 Systemic sclerosis (SSc) autoantibody profile and its more frequently associated clinical presentation. Although ~98% of SSc patients will have a (+) ANA, the diagnosis is still based on history and physical examination. The value of a (+) ANA lies in the subsequent identification of the patient's SSc-specific autoantibody. More than 90% will have one of nine SSc autoantibodies. The nine autoantibodies are mostly mutually exclusive and tend not to change with time.

DIFFERENTIAL DIAGNOSIS OF SCLERODERMOID CONDITIONS

Mucinoses
- Scleredema
- Scleromyxedema

Neurologic
- Reflex sympathetic dystrophy*
- Spinal cord injury

Immunologic
- Chronic GVHD*
- Eosinophilic fasciitis
- Generalized morphea*
- Fibroblastic rheumatism

Toxin-mediated
- Nephrogenic systemic fibrosis*
- Eosinophilia-myalgia syndrome (historic)
- Toxic oil syndrome* (historic)

Paraneoplastic
- POEMS syndrome
- Amyloidosis (primary systemic)**
- Carcinoid syndrome

Drug- or chemical-induced
- Bleomycin*
- Taxanes
- Vinyl chloride, chlorinated hydrocarbons*

Neoplastic
- Carcinoma *en cuirasse**

Venous insufficiency
- Lipodermatosclerosis*

Metabolic
- Diabetic cheiroarthropathy
- Porphyria cutanea tarda*,†

Other
- Silicosis
- Stiff skin syndrome*

*Can overlap with morpheaform disorders, which are listed in Table 36.2.
**Primary cutaneous amyloidosis can also occur in patients with systemic sclerosis and generalized morphea.
†May also be observed in patients with congenital erythropoietic porphyria and hepatoerythropoietic porphyria.
GVHD, graft-versus-host disease; POEMS, polyneuropathy, organomegaly, endocrinopathy, monoclonal gammopathy, and skin changes.

Table 35.4 Differential diagnosis of sclerodermoid conditions.

CLINICAL AND LABORATORY FEATURES OF PRIMARY AND SECONDARY RAYNAUD'S PHENOMENON

Feature	Primary Raynaud's	Secondary Raynaud's
Sex	F : M 20 : 1	F : M 4 : 1
Age at onset	Puberty	>25 years
Frequency of attacks	Usually <5 per day	5–10+ per day
Precipitants	Cold, emotional stress	Cold
Ischemic injury	Absent	Present
Abnormal capillaroscopy	Absent	>95%
Other vasomotor phenomena	Yes	Yes
Antinuclear antibodies	Absent/low titer	90–95%
Anticentromere antibody	Absent	50–60%
Anti-topoisomerase I (Scl-70) antibody	Absent	20–30%
In vivo platelet activation	Absent	>75%

Adapted from Hochberg MC, Silman AJ, Smolen JS, et al. (Eds.). Rheumatology, 3rd edn. Edinburgh: Mosby, 2003. © Elsevier 2003.

Table 35.5 Clinical and laboratory features of primary and secondary Raynaud's phenomenon.

DIFFERENTIAL DIAGNOSIS OF RAYNAUD'S PHENOMENON

Structural vasculopathies

Large and medium-sized arteries

- Thoracic outlet syndrome
- Brachiocephalic trunk disease (atherosclerosis, Takayasu's arteritis)
- Buerger's disease (thromboangiitis obliterans)*
- Crutch pressure

Small arteries and arterioles

- Systemic sclerosis
- Systemic lupus erythematosus
- Dermatomyositis
- Overlap syndromes
- Cold injury
- Vibration disease (hand–arm vibration syndrome, hypothenar hammer syndrome)
- Chemotherapy (bleomycin, vinca alkaloids, cisplatin, carboplatin)
- Vinyl chloride disease
- Arsenic poisoning

Normal blood vessels – abnormal blood elements

- Cryoglobulinemia (monoclonal or mixed)
- Cryofibrinogenemia
- Cold agglutinin disease
- Myeloproliferative disorders (e.g. essential thrombocythemia)

Normal blood vessels – abnormal vasomotion

- Primary (idiopathic) Raynaud's phenomenon
- Drug-induced (ergot alkaloids, bromocriptine, interferon, estrogen, cyclosporine, sympathomimetic agents, clonidine, cocaine, nicotine)
- Carpal tunnel syndrome
- Pheochromocytoma
- Carcinoid syndrome
- Reflex sympathetic dystrophy
- Other vasospastic disorders (migraine, Prinzmetal)

*Can also affect small arteries.
Adapted from Hochberg MC, Silman AJ, Smolen JS, et al. (Eds.). Rheumatology, 3rd edn. Edinburgh: Mosby, 2003. © Elsevier 2003.

Table 35.6 Differential diagnosis of Raynaud's phenomenon. Paraneoplastic acral vascular syndrome, which can present with Raynaud's phenomenon as well as acrocyanosis and gangrene, has been observed in patients with various solid tumors (e.g. lung or ovarian carcinoma).

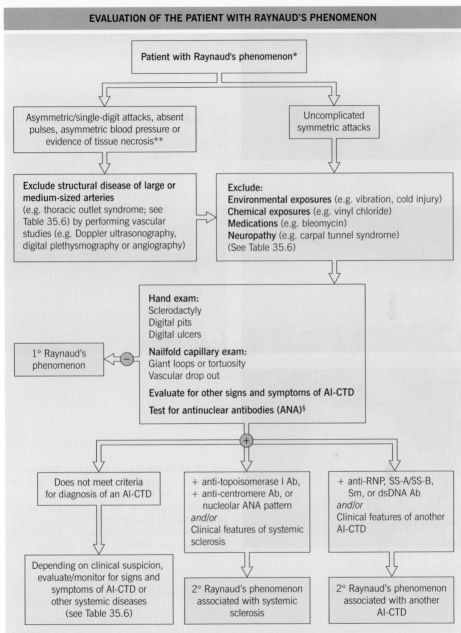

SYSTEMIC SCLEROSIS AND SCLERODERMOID DISORDERS

* Defined as a history of sensitivity to the cold and episodic pallor, cyanosis or both after cold exposure.
** Also consider evaluating for microvascular occlusion syndromes (e.g. cryoglobulinemia).
§ Positive predictive value for an associated autoimmune connective tissue disease (AI-CTD) is approximately 30%.

Fig. 35.8 Evaluation of the patient with Raynaud's phenomenon. RNP, ribonucleoprotein; Sm, Smith; ds, double-stranded.

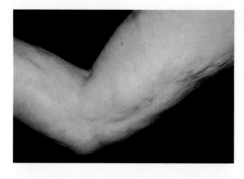

Fig. 35.9 Eosinophilic fasciitis. Induration of the skin with a dimpled or 'pseudo-cellulite' appearance, also referred to as rippling or puckering. *Courtesy, Joyce Rico, MD.*

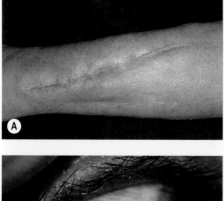

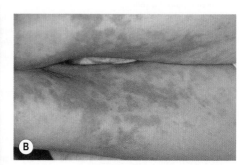

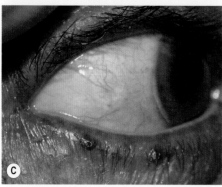

Fig. 35.10 Nephrogenic systemic fibrosis (NSF). Thickening and induration of the skin can be obvious **(A),** or lesions may present as purple-brown plaques **(B). C** Scleral plaques in a patient younger than 45 years of age is a minor criterion for NSF. *A, Courtesy, Jean L. Bolognia, MD; B, Courtesy, Kalman Watsky, MD.*

For further information see Ch. 43. From *Dermatology, Third Edition*.

Morphea and Lichen Sclerosus

36

Morphea (Localized Scleroderma)

• An uncommon fibrosing disorder that is limited to the skin, subcutaneous tissues, and occasionally the underlying bone; rarely, if present on the face and/or scalp, it can be associated with underlying CNS abnormalities.

• It is distinct from systemic sclerosis (SSc; see Chapter 35) in that morphea is not associated with sclerodactyly, Raynaud's phenomenon, nailfold capillary abnormalities, or internal organ involvement.

• Morphea does not transition into SSc, except for a few rare case reports.

• Equal prevalence in adults and children; more common in females and Caucasians.

• Pathogenesis unknown but thought to involve (like SSc) vascular damage, immune activation, and increased connective tissue production by fibroblasts.

• Approximately 2–5% of children and 30% of adults with morphea have a concomitant autoimmune disease (e.g. alopecia areata, vitiligo) as well as a family history of autoimmunity.

• Classified based on clinical presentation, with five major variants recognized (see Fig. 35.1; Table 36.1).

• Early morphea lesions present as erythematous to violaceous patches and plaques (Fig. 36.1); they then evolve into sclerotic (often ivory-colored), hairless, anhidrotic plaques with variable degrees of dyspigmentation (Fig. 36.2).

• *Circumscribed (plaque) morphea* is the most common variant in adults, presenting with ≤3 discrete indurated plaques; the latter favor the trunk and tend to develop in areas of pressure (e.g. hips, waist, and bra line in women); superficial and deep variants (morphea profunda) exist (Fig. 36.3).

• *Generalized morphea* is a rare variant that presents with >3 indurated plaques larger

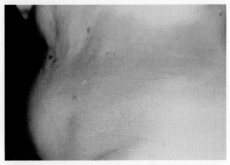

Fig. 36.1 Early inflammatory circumscribed morphea (morphea en plaque) of the trunk. Early stage lesion presenting as an erythematous edematous plaque. *Courtesy, Martin Rocken, MD, and Kamran Ghoreschi, MD.*

than 3 cm and/or involving ≥2 body sites; spares the face and hands (see Fig. 36.11); more likely to have a (+) ANA and systemic symptoms.

• *Linear morphea* is the most common variant in children and may cause a significant degree of morbidity because of ocular involvement and occasionally CNS involvement in the head variant (Fig. 36.4) or muscle atrophy, discrepancies in limb length, and joint contractures in the limb variant (Fig. 36.5).

• *Pansclerotic morphea* is the most debilitating, but very rare, variant; it affects the subcutaneous tissues down to and often including the bone; presents as expanding plaques that may eventually coalesce over the entire trunk or extend circumferentially down the extremities; increased risk of cutaneous SCC.

• *Mixed morphea* involves a combination of ≥2 other morphea variants and constitutes ~15% of all morphea cases; overlap with lichen sclerosus can also occur.

• Extracutaneous manifestations are most common in patients with generalized morphea

APPROACH TO THE TREATMENT OF MORPHEA

Morphea Variant	Treatment
Circumscribed morphea	First line* • Topical class I or intralesional CS • Topical tacrolimus Second line • Lesion limited phototherapy** *or* • Topical imiquimod *or* • Topical vitamin D analog under occlusion ± class I topical CS
Generalized morphea	*(Without joint contractures)* First line* • Phototherapy** (Fig. 36.11) Second line • Weekly methotrexate† ± systemic CS$
Linear morphea	*(Involving face or crossing joints)* First line* • Weekly methotrexate† ± systemic CS$ Second line • Phototherapy** *or* • CS-sparing agents
Pansclerotic morphea	*(Often poor response to treatment attempts)* First line • Weekly methotrexate† ± systemic CS$
Mixed morphea	Treatment as above, depending on variants

*If not improved after ~8 to 10 weeks, progress to next line of therapy.
**Phototherapy choice based on local availability (BB-UVA, UVA1, NB-UVB, PUVA); NB-UVB more effective for superficial lesions and UVA1 more effective for deeper lesions.
†Weekly methotrexate doses: adults, 15–25 mg/week; children, 0.3–0.4 mg/kg/week.
$Especially for early/progressive lesions; pulsed > daily dosing.
BB-UVA, broadband ultraviolet A light phototherapy; UVA1, narrowband ultraviolet A light phototherapy; NB-UVB, narrowband ultraviolet B light phototherapy; PUVA, psoralens plus ultraviolet A light phototherapy.

Table 36.1 Approach to the treatment of morphea. Treatment is most effective in active, inflammatory lesions. Topical monotherapy should not be used if any of the following are present: progressing functional impairment, joint contractures or involvement across joints, linear facial involvement.

and in children; arthralgia is the most common finding.

• Children with morphea involving the upper face should have regular ophthalmologic examinations to monitor for asymptomatic involvement that could potentially result in irreversible damage.

• **DDx:** morpheaform disorders (Table 36.2; see Table 35.4), SSc, lichen sclerosus, keloids (Fig. 36.6), atrophoderma of Pasini and Perini.

• Morphea and SSc cannot be differentiated by histopathologic examination.

• **Rx:** best utilized during the early, inflammatory stage (see Table 36.1); in general, therapy will not readily reverse established

sclerosis; however, the truncal plaques of circumscribed and generalized morphea often soften over a period of years, eventually resembling atrophoderma or completely resolving.

Lichen Sclerosus (LS)

• Formerly called lichen sclerosus et atrophicus.

• A clinically distinct inflammatory disease of the superficial dermis that leads to white, scar-like lesions with surface wrinkling due to epidermal atrophy.

• Most commonly affects female or male genitalia, less often nongenital skin.

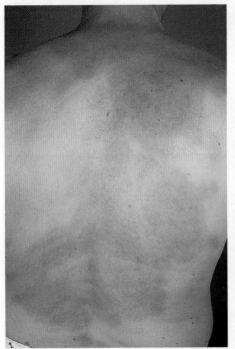

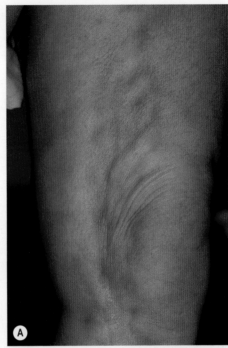

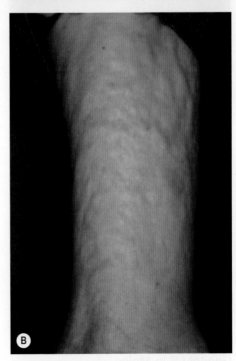

Fig. 36.2 Mid to later stage circumscribed morphea (morphea en plaque). Multiple, large hyperpigmented plaques, several of which have an inflammatory border.

• Approximately 80% of LS patients have IgG autoantibodies against extracellular matrix (ECM-1).

• Ultrapotent topical corticosteroids are highly effective for treatment of LS (see Fig. 36.12); other treatment options are listed in Table 36.3.

Genital LS in Females

• Bimodal presentation: 6th–7th decade and 8–13 years of age.

• Favors vulva and perianal regions; confluent involvement of the labial, perineal, and perianal areas has been likened to a 'figure 8 configuration'.

• **Early:** well-demarcated, erythematous thin plaque; ± erosions (Fig. 36.7).

• **Mid:** evolves into dry, hypopigmented sclerotic lesion.

• **Late:** obliteration of the labia minora and periclitoral structures; narrowing of the vaginal introitus.

Fig. 36.3 Comparison of deep morphea and eosinophilic fasciitis. A Note the 'pseudo-cellulite' appearance of the involved skin of the thigh in deep morphea. **B** In eosinophilic fasciitis, the level of fibrosis is also deep, resulting in a similar clinical appearance.

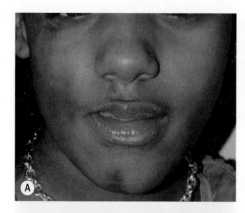

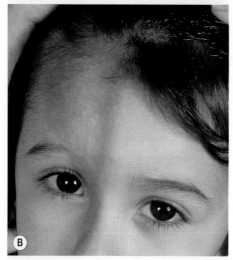

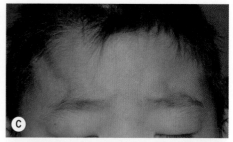

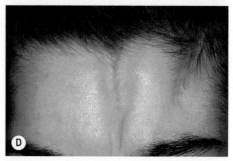

Fig. 36.4 Linear morphea, head variant.
A Parry–Romberg syndrome, demonstrating hyperpigmentation and loss of subcutaneous tissue, leading to facial asymmetry. **B–D** *En coup de sabre* with linear paramedian depressions and sclerosis – **(B)** (wide) and **(C)** (narrow) – being more common than midline involvement as in **(D).** Note the prominent veins and loss of the medial eyebrow in **(B).** *A and C, Courtesy, Julie V. Schaffer, MD; D, Courtesy, Martin Rocken, MD, and Kamran Ghoreschi, MD.*

• Purpura and perineal fissures are common findings and sometimes mistaken for sexual abuse.

• Associated symptoms: severe pruritus, soreness, dysuria, dyspareunia, and pain upon defecation.

• May be complicated by possible SCC development.

• **DDx:** vitiligo, erosive lichen planus, sexual abuse, intraepithelial neoplasia (see Chapter 60), SCC, extramammary Paget's disease.

Genital LS in Males

• Also known as balanitis xerotica obliterans.

• Bimodal presentation: older males and pre-pubertal males; more common if uncircumcised.

• Often presents with recurrent balanitis or acquired phimosis; rarely affects perianal region.

• **Early:** glans and inner foreskin have well-demarcated, erythematous thin plaques; ± erosions.

• **Mid:** evolves into atrophic, white, sclerotic, scar-like lesion (Fig. 36.8).

• **Late:** phimosis or complete occlusion of glans.

• Associated with pruritus and soreness, painful erections, dysuria, urinary obstruction, and possible development of SCC.

• **DDx:** SCC *in situ*, sexual abuse, erosive lichen planus, candidiasis, intraepithelial neoplasia (see Chapter 60), extramammary Paget's disease.

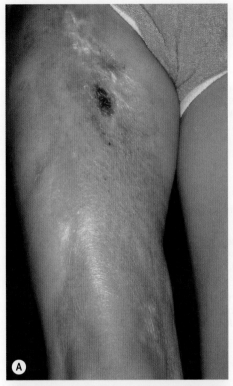

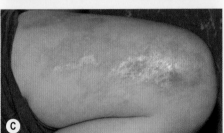

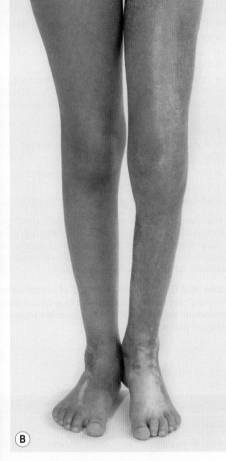

Fig. 36.5 Linear morphea, limb variant. A Linear morphea involving the leg; the differential diagnosis includes linear melorheostosis, which is associated with underlying candlewax-like linear hyperostosis. **B** Extensive induration of the left leg with hypoplasia and an obvious flexion contracture of the knee; there is also involvement of the right foot. **C** Linear distribution of coalescing sclerotic plaques on the thigh; note the lilac-colored border. *B, Courtesy, Martin Rocken, MD, and Kamran Ghoreschi, MD; C, Courtesy, Julie V. Schaffer, MD.*

Extragenital LS

• Affects all ages with slight female predominance.
• Favors the neck (Fig. 36.9), shoulders, trunk, proximal extremities, flexor wrists, and sites of trauma or pressure; associated xerosis and mild pruritus.
• **Early:** polygonal, white, shiny, elevated papules that often coalesce into plaques.

• **Mid:** evolve into scar-like, atrophic, wrinkled patches and plaques.
• **Late:** telangiectasias, follicular plugging (Fig. 36.10A), and occasional hemorrhagic bullae (Fig. 36.10B).
• **DDx:** localized morphea, scar; of note, LS may coexist with morphea and/or vitiligo.

DIFFERENTIAL DIAGNOSIS OF MORPHEAFORM SKIN LESIONS

- Morphea (circumscribed [superficial or deep*], linear, generalized*)
- Chronic graft-versus-host disease*
- Lichen sclerosus (may coexist with morphea)
- Lipodermatosclerosis*
- Sclerosis at injection sites** (e.g. vitamin K_1 or B_{12}, silicone or paraffin implants, intralesional bleomycin, interferon-β, glatiramer, enfuvirtide, opioids)
- Chemical/toxin exposures (e.g. aromatic/chlorinated hydrocarbons,* nephrogenic systemic fibrosis,* toxic oil syndrome*)
- Radiation-induced morphea
- Porphyria (e.g. porphyria cutanea tarda)
- H syndrome
- Stiff skin syndrome,* linear melorheostosis
- Reflex sympathetic dystrophy*
- Cutaneous metastases (e.g. carcinoma *en cuirasse*)

Can overlap with sclerodermoid disorders, which are outlined in Table 35.4; in particular, deep morphea and eosinophilic fasciitis may have a similar appearance (see Fig. 36.3).
**Systemic medications for which there have been reports of an association with morpheaform lesions include bleomycin, taxanes (e.g. paclitaxel, docetaxel), bromocriptine, ethosuximide, valproic acid, appetite suppressants, and penicillamine.*

Table 36.2 Differential diagnosis of morpheaform skin lesions. The location of the morpheaform lesions may offer a clue to the diagnosis, e.g. in lipodermatosclerosis lesions are located on the lower extremities, and in radiation-induced morphea lesions are within the radiation port site.

TREATMENT OPTIONS FOR LICHEN SCLEROSUS (LS)

Disease Severity	Treatment
Mild to moderate	Clearance: 6–12 weeks (may need to be repeated yearly if remains clinically active) • Topical class I CS* (Fig. 36.12) – daily • Topical calcineurin inhibitors* – daily • Intralesional CS – once to three times during clearance phase, depending upon extent and severity Maintenance • Topical petrolatum-based ointments – daily • Topical class VII CS* – daily • Topical class I CS* – occasional, e.g. twice weekly • Topical calcineurin inhibitors* – occasional, e.g. twice weekly
Severe or refractory	• Oral retinoids (acitretin 10–50 mg/day for ≥6 months) • Phototherapy** (e.g. bath PUVA, NB-UVB, UVA1)

Ointments are preferred over creams for genital LS because they are less irritating.
**Not recommended for genital LS because increases risk of genital SCC.*
PUVA, psoralens plus ultraviolet A light phototherapy; NB-UVB, narrowband ultraviolet B light phototherapy; UVA1, narrowband ultraviolet A light phototherapy.

Table 36.3 Treatment options for lichen sclerosus (LS). Some clinicians limit the use of calcineurin inhibitors for genital LS.

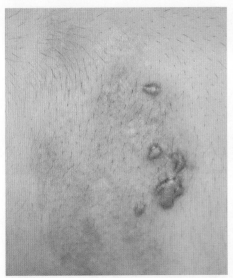

Fig. 36.6 Nodular (keloidal) morphea.
Elevated, firm pink papulonodules arising within an area of hyperpigmented induration. *Courtesy, Jean Bolognia, MD.*

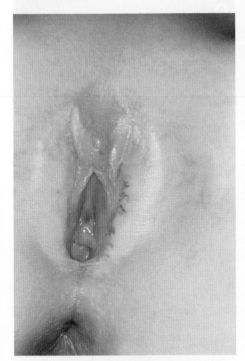

Fig. 36.7 Genital lichen sclerosus involving the vulva of a young female. Centrally, there is erythema with superficial erosion and purpura. More peripherally, white plaques with a wrinkled surface are seen. Note fissuring of the perineum. *Courtesy, Martin Rocken, MD, and Kamran Ghoreschi, MD.*

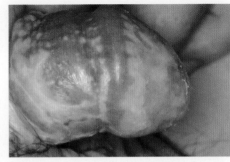

Fig. 36.8 Genital lichen sclerosus involving the penis (balanitis xerotica obliterans). Note the ivory color, erosion, and scarring.

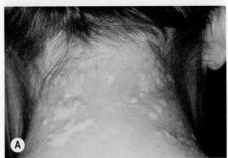

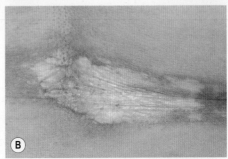

Fig. 36.9 Extragenital lichen sclerosus (LS).
LS of the neck presenting as white papules and small plaques **(A)** and as a large, shiny, ivory-colored plaque of the lower back **(B).** *Courtesy, Martin Rocken, MD, and Kamran Ghoreschi, MD.*

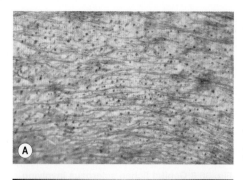

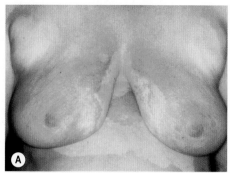

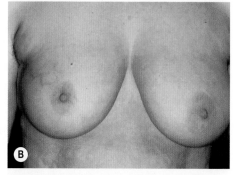

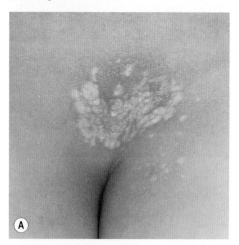

Fig. 36.11 Phototherapy of generalized morphea. Generalized morphea with trunk involvement before **(A)** and after PUVA bath photochemotherapy **(B).** Note that generalized morphea may involve the breasts but characteristically spares the nipples. *Courtesy, Martin Rocken, MD, and Kamran Ghoreschi, MD.*

Fig. 36.10 Extragenital lichen sclerosus (LS). **A** Follicular plugging in a plaque of LS on the back of a patient with chronic GVHD. **B** Hemorrhagic bullae on the leg. *A, Courtesy, Jean Bolognia, MD.*

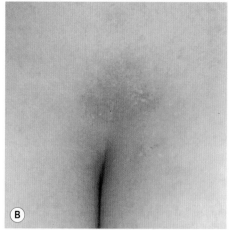

Fig. 36.12 Ultrapotent topical corticosteroids in the treatment of lichen sclerosus in a 12-year-old girl. Before **(A)** and after **(B)** topical application of clobetasol propionate 0.05% cream daily for 5 months. *Courtesy, Martin Rocken, MD, and Kamran Ghoreschi, MD.*

For further information see Ch. 44. From *Dermatology, Third Edition.*

Other Rheumatologic Diseases | 37

Systemic-Onset Juvenile Idiopathic Arthritis (SoJIA; Still's Disease) and Adult-Onset Still's Disease (AoSD)

• Among the major types of juvenile idiopathic arthritis (JIA; formerly juvenile rheumatoid arthritis [JRA]), cutaneous manifestations are most common in SoJIA, psoriatic arthritis (see Chapter 6), and rheumatoid factor (RF)-positive polyarthritis (rheumatoid nodules and other findings similar to rheumatoid arthritis [RA]; see below).

• SoJIA can develop at any age prior to 16 years and affects both sexes equally; AoSD has peaks in the second and fourth decades and affects women more often than men.

• Both SoJIA and AoSD are characterized by daily spiking fevers (especially in the late afternoon/early evening) accompanied by an *evanescent* eruption of salmon-pink macules and slightly edematous papules and plaques (Fig. 37.1A,B); these lesions are usually asymptomatic and favor sites of pressure or trauma, often occurring in a linear array.

• Less common skin findings include periorbital edema and persistent pruritic papules and plaques that are scaly, violaceous to reddish brown in color, and linear in configuration (Fig. 37.1C).

• Additional features include a prodromal sore throat and arthralgias/myalgias, arthritis (usually polyarticular; ± carpal ankylosis in AoSD), lymphadenopathy, hepatosplenomegaly, and serositis; occasionally patients may develop macrophage activation syndrome (also characterized by markedly elevated ferritin).

• Leukocytosis with neutrophilia, thrombocytosis, anemia, elevated ESR/CRP, and extremely high serum ferritin levels (e.g. >4000 mg/ml) are common laboratory findings, whereas ANA and RF are usually absent.

• **DDx:** infections (e.g. parvovirus B19), rheumatic fever, serum sickness-like reactions, urticarial vasculitis, Schnitzler's syndrome (in adults; see Chapter 14), other autoimmune connective tissue diseases, hereditary periodic fever syndromes (see Table 3.2).

• **Rx:** NSAIDs (for mild disease), systemic CS, methotrexate, antagonists of IL-1 (e.g. anakinra, canakinumab) or IL-6 (e.g. tocilizumab), and TNF inhibitors (the latter especially for arthritis).

Rheumatoid Arthritis

• Chronic inflammatory disorder characterized primarily by destructive arthritis.

• Affects 1–3% of adults, with a female : male ratio of 2–3 : 1 and a peak onset between 35 and 60 years of age.

• RF and anti-cyclic citrullinated peptide (CCP) antibodies represent serologic markers of RA.

• Cutaneous manifestations of RA are presented in Table 37.1 and Fig. 37.2; these findings can serve as diagnostic clues or signs of serious systemic disease.

Interstitial Granulomatous Dermatitis (IGD) and Palisaded Neutrophilic and Granulomatous Dermatitis (PNGD)

• Two clinicopathologic patterns of granulomatous dermatitis that occur in patients (women > men) with RA and other autoimmune disorders.

• *IGD* presents as annular erythematous plaques or linear cords ('rope sign') that favor the lateral and upper trunk, axillae, medial thighs, and buttocks (Fig. 37.3); patients often have RA or seronegative arthritis.

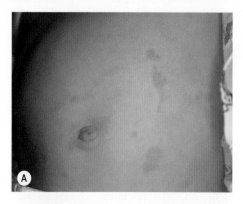

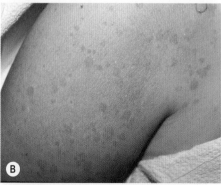

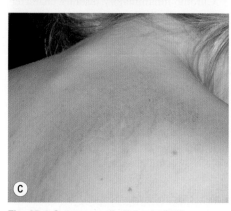

Fig. 37.1 Cutaneous findings in Still's disease. A Evanescent pink papules and plaques in a child. Note the linear array of some of the lesions. **B** Multiple pink macules and urticarial papules that developed during a fever spike in a woman. **C** Flagellate array of pinkish-tan, scaly persistent plaques on the upper back in a teenage girl. *A, Courtesy, Carlos Nousari, MD; B, Courtesy, Diane Davidson, MD; C, Courtesy, Julie V. Schaffer, MD.*

• *PNGD* presents as skin-colored to erythematous, umbilicated papulonodules that are often crusted and favor the elbows (see Fig. 19.11B) and extensor hands/fingers; associated with RA, SLE, and ANCA-positive systemic vasculitides (e.g. Churg–Strauss syndrome).

• Because interstitial granulomatous drug reactions can have clinical and histologic features similar to those of IGD and PNGD, a review of all medications should be performed; culprit drugs include calcium channel blockers, angiotensin-converting enzyme inhibitors, statins, and TNF inhibitors.

• Histologically, a dense pandermal infiltrate is seen in both entities; IGD features rosettes of palisading histiocytes surrounding tiny foci of degenerated collagen, while findings in PNGD range from a predominance of neutrophils with foci of leukocytoclastic vasculitis to well-developed palisaded granulomas surrounding basophilic degenerated collagen.

• **DDx:** interstitial granulomatous drug reaction (see above); *for IGD* – patch-type granuloma annulare (GA), morphea (inflammatory stage), mycosis fungoides and leprosy; *for PNGD* – papular GA, rheumatoid nodules/nodulosis, perforating disorders.

• **Rx:** high-potency topical or intralesional CS, dapsone (if prominent neutrophils); may improve with treatment of the underlying disorder.

Sjögren's Syndrome

• Autoimmune disorder primarily affecting the lacrimal and salivary glands, resulting in xerophthalmia and xerostomia; may coexist with other AI-CTDs (e.g. LE).

• Affects ~0.5% of the general population, with a female:male ratio of 9:1; peak onset is in the fourth and fifth decades of life, but can occur at any age.

• Cutaneous manifestations include xerosis, palpable purpura due to small vessel vasculitis (including cryoglobulinemic vasculitis), hypergammaglobulinemic purpura of Waldenström, urticarial vasculitis, annular erythema, and Raynaud's phenomenon.

• Additional features can include vaginal dryness, arthritis, peripheral neuropathy, internal organ involvement (e.g. kidneys), and

CUTANEOUS MANIFESTATIONS OF RHEUMATOID ARTHRITIS (RA)

Condition	Features
Palisading Granulomas	
Rheumatoid nodules	• Affect ~20% of RA patients, often associated with high-titer RF • Firm, semi-mobile papulonodules favoring periarticular locations (e.g. elbows; Fig. 37.2A) and other sites of repetitive trauma or pressure (e.g. the sacral region if bedridden) • **DDx:** subcutaneous granuloma annulare, gouty tophi, synovial hyperplasia/cysts (softer, painful) • Histologically, central zone of eosinophilic fibrin surrounded by palisaded histiocytes
Interstitial granulomatous dermatitis (IGD) and palisaded neutrophilic & granulomatous dermatitis (PNGD)	• See text; the PNGD spectrum includes *rheumatoid papules* (Fig. 37.2B) and *superficial ulcerating rheumatoid necrobiosis* (Fig. 37.2C)
Neutrophilic Dermatoses	
Rheumatoid neutrophilic dermatitis	• Erythematous papules and plaques that may be vesiculated or crusted; favors extensor extremities • Unlike Sweet's syndrome, *not* tender or associated with fevers and malaise
Sweet's syndrome and pyoderma gangrenosum (PG)*	• See Chapter 21; Fig. 37.2D
Neutrophilic lobular panniculitis	• Tender red nodules favoring the lower legs; may ulcerate with purulent drainage
Vasculitis and Vascular Reactions	
Bywater's lesions	• Punctate purpuric papules on the distal digits due to cutaneous small vessel vasculitis (Fig. 37.2E)

Rheumatoid vasculitis	• Associated with long-standing (often 'burnt out') joint disease, high-titer RF, and mononeuritis multiplex; may also affect the eyes and internal organs
	• Cutaneous involvement is usually the first manifestation
	  – *Small vessel vasculitis*: purpuric macules and papules
	  – *Medium-sized vessel vasculitis*: nodules, ulcers, digital gangrene, livedo reticularis, atrophie blanche-like scars
	• Systemic disease requires aggressive immunosuppressive therapy

Intravascular/intralymphatic histiocytosis	• Erythema, induration and papules in a reticular pattern overlying swollen joints, most often the elbows
Complications of Therapy for RA	
NSAIDs	• Pseudoporphyria, toxic epidermal necrolysis
Methotrexate > TNF inhibitors	• Accelerated rheumatoid nodulosis – sudden appearance of multiple papulonodules, especially on the hands (Fig. 37.2F)
TNF inhibitors	• Injection site reactions, urticaria, vasculitis, IGD, cutaneous LE, psoriasiform eruptions, palmoplantar pustulosis

'PG-like' leg ulcers are a feature of Felty syndrome, which is characterized by the triad of neutropenia, splenomegaly, and RA; Felty syndrome may be associated with T-cell large granular lymphocyte leukemia.

Table 37.1 Cutaneous manifestations of rheumatoid arthritis (RA).

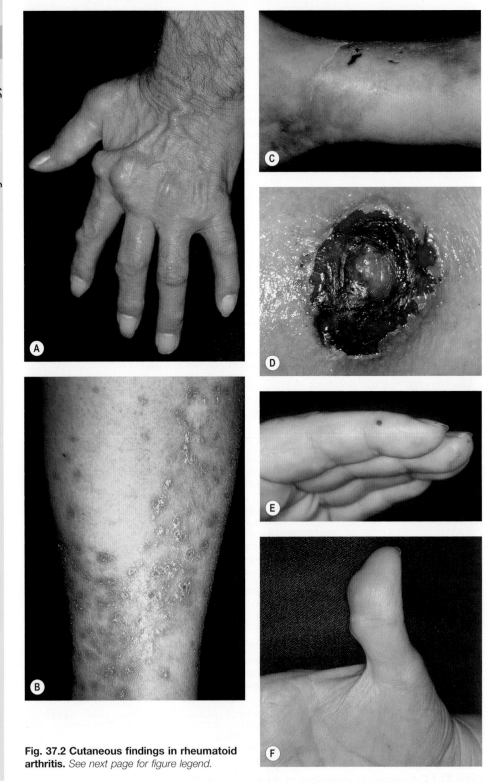

Fig. 37.2 Cutaneous findings in rheumatoid arthritis. *See next page for figure legend.*

development of B-cell lymphoma (often extra-nodal marginal zone).

• Majority of patients have anti-Ro/SS-A and anti-La/SS-B antibodies, a positive RF, and an elevated ESR.

• Diagnostic criteria for Sjögren's syndrome are presented in Table 37.2.

• **Rx:** mostly symptomatic – use of artificial tears and saliva (e.g. methylcellulose drops), chewing sugar-free gum, meticulous dental hygiene, and treatment of superimposed oral candidiasis; sicca symptoms may improve with cyclosporine eye drops or muscarinic receptor agonists (e.g. pilocarpine), and vasculitis or internal involvement often require systemic CS, conventional immunosuppressive agents, or rituximab.

Relapsing Polychondritis

• Uncommon autoimmune condition that affects cartilaginous structures; pathogenesis is thought to involve a reaction against type II collagen.

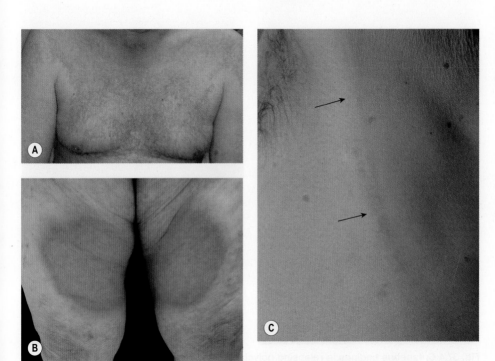

Fig. 37.3 Interstitial granulomatous dermatitis (IGD). A Large, symmetric pink patches and thin plaques that resemble patch-type granuloma annulare. **B** Annular lesions on the medial thighs. **C** Firm linear cord along the axillary line in a patient with rheumatoid arthritis. *A, C, Courtesy, Kathryn Schwarzenberger, MD; B, Courtesy, Jeffrey Callen, MD.*

Fig. 37.2 Cutaneous findings in rheumatoid arthritis. A Rheumatoid nodules in a periarticular location on the hands. **B** Rheumatoid papules presenting as coalescing red-brown lesions, some with scale-crust, on the lower extremity. **C** Superficial ulcerating rheumatoid necrobiosis manifesting as shiny, yellow-brown plaques with red-brown borders and areas of ulceration; these clinical findings are reminiscent of necrobiosis lipoidica, although both this entity and rheumatoid papules are categorized as forms of palisaded neutrophilic and granulomatous dermatitis. **D** Pyoderma gangrenosum resulting in recurrent ulcerations on the lower extremities. **E** Bywater's lesions. These tender purpuric papules on the distal fingers are characterized histologically by leukocytoclastic vasculitis. **F** Methotrexate-induced nodulosis. *A, Courtesy, Kalman Watsky, MD; B, C, E, Courtesy, Jeffrey Callen, MD; D, Courtesy, Carlos Nousari, MD; F, Courtesy, Jean L. Bolognia, MD.*

AMERICAN COLLEGE OF RHEUMATOLOGY 2012 CLASSIFICATION CRITERIA FOR SJÖGREN'S SYNDROME

Suggestive signs/symptoms (e.g. xerophthalmia, xerostomia) **plus ≥2 of the following:**

- + anti-SSA/Ro antibodies *or* + anti-SSB/La antibodies *or* + RF plus ANA titer ≥1:320
- Labial salivary gland biopsy showing focal lymphocytic sialadenitis with ≥1 focus/4 mm²
- Keratoconjunctivitis sicca with ocular staining score ≥3*

Using fluorescein and lissamine green to stain the cornea (score of 1–6) and conjunctiva (score of 1–3), respectively; other assessment methods include Schirmer and Rose Bengal tests.

Table 37.2 American College of Rheumatology 2012 classification criteria for Sjögren's syndrome. Other possible causes of similar findings include chronic GVHD, primary systemic amyloidosis, sarcoidosis, and radiation therapy of the head and neck.

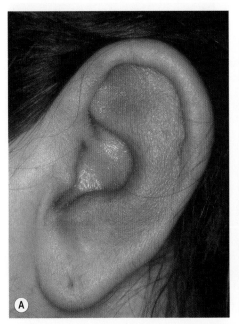

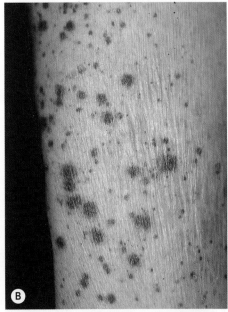

Fig. 37.4 Cutaneous findings in relapsing polychondritis. A Erythema and swelling of the ear with sparing of the earlobe. **B** Small vessel vasculitis presenting as palpable purpura in a patient who also had myelodysplastic syndrome. *A, Courtesy, Kalman Watsky, MD; B, Courtesy, Jean L. Bolognia, MD.*

- Most patients develop erythema, swelling and pain of the cartilaginous portion of the auricle, with sparing of the earlobe (Fig. 37.4A).
- Other manifestations include cutaneous small vessel vasculitis (Fig. 37.4B), aphthae (oral or genital; may overlap with Behçet's disease), nasal chondritis (potentially producing a saddle nose deformity), involvement of cartilage of the respiratory tract (e.g. larynx, trachea, bronchi) and costochondral junctions, arthritis, ocular inflammation, audiovestiblar damage, and myelodysplastic syndrome.
- **DDx:** *early phase* – erysipelas, cellulitis, infectious chondritis or zoster; *nasal destruction* – Wegener's granulomatosis, nasal natural killer/T-cell lymphoma, infections (e.g. mucocutaneous leishmaniasis) (see Table 19.3).
- **Rx:** prednisone (for acute flares), dapsone, immunosuppressive agents, TNF inhibitors; surgical repair of damaged cartilaginous structures.

Mixed Connective Tissue Disease (MCTD)

• Characterized by high-titer anti-U1 ribonucleoprotein (U1-RNP) antibodies plus a constellation of clinical features including arthritis, myositis, and findings of systemic sclerosis; the latter range from swollen hands and Raynaud's phenomenon to esophageal dysmotility and pulmonary hypertension (the most serious complication) or fibrosis (often mild).

• Favors women (female:male ratio ~9:1) in the second and third decades of life.

• Edema and erythema of the digits is an early manifestation; digital infarcts, periungual telangiectasias with dropout areas, sclerodactyly, and calcinosis cutis may also develop.

• Poikiloderma on the upper trunk and proximal extremities is common; photosensitivity, malar erythema, and subacute cutaneous LE occasionally occur.

• **DDx:** features overlap with those of systemic sclerosis, dermatomyositis/polymyositis, and SLE; for this reason, the debate continues regarding the distinction between MCTD (a specific entity requiring the presence of elevated U1-RNP) and less specific 'overlap syndromes' (features of two or more AI-CTDs in a single patient).

• **Rx:** varies depending on the organs involved and disease severity.

For further information see Ch. 45. From *Dermatology, Third Edition.*

38 | Mucinoses

In this group of disorders, there is deposition of glycosaminoglycans, previously referred to as mucopolysaccharides ('mucin'), within the skin, especially the dermis. Most frequently, the deposit is composed of hyaluronic acid. While several of the entities are idiopathic, underlying disorders include autoimmune thyroid disease, a monoclonal gammopathy, and diabetes mellitus.

Scleredema

- Symmetric diffuse induration of the skin, usually limited to the upper back and posterior neck, that may require palpation to be appreciated; a *peau d'orange* appearance may be present with prominent follicular orifices, and occasionally there is blanching erythema in the sites of involvement (Fig. 38.1).
- While scleredema is often asymptomatic, some patients may complain of tightness or decreased range-of-motion; occasionally there is also involvement of the face and upper extremities and rarely, the muscles, eyes, or heart.
- The three major types have different associations: type I – preceding streptococcal infections; type II – monoclonal gammopathy; and type III – diabetes mellitus, with men representing the majority of patients.
- **DDx:** systemic sclerosis (diffuse form), scleromyxedema, and other sclerodermoid disorders (see Table 35.4); occasionally, cellulitis if erythema is present.
- **Rx:** sometimes there is spontaneous resolution, especially with type I disease, but control of underlying diabetes mellitus does not lead to improvement; anecdotal therapies include phototherapy (e.g. UVA1, PUVA) and electron beam therapy.

Scleromyxedema/Papular Mucinosis

- A spectrum of clinical findings that varies from multiple linear arrays of firm, 2- to 3-mm, waxy, skin-colored papules (Fig. 38.2) to diffuse induration of the skin with thickened folds, including leonine facies (Fig. 38.3; Table 38.1); involvement is symmetric and often widespread.
- Associated with an underlying monoclonal gammopathy; in addition to skin stiffness, there can be decreased range-of-motion of joints and contractures as well as myositis, peripheral neuropathy, and encephalopathy (dermato-neuro syndrome).
- **DDx:** systemic sclerosis, scleredema; if primarily papules, primary systemic amyloidosis, lipoid proteinosis, and especially the various types of skin-limited (localized) mucinoses, e.g. acral persistent papular mucinosis, self-healing cutaneous mucinosis, the discrete papular form of lichen myxedematosus.
- **Rx:** similar to that of multiple myeloma (see primary systemic amyloidosis, Chapter 39), systemic retinoids, PUVA, UVA1.

Pretibial Myxedema

- In the vast majority of patients, associated with hyperthyroidism, primarily due to Graves' disease, an autoimmune disorder with circulating anti-thyroid-stimulating hormone receptor autoantibodies; lesions may appear following treatment of the thyroid disease, i.e. when the patient is euthyroid or hypothyroid.
- Favors the shins but can involve the foot and presents as indurated, waxy nodules or plaques that vary from skin-colored to red-brown (Fig. 38.4); there can be a prominence of follicular openings (*peau d'orange* appearance) and occasionally elephantiasis develops.
- Additional clinical findings include exophthalmos, goiter, and thyroid acropathy.
- **DDx:** obesity-associated lymphedematous mucinosis (no history of hyperthyroidism), lymphedema, lipedema, lichen amyloidosis.

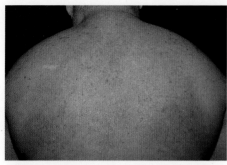

Fig. 38.1 Scleredema in association with diabetes mellitus. Diffuse induration of the upper back and neck with overlying erythema.

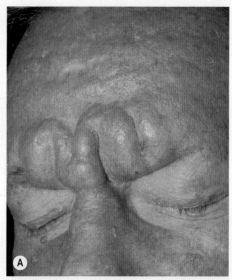

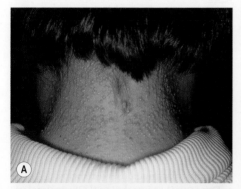

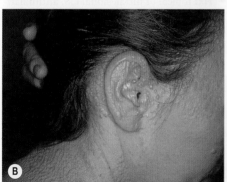

Fig. 38.2 Scleromyxedema/papular mucinosis. A, B Numerous monomorphic, firm, skin-colored papules which can have a linear arrangement (most obvious on the upper back).

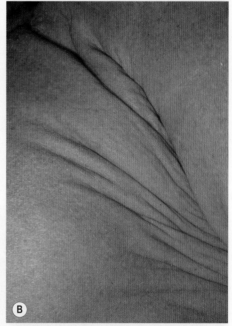

Fig. 38.3 Scleromyxedema/papular mucinosis. Thickening of the skin of the forehead **(A)** and trunk **(B)**, leading to deep furrows and folds. Scleromyxedema is one of the causes of leonine facies. *Courtesy, Joyce Rico, MD.*

Generalized Myxedema

• **Rx:** although lesions may clear spontaneously over a period of several years, treatment of the underlying thyroid disease usually has no effect; anecdotal therapies include topical and intralesional CS, pneumatic compression, surgical shave removal, octreotide.

• As a result of profound hypothyroidism, the skin is diffusely dry, cool, and pale, with a waxy appearance; the hair and nails can be brittle, leading to a diffuse non-scarring alopecia of the scalp and alopecia of the lateral eyebrows.

• Additional mucocutaneous findings include eczema craquelé, acquired ichthyosis, carotenoderma, and a puffiness of the hands and the face, including the eyelids; the tongue may be enlarged.

• In the congenital form, mental retardation, dwarfism, poor muscle tone, constipation, and somnolence are characteristic findings.

• Because the most common underlying disease in adults is Hashimoto's thyroiditis,

LEONINE FACIES – ASSOCIATED DERMATOLOGIC DISEASES
• Cutaneous lymphoma (T-cell, B-cell) • Lepromatous leprosy • Scleromyxedema/papular mucinosis • Actinic reticuloid form of chronic actinic dermatitis • Leishmaniasis • Leukemia cutis • Primary systemic amyloidosis • Lipoid proteinosis • Pachydermoperiostosis

Table 38.1 Leonine facies – associated dermatologic diseases. Additional causes include sarcoidosis, mastocytosis, multicentric reticulohistiocytosis, and progressive nodular histiocytosis.

women are more commonly affected; in addition to the skin changes outlined above, patients may gain weight, have cold intolerance and constipation, feel sluggish, and can occasionally develop cutaneous xanthomas.

• **Rx:** thyroid replacement.

Self-Healing Cutaneous Mucinosis

• Acute eruption of multiple firm papules and nodules favoring the face (especially the forehead and periorbital region), scalp, and periarticular areas.

• No underlying disorder and characterized by spontaneous resolution over months to years.

Reticular Erythematous Mucinosis (REM)

• Persistent erythematous papules of the central chest and central back that can form a net-like pattern and/or coalesce into plaques (Fig. 38.5); may be photo-aggravated.

• Overlaps with lupus erythematosus (LE) tumidus, Jessner's benign lymphocytic infiltrate (minimal to no dermal mucin), and papulonodular mucinosis (see below).

• **Rx:** topical or intralesional CS, antimalarials, e.g. hydroxychloroquine, chloroquine, sunscreens.

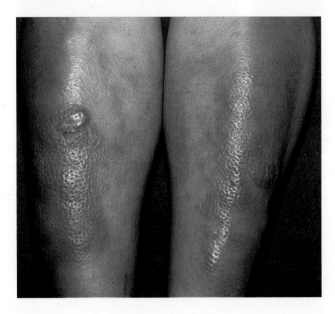

Fig. 38.4 Pretibial myxedema. Purple-brown plaques on the shins of a patient with Graves' disease. A *peau d'orange* appearance is present due to prominent follicular openings. *Courtesy, Franco Rongioletti, MD, and Alfredo Rebora, MD.*

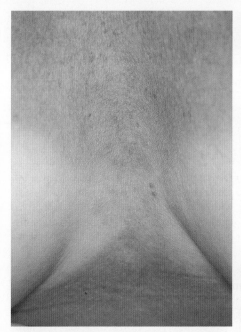

Fig. 38.5 Reticular erythematous mucinosis (REM). Grouped pink papules on the central chest with no surface changes; there is a subtle annular and reticulated configuration. Note the significant tan.

Cutaneous Lupus Mucinosis/ Papulonodular Mucinosis (of Gold)

- Occurs in the setting of autoimmune connective tissue diseases, with LE >> dermatomyositis or systemic sclerosis; ~75% of patients with LE who develop these lesions have systemic involvement.
- Skin-colored to erythematous papules and nodules that may require side-lighting to appreciate; favors the back, V of the chest and upper extremities (Fig. 38.6).
- Overlaps with LE tumidus, reticular erythematous mucinosis, and Jessner's benign lymphocytic infiltrate (minimal to no dermal mucin).
- **Rx:** antimalarials, e.g. hydroxychloroquine, chloroquine, topical or intralesional CS, sunscreens.

Follicular Mucinosis (Alopecia Mucinosis)

- In contrast to the other disorders in this chapter, here the mucin is deposited within

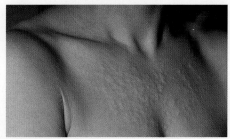

Fig. 38.6 Cutaneous lupus mucinosis/ papulonodular mucinosis. Skin-colored papules and nodules leading to a 'lumpy' appearance to the skin that is best appreciated by side-lighting. *Courtesy, Franco Rongioletti, MD, and Alfredo Rebora, MD.*

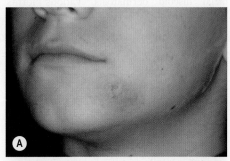

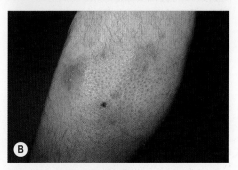

Fig. 38.7 Follicular mucinosis. A Pink plaque containing follicular papules in a young boy. **B** Grouped follicular papules on the leg of an older adult in association with violet-brown plaques; note the associated alopecia. The hemorrhagic crust is the site of a previous biopsy. *A, Courtesy, Lorenzo Cerroni, MD.*

the epithelium of hair follicles rather than in the dermis.

- In the primary form, there are pink to violet-brown plaques, primarily in the head and neck region, that have associated alopecia and sometimes scale (Fig. 38.7A); in some

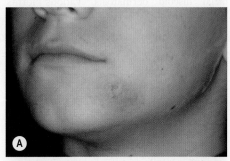

patients, there are grouped follicular papules (Fig. 38.7B), and in patients with darkly pigmented skin, lesions may be hypopigmented.

• The primary form most commonly occurs in children and young adults and represents a benign, self-limited disease; in older adults, especially when the lesions are more widespread and persistent, the possibility of coexisting mycosis fungoides needs to be considered.

• In addition to the characteristic histologic finding of mucin deposition within the follicular epithelium, it is important to comment on the presence or absence of atypical lymphocytes.

• **DDx:** cutaneous LE, tinea faciei or capitis, facial discoid dermatosis, various forms of dermatitis; if diagnosed histologically, consider an incidental finding (e.g. associated with atopic dermatitis).

• **Rx:** for primary, observation until spontaneous resolution, topical or intralesional CS, antimalarials; if associated with mycosis fungoides, treat the latter (see Chapter 98).

Other Entities

Digital mucous cyst is covered in Chapter 90. Cutaneous mucin deposits can also be seen within tumors (e.g. basal cell carcinomas, cutaneous metastases) and inflammatory disorders (e.g. granuloma annulare, cutaneous LE, dermatomyositis).

For further information see Ch. 46. From *Dermatology, Third Edition*.

Amyloidosis | 39

Amyloidosis encompasses a wide range of disorders, several of which have cutaneous manifestations. The common thread is the formation of extracellular deposits that are composed of a β-pleated sheet by x-ray crystallography. In general, amyloid deposits exhibit a red color with Congo red stain and demonstrate birefringence (apple green color) under polarized light. Precursor proteins of amyloid vary from keratin to immunoglobulin (Ig) light chains to gelsolin. If necessary, tandem mass spectrometry can be performed to characterize the specific protein.

In dermatology, the initial distinction is between amyloidosis that is systemic versus skin-limited (Fig. 39.1). The former is less common than the latter.

Systemic Amyloidosis

• *Primary systemic amyloidosis* is due to a plasma cell dyscrasia, but most patients do not fulfill the criteria for multiple myeloma (e.g. >10% plasma cells in a bone marrow biopsy, osteolytic bone lesions, anemia, hypercalcemia); the precursor protein is almost always Ig light chains (AL; lambda > kappa) rather than Ig heavy chains (AH).

• Firm skin-colored to pink to yellow-brown waxy papules or plaques occur most commonly on the face (Fig. 39.2); infiltration of the tongue can lead to macroglossia (Fig. 39.3), and occasionally there is diffuse waxy induration of the skin (sclerodermoid presentation); purpura due to trauma or pinching of the skin can also be seen and is due to the

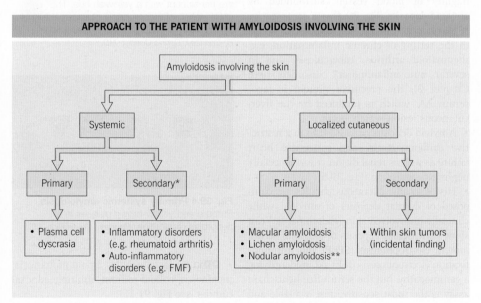

APPROACH TO THE PATIENT WITH AMYLOIDOSIS INVOLVING THE SKIN

Fig. 39.1 Approach to the patient with amyloidosis involving the skin. *Cutaneous lesions are rare; **A minority of patients may develop systemic amyloidosis. FMF, familial Mediterranean fever.

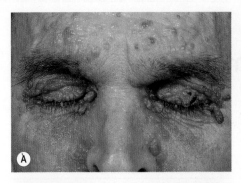

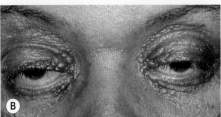

Fig. 39.2 Primary systemic amyloidosis.
A Numerous waxy translucent facial papules.
Some have a yellow to yellow-brown color.
B Some of the waxy papules have become
purpuric, but this may be difficult to appreciate
because of the pigmentation of the skin; the
periorbital region is a common site of
involvement. *A, Courtesy, Jean Bolognia, MD; B,
Courtesy, Judit Stenn, MD.*

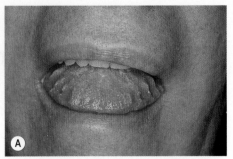

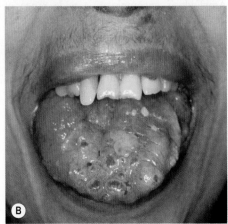

Fig. 39.3 Primary systemic amyloidosis.
A Macroglossia with dental impressions on the
tongue. **B** Papulonodues of the tongue and
external nares; some are purpuric while others
are translucent with a yellowish hue. The
combination of macroglossia plus carpal tunnel
syndrome is a classic clinical presentation.
B, Courtesy, Dennis Cooper, MD.

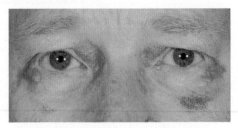

Fig. 39.4 Primary systemic amyloidosis.
Purpura and yellow-brown plaques in a
periorbital distribution. *Courtesy, Joyce Rico, MD.*

fragility of blood vessels surrounded by
amyloid deposits (Fig. 39.4).

• *Secondary systemic amyloidosis* develops
in the setting of chronic inflammation, e.g.
rheumatoid arthritis, tuberculosis, and in
several auto-inflammatory disorders (see
Chapter 3); the precursor protein is (apo)
serum AA, which is produced by the liver;
cutaneous lesions rarely occur.

• Amyloid deposits can also lead to a restric-
tive cardiomyopathy and congestive heart
failure as well as renal dysfunction, especially
nephrotic syndrome (Fig. 39.5).

• Histologically, cutaneous papules are composed of dermal deposits of amyloid while
clinically uninvolved skin (abdominal fat) can
show perivascular deposits of amyloid; serum
protein electrophoresis (SPEP) and immunofixation electrophoresis (IFE) aid in identifying
a gammopathy, but the serum free light-chain
assay is the most sensitive test available and
the presence of monoclonal free light chains is
required to establish the diagnosis.

• **DDx:** for facial papules, lipoid proteinosis,
mucinoses, colloid milium, multiple adnexal
tumors (see Fig. 91.15).

• **Rx:** for primary systemic amyloidosis, it is
similar to myeloma, e.g. dexamethasone,

EVALUATION OF A PATIENT WITH SUSPECTED PRIMARY SYSTEMIC AMYLOIDOSIS

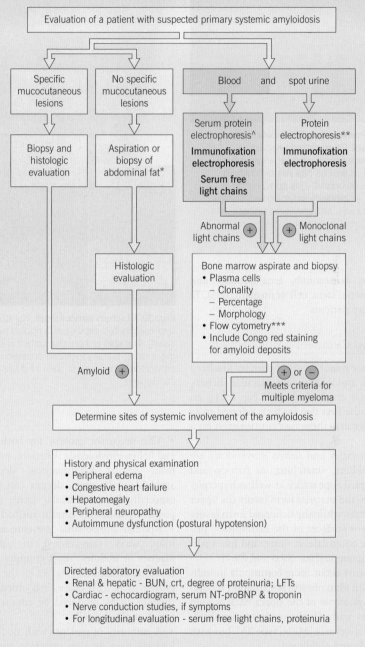

Fig. 39.5 Evaluation of a patient with suspected primary systemic amyloidosis. BUN, blood urea nitrogen; crt, creatinine; LFTs, liver function tests; NT-proBNP, N-terminal pro-brain natriuretic peptide.

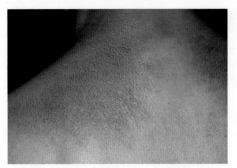

Fig. 39.6 Primary localized cutaneous amyloidosis. Characteristic rippled hyperpigmentation of macular amyloidosis (superiorly) as well as papules of lichenoid amyloidosis (inferiorly). This combination is referred to as biphasic amyloidosis. *Courtesy, Richard W. Groves, MD, and Martin M. Black, MD.*

melphalan, bortezomib, lenalidomide, and hematopoietic stem cell transplant (HSCT) (for younger patients).

Localized Cutaneous Amyloidosis

• The three major forms of *primary* localized cutaneous amyloidosis are macular, lichen, and nodular amyloidosis (see Fig. 39.1); an overlap of the first two forms is referred to as biphasic because these two entities exist on a spectrum.

• Both *macular* and *lichen amyloidosis* are due to rubbing, scratching, or friction and have a rippled appearance as well as hyperpigmentation; the macular form favors the upper back of adults while the lichenoid form favors the extensor surfaces of the extremities, primarily the anterolateral shins, and has a palpable component (Figs. 39.6 and 39.7).

• Both forms occur more commonly in individuals with skin phototypes III and IV; cutaneous amyloidosis of the upper back is seen in patients with Sipple syndrome (multiple endocrine neoplasia [MEN] type 2A), but with an onset during childhood.

• Mutations in two genes which encode the oncostatin M receptor β (a component of the IL-31 receptor) or the α subunit of the IL-31 receptor have been detected in patients with familial primary cutaneous amyloidosis; of note, IL-31 plays a role in pruritus.

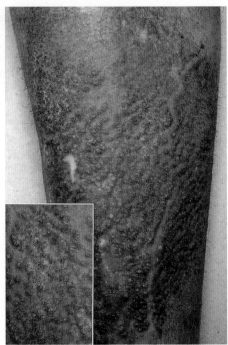

Fig. 39.7 Lichen amyloidosis. Keratotic hyperpigmented papules in a rippled pattern (see insert). The shin is the most common location for this form of primary localized cutaneous amyloidosis. *Courtesy, St. John's Institute of Dermatology.*

• The precursor protein for both macular and lichen amyloidosis is keratin, presumably from nearby keratinocytes; deposits of amyloid in the upper dermis can be subtle, especially in the macular form, and stain positively with anti-keratin antibodies.

• *Nodular amyloidosis* presents as one or more waxy skin-colored to pink-orange plaques or nodules, most commonly on the trunk or extremities (Fig. 39.8); the precursor protein is Ig light chains ± β_2-microglobulin, thought to be produced by cutaneous infiltrates of plasma cells.

• A minority of patients with nodular amyloidosis may develop systemic amyloidosis, so longitudinal evaluation is recommended.

• Occasionally, deposits of amyloid are seen in cutaneous tumors, e.g. basal cell carcinomas, dermatofibromas, intradermal melanocytic nevi, as an inconsequential *secondary* phenomenon.

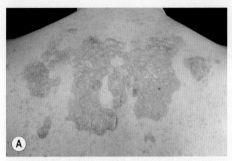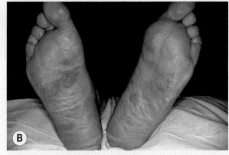

Fig. 39.8 Nodular amyloidosis. A, B Firm pink to pink-orange plaques on the back and plantar surface of the foot. *A, Courtesy, Richard W. Groves, MD, and Martin M. Black, MD.*

- **DDx:** back – notalgia paresthetica, lichen simplex chronicus (LSC) with post-inflammatory hyperpigmentation; lower extremity – LSC, hypertrophic lichen planus, pretibial myxedema; nodular – cutaneous lesions of systemic amyloidosis, pretibial myxedema, cutaneous lymphoma.

- **Rx:** difficult; can try topical antipruritics, e.g. pramoxine, topical or intralesional CS; physical coverings, e.g. zinc oxide-impregnated gauze (Unna boot) or hydrocolloid dressings, can lead to improvement but recurrences common when discontinued.

For further information see Ch. 47. From *Dermatology, Third Edition*.

40 | Deposition Disorders

A heterogeneous group of disorders in which there are deposits, usually of endogenous materials, within the skin. Entities belonging to this group that are covered in other chapters include mucinoses (Chapter 38), amyloidosis (Chapter 39), porphyrias (Chapter 41), and calcinosis cutis (Chapter 42).

Gout

• Metabolic disorder in which there is hyperuricemia due to increased production and/or decreased excretion of uric acid; often idiopathic but secondary causes include renal insufficiency and medications such as diuretics or cyclosporine; affects primarily adult men.
• Crystals of monosodium urate can deposit within the skin (tophi) as well as the joints and kidneys; when expressed from the skin or aspirated from the joints, the crystals are needle-like and exhibit negative birefringence under polarized light.
• Tophi present as firm skin-colored to white or yellow papules and nodules, usually around joints and on the helices of the ears (Fig. 40.1); in general, they appear ~10 years after the initial episode of acute arthritis and occur in ~10% of patients with gout.
• Tophi can become inflamed (Fig. 40.2), and they may or may not resolve following normalization of serum uric acid levels.
• **DDx:** rare cutaneous involvement in pseudogout (rhomboid crystals) as well as calcinosis cutis, xanthomas, and rheumatoid nodules.
• **Rx** for tophi: diet, allopurinol, febuxostat; for refractory disease, pegloticase, IL-1 antagonists (e.g. rilonacept).

Lipoid Proteinosis

• Autosomal recessive disease due to loss-of-function mutations in *ECM1*, which encodes extracellular matrix protein 1; the result is deposition of hyalin-like material in multiple sites, in particular the brain (seizures) and larynx (hoarseness), as well as the skin and oral mucosa.
• Skin-colored to yellowish waxy papules and nodules favor the face, including the eyelid margin, and the tongue (Fig. 40.3); atrophic scarring, verrucous changes (especially on the elbows and knees), and a diffuse waxy appearance are additional findings; during infancy, fragility, vesicles and crusting of the face, extremities and mouth can occur.
• **DDx:** mucinoses, erythropoietic protoporphyria, primary systemic amyloidosis, colloid milium, and in infants, hyaline fibromatosis syndrome.

Colloid Milium

• Two major variants – inherited juvenile form and acquired adult form; because the latter is related to cumulative photodamage, it occurs primarily in adults with lightly pigmented skin.
• Dermal deposits lead to dome-shaped, translucent to yellowish papules in chronically sun-exposed sites, in particular the face, ears, posterior neck, and dorsal aspect of the distal extremities; the lesions can become nodular or even pigmented if topical agents such as hydroquinone have been applied.
• **DDx:** similar to that of lipoid proteinosis (see above).
• **Rx:** laser, cryosurgery.

Mucopolysaccharidoses (MPS)

• Group of inherited metabolic disorders in which there is an accumulation of glycosaminoglycans (GAGs; previously referred to as mucopolysaccharides) due to deficiencies in lysosomal enzymes that break down sulfated GAGs (e.g. heparan sulfate, dermatan sulfate).

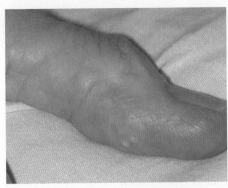

Fig. 40.1 Tophaceous gout of a digit. The deposits create a multilobulated appearance. A small incision over the yellow-white areas followed by microscopic examination of the expressed material would allow a bedside diagnosis.

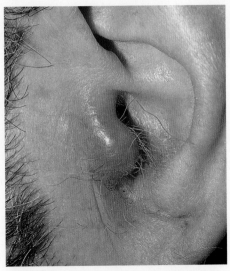

Fig. 40.2 Tophaceous gout of the tragus. The erythema reflects surrounding inflammation. *Courtesy, Harald Gollnick, MD.*

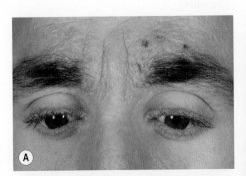

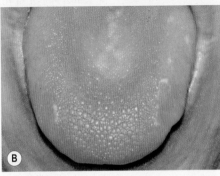

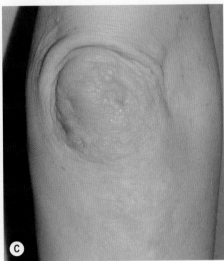

Fig. 40.3 Lipoid proteinosis. A Beaded eyelid papules, hemorrhagic crusts, and confluent waxy papules of the glabella leading to an early leonine facies. **B** A firm tongue with numerous tiny papules on its dorsal surface. **C** Skin-colored papulonodules of the elbow as well as irregular hypopigmented scars of the extensor forearm. *B, C, Courtesy, Julie V. Schaffer, MD.*

• The accumulation of GAGs can lead to mental retardation, hepatosplenomegaly, skeletal and joint disease, corneal clouding, and a coarse facies; in addition to thickening of the skin, some patients have hypertrichosis; in Hunter syndrome (MPS II), grouped skin-colored to white papules can develop in the scapular region ('pebbling'), and in Hurler syndrome (MPS I), patients may have dermal melanocytosis.

• Following measurement of urinary GAGs and examination of peripheral leukocytes or dermal fibroblasts for vacuoles, genetic analyses can be performed.

• **Rx:** for some of the types (MPS I, II, VI), enzyme replacement therapy is available; hematopoietic stem cell transplant (HSCT) is another option.

For further information see Ch. 48. From *Dermatology, Third Edition*.

Porphyrias 41

The porphyrias represent a group of metabolic disorders in which there is dysfunction of the enzymes involved in heme synthesis (Fig. 41.1). With the exception of acquired porphyria cutanea tarda (PCT), the underlying etiology is monogenetic mutations. Porphyrins absorb light energy (400–410 nm) and their accumulation within the skin can lead to photosensitization, with water-soluble porphyrins producing blisters and lipophilic porphyrins leading to acute burning and erythema. This chapter focuses on those porphyrias with cutaneous manifestations.

Porphyria Cutanea Tarda (PCT)

• The most common form of cutaneous porphyria; clinical findings typically appear during the 3rd to 4th decade of life.
• Dysfunction of uroporphyrinogen decarboxylase (UD) is usually acquired (type I) but can be inherited in an autosomal dominant manner (type II); the ratio of type I : type II is ~3 : 1.
• In type I PCT, the enzyme is only dysfunctional in the liver, rather than in all tissues; hepatotoxins (e.g. alcohol, iron overload), hepatitis C virus, HIV infection, or estrogens can precipitate or exacerbate PCT.
• In addition to photosensitivity, characteristic skin findings include fragility, erosions, vesicobullae, milia, and scars in sun-exposed areas, especially on the dorsal aspects of the hand (Fig. 41.2); hypertrichosis (malar region) and hyperpigmentation can develop on the face (Fig. 41.3); morpheaform plaques are seen less often (Fig. 41.4).
• Histologically, if a bulla is biopsied, there is a subepidermal split with minimal inflammation; thickened basement membranes around capillaries in the dermis with festooning of the dermal papillae are also seen.

• Diagnosis is based on the detection of elevated levels of *urinary* uro- and coproporphyrins (water-soluble) or elevated plasma uroporphyrins or fecal isocoproporphyrins; genetic analysis can be performed for type II PCT.
• Additional evaluation includes serum ferritin and if elevated, analysis of the hemochromatosis gene, screening for hepatitis B or C viral infection, and if risk factors, HIV infection.
• **DDx:** pseudoporphyria due to medications (Table 41.1) or in patients with chronic kidney disease and those undergoing dialysis; phototoxic drug eruption; epidermolysis bullosa acquisita (sites of trauma but not limited to sun-exposed sites); rare forms of porphyria with similar cutaneous findings plus neurologic manifestations similar to acute intermittent porphyria (AIP) – variegate porphyria (see below) and hereditary coproporphyria (elevated coproporphyrins in feces consistently and in urine when symptomatic) – and mild forms of congenital erythropoietic porphyria.
• **Rx:** photoprotection via clothing and sunscreens containing titanium dioxide and zinc oxide (blocks visible light); avoidance of exacerbating factors; phlebotomy, initially 500 ml every 2–3 weeks, depending on the hematocrit; oral antimalarials, but at much lower doses than are used for cutaneous lupus erythematosus (LE), i.e. hydroxychloroquine 200 mg twice weekly.
• In the setting of chronic kidney disease or renal dialysis and the associated anemia, the inability to use phlebotomy and/or antimalarials limits therapeutic options.

Erythropoietic Protoporphyria (EPP)

• Complaints of erythema, edema, and a painful burning sensation of the skin

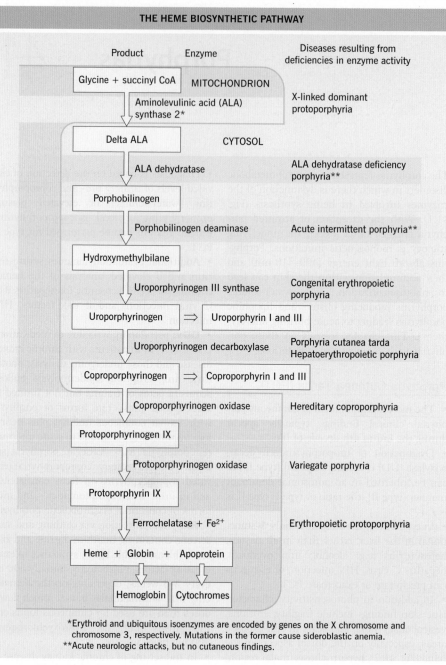

THE HEME BIOSYNTHETIC PATHWAY

Product   Enzyme

Diseases resulting from deficiencies in enzyme activity

Glycine + succinyl CoA   MITOCHONDRION

Aminolevulinic acid (ALA) synthase 2*

X-linked dominant protoporphyria

Delta ALA   CYTOSOL

ALA dehydratase

ALA dehydratase deficiency porphyria**

Porphobilinogen

Porphobilinogen deaminase

Acute intermittent porphyria**

Hydroxymethylbilane

Uroporphyrinogen III synthase

Congenital erythropoietic porphyria

Uroporphyrinogen $\Rightarrow$ Uroporphyrin I and III

Uroporphyrinogen decarboxylase

Porphyria cutanea tarda
Hepatoerythropoietic porphyria

Coproporphyrinogen $\Rightarrow$ Coproporphyrin I and III

Coproporphyrinogen oxidase

Hereditary coproporphyria

Protoporphyrinogen IX

Protoporphyrinogen oxidase

Variegate porphyria

Protoporphyrin IX

Ferrochelatase + Fe^{2+}

Erythropoietic protoporphyria

Heme + Globin + Apoprotein

Hemoglobin   Cytochromes

*Erythroid and ubiquitous isoenzymes are encoded by genes on the X chromosome and chromosome 3, respectively. Mutations in the former cause sideroblastic anemia.
**Acute neurologic attacks, but no cutaneous findings.

Fig. 41.1 The heme biosynthetic pathway. *Courtesy, Jorge Frank, MD, and Pamela Poblete-Gutiérrez, MD.*

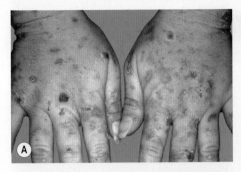

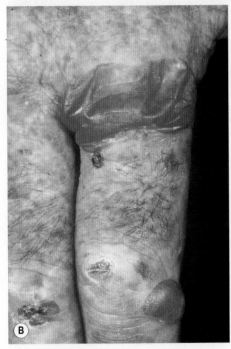

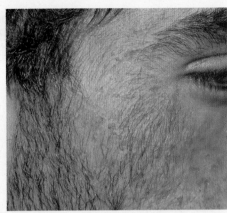

Fig. 41.3 Porphyria cutanea tarda.
Hypertrichosis of the malar region of the cheek.
Courtesy, Judit Stenn, MD.

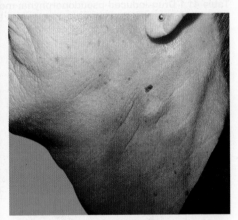

Fig. 41.4 Porphyria cutanea tarda presenting as yellow-brown morpheaform plaques. The plaques were in sun-exposed areas in this patient with a history of alcohol abuse.

Fig. 41.2 Porphyria cutanea tarda. A Marked fragility with multiple hemorrhagic crusts, erosions, and milia as well as scars. **B** Flaccid bulla and tense vesicle with clear fluid on the forefinger, accompanied by crusts and scars.
B, Courtesy, Jorge Frank, MD, and Pamela Poblete-Gutiérrez, MD.

following sun exposure usually begin during early childhood; purpura and crusts may also be seen and over time, a waxy texture and scarring develop in areas of greatest cumulative UV exposure, i.e. on the nose and dorsal hands (Fig. 41.5).

• Inherited primarily in a semidominant pattern (mutation in one allele and specific polymorphism in second allele); internal

manifestations include gallstones and cholestatic liver disease which can lead to liver failure (~5% of patients).

• Diagnosis is based on the detection of elevated levels of *red blood cell (RBC) free* protoporphyrins (lipophilic); elevated protoporphyrins are also present in the stool and genetic analysis can be performed; of note, zinc protoporphyrins are also elevated but this can be seen in other disorders, e.g. lead poisoning.

• **DDx:** solar urticaria, phototoxic or photoallergic contact dermatitis and drug reactions, hydroa vacciniforme, cutaneous LE,

DRUG-INDUCED PSEUDOPORPHYRIA: MOST COMMONLY INCRIMINATED MEDICATIONS	
NSAIDs*	**Diuretics**
Naproxen (proprionic acid derivative)** Nabumetone Ketoprofen (proprionic acid derivative) **Mefenamic acid** Diflunisal Celecoxib	**Furosemide** Hydrochlorothiazide/triamterene Chlorthalidone Bumetanide
	Retinoids
	Isotretinoin Acetretin/etretinate
Antibiotics	
Nalidixic acid Tetracycline, doxycycline Ciprofloxacin	**Miscellaneous**
	Amiodarone Voriconazole

NSAID, nonsteroidal anti-inflammatory drug.
*When caused by NSAIDs, consider prescribing diclofenac, indomethacin, or sulindac.
**Most frequently implicated NSAID.

Table 41.1 Drug-induced pseudoporphyria: most commonly incriminated medications. The most commonly incriminated medications are in bold. For a more complete list, see Table 49.5 in *Dermatology, Third Edition. Courtesy, Misty Sharp, MD.*

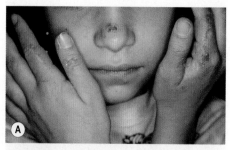

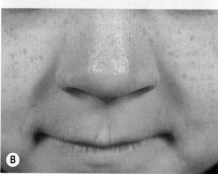

Fig. 41.5 Erythropoietic protoporphyria (EPP). A Erythema, edema, and hemorrhagic crusts on the nose as well as the fingers in a young girl. **B** Subtle scarring on the nose and linear scars on the upper cutaneous lip in a 6-year-old child. *B, Courtesy, Gillian Murphy, MD.*

other causes of early onset photosensitivity (e.g. xeroderma pigmentosum, Rothmund–Thomson syndrome), and a very rare form of porphyria with similar cutaneous and hepatic findings – X-linked dominant protoporphyria.
• **Rx:** photoprotection (see PCT), β-carotene, α-melanotide; cholestyramine or charcoal, if liver disease.

Variegate Porphyria (VP)

• Rare form of porphyria, except in South Africa; autosomal dominant inheritance pattern.
• While the cutaneous findings are similar to PCT, the systemic manifestations are similar to those of AIP, in particular acute attacks of abdominal pain, vomiting, paresthesias, motor and sensory neuropathies, and/or psychosis.
• Diagnosis is based on detection of elevated levels of urinary uro- and coproporphyrins (as in PCT) as well as elevated aminolevulinic acid and porphobilinogen (as in AIP), but these elevations may only be present during periods of symptomatic disease; elevated fecal porphyrins are present consistently and in the plasma, a characteristic peak fluorometric emission at 624–626 nm is observed in symptomatic patients; genetic analysis can also be performed.

- **DDx:** for cutaneous findings, PCT, pseudo-porphyria, epidermolysis bullosa acquisita (see PCT **DDx**).
- **Rx:** photoprotection (see PCT); avoidance of exacerbating factors (e.g. alcohol, fasting); for acute attacks, heme preparations.

Congenital Erythropoietic Porphyria (CEP)

- Rare severe form of porphyria in which erythema, edema, blisters, erosions, and scarring, as well as hyperpigmentation and hypertrichosis, develop in sun-exposed areas during infancy; autosomal recessive inheritance.
- Over time, the degree of scarring can become marked, leading to mutilation, e.g. mitten deformities of the hand (Fig. 41.6); additional manifestations include hemolytic anemia, hepatosplenomegaly, and pink-red urine stains and pink-red teeth (erythrodontia).
- Diagnosis is based on detection of elevated levels of uro- and coproporphyrins in the urine, RBCs, and plasma and elevated coproporphyrins in the stool; genetic analysis can also be performed.
- **DDx:** hepatoerythropoietic porphyria, which represents the rare autosomal recessive variant of PCT (Fig. 41.7); other causes of early onset photosensitivity (see EPP above).
- **Rx:** strict photoprotection (see PCT), blood transfusions plus iron chelators such

as oral deferasirox, hematopoietic stem cell transplantation.

Pseudoporphyria (Pseudo-PCT, Bullous Dermatosis of Dialysis)

- Clinical presentation similar to PCT but without abnormal elevation of porphyrins, although patients with renal disease can have borderline elevations in porphyrin levels.
- Seen in patients with chronic kidney disease and those undergoing dialysis, usually hemodialysis (Fig. 41.8); it is also associated with certain medications (Table 41.1).
- Can also occur following tanning bed use.
- **DDx:** see PCT.
- **Rx:** discontinue suspect drug; photoprotection (see PCT).

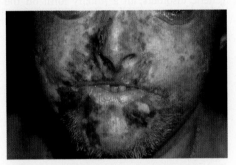

Fig. 41.7 Hepatoerythropoietic porphyria. Hypertrichosis and severe scarring are present, resulting in a clinical appearance similar to congenital erythropoietic porphyria. *Courtesy, José Mascaro, MD.*

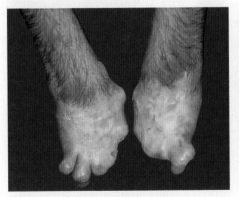

Fig. 41.6 Congenital erythropoietic porphyria. Severe mutilation of the hands due to scarring. *Courtesy, José Mascaro, MD.*

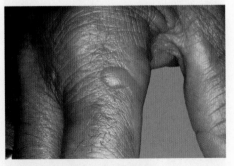

Fig. 41.8 Dialysis-associated pseudoporphyria. Vesicles filled with clear fluid formed on the dorsal aspects of the hand in this patient with chronic kidney disease. *Courtesy, Kalman Watsky, MD.*

For further information see Ch. 49. From *Dermatology, Third Edition.*

42

Calcinosis Cutis and Osteoma Cutis

There are four major forms of cutaneous calcification (calcinosis cutis): (1) *dystrophic* – locally within sites of pre-existing skin damage; (2) *metastatic* – due to systemic metabolic derangements; (3) *iatrogenic* – secondary to medical treatment or testing; and (4) *idiopathic*. Cutaneous ossification (osteoma cutis) occurs in the setting of several genetic disorders, in a miliary form on the face and within neoplasms and sites of inflammation (secondary).

Calcinosis Cutis

• Deposition of amorphous, insoluble calcium salts within the skin.

Calcinosis Cutis – Dystrophic

• Often seen in autoimmune connective tissue diseases (AI-CTDs), in particular the limited form of systemic sclerosis (also referred to as CREST syndrome) and childhood dermatomyositis (Figs. 42.1 and 42.2); in the former, hard, skin-colored to white papules overlie the bony prominences of the extremities (upper > lower), whereas in the latter the deposits are often larger and sometimes plate-like.

• Extrusion (transepidermal elimination or 'perforation'; see Ch. 79) of the calcium deposits appears as a white chalky material and it can be followed by a persistent ulceration.

• Other underlying causes are listed in Table 42.1.

• **Rx:** aggressive treatment of AI-CTDs, when possible, prior to the appearance of calcinosis cutis; excision of symptomatic

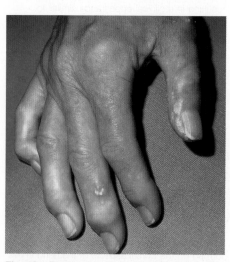

Fig. 42.1 Dystrophic form of calcinosis cutis. Note the cluster of small white papules in this patient with the limited form of systemic sclerosis (also referred to as CREST syndrome). *Courtesy, Janet Fairley, MD.*

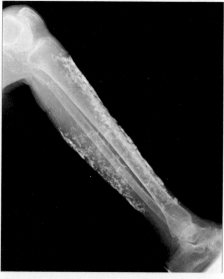

Fig. 42.2 Radiograph of calcinosis cutis in a patient with generalized morphea. Areas that were previously firm became rock-hard, and lesions of perforating calcinosis cutis (transepidermal elimination) developed on both legs. *Courtesy, Jean L. Bolognia, MD.*

DISORDERS OF CUTANEOUS CALCIFICATION

Dystrophic

- Autoimmune connective tissue diseases, especially dermatomyositis and the limited form of systemic sclerosis
- Cutaneous tumors or cysts, e.g. pilomatricomas, pilar cysts
- Infections, especially when cysts form around larvae or worms
- Trauma, including 'heel sticks' in neonates (Fig. 42.3), injection sites, surgical scars
- Panniculitis, e.g. pancreatic, lupus profundus, subcutaneous fat of the newborn
- Genetic disorders, e.g. pseudoxanthoma elasticum, Ehlers–Danlos syndrome (spherules)

Metastatic

- Chronic renal failure
  - Calciphylaxis*
  - Benign nodular calcification of renal disease
- Hypervitaminosis D
- Milk–alkali syndrome
- Sarcoidosis
- Tumoral calcinosis (familial; hyper- or normophosphatemic)
- Hyperparathyroidism
- Neoplasms (e.g. multiple myeloma, adult T-cell leukemia/lymphoma, SCC of the lung or head and neck)

Idiopathic

- Idiopathic calcified nodules of the scrotum
- Subepidermal calcified nodule (favors head and neck of children)
- Tumoral calcinosis (sporadic)
- Milia-like calcinosis

Iatrogenic

- Extravasation of intravenous solutions containing calcium or phosphate
- Application of calcium-containing electrode paste for EMGs and EEGs
- Application of calcium alginate dressings to denuded skin
- Organ transplantation, especially liver

*Can occasionally occur in the setting of severe primary hyperparathyroidism and, less often, in the absence of a clearly identifiable trigger.
EEG, electroencephalogram; EMG, electromyography; SCC, squamous cell carcinoma.

Table 42.1 Disorders of cutaneous calcification.

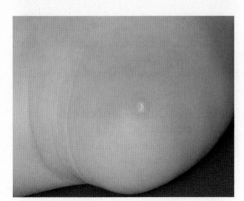

Fig. 42.3 Dystrophic calcification in an infant at the site of a previous 'heel stick' for obtaining blood. *Courtesy, Julie V. Schaffer, MD.*

localized deposits, if feasible; sodium thiosulfate and calcium channel blockers, e.g. diltiazem, may be effective in some patients.

Calcinosis Cutis – Metastatic

- The most common cause is end-stage renal disease with its associated hyperphosphatemia and decreased 1,25-dihydroxyvitamin D levels (Fig. 42.4).
- The two major presentations in patients with chronic kidney disease are: (1) *benign nodular calcification* in which deposits occur within otherwise normal skin, especially around joints; and (2) *calciphylaxis*, which is associated with significant morbidity and mortality.

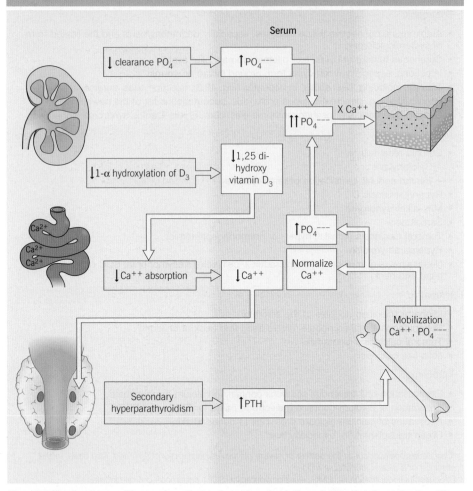

Fig. 42.4 Mechanisms of hyperphosphatemia and metastatic calcification in patients with chronic kidney disease.

• Calciphylaxis is characterized by cutaneous ischemia and necrosis which presents as markedly painful retiform purpura and ulcerations (Fig. 42.5); risk factors include obesity and hypercoagulability (e.g. protein C dysfunction); deposits of calcium within blood vessel walls of the subcutis are usually present, but not always, presumably due to sampling error.

• Other etiologies are listed in Table 42.1.

• **Rx** of calciphylaxis is difficult but includes aggressive wound care and normalization of the $Ca^{++}-PO_4^{---}$ product via the use of phosphate binders and sometimes

parathyroidectomy; drugs such as sodium thiosulfate and cinacalcet can also be tried as well as local injections of sodium thiosulfate.

Calcinosis Cutis – Iatrogenic and Idiopathic

• Iatrogenic causes and idiopathic forms are listed in Table 42.1.

• Calcification of epidermoid inclusion cysts is the major cause of calcified nodules of the scrotum.

• **Rx:** if symptomatic and feasible, surgical excision.

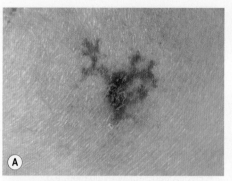 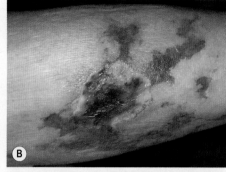

Fig. 42.5 Calciphylaxis in two patients with chronic kidney disease. A, B Characteristic painful reticulated purpuric plaques that can develop ulceration. *A, Courtesy, Kalman Watsky, MD.*

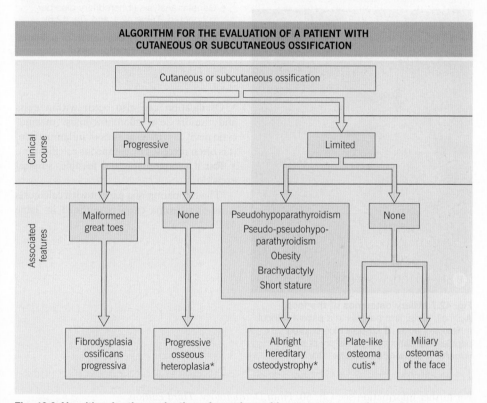

ALGORITHM FOR THE EVALUATION OF A PATIENT WITH CUTANEOUS OR SUBCUTANEOUS OSSIFICATION

Cutaneous or subcutaneous ossification

Clinical course

Progressive — Limited

Associated features

Malformed great toes | None | Pseudohypoparathyroidism / Pseudo-pseudohypo-parathyroidism / Obesity / Brachydactyly / Short stature | None

Fibrodysplasia ossificans progressiva | Progressive osseous heteroplasia* | Albright hereditary osteodystrophy* | Plate-like osteoma cutis* | Miliary osteomas of the face

Fig. 42.6 Algorithm for the evaluation of a patient with cutaneous or subcutaneous ossification. *Associated with mutations in *GNAS1*, which encodes the alpha subunit of the stimulatory G protein that regulates adenyl cyclase activity (thought to be negative regulator of bone formation); clinical phenotype may be a reflection of imprinting.

Osteoma Cutis

• Deposition of a protein matrix plus hydroxyapatite (Ca^{++}, PO_4^{---}) within the skin.
• The four genetic disorders that often have cutaneous or subcutaneous ossification are outlined in Fig. 42.6.

• Miliary osteomas of the face is a rather common entity; small hard papules, whose color can vary from white or skin-colored to blue (Fig. 42.7), gradually appear on the face of adult women > men; the role of pre-existing acne vulgaris and its treatment with oral antibiotics is debated.

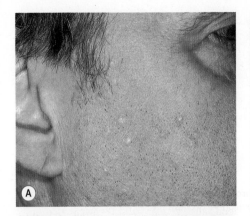

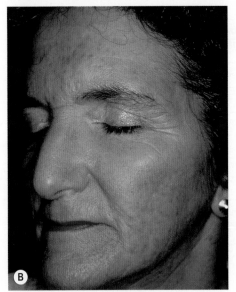

Fig. 42.7 Miliary osteomas of the face.
A Small, white, firm papules in a patient without a history of acne. **B** Multiple blue-colored papules in a patient with a history of acne vulgaris. *A, Courtesy, Janet Fairley, MD.*

LABORATORY EVALUATION OF PATIENTS WITH CUTANEOUS CALCIFICATION/OSSIFICATION

- Special histologic stains for calcium, e.g. von Kossa
- Serum levels of:
  - Calcium
  - Phosphate
  - Parathyroid hormone (PTH)
  - Vitamin D_3
- 24-Hour urinary calcium excretion (in some patients)
- Hypercoagulability evaluation, e.g. protein C activity (if calciphylaxis suspected)
- Genetic analysis (if hereditary disorder suspected; Table 42.1 and Fig. 42.6)

Table 42.2 Laboratory evaluation of patients with cutaneous calcification/ossification.

• Ossification can also occur within cysts and tumors (e.g. pilomatricomas, melanocytic nevi) as well as at sites of inflammation; it is often preceded by cutaneous calcification.

• **Rx:** if symptomatic and feasible, surgical excision.

The evaluation of a patient with calcinosis cutis or osteoma cutis is outlined in Table 42.2.

For further information see Ch. 50. From *Dermatology, Third Edition*.

Nutritional Disorders 43

Malnutrition

- Poor nutrition resulting from an insufficient or poorly balanced diet or from defective digestion or utilization of foods.
- Malnutrition encompasses both deficiencies and excesses (e.g. obesity) (Fig. 43.1; Tables 43.1 and 43.2).
- Primary or exogenous: related to the ingestion of food.
- Secondary or endogenous: inadequate or faulty absorption and/or defective metabolism of food and nutrients.
- In low-income populations, exogenous protein-energy malnutrition (marasmus), due to diminished or inadequate food ingestion, is often observed.
- In high-income populations, obesity due to excessive food consumption and primary or secondary deficiencies due to psychiatric or medical conditions are more commonly seen.

Marasmus (Protein-Energy Malnutrition)

- Affects infants, children, and adults (Fig. 43.2).
- Patients present with <60% of expected body weight due to prolonged deficiency of protein and calories.
- Is common in the setting of severe food deprivation, often in association with recurrent infections.

Kwashiorkor (Protein or Wet Malnutrition)

- Most commonly affects weaning children, who present with edema (Fig. 43.3) and are at 60–80% of expected body weight.
- Less often it is seen in children older than 5 years of age or adults.

- In developed countries, may occur in the setting of 'fad' diets or restrictions due to food allergy, e.g. infants given rice milk formula.
- May also be the presenting manifestation in infants with cystic fibrosis.

Vitamins

- Organic compounds that are biologically active and indispensable for normal physiologic functions.
- Serve as coenzymes of cellular metabolic processes essential for the adequate functioning and growth of tissues.
- Supplied exogenously.
- Both vitamin deficiency (hypovitaminosis) and excess (hypervitaminosis) can cause dermatologic abnormalities (see Tables 43.1 and 43.2; Figs. 43.4–43.9).
- Vitamin excess is more common with the fat-soluble vitamins (A, D, K, E).

Vitamin D

- Fat-soluble vitamin that regulates calcium and phosphate homeostasis and bone metabolism; also involved in gene regulation, cell differentiation, and the normal functioning of the innate and adaptive immune system.
- Initial step in synthetic pathway occurs in the skin (Fig. 43.10); many tissues, in addition to the kidney, have been shown to hydroxylate vitamin D precursors to produce the active form.
- Endogenous synthesis and exogenous sources (fortified foods and supplements) represent the major sources.
- Individual vitamin D requirements vary depending on an individual's age, skin pigmentation, underlying diseases, current medications, geographic location, and season of

MALNUTRITION – CLASSIFICATION AND CAUSES

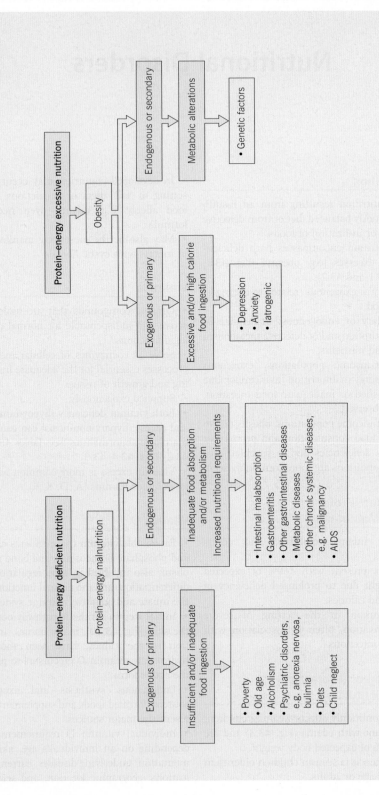

Fig. 43.1 Malnutrition. Classification and causes. *Courtesy, Ramón Ruiz-Maldonado, MD.*

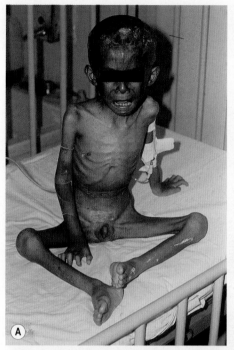

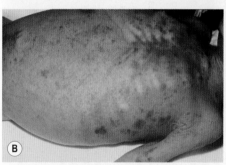

Fig. 43.2 Marasmus. A This child is emaciated and there is both hyperpigmentation and desquamation of the skin. **B** Multiple purpuric lesions are seen. *Courtesy, Ramón Ruiz-Maldonado, MD.*

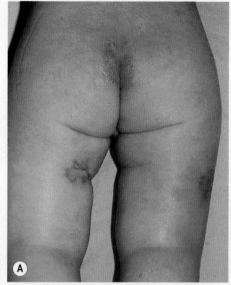

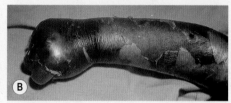

Fig. 43.3 Kwashiorkor. A This child's buttocks and legs show tense edema, scaling, and areas of erythema with desquamation. **B** This child's arm has edema and superficial epidermal necrosis with an 'enamel paint' appearance. *Courtesy, Ramón Ruiz-Maldonado, MD.*

the year; vitamin D receptor polymorphisms may play an important role in disease risk.

• Vitamin D body stores decline with age, during the winter months, and at higher latitudes.

• Phototypes V and VI require about three-fold more UVB exposure than phototypes I and II to maintain adequate vitamin D body stores.

• Oral glucocorticoids inhibit the vitamin D-dependent intestinal absorption of calcium.

• Vitamin D *insufficiency* is actually quite common and is thought to contribute to the development of osteoporosis; it has been associated with decreased immune function, bone pain, and possibly cardiovascular disease and certain malignancies.

• True vitamin D *deficiency* is more rare and results in rickets in children and osteomalacia in adults.

• Deficiency of vitamin D can result from inadequate dietary intake, fat malabsorption, lack of adequate UVB exposure, older age with its associated decrease in endogenous vitamin D production, impairment in liver and kidney hydroxylation of active vitamin D precursors, and end-organ resistance to vitamin D metabolites.

• Excess vitamin D, typically resulting from prolonged and excessive intake of vitamin D

MALNUTRITION-DEFICIENCY SYNDROMES WITH MUCOCUTANEOUS MANIFESTATIONS

Deficiency Syndrome	Mucocutaneous Features	Systemic Features
Marasmus (see Fig. 43.2) (protein-energy malnutrition)	Xerotic, thin, pale, lax, wrinkled skin Occasionally fine scaling and hyperpigmentation Follicular hyperkeratosis and folliculitis in adults Ulcerations Lanugo-like hair Slow-growing, thin hair that readily falls out Impaired nail growth and fissured nails Purpura	Emaciated appearance <60% expected body weight Loss of subcutaneous fat and muscle Suppression of growth 'Monkey facies' due to loss of buccal fat
Kwashiorkor (see Fig. 43.3) (protein or wet malnutrition)	Dyschromia. Pallor due to distention of skin and loss of pigment 'Enamel' or 'flaky paint' areas of superficial desquamation Erythema, petechiae, purpura, and ecchymoses Sparse, dry, lusterless, brittle hair with reddish tinge 'Flag sign' or alternating light- and dark-colored bands in hair, reflecting intermittent periods of malnutrition Soft and thin nails Cheilitis, xerophthalmia, vulvovaginitis	Edema At 60–80% expected body weight Moon facies Anorexia, irritability, apathy Growth retardation and failure to thrive Secondary infections Bilateral parotitis Hepatomegaly Diarrhea Decreased muscle mass
Essential fatty acids	Dry, scaly, leathery skin with underlying erythema Intertriginous erosions (Fig. 43.4) Alopecia and more lightly pigmented hair Increase in transepidermal water loss Petechiae	Growth failure Poor wound healing Impaired fertility Capillary fragility Neurologic damage Increased susceptibility to infections
Vitamin A (Fig. 43.5)	Phrynoderma manifests as follicular hyperkeratosis, favoring the extensor surfaces Xerosis Sparse, fragile hair	Ocular abnormalities, including night blindness, xerophthalmia, Bitot's spots (gray-white patches on the conjunctiva), keratomalacia, corneal scarring, and blindness Growth and mental retardation Low serum vitamin A (retinol) levels
Vitamin K	Purpura and ecchymoses	Bleeding diathesis Low plasma vitamin K levels

Vitamin C (ascorbic acid) Scurvy (Fig. 43.6)	Follicular hyperkeratosis Corkscrew hairs Perifollicular hemorrhages Petechiae and ecchymoses Gingival hypertrophy with erosions and bleeding gums	Subperiosteal hemorrhage Loose teeth Weakness, fatigue, pseudoparalysis Weight loss, diarrhea, anemia, depression, arthralgias Long-term: edema, hypotension, seizures, increased infections Low plasma vitamin C levels
Thiamine (vitamin B₁) Beriberi	Glossitis and glossodynia	Wernicke's encephalopathy* Korsakoff's syndrome** Leigh's syndrome†
Riboflavin (vitamin B₂) Oro-oculo-genital syndrome	Seborrheic dermatitis-like changes in periorificial sites (see Fig. 43.4) Painless scaly papules Indolent fissures and ulcers Depapillated glossitis Conjunctivitis and photophobia	Anemia Mental retardation Electroencephalographic changes Low serum and plasma riboflavin levels
Niacin/nicotinic acid (vitamin B₃) Pellagra (Fig. 43.7 and see Fig. 43.4) *Acquired* Dietary insufficiency, prolonged isoniazid therapy, carcinoid syndrome *Genetic* Hartnup disease	Dermatitis begins as a symmetric erythema in sun-exposed areas, that later becomes scarlet or hyperpigmented, with desquamation and crusting Casal's necklace is the photosensitive eruption forming a broad band around the neck Shellac-like appearance Perianal inflammation and erosions Painful fissures on palms and soles Mucosal membranes with edema, cheilitis, atrophic glossitis Buccal and vaginal mucosae susceptible to ulceration and secondary infection	Classic triad of diarrhea, dementia, and dermatitis Abdominal pain Achlorhydria Low plasma niacin level
Vitamin B₅ (pantothenic acid)		Fatigue Headaches Vomiting Paresthesias, dysesthesias 'Burning feet syndrome'

Table 43.1 Malnutrition-deficiency syndromes with mucocutaneous manifestations. *Continued*

Table 43.1 *Continued* **Malnutrition-deficiency syndromes with mucocutaneous manifestations.**

Deficiency Syndrome	Mucocutaneous Features	Systemic Features
Vitamin B$_6$ (pyridoxine)	Periorificial scaly, seborrheic dermatitis-like eruption (see Fig. 43.4) Glossitis Conjunctivitis Stomatitis	Anorexia, nausea, vomiting Hematologic abnormalities, e.g. sideroblastic anemia, lymphopenia, eosinophilia Neurologic changes, e.g. peripheral neuropathy, weakness, confusion, seizures Low plasma vitamin B$_6$ levels
Biotin (vitamin H; vitamin B$_7$) **Multiple carboxylase deficiency** ***Acquired*** – parenteral nutrition deficient in biotin, GI disorders, excessive intake of raw egg whites, chronic anticonvulsant therapy ***Genetic*** 1. Biotinidase deficiency (juvenile onset) 2. Holocarboxylase synthetase deficiency (neonatal onset)	Alopecia Blepharitis, conjunctivitis Secondary infections Eczematous dermatitis resembling acrodermatitis enteropathica (see Fig. 43.4)	Vomiting Metabolic acidosis Hypotonia, lethargy, seizures Developmental delay Optic atrophy, hearing loss Ataxia Low serum biotin levels
Folic acid (vitamin B$_9$)	Mucocutaneous features overlap with those seen with B$_{12}$ deficiency Cheilitis, glossitis, and mucosal erosions Gray-brown pigmentation in sun-exposed areas	Megaloblastic anemia, which may present with weakness or congestive heart failure Neuropsychiatric symptoms Low RBC folate levels
Vitamin B$_{12}$ (cyanocobalamin)	Smooth, red, painful tongue Generalized hyperpigmentation with accentuation in flexural areas, palms, soles, nails, and oral cavity Increased incidence of poliosis, vitiligo, and alopecia areata in patients with pernicious anemia	**Pernicious anemia** Megaloblastic anemia Pancytopenia If untreated can lead to degenerative neurologic disease Low serum B$_{12}$ levels[‡]
Zinc (Fig. 43.8) ***Acquired*** – low zinc in maternal milk, deficient parenteral nutrition, GI disorders, high-fiber diets, HIV infection	Acral and periorificial dermatitis with erythematous patches and plaques, secondary scaling and crust, erosions and possible vesicles and bulla (see Fig. 43.4) Chronic: may see rough, dry skin, seborrheic dermatitis-like eruptions, lichenified psoriasiform plaques, and poor wound healing	**Classic triad** of diarrhea, dermatitis, and alopecia Failure to thrive Apathy and irritability Photophobia Low serum zinc and alkaline phosphatase levels

Genetic (acrodermatitis enteropathica) – onset days–weeks after birth if bottle-fed or onset typically after weaning if breast-fed	Necrosis present in severe cases Stomatitis, glossitis, and cheilitis Pustular paronychia and nail dystrophy	
Copper **Acquired** – rare; excessive zinc intake, gastrointestinal surgeries, and malabsorptive syndromes **Genetic** (Menkes disease or kinky hair disease) (Fig. 43.9) – autosomal recessive; mutation in gene that encodes a copper transporting ATPase	**Acquired** May rarely see pigmentary dilution of hair and skin **Genetic** Onset age 2–3 months Diffuse cutaneous pigmentary dilution Characteristic facies with pudgy cheeks, cupid bow of upper lip, and horizontal eyebrows Light-colored, sparse, fragile, kinky hair Characteristic structural abnormalities of hair, e.g. pili torti, monilethrix, trichorrhexis nodosa Obligate female carriers – as a result of lyonization may see patches of swirled hypopigmentation or pili torti in Blaschko's lines	**Acquired** Anemia, neutropenia, bone marrow dysplasia Neuropathy Failure to thrive **Genetic** Failure to thrive Lethargy, hypotonia Hypothermia Seizures Mental retardation Osseous alterations Anemia Low serum copper levels
Selenium	Hypopigmentation of skin and hair White nails	Weakness Myalgias and elevated muscle enzymes Cardiomyopathy Low serum selenium levels
Iron	**May see prior to clinically evident anemia** Koilonychia, brittle nails Glossitis, angular cheilitis Pruritus Alopecia; dry, dull, and brittle hair **If significant anemia present** Skin and nail bed pallor	**Anemia and its associated symptoms** Lethargy, fatigue Decreased exercise tolerance Shortness of breath Congestive heart failure Restless legs syndrome Low serum iron and ferritin levels

*Wernicke's encephalopathy characterized by ophthalmoplegia, ataxia, confusion.

**Korsakoff's syndrome characterized by peripheral neuropathy, memory loss, confabulation.

†Leigh's syndrome characterized by subacute necrotizing encephalomyopathy; anorexia, weakness, constipation; congestive heart failure; low serum or plasma thiamine levels.

‡Elevated serum homocysteine and methylmalonic acid levels are more reliable indicators of B_{12} deficiency and are useful to obtain if B_{12} deficiency is strongly suspected but serum levels of B_{12} are low-normal.

MALNUTRITION-EXCESS SYNDROMES WITH MUCOCUTANEOUS MANIFESTATIONS

Excess Syndrome	Mucocutaneous Features	Systemic Features
Obesity	Plantar hyperkeratosis Acanthosis nigricans Acrochordons Striae distensae Intertrigo Frictional hyperpigmentation Hyperhidrosis Stasis dermatitis Leg ulcers, mostly venous > arterial Lipodermatosclerosis, including the pannus Stasis mucinosis	Body mass index >30 Hypertension Diabetes and insulin resistance Gastroesophageal reflux disease Atherosclerotic cardiovascular disease Steatorrhea
Vitamin A	Mucocutaneous findings similar to patients on oral retinoids Xerotic, rough, pruritic, and scaly skin Xerotic cheilitis Diffuse alopecia	Anorexia, weight loss, lethargy Elevated liver enzymes Painful swellings in limbs due to bony changes Radiographic bone changes, e.g. skeletal hyperostosis, extraspinal tendon and ligament calcification
Beta carotene (the natural pro-vitamin of vitamin A) **Carotenemia**	**Carotenoderma** (Fig. 43.11) – orange-yellow skin pigmentation primarily in sebaceous gland-rich areas (forehead, nasolabial fold) and in areas with a thicker stratum corneum (palms, soles) Differentiated from jaundice, which has prominent yellow discoloration of the sclerae and mucosae	
Copper **Acquired** – rare **Genetic** (Wilson's disease) – autosomal recessive; mutation in gene that encodes a copper transporting P-type ATPase	**Genetic** **Kayser–Fleischer** corneal rings	**Genetic** Liver disease and cirrhosis Dysarthria, dyspraxia, ataxia, and parkinsonian-like extrapyramidal signs
Iron **Acquired** – numerous blood transfusions; excess intake **Genetic** (type I hemochromatosis) – autosomal recessive; mutation in gene (*HFE*) that regulates absorption of iron; two most common mutations of *HFE* gene are C282Y and H63D	Generalized hyperpigmentation (bronzing)	Chronic fatigue Diabetes Liver disease, cirrhosis Arthritis Cardiac disease Impotence Hypothyroidism

Table 43.2 Malnutrition-excess syndromes with mucocutaneous manifestations.

supplements, can present with anorexia, vomiting, diarrhea, headaches, hypercalcemia, hypercalciuria, muscle weakness, and bone demineralization.

• No specific cutaneous features have been described with vitamin D deficiency or excess.

• The best indicator of vitamin D stores is a measurement of the *serum 25-OH vitamin*

D_3 *level*, and this laboratory value is frequently used to guide individual vitamin D requirements.

• Guidelines for vitamin D supplementation have been in flux, but oral supplementation is generally recommended for exclusively breast-fed infants, children who drink less than a liter of fortified milk per day, pregnant

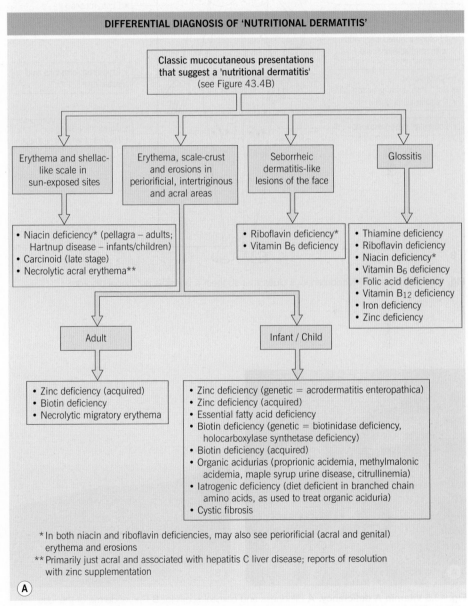

DIFFERENTIAL DIAGNOSIS OF 'NUTRITIONAL DERMATITIS'

Classic mucocutaneous presentations that suggest a 'nutritional dermatitis' (see Figure 43.4B)

Erythema and shellac-like scale in sun-exposed sites
• Niacin deficiency* (pellagra – adults; Hartnup disease – infants/children)
• Carcinoid (late stage)
• Necrolytic acral erythema**

Erythema, scale-crust and erosions in periorificial, intertriginous and acral areas

Seborrheic dermatitis-like lesions of the face
• Riboflavin deficiency*
• Vitamin B$_6$ deficiency

Glossitis
• Thiamine deficiency
• Riboflavin deficiency
• Niacin deficiency*
• Vitamin B$_6$ deficiency
• Folic acid deficiency
• Vitamin B$_{12}$ deficiency
• Iron deficiency
• Zinc deficiency

Adult
• Zinc deficiency (acquired)
• Biotin deficiency
• Necrolytic migratory erythema

Infant / Child
• Zinc deficiency (genetic = acrodermatitis enteropathica)
• Zinc deficiency (acquired)
• Essential fatty acid deficiency
• Biotin deficiency (genetic = biotinidase deficiency, holocarboxylase synthetase deficiency)
• Biotin deficiency (acquired)
• Organic acidurias (proprionic acidemia, methylmalonic acidemia, maple syrup urine disease, citrullinemia)
• Iatrogenic deficiency (diet deficient in branched chain amino acids, as used to treat organic aciduria)
• Cystic fibrosis

* In both niacin and riboflavin deficiencies, may also see periorificial (acral and genital) erythema and erosions
** Primarily just acral and associated with hepatitis C liver disease; reports of resolution with zinc supplementation

(A)

Fig. 43.4 Clinical approach to the patient with a presumed nutritional disorder. A Differential diagnosis of 'nutritional dermatitis.' *Continued*

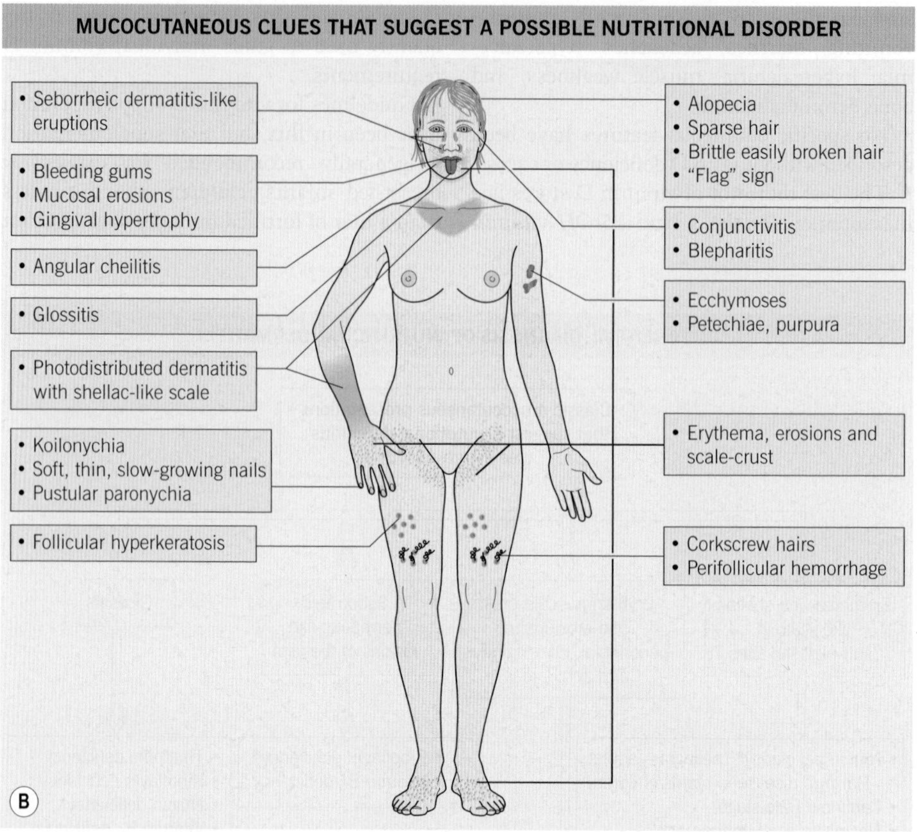

MUCOCUTANEOUS CLUES THAT SUGGEST A POSSIBLE NUTRITIONAL DISORDER

- Seborrheic dermatitis-like eruptions

- Bleeding gums
- Mucosal erosions
- Gingival hypertrophy

- Angular cheilitis

- Glossitis

- Photodistributed dermatitis with shellac-like scale

- Koilonychia
- Soft, thin, slow-growing nails
- Pustular paronychia

- Follicular hyperkeratosis

- Alopecia
- Sparse hair
- Brittle easily broken hair
- "Flag" sign

- Conjunctivitis
- Blepharitis

- Ecchymoses
- Petechiae, purpura

- Erythema, erosions and scale-crust

- Corkscrew hairs
- Perifollicular hemorrhage

B

Fig. 43.4 *Continued* **B** Mucocutaneous clues that suggest a possible nutritional disorder.

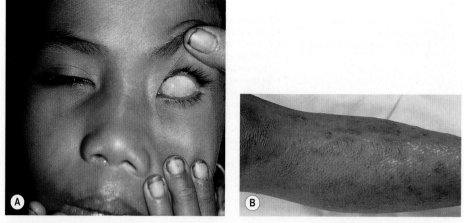

Fig. 43.5 Vitamin A deficiency. A Blindness and corneal scarring. **B** Phrynoderma of the legs. Multiple clusters of follicular papules with central keratotic plugs. *A, Courtesy, Peter Erhnstrom, MD; B, Courtesy, Chad M. Hivnor, MD.*

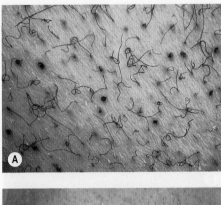

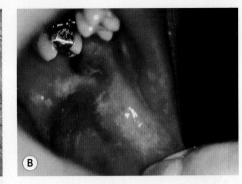

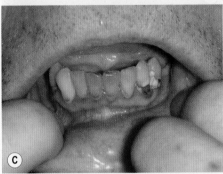

Fig. 43.6 Scurvy. A Corkscrew hairs and perifollicular hemorrhage on the lower extremities. **B** Hemorrhage beneath the buccal mucosa. **C** Gingival hypertrophy and infection, with loosened teeth. *C, Courtesy, Jeffrey Callen, MD.*

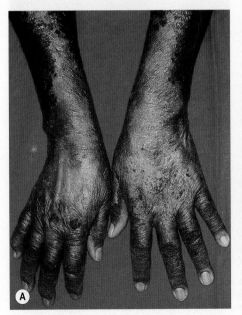

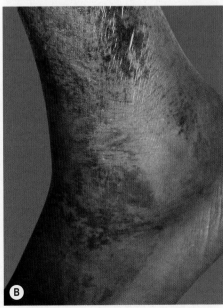

Fig. 43.7 Pellagra. A Hyperpigmentation with desquamation of the dorsal aspects of the hands and forearms. **B** Hyperpigmented desquamation of the distal lower extremity. Note the shiny shellac-like appearance on the lateral ankle.

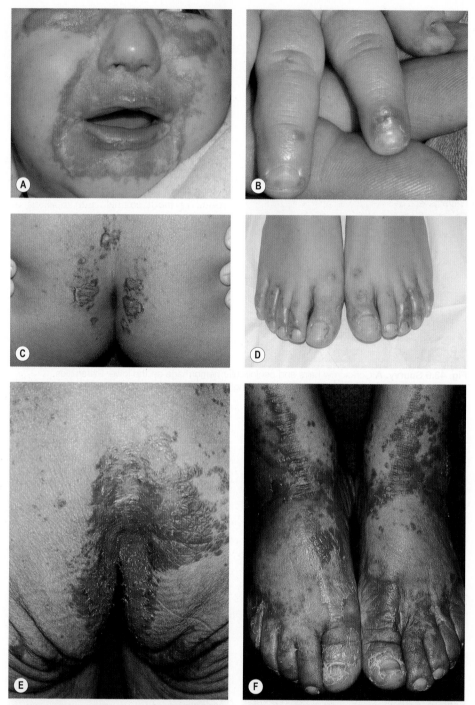

Fig. 43.8 Zinc deficiency. Genetic (acrodermatitis enteropathica) **(A–D)** and acquired **(E, F)** forms. Both have erythema with erosions **(A, E)** as well as crusting **(C, E, F)** and desquamation **(A, D–F)**. Lesions favor the acral and periorificial sites, and pustular paronychia may also be seen **(B)**. Acrodermatitis enteropathica most often presents in infancy **(A, B)**, but rarely, it is not diagnosed until later childhood, as in the case of this 11-year-old boy **(C, D)**. *A–D, courtesy, Julie V. Schaffer, MD.*

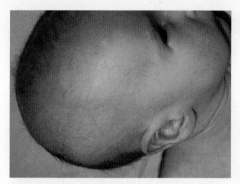

Fig. 43.9 Menkes disease. This child has the characteristic pale skin and sparse kinky hair. *Courtesy, Ramón Ruiz-Maldonado, MD.*

parenteral nutrition without lipid supplementation and with overly aggressive low-fat diets.

Anorexia/Bulimia

• Eating disorders that may lead to nutritional deficiencies.

• Associated cutaneous findings include xerosis, telogen effluvium, lanugo-like hair, brittle nails, carotenoderma, cheilitis, acrocyanosis, and worsening of chilblains.

• In addition, patients with bulimia may develop parotid and salivary gland swelling, erosion of tooth enamel, and abrasions or calluses on the dorsal fingers and knuckles (Russell's sign).

Carotenoderma

• Orange-yellow skin pigmentation (Fig. 43.11) that develops when carotene levels are 3–4 times normal (carotenemia).

• Can result from the high intake of carotenoid-rich foods (carrots) or the inability to convert ingested beta-carotene into vitamin A (some patients with diabetes, hypothyroidism, or anorexia nervosa).

• An excess intake of lycopene-rich foods (tomato, papaya) may induce lycopenemia and skin findings similar to carotenoderma.

Obesity

• Defined as a body mass index (BMI) > 30.

• Predisposing genetic syndromes that result in an earlier, childhood onset include Prader–Willi, Bardet–Biedl, Alström, and Wilson–Turner syndromes.

• Predisposing endocrine conditions include Cushing's disease, Cushing's syndrome, polycystic ovarian syndrome, and insulin resistance.

• Acquired obesity is at epidemic levels, especially in high-income populations.

• The cutaneous manifestations of obesity are outlined in Table 43.2.

• May have associated metabolic syndrome (see Chapter 45).

women, the elderly, most adults for the prevention of osteoporosis, and individuals on long-term oral glucocorticoids.

• Dermatologists recommend oral vitamin D supplementation over the practice of getting more UVB exposure to maintain adequate vitamin D stores.

Minerals

• Inorganic elements that constitute about 3–4% of body weight.

• Located primarily in the bones and muscle.

• Some are trace elements essential for human nutrition.

• The trace elements of dermatologic importance are zinc, copper, selenium, and iron (see Tables 43.1 and 43.2).

Essential Fatty Acids (EFAs)

• Unsaturated fatty acids that the body needs but cannot synthesize, and therefore must be obtained from the diet.

• The three major EFAs are linoleic, linolenic, and arachidonic acids.

• In most patients, EFA deficiency is seen along with other nutritional deficiencies.

• Isolated deficiencies of EFAs are uncommon but can be seen in patients receiving

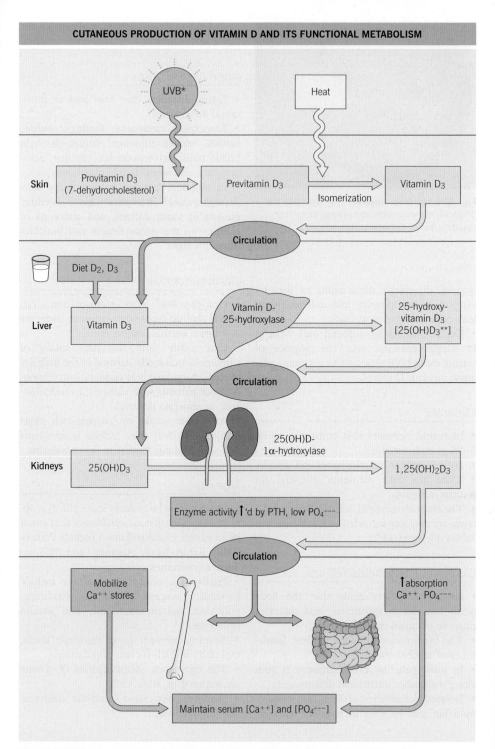

Fig. 43.10 Cutaneous production of vitamin D and its functional metabolism. *See next page for figure legend.*

Fig. 43.10 Cutaneous production of vitamin D and its functional metabolism. During exposure to ultraviolet B radiation, 7-dehydrocholesterol within the skin is converted to previtamin D_3, which is then immediately converted to vitamin D_3 in a heat-dependent process. Of note, the heat from excessive sunlight exposure can degrade previtamin D_3 and vitamin D_3 into inactive photoproducts. Both forms of vitamin D (D_3 and D_2) are biologically inactive and they require activation in the liver and then the kidney. After binding to carrier proteins, vitamin D is transported to the liver, where it is enzymatically hydroxylated to 25-hydroxyvitamin D [25(OH)D], the major circulating form of vitamin D. 25-Hydroxyvitamin D is then converted into its active form, 1,25-dihydroxyvitamin D [1,25(OH)$_2$D], within the kidney by the enzyme 1α-hydroxylase. Of interest, this final hydroxylation step can also occur in keratinocytes when the enzyme CYP27B1 is upregulated in response to wounding or by Toll-like receptor (TLR) activation from microbial-derived ligands. Serum levels of phosphate, calcium, and fibroblast growth factor 23 can either increase or decrease renal production of 1,25(OH)$_2$D. 1,25(OH)$_2$D decreases its own synthesis via feedback inhibition and decreases the synthesis and secretion of parathyroid hormone by the parathyroid glands. 1,25(OH)$_2$D also enhances intestinal calcium absorption in the small intestine by interacting with the vitamin D receptor–retinoic acid X receptor complex (VDR-RXR) to enhance the expression of the epithelial calcium channel and calbindin-D 9K, a calcium-binding protein. In addition, 1,25(OH)$_2$D is recognized by its receptor in osteoblasts, leading to a series of events that maintain calcium and phosphorus levels in the blood which in turn promotes mineralization of the skeleton. *Most effective wavelength = 300 ± 5 nm. **Measurement of this form most commonly done to assess vitamin D status.

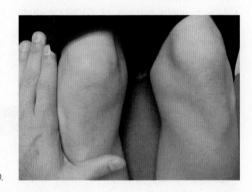

Fig. 43.11 Carotenoderma. Patient's legs are noticeably orange when compared to photographer's hand. *Courtesy, Chad M. Hivnor, MD.*

For further information see Ch. 51. From *Dermatology, Third Edition.*

44 | Graft-Versus-Host Disease

- Multiorgan disorder that most commonly results from the transfer of donor hematopoietic stem cells into a recipient via an allogeneic hematopoietic stem cell transplant (HSCT).
- Despite advances in HSCT procedures and post-transplantation immunosuppressive therapy, more than half of HSCT recipients develop chronic graft-versus-host disease (GVHD), which remains a major cause of morbidity and mortality.
- Table 44.1 lists risk factors for GVHD in HSCT recipients.
- Less frequent settings of GVHD include transfusion of non-irradiated blood products to an immunocompromised patient, maternal–fetal transmission to an immunodeficient neonate, and solid organ transplantation.

- Divided into acute and chronic forms based on clinical features.
- Pathogenesis of acute GVHD occurs in three steps: (1) HSCT conditioning regimen leads to epithelial cell injury and activation of *host* antigen presenting cells; (2) activation of *donor* T cells; (3) tissue destruction by cytotoxic T cells, natural killer cells, and soluble factors (e.g. tumor necrosis factor-α [TNF-α]).
- Chronic GVHD shares features (e.g. autoantibody production, cutaneous sclerosis) with autoimmune connective tissue diseases.
- Histologically, acute GVHD and epidermal involvement in chronic GVHD are characterized by variable degrees of keratinocyte necrosis (often accentuated in appendages), vacuolar degeneration of the basal layer, and a band-like lymphocytic infiltrate.

RISK FACTORS ASSOCIATED WITH THE DEVELOPMENT OF GRAFT-VERSUS-HOST DISEASE (GVHD)
Donor
HLA incompatibility with recipient Unrelated to recipient Female (especially multiparous) with male recipient Older age
Recipient
Age (elderly > middle aged > pediatric)
Stem Cell Source
Peripheral blood > bone marrow > cord blood T-cell replete graft
Transplantation Protocol
More intense (myeloablative) conditioning regimen (increases risk of acute GVHD) Less aggressive administration of prophylactic immunosuppressive agents
Clinical Course
Reduction of immunosuppression ± donor lymphocyte infusions if recurrence of malignancy Reduction of immunosuppression if decrease in donor chimerism
HLA, human leukocyte antigen.

Table 44.1 Risk factors associated with the development of graft-versus-host disease (GVHD).

Acute GVHD

• Most often arises 4–6 weeks after HSCT with traditional regimens.

• Persistent, recurrent, and late-onset variants of acute GVHD can occur during a time period (>100 days post-transplant) traditionally reserved for chronic GVHD, especially following interventions such as tapering of immunosuppression and donor lymphocyte infusions.

• Typically presents as a morbilliform exanthem, often with perifollicular accentuation.

• Initial predilection for acral sites (e.g. dorsal hands and feet, palms, soles, ears), forearms, and upper trunk.

• Clinical staging is based on the proportion of the cutaneous surface involved: Stage 1, <25%; Stage 2, 25–50%; and Stage 3, >50%. Stage 4 represents erythroderma with bullae/ epidermal detachment resembling toxic epidermal necrolysis (Fig. 44.1).

• Mucosal surfaces (including the conjunctiva), the gastrointestinal tract (nausea, diarrhea, abdominal pain), and the liver (transaminitis, cholestasis) are frequently affected.

• Histologic evaluation is helpful but not necessarily diagnostic, and clinicopathologic correlation is essential.

• **DDx:** drug eruption, viral exanthem, engraftment syndrome (nonspecific erythematous eruption, fever, pulmonary edema; onset day 10–14 post transplant), toxic erythema of chemotherapy (especially with palmoplantar or intertriginous involvement).

• **Rx:** topical CS if limited cutaneous involvement only; most patients require systemic CS, which are typically added to ongoing prophylactic treatment with a systemic calcineurin inhibitor; second-line treatments include other immunosuppressive agents (e.g. mycophenolate mofetil [MMF], TNF-α inhibitors).

Chronic GVHD

• Can occur as a continuation of acute GVHD, as a recurrence following a GVHD-free interval, or without a history of acute GVHD.

• Skin and mucosal involvement are extremely common and highly variable in their presentations (Table 44.2; Fig. 44.2A), and almost any organ system can be affected (Fig. 44.2B).

• Reticulate pink to violet papules with scale (*lichen planus-like*) favoring the dorsal hands and feet, forearms, and trunk represent one characteristic manifestation (Fig. 44.3A).

• The spectrum of sclerotic involvement includes.

  – *Lichen sclerosus-like* shiny, wrinkled, gray-white plaques, ± follicular plugging, favoring the upper trunk (Fig. 44.3B,C).

  – Localized or widespread *morphea-like* indurated, hyperpigmented to skin-colored plaques favoring the lower trunk (Fig. 44.3D).

  – *Eosinophilic fasciitis-like* presentations with acute edema and pain evolving into areas of firm skin with subcutaneous rippling ('pseudo-cellulite'; Fig. 44.3F) and linear depressions following a vein or between muscle groups (groove sign); favors the extremities (sparing the hands and feet) and may result in joint contractures.

• Often affects the nails and the oral and genital mucosa (Fig. 44.4; see Table 44.2).

• Other frequent sites of involvement include the eyes (keratoconjunctivitis sicca, blepharitis), salivary glands (sicca syndrome), esophagus (strictures), liver, pancreas (exocrine insufficiency), and lungs (bronchiolitis obliterans).

• **DDx:** drug eruption (e.g. lichenoid, photosensitive), autoimmune connective tissue diseases (e.g. lupus erythematosus, morphea), papulosquamous disorders.

• **Rx:** skin-directed with topical CS or calcineurin inhibitors (for superficial disease) or phototherapy (narrowband UVB, UVA1, PUVA); components of systemic combination therapy may include CS, calcineurin inhibitors, imatinib, acitretin, and rituximab; physical therapy (for joint mobility), sun protection, and regular skin examinations, especially if prolonged immunosuppression.

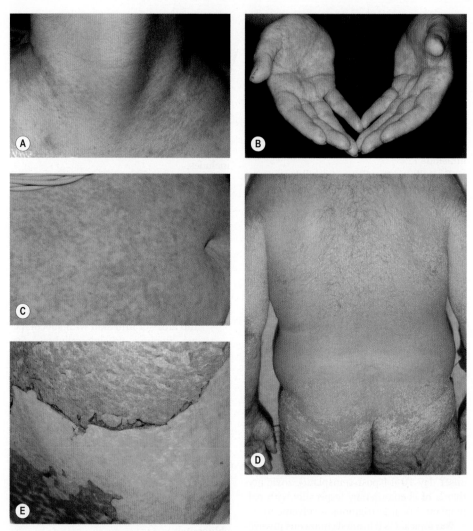

Fig. 44.1 Clinical spectrum of acute cutaneous graft-versus-host disease. A *Stage 1* – discrete and coalescing small pink papules on the upper chest and neck of a woman 6 weeks following allogeneic bone marrow transplant. **B, C** *Stage 2* – pink macules and papules of the palms that are becoming confluent 14 weeks post allogeneic bone marrow transplant and pink-violet macules and minimally elevated papules on the abdomen in a liver transplant recipient. **D** *Stage 3* – diffuse erythema with desquamation, but without bullae formation. **E** *Stage 4* – coalescence of bullae plus epidermal necrosis leading to large areas of denudation in a patient who had received an allogeneic bone marrow transplant; note the resemblance to toxic epidermal necrolysis. *A, D, Courtesy, Edward Cowen, MD; B, Courtesy, Dennis Cooper, MD; C, Courtesy, Julie V. Schaffer, MD.*

MUCOCUTANEOUS MANIFESTATIONS OF CHRONIC GRAFT-VERSUS-HOST DISEASE (GVHD)

Skin and Subcutaneous Tissues

Inflammatory manifestations
- **Lichen planus-like (lichenoid)**
- Photosensitive eruptions resembling lupus erythematosus or dermatomyositis
- Eczematous, psoriasiform, or panniculitis

Sclerotic manifestations
- **Lichen sclerosus-like**
- **Morphea-like (morpheaform)**
- **Fasciitis[†]**
- **Scleroderma-like (sclerodermoid)**
- Nodular fibromas

Skin breakdown*
- Bullae and ulcerations

Hyperkeratotic** and/or adnexal manifestations
- Eczema craquelé, keratosis pilaris-like, ichthyosiform
- Alopecia (often scarring)
- Impaired sweating

Vascular manifestations
- **Poikiloderma**
- Angiomatous papules

Pigmentary alterations
- Hypo- or depigmentation (e.g. vitiligo-like leukoderma, leukotrichia)
- Hyperpigmentation (e.g. leopard-like)

Nail changes
- Brittleness, longitudinal ridging/splitting, onycholysis
- Pterygium (dorsal)

Mucosa

Oral manifestations
- **Lichen planus-like** (e.g. lacy white plaques)
- **Keratotic plaques**
- Mucositis, gingivitis, erosions, ulcerations, pseudomembranes
- **Restriction of oral opening from sclerosis**
- Xerostomia

Genital manifestations
- **Lichen planus-like**
- Erosions, fissures (especially of the vulva)
- **Scarring, vaginal stenosis**

*Often overlying areas of cutaneous sclerosis.
[†]Magnetic resonance imaging can help to establish the diagnosis.
**May be related to destruction of eccrine glands.
Based on Filipovich AH, Weisdorf P, Pavletic S, et al. National Institutes of Health Consensus Development Project on Criteria for Clinical Trials in Chronic Graft-versus-Host Disease: I. Diagnosis and Staging Working Group report. Biol. Blood Marrow Transplant. 2005;11:945–956. For manifestations in other organs (including the eye), see this reference as well as the text.

Table 44.2 Mucocutaneous manifestations of chronic graft-versus-host disease (GVHD). Diagnostic features are in bold; other signs and symptoms listed are not considered sufficient to establish a diagnosis of chronic GVHD without further testing (e.g. histologic assessment) or evidence of other organ system involvement.

MANIFESTATIONS OF CHRONIC GRAFT-VERSUS-HOST DISEASE

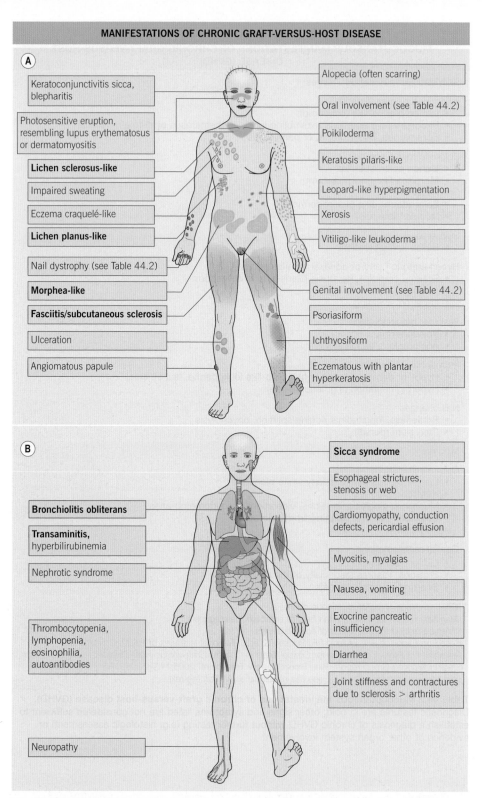

A

Keratoconjunctivitis sicca, blepharitis

Photosensitive eruption, resembling lupus erythematosus or dermatomyositis

Lichen sclerosus-like

Impaired sweating

Eczema craquelé-like

Lichen planus-like

Nail dystrophy (see Table 44.2)

Morphea-like

Fasciitis/subcutaneous sclerosis

Ulceration

Angiomatous papule

Alopecia (often scarring)

Oral involvement (see Table 44.2)

Poikiloderma

Keratosis pilaris-like

Leopard-like hyperpigmentation

Xerosis

Vitiligo-like leukoderma

Genital involvement (see Table 44.2)

Psoriasiform

Ichthyosiform

Eczematous with plantar hyperkeratosis

B

Bronchiolitis obliterans

Transaminitis, hyperbilirubinemia

Nephrotic syndrome

Thrombocytopenia, lymphopenia, eosinophilia, autoantibodies

Neuropathy

Sicca syndrome

Esophageal strictures, stenosis or web

Cardiomyopathy, conduction defects, pericardial effusion

Myositis, myalgias

Nausea, vomiting

Exocrine pancreatic insufficiency

Diarrhea

Joint stiffness and contractures due to sclerosis > arthritis

Fig. 44.2 Manifestations of chronic graft-versus-host disease. A Mucocutaneous findings. Lichen sclerosus-like lesions may be prominent on the back. Highly characteristic manifestations are in bold. **B** Internal involvement. The most common manifestations are in bold.

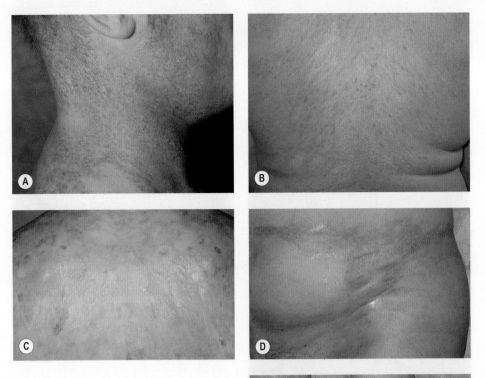

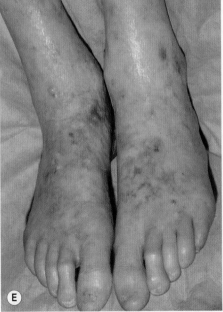

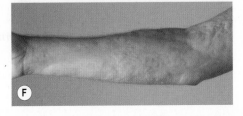

Fig. 44.3 Clinical spectrum of chronic cutaneous graft-versus-host disease.
A Lichen planus-like – thin pink-violet papules and plaques with scale, admixed with post-inflammatory hyperpigmentation. **B** Lichen sclerosus-like (early) – multiple gray-white thin plaques with obvious wrinkling are present on the mid back. **C** Lichen sclerosus-like (late) – thicker shiny white plaques on the upper back admixed with erosions. **D** Morphea-like (morpheaform) – shiny, hyperpigmented, sclerotic plaque extending circumferentially around the beltline and into the inguinal area. **E** Scleroderma-like (sclerodermoid) – the skin is shiny and bound-down with dyspigmentation, hair loss, and multiple erosions; nail loss, small angiomatous nodules, and marked reduction in range of motion of the ankles are also present. **F** Eosinophilic fasciitis-like – a rippled appearance and irregular nodular texture to the skin is indicative of involvement of subcutaneous tissues; extension of the elbow is limited. Especially in the earlier, more edematous phase, the presence of hypereosinophilia is a clue to the diagnosis. *A, D-F, Courtesy, Edward Cowen, MD; B, Courtesy, Dennis Cooper, MD; C, Courtesy, Joyce Rico, MD.*

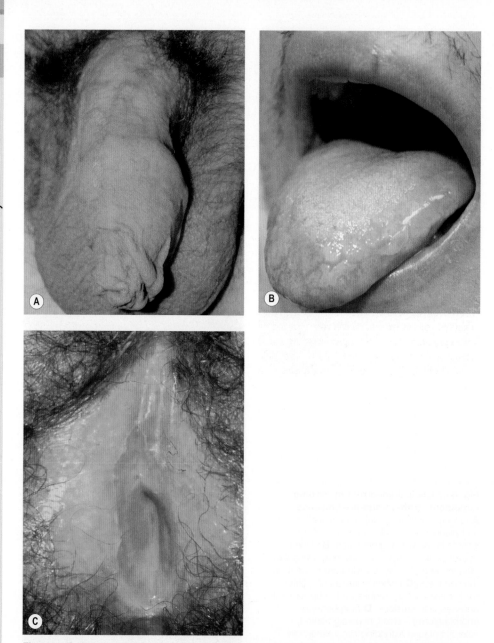

Fig. 44.4 Orogenital involvement in chronic cutaneous graft-versus-host disease. A, B Lichen planus-like – flat-topped violet papules on the penis and several ulcers on the tongue, also with a lacy white pattern on the upper vermilion lip and the distal dorsal tongue. **C** Severe erosive disease of the vulva, with nearly total resorption of the labia minora and agglutination of the lips of the clitoral hood. The vulvar introitus is also markedly narrowed. *A, C, Courtesy, Edward Cowen, MD. B, Courtesy, Jean L. Bolognia, MD.*

For further information see Ch. 52. From *Dermatology, Third Edition.*

Skin Signs of Systemic Disease

45

Introduction

• Recognizing the skin signs of systemic disease is an important aspect of dermatology; however, the vast number of cutaneous manifestations, combined with the infrequency with which each sign is encountered, can be daunting.

• The approach in this chapter is to provide several examples of the most commonly observed or most characteristic cutaneous findings, based on the organ system most often involved – for example, papulonodules of sarcoidosis (lung), diffuse induration of systemic sclerosis (kidney), and melanotic macules of Peutz–Jeghers syndrome (gastrointestinal tract).

• With the exception of endocrinologic disorders and paraneoplastic dermatoses, most of these skin signs have been discussed in other chapters – for example, pyoderma gangrenosum in Chapter 21, telangiectasias of hereditary hemorrhagic telangiectasia (Osler-Weber-Rendu syndrome) in Chapter 87, and sebaceous neoplasms of Muir–Torre syndrome in Chapters 52 and 91.

Pulmonary Disease and the Skin

• Table 45.1 and Fig. 45.1.

Cardiac Disease and the Skin

• Table 45.2 and Fig. 45.2.

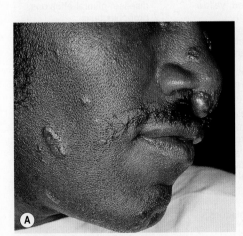

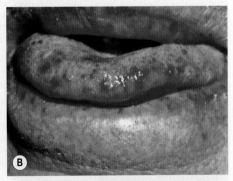

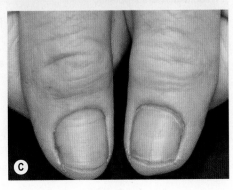

Fig. 45.1 Skin signs of pulmonary disease.
A Periorificial and facial papules of sarcoidosis. The presence of lesions on the nasal rim is often associated with granulomatous inflammation of the upper respiratory tract. **B** Hereditary hemorrhagic telangiectasia. Multiple small bright red macules and papules on the tongue and lips. **C** Yellow nail syndrome. *A, B, Courtesy, Jeffrey P. Callen, MD; C, Courtesy, Karynne O. Duncan, MD.*

EXAMPLES OF SKIN SIGNS OF PULMONARY DISEASE		
Disorder	**Cutaneous Findings**	**Pulmonary Disease**
Genetic		
Birt–Hogg–Dubé syndrome (see Chapter 91)	• Classic triad of fibrofolliculomas, trichodiscomas, and acrochordons	• Lung cysts, spontaneous pneumothoraces
Hereditary hemorrhagic telangiectasia (HHT) (see Chapter 87)	• Mucosal, facial, and acral telangiectatic macules and papules (Fig. 45.1B)	• Pulmonary AVMs
Inflammatory/Autoimmune		
Sarcoidosis (see Chapter 78)	• Acute: erythema nodosum • Chronic: papules, nodules (Fig. 45.1A), plaques, lupus pernio, lesions in scars and tattoos; acquired ichthyosis	• Acute: bilateral hilar lymphadenopathy • Chronic: fibrosis due to granulomatous inflammation
Wegener's granulomatosis (granulomatosis with polyangiitis; see Chapter 19)	• Vasculitic lesions (e.g. palpable purpura or nodules), cutaneous granulomas, pyoderma gangrenosum-like ulcers, 'strawberry gums' (see Fig. 59.16), oral ulcers (see Fig. 19.10B)	• Cavitating pulmonary nodules, vasculitis
Churg–Strauss syndrome (see Chapter 19)	• Palpable purpura, urticarial plaques, nodules, crusted papules of the elbows	• Asthma
Yellow nail syndrome (Fig. 45.1C)	• Thickened, slow-growing, excessively curved, yellow-to-green nails with onycholysis, transverse ridging, onychomadesis, and absent cuticles and lunulae	• Bronchopulmonary disease: pleural effusions, bronchiectasis • Lymphedema, sinusitis
Dermatomyositis (see Chapter 34)	• Gottron's papules, heliotrope, photodistributed poikiloderma (see Fig. 34.4)	• ILD, aspiration pneumonitis, hypoventilation
Systemic sclerosis (see Chapter 35)	• DcSSc: Raynaud's disease (sudden onset); more widespread sclerosis • LcSSc: Raynaud's disease (preceding long duration); limited, acrofacial sclerosis	• DcSSc: ILD > PAH • LcSSc: PAH > ILD (see Fig. 35.2)
Neoplastic/Paraneoplastic		
Lymphomatoid granulomatosis (see Chapter 99)	• Papulonodules, plaques, ulcers	• Angiocentric, angiodestructive infiltrate of atypical lymphocytes
Paraneoplastic pemphigus (see Chapter 23)	• See Table 45.9 and Fig. 23.8	• Bronchiolitis obliterans
Infectious		
Tuberculosis (see Chapter 62)	• Lupus vulgaris, scrofuloderma, orificial	• Apical infiltrates, cavitating infiltrates; nonproductive or productive cough

Table 45.1 Examples of skin signs of pulmonary disease. *Continued*

Table 45.1 *Continued* **Examples of skin signs of pulmonary disease.**

Disorder	Cutaneous Findings	Pulmonary Disease
Blastomycosis* (see Chapter 64)	• Verrucous or ulcerated plaques or nodules	• Patchy infiltrates or normal chest x-ray
Cryptococcosis (see Chapter 64)	• Variable cutaneous findings, from papulonodules and plaques to molluscum contagiosum-like lesions and cellulitis	• Varies from asymptomatic infection to severe pneumonia and acute respiratory distress syndrome
Aspergillosis (see Chapter 64)	• Cutaneous emboli: necrotic papules and plaques, often with ulceration and rapidly progressive	• In those with disseminated cutaneous emboli, cavitating infiltrates and nodules
Varicella (see Chapter 67)	• Lesions in various stages of development, including papules, papulovesicles, pustules, and hemorrhagic crusts	• Pulmonary involvement correlates with severity of skin involvement. Interstitial infiltrates or patchy airway disease leads to cough and dyspnea.
Other		
Toxic epidermal necrolysis (TEN) (see Chapter 16)	• Widespread necrosis and detachment	• Acute respiratory distress syndrome

Primary pulmonary infection also occurs in other systemic mycoses due to dimorphic pathogens, including coccidioidomycosis, histoplasmosis, and paracoccidioidomycosis.
AVM, arteriovenous malformation; DcSSc, diffuse cutaneous systemic sclerosis; LcSSc, limited cutaneous systemic sclerosis; ILD, interstitial lung disease; PAH, pulmonary arterial hypertension.

EXAMPLES OF SKIN SIGNS OF CARDIAC DISEASE	
Disorder	**Cardiac Disease**
Genetic	
Cardiofaciocutaneous syndrome	• Pulmonic stenosis, atrial septal defects, hypertrophic cardiomyopathy
Heritable connective tissue diseases: cutis laxa, Ehlers–Danlos syndrome (EDS), pseudoxanthoma elasticum, Marfan syndrome (see Chapter 80); cardiac disease varies from mitral valve prolapse to arterial/aortic aneurysms, dissection, and rupture	
Carney complex (NAME and LAMB syndromes) (see Chapter 92)	• Atrial myxomas
Tuberous sclerosis complex (TSC) (see Chapter 50)	• Cardiac rhabdomyomas, arrhythmias
Inflammatory/Autoimmune	
Psoriasis (see Chapter 6)	• Increased risk of cardiovascular disease
Systemic lupus erythematosus (see Chapter 33)	• Pericarditis, verrucous endocarditis (Libman–Sacks), coronary artery disease

Table 45.2 Examples of skin signs of cardiac disease. The cutaneous features of these disorders are discussed in the chapters cited. Cardiofaciocutaneous syndrome is characterized by generalized ichthyosis-like scaling, keratosis pilaris, café-au-lait macules, sparse curly hair, and developmental delay. *Continued*

Table 45.2 *Continued* **Examples of skin signs of cardiac disease.** The cutaneous features of these disorders are discussed in the chapters cited.

Disorder	Cardiac Disease
Neonatal lupus erythematosus (see Chapter 33)	• Congenital heart block
Rheumatic fever (see Chapter 15)	• Pancarditis in the acute phase; late manifestations include mitral and/or aortic valve dysfunction
Kawasaki disease (mucocutaneous lymph node syndrome) (see Chapter 3)	• Coronary arteritis, coronary artery aneurysms
Other	
Hyperlipidemia (see Chapter 77; Fig. 45.2)	• Coronary artery disease
Primary systemic amyloidosis (AL) (see Chapter 39)	• Restrictive cardiomyopathy, conduction disturbances
Endocarditis – bacterial or fungal (see Chapters 61 and 64)	• Vegetations and dysfunction of the valves
Exfoliative erythroderma (see Chapter 8)	• High-output cardiac failure

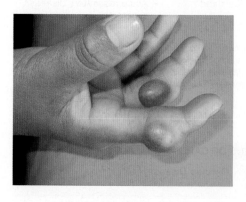

Fig. 45.2 Skin signs of cardiac disease. Multiple tendinous xanthomas in a patient with familial hypercholesterolemia. *Courtesy, Dermatology Department, Hospital Regional Honorio Delgado Espinoza de Arequipa Perú.*

Gastrointestinal Disease and the Skin

• Tables 45.3–45.5 and Figs. 45.3 and 45.4.

Liver Disease and the Skin

• Table 45.6 and Fig. 45.5.

Renal Disease and the Skin

• Table 45.7.

Skin Signs of Internal Malignancy

• Tables 45.8 and 45.9 and Figs. 45.6 and 45.7.

Skin Signs of Endocrine Disorders and Metabolic Disease

• Tables 45.10–45.14 and Figs. 45.8–45.12.

EXAMPLES OF SKIN SIGNS OF GASTROINTESTINAL (GI) DISEASE	
Disorder	**Gastrointestinal Disease/Other**
Genetic	
Hereditary hemorrhagic telangiectasia (HHT) (see Chapter 87; Table 45.1)	• Recurrent hemorrhage in the upper GI tract
Blue rubber bleb nevus syndrome (see Chapter 85; Fig. 45.3A)	• GI vascular malformations
Pseudoxanthoma elasticum (see Chapter 80; Table 45.2)	• Upper or lower GI hemorrhage
Ehlers–Danlos syndrome, vascular type (type IV) (see Chapter 80; Table 45.2)	• GI hemorrhage due to arterial rupture, intestinal perforation
Gardner syndrome (see Chapters 90, 91, and 95)	• Hemorrhage from adenomatous colonic polyps. Adenocarcinoma of the colon is universal if the colon is not removed • Congenital hypertrophy of the retinal pigment epithelium (CHRPE)
Peutz–Jeghers syndrome (see Chapter 92; Fig. 45.3B)	• Hamartomatous polyps throughout the GI tract. Intussusception or hemorrhage may occur
Cowden disease (multiple hamartoma syndrome; PTEN hamartoma syndrome) (see Chapters 52 and 91; Fig. 45.3C)	• Hamartomatous polyps throughout the GI tract. Bleeding is rare
Muir–Torre syndrome (see Chapter 91)	• Intestinal polyps in ≥25%; multiple, usually low-grade, visceral malignancies, including colorectal and genitourinary
Inflammatory/Autoimmune	
Ulcerative colitis (see Chapter 21; Table 45.4)	• Uniform and continuous inflammation of the large bowel. Rectal involvement is present in majority (>95%) of patients. Toxic megacolon may develop
Crohn's disease (see Chapter 21; Fig. 45.4; Table 45.4)	• Chronic inflammation, often granulomatous, of the bowel. Skip areas occur
Vasculitis (see Chapter 19)	• Ulcerations secondary to vasculitis of the vessels in the bowel. May be more common in IgA-associated vasculitis (Henoch–Schönlein purpura)
Malignant atrophic papulosis (Degos' disease) (see Chapter 18)	• Small infarctions in the GI mucosa; hemorrhage and intestinal perforation may result in death

Table 45.3 Examples of skin signs of gastrointestinal (GI) disease.

SKIN FINDINGS IN CROHN'S DISEASE AND ULCERATIVE COLITIS

- Erythema nodosum – often reflective of active bowel disease
- Urticaria
- Cutaneous small vessel vasculitis
- Cutaneous polyarteritis nodosa
- 'Pustular' vasculitis or bowel-associated dermatosis–arthritis syndrome-like lesions
- Pyoderma gangrenosum – primarily the classic (typical) ulcerative form (see Fig. 21.5) or peristomal lesions (Fig. 45.4B); a vegetative pustular variant (pyoderma vegetans) occasionally occurs. These lesions may or may not reflect activity of the bowel disease
- Other neutrophilic dermatoses, ranging from acneiform lesions to Sweet's syndrome and panniculitis
- Oral lesions
  - Granulomatous infiltrates (with Crohn's disease only)
  - Aphthosis
  - Angular cheilitis
  - Pyostomatitis vegetans (mucosal variant of pyoderma gangrenosum)
- Contiguous (anogenital) and 'metastatic' Crohn's disease (Fig. 45.4A)
- Fistulae (perianal and abdominal)
- Acquired acrodermatitis enteropathica-like lesions (patients with zinc deficiency and/or essential fatty acid deficiency)
- Epidermolysis bullosa acquisita
- Psoriasis

Table 45.4 Skin findings in Crohn's disease and ulcerative colitis.

PERISTOMAL SKIN DISORDERS

Skin Disorder	Comments
Irritant contact dermatitis	Most common cause of peristomal dermatitis, especially in patients with an ileostomy. Primarily attributed to exposure to feces or urine
Pre-existing skin disease (e.g. psoriasis, seborrheic dermatitis, atopic dermatitis)	Exclude primary contact dermatitis or infection or superimposed contact dermatitis
Cutaneous infection (*Candida* spp. dermatophyte, herpes-virus [primarily simplex], bacteria [especially *Staphylococcus aureus*])	Colonization with bacteria and/or yeast is common. Recent treatment with antibiotics predisposes to candidiasis. May initially improve and then worsen if treated inappropriately with topical corticosteroids
Allergic contact dermatitis	Relatively uncommon. Potential allergens include adhesive pastes, adhesive ring or wafer of stoma bag, ostomy bag, epoxy resin, rubber, lanolin, and fragrances. Patch test with both standardized allergens and patient's own products
Pyoderma gangrenosum	Infrequent cause of peristomal dermatitis; most common in patients with inflammatory bowel disease (Fig. 45.4B)
Pseudo-verrucous papules and nodules	Seen more commonly in association with urostomies; may be misdiagnosed as verrucae

Table 45.5 Peristomal skin disorders. Peristomal skin disorders are common and may limit use and efficacy of the stoma appliance. When the etiology is uncertain, evaluation can include KOH examination, microbial cultures, patch testing, and histologic examination. *Adapted from Lyon CC, Smith AJ, Griffiths CE, et al. The spectrum of skin disorders in abdominal stoma patients. Br. J. Dermatol. 2000;143:1248–1260.*

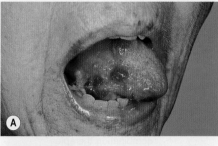

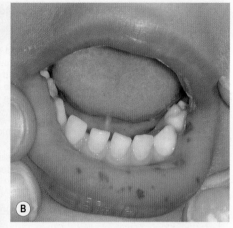

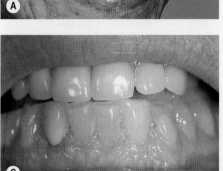

Fig. 45.3 Skin signs of gastrointestinal disease. A Blue rubber bleb nevus syndrome. Several venous malformations are evident on this patient's tongue. **B** Peutz–Jeghers syndrome. Multiple brown macules on the lips and oral mucosa. **C** Gingival cobblestoning in Cowden disease. This patient also had trichilemmomas and a 'Cowden's nodule' or sclerotic fibroma on the neck. *Courtesy, Jeffrey P. Callen, MD.*

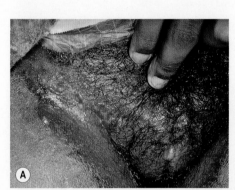

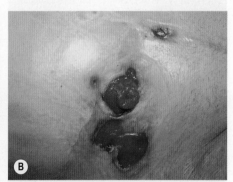

Fig. 45.4 Skin signs of inflammatory bowel disease. A 'Metastatic' Crohn's disease. Non-contiguous granulomatous inflammation of the skin manifested by deep inflammatory fissures in the inguinal folds. **B** Peristomal pyoderma gangrenosum in the setting of inflammatory bowel disease. Patients with ostomies, particularly ileostomies, are at risk for peristomal dermatoses, including pyoderma gangrenosum. *Courtesy, Jeffrey P. Callen, MD.*

EXAMPLES OF SKIN SIGNS OF LIVER DISEASE

Disorder	Cutaneous Findings	Other
Cirrhosis	• Spider angiomas and other telangiectasias, palmar erythema, Terry's and Muehrcke's nails (see Chapter 58), pruritus, jaundice	• Gynecomastia • Parotid enlargement
Hepatitis B and C viral infections	• See Table 68.4 • Anal pruritus is common side effect of telaprevir • Cutaneous sarcoidosis has been seen with interferon and/or ribavirin therapy	• Rx: dual- (peginterferon-α and ribavirin) and triple-combination therapies (peginterferon-α, ribavirin, and telaprevir or boceprevir); direct-acting antiviral agents under development
Hemochromatosis ('bronze diabetes')	• Generalized hyperpigmentation	• Due to mutations in *HFE*, most commonly C282Y. Phlebotomy to reduce iron stores or chelation (e.g. deferasirox)
Primary biliary cirrhosis (PBC)	• Jaundice, diffuse hyperpigmentation, pruritus, xanthomas (eruptive, planar, sometimes tuberous), may coexist with systemic sclerosis	• Cholestyramine, rifampin, ursodiol, and naloxone may help to relieve the pruritus

CSVV, cutaneous small vessel vasculitis; HCV, hepatitis C.

Table 45.6 Examples of skin signs of liver disease.

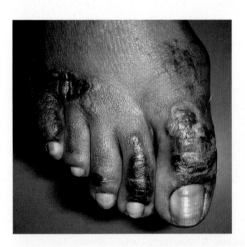

Fig. 45.5 Skin signs of liver disease.
Necrolytic acral erythema. This is a manifestation of hepatitis C viral infection. *Courtesy, Jeffrey P. Callen, MD.*

EXAMPLES OF SKIN SIGNS OF RENAL DISEASE

Disorder	Renal Disease/Other
Genetic	
Tuberous sclerosis complex (TSC) (see Chapter 50; Table 45.2)	• Renal hamartomas (angiomyolipomas). Polycystic kidney disease may occur in a contiguous gene syndrome with *TSC2*
Nail patella syndrome (see Chapter 58)	• Congenital nephrosis, glomerulonephritis

Table 45.7 Examples of skin signs of renal disease. *Continued*

Disorder	Renal Disease/Other
Birt–Hogg–Dubé syndrome (see Chapter 91; Table 45.1)	• Renal tumors, particularly chromophobe and hybrid oncocytic carcinomas
Familial cutaneous leiomyomatosis (see Chapter 95)	• Predisposition to develop renal carcinoma
Inflammatory/Autoimmune	
Systemic lupus erythematosus (see Chapter 33; Table 45.2)	• Glomerulonephritis – focal, membranous, or proliferative
Systemic sclerosis (see Chapter 35; Table 45.1)	• Malignant hypertension, rapidly progressive renal failure
Henoch–Schönlein purpura (see Chapter 19)	• IgA-associated glomerulonephritis
Polyarteritis nodosa (see Chapter 19)	• Renal artery aneurysms, hypertension
Wegener's granulomatosis (granulomatosis with polyangiitis; see Chapter 19; Table 45.1)	• Glomerulonephritis
Cutaneous small vessel vasculitis (CSVV) (see Chapter 19)	• Glomerulonephritis may occur but is less common than in the vasculitides mentioned previously
Other	
Primary systemic amyloidosis (AL) (see Chapter 39; Table 45.2)	• Proteinuria, including nephrotic syndrome, and renal insufficiency
Cutaneous changes of end-stage renal disease	1. Pale color, sallowness 2. Xerosis or acquired ichthyosis (see Fig. 4.2) 3. Pruritus (see Chapter 4) 4. Acquired perforating dermatosis (see Chapter 79 and Figs 4.2, 79.1, and 79.2) 5. Pseudoporphyria (see Chapter 41 and Fig. 41.8) 6. Calciphylaxis (see Chapter 42 and Fig. 42.5) 7. Uremic frost
Nephrogenic systemic fibrosis (NSF) (see Chapter 35 and Fig. 35.10)	• Occurs primarily in patients with chronic renal failure on dialysis > renal transplant recipients, patients with acute renal failure

CRITERIA USED TO ASSOCIATE A DERMATOSIS AND MALIGNANCY (CURTH'S POSTULATES)	
Concurrent onset	The neoplasm is discovered at the time of diagnosis of the dermatosis or shortly following diagnosis
Parallel course	Therapy of the malignancy results in disappearance of the dermatosis, and, if the malignancy recurs, then the dermatosis relapses
Uniform site or type of neoplasm	The neoplasm is of a specific cell type within a specific organ or tissue
Statistical association	
Genetic linkage	

Table 45.8 **Criteria used to associate a dermatosis and malignancy (Curth's postulates).**

PARANEOPLASTIC DERMATOSES		
Dermatoses	**Cutaneous Findings**	**Comments**
Disorders that are associated with cancer in most or all cases		
Bazex syndrome (acrokeratosis paraneoplastica)	Acral psoriasiform plaques, typically with involvement of the nose and helices; often the lesions are violaceous (Fig. 45.6A). Longitudinal and horizontal ridging of the nails occurs in 75% of patients	By definition, this condition is linked to malignancy, generally occurring in the upper aerodigestive tract (pharynx, larynx, or esophagus)
Carcinoid syndrome	Flushing and erythema of the head and neck. Pellagra-like dermatitis and sclerodermoid changes may develop in advanced disease	Flushing associated with ~10% of midgut tumors (small intestine, appendix, proximal colon) and liver metastases are required; type III gastric and bronchial carcinoid tumors are also associated with flushing (liver metastases are not required)
Erythema gyratum repens	Concentric erythematous lesions, often giving the appearance of grains of wood (Fig. 45.6B; see Chapter 15)	Variable sites and types of malignancy
Acquired hypertrichosis lanuginosa (malignant down)	Growth of fine lanugo hairs in a generalized distribution or localized to the face. With time, these hairs may become coarser (see Chapter 57)	Associated with a variety of internal malignancies, most often carcinoma of the lung, colon, or breast
AESOP syndrome	Large red to violet-brown patch	Patch overlies a plasmacytoma
Ectopic adrenocorticotropic hormone (ACTH) syndrome	Generalized hyperpigmentation	Production of ACTH by a tumor (often a small cell carcinoma of the lung) may result in hyperpigmentation and features of Cushing's syndrome
Glucagonoma syndrome	Necrolytic migratory erythema, angular cheilitis, glossitis	Due to a glucagon-secreting tumor of the pancreas. Patients are often treated for intertrigo before the syndrome is diagnosed. Weight loss and diabetes mellitus accompany the dermatosis
Paraneoplastic pemphigus	Erosive disease of the mucous membranes (see Fig. 23.8) and erythema multiforme-like, bullous pemphigoid-like, or lichenoid skin lesions (see Chapter 23)	Most often associated with non-Hodgkin lymphoma, chronic lymphocytic leukemia, or Castleman's disease (with the latter accounting for the majority of cases in children and Asian populations). Castleman's tumors have been shown to produce the autoantibodies responsible for paraneoplastic pemphigus, and their resection can lead to remission of mucocutaneous lesions. Bronchiolitis obliterans is a common complication

Table 45.9 Paraneoplastic dermatoses. *Continued*

Table 45.9 *Continued* **Paraneoplastic dermatoses.**

45

Dermatoses	Cutaneous Findings	Comments
POEMS syndrome (*polyneuropathy, organomegaly, endocrinopathy, M*-protein, and *skin* changes)	Although the glomeruloid hemangioma (Fig. 45.6C) is considered to be pathognomonic, it is present in a minority of patients. Other skin findings include cherry angiomas, hyperpigmentation, hypertrichosis, sclerodermatous thickening, hyperhidrosis, digital clubbing, plethora, acrocyanosis, and leukonychia	Osteosclerotic myeloma, Castleman's disease, and plasmacytomas have been reported in patients with POEMS. In addition to the findings designated in the acronym, patients may have peripheral edema, ascites, pulmonary effusions, papilledema, thrombocytosis, polycythemia, and increased serum levels of VEGF
Sign of Leser–Trélat	Rapid appearance or growth of multiple seborrheic keratoses; keratoses may be inflamed	Often these patients have acanthosis nigricans and generalized pruritus. Controversy continues regarding the existence of this sign in the absence of generalized pruritus and acanthosis nigricans, in part because determining whether seborrheic keratoses are eruptive can be difficult. Eruptive seborrheic keratoses can also develop in erythrodermic patients who do not have an underlying malignancy
Tripe palms	Ridged velvety lesions on the palms	May or may not be accompanied by acanthosis nigricans
Disorders that are strongly associated with cancer in a subset of cases		
Acanthosis nigricans	Rapid onset of hyperpigmented velvety changes of the flexural surfaces (e.g. neck, axillae, and groin). May also involve extensor surfaces (e.g. elbows, knees, and knuckles) and, in malignancy-associated cases, the lips, oral mucosa, and palms (see above, tripe palms). Glossitis is also frequently present in malignancy-associated acanthosis nigricans	Association with adenocarcinoma of the stomach or other sites within the GI or GU tracts; in this setting, acanthosis nigricans is often accompanied by weight loss. Acanthosis nigricans is more commonly associated with endocrinologic abnormalities, particularly insulin resistance (Figs 45.8 and 45.9); such patients are typically overweight, and the onset of the condition is usually insidious
Anti-epiligrin cicatricial pemphigoid (AECP)*	Oral ulcerations, conjunctival erosions, and scarring. Tense blisters and erosions of the skin may also develop	Roughly one-third of patients with AECP have or develop cancer within the first year following diagnosis. The cancer is usually an adenocarcinoma and is often at an advanced stage at the time of diagnosis, possibly accounting for the high mortality rate of AECP

Table 45.9 *Continued* **Paraneoplastic dermatoses.**

Dermatoses	Cutaneous Findings	Comments
Dermatomyositis (adult)*	Heliotrope, Gottron's papules, photodistributed poikiloderma, nailfold overgrowth with dilated capillary loops, pruritus and diffuse scaling of the scalp (see Chapter 34)	Population-based studies demonstrate an overrepresentation of ovarian, lung, colorectal, and pancreatic carcinomas and non-Hodgkin lymphoma in Caucasians
Neutrophilic dermatoses	Sweet's syndrome or pyoderma gangrenosum (particularly the atypical bullous form) (see Chapter 21)	Approximately 10–20% of cases are associated with hematologic disorders such as acute myelogenous leukemia or plasma cell dyscrasia (IgA). Underlying solid tumors are rare
Dermatoses that may be associated with cancer in a subset of patients		
Acquired angioedema due to C1 esterase inhibitor dysfunction	Acquired angioedema without associated wheals	Associated with B-cell lymphoproliferative disorders, including lymphomas, as well as monoclonal gammopathy of undetermined significance (MGUS)
Acquired ichthyosis	Resembles ichthyosis vulgaris; most often located on the legs	Lymphoma typically predates the diagnosis of the ichthyosis
Amyloidosis, primary systemic	Waxy, translucent, or purpuric papules; periorbital and pinch purpura; macroglossia	Monoclonal gammopathy due to plasma cell dyscrasia >> multiple myeloma; deposits composed of immunoglobulin light chain (AL)
Cryoglobulinemia, type I	Retiform purpura and necrosis that favors cooler acral sites; acral cyanosis; livedo reticularis	Monoclonal gammopathy due to lymphoplasmocytic disorders
Cutaneous small vessel vasculitis	Palpable purpura	Less than 1% of patients with vasculitis have an associated malignancy, most commonly hairy cell leukemia and chronic lymphocytic leukemia
Dermatitis herpetiformis (DH)	Pruritic erosions and blisters on extensor surfaces, scalp, and/or buttocks	Through the association of DH with gluten-sensitive enteropathy, enteropathy-associated T-cell lymphoma occasionally occurs
Exfoliative erythroderma	Diffuse, scaly, erythematous skin	May be associated with cutaneous T-cell lymphoma or, occasionally, with a systemic lymphoma or leukemia

Table 45.9 *Continued* **Paraneoplastic dermatoses.**

45

Dermatoses	Cutaneous Findings	Comments
Juvenile xanthogranulomas (JXGs) in the setting of neurofibromatosis 1 (NF1)	Pink-yellow to red-brown, dome-shaped papules and nodules, most often located on the head and neck	A triple association between JXGs, NF1, and JMML has been described
Multicentric reticulohistiocytosis	Nodular lesions, most often on the dorsal aspects of the hands (see Fig. 76.9)	A variety of associated malignancies have been reported, developing in approximately 25% of adult patients
Mycosis fungoides	Patch, plaque, or nodular disease	Some studies have demonstrated an increased risk of second malignancies
Necrobiotic xanthogranuloma	Indurated xanthomatous plaques with necrosis and ulceration, usually in a periorbital location	Paraproteinemia (>80% of cases, most often IgG with κ light chains); multiple myeloma or a lymphoproliferative disorder develop in a minority of patients
Normolipemic plane xanthoma	Yellowish patches and thin plaques that favor the skin folds, upper trunk, and periorbital area	Paraproteinemia, due to a plasma cell dyscrasia or lymphoproliferative disorder
Porphyria cutanea tarda (PCT)	Erosions, blisters, and scars on the dorsal aspect of the hands, hyperpigmentation, hypertrichosis, milia	Through its association with hepatitis C virus, PCT may also be associated with primary hepatocellular carcinoma (hepatoma)
Schnitzler's syndrome	Chronic urticaria	Associated with an IgM usually κ paraproteinemia; lymphoplasmacytic malignancies develop in approximately 15% of patients. Additional manifestations include fevers, arthralgias, and bone pain
Scleromyxedema	Sclerodermoid induration and a widespread eruption of firm, waxy papules arranged in linear arrays	Almost always associated with paraproteinemia (usually IgG with λ light chains); multiple myeloma develops in <10% of cases
Dermatoses that have been proven not to be associated with cancer		
Bowen's disease	Erythematous scaly plaque	The results of early studies that suggested an association with internal malignancy were likely explained by arsenic exposure in affected individuals and have not been replicated

Table 45.9 *Continued* **Paraneoplastic dermatoses.**

Familial cancer syndromes and the skin

- Cowden disease (breast, thyroid, and GI carcinomas), Muir–Torre syndrome (GI carcinoma), Gardner syndrome (GI carcinoma), Peutz–Jeghers syndrome (various malignancies) – see Table 45.3
- Werner syndrome (sarcomas and other malignancies)
- Birt–Hogg–Dubé syndrome, familial cutaneous leiomyomatosis (renal carcinoma) – see Tables 45.1 and 45.7
- Howel–Evans syndrome (esophageal carcinoma) – see Chapter 47
- Ataxia–telangiectasia (leukemia, lymphoma, breast cancer) – see Chapter 49 and Fig. 49.1
- Neurofibromatosis (malignant peripheral nerve sheath tumors, JMML, rhabdomyosarcoma, pheochromocytoma, carcinoid), tuberous sclerosis (renal carcinoma) – see Chapter 50
- Multiple endocrine neoplasia syndromes – see Chapter 52, Table 52.2, and Fig. 52.2
- Dyskeratosis congenita (leukemia, Hodgkin disease) – see Table 55.6 and Fig. 55.18
- Nevoid basal cell carcinoma syndrome (medulloblastoma, fibrosarcoma) – see Chapter 88
- Bloom syndrome (lymphoproliferative and GI malignancies), Rothmund–Thomson syndrome (osteosarcoma), xeroderma pigmentosum (sarcomas, leukemia, GI and lung carcinomas) – see Table 73.5
- Familial atypical mole and multiple melanoma syndrome (pancreatic carcinoma in a subset) – see Chapters 92 and 93

*Statistical association.
AESOP syndrome, adenopathy, extensive skin patch overlying (a) plasmacytoma; GI, gastrointestinal; GU, genitourinary; VEGF, vascular endothelial growth factor; JMML, juvenile myelomonocytic leukemia.*

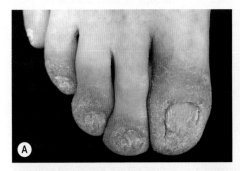
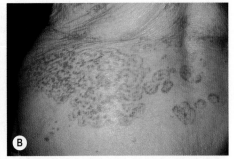
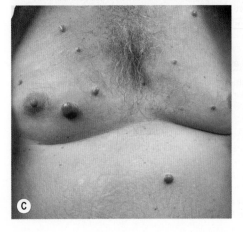

Fig. 45.6 Skin signs that are associated with an internal malignancy in most or all cases. A Bazex syndrome (acrokeratosis paraneoplastica). The patient had an SCC of the tonsillar pillar. **B** Erythema gyratum repens. This patient had cancer of the breast. **C** POEMS syndrome. Note the multiple angiomas (glomeruloid hemangiomas histologically) on the trunk. In addition, he had peripheral neuropathy, hypothyroidism, and peripheral edema. His underlying disorder was an osteosclerotic myeloma. *Courtesy, Jeffrey P. Callen, MD.*

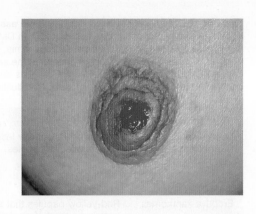

Fig. 45.7 Paget's disease of the breast.
A chronic, eroded erythematous plaque
surrounds the nipple and is due to epidermal
extension of an underlying ductal
adenocarcinoma of the breast. *Courtesy, Robert
Hartmann, MD.*

SELECTED DERMATOLOGIC ASSOCIATIONS OF DIABETES MELLITUS (DM)		
Dermatosis	**Clinical Description**	**Comments**
Acanthosis nigricans (AN)	Velvety hyperpigmentation of the intertriginous/flexural areas (Fig. 45.9A) and, less often, extensor surfaces (Fig. 45.9B)	Commonly associated with insulin resistance and most of the patients are obese. More common in Hispanics and individuals of African descent. Recent evidence strongly links AN in children with insulin resistance and diabetes
Acral dry gangrene	Necrosis of the fingertips or toes	Due to vascular disease in larger vessels
Acral erythema	Erysipelas-like blanching erythema of the hands and/or feet	May be due to small vessel occlusive disease with compensatory hyperemia
Carotenoderma	Diffuse orange-yellow skin color	Related to an increase in serum carotene level
Diabetic bullae (bullosis diabeticorum)	Tense non-inflammatory bullae on the lower extremities (Fig. 45.10A)	Unknown pathogenesis
Diabetic cheiroarthropathy	Thickened skin and limited joint mobility of the hands and fingers, leading to flexion contractures (starting with the fifth digit and progressing radially) and an inability to approximate the palmar surfaces of the hands and fingers (prayer sign)	Postulated to result from increased glycosylation of collagen in the skin. Associated with retinopathy, nephropathy, and duration (but not control) of the DM
Diabetic dermopathy	Brown atrophic macules and patches on the legs (Fig. 45.10B)	Possibly precipitated by trauma

Table 45.10 Selected dermatologic associations of diabetes mellitus (DM). Additional
cutaneous conditions associated with DM include hirsutism (e.g. related to polycystic ovary
syndrome or HAIR-AN – *h*yperandrogenemia, *i*nsulin *r*esistance, *a*canthosis *n*igricans; see
Chapter 57), necrolytic migratory erythema (in the setting of DM due to a glucagon-secreting
pancreatic tumor; see Table 45.9), and infections such as mucocutaneous candidiasis,
erythrasma (especially the disciform variant), cellulitis, and necrotizing fasciitis. *Continued*

Table 45.10 *Continued* **Selected dermatologic associations of diabetes mellitus (DM).**
Additional cutaneous conditions associated with DM include hirsutism (e.g. related to polycystic ovary syndrome or HAIR-AN – *h*yperandrogenemia, *i*nsulin *r*esistance, *a*canthosis *n*igricans; see Chapter 57), necrolytic migratory erythema (in the setting of DM due to a glucagon-secreting pancreatic tumor; see Table 45.9), and infections such as mucocutaneous candidiasis, erythrasma (especially the disciform variant), cellulitis, and necrotizing fasciitis.

Dermatosis	Clinical Description	Comments
Disseminated granuloma annulare	Erythematous annular lesions composed of papules	There is controversy about the exact relationship of disseminated granuloma annulare and DM (see Chapter 78)
Eruptive xanthomas	Red-yellow papules that appear over a period of weeks to months (Fig. 45.10C)	Associated with elevated serum triglycerides in patients with poorly controlled diabetes. Control of the DM results in a disappearance of the xanthomas (see Chapter 77)
Hemochromatosis	Bronzing of the skin due to an increase in melanin rather than iron	Excess of iron stores associated with cirrhosis and cardiac dysfunction as well as DM. Due to mutations in *HFE*, most commonly C282Y. Also risk factor for porphyria cutanea tarda
Necrobiosis lipoidica	Yellow atrophic patches, most often on the shins. A red-brown rim may indicate activity at the border (Fig. 45.10D). Ulceration can occur and is often slow to heal	Intralesional triamcinolone, aspirin, dipyridamole, and/or pentoxyfylline are possibly helpful. Not all patients have DM (see Chapter 78)
Neuropathic leg ulcers	Non-painful ulcerations at sites of pressure, most commonly on the foot, including the plantar surface (Fig. 45.10E); a keratotic rim is characteristic	Associated with sensory neuropathy (see Chapter 86)
Perforating disorders (e.g. acquired perforating dermatosis)	Keratotic papules, primarily on the extremities	Often occurs in African-American diabetic patients with chronic kidney disease on dialysis (see Chapter 79)
Rubeosis	Chronic, flushed appearance of the face, neck, and upper extremities	Improved by dietary diabetic control. Flares with vasodilator therapies
Scleredema (adultorum of Buschke)	Erythematous induration of the upper back and nape due to glycosaminoglycan deposition	Unknown etiology. No relationship to control of the DM

Adapted from Jorizzo JL, Callen JP. Dermatologic manifestations of internal disease. In: Arndt KA, Robinson JK, LeBoit PE, et al. (eds) Cutaneous Medicine and Surgery. Philadelphia: Saunders, 1996:1863–1889.

CRITERIA FOR THE DIAGNOSIS OF THE METABOLIC SYNDROME

- Elevated waist circumference (population- and country-specific definitions)
- Elevated triglycerides ($\geq$150 mg/dl)
- Reduced HDL (<40 mg/dl in males; <50 mg/dl in females)
- Elevated blood pressure (systolic $\geq$130 and/or diastolic $\geq$85 mmHg)
- Elevated fasting blood glucose ($\geq$100 mg/dl)

Table 45.11 Criteria for the diagnosis of the metabolic syndrome. Metabolic syndrome is identified by the presence of three of these five criteria. Drug treatment for dyslipidemia, hypertension, or hyperglycemia also fulfills the corresponding criterion. Most patients with type 2 diabetes mellitus meet criteria for metabolic syndrome.

DERMATOLOGIC MANIFESTATIONS OF THYROID DISEASE

	Hyperthyroidism	Hypothyroidism
Cutaneous changes	Fine, velvety, smooth skin Warm and moist due to increased sweating Hyperpigmentation – localized or generalized Pruritus	Dry, rough, coarse skin Cold and pale Boggy and edematous skin (myxedema) Yellow discoloration as a result of carotenemia Easy bruising (capillary fragility)
Cutaneous diseases	Pretibial myxedema,* thyroid acropachy Urticaria, dermatographism Increased incidence of vitiligo	Acquired ichthyosis and palmoplantar keratoderma Eruptive and/or tuberous xanthomas Increased incidence of vitiligo
Hair changes/diseases	Fine, thin Mild, diffuse alopecia Increased incidence of alopecia areata	Dull, coarse, brittle Slow growth (increase in telogen hair phase) Alopecia of the lateral third of the eyebrows Increased incidence of alopecia areata
Nail changes	Onycholysis Koilonychia Clubbing from thyroid acropachy	Thin, brittle, striated Slow growth Onycholysis (rare)

*Can persist when patient is treated and becomes euthyroid or can be associated with euthyroid Graves' disease.

Table 45.12 Dermatologic manifestations of thyroid disease. A serum thyroid-stimulating hormone (TSH) level is the most reliable test of thyroid function, and it is usually markedly suppressed in patients with hyperthyroidism. Additional laboratory findings in hyperthyroid patients include elevated free T3 and/or free T4 levels. Patients with primary hypothyroidism have elevated TSH levels and decreased free T4 levels. The detection of anti-thyroid peroxidase and/or anti-thyroglobulin antibodies points to autoimmune thyroid disease (Hashimoto's thyroiditis, Graves' disease), whereas the presence of anti-TSH receptor antibodies points to Graves' disease. Ascher's syndrome consists of blepharochalasis, double lip, and goiter.

DERMATOLOGIC MANIFESTATIONS OF CUSHING'S SYNDROME

Altered subcutaneous fat distribution
- Rounded facies
- Fullness of the cheeks ('moon' facies)
- Dorsal cervical vertebral fat deposition ('buffalo hump') (Fig. 45.11A)*
- Pelvic girdle fat deposition*
- Reduced fat in the arms and legs*

Skin atrophy
- Global atrophy with epidermal and dermal components affected
- Multiple striae on abdomen, flanks, arms and thighs (Fig. 45.11B)
- Cutaneous fragility and prolonged wound healing
- Purpura with minor trauma due to reduced connective tissue support

Cutaneous infections
- Tinea (pityriasis) versicolor
- Dermatophytosis and onychomycosis
- Candidiasis

Adnexal effects
- Corticosteroid-related acne
- Hirsutism

This same change is indicative of insulin resistance and occurs in HIV-associated lipodystrophy.

Table 45.13 Dermatologic manifestations of Cushing's syndrome. An overnight dexamethasone suppression test (8 a.m. plasma cortisol >140 nmol/l after receiving 1 mg at midnight) or 24-hour urine free cortisol determination (>140 nmol/24 h) can be used as a screen for Cushing's syndrome due to endogenous cortisol production. Elevated plasma adrenocorticotropic hormone (ACTH) levels are found in Cushing's disease (pituitary overproduction of ACTH) and ectopic ACTH syndrome, whereas ACTH levels are suppressed in patients with adrenal tumors.

SELECTED DERMATOLOGIC MANIFESTATIONS OF ADDISON'S DISEASE

- Hyperpigmentation (MSH-like effect due to secretion of ACTH)
  - Diffuse with accentuation in sun-exposed areas (Fig. 45.12)
  - Sites of trauma
  - Axillae, perineum, and nipples
  - Palmar creases
  - Melanocytic nevi
  - Mucous membranes
  - Hair
  - Nails
- Loss of ambisexual hair in postpubertal women
- Fibrosis and calcification of cartilage including the ear (rare)
- Associated findings in candidiasis endocrinopathy syndrome
  - Vitiligo
  - Chronic mucocutaneous candidiasis

MSH, melanocyte stimulating hormone.

Table 45.14 Selected dermatologic manifestations of Addison's disease. The rapid adrenocorticotropic hormone (ACTH) stimulation test (which assesses adrenal reserve) should be performed when adrenal insufficiency is suspected, because basal serum cortisol levels may be normal in patients with partial deficiencies. Plasma ACTH levels are elevated in primary adrenocortical insufficiency (Addison's disease) and suppressed in secondary adrenocortical insufficiency (e.g. due to exogenous glucocorticoid therapy).

Was AN apparent at birth or during early childhood and associated with skeletal abnormalities and/or short stature?	⇒	Consider autosomal dominant disorders due to FGFR defects, specially if AN is extensive: • Crouzon syndrome with AN (features craniosynostosis), SADDAN, and thanatophoric dysplasia (*FGFR3* mutations) • Beare-Stevenson cutis gyrata syndrome (features craniosynostosis; *FGFR2* mutations) • Consider Costello syndrome
Was AN apparent during childhood or adolescence and associated with loss/absence of subcutaneous fat?	⇒	Consider generalized lipodystrophy (more extensive AN with congenital variant) or partial lipodystrophy (familial > acquired) (see Ch. 84)
Was the onset sudden and accompanied by constitutional symptoms or weight loss?	⇒	Consider underlying malignancy, particularly if AN is extensive and involves sites such as the palms and soles. Restaging is required if AN recurs in a patient with a known malignancy
Is the patient overweight or obese?	⇒	Evaluate for associated insulin resistance states, especially diabetes mellitus. Consider evaluation for other underlying endocrinopathies, including thyroid disease
Does the patient have striae, hypertension, central obesity and/or a buffalo hump?	⇒	Evaluate for Cushing's syndrome
If female, does the patient have acne, hirsutism and/or irregular menses?	⇒	Evaluate for polycystic ovary syndrome and HAIR-AN syndrome (see Ch. 57)
Is the patient on medications such as niacin, human growth hormone, oral contraceptives, corticosteroids or protease inhibitors?	⇒	AN may be drug-induced

Fig. 45.8 Evaluation of the patient with acanthosis nigricans (AN). FGFR, fibroblast growth factor receptor; HAIR-AN, *h*yperandrogenemia, *i*nsulin *r*esistance, *a*canthosis *n*igricans; SADDAN, severe *a*chondrodysplasia with *d*evelopmental *delay* and *AN*.

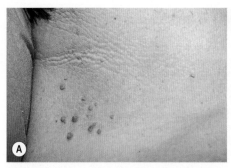

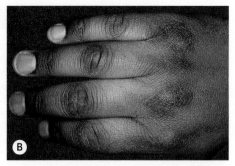

Fig. 45.9 Acanthosis nigricans (AN). A AN and acrochordons of the neck in the setting of insulin resistance and obesity. Note the velvety texture of the skin. **B** AN over the knuckles. AN can involve extensor surfaces as well as flexural areas. *A, Courtesy Jeffrey P. Callen; B, Courtesy, Jean L. Bolognia, MD.*

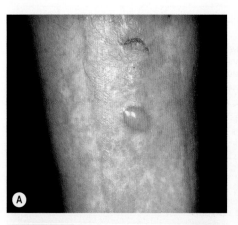

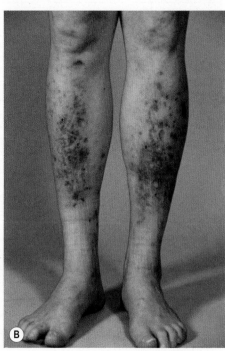

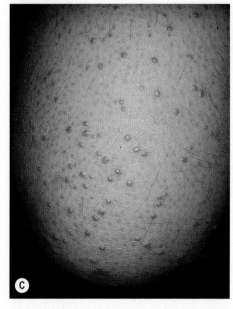

Fig. 45.10 Skin signs of diabetes mellitus.
A Bullosis diabeticorum (diabetic bullae) with non-inflammatory bullae on the lower extremity.
B Diabetic dermopathy characterized by brown macules and patches on the shins. **C** Eruptive xanthomas are frequently associated with poorly controlled diabetes mellitus. This patient was first discovered to have diabetes following the appearance of these yellow-red papules.
Continued

For further information see Ch. 53. From *Dermatology, Third Edition.*

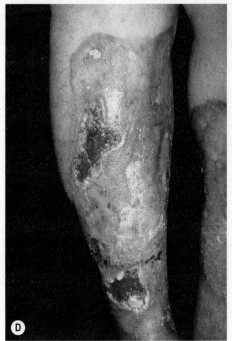

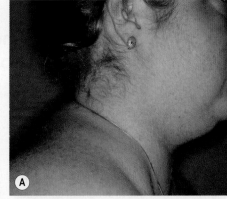

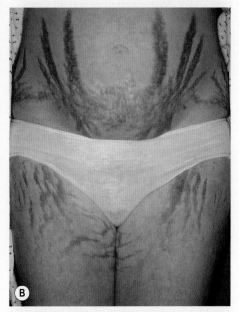

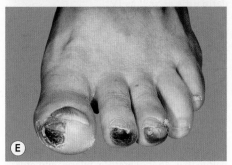

Fig. 45.10 *Continued* **D** Necrobiosis lipoidica. Controversy exists about the exact risk of diabetes mellitus in such patients, but it is more strongly associated with diabetes than is granuloma annulare. **E** Neuropathic ulcers on the toes of a patient with diabetic sensory neuropathy. *A, C–E, Courtesy, Jeffrey P. Callen, MD; B, Courtesy, Jean L. Bolognia, MD.*

Fig. 45.11 Skin signs of Cushing's disease. **A** 'Buffalo hump' of Cushing's syndrome due to fat redistribution. The patient also has evidence of hirsutism. **B** Cushing's syndrome with multiple striae. *Courtesy, Judit Stenn, MD.*

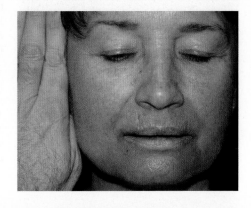

Fig. 45.12 Skin signs of Addison's disease. Diffuse hyperpigmentation (shown in contrast to the physician's hand) is accentuated in sun-exposed skin and can also involve sites of trauma, skin creases, and mucosae. *Courtesy, Jeffrey P. Callen, MD.*

46 | Ichthyoses and Erythrokeratodermas

- Ichthyoses and erythrokeratodermas represent a diverse group of disorders of cornification, which are characterized by a defective epidermal barrier due to abnormal differentiation and/or desquamation of keratinocytes.
- *Ichthyoses* feature diffuse scaling of the skin, often in a widespread distribution, whereas *erythrokeratodermas* present with circumscribed areas of hyperkeratosis without prominent scaling.
- These conditions usually have a genetic basis, with the occasional exception of acquired ichthyosis associated with disorders such as malnutrition, hypothyroidism, sarcoidosis, lymphoma, leprosy, or HIV infection.
- A thorough family history helps in recognizing the inheritance pattern; an affected parent suggests dominant inheritance, whereas inheritance in patients with unaffected parents may be autosomal recessive (especially with affected siblings or parental consanguinity), X-linked recessive (especially for a male patient with affected maternal male relatives), or dominant (e.g. due to a 'new' mutation or with incomplete penetrance).
- Clinical features that are useful in determining the type of ichthyosis include the time of presentation (e.g. at birth, ± a collodion membrane, vs. later in life), the quality and distribution of the scaling, other cutaneous manifestations (e.g. erythroderma, blistering, abnormal hair), and extracutaneous or laboratory findings (Table 46.1).
- A few ichthyoses have characteristic histologic features (e.g. epidermolytic ichthyosis; see below).
- For conditions with a known molecular etiology, genetic testing can confirm the diagnosis in the patient and affected relatives as well as provide the basis for prenatal/preimplantation testing.

Ichthyosis Vulgaris (IV)

- The most common disorder of cornification, with a prevalence of at least 1 in 200.
- Autosomal semidominant inheritance – mild ichthyosis with a heterozygous filaggrin (*FLG*) mutation and more severe ichthyosis with mutations in both *FLG* alleles.
- Filaggrin deficiency results in impaired formation of cornified keratinocytes, increased transepidermal water loss, and a propensity for an inflammatory response upon exposure to irritants or allergens; this explains the pathogenic role of *FLG* mutations in atopic dermatitis as well as IV.
- Typically becomes apparent during infancy or early childhood and improves by adulthood; worsens in a cold, dry environment.
- Mild to moderate scaling favors the extensor extremities (Fig. 46.1), ranging from fine white scales to larger adherent scales (especially on the lower legs); the trunk, scalp, and forehead are occasionally affected, and flexural sites are characteristically spared.
- Associated findings include hyperlinear palms (Fig. 46.2), keratosis pilaris, and atopic dermatitis (25–50% of patients, ± other atopic disorders such as asthma and allergic rhinitis).
- **DDx:** xerosis, acquired ichthyosis, X-linked ichthyosis.
- **Rx:** emollients (especially those containing ceramides + other lipids), humectants, and keratolytic agents (e.g. urea, lactic and salicylic acids); the latter group may be irritating in patients with coexistent atopic dermatitis.

X-Linked Recessive Ichthyosis (XLRI; Steroid Sulfatase Deficiency)

- Incidence of ~1 in 5000 male births; almost exclusively affects boys and men, with transmission by asymptomatic female carriers.

CLUES TO THE DIAGNOSIS OF ICHTHYOSES AND ERYTHROKERATODERMAS

Cutaneous Findings in Neonates

Collodion membrane: lamellar ichthyosis, CIE, 'self-healing' form >> SLS, TTD, NLSD, others (e.g. infantile Gaucher disease, ectodermal dysplasias)

Blisters/erosions/peeling: EI, superficial EI, Netherton syndrome, peeling skin syndromes

Erythroderma: EI, CIE, Netherton syndrome, ichthyosis en confetti > SLS, TTD, NLSD, KID, CHH (along Blaschko's lines)

Other Findings

Hair shaft abnormalities or hypotrichosis: Netherton, TTD, KID, IFAP

Ocular findings: X-linked recessive ichthyosis, SLS, NLSD, TTD, KID,[§] IFAP,[§] CHH (unilateral), Refsum

Sensorineural hearing impairment: KID, NLSD > Refsum, CHH, CHILD

Neurologic abnormalities/developmental delay: SLS, NLSD, TTD, IFAP, Refsum

Severe pruritus: ichthyosis vulgaris (with atopic dermatitis), Netherton, SLS, inflammatory peeling skin syndrome

Initial Evaluation of a Neonate/Infant with a Collodion Membrane or Other Signs of Ichthyosis

- Complete blood count, electrolytes,* hepatic panel,** IgE level[†]
- Peripheral blood smear (to evaluate for leukocyte vacuoles of NLSD)
- Light microscopic evaluation of clipped hairs (scalp and eyebrows)
- ± Skin biopsy – e.g. if bullae (to assess for EI) or after resolution of collodion membrane (e.g. for TGM-1 immunostaining)
- Ophthalmologic examination, hearing screen, ± x-rays of epiphyses (if mosaic distribution, for stippling of CHH > CHILD)

[§]*Keratitis has variable onset.*
**Hypernatremic dehydration occurs primarily in collodion babies and neonates with Netherton syndrome, EI, or Harlequin ichthyosis.*
***Elevated transaminases are common in NLSD.*
[†]*Increased in Netherton and inflammatory peeling skin syndromes.*
CIE, congenital ichthyosiform erythroderma; CHH, Conradi–Hünermann–Happle syndrome; EI, epidermolytic ichthyosis; CHILD, congenital hemidysplasia with ichthyosiform nevus and limb defects; IFAP, ichthyosis follicularis with atrichia and photophobia; KID, keratitis–ichthyosis–deafness syndrome; NLSD, neutral lipid storage disease; SLS, Sjögren–Larsson syndrome; TGM-1, transglutaminase-1; TTD, trichothiodystrophy.

Table 46.1 Clues to the diagnosis of ichthyoses and erythrokeratodermas. The disorders in this table are discussed in greater detail in the text or Table 46.2. Other rare ichthyoses and related disorders can also present with these findings.

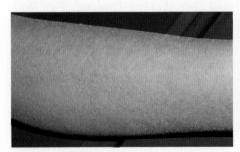

Fig. 46.1 Ichthyosis vulgaris. Fine white scales on the lower extremities. *Courtesy, Julie V. Schaffer, MD.*

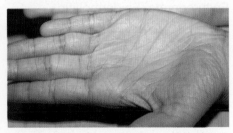

Fig. 46.2 Hyperlinear palms in ichthyosis vulgaris. *Courtesy, S. J. Bale, PhD, and J. J. DiGiovanna, MD.*

• The underlying steroid sulfatase deficiency is caused by deletion of the entire *STS* gene on chromosome Xp22 in ~90% of patients; XLRI is occasionally part of a contiguous Xp microdeletion syndrome that also includes Kallman syndrome (hypogonadotropic hypogonadism with anosmia) and X-linked recessive chondrodysplasia punctata.

• Affected neonates may have generalized exfoliation of translucent scales, followed during infancy by the development of characteristic dark brown, polygonal, adherent scales favoring the neck, preauricular area, scalp (especially in young children), extremities, and trunk; the palms, soles, and flexural sites tend to be spared (Fig. 46.3).

• Often improves substantially in the summer.

• Associated findings include a perinatal history of prolonged labor due to low placental estrogen production (frequently resulting in birth via cesaren section), cryptorchidism, and asymptomatic corneal opacities.

• Dx: fluorescence *in situ* hybridization (FISH) detects the underlying deletion in most patients; other methods include measurement of leukocyte STS activity, array comparative genomic hybridization (CGH), and molecular genetic testing.

• Prenatal findings include decreased unconjugated estriol levels in maternal serum and the presence of nonhydrolyzed sulfated steroids in maternal urine.

• **Rx:** topical humectants, keratolytics, and retinoids.

Epidermolytic Ichthyosis (EI; Bullous Congenital Ichthyosiform Erythroderma, Epidermolytic Hyperkeratosis [EHK])

• Uncommon autosomal dominant disorder due to mutations in the keratin 1 (*KRT1*) or keratin 10 (*KRT10*) gene; occasionally occurs in the offspring of an individual with an epidermolytic epidermal nevus due to a mosaic *KRT1/10* mutation that involves the gonads as well as the skin.

• Presents at birth with erythroderma, peeling skin, and erosions (Fig. 46.4A); sepsis, dehydration, and electrolyte imbalances may occur.

• Skin fragility decreases over time, with development of widespread hyperkeratosis

that forms corrugated ridges in flexures and a cobblestone pattern on extensor surfaces of joints (Fig. 46.4B–D); palmoplantar keratoderma (PPK) is seen in patients with *KRT1* mutations.

• Other manifestations include episodic blistering, secondary skin infections, and a pungent body odor.

• Characteristic histologic changes of epidermolytic hyperkeratosis (e.g. keratinocyte vacuolization and clumped keratin filaments) help to establish the diagnosis.

• **DDx:** *in neonates* – epidermolysis bullosa, staphylococcal scalded skin syndrome, other erosive disorders (see Chapter 28); *in children/adults* – superficial EI, ichthyosis hystrix of Curth–Macklin, other ichthyoses with non-scaling hyperkeratosis (e.g. Sjögren–Larsson and KID syndromes).

• **Rx in neonates:** protective isolation, emollients, and monitoring.

• **Rx in children and adults:** emollients/humectants, mechanical exfoliation of hyperkeratotic areas, antiseptic washes (e.g. dilute sodium hypochlorite baths), antimicrobial therapy for superinfections; keratolytics and retinoids (topical or oral) can improve hyperkeratosis but may lead to irritation and exacerbate skin fragility; widespread application of concentrated salicylic acid preparations should be avoided due to risk of salicylism.

• ***Superficial epidermolytic ichthyosis (ichthyosis bullosa of Siemens)*** is a related autosomal dominant condition due to mutations in the keratin 2 gene (*KRT2*), which is expressed only in the upper epidermis; affected individuals have milder, more superficial skin shedding ('molting'; Fig. 46.5), minimal erythema, and no PPK.

• ***Ichthyosis hystrix of Curth–Macklin***, which is caused by specific *KRT1* mutations, features hyperkeratosis (sometimes severe and spiky) and PPK similar to epidermolytic ichthyosis, but no skin fragility or histologic evidence of epidermolysis.

Nonsyndromic Autosomal Recessive Congenital Ichthyosis (ARCI): Lamellar Ichthyosis and Congenital Ichthyosiform Erythroderma (CIE)

• Lamellar ichthyosis and CIE exist on a phenotypic spectrum, and nonsyndromic

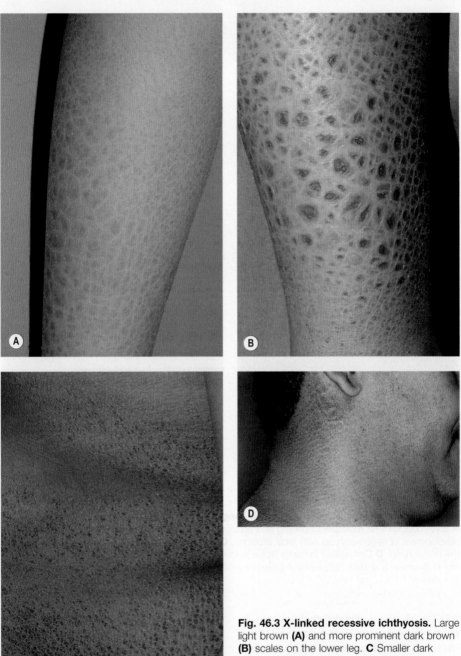

Fig. 46.3 X-linked recessive ichthyosis. Large light brown **(A)** and more prominent dark brown **(B)** scales on the lower leg. **C** Smaller dark brown scales on the trunk, with sparing of the skin folds. **D** Dark scales on the neck, sometimes referred to as a 'dirty neck.' *A–C, Courtesy, Julie V. Schaffer, MD; D, Courtesy, Gabriele Richard, MD, and Franziska Ringpfeil, MD.*

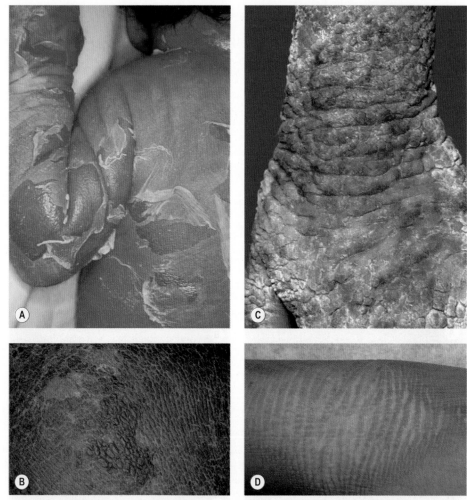

Fig. 46.4 Epidermolytic ichthyosis (bullous congenital ichthyosiform erythroderma).
A Erythroderma with widespread peeling and erosions during the neonatal period. **B** Later development of hyperkeratosis with focal erosions. **C** Hyperkeratosis with a cobblestone pattern on the dorsal hand. **D** Corrugated hyperkeratosis in the antecubital fossa. *A, B, Courtesy, Eugene Mirrer, MD; C, Courtesy, S. J. Bale, PhD, and J. J. DiGiovanna, MD; D, Courtesy, Julie V. Schaffer, MD.*

ARCI with these clinical findings can be caused by mutations in at least seven different genes, including those encoding transglutaminase 1 (*TGM1*; most common), two lipoxygenases (*ALOX12B, ALOXE3*), and an ABC lipid transporter (*ABCA12*).

Collodion Baby

• Infants with ARCI (and occasionally other ichthyoses; see Table 46.1) are often born covered by a taut, shiny, transparent membrane resembling plastic wrap, which leads to ectropion, eclabium, and distortion of the nose and ears (Fig. 46.6).

• Neonatal complications can include impaired sucking, restricted ventilation, fluid and electrolyte imbalances, skin infections, and sepsis.

• **Rx:** humidified incubator, emollients, and monitoring for complications; keratolytic agents and manual debridement of the membrane are *not* advised due to risk of systemic absorption and infection, respectively.

• Within 2 weeks, the membrane peels off in sheets and a transition to the underlying disease phenotype takes place; a subset of collodion babies with underlying mutations in *TGM1*, *ALOX12B*, or *ALOXE3* have a 'self-healing' phenotype where the skin is fairly normal in appearance when the membrane resolves.

Lamellar Ichthyosis

• Characterized by large, brown, plate-like scales with little or no associated erythema (Fig. 46.7).

• Usually generalized, although involvement is limited to the trunk and scalp in the South African 'bathing suit ichthyosis' variant (due to a particular *TGM1* mutation).

• Associated findings can include ectropion (which may result in conjunctivitis or keratitis), eclabium, scarring alopecia (especially of the peripheral scalp), PPK, nail dystrophy, and heat intolerance due to disruption of sweat ducts.

• **Rx:** oral retinoids (e.g. acitretin) for severe disease; use of topical retinoids (e.g. tazarotene) and keratolytics is limited by irritation and (for the latter agents) potential systemic absorption if applied to an extensive area;

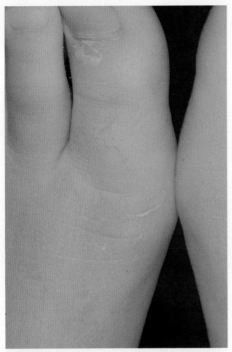

Fig. 46.5 Superficial epidermolytic ichthyosis. Increased skin markings and 'collarettes' where the skin has been superficially shed ('Mauserung'). *Courtesy, Anthony Mancini, MD.*

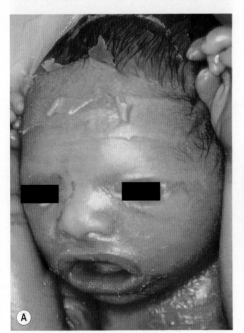

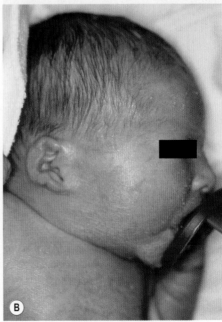

Fig. 46.6 Collodion baby. A Day 1 with ectropion and eclabium. **B** Day 8 with erythema and diffuse mild scaling and misshapen ears.

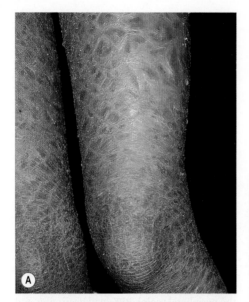

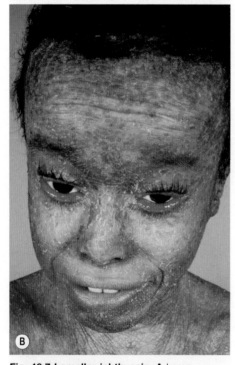

Fig. 46.7 Lamellar ichthyosis. A Large, plate-like scales on the lower extremities forming a mosaic pattern. **B** Obvious ectropion as well as plate-like scales. *A, Courtesy, Gabriele Richard, MD, and Franziska Ringpfeil, MD.*

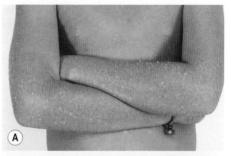

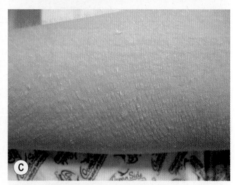

Fig. 46.8 Congenital ichthyosiform erythroderma. The differential diagnosis may include other causes of erythroderma (see Chapter 8). **A** Intense redness and fine, flaky, white scale on the trunk and arms. Close-up of fine white **(B)** and coarser yellowish **(C)** scale in a background of prominent erythema. *A, B, Courtesy, S. J. Bale, PhD, and J. J. DiGiovanna, MD.*

longitudinal ophthalmologic care can help to prevent complications of ectropion.

Congenital Ichthyosiform Erythroderma

- Characterized by erythroderma and small white scales, often with a powdery consistency, in a generalized distribution (Fig. 46.8).
- The degree of erythema and type of scale varies, and phenotypic overlap with lamellar

ichthyosis is often observed; for example, larger, darker scales may be evident, especially on the lower extremities, and some patients have relatively small scales but little associated erythema.

- PPK and nail dystrophy are frequently present, but ectropion and scarring alopecia are less common than in lamellar ichthyosis; severe exfoliative erythroderma represents a substantial metabolic stress that can result in poor growth and failure to thrive in children.
- **Rx:** similar to lamellar ichthyosis, although oral retinoids are more beneficial for scaling

than the associated erythema; increased intake of fluids, calories, and protein is required for erythrodermic patients.

Other Ichthyoses and Erythrokeratodermas

- Major features of several additional ichthyoses and erythrokeratodermas are summarized in Table 46.2 (Figs. 46.9–46.15); many other rare disorders of cornification with diverse cutaneous and extracutaneous manifestations also exist.

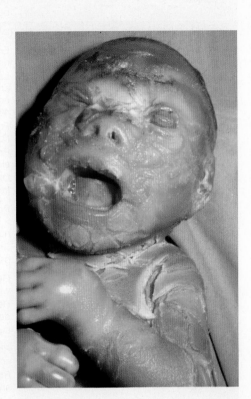

Fig. 46.9 Harlequin ichthyosis. Severe hyperkeratosis with fissuring as well as eclabion and ectropion. *Reproduced from Morillo M, Novo R, Torrelo A, et al. Feto arlequin.* Actas Dermosifiliogr. *1999;90:185–187.*

MAJOR FEATURES OF OTHER SELECTED ICHTHYOSES AND ERYTHROKERATODERMAS

Diagnosis	Gene, Inheritance Pattern	Major Features
Other Nonsyndromic Ichthyoses		
Harlequin ichthyosis	*ABCA12*, AR	• Extremely thick, armor-like plates of scale with deep fissures encase the neonate (Fig. 46.9) • Extreme ectropion, eclabium, and deformities of the ear, nose, and hands/feet • Often premature birth and neonatal death due to sepsis or respiratory insufficiency • Acitretin therapy may allow survival with a severe CIE-like phenotype
Ichthyosis en confetti	*KRT10*, AD	• CIE phenotype at birth, followed by progressive development of small 'islands' of normal skin reflecting revertant mosaicism
Syndromic Ichthyoses Presenting in the Neonatal Period		
Netherton syndrome	*SPINK5*, AR	• Erythroderma and peeling in neonates, with risk of hypernatremic dehydration and FTT • Later ichthyosis linearis circumflexa (circinate erythematous plaques bordered with double-edged scale) or a CIE-like phenotype (Fig. 46.10A–C) • Fragile hair with trichorrhexis invaginata ('bamboo hair'; eyebrow > scalp) (Fig. 46.10D) • Pruritus, eczematous dermatitis, food allergies, elevated serum IgE, recurrent infections • **DDx:** inflammatory peeling skin syndrome (corneodesmosin mutations)
Sjögren–Larsson syndrome (SLS)	*ALDH3A2*, AR	• Pruritic nonscaling hyperkeratosis (Fig. 46.11) > scaling (fine to plate-like); favors abdomen, neck, flexures • Spastic di- and tetraplegia, mental retardation, perifoveal glistening white dots
Neutral lipid storage disease with ichthyosis (NLSD)	*ABHD5*, AR	• Generalized scaling (fine, plate-like on legs) with variable erythema • Hepatomegaly, myopathy, developmental delay, hearing impairment, cataracts • Lipid-containing vacuoles in leukocytes
Trichothiodystrophy (TTD; Tay syndrome, [P] IBIDS)	*ERCC2* > *ERCC3* > *GTF2H5*, AR	• *Photosensitivity; Ichthyosis:* generalized scaling with minimal erythema beyond infancy • *Brittle hair* (tiger-tail banding, trichoschisis) and nails • *Intellectual impairment, Decreased fertility, Short stature,* cataracts (occasionally)
Refsum disease	*PHYH* or *PEX7*, AR	• Whitish scales develop on trunk and extremities in childhood or adolescence; ± PPK or hyperlinear palms • Neuropathy, cerebellar dysfunction, hypo-/anosmia, atypical retinitis pigmentosa, deafness

Table 46.2 **Major features of other selected ichthyoses and erythrokeratodermas.** *Continued*

Table 46.2 *Continued* **Major features of other selected ichthyoses and erythrokeratodermas.**

Diagnosis	Gene, Inheritance Pattern	Major Features
Syndromic X-Linked Dominant Ichthyosiform Conditions		
CHILD syndrome	*NSDHL*, X-D	• Unilateral erythematous, thickened skin with striking midline demarcation and a waxy surface or adherent scale in neonates (Fig. 46.12) • Later less erythematous and more verrucous, with affinity for skin folds • Ipsilateral skeletal abnormalities and organ hypoplasia
Conradi–Hünermann–Happle syndrome (CHH)	*EBP*, X-D	• Ichthyosiform erythroderma with feathery, adherent scale along Blaschko's lines in neonates (Fig. 46.13) • Later follicular atrophoderma along Blaschko's lines and patchy scarring alopecia • Unilateral cataracts, asymmetric skeletal abnormalities, chondrodysplasia punctata (infants)
Erythrokeratodermas		
Keratitis–ichthyosis–deafness (KID) syndrome	*GJB2*, AD	• Transient neonatal erythroderma; later well-demarcated, erythematous, furrowed hyperkeratotic plaques favoring the face and extremities (Fig. 46.14A) > diffusely thickened, grainy skin • Cheilitis, stippled PPK (Fig. 46.14B), follicular keratoses, follicular occlusion triad, cysts • Congenital sensorineural hearing impairment; progressive keratitis and conjunctivitis • Recurrent mucocutaneous infections (especially candidiasis); risk of SCC (oral and cutaneous) • DDx: *Ichthyosis Follicularis, Atrichia* and *Photophobia* (IFAP) syndrome (*MBTPS2*)
Erythrokeratodermia variabilis (EKV)	*GJB3* or *GJB4*, AD	• Transient erythematous patches (Fig. 46.15A), especially in childhood (occasionally circinate) • Fixed, geographic hyperkeratotic plaques on extremities and trunk (Fig. 46.15B); ± PPK • DDx: progressive symmetric erythrokeratoderma (no transient lesions, often affects face)

ABCA12, ATP-binding cassette, subfamily A, member 12; ABHD5, abhydrolase domain-containing 5; AD, autosomal dominant; ALDH3A2, aldehyde dehydrogenase 3A2; AR, autosomal recessive; CHILD, congenital hemidysplasia with ichthyosiform nevus and limb defects; CIE, congenital ichthyosiform erythroderma, EBP, emopamil binding protein (sterol isomerase); ERCC2/3, excision repair cross-complementing 2/3; FTT, failure to thrive; GJB2/3/4, gap junction β2/3/4 (encoding connexins 26/31/30.3); GTF2H5, general transcription factor IIH, polypeptide 5; KRT10, keratin 10; NSDHL, NAD(P)-dependent steroid dehydrogenase-like; PEX7, peroxisome biogenesis factor 7; PHYH, phytanoyl-CoA hydroxylase; PPK, palmoplantar keratoderma; SCC, squamous cell carcinoma; SPINK5, serine protease inhibitor Kazal type 5; X-D, X-linked dominant.

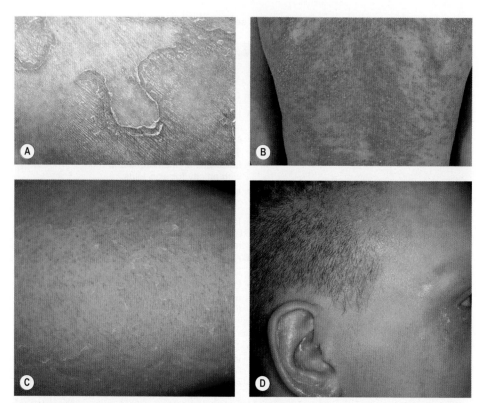

Fig. 46.10 Netherton syndrome. A Ichthyosis linearis circumflexa. Note the double-edged scale. **B** Generalized involvement with features of congenital ichthyosiform erythroderma. **C** Close-up showing 'peeling' quality of the scale. **D** Short, thin hair on the scalp, sparse eyebrows, and a lack of eyelashes. *A, Courtesy, Gabriele Richard, MD, and Franziska Ringpfeil, MD.*

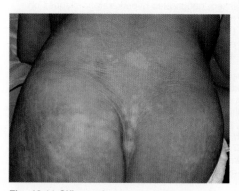

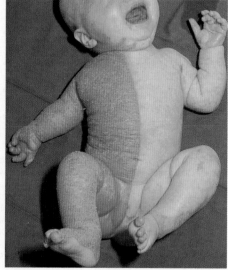

Fig. 46.11 Sjögren–Larsson syndrome. Yellowish-brown hyperkeratosis, accentuated skin markings, and areas of scaling on the lower back and buttocks. *Courtesy, Julie V. Schaffer, MD.*

Fig. 46.12 CHILD syndrome. Note the sharp midline demarcation on the trunk. *From Happle R, Mittag H, Kuster W. Dermatology 1995;191:210–216, with permission. Courtesy, Rudolph Happle, MD.*

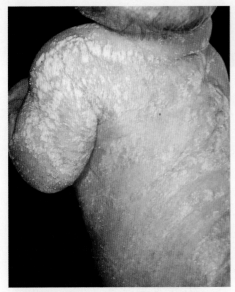

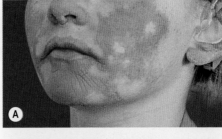

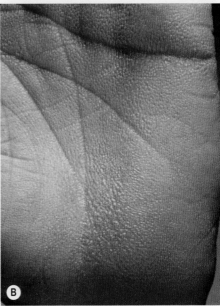

Fig. 46.13 Conradi–Hünermann–Happle syndrome. Erythroderma and linear streaks and whorls of hyperkeratosis. *Courtesy, Rudolph Happle, MD.*

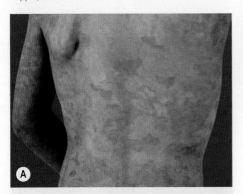

Fig. 46.14 KID syndrome. A Erythematous plaques around the mouth have characteristic radial furrows. **B** Palmar keratoderma with a grainy surface. *A, Courtesy, L. Russell, MD, and S. J. Bale, PhD; B, Courtesy, Gabriele Richard, MD, and Franziska Ringpfeil, MD.*

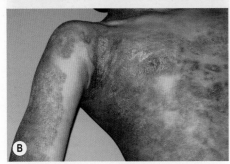

Fig. 46.15 Erythrokeratodermia variabilis. A Transient erythematous patches and generalized brownish hyperkeratosis. **B** Symmetrically distributed hyperkeratotic plaques with hypertrichosis. *Courtesy, Gabriele Richard, MD, and Franziska Ringpfeil, MD.*

For further information see Ch. 57. From *Dermatology, Third Edition.*

47 Keratodermas

- Palmoplantar keratodermas (PPKs) represent a group of hereditary and acquired disorders characterized by hyperkeratosis of the skin on the palms and soles.
- Three major types of involvement.
  - *Diffuse PPK*: confluent over the entire palmoplantar surface; onset by early childhood in hereditary forms, with initial erythema evolving into thick, yellow hyperkeratosis that may be waxy or verrucous (Fig. 47.1).
  - *Focal PPK*: primarily in areas of friction or pressure; the *areata/nummular* (oval) pattern affects the soles (Fig. 47.2A) > palms; the *striate* (linear) pattern extends from the palms to the volar fingers (Fig. 47.2B).
  - *Punctate PPK*: small (≤1 cm) keratotic papules on the palms and soles; onset is usually in adolescence or early adulthood, with initial pinhead-sized translucent papules that may become larger and callus-like (Fig. 47.3).
- Other possible features include hyperhidrosis, an erythematous border (see Fig. 47.1C), extension beyond the palmoplantar

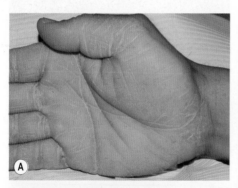
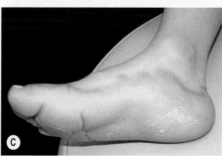
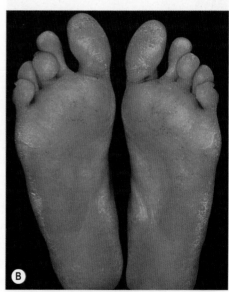

Fig. 47.1 Diffuse palmoplantar keratoderma. A Non-epidermolytic keratoderma with sharp demarcation at the wrist and side of the thumb. **B** Non-epidermolytic keratoderma with greater thickness in sites of pressure. **C** Epidermolytic keratoderma with prominent erythema at the border. In general, epidermolytic and non-epidermolytic forms cannot be distinguished clinically. *A, Courtesy, Julie V. Schaffer, MD; B, C, Courtesy, Alfons L. Krol, MD, and Dawn Siegel, MD.*

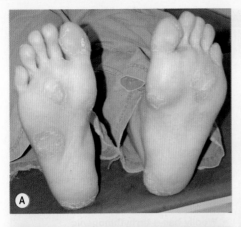

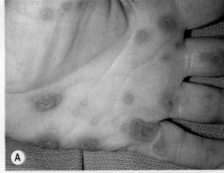

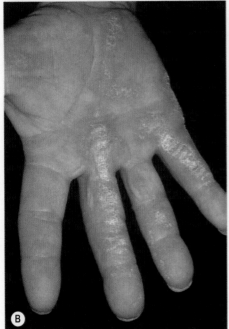

Fig. 47.3 Punctate palmoplantar keratoderma. Keratotic papules, some coalescing to form plaques, on the palm **(A)** and sole **(B)**. *A, Courtesy, Kalman Watsky, MD.*

Fig. 47.2 Focal palmoplantar keratoderma. **A** Areata type on the soles. **B** Striate type on the palm. *A, Courtesy, Alfons L. Krol, MD, and Dawn Siegel, MD.*

skin (e.g. onto dorsal hands/feet; 'transgrediens'), digital constriction bands (pseudoainhum; see Fig. 47.4B), and the histologic finding of epidermolytic hyperkeratosis ('epidermolytic PPK').

• Table 47.1 outlines major forms of PPK, either isolated or associated with additional cutaneous and extracutaneous manifestations (Figs. 47.4–47.11; Table 47.2).

• **Rx:** keratolytics (e.g. salicylic acid 4–6% in petrolatum, urea 40%), mechanical debridement, topical or oral retinoids; treatment of secondary fungal and bacterial infections.

MAJOR FORMS OF PALMOPLANTAR KERATODERMA (PPK)	
Forms with Primarily Cutaneous Manifestations	**Forms with Adnexal and/or Extracutaneous Manifestations**
Hereditary Diffuse PPK	
• **Isolated epidermolytic PPK:** *Vörner type* (AD, keratin 9 > 1) • **Isolated non-epidermolytic PPK:** *Unna–Thost type* (AD) • Other: e.g. ichthyoses and erythrokeratodermas (see Chapter 46), epidermolysis bullosa simplex (see Figure 26.3B), Mal de Meleda (malodorous transgredient PPK)	• **Deafness* + 'honeycombed' PPK** (AD, connexin 26) (Figure 47.4) • **Hypotrichosis + nail dystrophy:** *hidrotic ectodermal dysplasia (Clouston syndrome)* (Figure 47.5; see Chapter 52) • **Mutilating PPK + periorificial plaques:** *Olmsted syndrome* • **Periodontitis + psoriasiform plaques + pyogenic infections:** *Papillion–Lefèvre syndrome*
Hereditary Diffuse *or* Focal PPK (with infantile onset)	• **Woolly hair + arrhythmogenic cardiomyopathy†:** *Naxos disease* (**diffuse PPK**; AR, plakoglobin), *Carvajal syndrome* (**striate PPK**; AR >> AD, desmoplakin)
Hereditary Focal PPK	
• **Isolated striate/areata PPK:** onset usually in childhood, increased severity with repetitive friction (AD; desmoglein 1, desmoplakin, keratin 1 or 6c)	• **Hypertrophic nail dystrophy + painful areata PPK** (Figure 47.6) ± other findings (Table 47.2): *pachyonychia congenita* • **Esophageal carcinoma** (in adulthood) + **areata PPK** (Figure 47.7) + **oral leukokeratosis + follicular keratoses:** *Howel–Evans syndrome* (AD, *RHBDF2*) • **Dendritic keratitis** (in infancy) + **areata PPK** (Figure 47.8) + **mental retardation:** *Richner–Hanhart syndrome*
Hereditary Punctate PPK	
• **Isolated punctate PPK*** (AD, *AAGAB*) • **Punctate keratoses of the palmar creases*** (Figure 47.9) • **Small papules at margins of hands/feet** (Figure 47.10): *acrokeratoelastoidosis/focal acral hyperkeratosis* (AD)	• **Other:** e.g. Darier disease** (see Chapter 48), PTEN hamartoma-tumor syndrome** (see Chapter 52) • **DDx:** warts, punctate porokeratosis** (see Chapter 89), arsenical keratoses (see Chapter 74)
Acquired PPK	
• **Focal PPK on heels/weight-bearing areas of soles, especially in women > 45 years of age:** *keratoderma climactericum*; associated with obesity, cold climate, backless shoes • **DDx:** see Table 13.1 and Figure 13.1	• Associations: **hypothyroidism, cancer** (e.g. lung, GI), **drugs** (e.g. sorafenib) • **Thickening + white/translucent 'pebbling' of palms > soles upon water immersion** (Figure 47.11): *aquagenic PPK*; usually isolated, but affects >50% of cystic fibrosis patients

*Deafness + PPK may also occur in mitochondrial disorders.
†Cardiac disease usually becomes evident after puberty and can present with sudden death; desmocollin 2 mutations have also been described
**May leave a pit upon removal of the keratotic plug; DDx of palmoplantar pits also includes pitted keratolysis (see Chapter 61) and nevoid BCC syndrome (see Chapter 88).
AAGAB, α- and γ-adaptin binding protein; AD, autosomal dominant; AR, autosomal recessive; RHBDF2, rhomboid 5 homolog 2 protease.

Table 47.1 Major forms of palmoplantar keratoderma (PPK). The most common types in children and adults are shaded pink and blue, respectively. Selected genetic etiologies are in parentheses.

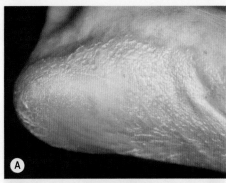

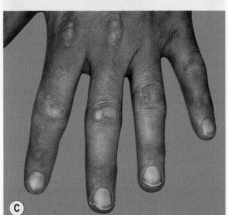

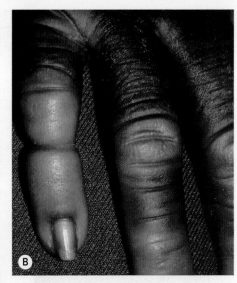

Fig. 47.4 Palmoplantar keratoderma associated with deafness due to connexin 26 mutations. A Diffuse 'honeycombed' keratoderma on the sole. **B** Pseudoainhum formation in Vohwinkel syndrome, which can also feature 'starfish' keratoses on the knuckles. **C** Leukonychia and knuckle pads in Bart–Pumphrey syndrome. *A, C, Courtesy, Alfons L. Krol, MD, and Dawn Siegel, MD.*

Fig. 47.5 Hidrotic ectodermal dysplasia (Clouston syndrome). Note the 'pebbled' skin on the dorsal aspect of the toes as well as the dystrophic nail plates. *Courtesy, D. Sasseville, MD, and R. Wilkinson, MD.*

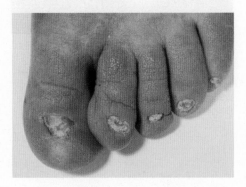

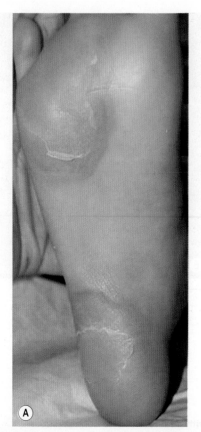

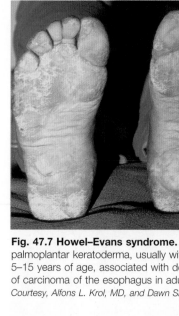

Fig. 47.7 Howel–Evans syndrome. Focal palmoplantar keratoderma, usually with onset at 5–15 years of age, associated with development of carcinoma of the esophagus in adulthood. *Courtesy, Alfons L. Krol, MD, and Dawn Siegel, MD.*

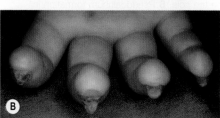

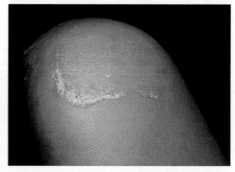

Fig. 47.6 Pachyonychia congenita. A Painful focal plantar keratoderma with associated erythema and blistering. **B** Thickening of palmar skin and hypertrophic nail dystrophy with wedge-shaped subungual hyperkeratosis. *A, Courtesy, Alfons L. Krol, MD, and Dawn Siegel, MD.*

Fig. 47.8 Richner–Hanhart syndrome (tyrosinemia II). Focal painful keratoses on the plantar surface in a patient with corneal ulcers and mental retardation. In this disorder, the onset of keratoderma ranges from early childhood to adolescence. *Courtesy, Jean L. Bolognia, MD.*

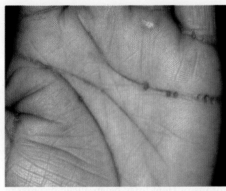

Fig. 47.9 Punctate keratoses of the palmar creases in an African-American.

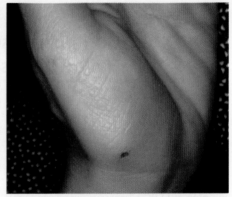

Fig. 47.10 Focal acrokeratoelastoidosis. Multiple skin-colored papules at the margin of the palmar skin.

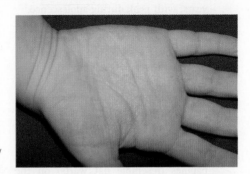

Fig. 47.11 Aquagenic keratoderma. White 'pebbly' changes on the palm following immersion in water for a few minutes in a healthy teenage girl. *Courtesy, Julie V. Schaffer, MD.*

CLINICAL FEATURES OF PACHYONYCHIA CONGENITA (PC)		
Feature	PC-6a/16 (Formerly PC-1)	PC-6b/17 (Formerly PC-2)
Painful focal palmoplantar keratoderma* (Fig. 47.6A)	++	++
Hypertrophic nail dystrophy† (Fig. 47.6B)	++	++
Oral leukokeratosis — leukoplakia	++	+
Follicular keratoses	++	++
Steatocystoma multiplex and vellus hair cysts	+ (uncommon)	++
Natal/prenatal teeth	–	+ (primarily in PC-17)
Pili torti/other hair abnormalities**	+ (uncommon)	+

*Soles (median onset at age 2 years) > palms; hyperhidrosis is common, and acral blistering may occur.
†Wedge-shaped subungual hyperkeratosis as well as thickened, omega-shaped nail plates.
**For example, coarse, brittle, and/or curly hair.

Table 47.2 Clinical features of pachyonychia congenita (PC). ++, present in majority of patients; + present in minority of patients. PC-6a/16 and PC-6b/17 are caused by mutations in the genes encoding keratin 6a or 16 and keratin 6b or 17, respectively.

For further information see Ch. 58. From *Dermatology, Third Edition.*

48 Darier Disease and Hailey–Hailey Disease

Darier Disease (Keratosis Follicularis)

- Autosomal dominant.
- Mutation in the *ATP2A2* gene causing dysfunction of SERCA2 protein, interfering with cellular calcium signaling.
- Clinical features.
    - Onset usually between ages 6 and 20 years, with peak during adolescence.
    - Chronic course, often worse in summer.
    - Crusted, pink-red to brown papules that may coalesce into plaques (Fig. 48.1) in a 'seborrheic' and sometimes intertriginous distribution (Fig. 48.2).
    - Hypopigmented macules may be the predominant feature, especially in darker skin types (Fig. 48.3).
    - Itching and malodor can be prominent.
    - Flat-topped skin-colored to brown papules (resemble flat warts) on the dorsal hands and feet (Fig. 48.4).
    - Palmoplantar keratotic papules (Fig. 48.5).
    - Nail changes, e.g. distal notching with longitudinal erythronychia (see Chapter 58).
    - Whitish papules of the oral mucosa (Fig. 48.6).
- Rare subtypes – acral hemorrhagic, segmental (see Chapter 51).
- Exacerbating factors include sunlight, heat, occlusion, sweat, bacterial colonization.
- There may be an association with neuropsychiatric disease (e.g. major depression).
- Complications include bacterial (e.g. *Staphylococcus aureus*), fungal (e.g. tinea corporis), viral (e.g. herpes simplex virus [HSV]) infections; consider Kaposi's varicelliform eruption due to HSV in a patient with sudden onset of uniform hemorrhagic crusts, fever, and malaise (Fig. 48.7).
- Histologic features – acantholytic dyskeratosis above suprabasilar clefting.
- **DDx:** mild forms – severe seborrheic dermatitis, Grover's disease; predominantly intertriginous – Hailey–Hailey disease, pemphigus vegetans, blastomycosis-like pyoderma, papular acantholytic dyskeratosis (vulvar); acral lesions – acrokeratosis verruciformis of Hopf (may be an allelic disorder or forme fruste; Fig. 48.8), flat warts, stucco keratosis, Flegel's disease.
- **Rx:**
    - General measures: lightweight clothing, sunscreen, antimicrobial cleansers, keratolytic emollients.
    - For symptomatic disease: topical retinoids ± topical CS (to decrease irritation from the former), oral retinoids (e.g. isotretinoin).
    - As-needed basis: topical and oral antibiotics and antifungals, systemic antivirals (e.g. acyclovir) for Kaposi's varicelliform eruption, destructive modalities (e.g. laser treatment) for refractory lesions.

Hailey–Hailey Disease (Familial Benign Chronic Pemphigus)

- Autosomal dominant.
- Mutation in the *ATP2C1* gene causing dysfunction of a Golgi-associated protein, interfering with cellular calcium signaling.
- Clinical features.
    - Onset in the second or third decade but sometimes delayed into the fourth or fifth decade.
    - Variable course with remissions and flares.
    - Mainly affects the major body folds (Fig. 48.2), including inframammary in women (Fig. 48.9); sometimes other sites affected (Fig. 48.10).
    - Moist, malodorous plaques, with erosions, fissures, and flaccid blisters (Fig. 48.9); circinate plaques with eroded/crusted borders (Fig. 48.10).
- Rare subtype – segmental (see Chapter 51).

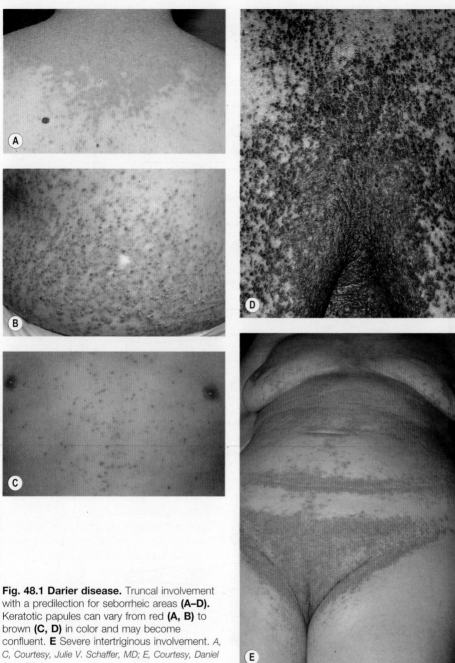

Fig. 48.1 Darier disease. Truncal involvement with a predilection for seborrheic areas **(A–D)**. Keratotic papules can vary from red **(A, B)** to brown **(C, D)** in color and may become confluent. **E** Severe intertriginous involvement. *A, C, Courtesy, Julie V. Schaffer, MD; E, Courtesy, Daniel Hohl, MD.*

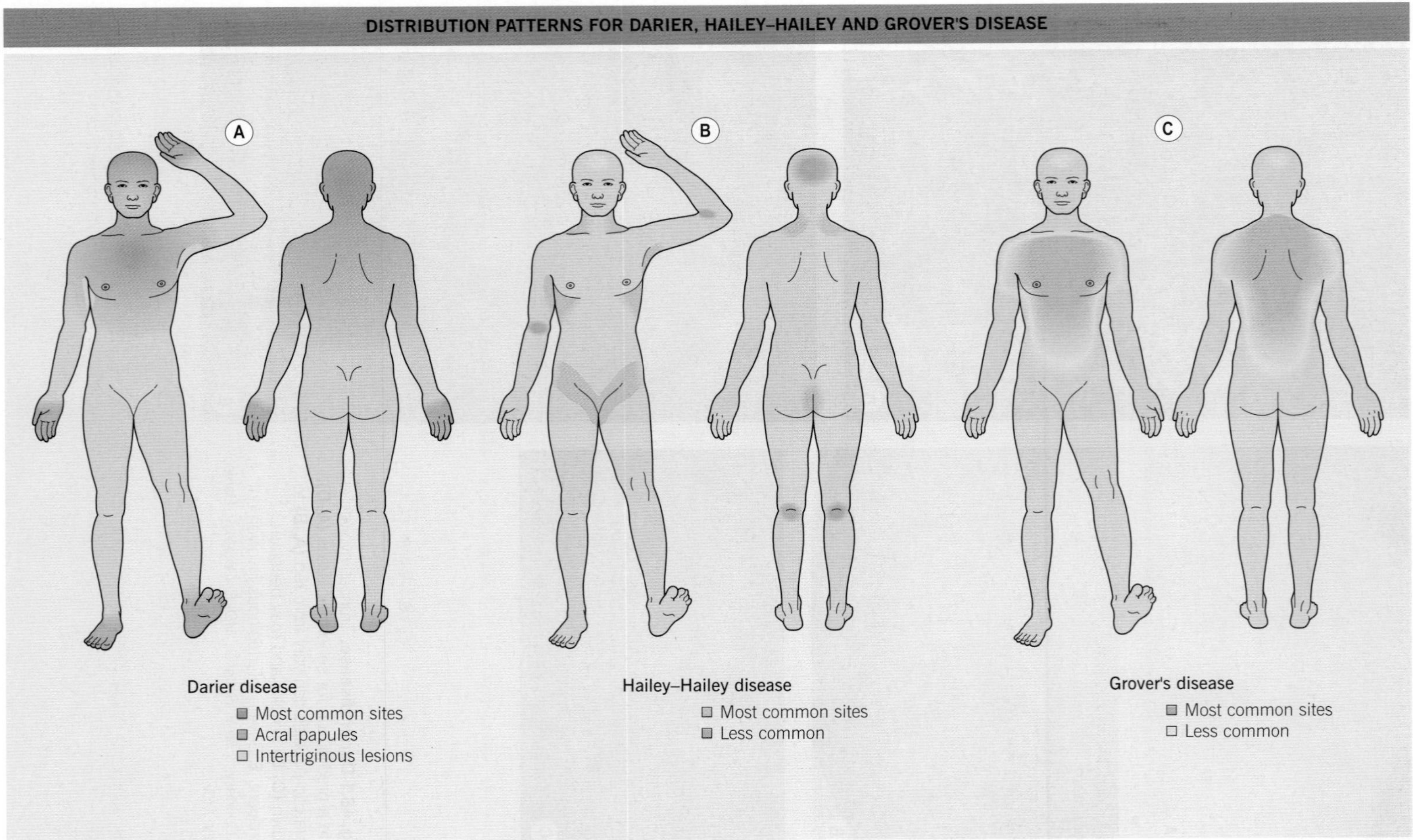

DISTRIBUTION PATTERNS FOR DARIER, HAILEY–HAILEY AND GROVER'S DISEASE

Darier disease
- Most common sites
- Acral papules
- Intertriginous lesions

Hailey–Hailey disease
- Most common sites
- Less common

Grover's disease
- Most common sites
- Less common

Fig. 48.2 Distribution patterns for Darier, Hailey–Hailey, and Grover's disease.

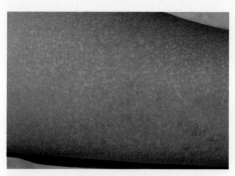

Fig. 48.3 Darier disease. Observed most commonly in individuals with darkly pigmented skin, a guttate leukoderma may be seen in patients with Darier disease, including the segmental form. *Courtesy, Julie V. Schaffer, MD.*

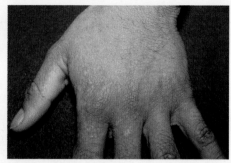

Fig. 48.4 Darier disease. Multiple flat-topped papules on the dorsal aspect of the hand. *Courtesy, Daniel Hohl, MD.*

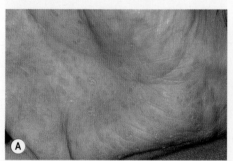

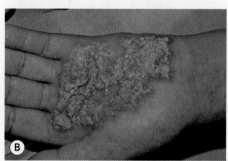

Fig. 48.5 Palmar involvement in Darier disease. A Both keratotic papules and keratin-filled depressions are seen. **B** Less commonly, a thick, spiked focal keratoderma is observed. *A, Courtesy, Kalman Watsky, MD; B, Courtesy, Julie V. Schaffer, MD.*

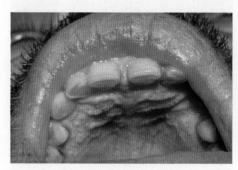

Fig. 48.6 Oral mucosal Darier disease. Whitish papules on the palate. *Courtesy, Daniel Hohl, MD.*

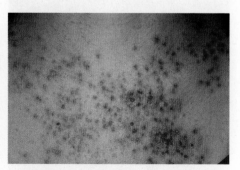

Fig. 48.7 Darier disease with superimposed HSV infection (Kaposi's varicelliform eruption). Multiple hemorrhagic crusts of a similar size are seen.

- Exacerbating factors include friction, heat, sweat, bacterial colonization, application of adhesive tape; complications the same as for Darier disease (see above).
- Histologic features – acantholysis of the majority of the epidermis.
- **DDx:** intertrigo, irritant contact dermatitis, cutaneous candidiasis, pemphigus vegetans, Darier disease.
- **Rx:**
  - General measures: lightweight clothing, antimicrobial cleansers.

  - For symptomatic disease: intermittent topical/intralesional CS.
  - As-needed basis: topical and oral antibiotics and antifungals, destructive modalities (e.g. surgical excision, laser treatment) for refractory lesions.

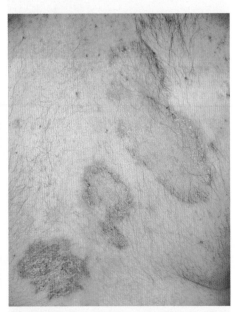

Fig. 48.10 Hailey–Hailey disease. Circinate plaques on the back with erosions and crusting in the active borders. *Courtesy, Louis A. Fragola, Jr., MD.*

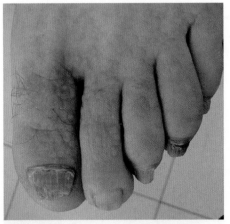

Fig. 48.8 Acrokeratosis verruciformis of Hopf. Involvement of the dorsal aspect of the foot with flat-topped papules.

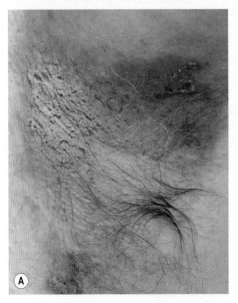

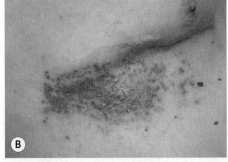

Fig. 48.9 Hailey–Hailey disease.
A Erythematous, eroded plaque in the axilla. Note the intact flaccid vesicles at 2 and 7 o'clock. **B** Chronic submammary lesion with erosions in a worm-eaten pattern.

For further information see Ch. 59. From *Dermatology, Third Edition.*

Primary Immunodeficiencies | 49

• Heterogeneous group of disorders characterized by immune system defects that result in increased susceptibility to various infections, often with additional manifestations such as autoimmunity, allergy, and risk of malignancy.

• The genetic basis has been determined for >150 primary immunodeficiencies.

• Many immunodeficiency syndromes present with dermatologic findings that can facilitate early diagnosis (Table 49.1; Figs. 49.1–49.8); these features may be divided into three categories:

   – Recurrent, severe, atypical or recalcitrant mucocutaneous infections, most often with *Staphylococcus aureus*, *Candida* spp., and human papillomaviruses.

   – Patterns of cutaneous inflammation that are shared by several immunodeficiencies, e.g. eczematous dermatitis, non-infectious granulomas, lupus erythematosus-like lesions, small vessel vasculitis, and ulcers.

   – More specific skin findings suggestive of particular disorders, e.g. oculocutaneous telangiectasias in ataxia telangiectasia and maternofetal GVHD in severe combined immunodeficiencies (SCID).

• In addition to extracutaneous infections with unusual organisms and increased frequency (e.g. pneumonia ≥2 times or otitis media ≥4 times yearly) or severity, signs of immunodeficiency in children may include

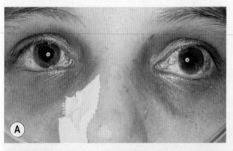
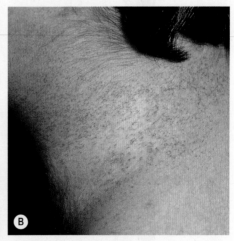
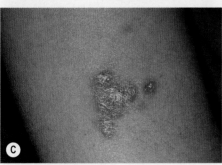

Fig. 49.1 Ataxia–telangiectasia. A Characteristic linear telangiectasias on the bulbar conjunctivae. **B** Extensive telangiectasias on the neck of a young woman. **C** Persistent granulomatous plaques on the leg of a child. These lesions often ulcerate and are difficult to manage. *A, Courtesy, Jean L. Bolognia, MD; B, C, Courtesy, Amy Paller, MD.*

425

CUTANEOUS FINDINGS IN PRIMARY IMMUNODEFICIENCY (ID) DISORDERS

Disorder	S. aureus Infections*	CMC	Warts**	Eczematous Dermatitis	Granulomas***	LE	SVV	Ulcers (PG-like)	Additional Mucocutaneous Findings	Other Major Clinical Features
Ataxia-telangiectasia (Fig. 49.1)	+			+ (facial)	+ (often ulcerates)				Oculocutaneous telangiectasias (onset age 3–6 years; favor ears, cheeks), CALMs, progeric changes	Cerebellar ataxia (onset age 1–2 years), sinopulmonary infections, leukemia/lymphoma, sensitivity to IR
Chédiak–Higashi syndrome (DDx includes Griscelli syndrome type 2; see Chapter 54)	+							+	Pigmentary dilution, hyper- or dyspigmentation in sun-exposed sites, silvery hair, gingivitis	Bleeding diathesis, lymphoproliferative 'accelerated phase,' neurologic degeneration
Chronic granulomatous disease (XR > AR) (Fig. 49.2)	++	+		+	++ (nodular, necrotic)	+		+	Sweet's syndrome, oral ulcers; DLE in female carriers	LAN (often suppurative), HSM, internal granulomas, pneumonias
CMC syndromes (Fig. 49.3)		++			(++) (candidal)				See text	See text
Complement deficiencies	+	+				++	+	+	See Table 59.3	See Table 59.3
DiGeorge (22q11.2 deletion) syndrome (Fig. 49.3D)		+		+	+				Erythroderma	Thymic hypoplasia, ↓ Ca^{+2} due to hypoparathyroidism, congenital heart defects, craniofacial anomalies
Hyper-IgE syndromes (Figs. 49.4 and 49.5)	++	+	+ (AR)	++					See text	See text

Immunoglobulin Deficiencies

						Non-infectious	Infectious
• Agammaglobulinemia (XR > AR)	+		+	+	+	Dermatomyositis-like (due to echovirus); ecthyma gangrenosum	Bacterial and viral infections (e.g. lungs, GI)
• Hyper-IgM syndromes (Fig. 49.6)	+	+	+	+	+	Oral and anogenital ulcers	Infections (e.g. lungs, GI), autoimmunity
• Common variable ID (CVID)	+	+	++	++	+	Dermatophyte infections, vitiligo, alopecia areata	Variable infections (e.g. lungs, GI), autoimmunity (e.g. cytopenias), granulomas
• IgA deficiency†	+	+	+	+	+	Vitiligo, lipodystrophy	Similar to CVID but milder
• Leukocyte adhesion deficiency (Fig. 49.7)	++ (necrotic, little pus)		++		++	Poor wound healing, delayed umbilical stump separation, gingivitis	Pneumonias > severe bacterial or fungal infections
• Severe combined ID (SCID)	+	+	+***	+	+	GVHD, erythroderma, Omenn syndrome‡	Severe infections, diarrhea, failure to thrive
• Wiskott-Aldrich syndrome (XR) (Fig. 49.8)	++		+	+		Petechiae, ecchymoses	Platelet dysfunction, sinopulmonary infections, autoimmunity, atopy, LAN, HSM, lymphoma

*Including abscesses and superficial pyoderma.

**Extensive warts are also a characteristic finding in warts, hypergammaglobulinemia, infections, and myelokathexis (WHIM) syndrome.

***Non-infectious unless otherwise noted; extensive granulomas (including destructive mid-facial lesions) are associated with hypomorphic RAG1 or RAG2 mutations.

†Prevalence of ~1:500, with clinical manifestations in only ~15% of affected individuals; profound IgA deficiency is occasionally associated with reactions to blood products containing IgA.

‡Neonatal onset of erythrodermic eczematous dermatitis, alopecia, lymphadenopathy, hepatosplenomegaly, and peripheral eosinophilia.

+, occasional finding; ++, common finding.

AR, autosomal recessive; CALMs, café-au-lait macules; CMC, chronic mucocutaneous candidiasis; DLE, discoid lupus erythematosus; HSM, hepatosplenomegaly; IR, ionizing radiation; LAN, lymphadenopathy; LE, lupus erythematosus; PG, pyoderma gangrenosum; SVV, small vessel vasculitis; XR, X-linked recessive (affects primarily boys/men).

Table 49.1 Cutaneous findings in primary immunodeficiency (ID) disorders. Infectious conditions are in darker blue shading and non-infectious conditions in lighter blue shading.

failure to thrive, chronic diarrhea, lymphadenopathy (or lack of expected lymph nodes), and hepatosplenomegaly.

• The primary feature of some immunodeficiency disorders is lymphoproliferation due to immune dysregulation (e.g. familial hemophagocytic lymphohistiocytosis,

X-linked and autoimmune lymphoproliferative syndromes), whereas others involve predisposition to a specific type of infection, such as severe mycobacterial infections with defects in the IL-12/interferon-γ axis.

• Initial laboratory evaluation for patients suspected to have an immunodeficiency is outlined in Table 49.2.

Chronic Mucocutaneous Candidiasis (CMC)

• Group of immunodeficiencies characterized by recurrent and severe infections of the skin, nails, and mucous membranes with *Candida albicans*, together with variable autoimmunity and susceptibility to other infections (see Table 49.1).

• These disorders share an underlying impairment in Th17 responses, e.g. due to autoantibodies neutralizing Th17 cytokines in APECED (see below) and mutations in the genes encoding IL-17F, the IL-17 receptor A or STAT1 (*s*ignal *t*ransducer and *a*ctivator of *t*ranscription *1*) in other forms of CMC.

• Clinical manifestations include recalcitrant oral thrush, dystrophic nails, and granulomatous plaques with scale-crust favoring the scalp, face, and skin folds (see Fig. 49.3).

• The *a*utoimmune *p*oly*e*ndocrinopathy–*c*andidiasis–*e*ctodermal *d*ystrophy syndrome (APECED) is caused by mutations (usually with autosomal recessive inheritance) in the *a*uto*i*mmune *r*egulator gene (*AIRE*), which result in failure to delete autoreactive T cells

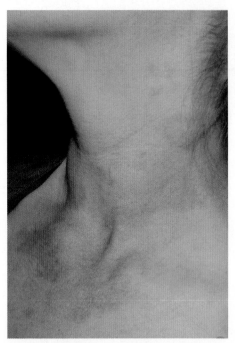

Fig. 49.2 Chronic granulomatous disease. Lupus erythematosus-like annular plaques on the neck. *Courtesy, Edward Cowen, MD.*

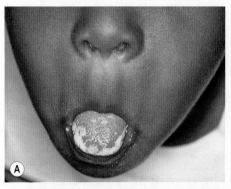

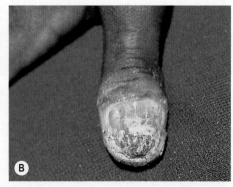

Fig. 49.3 Chronic mucocutaneous candidiasis (CMC). Non-syndromic CMC presenting as **(A)** extensive, recalcitrant thrush on the tongue of a 5-year-old child; **(B)** marked onychodystrophy with significant paronychial swelling and erythema. *A, B, Courtesy, Amy Paller, MD. Continued*

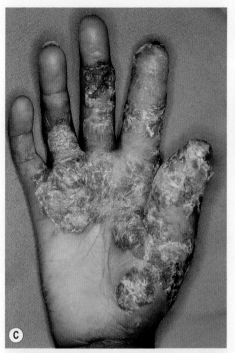

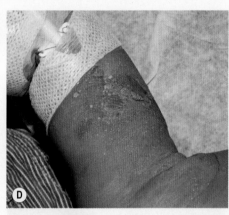

Fig. 49.3 *Continued* **C** Non-syndromic CMC presenting as crusted granulomatous plaques on the palm. **D** Recurrent cutaneous candidiasis in an infant with DiGeorge syndrome. Note the erythema, pustules, and scale-crust near the site of an intravenous line on the arm. *D, Courtesy, Julie V. Schaffer, MD.*

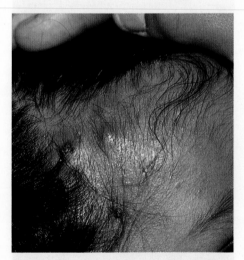

Fig. 49.4 Classic hyperimmunoglobulin E syndrome. Several mildly erythematous, slightly purulent 'cold' abscesses on the forehead and scalp of an infant. *Courtesy, Amy Paller, MD.*

in the thymus; patients present with a variety of autoimmune disorders (e.g. hypoparathyroidism, hypoadrenocorticism, alopecia areata) in addition to CMC.

Complement Disorders

• Clinical manifestations of various complement deficiencies are presented in Table 49.3.

Hyperimmunoglobulin E Syndromes (HIESs)

• HIESs feature eczematous dermatitis, recurrent staphylococcal skin (including 'cold' abscesses and impetigo) and respiratory tract infections, and markedly elevated serum IgE levels (usually > 2000 IU/ml) (see Figs. 49.4 and 49.5A).

• *Classic HIES* has autosomal dominant inheritance and is caused by mutations in the *STAT3* gene, which encodes a signaling protein that promotes production of cytokines

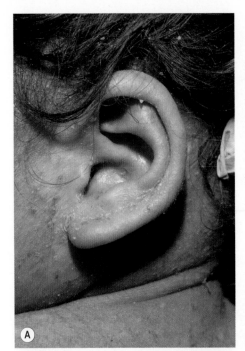

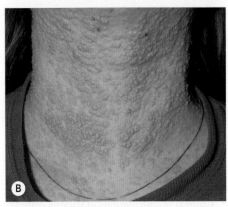

Fig. 49.5 Autosomal recessive hyperimmunoglobulin E syndrome due to *DOCK8* deficiency. A Widespread eczematous dermatitis. **B** Extensive molluscum contagiosum. *Courtesy, Edward Cowen, MD.*

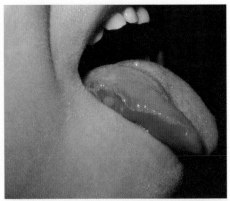

Fig. 49.6 Hyperimmunoglobulin M syndrome. Painful oral ulceration. *Reprinted with permission from Schachner L, Hansen R (Eds.).* Pediatric Dermatology, *4th edn. London: Mosby, 2011.*

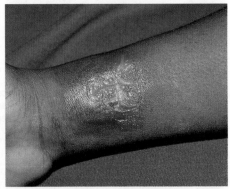

Fig. 49.7 Leukocyte adhesion deficiency type I. This 7-year-old boy was scratched by his sister, resulting in a large gaping wound that healed poorly. *Reprinted with permission from Schachner L, Hansen R (Eds.).* Pediatric Dermatology, *4th edn. London: Mosby, 2011.*

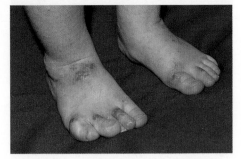

Fig. 49.8 Wiskott–Aldrich syndrome. This young boy presented with widespread, severe atopic dermatitis. Following successful treatment with hematopoietic stem cell transplantation, his dermatitis virtually cleared. *Reprinted with permission from Schachner L, Hansen R (Eds.).* Pediatric Dermatology, *4th edn. London: Mosby, 2011.*

INITIAL LABORATORY EVALUATION FOR A PATIENT SUSPECTED TO HAVE A PRIMARY IMMUNODEFICIENCY (ID)		
Test	**Potential Finding**	**Examples of Disorders Identified**
Complete blood count with differential, platelet count, and examination of smear	• Giant granules within neutrophils, ± neutropenia	• Chédiak–Higashi syndrome
	• Neutrophilia	• Leukocyte adhesion deficiency
	• Small platelets, thrombocytopenia, eosinophilia	• Wiskott–Aldrich syndrome
	• Marked eosinophilia	• Hyper-IgE syndromes • Omenn syndrome
Quantitative immunoglobulins	• All Ig ↓ • IgA ↓, IgG ↓, ± IgM ↓ • IgA ↓ or IgM ↓ • IgM ↑, other Ig ↓ • IgA ↓, IgE ↓, IgG$_{2,4}$ ↓ • IgE ↑↑ • IgM ↓, ± IgG ↓, IgA ↑, IgE ↑	• Agammaglobulinemia • Common variable ID • IgA or IgM deficiency • Hyper-IgM syndrome • Ataxia telangiectasia • Hyper-IgE syndromes • Wiskott–Aldrich syndrome
Total hemolytic complement (CH50)	• Marked ↓	• Various complement deficiencies
Nitroblue tetrazolium (NBT) reduction assay	• <10% of normal NBT reduction	• Chronic granulomatous disease
T- and B-cell analysis by flow cytometry	• Lack of T cells ± B cells	• Severe combined ID
Hair shaft examination (if silvery hair color)	• Small, regular melanin clumps	• Chédiak–Higashi syndrome
	• Large, irregular melanin clumps	• Griscelli syndrome

Table 49.2 **Initial laboratory evaluation for a patient suspected to have a primary immunodeficiency (ID).**

(e.g. IL-6, IL-10, IL-17, IL-22) important to fighting infections at epithelial surfaces and controlling inflammation.

- Usually presents in the first month of life with a non-infectious papulopustular eruption on the face, scalp, and diaper area.
- Other findings include progressive facial coarsening with pitted scarring, retention of primary teeth, a high-arched palate, osteopenia with minimal-trauma fractures, scoliosis, pneumatocele formation, and increased risk of B-cell lymphomas.
- Absent Th17 cells.

• An *autosomal recessive form of HIES (AR-HIES)* can be caused by mutations in the *dedicator of cytokinesis 8 (DOCK8)* gene.

- Characterized by severe viral (e.g. warts, molluscum contagiosum, HSV, VZV; see Fig. 49.5B) and opportunistic infections, other atopic manifestations, CNS vasculitis, and increased risk of mucocutaneous SCC as well as lymphoma.
- Decreased CD4+ T cells and low IgM levels.

• **DDx:** atopic dermatitis; Wiskott–Aldrich, Netherton, Omenn, and IPEX (*i*mmune dys*r*egulation, *p*olyendocrinopathy, *e*nteropathy, *X*-linked) syndromes.

COMPLEMENT DISORDERS

Complement Component(s)	Susceptibility to Infectious Agents	Autoimmune/Inflammatory Disorders
Classical Pathway		
C1q/r/s, C4, C2*	Encapsulated bacteria (especially *Streptococcus pneumoniae*) > *Candida* (C1q)	• **SLE:** risk with C1q (~90%) > C4** > C1r/s > C2 (~20%) – C1q/r/s or C4: often childhood onset (F = M); photosensitivity, renal disease – C2: usually adult onset (median age ~30 years; ~8 F:1 M); photosensitivity, SCLE > DLE, oral ulcers – ANA may be – or low-titer; anti-Ro/SSA usually + • Uncommon associations include dermatomyositis, Henoch–Schönlein purpura, urticaria, and atrophoderma
C1 inhibitor		• Hereditary angioedema (see Chapter 14)
Lectin Pathway		
Mannose-binding lectin (MBL)§	Encapsulated bacteria (in young children and immunocompromised individuals)	• SLE, dermatomyositis
C3 and Alternative Pathway		
C3, factor H, factor I	Encapsulated bacteria (severe for C3)	• SLE, vasculitis, partial lipodystrophy (C3), glomerulonephritis, atypical HUS • 'Leiner phenotype' (C3): erythroderma, failure to thrive, chronic diarrhea, recurrent infections
Properdin¶, factor D	***Neisseria* spp. (fulminant)**	
Membrane Attack Complex		
C5, C6, C7, C8, C9†	***Neisseria* spp. (recurrent)**	• SLE (rarely); 'Leiner phenotype' (C5)

*C2 deficiency is the most common homozygous complement disorder.
**For complete deficiency of C4A and C4B; homozygous C4A deficiency is associated with an increased (but lower) risk of SLE.
§Very low penetrance.
¶X-linked recessive, so occurs primarily in male patients.
†Prevalence of ~1:1000 in Japan; milder than other etiologies.
DLE, discoid lupus erythematosus; F, female; HUS, hemolytic–uremic syndrome; M, male; SCLE, subacute cutaneous lupus erythematosus.

Table 49.3 Complement disorders. Unless otherwise specified, refers to homozygous/biallelic deficiencies.

For further information see Ch. 60. From *Dermatology, Third Edition.*

Neurofibromatosis and Tuberous Sclerosis

50

- Neurofibromatosis (NF) and tuberous sclerosis (TS) are neurocutaneous disorders (phacomatoses) characterized by skin lesions as well as neoplasms of the central and peripheral nervous systems.
- Cutaneous manifestations (especially pigmentary findings) are often the first clinical signs of NF type 1 (NF1) and TS.
- Both disorders have autosomal dominant inheritance, although ~30–50% of patients have unaffected parents and harbor new, spontaneous mutations.
- Education of patients/parents about the condition, attention to psychosocial concerns, and genetic counseling represent important components of care.

Neurofibromatosis Type 1 (von Recklinghausen Disease)

- Incidence of approximately 1 in 3000 births.
- The *NF1* tumor suppressor gene encodes the neurofibromin protein, which negatively regulates the RAS-mitogen-activated protein kinase (MAPK) pathway that promotes cell survival and proliferation.
- Patients with NF1 have a constitutive (germline) *NF1* mutation plus a somatic 'second hit' mutation inactivating the other copy of the gene in affected tissues (e.g. Schwann cells in neurofibromas, melanocytes in café-au-lait macules [CALMs]).
- The major clinical features of NF1 are outlined in Table 50.1 and depicted in Figs. 50.1–50.5; Fig. 50.6 shows the time course of their development.
- The NIH diagnostic criteria for NF1 (Table 50.2) are met in 97% of patients by age 8 years.
- An approach to infants or young children with ≥6 CALMs is presented in Fig. 50.7.

- Comprehensive *NF1* gene analysis with ≥95% sensitivity is available; this can help to establish the diagnosis in atypical presentations or young children not yet meeting criteria.
- **DDx:** other disorders that can manifest with multiple CALMs are summarized in Table 50.3.
- Management of NF1 requires a multidisciplinary approach (Table 50.4).

Tuberous Sclerosis

- Incidence of approximately 1 in 10 000 births.
- Hamartomatous disorder caused by mutations in either the *TSC1* or *TSC2* gene; both encode proteins (hamartin and tuberin, respectively) that negatively regulate the mammalian target of rapamycin (mTOR) pathway that promotes cell growth.
- *TSC2* mutations are associated with more severe disease and are threefold more common than *TSC1* mutations in TS patients overall.
- Fig. 50.9 shows the time course for the development of cutaneous findings in TS.
- Hypomelanotic macules may be very subtle or inapparent in individuals with lightly pigmented skin, and a Wood's light can help to identify them.
- The hypomelanotic macules in TS patients vary in number (few to >100) and size (<1 to >10 cm); their shapes are polygonal more often than resembling an 'ash leaf' – rounded at one end, tapered at the other (Fig. 50.10A).
  - **DDx:** nevus depigmentosus is a common (1–5% of healthy children) cause of one or two hypopigmented macule(s) or patch(es); Fig. 50.11 presents an approach to infants/young children with ≥3 hypomelanotic macules.

MAJOR CLINICAL FEATURES OF NEUROFIBROMATOSIS TYPE 1 (NF1)

Cutaneous findings

- Café-au-lait macules (CALMs) (>90%; often evident within first year of life)
  - Tan to dark brown, uniformly pigmented macules/patches with regular borders (Fig. 50.1A–C)
  - Most patients have ≥6 by early childhood
- Axillary and/or inguinal freckling (Crowe's sign) (~80%; usually present by 4–6 years of age)
  - 1- to 3-mm brown macules, more akin to lentigines than ephelides
  - Favor intertriginous sites (Fig. 50.1B) and the neck, but may be widespread (Fig. 50.1C,D)
- *Cutaneous* neurofibromas (70–90%; typically begin to appear around puberty)
  - Skin-colored to pink-tan, soft papulonodules that invaginate with gentle pressure ('buttonhole' sign); dome-shaped, pedunculated, or barely elevated (early lesions) (Figs. 50.2 and 50.3)
  - Range from a few millimeters to several centimeters in diameter and <10 to >1000 in number
- *Plexiform* neurofibromas (PNF) (25%; congenital origin, enlarge during first 4–5 years of life)
  - Deeper nodules or masses resembling a 'bag of worms' upon palpation (Fig. 50.4)
  - May have overlying hyperpigmentation (Fig. 50.4A) ± hypertrichosis and associated soft tissue overgrowth
- Juvenile xanthogranuloma (JXG) (~15%; typically develops in first 3 years of life)
  - Pink (early) to yellow-brown papule/nodule (see Chapter 76); in NF1 patients, associated with increased risk of JMML
- Glomus tumors of the fingers and toes (see Chapter 94)

Ocular Lesions

- Lisch nodules (iris hamartomas) (>90% by 20 years of age; begin to appear at ~3 years of age)
  - 1- to 2-mm yellow-brown papules, best seen on slit-lamp examination (Fig. 50.5)

Skeletal Anomalies

- *Cranial*: macrocephaly (20–50%), hypertelorism (25%), sphenoid wing dysplasia (<5%)
- *Spinal*: scoliosis (5–10%)
- *Limbs*: cortical thinning ± pseudoarthrosis (2%; e.g. tibial bowing)

Extracutaneous Tumors

- Optic glioma (10–15%; childhood) (± precocious puberty), other CNS tumors (~5%)
- Malignant peripheral nerve sheath tumor (3–15%, peak in young adults, usually arising from a PNF)
  - Rapid growth, increased firmness, or persistent pain in established PNF; new neurologic deficit
- Other, e.g. pheochromocytoma (1%), JMML, GIST, rhabdomyosarcoma (especially GU), breast cancer

Neurologic Manifestations

- Unidentified bright objects (UBO) on MRI (50–75%)
- Learning difficulties (30–50%), ADD, mental retardation (severe in <5%), seizures (~5%)

Cardiovascular Manifestations

- Hypertension (~30%): essential > from renal artery stenosis (~2%) or pheochromocytoma (1%)
- Pulmonic stenosis (~1%), cerebrovascular anomalies (2–5%)

ADD, attention deficit disorder; GIST, gastrointestinal stromal tumors; GU, genitourinary; JMML, juvenile myelomonocytic leukemia.

Table 50.1 Major clinical features of neurofibromatosis type 1 (NF1).

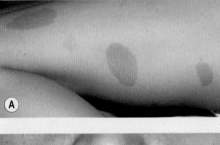

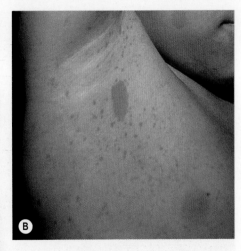

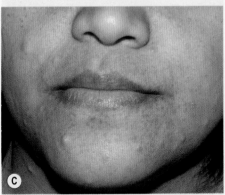

Fig. 50.1 Café-au-lait macules and 'freckling'. Oval-shaped, light-to medium-brown patches with regular borders and uniform pigmentation **(A, B)**. Numerous 1- to 3-mm lentigines are most commonly found in the axilla (Crowe's sign) **(B)** but can also develop in other sites such as the perioral region **(C)**. *A, C, Courtesy, Julie V. Schaffer, MD.*

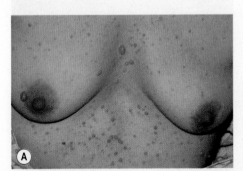

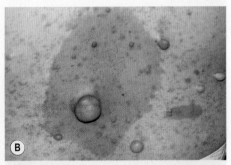

Fig. 50.2 Multiple cutaneous neurofibromas. Soft, skin-colored to pinkish tan, dome-shaped or polypoid, well-demarcated papules and nodules of various sizes **(A, B)** in patients with NF1. Neurofibromas may be superimposed on café-au-lait macules and lentigines **(B)**. *Courtesy, Julie V. Schaffer, MD.*

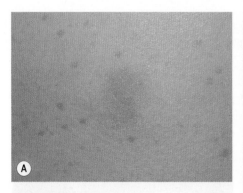

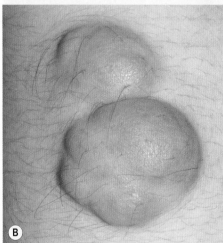

Fig. 50.3 Spectrum of cutaneous neurofibromas. Lesions range from subtle blue-red macules **(A)** to exophytic nodules with associated hypertrichosis **(B)**. *Courtesy, Julie V. Schaffer, MD.*

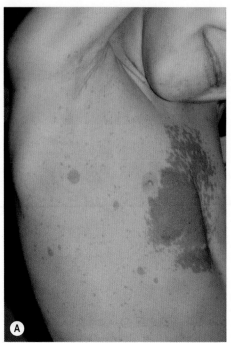

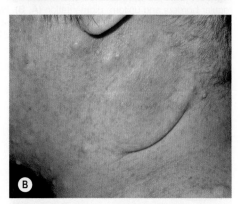

Fig. 50.4 Plexiform neurofibromas.
A A hyperpigmented plaque that may be misdiagnosed as a congenital melanocytic nevus or (if not palpated) a café-au-lait macule. Note the widespread 'freckling' on the trunk. **B** A poorly circumscribed, sagging pink mass. *Courtesy, Julie V. Schaffer, MD.*

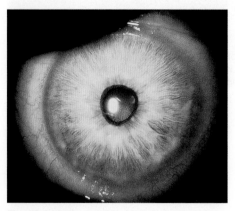

Fig. 50.5 Lisch nodules. Multiple yellow-brown papules of the iris.

DEVELOPMENT OF CLINICAL FEATURES IN NEUROFIBROMATOSIS TYPE 1

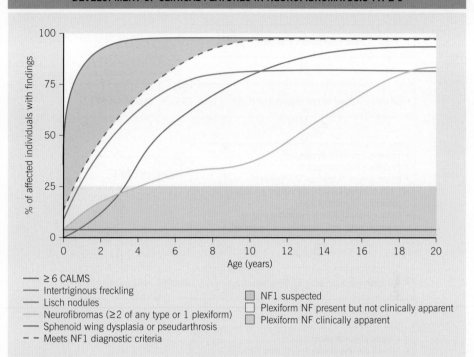

Legend:
— ≥ 6 CALMS
— Intertriginous freckling
— Lisch nodules
— Neurofibromas (≥2 of any type or 1 plexiform)
— Sphenoid wing dysplasia or pseudarthrosis
- - Meets NF1 diagnostic criteria

☐ NF1 suspected
☐ Plexiform NF present but not clinically apparent
☐ Plexiform NF clinically apparent

Fig. 50.6 Development of clinical features in neurofibromatosis type 1. The time course of major diagnostic lesions that develop in NF1. During the first few years of life, a child may have only café-au-lait macules. *Adapted from DeBella K, Szudek J, Friedman JM. Use of the National Institutes of Health criteria for diagnosis of neurofibromatosis 1 in children. Pediatrics 2000;105:608–614.*

CLASSIC DIAGNOSTIC CRITERIA FOR NEUROFIBROMATOSIS TYPE 1 (NF1)

Two or more of the following must be present:
• Six or more café-au-lait macules (>5 mm if prepubertal, >15 mm if postpubertal)
• Two or more neurofibromas of any type or one plexiform neurofibroma
• 'Freckling' in the axillary or inguinal regions
• Optic gliomas
• Two or more Lisch nodules
• Typical osseous lesion, e.g. sphenoid wing dysplasia, thinning of long bone cortex ± pseudarthrosis
• First-degree relative (parent, sibling, or offspring) with NF1 by the above criteria

Reproduced with permission from NIH Conference: Neurofibromatosis Statement. Arch. Neurol. 1988;45:575–578.

Table 50.2 Classic diagnostic criteria for neurofibromatosis type 1 (NF1).

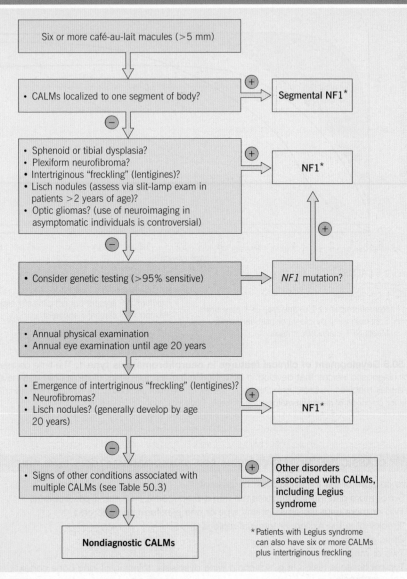

Fig. 50.7 Approach to a young child with six or more café-au-lait macules (CALMs).
More than half of these patients will eventually be diagnosed with NF1 or, less often, another CALM-associated syndrome (see Table 50.3). The latter should be considered if other signs of NF1 do not develop.

OTHER DISORDERS ASSOCIATED WITH MULTIPLE CAFÉ-AU-LAIT MACULES (CALMs)	
Disorder	**Additional Features**
Mosaic Conditions	
Segmental NF1[†]	CALMs ± 'freckling' in a segmental distribution (e.g. block-like; can also have neurofibromas (Fig. 50.8); postzygotic *NF1* mutations – if in gonads, could potentially pass on generalized NF1 to offspring
McCune–Albright syndrome	CALMs often block-like or in broad bands along Blaschko's lines with midline demarcation and irregular ('coast of Maine') borders; polyostotic fibrous dysplasia; endocrine hyperfunction (e.g. precocious puberty); activating *GNAS1* mutations (encodes $G_s\alpha$) in affected tissues
'Pigmentary mosaicism' due to chromosomal anomalies	CALMs often have irregular borders; may be segmental or follow Blaschko's lines (see Chapter 51)
Other RASopathies (Characterized by Increased MAPK Signaling)	
Legius (NF1-like) syndrome	AD; ≥6 CALMs in >80% ± intertriginous 'freckling' (~50%); *lacks* neurofibromas, Lisch nodules, and optic gliomas; often macrocephaly, learning disabilities; loss-of-function *SPRED1* mutations
Noonan syndrome*	AD; lymphedema, webbed neck; KP (atrophicans); nevi; short stature, characteristic facies, developmental delay; cardiac defects, especially pulmonic stenosis; activating mutations in *PTPN11* > *SOS1*, *RAF1* > *KRAS*, *NRAS*; Noonan-like: *SHOC12* (loose anagen hair), *CBL* (JMML)
LEOPARD syndrome	Called 'café noir' macules due to dark color; *PTPN11* mutations
Disorders Characterized by Genomic Instability	
Constitutional mismatch repair deficiency syndrome	AR; multiple CALMs, axillary freckling, neurofibromas, CNS gliomas (similar to NF1); also other malignancies (e.g. hematologic, colorectal)
Fanconi anemia* (see Chapter 55), Bloom syndrome* (see Chapter 73), ataxia telangiectasia* (see Chapter 49)	
Other Tumor Predisposition Syndromes	
Neurofibromatosis type 2*	AD; cutaneous and bilateral vestibular schwannomas; meningiomas, spinal tumors; *NF2* gene
Tuberous sclerosis*	See text
PTEN hamartoma-tumor syndrome*, MEN1*, and MEN2B* (see Chapter 52)	
Disorders of Pigmentation	
Piebaldism (CALMs in leukodermic and uninvolved skin; see Chapter 54), familial progressive hyper- and hypopigmentation (see Chapter 55)	

[†]*DDx may include a large speckled lentiginous nevus (nevus spilus) or partial unilateral lentiginosis (see Chapter 92).*
Multiple CALMs in small minority of affected individuals.
AD, autosomal dominant; AR, autosomal recessive; JMML, juvenile myelomonocytic leukemia; KP, keratosis pilaris; LEOPARD, lentigines/electrocardiogram abnormalities/ocular hypertelorism/pulmonary stenosis/abnormalities of genitalia/retardation of growth/deafness syndrome; MAPK, mitogen-activated protein kinase; NF1, neurofibromatosis type 1.

Table 50.3 Other disorders associated with multiple café-au-lait macules (CALMs). Of note, approximately 30% of the general population has at least one CALM.

EVALUATION AND MANAGEMENT OF NEUROFIBROMATOSIS 1 (NF1) PATIENTS

At time of diagnosis and annually

Dermatologic examination (especially if a plexiform neurofibroma [PNF] is present)
- Surgical consultation if painful or disfiguring neurofibromas
- PET/CT if rapid growth, increased firmness, or persistent pain in an established PNF

Neurologic examination
- MRI and/or other studies (e.g. PET/CT if related to a PNF) if neurologic signs/symptoms*

Cardiac assessment (*at initial diagnosis*) and measurement of blood pressure
- Renal arteriography and 24-hour urine collection for catecholamines and metanephrines if hypertension

At the time of diagnosis and annually, *depending on the age of the patient*

Evaluation for scoliosis and other bony defects (e.g. tibial bowing) (*annually only in children/ adolescents*)

Neurodevelopmental/behavioral evaluation (*annually only in children/adolescents*)

Ophthalmologic examination with visual assessment (*prior to 8 years of age*)
- Orbital/brain MRI if signs/symptoms of optic glioma (e.g. visual compromise, proptosis)

Assessment for precocious pubertal development (*prior to ~8 years of age*)

Measurement of head circumference (*in young children*)

Screening for breast cancer with clinical examination + mammography ± MRI (*in women, beginning by age 40 years*)

*The role of neuroimaging in asymptomatic patients is controversial.
PET/CT, positron emission tomography/computed tomography.

Table 50.4 Evaluation and management of neurofibromatosis 1 (NF1) patients.

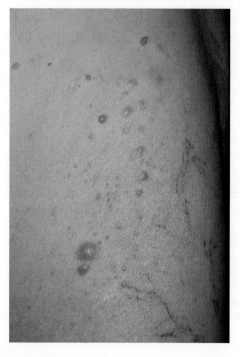

Fig. 50.8 Segmental neurofibromatosis. A cluster of soft, pink to pink-brown papules limited to the thigh. There were no associated café-au-lait macules. *Courtesy, Jean L. Bolognia, MD.*

DEVELOPMENT OF CUTANEOUS FEATURES IN TUBEROUS SCLEROSIS

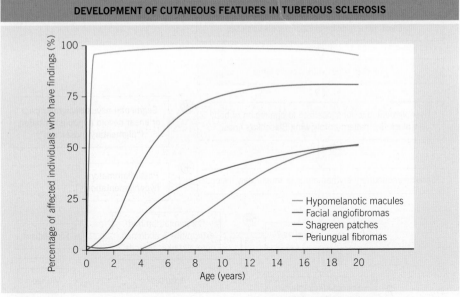

Legend:
- Hypomelanotic macules
- Facial angiofibromas
- Shagreen patches
- Periungual fibromas

y-axis: Percentage of affected individuals who have findings (%)
x-axis: Age (years)

Fig. 50.9 Development of cutaneous features in tuberous sclerosis. Hypomelanotic macules are usually the only cutaneous finding at birth.

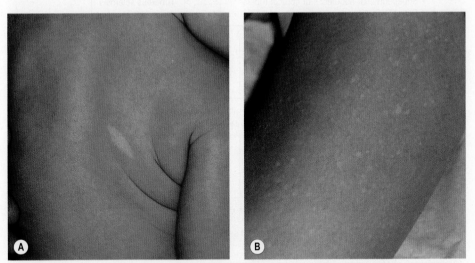

Fig. 50.10 Hypopigmentation in tuberous sclerosis. A Ash leaf macule. **B** 'Confetti' macules of guttate leukoderma. *B, Courtesy, Jean L. Bolognia, MD.*

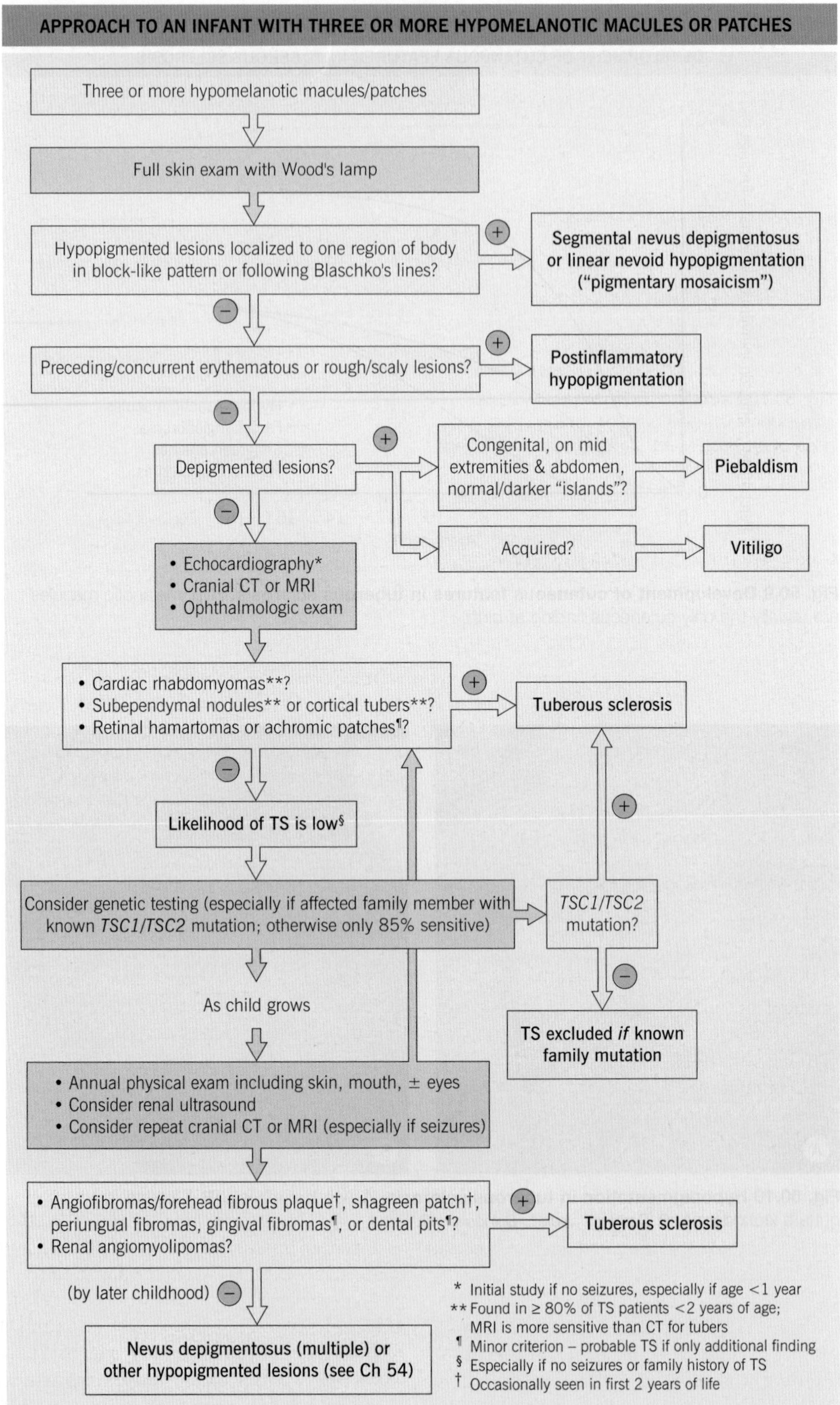

Fig. 50.11 Approach to an infant with three or more hypomelanotic macules or patches. A child with fewer than three macules and no family history of tuberous sclerosis (TS) has an extremely low likelihood of having this disease.

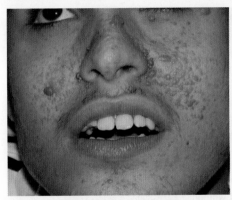

Fig. 50.12 Facial angiofibromas. Multiple shiny, dome-shaped papules on the cheeks and nose of an adolescent. *Courtesy, Julie V. Schaffer, MD.*

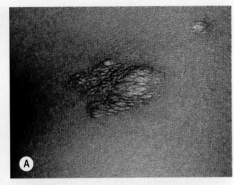

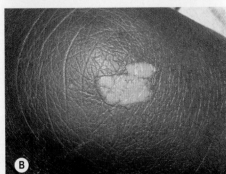

Fig. 50.14 Connective tissue nevi (shagreen patches) in tuberous sclerosis. These plaques can be hyperpigmented **(A)** or hypopigmented **(B)** relative to the patient's background skin. The surface is said to resemble leather or pigskin.
B, Courtesy, Julie V. Schaffer, MD.

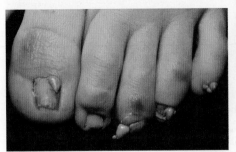

Fig. 50.13 Periungual fibromas of tuberous sclerosis. Multiple fibromas of the toes arising in a periungual location.

• Numerous small, confetti-like hypopigmented macules (especially on the extremities) represent a relatively specific finding for TS (Fig. 50.10B).

• Angiofibromas (formerly known as 'adenoma sebaceum') are smooth, dome-shaped, pink to red-brown papules (Fig. 50.12); they favor the central face and sometimes coalesce to form plaques.

  – **DDx:** multiple facial angiofibromas can occur in multiple endocrine neoplasia type 1 (MEN1) and Birt–Hogg–Dubé syndrome (see Chapter 91).

• Variants of angiofibromas include cephalic fibrous plaques (e.g. on forehead), ungual fibromas (Koenen tumors; toes > fingers) (Fig. 50.13), and molluscum pendulum (resembling large skin tags) in flexural sites.

• Shagreen patches are connective tissue nevi with a predilection for the lower back; they present as skin-colored, hyperpigmented or (less often) hypopigmented plaques with an uneven, pigskin-like surface (Fig. 50.14).

• Infantile spasms affect ~70% of TS patients, typically beginning at 3–6 months of age; mental deficiency and neuropsychiatric conditions (e.g. autism, attention deficit disorder) are common.

• Additional extracutaneous manifestations and diagnostic criteria are listed in Table 50.5.

• Recommendations for evaluation and management are presented in Table 50.6.

• **Rx:** systemic administration of mTOR inhibitors (rapamycin [sirolimus], everolimus) for astrocytomas, renal angiomyolipomas, and pulmonary lymphangioleiomyomas; topical rapamycin, lasers (pulsed dye or ablative), and electrosurgery to treat angiofibromas.

REVISED CRITERIA FOR TUBEROUS SCLEROSIS COMPLEX

Major Features

Hypomelanotic macules (≥3, each ≥5 mm in diameter) (≥90%)

Facial angiofibromas (≥3) (~80%) or fibrous cephalic plaque (~20%)

Nontraumatic ungual fibromas (≥2) (30–60%)

Shagreen patch (40–50%)

Multiple retinal nodular hamartomas (~40%)

Cortical dysplasias* (>90%), subependymal nodules (>80%), subependymal giant cell astrocytoma

Renal angiomyolipomas (≥2) (75–90%)

Cardiac rhabdomyoma (~80% during infancy, with subsequent involution)

Pulmonary lymphangioleiomyomatosis (~30% of women)

Minor Features

'Confetti' hypopigmented skin lesions (~5%)

Dental enamel pits (≥3) (>90%)

Intraoral fibromas (≥2) (up to 70%)

Retinal achromic patch (~40%)

Multiple renal cysts

Nonrenal hamartomas

Definite clinical diagnosis
- Either two major features† *or* one major feature plus two minor features

Possible clinical diagnosis
- One major feature or two minor features

Definite genetic diagnosis
- Identification of a pathogenic mutation in either *TSC1* or *TSC2* in DNA from normal tissue**

Including tubers and white matter radial migration lines.
†*With the exception of lymphangioleiomyomatosis plus angiomyolipomas.*
**10–25% of patients with TSC have no identifiable mutation, so a normal result does not exclude TSC unless there is a known pathogenic mutation in an affected relative.*

Table 50.5 Revised diagnostic criteria for tuberous sclerosis complex. In contrast to NF1, café-au-lait macules are found in a minority of patients and are usually few in number. Green background = cutaneous lesions.

EVALUATION AND MANAGEMENT OF TUBEROUS SCLEROSIS PATIENTS

Neurodevelopmental/behavioral evaluation (especially for children): *at diagnosis, at school entry, and if educational/behavioral concerns*

Ophthalmologic examination: *at diagnosis*

Cranial CT or MRI*: *at diagnosis and every 1–3 years during childhood/adolescence*

Electroencephalogram (EEG): *at diagnosis if history of seizures; later if seizures or cognitive decline*

Electrocardiogram (ECG)†: *at diagnosis*; echocardiography *if cardiac symptoms or ECG abnormalities*

Renal ultrasonography: *at diagnosis to detect polycystic kidney disease, every 1–3 years if no renal lesions, twice yearly if angiomyolipomas¶*

Chest CT to assess for lymphangioleiomyomatosis: *in adult women at diagnosis and if pulmonary symptoms develop*

Findings may correlate with seizure activity and cognitive deficits; assess for enlarging lesions suggestive of giant cell astrocytomas (most common during childhood).
†*Arrhythmias are more common in patients with TS than the general population.*
¶*Angiomyolipomas >3.5–4 cm in diameter should be assessed with CT or MRI.*

Table 50.6 Evaluation and management of tuberous sclerosis patients.

For further information see Ch. 61. From *Dermatology, Third Edition*.

Mosaic Skin Conditions   51

- A mosaic organism is composed of ≥2 genetically distinct cell populations derived from a homogeneous zygote.
  - *Genomic mosaicism* results from alteration in the DNA sequence (affecting genes or chromosomes).
  - *Functional (epigenetic) mosaicism* results from changes in gene expression (but not the DNA sequence) that are passed on during cellular replication; an important example is *lyonization* in female embryos, where random inactivation of one of the two X chromosomes occurs in each cell during early development.
- Clinical findings in mosaic skin conditions depend not only on the underlying genetic alteration but also on the timing of its origin (with earlier onset generally leading to more widespread involvement) and the cells or tissues affected (cutaneous ± extracutaneous).
  - For example, mosaicism for an activating *HRAS* mutation can produce the combination of a nevus sebaceus (keratinocytes affected), speckled lentiginous nevus (melanocytes affected), and occasionally CNS abnormalities (nerve cells affected) in patients with phakomatosis pigmentokeratotica, a form of 'twin spotting'.
- The accessibility of the skin allows visualization of mosaic patterns.
  - *Blaschko's lines* are streaks and swirls that represent pathways of epidermal cell (e.g. keratinocyte or melanocyte) migration during embryonic development (Fig. 51.1).
  - Block-like, segmental, and dermatomal patterns can also reflect cutaneous mosaicism, typically involving melanocytes, mesodermal cells, and nerve cells, respectively.
- Types of cutaneous lesions that can follow Blaschko's lines or have a block-like/segmental pattern are outlined in Tables 51.1 and 51.2, respectively (Fig. 51.2).
- In *chimerism*, different cell populations reflect a genetically heterogeneous zygote (e.g. fusion of two zygotes or fertilization of one egg by two sperm); this may manifest with a block-like, linear, or irregular pattern of pigmentary variation.

Epidermal Nevi and 'Epidermal Nevus Syndromes'

- Epidermal nevi (see Chapter 89) present as streaks and swirls of thickened (e.g. verrucous, hyperkeratotic, or velvety) skin along Blaschko's lines, usually with hyperpigmentation and sometimes with adnexal involvement (e.g. in a nevus sebaceus or nevus comedonicus) (Fig. 51.3).
- The heterogeneous genetic etiologies and potential systemic associations ('epidermal nevus syndromes') of various types of epidermal nevi are presented in Table 51.3 (Fig. 51.4).

Mosaicism in Autosomal Dominant Skin Conditions

- When evaluating a patient with skin lesions in a mosaic pattern, it can be helpful to consider whether the findings would resemble an autosomal dominant genodermatosis if present in a more generalized distribution.
- Type 1, type 2, and revertant forms of mosaicism occurring in autosomal dominant skin disorders are summarized in Fig. 51.5.

BLASCHKO'S LINES

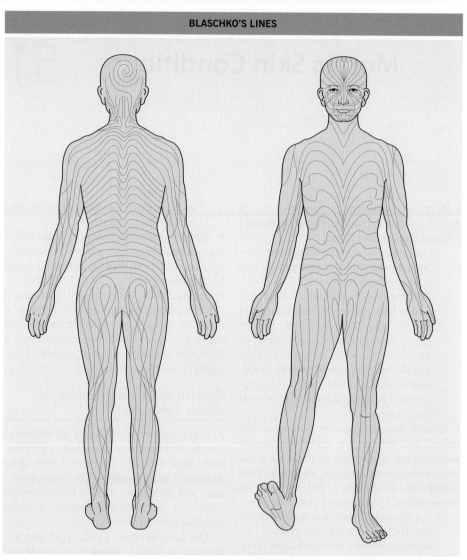

Fig. 51.1 Blaschko's lines. Note the S-shape of lines on the abdomen, the V-shape on the central back, perpendicular lines on the face, and swirls on the posterior scalp.

SKIN FINDINGS THAT CAN OCCUR ALONG BLASCHKO'S LINES	
Inflammation	
Examples	*Clinical Clues*
Lichen striatus	• Pink to hypopigmented flat-topped papules; common in children (see Chapter 9)
Linear lichen planus (Fig. 51.2A)	• Violaceous flat-topped papules with Wickham's striae; often in adults
'Blaschkitis'	• Pruritic erythematous papulovesicles in multiple streaks on the trunk; usually develops in adults and often recurs

Table 51.1 Skin findings that can occur along Blaschko's lines. *Continued*

Table 51.1 *Continued* **Skin findings that can occur along Blaschko's lines.**

Inflammation	
Examples	*Clinical Clues*
Inflammatory linear verrucous epidermal nevus (ILVEN) (Fig. 51.2B)	• Scaly, erythematous psoriasiform plaques with prominent pruritus and lack of response to therapy; onset usually by childhood
Linear psoriasis (Fig. 51.2C)	• Psoriasiform plaques, often responding to therapy; ± psoriasis elsewhere

Other conditions resembling lichen planus: linear GVHD, lupus erythematous > dermatomyositis, drug eruptions

Other conditions with a keratotic and/or vesiculobullous component:
• Variable onset: linear Darier (Fig. 51.2D) and Hailey–Hailey (Fig. 51.2E) diseases
• Early onset: linear porokeratosis (see Fig. 89.7E), PEODDN, IP* stages 1–2 (see Figs. 28.9 and 51.7A), epidermolytic epidermal nevus*, Conradi–Hünermann–Happle syndrome* (see Fig. 46.13)

Verrucous lesions – e.g. epidermal/sebaceous nevi (Table 51.3; Fig. 51.3), IP stage 2 (Fig. 51.7A,B)

Spines/comedones – e.g. nevus comedonicus (Table 51.3), PEODDN (favors palms/soles), linear lichen planopilaris (later onset; see Fig. 9.4H)

Hypopigmentation (see Table 54.3)

Hyperpigmentation (see Table 55.4)

Hairlessness – e.g. X-linked hypohidrotic ectodermal dysplasia (female 'carriers'; Fig. 51.6), Goltz syndrome, IP stage 4 (Fig. 51.7C)

Atrophy – e.g. linear lichen sclerosus (epidermal wrinkling), linear atrophoderma of Moulin (hyperpigmented and depressed), Goltz syndrome (Fig. 51.8A,B), IP stage 4, Conradi– Hünermann–Happle syndrome (follicular atrophoderma)

Papulonodular lesions** – e.g. adnexal neoplasms (e.g. trichoepitheliomas), BCCs, basaloid follicular hamartomas

*Inflammatory manifestations occur primarily during infancy.
**In addition to conditions with inflammatory or verrucous papulonodules noted above.
GVHD, graft-versus-host disease; IP, incontinentia pigmenti; PEODDN, porokeratotic eccrine ostial and dermal duct nevus.*

SKIN FINDINGS THAT CAN HAVE A BLOCK-LIKE OR SEGMENTAL PATTERN THAT REFLECTS MOSAICISM
Hypopigmentation – e.g. nevus depigmentosus, segmental vitiligo (see Chapter 54)
Hyperpigmention ± hypertrichosis – e.g. CALM, Becker's nevus/smooth muscle hamartoma (see Table 50.3 and Chapter 55)
Hypertrichosis – e.g. X-linked congenital generalized hypertrichosis (female 'carriers')
Vascular lesions – e.g. port wine stain,† CMTC, unilateral nevoid telangiectasia, venous malformation,* plaque-type glomuvenous malformation,** segmental infantile hemangioma (see Chapter 85)
Papulonodular lesions – e.g. segmental leiomyomas** or neurofibromas**

*†Associated with mosaic activating mutations in the GNAQ gene encoding the Q-class G protein α-subunit; mutations in this gene have also been associated with dermal melanocytosis, which occurs as 'twin spots' with port wine stains in phakomatosis pigmentovascularis.
*Type 1 segmental manifestation of an autosomal dominant disorder (Fig. 51.5).
**Type 2 segmental manifestation of an autosomal dominant disorder (Fig. 51.5).
CALM, café-au-lait macule; CMTC, cutis marmorata telangiectatica congenita.*

Table 51.2 Skin findings that can have a block-like or segmental pattern that reflects mosaicism.

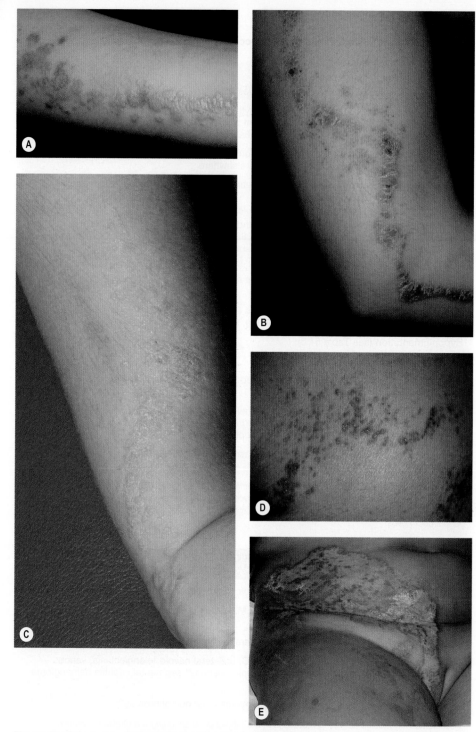

Fig. 51.2 Inflammatory lesions along Blaschko's lines. A Linear lichen planus presenting as a band of coalescing violaceous papules and plaques with Wickham's striae on an extremity. Note the postinflammatory hyperpigmentation proximally. **B** Inflammatory linear verrucous epidermal nevus (ILVEN) featuring persistent, extremely pruritic, scaly psoriasiform plaques. **C** Linear psoriasis with erythema and scale that responded to treatment with a high-potency topical CS. **D** Linear Darier disease presenting with keratotic papules in an adult, representing type 1 mosaicism (see Fig. 51.5A). **E** Linear Hailey–Hailey disease presenting with recurrent blistering and erosions in a young girl, representing type 2 mosaicism with earlier and more severe involvement in the affected region due to a 'second hit' mutation (see Fig. 51.5B). *A, Courtesy, Joyce Rico, MD; C, E, Courtesy, Julie V. Schaffer, MD.*

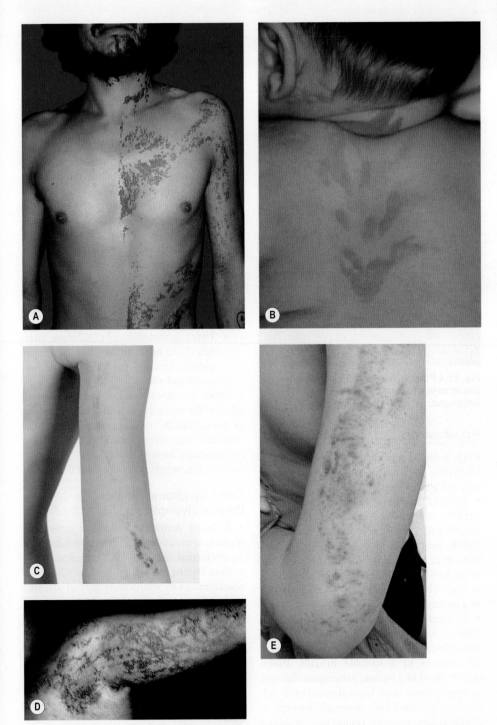

Fig. 51.3 Epidermal nevi. A Extensive lesion with especially verrucous areas on the neck. **B** V-shaped pattern on the mid back. **C** Lesion due to a *FGFR3* mutation, representing a mosaic counterpart of the acanthosis nigricans in thanatophoric dysplasia, an autosomal dominant neuroskeletal syndrome. This explains the flexural accentuation of the epidermal nevus. **D** Epidermolytic epidermal nevus. Note the shedding of scale and associated hypopigmentation. **E** Nevus comedonicus with inflammatory papulonodules as well as comedones in an adolescent. The lesion initially presented as a congenital hypopigmented streak. *C, Courtesy, Celia Moss, MD; E, Courtesy, Julie V. Schaffer, MD.*

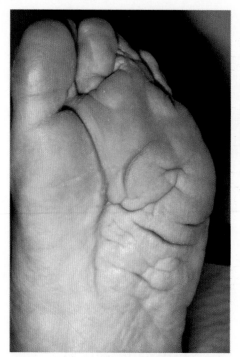

Fig. 51.4 Plantar cerebriform connective tissue nevus in a man with Proteus syndrome. *Courtesy, Odie Enjolras, MD.*

Mosaicism in X-Linked Conditions

• In X-linked disorders, functional mosaicism due to lyonization occurs in female patients and carriers.

• *X-linked dominant* conditions are typically lethal in male embryos and are therefore seen almost exclusively in a mosaic pattern in female patients with a heterozygous mutation; male patients occasionally survive due to underlying mosaicism, e.g. in the setting of Klinefelter syndrome (47,XXY karyotype) or a postzygotic mutation.

• In conditions traditionally referred to as *X-linked recessive*, male patients have generalized disease and female patients or 'carriers' are affected to a variable (usually lesser) degree, often in a mosaic pattern; an example is hypohidrosis and hyperpigmentation following Blaschko's lines in female 'carriers' of X-linked hypohidrotic ectodermal dysplasia (Fig. 51.6).

Incontinentia Pigmenti (IP)

• X-linked dominant disorder caused by mutations in the NF-κB essential modulator (*NEMO*)

gene, which encodes a protein that protects against TNF-α-induced apoptosis; male patients with milder *NEMO* mutations may present with hypohidrotic ectodermal dysplasia with immune deficiency (see Table 52.5).

• IP has four stages, which may be absent or overlapping, of cutaneous findings that follow Blaschko's lines (with the exception of stage 4) (Fig. 51.7; see Fig. 28.9):

- *Vesicular* streaks favoring the extremities and scalp in neonates, often associated with peripheral blood leukocytosis and eosinophilia; may recur during childhood febrile illnesses.
- *Verrucous* linear plaques favoring the extremities in infants; acral keratotic nodules sometimes develop after puberty.
- *Hyperpigmented* grayish-brown streaks and swirls favoring the trunk and intertriginous areas from infancy through adolescence.
- *Hypopigmented/atrophic* 'Chinese character'-like bands lacking hair and sweat glands, favoring the calves in adolescents and adults.

• Other manifestations can include alopecia (often at the vertex in a swirled pattern), missing or conical teeth, retinal vascular anomalies (requires monitoring with ophthalmologic examinations during infancy), and CNS abnormalities (e.g. seizures, developmental delay).

Goltz Syndrome (Focal Dermal Hypoplasia)

• X-linked dominant condition caused by mutations in the *PORCN* gene, which encodes a protein that regulates Wnt signaling.

• Skin lesions following Blaschko's lines are characterized by vermiculate dermal atrophy, outpouchings of fat, telangiectasias, and hypo- > hyperpigmentation (Fig. 51.8).

• Additional features include periorificial raspberry-like papillomas, dystrophic nails, sparse hair, abnormal teeth, split hand/foot ('lobster claw') malformations, ocular abnormalities (e.g. microphthalmia), and the radiographic finding of osteopathia striata in long bones.

X-Linked Dominant Ichthyosiform Conditions

• Examples include congenital hemidysplasia with ichthyosiform nevus and limb defects

VARIANTS OF EPIDERMAL NEVI (EN) AND POSSIBLE ASSOCIATED FINDINGS

Type of EN	Features of the EN	Gene(s)	Corresponding AD Condition(s) [Type of Mosaicism (See Fig. 51.5)]	Possible Associated Features
Keratinocytic EN (non-epidermolytic) (Fig. 51.3A-C)	Velvety or papillomatous to thin keratotic plaques; often more pronounced in body folds	*FGFR3* or *HRAS* > *PIK3CA*,* *NRAS* or *KRAS*	*FGFR3*: thanatophoric dysplasia (with acanthosis nigricans) [1] *RAS* genes**: Costello (with acanthosis nigricans), Noonan and cardiofaciocutaneous syndromes [1]	*FGFR3* or *RAS* genes: craniofacial/skeletal and CNS anomalies *PIK3CA*: CLOVES, M-CM, lipomatosis Risk of bladder carcinoma and (for *RAS* genes) rhabdomyosarcoma
Nevus sebaceus (see Chapter 91)	Waxy, hairless yellow-orange plaques that become verrucous at puberty; favors head and neck	*HRAS** > *KRAS**	None – lethal mutations rescued by mosaicism	*Schimmelpenning syndrome*: CNS, ocular and skeletal anomalies *Phakomatosis pigmentokeratotica* (HRAS): SLN; occasionally neurologic abnormalities, hypophosphatemic vitamin D-resistant rickets
Epidermolytic EN (Fig. 51.3D)	Verrucous keratotic plaques with epidermolytic hyperkeratosis histologically; may be spiny or have shedding of scale; ± palmoplantar involvement (especially with *KRT1*)	*KRT1* or *KRT10*	Epidermolytic ichthyosis [1]	None; affected individuals (presumably with mosaicism involving their gonads) occasionally have offspring with generalized epidermolytic ichthyosis

Table 51.3 Variants of epidermal nevi (EN) and possible associated findings. *Continued*

Table 51.3 *Continued* **Variants of epidermal nevi (EN) and possible associated findings.**

Type of EN	Features of the EN	Gene(s)	Corresponding AD Condition(s) [Type of Mosaicism (See Fig. 51.5)]	Possible Associated Features
PTEN ('Cowden') nevus	Thick, rough, papillomatous plaques (similar appearance to keratinocytic EN)	*PTEN*	Cowden disease/PTEN hamartoma–tumor syndrome [2]	Segmental overgrowth, *lipomas*, arteriovenous malformations, EN (SOLAMEN); macrocephaly; later features of Cowden disease (see Chapter 52)
Proteus syndrome	Thin plaques (similar appearance to keratinocytic EN)	*AKT1**	None – lethal mutations rescued by mosaicism	Progressive, asymmetric, disproportionate overgrowth; cerebriform connective tissue nevi on palms/soles (Fig. 51.4), vascular malformations, dysregulated adipose tissue
Nevus comedonicus/ acneiform nevus	Comedones ± inflammatory acne lesions, often with hypopigmented background	*FGFR2*	Apert syndrome (with widespread, severe, early onset acne) [1]	Skeletal and CNS anomalies
ILVEN (Fig. 51.2B)	Intensely pruritic, recalcitrant psoriasiform plaques	?	?	Limb reductions

*The underlying mosaic mutations are generally not compatible with life if present in all the cells of the body.
**Usually but not always different (e.g. more severe) mutations within the EN than in the AD disorder.
AD, autosomal dominant; CLOVES, congenital lipomatous overgrowth with vascular, epidermal, and skeletal anomalies; FGFR, fibroblast growth factor receptor; ILVEN, inflammatory linear verrucous epidermal nevus; KRT, keratin; M-CM, megalencephaly (macrocephaly)–capillary malformation syndrome; PIK3CA, phosphoinositide-3-kinase, catalytic α-polypeptide; SLN, speckled lentiginous nevus.

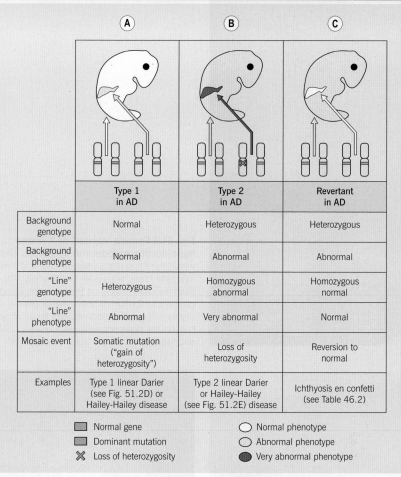

	Type 1 in AD	Type 2 in AD	Revertant in AD
Background genotype	Normal	Heterozygous	Heterozygous
Background phenotype	Normal	Abnormal	Abnormal
"Line" genotype	Heterozygous	Homozygous abnormal	Homozygous normal
"Line" phenotype	Abnormal	Very abnormal	Normal
Mosaic event	Somatic mutation ("gain of heterozygosity")	Loss of heterozygosity	Reversion to normal
Examples	Type 1 linear Darier (see Fig. 51.2D) or Hailey-Hailey disease	Type 2 linear Darier or Hailey-Hailey (see Fig. 51.2E) disease	Ichthyosis en confetti (see Table 46.2)

▨ Normal gene	◯ Normal phenotype
▨ Dominant mutation	◯ Abnormal phenotype
✖ Loss of heterozygosity	⬤ Very abnormal phenotype

Fig. 51.5 Mosaicism for autosomal dominant (AD) traits. A *Type 1 mosaicism* features a linear distribution of the skin lesions that characterize an AD genodermatosis in the absence of involvement elsewhere on the body. This results from a postzygotic heterozygous mutation in the underlying gene that is only present in the affected region. **B** *Type 2 mosaicism* presents with a more severe linear lesion superimposed on the background of a generalized AD genodermatosis. This reflects a constitutional (in all the cells of the body) heterozygous mutation plus a 'second hit' in the other allele of the gene within the more severely affected region. **C** In *revertant mosaicism*, an area of normal-appearing skin occurs in the background of a generalized AD genodermatosis due to a reversion to normal or other correction of the underlying heterozygous mutation in that region.

(CHILD) and Conradi–Hünermann–Happle syndromes (see Table 46.2).

Lethal Disorders Rescued by Mosaicism

• Some mutations in autosomal genes are only observed in a mosaic state, as they would not be compatible with life if present in all the cells of the body.

• Examples include Proteus and Schimmelpenning syndromes presenting with epidermal and sebaceous nevi (see Table 51.3), Sturge–Weber syndrome (see Table 51.2 and Chapter 85), and forms of 'pigmentary mosaicism' including McCune–Albright syndrome (see Table 50.3 and Chapters 54 and 55).

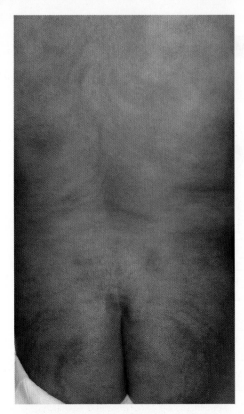

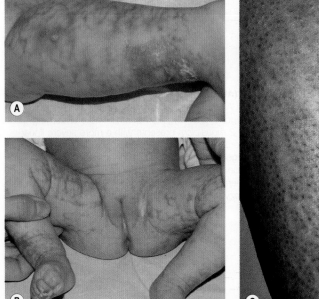

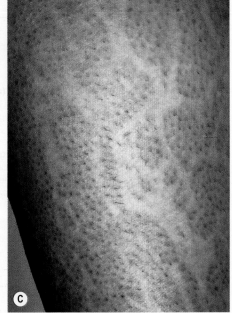

Fig. 51.6 Female 'carrier' of X-linked hypohidrotic ectodermal dysplasia. The skin within the hyperpigmented streaks and swirls following Blaschko's lines is extremely smooth. Starch-iodide testing on the back disclosed a patchy distribution of active sweat glands. This 2-year-old girl also had whorled areas of sparse hair on the posterior scalp and several cone-shaped teeth. *Courtesy, Julie V. Schaffer, MD.*

Fig. 51.7 Incontinentia pigmenti. A, B Stages 2 (verrucous) and 3 (hyperpigmented). Note the erythematous background of the keratotic papules and plaques on the leg **(A)** and the remaining keratotic lesions on the toes **(B).** The scalloped edges of the hyperpigmented streaks reflect growth of normal keratinocytes into areas of apoptosis. **C** Stage 4 (atrophic and hypopigmented). Note the absence of hairs within the streaks on the calf. *A and B, Courtesy, Julie V. Schaffer, MD.*

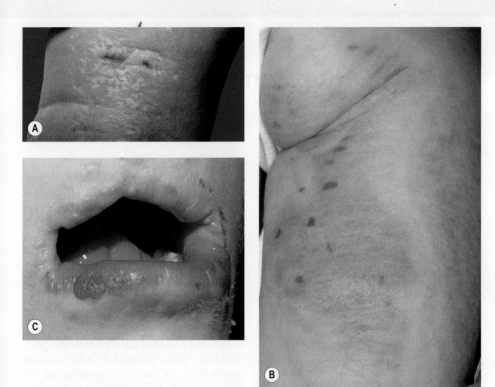

Fig. 51.8 Goltz syndrome. A Hypopigmented streaks of vermiculate atrophy and fat 'herniation.' **B** Bands of telangiectatic erythema, dermal atrophy with fat 'herniation,' and hyperpigmented macules on the posterior thigh. **C** Raspberry-like papules on the lower lip. Similar lesions can occur in the anogenital region and may be confused with warts. *B, C, Courtesy, Julie V. Schaffer, MD.*

Mosaic Manifestations of Acquired Skin Conditions

• Multifactorial skin disorders with environmental as well as genetic components occasionally occur along Blaschko's lines or in a segmental distribution, presumably reflecting mosaicism for a 'susceptibility' mutation; as a result, such conditions often develop in older children or adults following an environmental trigger, and they are sometimes superimposed on a pre-existing mosaic lesion (e.g. psoriasis within an epidermal nevus).

• Examples include linear lichen planus, linear GVHD, and segmental vitiligo.

For further information see Ch. 62. From *Dermatology, Third Edition.*

52 | Other Genodermatoses

This chapter discusses genetic skin diseases that are not covered in other chapters, including conditions featuring extracutaneous tumorigenesis, enzyme deficiencies, premature aging, and ectodermal dysplasia.

Disorders Featuring Extracutaneous Tumorigenesis

Cowden Disease and Other Forms of *PTEN* Hamartoma Tumor Syndrome

• Spectrum of autosomal dominant multisystem disorders that feature characteristic skin findings (Fig. 52.1), macrocephaly, hamartomatous overgrowth of a variety of tissues, and a predisposition to certain cancers (Table 52.1).

• Due to mutations in the phosphatase and tensin homolog tumor suppressor gene (*PTEN*), which negatively regulates the AKT/mammalian target of rapamycin (mTOR) pathway of increased cellular growth and survival.

Multiple Endocrine Neoplasia Syndromes

• Group of autosomal dominant disorders associated with neoplasia or hyperplasia in two or more endocrine organs, often presenting with mucocutaneous findings that serve as clues to the diagnosis (Table 52.2; Fig. 52.2).

Muir–Torre Syndrome (MTS)

• Subtype of hereditary nonpolyposis colorectal cancer (Lynch) syndrome characterized by sebaceous neoplasms (e.g. sebaceous adenoma, sebaceoma, sebaceous carcinoma; Fig. 52.3, see Table 91.2) and keratoacanthomas (± sebaceous differentiation) as well as internal malignancies (Table 52.3).

• Caused by heterozygous constitutional mutations in a DNA mismatch repair gene, e.g. *MSH2* (~90% of patients), *MLH1*, and *MSH6*.

• Cutaneous findings develop at a mean age of ~55 years, presenting as yellow to pink papulonodules on the face (the usual site of sebaceous neoplasms outside of MTS) or trunk > extremities.

Gardner Syndrome

• Variant of familial adenomatous polyposis syndrome with prominent extraintestinal involvement as well as premalignant GI polyps (typically by age 20 years) and colorectal carcinoma (usually by age 40 years); caused by heterozygous mutations in the adenomatous polyposis coli gene (*APC*).

• Epidermoid cysts often develop during childhood; pilomatricomas, fibromas, desmoid tumors (e.g. within abdominal scars), lipomas, and jaw osteomas are additional manifestations.

• *C*ongenital *h*ypertrophy of the *r*etinal *p*igment *e*pithelium (CHRPE) is an early sign.

Birt–Hogg–Dubé Syndrome

• Autosomal dominant genodermatosis caused by mutations in the folliculin gene (*FLCN*).

• Onset during early adulthood of multiple fibrofolliculomas > trichodiscomas, presenting as small whitish papules on the face, ears, and neck (see Figs. 91.4 and 91.15); also flexural acrochordons.

• Increased risk of spontaneous pneumothoraces and renal cell carcinoma (especially oncocytic and chromophobe subtypes).

Reed Syndrome (Hereditary Leiomyomatosis and Renal Cell Cancer Syndrome)

• Discussed in Chapter 95.

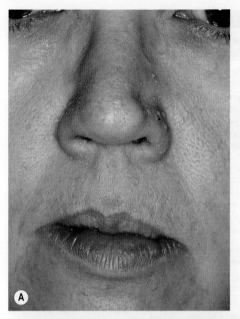

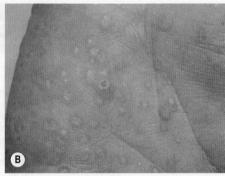

Fig. 52.1 Cowden disease. A Multiple skin-colored papules on the face, especially the nose, some of which are verrucous. **B** Multiple palmar keratoses, many with a glassy appearance or depression centrally. *A, Courtesy, Kalman Watsky, MD; B, Courtesy, Joyce Rico, MD.*

MAJOR CLINICAL MANIFESTATIONS OF *PTEN* HAMARTOMA TUMOR SYNDROME		
	Onset at Birth or in Childhood – Classic Features of BRR	**Onset in Adolescence or Adulthood – Classic Features of Cowden Disease**
Mucocutaneous	• Pigmented genital macules (penis > vulva) • Lipomas • Vascular anomalies* • Epidermal nevi • Café-au-lait macules • Neuromas (acrofacial, mucosal)	• Multiple facial trichilemmomas (Fig. 52.1A; see Chapter 91) and other verrucous papules (especially periorificial and on ears) • Multiple oral papillomas (lips, tongue) • Acral/palmoplantar keratoses (Fig. 52.1B) • Sclerotic fibromas • Multiple acrochordons, acanthosis nigricans
Extracutaneous	• Macrocephaly, intracranial developmental venous anomalies • High-arched palate, adenoid facies • Scoliosis/kyphosis, pectus excavatum • GI: ganglioneuromas, hamartomatous polyps • CNS: developmental delay, autism	• Breast: fibrocystic disease, fibroadenomas, carcinoma (25–50% of women, mean age = 40 years; occasionally in men) • Thyroid: goiter, adenomas, carcinoma (10–15% of patients; often follicular) • GU: testicular lipomatosis, ovarian cysts, uterine leiomyomas, endometrial carcinoma (5–10% of women), renal cell carcinoma • GI: colon carcinoma • CNS: Lhermitte–Duclos disease†

*Typically with fast-flow channels, intramuscular involvement, and ectopic fat; may have capillary, venous, and/or lymphatic components and associated soft tissue/bony overgrowth.
†Hamartomatous dysplastic gangliocytoma of the cerebellum.
BRR, Bannayan–Riley–Ruvalcaba syndrome.

Table 52.1 Major clinical manifestations of *PTEN* hamartoma tumor syndrome. This categorization reflects general tendencies, as the age of onset or recognition of these findings can vary. Criteria for *PTEN* gene testing and guidelines for surveillance in patients suspected to have Cowden disease are available at http://www.nccn.org/professionals/physician_gls/PDF/genetics_screening.pdf.

CLASSIC MULTIPLE ENDOCRINE NEOPLASIA (MEN) SYNDROMES

MEN Type	Gene	Major Extracutaneous Features	Cutaneous Features
1 (Wermer)	*MEN1* (*MENIN*)	• **Pituitary** neoplasia (e.g. prolactinoma) • **Parathyroid** hyperplasia/adenoma • **Pancreatic** islet cell hyperplasia/adenoma/carcinoma	• Multiple facial angiofibromas • Collagenomas (Fig. 52.2A), lipomas • Multiple gingival papules • Guttate hypopigmented macules
2A (Sipple)	*RET* (especially codon 634)	• **Parathyroid** hyperplasia/adenoma • **Thyroid** medullary carcinoma • **Adrenal** pheochromocytomas	• Pruritus/notalgia paresthetica → macular or lichen amyloidosis on the upper back (often with childhood onset)
2B (multiple mucosal neuroma syndrome)	*RET* (especially codon 918)	• **Thyroid** medullary carcinoma • **Adrenal** pheochromocytoma • **GI ganglioneuromatosis** • **Marfanoid** habitus	• Multiple mucosal neuromas (especially on eyelid margins/conjunctiva, lips, tongue; Fig. 52.2B); rarely neuromas of perinasal skin

Table 52.2 Classic multiple endocrine neoplasia (MEN) syndromes.

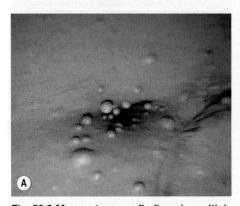
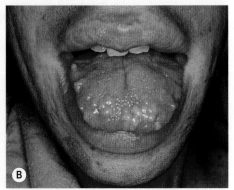

Fig. 52.2 Mucocutaneous findings in multiple endocrine neoplasia (MEN). A Multiple collagenomas in a patient with MEN type 1. **B** Enlarged nodular lips and multiple mucosal neuromas on the lateral and distal tongue in a patient with MEN type 2B. *A, Courtesy, Susan Bayliss, MD.*

Enzyme Deficiency Disorders

Alkaptonuria

• Rare autosomal recessive disorder due to homogentisic acid oxidase deficiency.

• Urine that darkens on standing and brown-black cerumen represent early findings.

• Blue-gray discoloration of the axillary skin, ear (Fig. 52.4), and sclera typically appears during early adulthood, when arthritis and valvular heart disease often develop.

Fabry Disease

• X-linked lysosomal storage disorder due to α-galactosidase A deficiency, which leads to glycosphingolipid accumulation within endothelial cells and results in progressive renal, coronary, and cerebrovascular insufficiency.

• Female heterozygotes have variable clinical manifestations, often with later onset than those in affected men.

• *Angiokeratoma corporis diffusum* presents as punctate dark red macules and papules

FACTORS ASSOCIATED WITH A GREATER LIKELIHOOD OF MUIR–TORRE SYNDROME (MTS)
Clinicopathologic Characteristics of Sebaceous Lesions
• Multiple sebaceous neoplasms (rather than a single lesion or sebaceous hyperplasia)
• Some located outside of the head and neck region (rather than only in sun-damaged facial skin)
• MTS-specific neoplasm, e.g. keratoacanthoma with sebaceous differentiation
• IHC staining showing loss of MSH2, MLH1, MSH6, and/or PMS2 expression*[†]
• Evidence of microsatellite instability (MSI) in cutaneous neoplasms* (more specific)
Characteristics of Patient and Family History
• Personal history of colorectal cancer, especially if before age 50 years or with 'MSI-high' histology
• Personal history of other HNPCC-related malignancies**
• Multiple diagnoses of colorectal cancer/other HNPCC-related malignancies in first-degree relatives, especially before age 50 years

*Testing can be performed on paraffin-embedded tissue; diagnostic yield may be higher for colonic lesions.
**For example, other GI cancers (small bowel, gastric, biliary, pancreatic), genitourinary cancers (endometrial, bladder, ureteral, renal), and glioblastoma.
[†]Sensitivity and specificity have varied and the overall utility is debated.
IHC, immunohistochemical; HNPCC, hereditary nonpolyposis colorectal cancer.

Table 52.3 Factors associated with a greater likelihood of Muir–Torre syndrome (MTS).

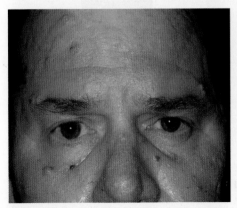

Fig. 52.3 Muir–Torre syndrome with multiple sebaceous neoplasms. *Courtesy, Dan Ring, MD.*

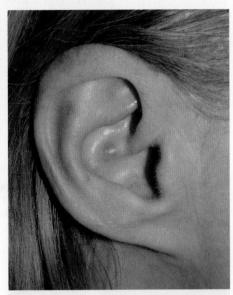

Fig. 52.4 Blue-gray discoloration of the pinna in a woman with alkaptonuria. *Courtesy, Julie V. Schaffer, MD.*

clustered between the umbilicus and knees ('bathing trunk' distribution); serves as an early sign of Fabry disease, typically developing in childhood or adolescence along with paresthesias of the extremities, hypohidrosis, and whorled corneal opacities.

• Fig. 52.5 compares the clinical features of Fabry disease and *fucosidosis*, one of several other lysosomal storage disorders associated with angiokeratomas.

• **Rx:** intravenous α-galactosidase A replacement therapy.

Phenylketonuria

• Autosomal recessive disorder due to phenylalanine hydroxylase deficiency.

• Cutaneous findings can include diffuse pigmentary dilution (skin, hair, eyes),

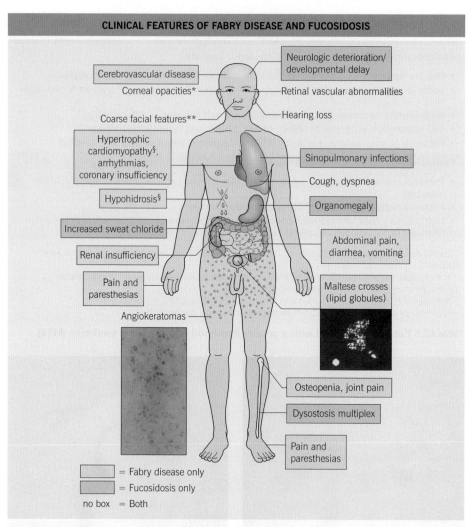

Fig. 52.5 Clinical features of Fabry disease and fucosidosis. *Also lenticular in Fabry disease. **Milder in Fabry disease. §Occasionally observed in fucosidosis. *Angiokeratomas of Fabry disease, courtesy, Julie V. Schaffer, MD; photomicrograph of urinary sediment demonstrating Maltese crosses (via polarization), courtesy, Robert J. Desnick, MD, PhD.*

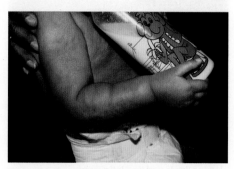

Fig. 52.6 Phenylketonuria (PKU). Infant with PKU and sclerodermoid skin changes. *Courtesy, New York Medical College.*

eczematous dermatitis, sclerodermatous skin changes favoring the proximal extremities (Fig. 52.6), and sweat with a musty odor; pigmentary banding of the hair can occur as a reflection of nonadherence to the diet.

• Newborn screening allows prevention of mental retardation and skin changes through early nutritional intervention (e.g. a phenylalanine-restricted diet).

Mitochondrial Disorders

• This heterogeneous group of conditions can present with a wide variety of cutaneous

CUTANEOUS MANIFESTATIONS OF MITOCHONDRIAL RESPIRATORY CHAIN DISORDERS
• Alopecia
• Hair shaft abnormalities – trichoschisis, pili torti, longitudinal grooving, trichorrhexis nodosa
• Hypertrichosis
• Pigmentary abnormalities – mottled or reticulated pigmentation
• Palmoplantar keratoderma (linked with deafness)
• Hypoplastic nails
• Lipomas
• Acrocyanosis

Table 52.4 Cutaneous manifestations of mitochondrial respiratory chain disorders.

manifestations (Table 52.4) as well as neuromuscular and visceral dysfunction.

Premature Aging Disorders

Hutchinson–Gilford Progeria Syndrome

• Accelerated aging due to heterozygous mutations in the *LMNA* gene; the mutant lamin A protein ('progerin') remains farnesylated and disrupts nuclear scaffolding.

• Onset during infancy of growth failure, facial findings (e.g. frontal bossing, protruding eyes, prominent veins), decreased subcutaneous fat, and cutaneous manifestations such as thin dry skin, acral wrinkling, mottled hyperpigmentation, sclerodermoid changes (especially on the lower trunk and thighs), and alopecia.

• Progressive atherosclerosis results in a median life span of 12 years.

• **Rx:** inhibitors of farnesylation and related processes may be of benefit.

Werner Syndrome

• Autosomal recessive disorder characterized by premature aging beginning in the second decade of life; caused by mutations in the *RECQL2* gene, which encodes a DNA helicase.

• Cutaneous findings include atrophy, mottled hyperpigmentation, sclerodermoid changes, keratoses and ulcers over pressure points (especially acrally), and premature graying of hair.

• Short stature, characteristic facies (e.g. thin with beaked nose; Fig. 52.7), atherosclerosis, osteoporosis, diabetes mellitus, and an

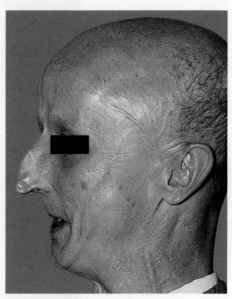

Fig. 52.7 Werner syndrome. Characteristic features include a beaked nose, tautness of the skin, prominent veins, and micrognathia. *Courtesy, Ronald P. Rapini, MD.*

increased risk of sarcomas are additional features; median survival ~50 years.

Ectodermal Dysplasias

• Large, heterogeneous group of genetic disorders characterized by abnormalities in ≥2 major ectodermal structures (hair, sweat glands, nails, teeth); other ectodermal structures (e.g. sebaceous or mucous glands) may also be affected.

• Major features of several classic forms of ectodermal dysplasia are presented in Table 52.5 and Figs. 52.8–52.11.

For further information see Ch. 63. From *Dermatology, Third Edition.*

SELECTED ECTODERMAL DYSPLASIA (ED) SYNDROMES

Syndrome	Inheritance (Gene)	Scalp Hair	Sweating	Nails	Teeth	Other Features
Hypohidrotic ED (Figs. 52.8 and 52.9)	XLR (*EDA*)* > AD, AR (*EDAR* > *EDARADD*)	Sparse–absent; often lightly pigmented in childhood	↓↓, often leads to hyperpyrexia	Normal	Hypodontia, conical	• Frontal bossing, saddle nose, everted lips, periorbital wrinkling/ hyperpigmentation, sebaceous hyperplasia • ± Collodion-like membrane at birth; eczema later • Frequent respiratory tract infections, thick cerumen
Hypohidrotic ED-immune deficiency	XLR (*NEMO*)** > AD (*NFKBIA*)	Sparse	→	Normal	Hypodontia, conical	• Intertrigo, seborrheic-like dermatitis, erythroderma • Colitis; recurrent infections (pyogenic, opportunistic); ↑IgM, IgA; ↓ IgG • Rare osteopetrosis, lymphedema
Hidrotic ED (Clouston syndrome) (Fig. 52.10)	AD (*GJB6*), most common in French Canadians	Wiry/brittle, variable alopecia	Normal	White in infants→ thickened with distal separation	Normal	• Diffuse PPK, 'pebbled' skin on dorsal digits with EFSA • Blepharitis, conjunctivitis

		Hair		Nails	Teeth	Other features
WNT10A-associated ED†	AR > AD (WNT10A)	Thin, sparse	±↓	Dystrophic or absent	Hypodontia	• Facial telangiectasias, reticulated erythema, atrophy • PPK with ESFA, xerosis
AEC (Hay–Wells) syndrome‡ (Fig. 52.11)	AD (p63, SAM domain)	Wiry/coarse, lightly pigmented, patchy alopecia	±↓	Thickened > absent	Hypodontia, often conical	• Neonatal erythroderma with peeling skin/erosions • Erosive scalp dermatitis • Ankyloblepharon • Cleft palate ± lip; GER • ± Syndactyly
EEC syndrome	AD (p63, DNA-binding domain)	Coarse, lightly pigmented, ± sparse	Usually normal	Transverse ridges, pitting	Hypodontia, premature loss	• PPK, xerosis • Cleft palate + lip • Ectrodactyly > syndactyly

*Variable phenotype with mosaic pattern (e.g. hypohidrosis and hyperpigmentation along Blaschko's lines) in female 'carriers' of XLR form.

**Female carriers may have mild features of incontinentia pigmenti (see Chapter 51).

†Includes odonto-onycho-dermal dysplasia and Schöpf–Schulz–Passarge syndrome, which also features eyelid hidrocystomas.

‡Rapp–Hodgkin syndrome is now included in the AEC spectrum.

AD, autosomal dominant; AEC, ankyloblepharon-ED-clefting; AR, autosomal recessive; EDA, ectodysplasin A; EDAR, EDA receptor; EDARADD, EDAR-associated death domain; EEC, ED-ectrodactyly-clefting; ESFA, eccrine syringofibroadenomatosis; GER, gastroesophageal reflux; GJB6, gap junction β6 (encodes connexin 30); NEMO, NF-κB essential modulator; NFKBIA, NF-κB inhibitor-α; PPK, palmoplantar keratoderma; XLR, X-linked recessive.

Table 52.5 Selected ectodermal dysplasia (ED) syndromes.

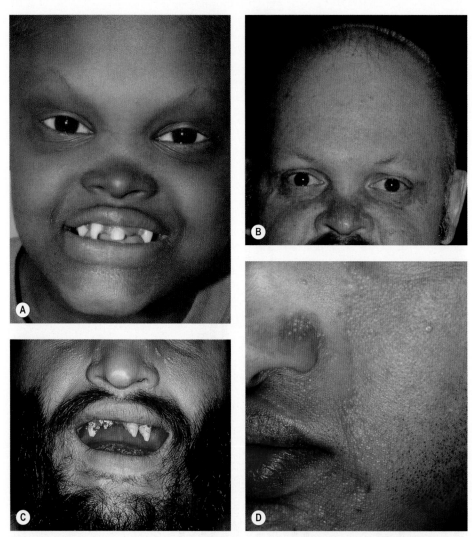

Fig. 52.8 Male patients with hypohidrotic ectodermal dysplasia. Note the flat nasal bridge, depressed nasal tip, sparse hair (scalp, eyebrows, eyelashes), peg-shaped teeth, full lips, and sebaceous hyperplasia. Also note the normal secondary hair in adults. *A, Courtesy, Julie V. Schaffer, MD; B, D, Courtesy, Mary Williams, MD.*

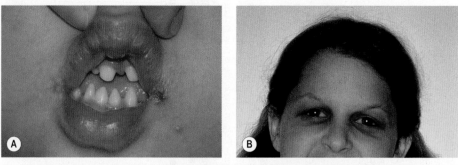

Fig. 52.9 Female patients with X-linked hypohidrotic ectodermal dysplasia. A Full lips, peg-shaped teeth, and hypodontia. **B** Periorbital hyperpigmentation. *A, Courtesy, Julie V. Schaffer, MD.*
Continued

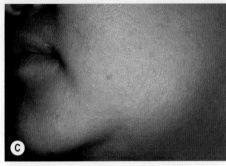

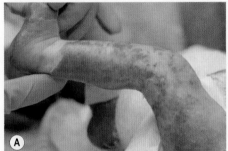

Fig. 52.9 *Continued* **C** Sebaceous hyperplasia.

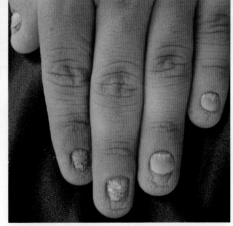

Fig. 52.10 Hidrotic ectodermal dysplasia (Clouston syndrome). Note the thickened, shortened nails with distal separation and the tiny papules in a regular distribution on the dorsal fingertips. *Courtesy, Virginia Sybert, MD, and Alanna Bree, MD.*

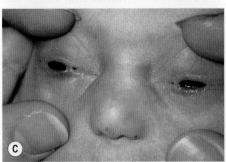

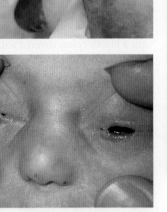

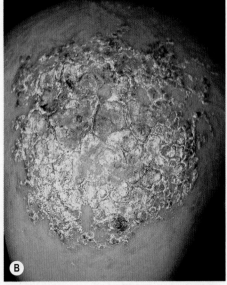

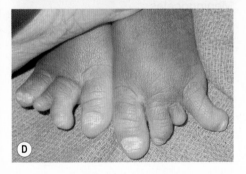

Fig. 52.11 Ankyloblepharon–ectodermal dysplasia–clefting syndrome. A Extensive erosions in an infant who succumbed to sepsis. **B** Chronic erosive scalp dermatitis with thick scale-crust and alopecia. **C** Strands of tissue between the eyelids (ankyloblepharon filiforme adnatum). **D** Digital abnormalities (including syndactyly) and nail dystrophy. *A, C, D, Courtesy, Virginia Sybert, MD, and Alanna Bree, MD; B, Courtesy, Jean L. Bologna, MD.*

53 | Developmental Anomalies

Developmental anomalies are a diverse group of congenital disorders that result from faulty *in utero* morphogenesis. When they affect the skin, developmental anomalies can range in severity from isolated minor physical findings to potentially life-threatening conditions or cutaneous signs of significant extracutaneous defects.

Midline Lesions of the Nose or Scalp

• A midline mass or pit on the nose or scalp due to a dermoid cyst, cephalocele, nasal glioma, or other heterotopic brain/meningeal tissue (Fig. 53.1) may have a deeper component with intracranial extension.
• These lesions are typically apparent at birth or during early childhood.
• *Hair collar sign*: a peripheral ring of long, dark hair often surrounds ectopic neural tissue or membranous aplasia cutis congenita (ACC) on the scalp (Figs. 53.2 and 53.3); the latter is thought to represent a forme fruste of a neural tube defect.
• **DDx:** outlined in Table 53.1 for nasal masses; epidermoid and pilar cysts for scalp masses (especially in older children and adults).
• **Rx:** avoid biopsy or aspiration, which could lead to a CNS infection (e.g. meningitis); MRI or CT is required to assess extent prior to surgical intervention, which should include exploration to exclude intracranial extension and repair of any bony/dural defects.

Dermoid Cysts

• Result from sequestration of ectodermal tissue along embryonic fusion planes.
• Recognized at birth or when they enlarge or become inflamed during infancy or childhood.

• Firm, noncompressible, skin-colored to pink subcutaneous nodules that often reach a size of 1–4 cm in diameter; some have a sinus ostium, which may be heralded by protruding hairs.
• Most often located around the eyes, especially the lateral eyebrow region (Fig. 53.4); midline lesions on the nose, scalp, or back may have intracranial extension.
• **Rx:** surgical excision, following imaging if midline.

Cephaloceles

• Neural tube defect characterized by congenital herniation of brain + meninges (*encephalocele*) or meninges (*cranial meningocele*) through a skull defect (see Fig. 53.3).
• Midline or paramedian location at the occiput or vertex > nasal region.
• Soft, compressible, pulsatile mass, often with a bluish color; covered with normal skin or a glistening membrane.
• Clues to the diagnosis include transillumination and transient expansion with crying or the Valsalva maneuver; nasal lesions may present with cerebrospinal fluid (CSF) rhinorrhea or a broad nasal bridge.
• **Rx:** MRI followed by neurosurgical repair.

Nasal Gliomas, Other Heterotopic Brain Tissue, and Rudimentary Meningoceles

• A *nasal glioma* is a congenital mass of heterotopic brain tissue (HBT) at the nasal root/glabella > intranasally; the skin overlying this firm, noncompressible nodule tends to be red with prominent telangiectasias (mimicking an infantile hemangioma) (Fig. 53.5).
• Other HBT and rudimentary meningoceles typically present as a solid or cystic

COMMON SITES OF DEVELOPMENTAL ANOMALIES OF THE FACE AND NECK

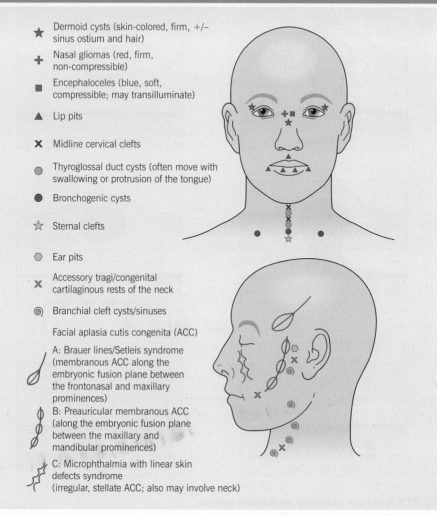

★ Dermoid cysts (skin-colored, firm, +/– sinus ostium and hair)

✛ Nasal gliomas (red, firm, non-compressible)

■ Encephaloceles (blue, soft, compressible; may transilluminate)

▲ Lip pits

✕ Midline cervical clefts

● Thyroglossal duct cysts (often move with swallowing or protrusion of the tongue)

● Bronchogenic cysts

☆ Sternal clefts

◯ Ear pits

✕ Accessory tragi/congenital cartilaginous rests of the neck

◎ Branchial cleft cysts/sinuses

Facial aplasia cutis congenita (ACC)

A: Brauer lines/Setleis syndrome (membranous ACC along the embryonic fusion plane between the frontonasal and maxillary prominences)

B: Preauricular membranous ACC (along the embryonic fusion plane between the maxillary and mandibular prominences)

C: Microphthalmia with linear skin defects syndrome (irregular, stellate ACC; also may involve neck)

Fig. 53.1 Common sites of developmental anomalies of the face and neck. *Courtesy, Julie V. Schaffer, MD.*

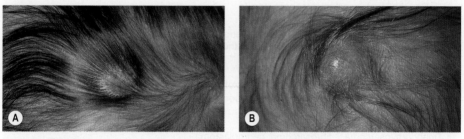

Fig. 53.2 Hair collar sign in membranous aplasia cutis congenita. Note the associated capillary malformation **(A)** and the bullous appearance **(B).** *A, Courtesy, Kalman Watsky, MD.*

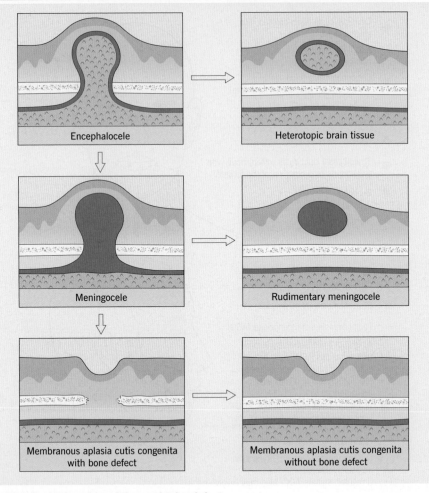

SPECTRUM OF CRANIAL NEURAL TUBE DEFECTS

Encephalocele

Heterotopic brain tissue

Meningocele

Rudimentary meningocele

Membranous aplasia cutis congenita with bone defect

Membranous aplasia cutis congenita without bone defect

Fig. 53.3 Spectrum of cranial neural tube defects.

THE DIFFERENTIAL DIAGNOSIS OF NASAL MASSES PRESENTING AT BIRTH OR DURING INFANCY
Cysts and developmental defects
Midline lesions (see Fig. 53.1) • Dermoid cyst, nasal glioma, cephalocele *Other lesions* • Vascular malformation (e.g. lymphatic, venous; see Chapter 85) • Epidermoid cyst (see Chapter 90), pilomatricoma (see Chapter 91), nasolacrimal duct cyst
Benign neoplasms and hamartomas
• Infantile hemangioma (see Chapter 85), neurofibroma (see Chapter 95) • Hamartomas (e.g. chondromesenchymal, lipomatous), teratoma*
Malignant neoplasms
• Rhabdomyosarcoma > fibrosarcoma, neuroblastoma
*May also be malignant.

Table 53.1 The differential diagnosis of nasal masses presenting at birth or during infancy.

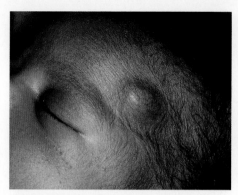

Fig. 53.4 Dermoid cyst. This dermoid cyst presented in an infant as a firm subcutaneous nodule superior to the lateral left eyebrow. *Courtesy, Kalman Watsky, MD.*

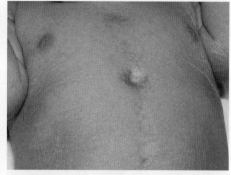

Fig. 53.6 Sternal cleft. Note the atrophic skin overlying the defect and prominent veins in the midline chest. Generalized desquamation is also evident in this 1-day-old post-term neonate. She did not develop an infantile hemangioma and had no cardiac defects or other features of PHACE(S) syndrome. *Courtesy, Julie V. Schaffer, MD.*

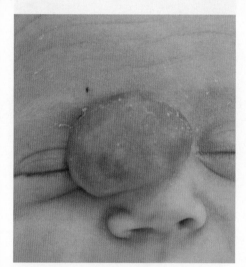

Fig. 53.5 Nasal glioma. A mass was noted on prenatal ultrasound, and this reddish, slightly pedunculated, rubbery nodule was evident at birth. *Courtesy, Mary Chang, MD.*

Midline Cervical, Sternal, and Supraumbilical Clefts

• A *midline cervical cleft* is a vertical band of atrophic skin on the mid anterior neck, often with a sinus tract inferiorly and a protuberance overlying a fibrous cord superiorly; surgical correction is needed to prevent neck contracture.

• A *sternal cleft* or *supraumbilical raphe* presents with a band of atrophic (Fig. 53.6), scarred or ulcerated skin; may occur in the setting of PHACE(S) syndrome (*p*osterior fossa malformations; *h*emangiomas; *a*rterial, *c*ardiac, and *e*ye anomalies; *s*ternal cleft/ *s*upraumbilical raphe; see Chapter 85).

Midline Lesions Overlying the Spine

• Midline cutaneous lesions serve as a valuable marker for 'occult' spinal dysraphism and are present in ~80% of affected individuals (most of whom have >1 type of skin lesion), compared to <3% of the general population; shallow coccygeal dimples and deep gluteal clefts, which are considered as normal variants, occur in an additional 4% of infants.

• Skin lesions associated with spinal dysraphism are presented in Table 53.2 and Fig. 53.7.

• **Rx:** Fig. 53.8 outlines an approach to patients with skin signs of spinal dysraphism.

subcutaneous nodule on the midline scalp, often with a blue-red hue, overlying alopecia and a surrounding hair collar (see above); a rudimentary meningocele may have a bullous appearance and can also be located over the spine.

• May have a vestigial fibrous stalk extending into the intracranial space, but lack a connection with the intracranial leptomeninges or CSF (see Fig. 53.3).

• **Rx:** MRI followed by surgical excision.

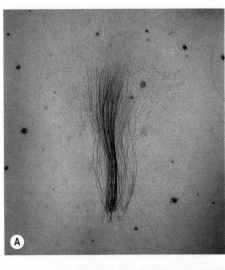

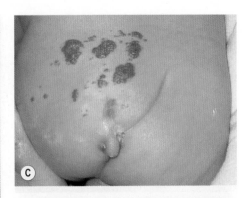

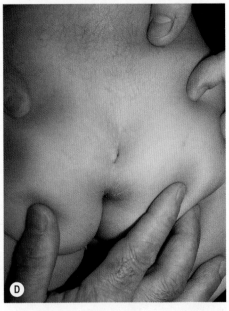

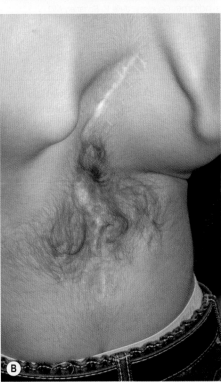

Fig. 53.7 Skin findings associated with spinal dysraphism. A Circumscribed midline
hypertrichosis overlying the lower thoracic spine in a patient with occult dysraphism. The patient
periodically clips the distal ends. **B** V-shaped patch of long, coarse hair on the mid back in a boy
born with a large thoracic myelomeningocele. Severe scoliosis remains after multiple surgeries.
C This infant with segmental infantile hemangiomas, a dimple, a pseudotail, and a deviated gluteal
cleft had an underlying lipomyelomeningocele. **D** Midline deep sacral dimple located above the gluteal
cleft in association with a small pseudotail. In contrast, a shallow dimple within the gluteal cleft is a
common finding and not a sign of spinal dysraphism. *A, Courtesy, Jean L. Bolognia, MD; B, Courtesy, Julie
V. Schaffer, MD; C, Courtesy, Richard Antaya, MD; D, Courtesy, Seth Orlow, MD.*

SKIN LESIONS OF THE SPINAL AXIS ASSOCIATED WITH DYSRAPHISM	
Lesion	**Features**
Hypertrichosis	A V-shaped patch of long, coarse or silky hair (see Fig. 53.7A,B); 'faun tail'
Lipomas	Soft subcutaneous mass, asymmetric buttocks, curved gluteal cleft (see Fig. 53.7C); most common sign of spinal dysraphism
Dimples	Above the gluteal cleft or >2.5 cm from the anal verge in neonates (see Fig. 53.7C,D); >0.5 cm in size or deep*
Dermal sinuses	Hair may be present at the ostium*
Acrochordons	May be associated with a dimple or dermal sinus
Pseudotails	Caudal protrusion due to prolonged vertebrae or hamartomatous elements, e.g. adipose tissue or cartilage (see Fig. 53.7C,D)
True tails	Persistent vestigial appendage with a central core of mature adipose tissue, muscle, blood vessels, and nerves May be capable of spontaneous or reflex motion
Infantile hemangiomas	Usually superficial with a segmental pattern (see Fig. 53.7C) and often ulcerated; represents a component of LUMBAR syndrome
Telangiectasias	May represent an early, minimal/arrested growth or regressed infantile hemangioma
Capillary malformations (CM)**	Typically found together with other skin lesions Cobb syndrome: segmental lesions mimicking a CM or angiokeratomas are part of a metameric arteriovenous malformation involving the spine
Aplasia cutis congenita (ACC)	Ulcer, scar, or atrophic skin
Connective tissue nevus	Typically found together with other skin lesions
Hypo/depigmentation	May represent a nevus depigmentosus (typically found together with other skin lesions) or the residua of ACC
Hyperpigmentation	Typically found together with other skin lesions
Congenital melanocytic nevi	Spinal dysraphism has been reported in patients with neurocutaneous melanosis
Subcutaneous masses	May represent (lipomyelo)meningoceles or teratomas

*Due to a potential risk of meningitis, these lesions should not be probed.
**The common occipital nevus simplex ('stork bite') and lumbosacral capillary stains in the setting of other nevus simplex lesions of the head/neck (but no other lumbosacral skin lesions) are generally not considered to be signs of spinal dysraphism.
LUMBAR, lumbosacral hemangiomas and lipomas; urogenital anomalies and ulceration, myelopathy, bony deformities, anorectal and arterial malformations, renal anomalies.

Table 53.2 Skin lesions of the spinal axis associated with dysraphism. The presence of two or more types of lesions increases the risk of a spinal anomaly.

DEVELOPMENTAL ANOMALIES

APPROACH TO PATIENTS WITH CUTANEOUS SIGNS OF SPINAL DYSRAPHISM

Cutaneous stigmata present

↓

Evaluate for associated features:
- Palpable vertebral defects
- Obvious urogenital or anorectal abnormalities
- History of meningitis

↓

Evaluate for clinical manifestations of the tethered cord syndrome:

By history	By physical examination
• Back or leg pain	• Abnormal strength, sensation, reflexes or tone
• Leg weakness (often asymmetric)	• Trophic ulcers
• Urinary or fecal incontinence	• Muscular atrophy or asymmetry of legs
• Recurrent urinary tract infections	• Foot deformities
	• Scoliosis
	• Abnormal gait

↓

- < 3-5 months of age and low clinical suspicion*

- ≥ 3-5 months of age *or*
- Either high clinical suspicion* or a bulky overlying skin lesion**

↓

Spinal ultrasonography → (+) or insufficient visualization → Spinal MRI

(−) → No further work-up required

(−) → Isolated posterior spina bifida

(+) → Potentially significant form of dysraphism†, whether symptomatic or asymptomatic

Isolated posterior spina bifida:
- Asymptomatic and no other clinical findings
- Symptomatic or other clinical findings

Asymptomatic and no other clinical findings:
- MRI finding likely not clinically significant
- Depending on clinical suspicion, consider referral to neurologist

Symptomatic or other clinical findings:
Referral to neurologist or neurosurgeon for evaluation

Potentially significant form of dysraphism:
Referral to neurosurgeon for evaluation and to plan intervention‡

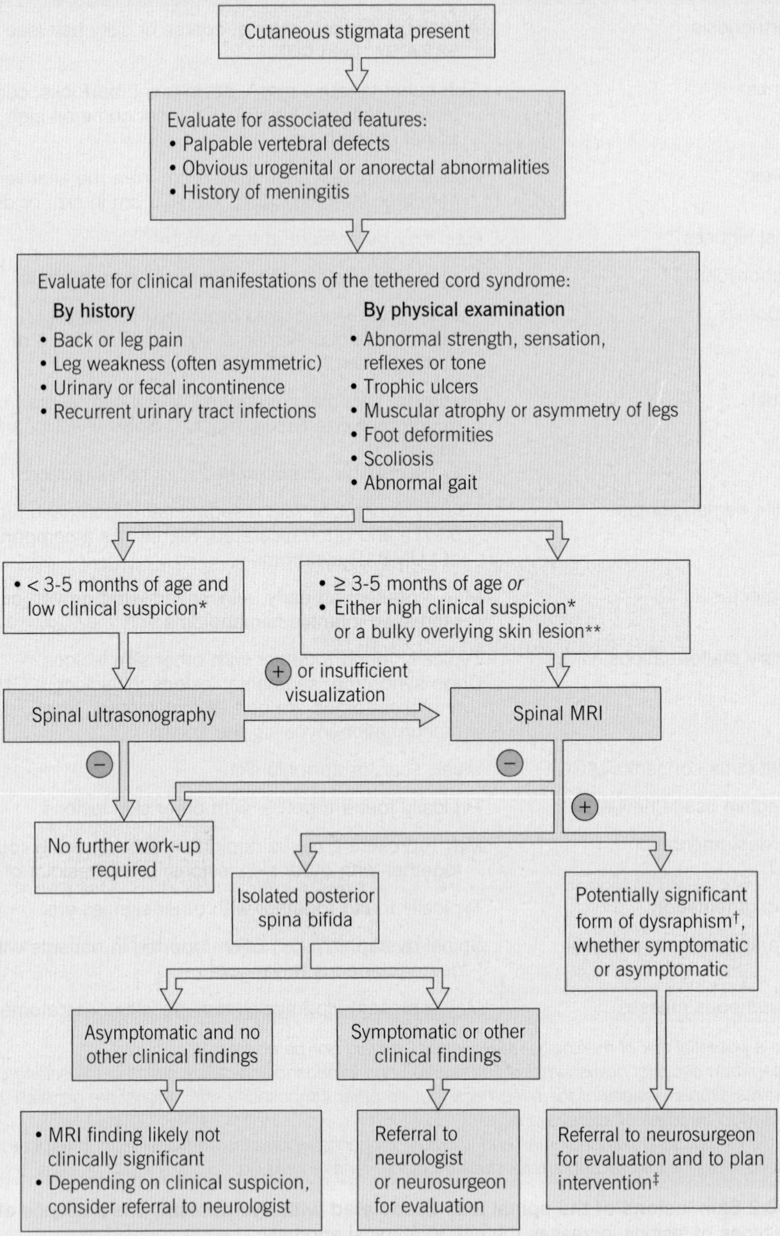

* The presence of two or more types of skin lesions increases the risk of dysraphism
** Visualization of spinal structures may be suboptimal in the setting of a bulky overlying skin lesion
† E.g., meningocele, intraspinal lipoma, lipomyelomeningocele, diastematomyelia (split cord), syringomyelia (fluid within the cord), tight filum terminale, dermoid cyst/dermal sinus
‡ If indicated, surgery should be performed prior to the development of symptoms, as neurologic damage may be reversible

Fig. 53.8 Approach to patients with cutaneous signs of spinal dysraphism. *Courtesy, Julie V. Schaffer, MD.*

Aplasia Cutis Congenita (Congenital Absence of Skin)

- ACC is a physical finding: areas of skin (localized or widespread) that are absent or scarred at birth.
- Possible causes of ACC include genetic factors, vascular compromise, trauma, teratogens and intrauterine infections.
- The morphology and distribution of the skin defects (Figs. 53.9 and 53.10) and the presence or absence of associated abnormalities represent clues to the etiology of ACC (Table 53.3).
- The most common form is *membranous ACC*, which favors the scalp (especially the vertex) and presents as a sharply marginated, round to oval defect that is covered by a thin translucent membrane and often surrounded by a hair collar (see Fig. 53.2 and above); may have a bullous appearance in neonates, evolving into an atrophic scar.
- Another morphology of ACC is stellate or angulated ulcerations and scars, which may result from vascular abnormalities and/or intrauterine ischemic events (see Table 53.3).
- **DDx:** obstetric trauma, rudimentary meningocele (especially if bullous).
- Imaging is recommended for irregular and membranous lesions on the scalp, in particular those that are large and/or deep, to assess for underlying skull defects and vascular anomalies.
- **Rx:** topical antibiotic ointment until re-epithelialization occurs; early surgical repair of large, deep stellate scalp lesions to prevent life-threatening hemorrhage, thrombosis, or meningitis.

Congenital Lip and Ear Pits

- *Commissural lip pits*: most common form of lip pits (1–2% of newborns), found bilaterally at angles of mouth (Fig. 53.11A); usually isolated, occasionally associated with branchio-otic syndrome (preauricular pits, deafness).
- *Lower lip pits*: typically bilateral at apex of conical elevation (Fig. 53.11B); isolated > associated with Van der Woude (cleft lip/palate, hypodontia) or popliteal pterygium syndrome.
- *Upper lip pits*: along philtrum; isolated > associated findings (e.g. hypertelorism).
- *Ear pits*: affect 0.5–1% of newborns, presenting as an invagination (Fig. 53.11C) > cystic nodule in the upper preauricular area (unilateral > bilateral); usually isolated (± autosomal dominant inheritance), occasionally associated with hearing impairment or malformation syndromes (e.g. branchio-oto-(±) renal syndrome, hemifacial microsomia).

Accessory Tragi (Preauricular Tags)

- Congenital anomalies of the first branchial arch that are found in ~5 per 1000 newborns.
- Soft or firm (due to a cartilaginous core) skin-colored papules or nodules covered by vellus hairs.
- Located in preauricular area > mandibular cheek (Fig. 53.12) or anterolateral neck (*congenital cartilaginous rests of the neck* or *'wattles'*).
- Usually an isolated finding; occasionally associated with hearing impairment or malformation syndromes (e.g. hemifacial microsomia).
- **Rx:** assessment of hearing; excision, with care to remove any cartilaginous component.

Branchial Cleft Cysts, Sinuses, and Fistulae

- Located on the neck along the anterior border of the sternocleidomastoid muscle or in the mandibular or preauricular region (see Fig. 53.1).
- *Branchial cleft cysts* lack a primary cutaneous opening and typically present in older children and adults when they become infected or inflamed.
- *Branchial cleft sinuses/fistulae* usually have a sinus ostium with mucus discharge that is evident at birth or during the first few years of life.
- Usually an isolated anomaly, but occasionally associated with branchio-oto-(±)renal and branchio-oculo-facial (with eroded/'hemangiomatous' overlying skin) syndromes.
- **Rx:** surgical excision after delineation of extent with MRI or fistulography (via CT or intraoperatively).

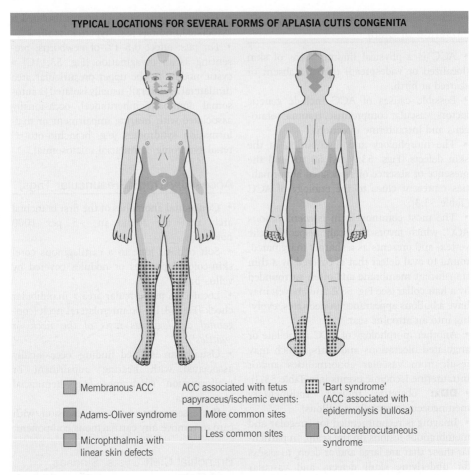

TYPICAL LOCATIONS FOR SEVERAL FORMS OF APLASIA CUTIS CONGENITA

☐ Membranous ACC

☐ Adams-Oliver syndrome

☐ Microphthalmia with linear skin defects

ACC associated with fetus papyraceus/ischemic events:

☐ More common sites

☐ Less common sites

▦ 'Bart syndrome' (ACC associated with epidermolysis bullosa)

☐ Oculocerebrocutaneous syndrome

Fig. 53.9 Typical locations for several forms of aplasia cutis congenita (ACC). See Fig. 53.1 for Brauer lines/Setleis syndrome and preauricular membranous ACC. *Courtesy, Julie V. Schaffer, MD.*

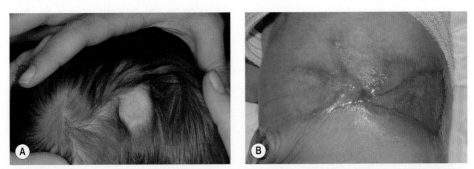

Fig. 53.10 Aplasia cutis congenita (ACC). A This hairless, round, scarred plaque on the scalp of a 6-month-old was present at birth. **B** Stellate ACC on the lateral trunk of a neonate born of an initial sextuplet gestation for which fetal reduction was performed. The lesions had a bilateral, symmetric distribution. *Continued*

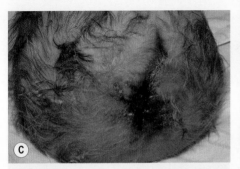
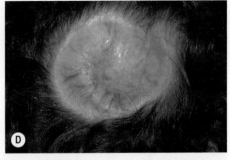

Fig. 53.10 *Continued* **C** Stellate ACC on the midline scalp of a neonate with mosaic trisomy 13. This hemorrhagic lesion was associated with an underlying skull defect and cerebrovascular anomalies. **D** Membranous ACC associated with a large defect of the underlying skull in a patient with Goltz syndrome. *A, Courtesy, Anthony J. Mancini, MD; B–D, Courtesy, Julie V. Schaffer, MD.*

CLASSIFICATION SCHEME FOR APLASIA CUTIS CONGENITA (ACC)		
Group	**Inheritance**	**Location, Features, and Associated Abnormalities**
1. Isolated scalp ACC (see Figs. 53.2 and 53.10A)	Sporadic > AD	• Favors vertex: membranous with hair collar
	Often AD	• Favors vertex: irregular and scar-like
2. Scalp ACC associated with Adams–Oliver syndrome (limb reductions, CMTC)	AD > AR	• Large, irregular lesions on midline scalp • Frequent skull defect and dilated scalp veins
3. Scalp ACC associated with epidermal, sebaceous, and/or large congenital melanocytic nevi	Sporadic	• Scalp, often unilateral and membranous • ± Ipsilateral ophthalmologic or CNS abnormalities
4. ACC overlying embryologic malformations	Variable	• Scalp with hair collar (heterotopic brain/meningeal tissue) • Lumbosacral (spinal dysraphism) • Anterior trunk (sternal defect, omphalocele)
5. ACC associated with fetus papyraceus* (see Fig. 53.10B), placental infarct, or other ischemic events	Sporadic	• Scalp, chest, flanks, axillae, extremities • Multiple, symmetric • Stellate/angulated morphology
6. ACC associated with epidermolysis bullosa (simplex, junctional, or dystrophic; see Chapter 26)	AD or AR	• Lower extremities ('Bart syndrome') or widespread
7. ACC localized to extremities without blistering	Variable	• Pretibial areas, extensor forearms (± radial dysplasia), dorsal hands/feet
8. ACC caused by teratogens (e.g. methimazole), maternal conditions (e.g. antiphospholipid syndrome), or intrauterine infections (e.g. varicella, HSV)	Not inherited	• Scalp with drugs • Any site with congenital infections
9. ACC associated with malformation syndromes	Variable	• Favors scalp, e.g. in trisomy 13 (see Fig. 53.10C), 4p- syndrome and Goltz syndrome (see Fig. 53.10D)

Due to second trimester death of a co-twin/triplet.
CMTC, cutis marmorata telangiectatica congenita.

Table 53.3 Classification scheme for aplasia cutis congenita (ACC).

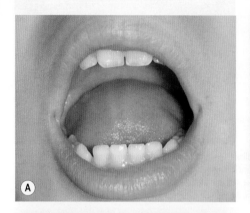

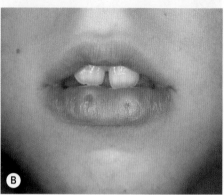

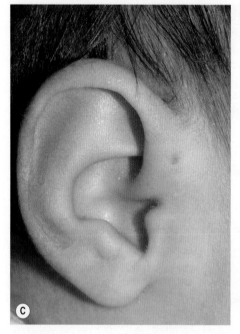

Fig. 53.11 Lip and ear pits. A Bilateral commissural lip pits. **B** Bilateral paramedian lower lip pits, each located on the apex of a conical elevation. **C** Ear pit. In all of these patients, the pits represented an isolated, asymptomatic finding. *B, Courtesy, Richard Antaya, MD; C, Courtesy, Julie V. Schaffer, MD.*

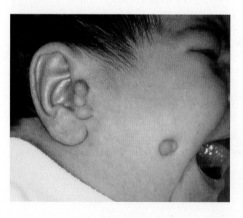

Fig. 53.12 Accessory tragi. Multiple skin-colored papulonodules in a typical preauricular location as well as on the mandibular cheek.

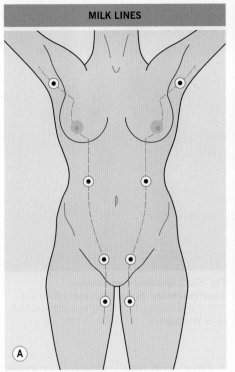

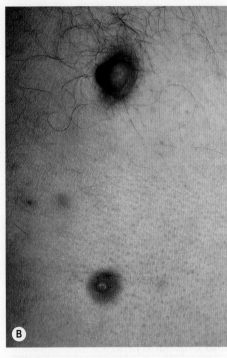

MILK LINES

Fig. 53.13 Supernumerary nipples. A Supernumerary nipples and other forms of accessory mammary tissue represent focal remnants of the embryologic mammary ridges ('milk lines') that extend from the anterior axillary fold to the upper medial thigh bilaterally. **B** Supernumerary nipple with a surrounding areola in a typical location on the inframammary chest. *B, Courtesy, Jean L. Bolognia, MD.*

Thyroglossal Duct Cysts and Bronchogenic Cysts (See Fig. 53.1)

• *Thyroglossal duct cysts* present in children and young adults as a nodule on the mid anterior neck that moves with swallowing.

• *Cutaneous bronchogenic cysts* typically appear as a congenital papule or nodule, most often in the suprasternal notch or surrounding areas; mucus discharge is sometimes noted.

• **Rx:** surgical excision.

Supernumerary Nipples and Other Accessory Mammary Tissue

• Present in 2–5% of the population, representing remnants of the embryonic 'milk lines' (Fig. 53.13A).

• Equally prevalent in men and women, but often become more prominent at puberty or during pregnancy in female patients.

• Found on the inframammary chest > axilla, vulva, or upper medial thigh.

• Small, soft, pink or brown papules, with or without a surrounding areola (Fig. 53.13B); ectopic glandular breast tissue is occasionally present (± a nipple/areola), especially in the axilla or vulva.

• Usually an isolated finding; controversial potential association with malformations of the kidneys or urinary tract, and occasionally seen together with a Becker's nevus or malformation syndrome.

• **Rx:** excision if symptomatic or cosmetically undesirable; accessory mammary tissue can develop the same disorders as normal

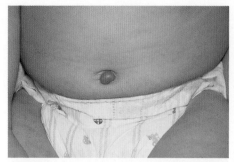

Fig. 53.14 Omphalomesenteric duct cyst.
The pink papule in the umbilicus of this infant
showed gastrointestinal epithelium histologically.
Courtesy, Mary S. Stone, MD.

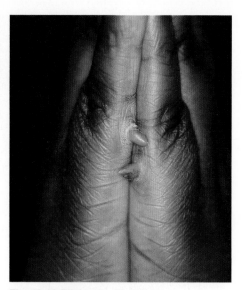

**Fig. 53.15 Bilateral rudimentary
supernumerary digits.** The ulnar side of the
fifth digit is the most common location (referred
to as postaxial).

breasts and requires periodic breast cancer
screening.

Omphalomesenteric Duct Cysts and Urachal Cysts

• Defective closure of the omphalomesenteric duct, the embryonic connection between the midgut and yolk sac, can result in an umbilical-enteric fistula, umbilical sinus or *omphalomesenteric duct cyst*, which typically presents as an umbilical polyp (Fig. 53.14).

• A patent urachus, which connects the fetal bladder to the umbilicus, results in leakage of urine from the umbilicus; in contrast, a *urachal cyst* typically presents with an umbilical mass, often in the setting of a secondary infection.

• **DDx:** umbilical granuloma (persistent granulation tissue after cord separation).

• **Rx:** excision after radiographic studies to determine extent.

Rudimentary Supernumerary Digits (Rudimentary Polydactyly)

• Found in 0.5–1 : 1000 white newborns and 5–10 : 1000 black newborns.

• Soft-tissue duplications without a skeletal component, usually arising from the ulnar side of the fifth finger (postaxial location) (Fig. 53.15).

• Range from small, fleshy or wart-like papules to pedunculated nodules that may contain cartilage or a vestigial nail; frequently bilateral.

• Typically an isolated finding, often with an autosomal dominant inheritance pattern.

• **Rx:** surgical excision; removal via ligation with suture material increases risk of infection and often leaves a residual papule that becomes a painful neuroma.

Amniotic Band Sequence and Disorganization Syndrome

• Various congenital anomalies of the limbs, head, body wall, and viscera with asymmetric, seemingly haphazard distribution patterns.

• Characterized by fibrous bands that form constriction rings and lead to amputations of limbs/digits.

• Extrinsic (entanglement in torn amnion) and intrinsic (endogenous 'disorganization syndrome') hypotheses for its pathogenesis; latter is favored by the presence of duplicated structures and internal malformations.

• **Rx:** surgical release of constriction bands.

For further information see Ch. 64. From *Dermatology, Third Edition.*

Vitiligo and Other Disorders of Hypopigmentation

54

Introduction/Definitions

• **Leukoderma** and **hypopigmentation**: areas of skin are lighter in color than uninvolved skin, due primarily to a decrease in melanin; decreased blood supply to the skin (e.g. nevus anemicus) can be another cause of leukoderma.

• **Hypomelanosis**: an absence or reduction of melanin in the skin that may be due to any one or a combination of the following:
1. A decrease in the number of melanocytes (e.g. vitiligo).
2. A decrease in melanin synthesis by a normal number of melanocytes (e.g. albinism).
3. A decrease in the transfer of melanin to keratinocytes (e.g. postinflammatory hypopigmentation).

• **Amelanosis**: total absence of melanin in the skin.

• **Depigmentation**: usually implies a total loss of skin color (e.g. as in vitiligo).

• **Pigmentary dilution**: a generalized lightening of the skin, hair, and eyes (e.g. oculocutaneous albinism); sites of melanin production include the epidermis, hair follicles, pigmented retinal epithelium, and uveal tract.

• **Poliosis**: a lock of scalp hair, eyebrows, or eyelashes that is white or lighter in color.

• **Canities**: generalized depigmentation of scalp hair.

• **Wood's lamp examination**: the greater the loss of epidermal pigmentation, the more marked the contrast with uninvolved skin on Wood's lamp examination.

• All disorders of hypopigmentation are more easily observed in darkly pigmented individuals or after a suntan.

Approach to Disorders of Hypopigmentation

• Assess the following parameters:
1. Age of onset (e.g. birth/infancy vs. childhood vs. adulthood).
2. Presence or absence of preceding inflammation.
3. Distribution pattern (see below) and anatomic location.
4. Degree of pigment loss.

• The distribution patterns can be divided into *circumscribed* (e.g. vitiligo), *diffuse* (e.g. albinism), *linear*, or *guttate* (e.g. idiopathic guttate hypomelanosis).

• An approach to leukoderma is outlined in Fig. 54.1.

Vitiligo

• An acquired disease, due to autoimmune destruction of melanocytes, that is characterized by circumscribed, amelanotic macules or patches of the skin and mucous membranes (Fig. 54.2); hairs within involved areas may be depigmented or pigmented; the uveal tract and retinal pigmented epithelium can also be affected.

• Two major subtypes of vitiligo: *generalized* (most common) and *localized* (Fig. 54.3).

• A polygenic disorder, i.e. involving multiple susceptibility genes, plus environmental factors (mostly unknown); increased incidence of other autoimmune disorders, either in the individual with vitiligo (*generalized* > *localized*) or in family members.

• 10–15% of patients with generalized vitiligo have systemic autoimmune diseases, in particular thyroid disease (Hashimoto's thyroiditis or Grave's disease), pernicious

APPROACH TO DISORDERS OF HYPOPIGMENTATION

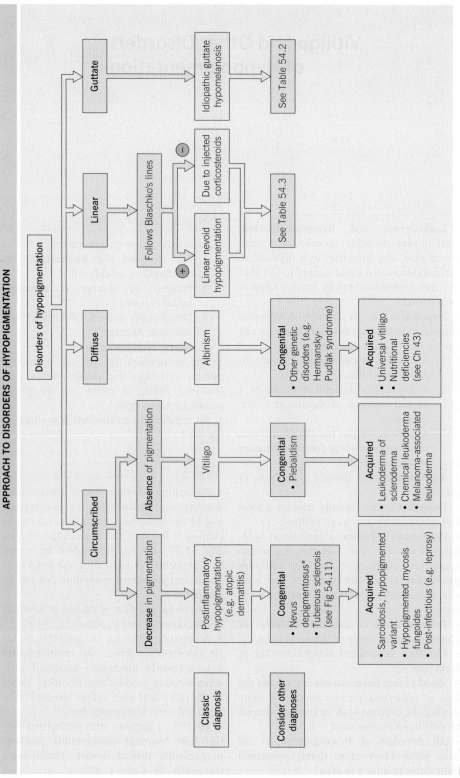

Fig. 54.1 Approach to disorders of hypopigmentation. *May also present in a block-like pattern.

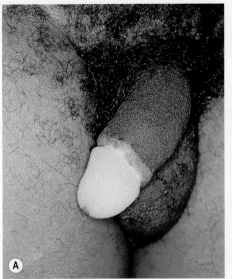
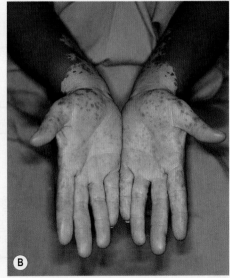

Fig. 54.2 Vitiligo. A Complete loss of pigment of the glans penis. Note the lack of any secondary changes. **B** Depigmentation of the volar wrists as well as the palmar surfaces; easily recognizable in darkly pigmented individuals. *Courtesy, Jean L. Bolognia, MD.*

anemia, Addison's disease, and AI-CTD (e.g. SLE); associated cutaneous disorders include halo melanocytic nevi, alopecia areata, and lichen sclerosus.

- *Generalized vitiligo.*
  - Includes acrofacial, vulgaris, and universal (see Fig. 54.3); occasionally an inflammatory edge is seen (Fig. 54.4).
  - Affects ~1% of the population worldwide; males = females; onset in ~50% before age 20 years; onset after age 50 years is unusual and prompts widening of the **DDx** (see below).
  - The typical lesion is an asymptomatic, amelanotic macule or patch that is milk or chalk-white in color; early on the pigment loss may not be complete; margins are fairly discrete and convex.
  - Course is unpredictable, but often progressive.
- *Segmental vitiligo.*
  - Usually begins in childhood; typically presents in a unilateral, segmental pattern that respects the midline and usually remains stable in size after 1–2 years (Fig. 54.5).
  - **DDx:** nevus depigmentosus (decreased but not total loss of pigment).

- **DDx** of depigmented lesion(s).
  - **In a child:** if 1–2 isolated circular or oval macules, stage 3 halo nevus; piebaldism, Waardenburg syndrome (see below).
  - **In an adult:** chemical leukoderma, melanoma-associated leukoderma, leukoderma of scleroderma, Vogt–Koyanagi–Harada syndrome, onchocerciasis, and postinflammatory *de*pigmentation (see below).
  - With the exception of onchocerciasis, or in areas of sclerosis or inflammation, a biopsy is not particularly helpful.
- **Vitiligo and ocular disease**.
  - Uveitis is the most significant ocular abnormality; asymptomatic depigmented areas of the ocular fundus can also be seen.
  - Uveitis is a major component of the *Vogt–Koyanagi–Harada syndrome*, in which patients also develop aseptic meningitis, otic involvement (e.g. dysacousia), poliosis, and vitiligo, especially of the head and neck region.
  - *Alezzandrini syndrome* is a rare disorder characterized by unilateral facial vitiligo, poliosis, and ipsilateral ocular involvement.

DISTRIBUTION PATTERN OF AMELANOTIC SKIN LESIONS IN VITILIGO

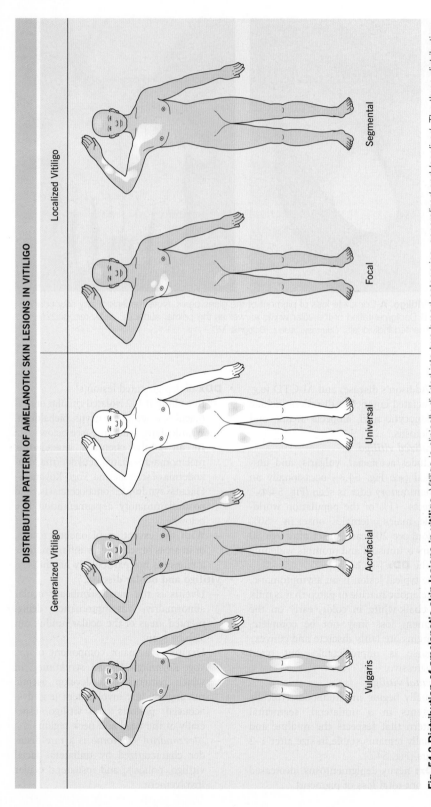

Fig. 54.3 Distribution of amelanotic skin lesions in vitiligo. Vitiligo is clinically divided into two broad categories: *generalized* and *localized*. The three distribution patterns in *generalized* vitiligo include *vulgaris*, *acrofacial*, and *universal*. In *focal* vitiligo, the amelanotic macules or patches are limited to one or only a few areas, but not necessarily in a segmental pattern, as in *segmental* vitiligo, which is also unilateral and respects the midline. *Adapted with permission from Le Poole C, Boissy RE. Vitiligo. Semin. Cutan. Med. Surg. 1997;16:3–14.*

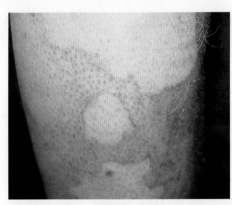

Fig. 54.4 Inflammatory vitiligo. There is a figurate outline to the inflammatory border, which is sometimes misdiagnosed as tinea corporis. *Courtesy, Jean-Paul Ortonne, MD.*

- **Rx:** primarily directed at repigmentation of patient-desired areas (Fig. 54.7).
    - The efficacy of treatment depends on four variables.
        1. **Site**: face, neck, mid extremities > acral, mucosal (i.e. sites without hairs).
        2. **Extent of involvement**: small area > large area.
        3. **Stability**: stable > active or progressive.
        4. **Pigmented hairs within the vitiligo patch**: presence > absence.
    - Repigmentation usually appears in a perifollicular pattern (Fig. 54.6) and/or from the periphery of lesions.

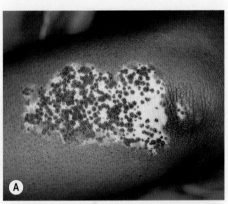

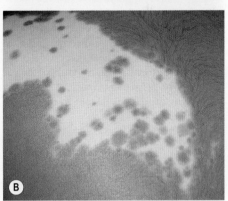

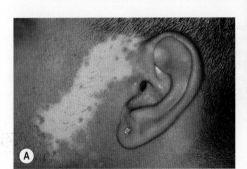

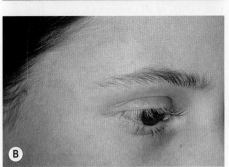

Fig. 54.5 Segmental vitiligo. A Unilateral band of depigmentation on the face, the most common location for segmental vitiligo. Note the pigmented and depigmented hairs within the affected area. **B** Under normal light, vitiligo can be subtle in lightly pigmented individuals. The clue to the diagnosis is the poliosis of the eyelashes. *A, Courtesy, Kalman Watsky MD; B, Courtesy, Jean L. Bolognia, MD.*

Fig. 54.6 Perifollicular repigmentation. Vitiligo on the elbow **(A)** and segmental vitiligo on the back **(B)** responding to PUVA and narrowband UVB therapy, respectively, with repigmentation in a prominent perifollicular pattern as well as from the periphery. The areas of repigmentation are darker in color than the uninvolved skin in **(A)**. *A, Courtesy, Jean L. Bolognia, MD; B, Courtesy, Julie V. Schaffer, MD.*

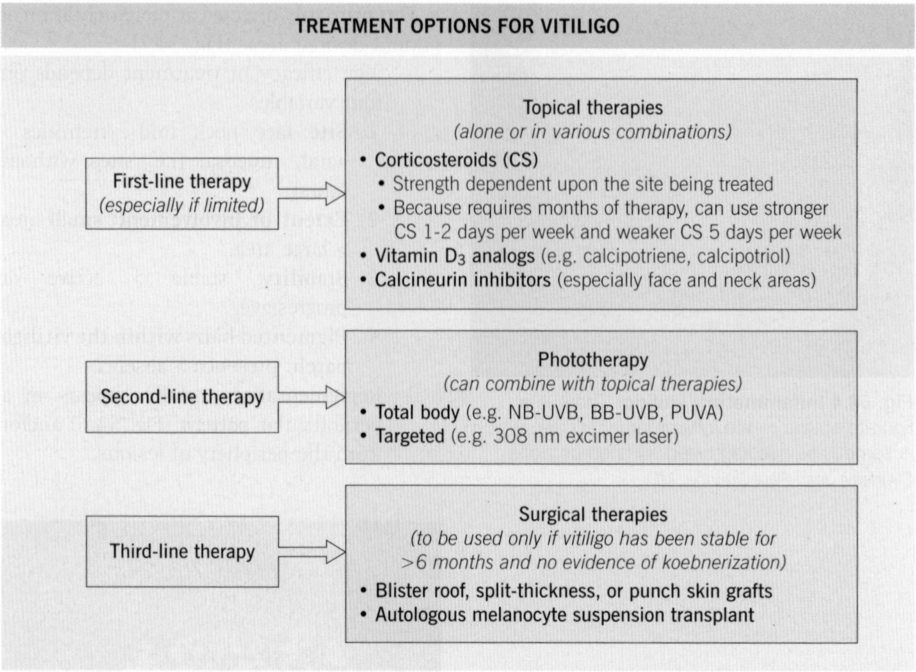

TREATMENT OPTIONS FOR VITILIGO

| First-line therapy
(especially if limited) | → | **Topical therapies**
(alone or in various combinations)
• **Corticosteroids (CS)**
  • Strength dependent upon the site being treated
  • Because requires months of therapy, can use stronger CS 1-2 days per week and weaker CS 5 days per week
• **Vitamin D₃ analogs** (e.g. calcipotriene, calcipotriol)
• **Calcineurin inhibitors** (especially face and neck areas) |

| Second-line therapy | → | **Phototherapy**
(can combine with topical therapies)
• **Total body** (e.g. NB-UVB, BB-UVB, PUVA)
• **Targeted** (e.g. 308 nm excimer laser) |

| Third-line therapy | → | **Surgical therapies**
(to be used only if vitiligo has been stable for >6 months and no evidence of koebnerization)
• Blister roof, split-thickness, or punch skin grafts
• Autologous melanocyte suspension transplant |

Fig. 54.7 Treatment options for vitiligo. Treatment of vitiligo is directed at repigmentation of patient-desired areas. Camouflage can be offered to all patients for temporary (e.g. makeup, self-tanners) or more permanent (e.g. tattoos) cosmetic relief. Referral to a support group [e.g. National Vitiligo Foundation (www.mynvfi.org)] may also be helpful. 10–20% monobenzyl ether of hydroquinone (MBEH) is sometimes used as depigmentation therapy for widespread or treatment-resistant vitiligo, but it can be permanent and lead to loss of pigment in areas distant to the sites of application. NB-UVB, narrowband ultraviolet B; BB-UVB, broadband UVB; PUVA, psoralens plus ultraviolet A.

– 10–20% monobenzyl ether of hydroquinone (MBEH) is sometimes used as depigmentation therapy for widespread or treatment-resistant vitiligo, but it can be permanent and lead to loss of pigment in areas distant to the sites of application.

Hereditary Hypomelanosis

Oculocutaneous Albinism (OCA)

• A group of genetic disorders characterized by pigmentary dilution due to a partial or total absence of melanin within the skin, hair follicles, and eyes; the number of melanocytes is normal.

• Estimated frequency is 1 : 20 000, but may be 1 : 1500 in areas of Africa.

• Four subtypes of OCA (Table 54.1) exist; nearly always inherited in an autosomal recessive manner; OCA1 and OCA2 constitute ~90% of all cases of OCA.

• The ocular manifestations are due to a decrease of melanin within eye structures (e.g. photophobia, reduced visual acuity) or the misrouting of optic nerve fibers during development (e.g. strabismus, nystagmus, lack of stereoscopic vision).

• Early ophthalmologic consultation and strict photoprotection are mandatory; the development of aggressive SCCs (Fig. 54.8A) is a significant cause of morbidity and mortality.

Disorders of Melanocyte Development

PIEBALDISM

• A rare autosomal dominant congenital disorder resulting from mutations in the *KIT* proto-oncogene, causing abnormal melanocyte development.

CLASSIFICATION OF OCULOCUTANEOUS ALBINISM (OCA)

Type/Gene Mutation	Clinical Features
OCA1A *TYR* gene (*absent* tyrosinase activity)	• **At birth:** white hair, milk-white skin, blue-gray eyes, pink nevi • No increase in pigmentation over time, except for the denaturing (yellow color) of hair • Most severe ocular abnormalities (see text)
OCA1B *TYR* gene (*reduced* tyrosinase activity)	• **At birth:** similar to OCA1A • Majority acquire some pigmentation of hair and skin during first two decades of life • Ocular abnormalities less severe than in OCA1A
OCA2 *OCA2* gene (previously known as *P*, 'pink-eyed' dilution)	• **At birth:** more pigmentation compared to OCA1A • Over time, pigmented nevi may develop and large, stellate lentigines appear in photodistributed sites (Fig. 54.8B)
OCA3 *TYRP1* gene	• Red-bronze skin, ginger-red hair, blue or brown irides
OCA4 *SLC45A2* gene (formerly *MATP* gene)	• Similar clinical presentation as OCA2, with variability in pigmentation

TYR, *tyrosinase;* OCA, *oculocutaneous albinism;* TYRP1, *tyrosinase-related protein-1;* SLC45A2, *solute carrier family 45 member 2.*

Table 54.1 Classification of oculocutaneous albinism (OCA).

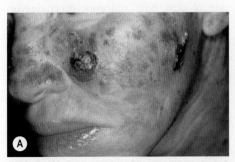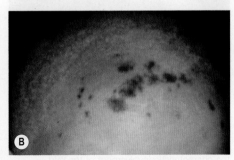

Fig. 54.8 Oculocutaneous albinism type 2 (OCA2). A African patient with obvious squamous cell carcinomas on the cheek as well as multiple pigmented lentigines. **B** African patient with hypopigmented hair and large pigmented lentigines. *Courtesy, James Nordlund, MD.*

• Presents at birth with poliosis of the mid frontal scalp and stable circumscribed areas of amelanosis in a characteristic distribution pattern, favoring the anterior trunk, mid extremities, and central forehead (Fig. 54.9).

• Areas of amelanosis contain normally pigmented and hyperpigmented macules and patches within them (see Fig. 54.9); the latter can be seen in uninvolved skin.

• **Rx:** amenable to autologous skin grafting given its stability.

WAARDENBURG SYNDROME (WS)

• A rare autosomal dominant or recessive disorder characterized by.

– Skin lesions resembling piebaldism, including the white forelock.

– Congenital deafness (10–40%).

– Partial or total heterochromia iridis.

– Medial eyebrow hyperplasia (synophrys).

– Broad nasal root.

– Dystopia canthorum (increase in the distance between the inner canthi with normal interpupillary distance).

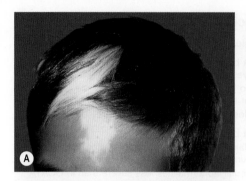

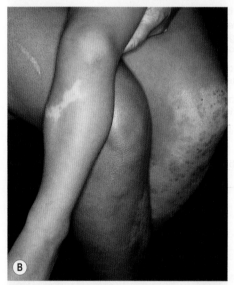

Fig. 54.9 Piebaldism. A White forelock (poliosis) and characteristic triangular amelanotic patch on the mid-forehead. Note the normally pigmented macules of varying sizes within the leukoderma, primarily at the periphery. **B** Mother and son with the characteristic involvement of the mid-extremities. Note the normally pigmented macules within the leukoderma. *A, Courtesy Diane Davidson, MD; B, Courtesy, Jean L. Bolog17a, MD.*

- Four clinical subtypes have been described.
  - WS1: classic form.
  - WS2: lacks dystopia canthorum (Fig. 54.10).
  - WS3: associated limb abnormalities.
  - WS4: associated with Hirschsprung disease.

Disorders of Melanosome Biogenesis

- Because biosynthesis of lysosome-related organelles, e.g. platelet-dense granules and

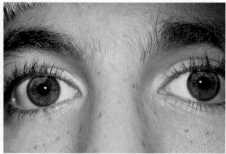

Fig. 54.10 Waardenburg syndrome type 2. Heterochromia iridis in the absence of dystopia canthorum. The white forelock is seen in the upper left corner. *Courtesy, Daniel Albert, MD.*

lytic granules of cytotoxic lymphocytes and natural killer cells, are also affected, patients can have a bleeding diathesis and immunodeficiency.

HERMANSKY–PUDLAK SYNDROME (HPS)

- Autosomal recessive inheritance; eight subtypes; HPS1 and HPS3 are the most common subtypes seen in Puerto Ricans.
- Characterized by variable pigmentary dilution of skin, hair, and eyes, depending on ethnicity; ocular manifestations of OCA; bleeding tendency; normal platelet count with a prolonged bleeding time.
- Depending on HPS subtype, may develop fatal pulmonary fibrosis and/or granulomatous colitis; average life span is 30–50 years.
- No specific treatment other than platelet transfusions prior to surgery.

CHEDIAK–HIGASHI SYNDROME (CHS)

- Characterized by silvery hair, OCA skin and ocular findings, bleeding diathesis, progressive neurologic dysfunction, and infections due to severe immunodeficiency.
- Giant lysosomes within neutrophils seen on peripheral blood smear.
- Death is often in childhood secondary to infection, bleeding, or an accelerated lymphoma-like phase.
- **Rx:** hematopoietic stem cell transplant.

Disorders of Melanosome Transport and/or Transfer to Keratinocytes

- Consequences of this disrupted transport are pigmentary dilution and silvery hair (which contains melanin clumps in the hair shafts).

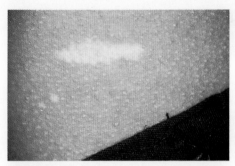

Fig. 54.11 Tuberous sclerosis. Two types of hypomelanotic macules, lance-ovate (ash leaf) and confetti (idiopathic guttate hypomelanosis-like). *Courtesy, David Strobel, MD.*

GRISCELLI SYNDROME (GS)

• Autosomal recessive; three subtypes, based on sites of expression of three mutated genes; all characterized by silvery hair and pigmentary dilution; patients can also have neurologic impairment (GS1) or immune abnormalities and hemophagocytic syndrome (GS2).

Other

TUBEROUS SCLEROSIS (TS)

(See Chapter 50)

• Hypomelanotic macules are often the first sign of TS.

• These hypomelanotic macules are typically multiple in number; polygonal is the most common shape, followed by lance-ovate or 'ash leaf' (Fig. 54.11); less often, the macules are 'thumbprint'-like, guttate/confetti, or segmental (see Fig. 54.11; Table 54.2); lesions favor the trunk or extremities.

Hypopigmentation in Mosaic Patterns

• Several patterns of hypopigmentation can result from a mosaic 'clone' of skin cells with decreased potential for pigment production ('pigmentary mosaicism').

• Hypopigmented areas may be apparent at birth or become evident during childhood, especially in patients with fair skin.

LINEAR NEVOID HYPOPIGMENTATION

• Localized or widespread streaks and swirls of hypopigmentation that follow Blaschko's lines, which represent pathways of epidermal

DIFFERENTIAL DIAGNOSIS OF GUTTATE LEUKODERMA
• Idiopathic guttate hypomelanosis*
• Pityriasis lichenoides chronica
• Lichen sclerosus
• Confetti-like lesions of tuberous sclerosis
• Early tinea versicolor (especially face)
• Achromic verruca plana**
• Frictional lichenoid dermatosis†
• Clear cell papulosis†
• Vitiligo ponctué
• Darier's disease
• Xeroderma pigmentosum
• In association with chromosomal abnormalities
• Following PUVA therapy

Seen in adults.
**Minimally elevated flat-topped papules.*
†Often papular.*
Adapted from Bolognia JL, Shapiro PE. Albinism and other disorders of hypopigmentation. In Arndt KA, et al. (Eds.), Cutaneous Medicine and Surgery. *Philadelphia: Saunders, 1995.*

Table 54.2 Differential diagnosis of guttate leukoderma. The size of the lesions in guttate leukoderma is smaller than in guttate psoriasis. Guttate hypopigmentation may also be seen in the setting of dyschromatoses (see Chapter 55).

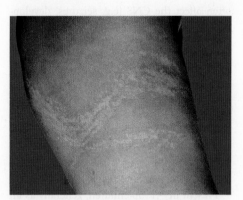

Fig. 54.12 Linear nevoid hypopigmentation. Note the S-shaped pattern of the hypopigmented streaks along Blaschko's lines.

cell migration during embryogenesis (Fig. 54.12; see Fig. 51.1).

• ~10–30% of affected individuals have associated extracutaneous abnormalities, which usually develop during infancy and most

DIFFERENTIAL DIAGNOSIS OF LINEAR HYPOPIGMENTATION

Disorder	Clinical Clues
Lesions Follow Blaschko's Lines	
Linear nevoid hypopigmentation	• Macular, early onset
Lichen striatus (Fig. 54.15D)	• Subtle elevation, favors children
Epidermal nevus	• Subtle elevation, early onset
Nevus comedonicus	• Superimposed comedones, early onset
Linear lichen sclerosus	• Shiny wrinkled surface, follicular plugging
Goltz syndrome	• Dermal atrophy, fat 'herniation,' early onset
Menkes disease (female carrier)	• Pili torti on scalp, early onset
Linear Darier disease	• Guttate hypopigmented macules, crusted papules
Lesions Occasionally Follow Blaschko's Lines	
Segmental vitiligo* (Fig. 54.5)	• Depigmented
Incontinentia pigmenti stage 4** (Fig. 54.14)	• Hairless and atrophic, favors calves
Lesions Do Not Follow Blaschko's Lines	
Due to injected corticosteroids (Fig. 54.22A)	• Irregular outline, along lymphatics
Pigmentary demarcation lines, type C	• Vertical or curved on mid chest (see Chapter 55)

*More often in a unilateral band or block-like configuration.
**Linear streaks typically resemble Chinese characters.

Table 54.3 Differential diagnosis of linear hypopigmentation.

often affect the CNS (e.g. seizures, developmental delay), eyes, or musculoskeletal system; evaluation is directed by clinical findings.
• The term *hypomelanosis of Ito* has been used in studies focusing on linear nevoid hypopigmentation associated with systemic manifestations, and it should be reserved for this subset of patients.
• **DDx:** outlined in Table 54.3 (see Fig. 54.14).

NEVUS DEPIGMENTOSUS
• Present in ~1:50 children, generally as an isolated finding.
• Lesions are typically hypopigmented, not depigmented as implied by the name.
• *Classic form*: ovoid or irregular hypopigmented patch, often breaking up into smaller macules at its periphery (Fig. 54.13).
• *Segmental form* (hypopigmented variant of 'segmental pigmentation disorder'): block-like hypopigmented patch with midline demarcation and less distinct lateral borders.

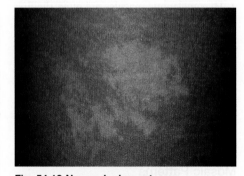

Fig. 54.13 Nevus depigmentosus.
Hypomelanotic patch with a decrease, but not absence, of pigmentation. Note how the lesion breaks apart into smaller macules at its periphery, resembling a 'splash of paint.'

PHYLLOID HYPOMELANOSIS
• Leaf-shaped and oblong hypopigmented macules and patches in an arrangement resembling a floral ornament, usually in the setting of mosaic trisomy 13 and associated with CNS abnormalities.

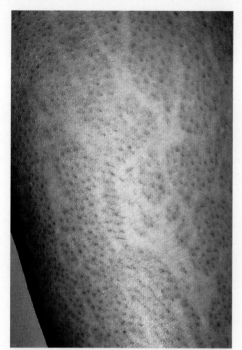

Fig. 54.14 Stage 4 of incontinentia pigmenti. Note the absence of hairs within the streaks on the calf.

Postinflammatory Hypomelanoses

• Inflammatory skin conditions can potentially result in postinflammatory *hypo*pigmentation or *hyper*pigmentation or both (see Chapter 55).

• Postinflammatory hypopigmentation is a very common skin disorder that follows a wide variety of dermatoses, most commonly atopic dermatitis, seborrheic dermatitis, and psoriasis, as well as pityriasis lichenoides chronica, lichen striatus, and lichen sclerosus (Fig. 54.15).

• It typically coexists or co-localizes with the inflammatory lesions, but occasionally only hypopigmented lesions are seen; the size, shape, and distribution pattern often provide clues to the underlying inflammatory dermatosis.

• Most commonly there is a decrease in pigmentation; rarely there is an absence (e.g. severe atopic dermatitis).

• Histopathologic examination is often non-specific, but in certain diseases (e.g. sarcoidosis and hypopigmented mycosis fungoides) can be diagnostic.

• **Rx** of underlying dermatosis is followed by gradual resolution.

Pityriasis Alba (See Chapter 10)

• A very common, asymptomatic disorder seen primarily during childhood and adolescence.

• On the malar region of the face, one to several slightly scaly, hypopigmented macules and patches are seen; the lesions are usually ill-defined and occasionally there is associated mild inflammation.

• The hypomelanosis often remains stationary and unchanged for several years; emollients, sunscreens, or low-strength topical CS (e.g. hydrocortisone 2.5%) may be helpful.

• **DDx:** tinea versicolor, early vitiligo, and postinflammatory hypopigmentation from seborrheic dermatitis or atopic dermatitis.

Sarcoidosis

• Sarcoidosis occurs more commonly in African-Americans, and the hypopigmented variant of cutaneous sarcoidosis may go undiagnosed; this form has no associated prognostic significance and may spontaneously repigment.

• Hypopigmented papules, plaques, or sometimes nodules are seen; range in size from 1 to several cm.

• Histopathology reveals noncaseating granulomas.

Hypopigmented Mycosis Fungoides (MF) (See Chapter 98)

• A variant of early stage MF that is most commonly observed in darkly pigmented individuals (see Fig. 54.15E); seen in adults, as well as children and adolescents.

• Atrophy often observed within the hypopigmented patches.

• Histopathology reveals typical features of MF.

• **DDx:** hypopigmented parapsoriasis, pityriasis lichenoides chronica (PLC).

Cutaneous Lupus Erythematosus (LE) (See Chapter 33)

• In discoid LE (DLE), hypomelanosis is often seen centrally within well-developed

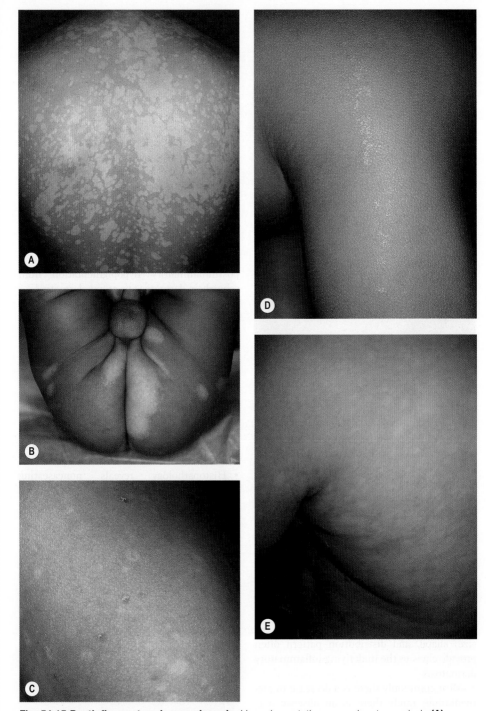

Fig. 54.15 Postinflammatory hypomelanosis. Hypopigmentation secondary to psoriasis **(A),** seborrheic dermatitis in an infant **(B),** pityriasis lichenoides chronica **(C),** lichen striatus (note the flat-topped papules) **(D),** and hypopigmented mycosis fungoides **(E).** *B, Courtesy, Jean L. Bolognia, MD. Continued*

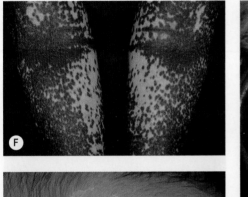

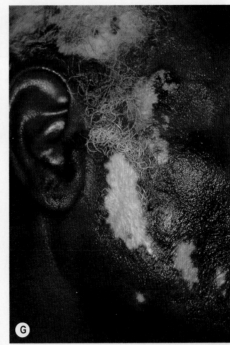

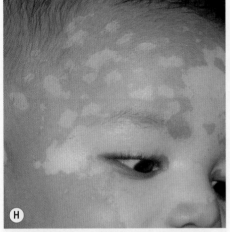

Fig. 54.15 *Continued* Complete pigment loss in patients with severe atopic dermatitis **(F)**, discoid lupus erythematosus **(G)**, and neonatal lupus erythematosus **(H)**. *H, Courtesy, Julie V. Schaffer, MD.*

lesions and the lesions also have cutaneous atrophy, scarring, and a hyperpigmented rim; pigmentary changes tend to be persistent (see Fig. 54.15G).

• In subacute cutaneous LE (SCLE), hypomelanosis typically occurs within the center of annular lesions and is usually reversible.

Systemic Sclerosis (SSc or Generalized Scleroderma)
(See Chapter 35)

• Patients with SSc can develop several pigmentary abnormalities, including diffuse hypermelanosis with photoaccentuation, mixed hyper- and hypopigmentation in areas of chronic sclerosis, and a characteristic leukoderma in both sclerotic and nonsclerotic skin (Fig. 54.16).

• This 'leukoderma of scleroderma' presents as circumscribed areas of depigmentation but with perifollicular and supravenous retention of pigment (see Fig. 54.16).

• This peculiar leukoderma is rather specific for SSc as it occasionally occurs in two other clinical settings, an overlap syndrome (that includes SSc) and scleromyxedema.

• Although clinically similar to the perifollicular repigmentation seen in treatment-responsive vitiligo, it is different in that in vitiligo the perifollicular macules represent *new* pigmentation, whereas in SSc the macules represent *old* or retained pigmentation.

Lichen Sclerosus (LS)
(See Chapter 36)

• Genital and extragenital lesions of LS are often hypopigmented, but in addition display cutaneous atrophy, follicular plugging (extragenital), and purpura (genital).

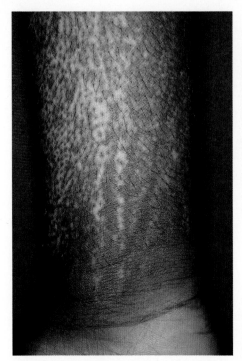

Fig. 54.16 Leukoderma of scleroderma.
Uniform retention of perifollicular pigment within areas of leukoderma. Hyperpigmentation is also seen overlying a superficial vein.

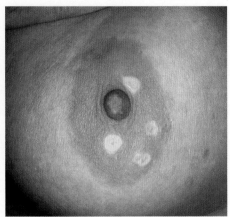

Fig. 54.17 Guttate lichen sclerosus involving the areolae.

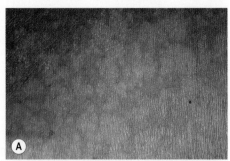

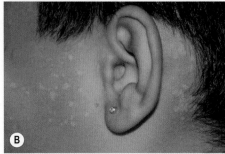

Fig. 54.18 Tinea (pityriasis) versicolor.
A Hypopigmented variant with obvious scale.
B Guttate hypopigmented lesions on the cheek; note the classic scaly lesions in the posterior auricular area. *B, Courtesy, Julie V. Schaffer, MD.*

• Occasionally extragenital LS presents as guttate leukoderma (Fig. 54.17; see Table 54.2).

Infectious and Parasitic Hypomelanosis

Tinea (Pityriasis) Versicolor
(See Chapter 64)

• A very common superficial cutaneous mycosis caused by *Malassezia* spp.; although there is usually minimal inflammation, this infection can lead to both hyper- and hypopigmentation.
• Typically presents symmetrically on the upper trunk and shoulders or flexural areas (e.g. groin and inframammary) as round to oval macules or thin papules that coalesce into patches or thin plaques; the lesions vary in color from pink to light tan to brown, hence the term *versicolor* (Fig. 54.18).
• Lesions often coalesce and when untreated, there is usually a subtle overlying fine scale

that is more readily apparent upon scratching or stretching the skin.
• Diagnosis is easily confirmed by KOH examination of the associated scale.
• Hypomelanosis without any scaling may remain for months after treatment.

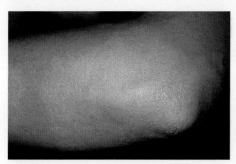

Fig. 54.19 Tuberculoid leprosy. Large thin hypopigmented plaque on the elbow with a raised light pink border.

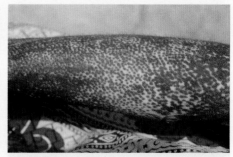

Fig. 54.20 Onchocerciasis (leopard skin). Depigmentation of the shin with follicular repigmentation or retention of perifollicular pigment, a common site for the associated leukoderma. Clinically resembles repigmenting vitiligo or the leukoderma of scleroderma. *Courtesy, Jean-Paul Ortonne, MD.*

Leprosy (See Chapter 62)

• *Tuberculoid leprosy* (Fig. 54.19): fewer larger hypopigmented patches with discrete, often raised, borders; favor posterolateral aspects of extremities, back, buttocks, face; associated anhidrosis, alopecia, and loss of sensation.
• *Borderline leprosy*: occasionally, ill-defined hypomelanotic macules are seen.
• *Indeterminate leprosy*: erythematous to hypomelanotic macules asymmetrically distributed on exposed sites; normal hair.
• *Lepromatous leprosy*: hypomelanotic macules may be the earliest manifestation; often small, multiple, subtle, and ill-defined; favor the face, extremities, and buttocks; minimal or no anhidrosis or loss of sensation.

Treponematoses (See Chapters 61 and 69)

• Non-venereal treponematoses (e.g. pinta, yaws, bejel) and venereal syphilis may be associated with hypomelanosis, especially during their untreated phase.

Onchocerciasis (River Blindness) (See Chapter 70)

• A filarial infestation that predominantly affects cutaneous and ocular tissues and is caused by the transmission of *Onchocerca volvulus* from the bite of a black fly in tropical areas of Africa > Central and South America.
• A later cutaneous finding is leukoderma of the shins with follicular pigmentation, resembling leopard skin (Fig. 54.20).

• **DDx:** atopic dermatitis with postinflammatory depigmentation, or atopic dermatitis plus vitiligo with Koebner phenomenon.

Other

• Hypopigmentation may also result from cutaneous bacterial or viral infections, e.g. herpes zoster.

Melanoma-Associated Leukoderma (See Chapter 93)

• Vitiligo-like depigmentation can occur in patients with cutaneous or ocular melanoma, either spontaneously or in the setting of immunotherapy (e.g. interleukin-2, interferon, ipilimumab, lambrolizumab, nivolumab).
• Thought to result from an immune reaction directed against shared antigens on normal and malignant melanocytes (Fig. 54.21).
• Whereas the spontaneous form points to the need for re-staging, the treatment-associated form can portend a better prognosis.

Chemical Leukoderma

• Contact with a number of chemical agents can lead to hypomelanosis of the skin and hair (Fig. 54.22).
• Depigmenting compounds have chemical structures that are similar to melanin

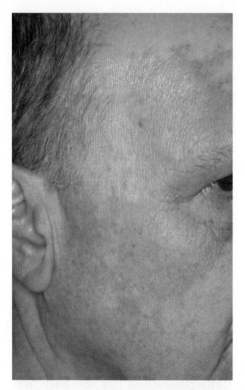

Fig. 54.21 Melanoma-associated leukoderma. Vitiligo-like leukoderma associated with ipilimumab, i.e. anti-cytotoxic T-lymphocyte-associated antigen-4 (CTLA-4) therapy for metastatic melanoma. *Courtesy, Jean L. Bolognia, MD.*

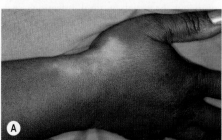
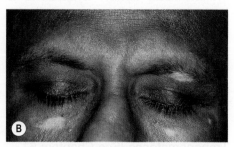

Fig. 54.22 Chemical leukoderma. A Hypopigmentation due to injection of corticosteroids into the anatomic snuff box. The outline is both stellate and linear. Typically appears several weeks to months after the injection. In most cases repigmentation occurs within one year after stopping the injections. **B** Depigmentation developed at sites of contact with rubber swimming goggles. *B, Courtesy, Kalman Watsky, MD.*

precursors; they include catechols, phenols, or quinones (e.g. hydroquinone [HQ] or monobenzyl ether of HQ [MBEH]).
• HQ induces a reversible hypopigmentation, whereas MBEH depigmentation is often permanent and occurs not only at the site of application but also at distant sites.
• Topical and injected CS can also lead to hypopigmentation (see Fig. 54.22).

Miscellaneous

Idiopathic Guttate Hypomelanosis (IGH)

• A very common disorder that increases in incidence with age; occurs in all races and skin types (Fig. 54.23).
• Typically presents as multiple, asymptomatic, small (guttate), well-circumscribed white macules on the extensor forearms and shins; the surface is smooth, often with accentuation of the skin markings.

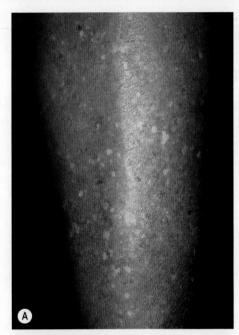

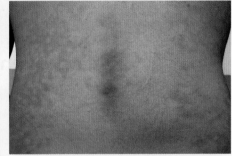

Fig. 54.24 Progressive macular hypomelanosis. Note the coalescence of the non-scaly hypopigmented macules on the center of the back. *Courtesy, Jean-Paul Ortonne, MD.*

• **DDx:** other guttate leukodermas (see Table 54.2).

Progressive Macular Hypomelanosis of the Trunk (PMH)

• Characterized by asymptomatic, poorly defined, small, round to oval, non-scaly, hypopigmented macules and patches, primarily on the trunk and proximal upper extremities, often with confluence of lesions (Fig. 54.24).

• A less common variant is seen in Afro-Caribbean females as larger patches.

• **DDx:** previously treated tinea versicolor.

Hair Hypomelanosis

• Circumscribed (poliosis) versus generalized (canities).

• Graying of hair, either localized or generalized, is characterized by an admixture of normally pigmented, hypomelanotic and amelanotic hairs.

• Whitening of hair is the endpoint of graying of hair, and both are due to defective maintenance of melanocyte stem cells.

• Premature graying of the hair has been associated with a number of genetic disorders (e.g. Werner syndrome, piebaldism) as well as vitiligo.

• Diffuse hypomelanosis of hair has been associated with both hereditary (e.g. Fanconi syndrome) and acquired causes (e.g. tyrosine kinase inhibitors, antimalarials).

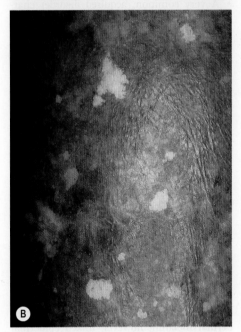

Fig. 54.23 Idiopathic guttate hypomelanosis.
A Typical 1- to 5-mm macules on the shin.
B Occasionally there is an admixture of larger lesions.

For further information see Chs. 65 and 66. From *Dermatology, Third Edition.*

55

Disorders of Hyperpigmentation

Definitions

• **Hyperpigmentation**: a term used to describe disorders characterized by darkening of the skin; encompasses hypermelanosis.
• **Hypermelanosis**: a more specific term that denotes an increase in the melanin content of the skin; typically due to an increase in melanin production but occasionally from an increase in the density of active melanocytes.
• **Discoloration**: a term used to describe an abnormal color of the skin; may be due to deposition of substances such as drugs, drug complexes (e.g. with melanin or iron), or heavy metals within the dermis.
• **Dyschromatosis**: a disorder characterized by the presence of both hypo- and hyperpigmentation.
• **Pigment incontinence**: the presence of melanin within dermal macrophages (melanophages); the source of the melanin is the epidermis, and this typically results from inflammation at the dermal–epidermal junction.
• **Epidermal pigmentation**: denotes increased melanin within the epidermis, which typically leads to a light brown to dark brown color.
• **Dermal pigmentation**: denotes increased melanin in the dermis, primarily within melanophages; characteristically presents as a gray-blue to gray-brown color.

Approach to Disorders of Hyperpigmentation

• Disorders of hyperpigmentation usually result from an increase in melanin production and occasionally from an increase in the density of active melanocytes.
• The clinical approach to these disorders is simplified by dividing them into four patterns, namely *circumscribed, diffuse, linear,* and *reticulated* (Fig. 55.1).

• The most common clinical pattern is *circumscribed*; observation of the sites of involvement, shape, configuration, and size can provide clues to the diagnosis.
• The dyschromatoses are discussed separately.

Circumscribed Hyperpigmentation

• The three major entities in this category are melasma, postinflammatory hyperpigmentation, and drug-induced hyperpigmentation.

MELASMA
• A very common, acquired disorder characterized by symmetric, hyperpigmented patches with irregular borders, resulting from an increase in epidermal and/or dermal melanin; favors the face (see below) > mid-upper chest and extensor forearms.
• Seen primarily in women; increased prevalence in individuals with skin phototypes III–IV.
• Pathogenesis thought to be related to hyperfunctional melanocytes that are stimulated by exacerbating factors, such as sun exposure and hormones (e.g. pregnancy, oral contraceptives).
• Three classic clinical patterns based on distribution: centrofacial (most common), malar, and mandibular (Fig. 55.2).
• Classically, melasma was also classified based on findings from Wood's lamp examination: lesions that enhance imply an increase in epidermal melanin and lesions that do not enhance imply an increase in dermal melanin; however, mixed epidermal and dermal melasma patterns are common.
• In northern latitudes, lesions tend to fade during the winter months; melasma tends to be more persistent in darkly pigmented individuals.
• **DDx:** postinflammatory hyperpigmentation, drug-induced (e.g. minocycline, amiodarone), acquired bilateral nevus of Ota-like

APPROACH TO DISORDERS OF HYPERPIGMENTATION

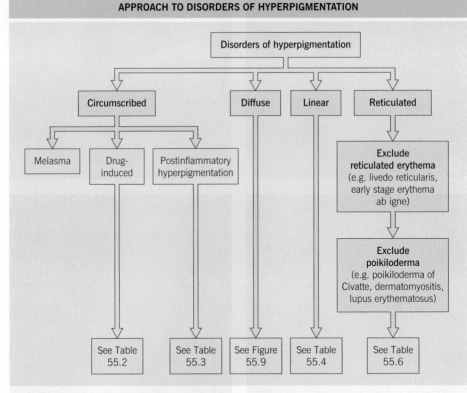

Fig. 55.1 Approach to disorders of hyperpigmentation.

macules (especially in Asian women), actinic lichen planus, pigmented contact dermatitis, exogenous ochronosis due to the application of hydroquinone-containing bleaching agents, erythromelanosis faciei.

• These other disorders are distinguished from melasma based on historical aspects (e.g. drug ingestion, application of topical medications or cosmetics, previous inflammation), color (e.g. clusters of nevus of Ota-like macules are typically blue-gray in color), distribution pattern, histologic features, and primary lesions, if present.

• Treatment options are outlined in Table 55.1; typically epidermal hyperpigmentation responds best to treatment.

DRUG-INDUCED CIRCUMSCRIBED HYPERPIGMENTATION AND DISCOLORATION

• A wide range of medications and chemicals can cause hyperpigmentation or discoloration

in circumscribed, diffuse, and even linear patterns; longitudinal or horizontal melano-nychia may also be present.

• The most common culprits of drug-induced circumscribed hyperpigmentation and discoloration are minocycline and the antimalarials (Table 55.2; Figs. 55.3–55.6).

• The pathogenesis involves varying mechanisms, from increased melanin production to deposition of drug complexes or heavy metals within the dermis.

• The hyperpigmentation or discoloration typically resolves upon discontinuation of the offending drug, but the course may be prolonged.

POSTINFLAMMATORY HYPERPIGMENTATION

• Represents an acquired excess of melanin pigment following cutaneous inflammation (e.g. acne, psoriasis) or injury (e.g. burns or friction).

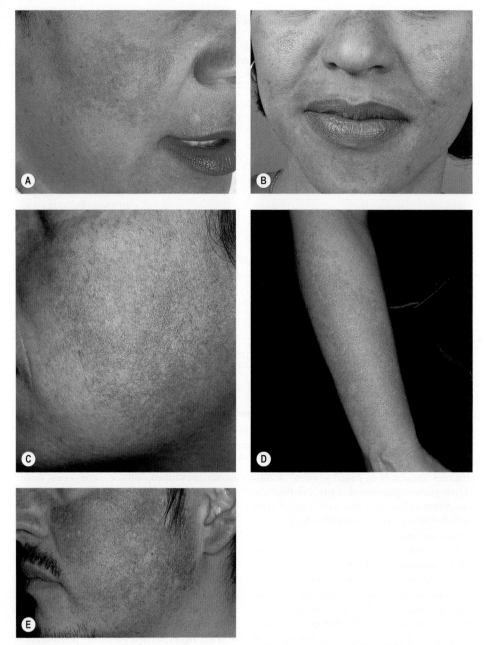

Fig. 55.2 Various forms of melasma and melasma-like hyperpigmentation. A Malar variant.
B Mild centrofacial type with sparing of the philtrum. **C** Extension of the hyperpigmentation onto the
mandible. **D** Involvement of the extensor forearm; note the same irregular outline as seen on the
face. **E** Melasma-like appearance in a patient with previous acute cutaneous lupus erythematosus.
C–E, Courtesy, Jean L. Bolognia, MD.

SUGGESTED TREATMENT OPTIONS FOR MELASMA

Recommendations for All Patients

- Avoidance of sun exposure and tanning beds
- Daily use of broad-spectrum sunscreen (ideally SPF ≥30 with physical blocker such as zinc oxide or titanium dioxide)
- Sun-protective hats and clothing
- Camouflage makeup
- Discontinue oral contraceptives, if possible

Active/Intense Treatment Options*,*

First-line topical therapies
- Triple combination of HQ + retinoid + CS† at bedtime
- 4% HQ daily, typically at bedtime
- Azelaic acid (15–20%)

Adjunctive topical therapy
- L-ascorbic acid (10–15%)
- Kojic acid (1–4%)

Second-line therapies
- Glycolic (typically start at 30% and increase as tolerated) or salicyclic acid peels every 4–6 weeks

Third-line therapies‡
- Fractional laser therapy
- Intense pulsed light therapy (IPL)

Long-Term Maintenance Recommendations

- Daily sunscreen and sun protective measures (see above)
- Topical retinoid
- Topical α-hydroxy acid (e.g. glycolic acid cream)
- Other topicals (e.g. L-ascorbic acid [10–15%], azelaic acid [15–20%], or kojic acid [1–4%])

*Results from topical treatments may take up to 6 months to appreciate; depending on the patient, HQ and combination HQ + retinoid + CS are typically used daily for 2–4 months and then decreased in frequency to 1–2 times per week; prolonged daily use can result in side effects such as perioral dermatitis, telangiectasias, and atrophy (CS) and ochronosis (HQ).
**While topical HQ can cause an allergic contact dermatitis, all topical agents may cause an irritant contact dermatitis, which can result in worsening of the dyspigmentation; if this is a concern, a small, nonfacial site test can be performed prior to widespread facial application.
†Typically a Class 5–7 topical CS is used (see Appendix).
‡Potential risk of post-procedural dyspigmentation; a site test should be performed prior to widespread facial laser or light therapy.
HQ, hydroquinone.

Table 55.1 Suggested treatment options for melasma.

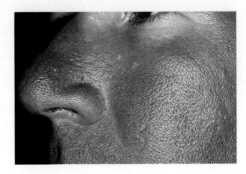

Fig. 55.3 Gray-violet discoloration of the face due to amiodarone. Note the sparing of the lower eyelid. *Courtesy, Jean L. Bolognia, MD.*

DRUGS AND CHEMICALS ASSOCIATED WITH CIRCUMSCRIBED HYPERPIGMENTATION OR DISCOLORATION

Drug or Chemical	Clinical Features
Chemotherapeutic Agents	
BCNU (carmustine), mechlorethamine (nitrogen mustard)	• Hyperpigmentation at sites of topical application
Bleomycin (intravenous or intralesional)	See text
Anthracyclines (e.g. daunorubicin, doxorubicin)	• Hyperpigmentation of sun-exposed areas • Hyperpigmentation overlying the small joints of the hand and involving the palms (especially the creases), soles, and oral mucosa (buccal, tongue) • Transverse brown-black melanonychia
5-Fluorouracil	• Hyperpigmentation in sun-exposed areas (~5% of patients treated systemically; often follows an erythematous photosensitivity reaction) • Hyperpigmentation of skin overlying veins in which the drug was infused • Other sites include the dorsal aspects of the hands, palms/soles, and radiation ports • Transverse or diffuse melanonychia; lunular pigmentation
Antimalarials	
Chloroquine, hydroxychloroquine, quinacrine	• Gray to blue-black discoloration, usually pretibial, with (hydroxy)chloroquine; face, hard palate, sclerae, and subungual areas may be involved • Diffuse yellow to yellow-brown discoloration with quinacrine • Discoloration affects up to 25% of patients
Heavy Metals	
Arsenic	• Areas of bronze hyperpigmentation ± superimposed 'raindrops' of lightly pigmented skin; favors axillae, groin, palms, soles, nipples, and pressure points (see Fig. 74.7A) • See Chapter 74
Bismuth	• Generalized blue-gray discoloration of the face, neck, and dorsal hands • Oral mucosa and gingivae may be involved
Gold (chrysiasis)	• Permanent blue-gray discoloration in sun-exposed areas, mostly around the eyes
Iron	• Permanent brown discoloration at injection sites or in areas of application of ferric subsulfate (Monsel's) solution as a hemostatic agent • Dermal hemosiderin deposits (due to lysis of extravasated red blood cells and release of their iron stores) are commonly observed in the setting of venous hypertension, in pigmented purpuric dermatoses, at sites of previous solar purpura, and as a side effect of sclerotherapy of superficial veins
Lead	• 'Lead line' in gingival margin • Nail discoloration
Mercury	• Slate-gray discoloration, particularly in skin folds

Table 55.2 Drugs and chemicals associated with circumscribed hyperpigmentation or discoloration. Diffuse hyperpigmentation and discoloration is discussed in Fig. 55.9. *Continued*

Table 55.2 *Continued* **Drugs and chemicals associated with circumscribed hyperpigmentation or discoloration.** Diffuse hyperpigmentation and discoloration is discussed in Fig. 55.9.

Drug or Chemical	Clinical Features
Silver (argyria)	• Sites of topical application (e.g. of silver sulfadiazine to burns or ulcers) • Diffuse slate-gray discoloration, increased in sun-exposed areas; occurs in settings of occupational exposure, alternative medications, or systemic absorption from use of silver sulfadiazine on extensive burns/wounds • The nail unit (diffuse or localized to the lunulae) and sclerae may also be affected
Hormones	
Oral contraceptives, hormone replacement therapy	• Melasma; increased pigmentation of nipples and nevi
Miscellaneous Compounds	
Amiodarone	• Slate-gray to violaceous discoloration of sun-exposed skin, especially the face (less common than erythema from photosensitivity; Fig. 55.3) • Fair-skinned patients after long-term, continuous therapy; usually fades over months to years after discontinuation of the drug, but may persist
Azidothymidine (zidovudine, AZT)	• Longitudinal > transverse and diffuse melanonychia (up to 10% of patients); blue lunulae • Mucocutaneous hyperpigmentation (e.g. widespread diffuse, acral, oral macules); most common in patients with darkly pigmented skin, and may be accentuated in areas of friction or sun exposure
Clofazimine	• Violet-brown to blue-gray discoloration, especially lesional skin (Figs. 55.4 and 62.6B) • Diffuse red to red-brown discoloration of skin, conjunctivae
Diltiazem	• Slate-gray to gray-brown discoloration of sun-exposed skin in patients with skin phototypes IV–VI (see Fig. 73.11); perifollicular accentuation and a reticular pattern may be observed
Hydroquinone	See text and Fig. 55.5
Minocycline	• *Type I*: blue-black discoloration in sites of inflammation and scars, including those due to acne (Fig. 55.6C) • *Type II*: blue-gray macules/patches (1 mm–10 cm in size) within previously normal skin, most often on the shins (Fig. 55.6A,B); sometimes misdiagnosed as ecchymoses • *Type III*: diffuse 'muddy brown' pigmentation that is most prominent in sun-exposed areas • Blue-black discoloration may also involve nails, sclerae, oral mucosa, bones, thyroid, and teeth
Psychotropic drugs (e.g. chlorpromazine, amitriptyline)	• Slate-gray discoloration in sun-exposed areas

BCNU, 1,3-bis (2-chloroethyl)-1-nitrosourea.

DISORDERS OF HYPERPIGMENTATION

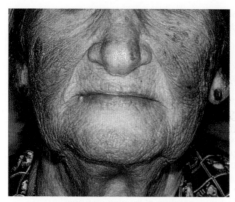

Fig. 55.4 Blue-violet discoloration of previous leprosy lesions in a patient treated with clofazimine. *Courtesy, Anne Burdick, MD.*

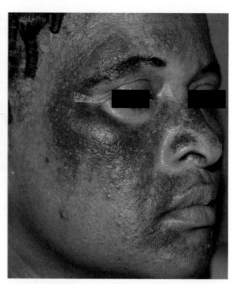

Fig. 55.5 Exogenous ochronosis secondary to topical hydroquinone. This cause of progressive darkening is seen more commonly in Africa. *Courtesy, Regional Dermatology Training Centre, Moshi, Tanzania.*

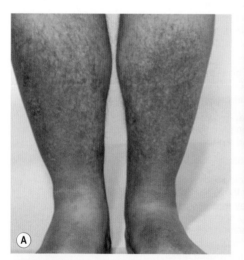

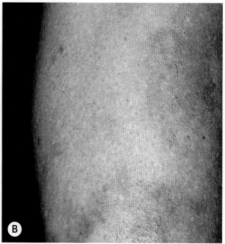

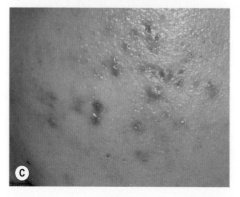

Fig. 55.6 Minocycline-induced discoloration.
A The distribution on the shins and the gray-blue color can be similar to that seen with antimalarials. **B** Sometimes the discoloration is misdiagnosed as ecchymoses, but the subsequent color changes of green and yellow do not occur. **C** Blue-black pigmentation within acne scars and inflammatory papules.
A, Courtesy, Mary Wu Chang, MD; C, Courtesy, Richard Antaya, MD.

- Depending on the disorder, postinflammatory hypopigmentation may also occur and is discussed in Chapter 54.
- Can occur anywhere on the body, including the mucosae or nail unit; increased pigmentation is localized to areas of inflammation and becomes more apparent once the associated erythema resolves (likened to 'a shadow left behind').
- The preceding inflammation may be obvious, transient, or subclinical (Table 55.3; Fig. 55.7).

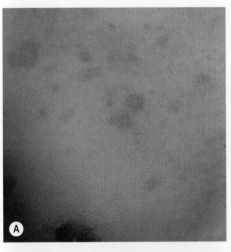

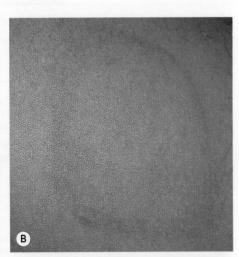

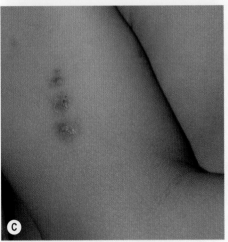

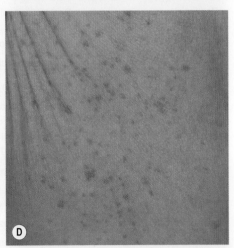

Fig. 55.7 Epidermal postinflammatory hyperpigmentation. The lesions were due to pemphigus foliaceus **(A)**, contact dermatitis from a contraceptive patch **(B)**, insect bites **(C)**, and transient neonatal pustular melanosis **(D)**. Note the residual inflammation and 'breakfast–lunch–dinner' configuration in **(C)**. **E** Linear epidermal postinflammatory hyperpigmentation due to phytophotodermatitis, which requires contact with a plant (e.g. lime) containing a photosensitizing chemical followed by UVR exposure. The desquamation is at the site of a previous bulla. *A, C, D, Courtesy, Julie V. Schaffer, MD; B, Courtesy, Andrew Alexis, MD, MPH.*

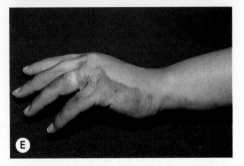

DISORDERS ASSOCIATED WITH POSTINFLAMMATORY HYPERPIGMENTATION

Inflammatory Disease	Clinical Clues
Common	
Acne vulgaris	Head/neck region, upper trunk; <1 cm; perifollicular
Atopic dermatitis	Atopic diathesis; face and extensor extremities in infants, then later flexural involvement; excoriations; atopic pleats; xerosis; lichenification; transverse nasal crease ('allergic salute')
Lichen simplex chronicus	Common locations: posterior neck, ankle, scrotum
Transient neonatal pustular melanosis (Fig. 55.7D)	Black newborns; pustules may precede pigmentation
Impetigo	Favors face; most common in children
Insect bites (Fig. 55.7C)	Favor exposed areas; usually <1 cm; lower extremities common with flea bites; clustered and sometimes linear patterns ('breakfast–lunch–dinner')
Linear trauma (Fig. 55.16)	Often a preceding history of trauma or injury; may have an angular or irregular shape or configuration
Less Common	
Irritant and allergic contact and photocontact dermatitis (Fig. 55.7B,E)	Sites determined by etiologic agent and form of exposure; phytophotodermatitis leads to irregularly shaped or linear hyperpigmentation in sun-exposed areas
Pityriasis rosea	Favors trunk and proximal extremities; lesions follow skin cleavage lines; oval-shaped
Psoriasis	Scalp/nail involvement; knees/elbows most common sites
Polymorphic light eruption	Extensor upper extremities, mid upper chest, face; seasonal (e.g. spring or early summer)
Discoid lupus erythematosus	Face and conchal bowls, with follicular plugging in latter site; oral lesions; in scarred lesions, central hypopigmentation with rim of hyperpigmentation
Lichen planus (LP; Fig. 55.8B)	Wrists, shins, and presacral area in classic LP; face, neck and intertriginous sites in LP pigmentosus; nail/oral involvement
Erythema dyschromicum perstans (ashy dermatosis) (Fig. 55.8A)	Neck, proximal upper extremities, trunk; round or oval in shape with gray-brown to blue-gray color; long axis can follow skin cleavage lines (similar to pityriasis rosea); less commonly observed in fair-skinned individuals
Fixed drug eruption (see Fig. 17.11F)	Circular; favors perioral, acral, and genital sites; recurrence at same site(s) with repeated exposure
Morbilliform drug eruption	Widespread; usually discrete lesions; history of drug exposure
Viral exanthem	Widespread; usually discrete lesions; history of associated symptoms
Morphea	Trunk or extremities; large-sized except in guttate variant; may be linear; induration and later dermal atrophy
Atrophoderma of Pasini and Pierini	Trunk; large-sized; depressed with 'cliff sign' at periphery; no induration
Neurotic (psychogenic) excoriation, acne excoriée	Favors face, scalp, extensor surface of arms, upper back (reachable areas); linear or angular shapes; multiple stages of evolution, from erosions/ulcerations to scars

Table 55.3 Disorders associated with postinflammatory hyperpigmentation. Disorders with a green background are characterized by inflammation at the dermal–epidermal junction. Such inflammation can lead to dermal melanin within melanophages (pigment incontinence), which can be resistant to treatment and take longer to resolve. Most disorders result in epidermal hyperpigmentation and eventually resolve if the underlying disorder is treated effectively. *Adapted from Bolognia JL. Disorders of hypopigmentation and hyperpigmentation. In: Harper J, Oranje A, Prose N (Eds.), Textbook of Pediatric Dermatology, 2nd edn. Oxford: Blackwell Science, 2006;997–1040.*

• The hyperpigmented macules and patches can range in color from light brown to dark brown (epidermal melanin) or gray-blue to gray-brown (dermal melanin).

• In general, postinflammatory epidermal pigmentation eventually resolves as long as the underlying disorder is treated effectively, but this may take months or even years; postinflammatory dermal pigmentation can be persistent.

• May also be exacerbated by UVR exposure, and photoprotection is an important part of treatment.

• **DDx:** see Table 55.3; occasionally a skin biopsy will assist in establishing the diagnosis.

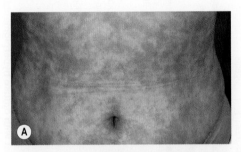

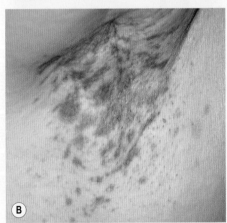

Fig. 55.8 Dermal postinflammatory hyperpigmentation. A Erythema dyschromicum perstans (EDP or ashy dermatosis). Multiple gray-brown macules and patches on the abdomen. The 'ashy' color is characteristic. **B** Lichen planus pigmentosus. Multiple coalescing brown to gray-brown macules in the axilla of a middle-aged woman.

• Causes of postinflammatory hyperpigmentation that often present without obvious prior inflammation.

- *Primary (localized) cutaneous amyloidosis* (see Chapter 39 and Figs. 39.6 and 39.7).
- *Erythema dyschromicum perstans (EDP or ashy dermatosis)* (see Chapter 9 and Figs. 9.9 and 55.8A).
- *Lichen planus pigmentosus (LPP)* (see Chapter 9, Table 9.1, and Figs. 9.4G and 55.8B).
- *Mastocytosis* (see Chapter 96 and Fig. 96.4).
- *Tinea (pityriasis) versicolor* (see Chapters 54 and 64 and Fig. 64.1).
- *Atrophoderma of Pasini and Pierini* (see Chapter 36).
  • There is some debate as to whether this represents a distinct entity or is an end-stage (i.e. 'burned-out' stage) of morphea.
  • Typically seen in young healthy adults as several 3- to 6-cm, oval, hyperpigmented, minimally depressed patches on the posterior trunk.
  • Lacks an inflammatory phase.

• **Rx:** In addition to treating the underlying inflammatory disorder and photoprotection, the following topical agents may be used: hydroquinone 2–4%; a combination of hydroquinone, tretinoin, and a low-strength CS; azelaic acid 15%; α-hydroxy acids (e.g. glycolic acid).

Diffuse Hyperpigmentation

• Diffuse hyperpigmentation has multiple causes, including drug-induced, metabolic and endocrine abnormalities, nutritional deficiencies, exposure to heavy metals, and inherited syndromes.

• May be accentuated in sun-exposed sites.

• An approach to the patient with diffuse hyperpigmentation is presented in Fig. 55.9.

Linear Hyperpigmentation

• Linear hyperpigmentation, like linear hypopigmentation (see Chapter 54), can result from multiple etiologies; one of the initial steps is determining if the lesions do

DIFFERENTIAL DIAGNOSIS AND CLINICAL APPROACH TO THE PATIENT WITH DIFFUSE HYPERPIGMENTATION OR DISCOLORATION

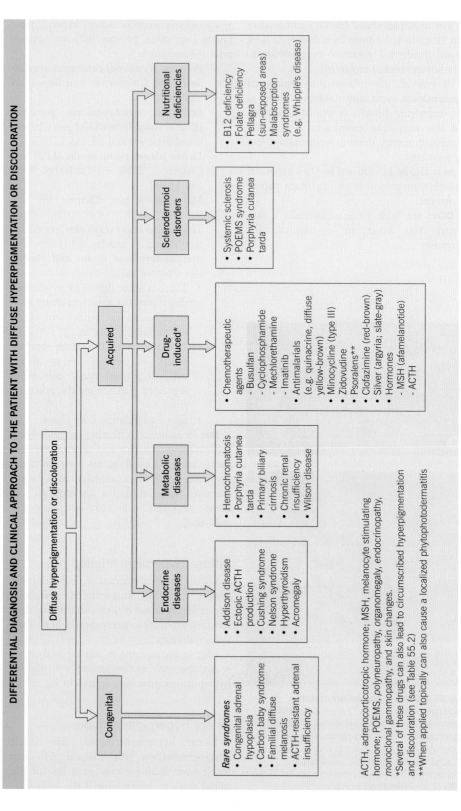

ACTH, adrenocorticotropic hormone; MSH, melanocyte stimulating hormone; POEMS, polyneuropathy, organomegaly, endocrinopathy, monoclonal gammopathy, and skin changes.

*Several of these drugs can also lead to circumscribed hyperpigmentation and discoloration (see Table 55.2)

**When applied topically can also cause a localized phytophotodermatitis

Fig. 55.9 Differential diagnosis and clinical approach to the patient with diffuse hyperpigmentation or discoloration.

or do not follow Blaschko's lines (see Chapter 51).
• The differential diagnosis of linear hyperpigmentation is presented in Table 55.4 (Figs. 55.10–55.16).

HYPERPIGMENTATION ALONG BLASCHKO'S LINES AND IN OTHER MOSAIC PATTERNS

• Hyperpigmentation can follow the lines of Blaschko or have other mosaic patterns (e.g. block-like [see Chapter 51]).
• Hyperpigmented streaks along Blaschko's lines has been termed *'linear and whorled nevoid hypermelanosis' (LWNH)* or linear nevoid hyperpigmentation, and they reflect pigmentary mosaicism (Fig. 55.10).
• In a minority of patients, LWNH is associated with systemic abnormalities (e.g. CNS,

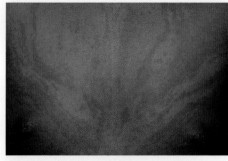

Fig. 55.10 Linear and whorled nevoid hypermelanosis (LWNH) on the trunk. This young African-American girl had developmental delay. Note the distribution along the lines of Blaschko. *Courtesy, Julie V. Schaffer, MD.*

DISORDERS WITH LINEAR LESIONS OF HYPERPIGMENTATION	
Lesions Follow Blaschko's Lines (*early onset, often during infancy*) (see Chapter 51)	**Additional Clues to the Diagnosis**
• Linear and whorled nevoid hypermelanosis (LWNH) (Fig. 55.10)	• Only hyperpigmentation within the affected skin
• Early stage or subtle epidermal nevus	• Slightly elevated papules (visible with side-lighting)
• Third stage of incontinentia pigmenti (see Figs. 55.11 and 51.7)	• Preceded by vesiculobullous and keratotic stages • Gray-brown hue due to melanin within the dermis
• Goltz syndrome (focal dermal hypoplasia)	• Streaks also contain cribriform dermal hypoplasia, hypopigmentation, telangiectasias and herniations of fat • Hyperpigmentation tends to be circular in shape within the streaks
• X-linked hypohidrotic ectodermal dysplasias	• Depression and lack of adnexae
Lesions Follow Blaschko's Lines (*acquired and often later age at onset*)	
• Linear lichen planus • Linear lichen planus pigmentosus • Linear fixed drug eruption • Linear atrophoderma of Moulin (Fig. 55.12) • Postinflammatory hyperpigmentation due to Blaschkitis	
Lesions Do Not Follow Blaschko's Lines	
• Pigmentary demarcation lines (Figs. 55.13 and 55.14; Table 55.5) • Linear postinflammatory hyperpigmentation (e.g. trauma, phytophotodermatitis, following allergic contact dermatitis [most often to plants]) • Flagellate hyperpigmentation (e.g. bleomycin [Fig. 55.15], mushroom dermatitis) • Hyperpigmentation overlying veins (e.g. phlebitis, intravenous drug abuse, systemic sclerosis)	

Table 55.4 Disorders with linear lesions of hyperpigmentation.

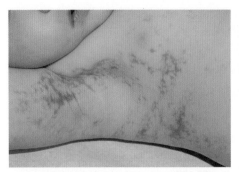

Fig. 55.11 Stage 3 incontinentia pigmenti in a 2-year-old child. Note the characteristic gray-brown color, and the distribution along the lines of Blaschko. *Courtesy, Julie V. Schaffer, MD.*

musculoskeletal, or ocular); hyperpigmented streaks usually appear in infancy.

• Patients presenting with hypo- or hyperpigmented streaks along Blaschko's lines can be approached in a similar fashion, with a physical examination and further evaluation (e.g. genetic) directed by clinical findings.

• Hyperpigmentation can also occur in a block-like configuration, also referred to as segmental pigmentation disorder; the **DDx** includes Becker's nevus and segmental CALM, either isolated or syndromic (e.g. McCune–Albright syndrome [see Table 50.3]); in the latter, the CALM may be more geographic in configuration.

LINEAR HYPERPIGMENTATION THAT IS NOT ALONG BLASCHKO'S LINES

• *Pigmentary demarcation lines*.
  – In humans, the dorsal skin surfaces are relatively hyperpigmented compared to the ventral surfaces.
  – In patients with darker pigmentation, visible lines of demarcation between dorsal and ventral surfaces are more apparent.
  – These demarcation lines are present from infancy and persist throughout life; they are most prevalent on the anterolateral upper arm and posteromedial thigh (Fig. 55.13).
  – Several forms of pigmentary demarcation lines exist and are presented in Table 55.5 and Fig. 55.14.
• *Flagellate pigmentation from bleomycin*.
  – Occurs in ~10–20% of patients treated with systemic bleomycin.

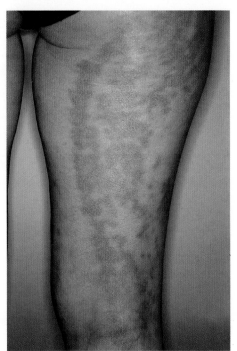

Fig. 55.12 Linear hyperpigmentation due to atrophoderma of Moulin. Note the subtle depression of the lesions on the upper lateral thigh. *Courtesy, Jean L. Bolognia, MD.*

  – Pathogenesis is not well understood.
  – Presents as linear hyperpigmented streaks on the chest, back, and occasionally extremities (Fig. 55.15); typically in a configuration that suggests a relationship to scratching, but attempts to reproduce lesions by scratching have in general been unsuccessful; an erythematous phase, which is typically pink in light-skinned individuals, can precede the hyperpigmentation.
  – The hyperpigmentation is usually reversible once the bleomycin is discontinued, but may take 3–4 months to fade.
  – Other skin findings can include circumscribed hyperpigmentation overlying the small joints of the hands as well as sclerodermoid changes.
• *Flagellate mushroom dermatitis*.
  – Occurs after eating large amounts of raw or partially cooked shiitake mushrooms.

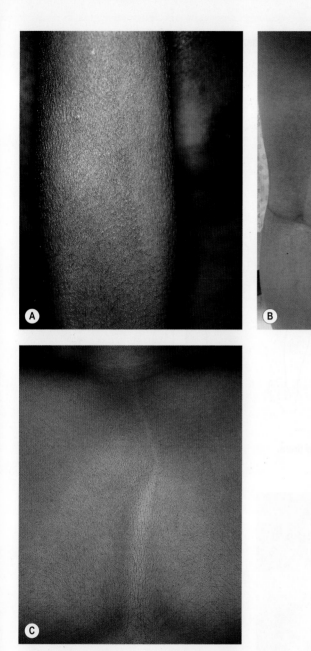

Fig. 55.13 Pigmentary demarcation lines (PDLs). A The most common PDL (Type A) is on the upper arm, with relative hypopigmentation on the ventral surface. **B** Type B PDLs on the posterior thighs, with relative hypopigmentation medially. **C** Type C PDL (composed of parallel lines) may be confused with hypopigmentation along Blaschko's lines. *A, C, Courtesy, Jean L. Bolognia, MD; B, Courtesy, Justin Finch, MD.*

PIGMENTARY DEMARCATION LINES

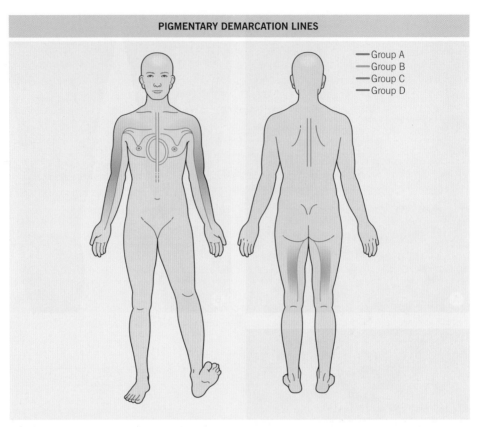

Group A
Group B
Group C
Group D

Fig. 55.14 Pigmentary demarcation lines.

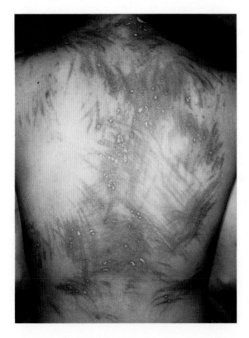

Fig. 55.15 Flagellate pigmentation. This young man had received bleomycin as a treatment for his lymphoma. Note the linear excoriations. *Courtesy, David E. Cohen, MD, MPH.*

FIVE MAJOR FORMS OF PIGMENTARY DEMARCATION LINES	
Type	**Description**
A	A vertical line along the anterolateral portion of the upper arm that may extend into the pectoral region (most commonly observed type)
B	A curved line on the posteromedial thigh that extends from the perineum to the popliteal fossa and occasionally to the ankle
C	A vertical or curved hypopigmented band on the mid chest that results from two parallel pigmentary demarcation lines
D	A vertical line in a pre- or paraspinal location
E	Bilateral chest markings (hypopigmented macules and patches) in a zone that runs from the mid third of the clavicle to the periareolar skin

Table 55.5 Five major forms of pigmentary demarcation lines.

- A second form occurs in persons who cultivate shiitake mushrooms.
- Presents initially with pruritic papules and vesicles that develop on the face, scalp, trunk, and proximal extremities; scratching of these lesions then leads to long, flagellate streaks composed of petechiae or papules, followed finally by linear patterns of discoloration (due to hemosiderin) or postinflammatory hyperpigmentation.

LINEAR HYPERPIGMENTATION THAT MAY OR MAY NOT BE ALONG BLASCHKO'S LINES

• *Linear postinflammatory hyperpigmentation*.
  - More common in individuals with darkly pigmented skin.
  - Occurs after linear trauma (e.g. burn, abrasion, dermatitis artefacta [Fig. 55.16]) and along veins (e.g. phlebitis, intravenous drug abuse, systemic sclerosis); also follows linear inflammatory dermatoses, most often allergic contact dermatitis due to plants (e.g. poison ivy/oak dermatitis) or phytophotodermatitis, which requires both plant exposure and UVR (see Fig. 55.7E).
  - Occasionally, postinflammatory hyperpigmentation may follow Blaschko's lines due to the configuration of the antecedent inflammatory dermatosis (e.g. linear lichen planus, Blaschkitis).

Reticulated Hyperpigmentation

• Disorders characterized by true reticulated macular hyperpigmentation are unusual and

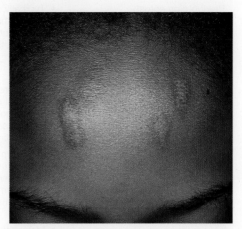

Fig. 55.16 Dermatitis artefacta resulting in linear postinflammatory hyperpigmentation of the forehead. The lesions were due to excoriations. *Courtesy, Mary Wu Chang, MD.*

are primarily rare genodermatoses (Table 55.6; Figs. 55.17–55.20).

• It is more common to encounter disorders where the reticulated hyperpigmentation represents just one of several components; as an example, confluent and reticulated papillomatosis (CARP) of Gougerot and Carteaud also has papillomatosis and slight hyperkeratosis.

• In addition, it is necessary to exclude cutaneous disorders characterized by reticulated erythema (e.g. livedo reticularis) or poikiloderma (e.g. poikiloderma of Civatte).

• Reticulated hyperpigmentation can also correspond to the pattern of the venous plexus (e.g. later stage of erythema ab igne); the clinical clue is a wider spacing than in genodermatoses.

DISORDERS CHARACTERIZED BY RETICULATED HYPERPIGMENTATION

Disorder	Key Features
Reticulated Hyperpigmentation with Additional Cutaneous Features	
Confluent and reticulated papillomatosis (CARP) of Gougerot and Carteaud (Fig. 55.17)	• Elevated, favors neck and upper trunk; treated with minocycline • Often appears during adolescence
Erythema ab igne (later stage) (Fig. 74.3)	• Widely spaced net that corresponds to vascular pattern • Due to heat injury, including from heating pads (back) or laptop computer batteries (anterior thighs)
Atopic dirty neck	• Anterolateral neck • Favors children
Epidermolysis bullosa simplex (EBS) herpetiformis (Dowling–Meara) and EBS with mottled pigmentation*	• 'Mottled' appearance; due to mutations in the genes that encode keratin 5 and 14 • Onset during early childhood
Prurigo pigmentosa	• Typically young Asian women • Favors the back, neck, and chest • Recurrent crops of pruritic papulovesicles that resolve with a reticulated pattern of hyperpigmentation
True Reticulated Macular Hyperpigmentation – Onset in Infancy or Early Childhood	
X-linked reticulate pigmentary disorder	• XLR • *Males* present with generalized reticulated pigmentation, neonatal colitis, recurrent pneumonia, hypohidrosis, photophobia, ± amyloid deposits in adults • *Female carriers* present with hyperpigmented streaks along Blaschko's lines
Dyskeratosis congenita* (Fig. 55.18)	• XLR form more common than AD and AR forms • ~50% due to mutations in the *TERT, TERC, DKC1,* or *TINF2* genes • Pterygium, leukoplakia, pancytopenia, mucosal squamous cell carcinoma, leukemia
Fanconi anemia*	• AR • More diffuse hyperpigmentation, radial ray bony defects, pancytopenia, leukemia
Dermatopathia pigmentosa reticularis (Fig. 55.19)	• AD; mutation in the gene that encodes keratin 14 • Persistent hyperpigmentation, alopecia, nail dystrophy; absent dermatoglyphics in some patients
Naegeli–Franceschetti–Jadassohn syndrome	• AD; mutations in the gene that encodes keratin 14 • Fading hyperpigmentation, hypohidrosis, dental anomalies, palmoplantar hyperkeratosis, reduced/missing dermatoglyphics, nail dystrophy
True Reticulated Macular Hyperpigmentation – Onset in Adolescence or Adulthood	
Dowling–Degos disease (DDD) (Fig. 55.20)	• AD; due to loss-of-function mutations in the gene that encodes keratin 5 • Reticulated hyperpigmentation of major flexures, comedones on the back and neck, pitted facial scars
Galli–Galli disease	• Acantholytic variant of DDD
Haber's syndrome	• Rosacea-like facial eruption plus the clinical features of DDD
Pigmentatio reticularis faciei et colli	• Possible variant of DDD • Hyperpigmentation of the face and neck plus multiple epidermoid cysts
Reticulate acropigmentation of Kitamura	• Primarily AD; caused by mutations in *ADAM10* • Atrophic, acral lentigo-like lesions, palmoplantar and dorsal phalangeal pitting

*Also dyschromatosis.
XLR, X-linked recessive; AD, autosomal dominant; AR, autosomal recessive.

Table 55.6 Disorders characterized by reticulated hyperpigmentation.

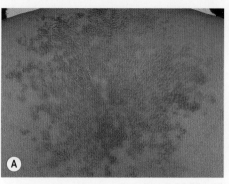

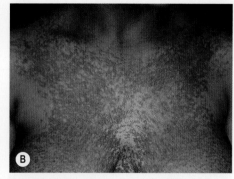

Fig. 55.17 Confluent and reticulated papillomatosis of Gougerot and Carteaud. A On the neck and back of a teenage girl. **B** On the chest of an older woman. *A, Courtesy, Seth Orlow, MD, PhD.*

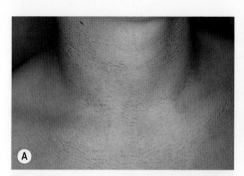

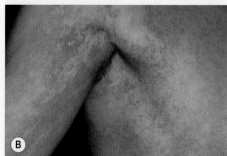

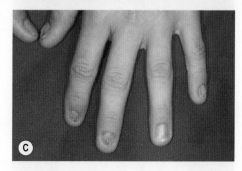

Fig. 55.18 Dyskeratosis congenita.
A Reticulated hyperpigmentation on the chest and neck of a teenage boy. **B** More pronounced reticulated and confluent hyperpigmentation on the shoulder and axilla. **C** Longitudinal ridging, splitting, and early pterygium formation in another teenage boy. *A, Courtesy, Seth Orlow, MD, PhD; B, Courtesy, Eugene Mirrer, MD; C, Courtesy, Anthony Mancini, MD.*

Dyschromatoses

- The dyschromatoses are characterized by the presence of both hypo- and hyperpigmentation; often at least one component of the dyspigmentation is guttate in configuration.
- These disorders can be divided into three groups:
  - *Genetic* (e.g. dyschromatosis symmetrica hereditaria [Fig. 55.21] and dys-chromatosis universalis hereditaria [Fig. 55.22]).
  - *Exposure-induced* (e.g. arsenic [see Fig. 74.7A], monobenzyl ether of hydroquinone [MBEH], diphenylcyclopropenone [DPCP], betel leaf).
  - *Infection-related* (e.g. secondary syphilis, pinta [see Chapter 61]).
- There is also a variant of cutaneous amyloidosis that is dyschromic.

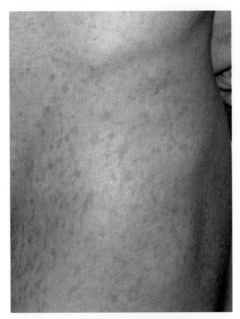

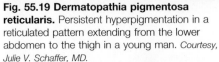

Fig. 55.19 Dermatopathia pigmentosa reticularis. Persistent hyperpigmentation in a reticulated pattern extending from the lower abdomen to the thigh in a young man. *Courtesy, Julie V. Schaffer, MD.*

Fig. 55.20 Dowling–Degos disease. Hyperpigmented macules forming a reticulated pattern in the axilla. *Courtesy, Thomas Schwarz, MD.*

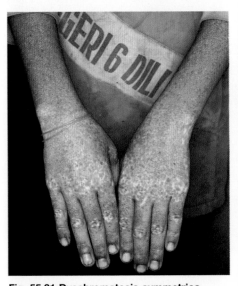

Fig. 55.21 Dyschromatosis symmetrica hereditaria. An autosomal dominant disorder characterized by mutations in *DSRAD* (encodes an adenosine deaminase) and mixed hypo- and hyperpigmentation on the distal hands and feet. Note that the hands are more involved than the forearms. *Courtesy, Peter Ehrnstrom, MD.*

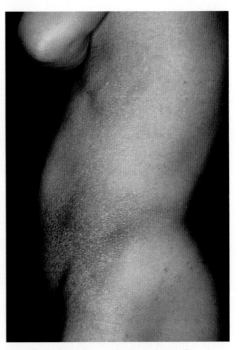

Fig. 55.22 Dyschromatosis universalis hereditaria. Widespread distribution of both hypo- and hyperpigmented macules. *With permission from Urabe K, Hori Y. Dyschromatosis. Semin Cutan Med Surg. 1997;16:81–85.*

For further information see Ch. 67. From *Dermatology, Third Edition.*

Alopecias | 56

• In a normal scalp, 90–95% of hairs are in anagen phase, 5–10% in telogen phase (Fig. 56.1).
• About 50–100 hairs normally shed daily.
• Alopecias can be categorized as diffuse vs. circumscribed, patterned vs. non-patterned, and non-scarring vs. scarring loss (Fig. 56.2).

Non-Scarring Alopecias

Male and Female Pattern Hair Loss (Androgenetic Alopecia)

• 80% of Caucasian men are affected by age 70 years.
• Women are less likely than men to have a family history of the disorder.
• Related to hormonal effects of dihydrotestosterone (DHT), converted from testosterone by 5-alpha reductase.
• Sensitivity of scalp hair to androgen hormones causes gradual miniaturization of hairs on the frontal/midline/vertex regions of men and the midline and crown of women (Fig. 56.3).
• In women, the frontal hairline is spared (except in the setting of virilization) and a Christmas tree pattern of widening of the hair part may be seen.
• May first become clinically apparent with superimposed telogen effluvium >> alopecia areata, especially in women.
• Should exclude hyperandrogenism (e.g. ovarian or adrenal source) in younger women or in women with signs of virilization (see Chapter 57).
• **Rx:** topical minoxidil 2% or 5%, finasteride (inhibits 5-alpha reductase) in men, hair transplantation (using occipital hair as the source).

Telogen Effluvium

• Sometimes a definable precipitating event ~3 months prior precedes diffuse shedding, leading to a reduced density of hair on the entire scalp and occasionally other areas of body hair (Table 56.1).
• Shed hairs are predominantly telogen hairs (Fig. 56.1).

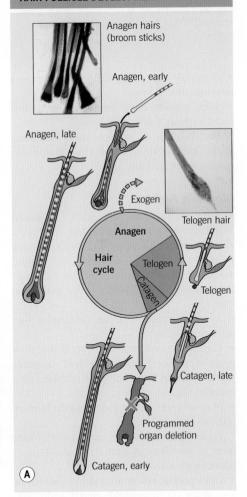

HAIR FOLLICLE DEVELOPMENT AND CYCLING

Anagen hairs (broom sticks)

Anagen, early

Anagen, late

Exogen

Telogen hair

Anagen

Hair cycle

Telogen

Catagen

Telogen

Catagen, late

Programmed organ deletion

(A) Catagen, early

Fig. 56.1 General concepts. A Hair follicle development and cycling. *A, Courtesy, Ralf Paus, MD; Anagen hairs, Courtesy, Maria K. Hordinsky, MD; Telogen hair, Courtesy, Leonard C. Sperling, MD.* *Continued*

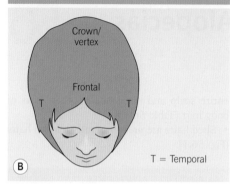

SCHEMATIC OF THE SCALP, SHOWING FRONTAL, TEMPORAL, AND CROWN/VERTEX REGIONS

Crown/vertex

Frontal

T

T

T = Temporal

B

Fig. 56.1 *Continued* **B** Schematic of the scalp, showing frontal, temporal, and crown/vertex regions.

• Generally complete hair regrowth occurs after months to years.

• Some women have chronic telogen effluvium without a definable cause.

• **Rx:** discontinue any potentially offending drugs, exclude thyroid abnormality and etiologies listed in Table 56.1.

Alopecia Areata

• Autoimmune disease with increased T-cells present in the hair matrix.

• Associated with atopy and other autoimmune diseases (e.g. autoimmune thyroid disease, vitiligo, inflammatory bowel disease, autoimmune polyendocrinopathy syndrome type 1).

• Average lifetime risk for developing this disease is 1–2%.

• Circular to oval areas of alopecia that may progress to total scalp hair loss (alopecia totalis) or total body hair loss (alopecia universalis) (Fig. 56.4).

• May see exclamation point hairs at borders (Fig. 56.4).

• Positive pull test (easily extractable telogen hairs at periphery of oval areas of loss) correlates with active disease.

• Ophiasis pattern is a band-like pattern of loss along the temporal/occipital scalp (Fig. 56.4) that may be less responsive to therapy.

• Associated nail findings = nail pitting, trachyonychia >> brittle nails, onycholysis, koilonychia, onychomadesis.

• **Rx** *(for regrowth of hair)*: high-potency topical or intralesional CS (e.g. 5 mg/cc); topical irritants (e.g. anthralin or tazarotene), topical immunotherapy (e.g. squaric acid dibutyl ester); in rapidly progressive disease, occasionally oral CS are given for a limited trial period (e.g. pulsed therapy over 2–3 months), topical minoxidil 5%.

Trichotillomania

• Self-induced twirling, pulling, and/or breaking of hair.

• May be related to a psychologic disorder or stress.

• Plucking of scalp hair results in patchy >> diffuse alopecia, sometimes in a wave-like pattern or centrifugally; hairs tend to be of different lengths.

• Occiput often spared.

• In difficult cases, can distinguish from alopecia areata by shaving a defined area of involvement and observing for regrowth.

• **Rx:** counseling and treat any underlying psychiatric illness (see Chapter 5).

Postoperative (Pressure-Induced Alopecia)

• Most commonly secondary to a long surgical procedure.

• Generally alopecia seen on occiput as a solitary, oval patch.

• Usually hair regrows completely.

Drug-Induced Alopecia

• Chemotherapeutic agents (e.g. cyclophosphamide, doxorubicin, paclitaxel, etoposide) are common causes of anagen effluvium.

• Anagen effluvium can also be secondary to exposure to metals, e.g. arsenic, gold.

• Telogen effluvium can be drug-induced (see Table 56.1).

Secondary Syphilis

• Patchy, 'moth-eaten' alopecia in 7% of patients with secondary syphilis.

• Telogen effluvium has also been described.

Scarring (Cicatricial) Alopecias

• Classically defined as loss of hair follicles with scarring (e.g. lupus erythematosus,

APPROACH TO ALOPECIA

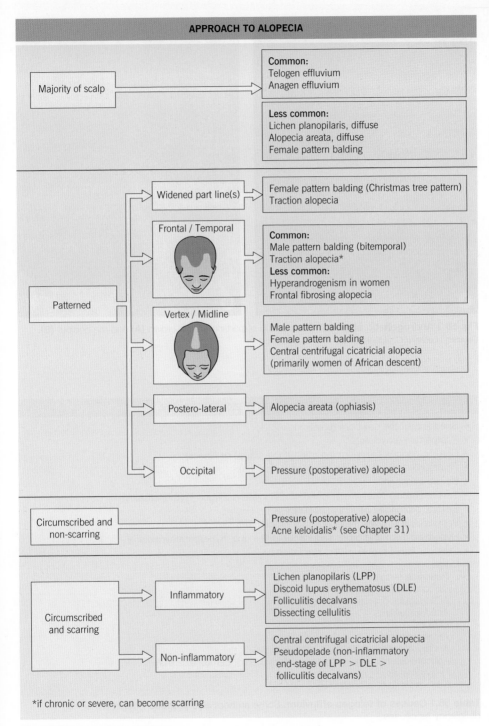

Fig. 56.2 Approach to alopecia.

The diagram shows:

Majority of scalp →
- **Common:** Telogen effluvium, Anagen effluvium
- **Less common:** Lichen planopilaris, diffuse; Alopecia areata, diffuse; Female pattern balding

Patterned →
- **Widened part line(s)** → Female pattern balding (Christmas tree pattern), Traction alopecia
- **Frontal / Temporal** → **Common:** Male pattern balding (bitemporal), Traction alopecia*; **Less common:** Hyperandrogenism in women, Frontal fibrosing alopecia
- **Vertex / Midline** → Male pattern balding, Female pattern balding, Central centrifugal cicatricial alopecia (primarily women of African descent)
- **Postero-lateral** → Alopecia areata (ophiasis)
- **Occipital** → Pressure (postoperative) alopecia

Circumscribed and non-scarring → Pressure (postoperative) alopecia, Acne keloidalis* (see Chapter 31)

Circumscribed and scarring →
- **Inflammatory** → Lichen planopilaris (LPP), Discoid lupus erythematosus (DLE), Folliculitis decalvans, Dissecting cellulitis
- **Non-inflammatory** → Central centrifugal cicatricial alopecia, Pseudopelade (non-inflammatory end-stage of LPP > DLE > folliculitis decalvans)

*if chronic or severe, can become scarring

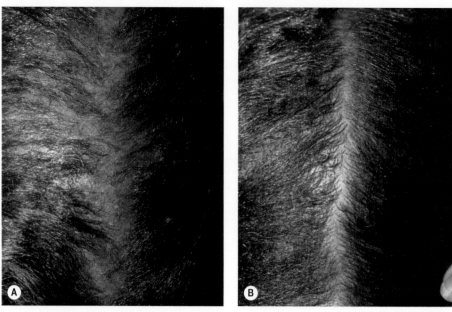

Fig. 56.3 Androgenetic alopecia. Comparison of partline on the crown **(A)** and the occiput **(B)**.
Courtesy, Leonard C. Sperling, MD.

CAUSES OF TELOGEN EFFLUVIUM
• Shedding of the newborn (physiologic)
• Postpartum (physiologic)
• Chronic telogen effluvium (no attributable cause or illness)
• Postfebrile (extremely high fevers, e.g. malaria)
• Severe infection
• Severe chronic illness (e.g. HIV disease, systemic lupus erythematosus)
• Severe, prolonged psychological stress
• Postsurgical (implies major surgical procedure)
• Hypothyroidism and other endocrinopathies (e.g. hyperparathyroidism)
• Crash or liquid protein diets; starvation
• Drugs
Retinoids (acitretin, isotretinoin)
Discontinuation of birth control pills
Anticoagulants (especially heparin)
Antidepressants
Lithium
Amphetamines
Antithyroid (propylthiouracil, methimazole)
Anticonvulsants (e.g. phenytoin, valproic acid, carbamazepine)
Heavy metals
β-blockers (e.g. propranolol)

Table 56.1 Causes of telogen effluvium. Some authors also propose vitamin B$_{12}$ or iron deficiency as causes.

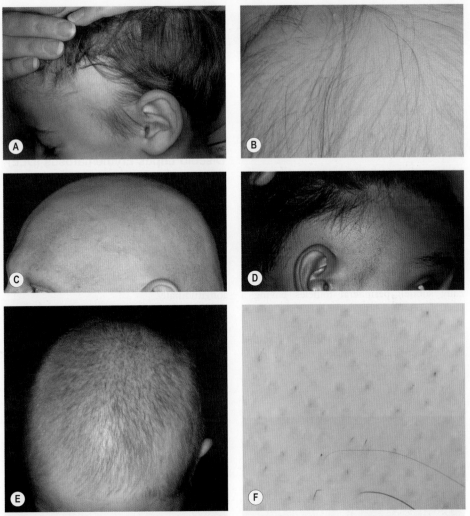

Fig. 56.4 Alopecia areata. A Circular area of alopecia in a child. **B** Exclamation point hair with the distal end broader than the proximal end. **C** Total alopecia of scalp, eyebrows, and eyelashes in a patient with alopecia universalis. **D** Ophiasis with a band-like pattern of hair loss along the periphery of the temporal and occipital scalp. **E** Diffuse variant of alopecia areata. **F** Typical yellow dots seen dermoscopically in alopecia areata. *B, Courtesy, Julie V. Shaffer, MD; C, Courtesy, Leonard C. Sperling, MD; E, Courtesy, Maria K. Hordinsky, MD. F, Courtesy, Iris Zalaudek, MD.*

lichen planopilaris) *or* an alopecia in which hair does not grow back (e.g. chronic, long-standing traction alopecia).

• Non-scarring alopecias that may eventually result in permanent hair loss include male and female pattern hair loss > alopecia areata.

• In *secondary* scarring alopecia, the hair is destroyed nonspecifically, i.e. secondary to burns, radiation dermatitis, cutaneous

malignancy (see Chapter 100), sarcoidosis, morphea, necrobiosis lipoidica, infections (e.g. severe kerion), mucous membrane (cicatricial) pemphigoid.

Central Centrifugal Cicatricial Alopecia (CCCA)

• Most commonly observed in black women.

• May be related to the use of chemical hair relaxers or thermal relaxers (e.g. flat iron).

- Slowly progressive; centered on the crown/vertex and midline (Fig. 56.5).
- Symptoms may be mild or absent.
- Occasionally patients have secondary changes, especially crusting or pustules.
- **Rx:** mild disease – oral tetracycline plus potent topical CS; severe disease – oral rifampin plus oral clindamycin; occasionally intralesional CS if an inflammatory component is present.

Lichen Planopilaris

- Women > men, more common in Caucasians.
- 50% may have associated lichen planus involving the skin, mucous membranes, or nails (see Chapters 9 and 58).
- Usually several foci of alopecia with loss of follicles and scarring centrally (may be clinically subtle); peripheral follicles having a central, keratotic plug and a rim of inflammation (pink to violet in color) (Fig. 56.6).
- Centered on the crown/vertex or midline, or predominantly affecting the frontal hairline and eyebrows ('frontal fibrosing alopecia') (Fig. 56.7), or rarely a diffuse pattern.
- Graham–Little syndrome = scalp alopecia, alopecia of axillary/pubic areas, and grouped spinous follicular papules on trunk/extremities.
- **Rx:** topical or intralesional CS, oral doxycycline, oral antimalarials (e.g. hydroxychloroquine), oral retinoids, oral mycophenolate mofetil (if severe).

Discoid Lupus Erythematosus (DLE)

- A type of chronic cutaneous lupus erythematosus.
- More common in adult women, especially black women.
- Minority of patients fulfill the criteria for systemic lupus erythematosus (see Chapter 33), but patients need to be evaluated at the time of diagnosis of DLE and followed longitudinally.
- Circular lesions of erythema, atrophy, dilated/plugged follicles, and scale as well as alopecia.

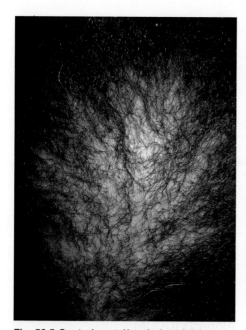

Fig. 56.5 Central centrifugal cicatricial alopecia in an African-American woman. Alopecia is most prominent on the crown/vertex and the midline. *Courtesy, Leonard C. Sperling, MD.*

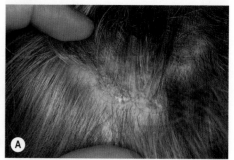

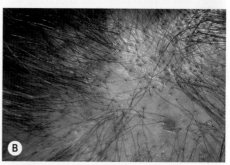

Fig. 56.6 Lichen planopilaris. A Perifollicular erythema in association with scale. **B** Later stage showing scarring with loss of follicular openings, but less erythema. Some of the follicles still have a rim of inflammation. *A, Courtesy, Jean L. Bolognia, MD.*

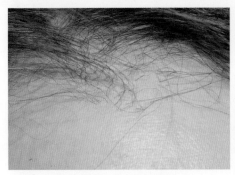

Fig. 56.7 Frontal fibrosing alopecia.
Progressive hair loss along the anterior hairline in an elderly woman. *Courtesy, Kalman Watsky, MD.*

- As lesions age, central hypopigmentation and peripheral hyperpigmentation may appear, along with scarring (Fig. 56.8).
- May see similar-appearing lesions elsewhere (especially face and ears).
- **Rx:** discussed in Chapter 33.

Acne Keloidalis

- Favors young black men (see Chapter 31).
- Occipital scalp most common site, but sometimes involves the crown/vertex.
- Smooth, firm papules > pustules.
- Initial lesions resolve with alopecia and/or protuberant papules.
- Coalescence of lesions leads to alopecia.
- **Rx:** intralesional CS, oral antibiotics, excision (see Table 31.6).

Dissecting Cellulitis

- May be associated with 'follicular occlusion tetrad,' which includes this entity, hidradenitis suppurativa, acne conglobata, and pilonidal cyst/sinus.
- Affects young adult men, especially black men.
- Multiple, firm scalp nodules over crown/vertex/occiput that become boggy and fluctuant with purulent discharge; often interconnecting.
- Sometimes little pain.
- **Rx:** intralesional CS, antibiotics based on cultures, incision and drainage, excision.

Folliculitis Decalvans

- Inflammatory scarring alopecia with perifollicular papules and pustules.

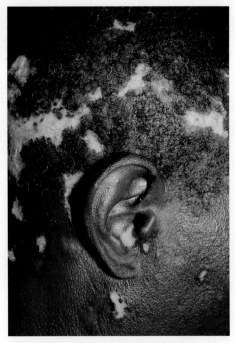

Fig. 56.8 Discoid lupus erythematosus.
Alopecia with dyspigmentation on the scalp and face. Note involvement of the conchal bowl. *Courtesy, Joyce Rico, MD.*

- **Rx:** dapsone, oral antibiotics (e.g. tetracycline or doxycycline for anti-inflammatory effects).

Pseudopelade

- Considered by most to be the end-stage, burned-out phase of different scarring alopecias (Fig. 56.9), especially lichen planopilaris.

Traction Alopecia (Late-Stage)

- Occurs after years of hair styling that causes traction.
- Generally seen in black women on the bitemporal/frontal scalp line (Fig. 56.10).

Hair Shaft Abnormalities

- Four main categories: (1) *fractures* (trichorrhexis nodosa and invaginata, trichoschisis); (2) *irregularities* (monilethrix); (3) *twisting*

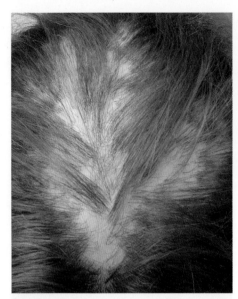

Fig. 56.9 Pseudopelade (end-stage scarring alopecia). Smooth, oval areas of alopecia resembling 'footprints in the snow.' *Courtesy, Kalman Watsky, MD.*

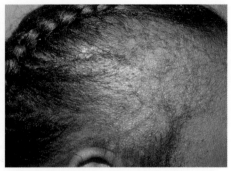

Fig. 56.10 Traction alopecia. Favors frontotemporal area in African-American women and is due to traumatic types of hair styling. *Courtesy, Leonard C. Sperling, MD.*

(pili torti, woolly hair, trichonodosis); and (4) *extraneous matter* (Fig. 56.11).

• Can also divide into *increased breakage* (bubble hair, monilethrix, pili torti, trichorrhexis invaginata and nodosa, trichothiodystrophy) and *no increased breakage* (loose anagen, pili annulati, spun-glass hair, woolly hair).

• Trichorrhexis nodosa – common hair shaft abnormality that leads to increased breakage; hair shaft fractured with the appearance of two brushes pushing against each other; seen with hair straightening.

• Loose anagen hair syndrome – common cause of sparse, short hair especially in young children, with improvement over time; anagen hairs are poorly anchored and therefore easily shed or pulled, but breakage is not increased.

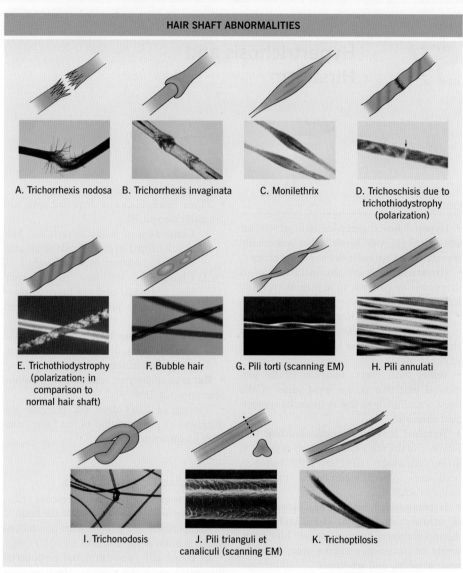

A. Trichorrhexis nodosa   B. Trichorrhexis invaginata   C. Monilethrix   D. Trichoschisis due to trichothiodystrophy (polarization)

E. Trichothiodystrophy (polarization; in comparison to normal hair shaft)   F. Bubble hair   G. Pili torti (scanning EM)   H. Pili annulati

I. Trichonodosis   J. Pili trianguli et canaliculi (scanning EM)   K. Trichoptilosis

Fig. 56.11 Schematic drawings and microscopic appearance of hair shaft abnormalities.
A Trichorrhexis nodosa. **B** Trichorrhexis invaginata. **C** Monilethrix. **D** Trichoschisis (due to trichothiodystrophy). **E** Trichothiodystrophy (polarization; in comparison to normal hair shaft). **F** Bubble hair. **G** Pili torti (scanning electron microscopy [EM]). **H** Pili annulati. **I** Trichonodosis. **J** Pili trianguli et canaliculi ('spun glass hair'). **K** Trichoptilosis. Some of the hair shaft abnormalities are seen in genetic syndromes (e.g. trichorrhexis invaginata in Netherton syndrome, trichoschisis in trichothiodystrophy). *A, B, Courtesy, Maria K. Hordinsky, MD; F, Courtesy, Jean L. Bolognia, MD.*

For further information see Ch. 69. From *Dermatology, Third Edition*.

57 | Hypertrichosis and Hirsutism

Definitions

• **Hypertrichosis**: excessive hair growth on any area of the body, beyond what is normally expected for a patient's demographic group.
• **Hirsutism**: excessive terminal hair growth in women or children in a pattern typically seen in adult men.
• **Lanugo hair**: long fine hair that is grown *in utero*, covers the fetus, and is normally shed either *in utero* or during the first few weeks of life.
• **Vellus hair**: short, non- or lightly pigmented hair that covers most areas of the body; occasionally so fine as to not be appreciated clinically.
• **Terminal hair**: thick pigmented hair that is typical of the scalp and androgen-dependent areas, such as the axillae and pubic region in both sexes, as well as the beard, trunk, and limbs in adult males.
• **Hyperandrogenism**: elevated serum levels of testosterone, DHEAS, and/or androstenedione; cutaneous findings include hirsutism, severe or treatment-resistant acne, androgenetic alopecia, and seborrhea.
• **Virilization**: in women, clinical features of hyperandrogenism plus clitoromegaly, deepened voice, increased muscle mass, breast atrophy, and increased libido.
• **Depilation**: removal of a portion of the hair at some point along its shaft.
• **Epilation**: removal of the entire hair shaft.

Hypertrichosis

• Can be classified based on the **distribution** (generalized vs. localized), **age of onset** (congenital or early onset vs. acquired), and **type of hair** (lanugo vs. vellus vs. terminal).

• Three mechanisms of hypertrichosis are generally recognized:
  1. Conversion of vellus to terminal hair (e.g. localized hypertrichosis in an area of chronic rubbing or scratching).
  2. Changes in the hair growth cycle (e.g. intranasal and ear hairs in older males due to prolongation of anagen phase).
  3. Increase in hair follicle density beyond what is normal for a given site (e.g. congenital melanocytic nevus).
• **Rx:** treat underlying condition, if possible, otherwise see Table 57.2.
• Shaving of hairs does not increase the thickness or pigmentation of the hairs, contrary to common belief.

Generalized Hypertrichosis

• The presence of lanugo hair, excess vellus hair, or terminal hair on most of the body.
• An approach to a patient with *generalized hypertrichosis* is presented in Fig. 57.1.
• In young girls, constitutional prepubertal hypertrichosis is the most common form of generalized hypertrichosis.

Localized Hypertrichosis

• Most often involves a switch from vellus to terminal hair in sites that normally do not have terminal hairs.
• *Congenital localized hypertrichosis* is usually related to an underlying hamartoma or occurs at a specific anatomic site (Table 57.1; Figs. 57.2–57.6).
• *Acquired localized hypertrichosis* most often develops after repeated trauma, friction, irritation, or inflammation (see Table 57.1).

APPROACH TO THE PATIENT WITH GENERALIZED HYPERTRICHOSIS

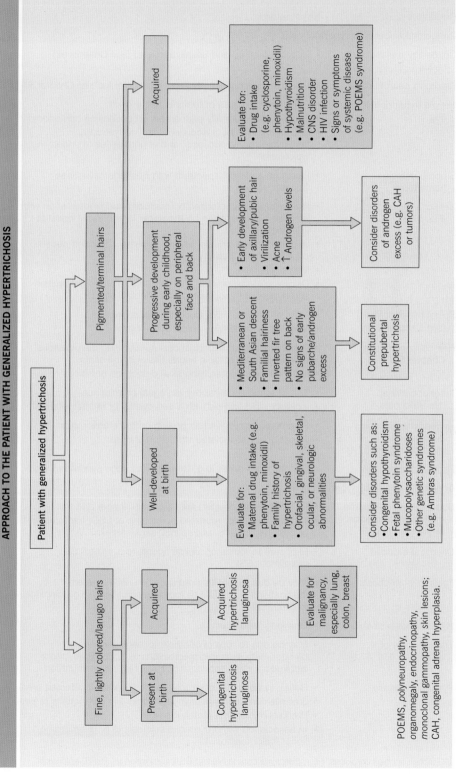

Fig. 57.1 Approach to the patient with generalized hypertrichosis. Acquired hypertrichosis lanuginosa occasionally may involve only the face.

POEMS, polyneuropathy, organomegaly, endocrinopathy, monoclonal gammopathy, skin lesions; CAH, congenital adrenal hyperplasia.

CLASSIFICATION AND KEY FEATURES OF SELECTED DISORDERS OF LOCALIZED HYPERTRICHOSIS

Condition	Key Features
Congenital Localized Hypertrichosis	
Congenital melanocytic nevus	• Hyperpigmented and usually elevated (see Chapter 92)
Plexiform neurofibroma	• Palpable component and often hyperpigmented (see Chapter 50)
Nevoid hypertrichosis (Fig. 57.2)	• Circumscribed area of terminal hair growth • *Primary*: skin normally pigmented; no underlying hamartoma • *Secondary*: can be associated with lipodystrophy, hemihypertrophy, scoliosis, and abnormalities of underlying vasculature
Smooth muscle hamartoma	• Exists on a clinical spectrum with Becker's nevus (see Chapter 95)
Becker's nevus (Fig. 57.3)	• Hamartoma characterized by macular hyperpigmentation with irregular borders; often on the upper lateral trunk; onset in first decade of life • Hypertrichosis (variable) usually appears in second decade, correlating with puberty • Males > females • Occasionally associated with asymmetry of the extremities and hyper- or hypoplasia of the affected areas
Spinal hypertrichosis (see Chapter 53)	• Tufts of terminal hairs along the dorsal midline • May signify underlying *spinal dysraphism*
Hair collar sign (see Chapter 53)	• Peripheral ring of hypertrichosis surrounding membranous aplasia cutis or ectopic neural tissue in the scalp • MRI can detect underlying skull defect; do *not* biopsy
Anterior cervical hypertrichosis	• Tuft of terminal hair above laryngeal prominence • Isolated > associated with a neuropathy or mental retardation
Hypertrichosis cubiti (hairy elbow syndrome) (Fig. 57.4)	• Symmetric excessive hair growth on the elbow region • Occasionally associated with short stature
Facial hypertrichosis	• Genetic syndromes (e.g. Cornelia de Lange syndrome)
Acquired Localized Hypertrichosis	
Due to repeated trauma, friction, inflammation, or irritation (Fig. 57.5)	• Hair within the affected area becomes longer and thicker • Typical scenarios: repeated scratching or LSC; fractured limb or orthopedic casts and splints; sack carriers
Chemical-induced	• Exposure to iodine or topical agents (e.g. minoxidil, tacrolimus, CS)
Facial hypertrichosis	• May be due to familial predisposition, PCT, systemic medications (e.g. CSA) or topical medications (e.g. minoxidil), malnutrition
Hypertrichosis singularis	• One long 'wild' hair
Trichomegaly of eyelashes (Fig. 57.6)	• May be due to topical ophthalmic medications (e.g. bimatoprost), systemic medications (e.g. EGFR inhibitors, zidovudine, CSA, topiramate), HIV infection, malnutrition
Systemic disease	• Reflex sympathetic dystrophy (hypertrichosis in affected area) • Juvenile dermatomyositis (hypertrichosis in infrapatellar region) • Pretibial myxedema (anterior shins) • In association with cutaneous sclerosis (e.g. H syndrome, linear melorheostosis)

LSC, lichen simplex chronicus; PCT, porphyria cutanea tarda; CSA, cyclosporine; EGFR, epidermal growth factor receptor.

Table 57.1 Classification and key features of selected disorders of localized hypertrichosis.

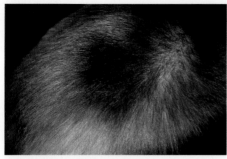

Fig. 57.2 Nevoid hypertrichosis in the scalp of a young boy. There was no underlying melanocytic nevus or hyperpigmentation. *Courtesy, Jean L. Bolognia, MD.*

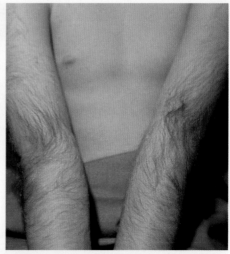

Fig. 57.4 Hypertrichosis cubiti. Multiple terminal hairs on both elbows in a child. *Courtesy, Francisco M. Camacho Martinez, MD.*

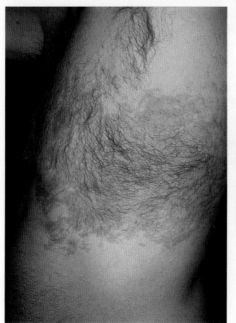

Fig. 57.3 Hypertrichosis in association with a Becker's nevus. *Courtesy, Jean L. Bolognia, MD.*

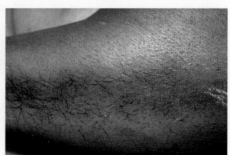

Fig. 57.5 Acquired localized hypertrichosis. Hypertrichosis, hyperpigmentation, and epidermal hyperplasia at the site of friction.

Hirsutism

- Affects ~5–10% of females of reproductive age; can also affect postmenopausal women.
- Due to hyperandrogenism (exogenous or endogenous) or increased sensitivity of the hair follicle to normal androgen levels and is the most commonly used clinical criterion of androgen excess.
- Quantified using the modified Ferriman and Gallwey (mFG) method (Fig. 57.7).

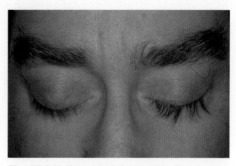

Fig. 57.6 Unilateral trichomegaly. Bimatoprost ophthalmic solution (0.03%) was applied to one eye to treat glaucoma. *Courtesy, Jean L. Bolognia, MD.*

TREATMENT OPTIONS FOR HYPERTRICHOSIS AND UNWANTED HAIR		
Camouflage	**Hair Removal Techniques**	**Retardation of Hair Growth**
• Make-up • Lightening of hair color with commercial bleach or 6–12% hydrogen peroxide	**Depilation** ***Chemical*** 1. Barium sulfate creams* 2. Calcium thioglycolate creams ***Mechanical*** 1. Hair trimming 2. Shaving	• Eflornithine hydrochloride cream (*best used in conjunction with other hair removal techniques*)
	Epilation • Tweezing • Waxing • Electrolysis** • Thermolysis** • Lasers or other light sources** (e.g. Nd:YAG, diode, alexandrite, IPL)	

More effective than calcium thioglycolate but more irritating and odiferous.
**These epilatory methods are operator-dependent and have the potential for permanent hair removal results.*
IPL, intense pulsed light.

Table 57.2 Treatment options for hypertrichosis and unwanted hair. Epilation technique results typically last longer than those of depilation. Chemical depilatories work by dissolving hair shafts, specifically by breaking disulfide bonds.

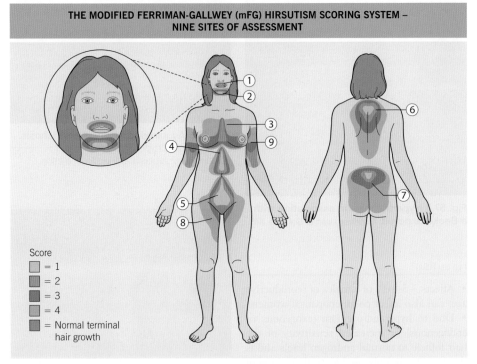

THE MODIFIED FERRIMAN-GALLWEY (mFG) HIRSUTISM SCORING SYSTEM – NINE SITES OF ASSESSMENT

Score
☐ = 1
▨ = 2
▩ = 3
☐ = 4
■ = Normal terminal hair growth

Fig. 57.7 The modified Ferriman–Gallwey (mFG) hirsutism scoring system. In this system, nine body areas are evaluated for the amount of terminal hair growth. A score of '0' (no terminal hair growth) up to '4' (frankly virile) is given to each of the nine areas and these are added together to compute a hormonal hirsutism score (mFG score). A total score <2–3 is considered normal for East Asian and Native American females, whereas <6–8 is considered normal in other populations.

2. Clinical and/or biochemical signs of hyperandrogenism (Fig. 57.11).

3. Polycystic ovaries (pelvic ultrasound).

• Occurs only during the reproductive years, and although the majority of patients are obese, some are of normal weight.

• Other associated findings may include acanthosis nigricans and insulin resistance; patients are at increased risk for the metabolic syndrome (see Table 45.11), infertility, obstructive sleep apnea, and possibly endometrial carcinoma.

• **Rx** of hirsutism: hormonal agents (Table 57.3) as well as general hair removal methods (see Table 57.2).

Idiopathic Hirsutism

• Usually characterized by mild hirsutism, regular ovulation, and normal testosterone levels.

• Diagnosis of exclusion.

Nonclassic Congenital Adrenal Hyperplasia (NC-CAH)

• Autosomal recessive disorder due to partial deficiency in 21-hydroxylase activity (mutations in *CYP21A2*), leading to increased 17-hydroxyprogesterone (17-OHP) levels.

• More prevalent in Ashkenazi Jews, Hispanics, and Slavics.

• Usually presents in the peripubertal and young adult years with hirsutism, menstrual irregularities, infertility, androgenetic alopecia, and acne.

• Initial testing includes measuring an early morning 17-OHP level during the follicular phase of menstrual cycle; if equivocal, a high-dose ACTH stimulation test and/or genotyping for *CYP21A2* can be performed.

• **Rx** of hirsutism: overlaps with that of PCOS, but may also include systemic CS (see Tables 57.2 and 57.3).

Ovarian Hyperthecosis

• Occurs in both premenopausal and postmenopausal females.

• Due to the differentiation of ovarian interstitial cells into steroidogenically active luteinized stromal cells, resulting in greater production of androgens.

• Clinical features are similar to those of PCOS but with more pronounced and

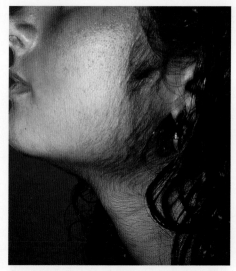

Fig. 57.8 Facial hirsutism in a young female. This can be due to hyperandrogenism or end-organ sensitivity. *Courtesy, Francisco M. Camacho Martinez, MD.*

• Defined as an mFG score of >2–3 in women from East Asia as well as Native Americans or an mFG score of ≥6–8 in other populations.

• Etiologies of hyperandrogenism and hirsutism in *premenopausal* females include.

– *Most common*: polycystic ovary syndrome (PCOS), idiopathic (end-organ sensitivity; Fig. 57.8).

– *Less common*: nonclassic congenital adrenal hyperplasia, ovarian hyperthecosis, tumoral.

– *Must exclude*: pregnancy; drugs (e.g. androgens, oral contraceptives with androgenic progestins, anabolic steroids, valproic acid).

• Etiology in *postmenopausal* women (new onset) is most likely ovarian hyperthecosis or tumoral hirsutism.

• Suggested algorithms for the evaluation of hirsutism and for hyperandrogenism are shown in Figs. 57.9 and 57.10, respectively.

Polycystic Ovary Syndrome (PCOS)

• Diagnosed by the presence of ≥2 of the following criteria *and* the exclusion of other possible etiologies (see Fig. 57.10):

1. Oligo- or anovulation (<8 menses/year or cycles >35 days).

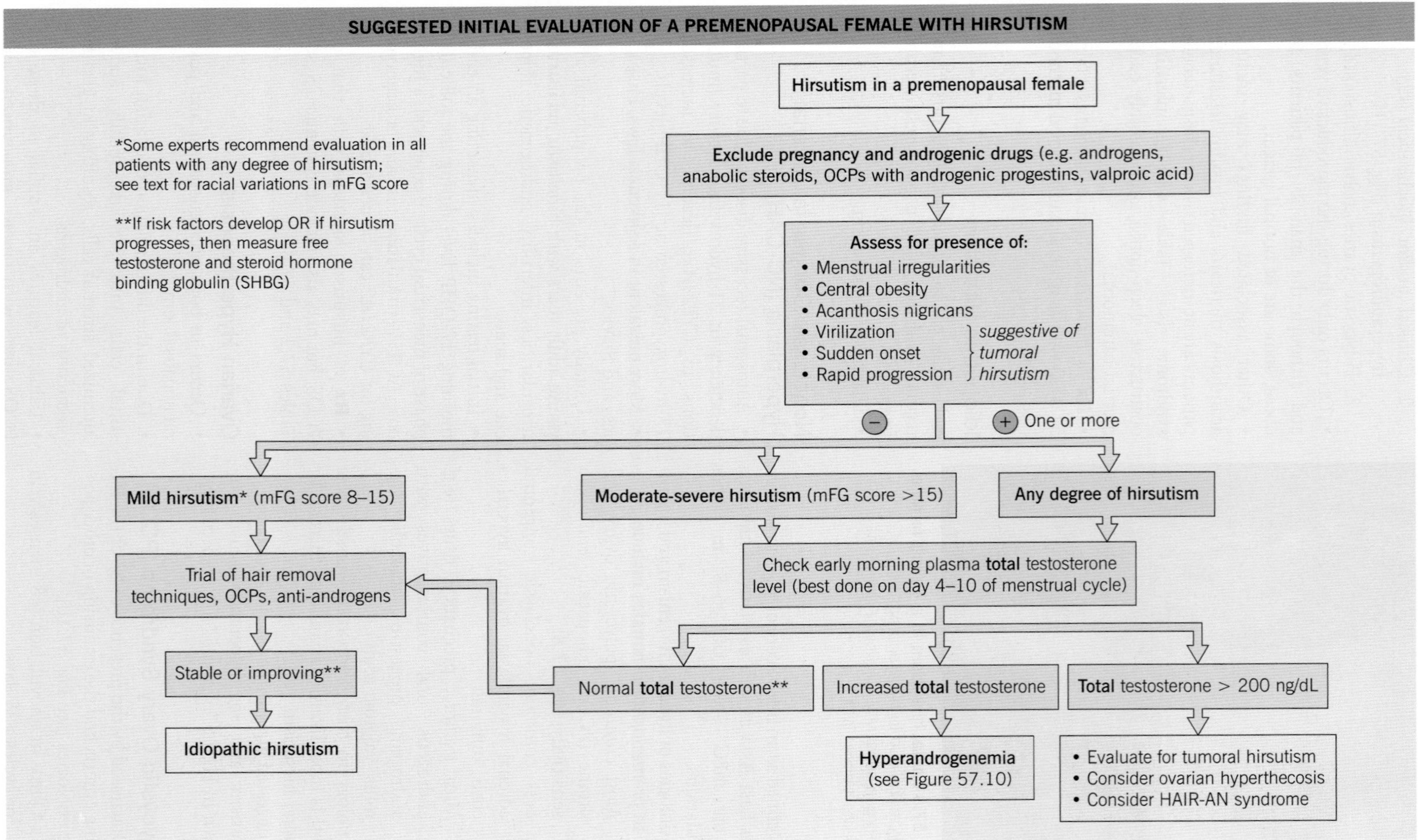

SUGGESTED INITIAL EVALUATION OF A PREMENOPAUSAL FEMALE WITH HIRSUTISM

Hirsutism in a premenopausal female

Exclude pregnancy and androgenic drugs (e.g. androgens, anabolic steroids, OCPs with androgenic progestins, valproic acid)

Assess for presence of:
- Menstrual irregularities
- Central obesity
- Acanthosis nigricans
- Virilization } *suggestive of tumoral hirsutism*
- Sudden onset
- Rapid progression

(−)　　　(+) One or more

Mild hirsutism* (mFG score 8–15)

Moderate-severe hirsutism (mFG score >15)　　Any degree of hirsutism

Trial of hair removal techniques, OCPs, anti-androgens

Check early morning plasma **total** testosterone level (best done on day 4–10 of menstrual cycle)

Stable or improving**

Normal **total** testosterone**　　Increased **total** testosterone　　Total testosterone > 200 ng/dL

Idiopathic hirsutism

Hyperandrogenemia (see Figure 57.10)

- Evaluate for tumoral hirsutism
- Consider ovarian hyperthecosis
- Consider HAIR-AN syndrome

*Some experts recommend evaluation in all patients with any degree of hirsutism; see text for racial variations in mFG score

**If risk factors develop OR if hirsutism progresses, then measure free testosterone and steroid hormone binding globulin (SHBG)

Fig. 57.9 Suggested initial evaluation of a premenopausal female with hirsutism (based on 2008 Endocrine Society clinical practice guidelines). OCP, oral contraceptive pills; mFG, modified Ferriman–Gallwey score (see Fig. 57.7); HAIR-AN, *hyperandrogenism, insulin resistance, acanthosis nigricans* syndrome.

SUGGESTED EVALUATION OF HYPERANDROGENISM IN A PREMENOPAUSAL FEMALE

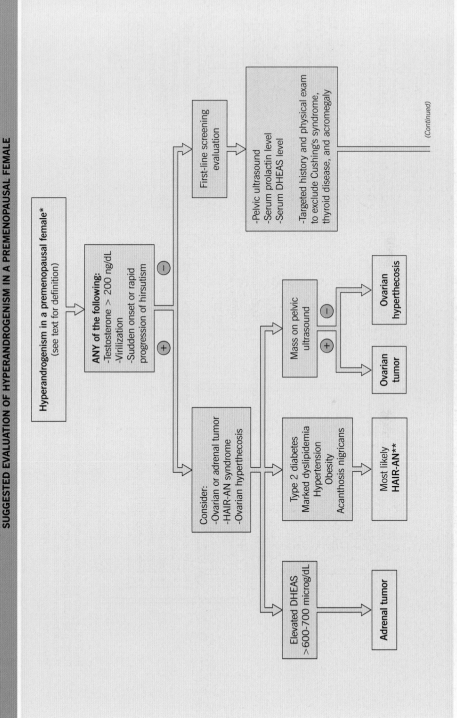

Fig. 57.10 **Suggested evaluation of hyperandrogenism in a premenopausal female.** *Continued*

SUGGESTED EVALUATION OF HYPERANDROGENISM IN A PREMENOPAUSAL FEMALE

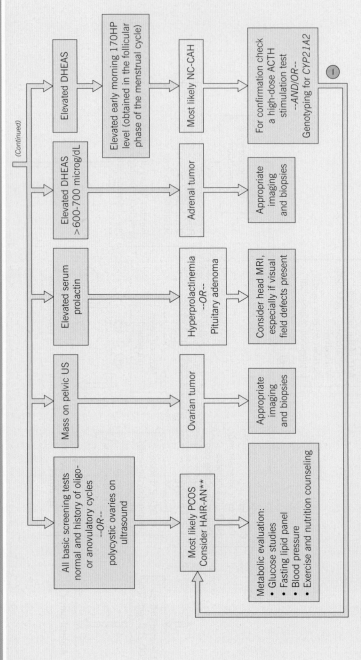

HAIR-AN, hyperandrogenism, insulin resistance, and acanthosis nigricans; 17OHP, 17-hydroxyprogesterone; PCOS, polycystic ovarian syndrome; NC-CAH, nonclassic congenital adrenal hyperplasia

*Exclude pregnancy and drugs

**HAIR-AN is more likely than PCOS to present with an obvious metabolic syndrome

Fig. 57.10 *Continued* **Suggested evaluation of hyperandrogenism in a premenopausal female.**

SYSTEMIC AGENTS AND PRACTICAL TREATMENT RECOMMENDATIONS FOR HIRSUTISM AND HYPERANDROGENISM		
Systemic Agents for Treating Hirsutism and Hyperandrogenism		
Oral contraceptives (OCPs)* (usually contain a combination of ethinyl estradiol [EE] plus a low androgenicity or antiandrogenic progestin; ***Avoid*** OCPs with the androgenic progestins levonorgestrel or norgestrel) • **Antiandrogenic progestins** (e.g. drospirenone, cyproterone acetate [CPA]**) • **Low androgenicity progestins** (e.g. norgestimate, desogestrel) **Antiandrogens***** • Spironolactone 100–200 mg/day (usually given in divided doses, twice daily) • CPA (given on days 5–15 of menstrual cycle)** • Finasteride > flutamide **GnRH agonists** (risk of severe estrogen deficiency) **Insulin-lowering agents** (e.g. metformin > thiazolidinediones; improves metabolic syndrome and reproductive function but not hirsutism as a single agent) **Glucocorticoids** (e.g. low-dose hydrocortisone [children], prednisone or dexamethasone [adolescents and adults]; *restricted to second-line treatment of women with NC-CAH or for those seeking ovulation induction*)		
Clinical Scenario of Hirsutism and Hyperandrogenism and Recommended Treatment†		
Premenopausal female	**First-line:** OCP **Second-line:** OCP + spironolactone or CPA**	**Severe or refractory:** Finasteride, flutamide, or GnRH agonist; plus an OCP if premenopausal
Postmenopausal female	**First-line:** Spironolactone or CPA**	
NC-CAH	**First-line:** OCP ± spironolactone or CPA** **Second-line or if seeking ovulation induction:** Glucocorticoids	

*Should avoid in females who smoke or who have risk factors for hypercoagulability and thrombosis.
**CPA is not available in the United States.
***Requires concomitant reliable contraceptive method because of the risk of feminization of the male fetus.
†A waiting period of 6–9 months is recommended after initiating a treatment and before adding or changing medications.
NC-CAH, nonclassic congenital adrenal hyperplasia.

Table 57.3 Systemic agents and practical treatment recommendations for hirsutism and hyperandrogenism.

long-standing hirsutism, an increased likelihood of virilization (Fig. 57.12), and the occurrence postmenopause.
• Testosterone levels are often quite elevated (>200 ng/dl); DHEAS can be normal or increased (see Fig. 57.10).
• Compared to tumoral hirsutism, a slower onset of symptoms and more gradual worsening over years.
• Increased risk of insulin resistance, type 2 diabetes, and endometrial carcinoma.

Tumoral Hirsutism

• Can be caused by a variety of benign or malignant ovarian or adrenal androgen-secreting tumors.

• Typically presents with either sudden onset or rapid progression of hirsutism and other clinical features of hyperandrogenism; virilization more likely.
• Diagnostic clues are extremely elevated levels of testosterone (>200 ng/dl, seen in ovarian and adrenal tumors) or DHEAS (>600–700 microg/dl, seen in adrenal tumors).
• If suspected, an appropriate imaging study is recommended (e.g. CT scan, MRI, and/or ultrasound).

HAIR-AN Syndrome

• **H**yperandrogenism, **i**nsulin **r**esistance, and **a**canthosis **n**igricans syndrome.

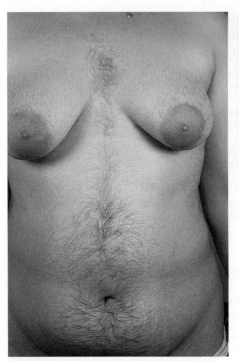

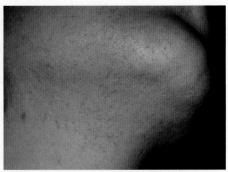

Fig. 57.12 Facial hirsutism (mFG score 4) due to ovarian hyperthecosis. *Courtesy, Robert Hartman, MD.*

Fig. 57.11 Hirsutism in a young woman with polycystic ovarian syndrome (PCOS). Modified Ferriman–Gallwey (mFG) score of 9 based on three sites: chest, upper abdomen, and lower abdomen.

• Marked insulin resistance leads to secondary increased insulin levels and resultant increased ovarian androgen production.

• More likely than PCOS to have overt type 2 diabetes, hypertension, and cardiovascular disease.

• Marked hyperandrogenism and often frank virilization; total testosterone levels are often markedly increased.

• Evaluation involves excluding an androgen-secreting tumor and PCOS.

Hirsutism Associated with Other Endocrine Abnormalities

• Cushing's syndrome, hyperprolactinemia, pituitary adenoma, acromegaly, and thyroid dysfunction may present with hirsutism and other signs of hyperandrogenism, but typically manifest with other distinguishing and diagnostic features specific to the underlying disease (see Chapter 45).

For further information see Ch. 70. From *Dermatology, Third Edition*.

Nail Disorders | 58

- The nail matrix, which is the growth area, has proximal and distal components (Fig. 58.1).
  - The proximal nail matrix forms the top (surface) of the nail plate.
  - The distal nail matrix forms the underside of the nail plate; therefore, biopsies of the distal matrix are less likely to produce a deformity of the surface of the nail plate.

- Fingernails grow ~1 mm per month and are replaced every 6 months.
- Toenails grow ~0.5 mm per month and are replaced every 12 months.
- Therefore, nail plate abnormalities such as Beau's lines that are due to insults to the nail matrix can be dated by their distance from the cuticle.
- **Rx** of common nail disorders is given in Table 58.1.

TREATMENT OF COMMON NAIL DISORDERS	
Disorder	**Treatment**
Psoriasis	Systemic treatment of psoriasis may be helpful Topical vitamin D analogues or tazarotene Injection of CS into nail matrix or nail bed Topical CS under occlusion
Lichen planus	Injection of CS into nail matrix
Beau's lines, Onychomadesis	Await spontaneous resolution
Paronychia, acute	Incision and drainage (may have occurred spontaneously) If mild, topical mupirocin or retapamulin Oral antibiotics (directed against *Staphylococcus aureus*)
Paronychia, chronic	Avoid trauma to cuticle Strict avoidance of irritants Topical CS for 2–3 weeks
Onycholysis*	Keep nails short, reduce trauma and friction to nail Strict avoidance of irritants Can consider topical antifungal solution If due to psoriasis, see above
Green nails*	1% acetic acid solution soaks Topical antibiotic (e.g. gentamycin, tobramycin, or ciprofloxacin ophthalmic solution)
Onychorrhexis	Topical 20% urea, 12% lactic acid, or retinoids; nail hardener; and/or biotin (2.5 mg PO daily)
Ingrown toenails	Correct predisposing factors (e.g. change to a larger toebox) Trim nail properly (straight across) Elevate lateral border of nail with piece of gauze, cotton, or dental floss Warm soaks If severe, matrixectomy (partial or total)

Table 58.1 Treatment of common nail disorders. *Cut back portions of detached nail plate.

NAIL UNIT ANATOMY

Free edge of the nail
Hyponychium
Onychodermal band
Nail plate
Lateral nail fold
Lunula
Eponychium (cuticle)
Proximal nail fold

Lateral nail fold — Lunula — Proximal nail fold
Onychodermal band
Distal nail edge
Proximal nail edge
Eponychium (cuticle)
Nail plate
Distal groove
Proximal nail fold
Hyponychium
Eponychium (cuticle)
Distal nail matrix
Eponychium (cuticle)
Proximal nail fold
Nail bed
Hyponychium
Collagen bundles
Distal phalanx
Proximal nail matrix
Joint
Tendon

Fig. 58.1 Nail unit anatomy.

Onycholysis

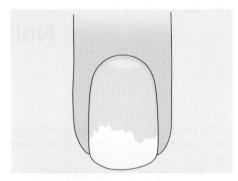

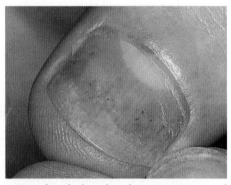

- Distal nail plate detachment, causing nail to look white to yellow-white (Fig. 58.2).
- Chronic exposure to water and irritants (e.g. soaps) is a common cause.
- Associated with psoriasis, onychomycosis, hyperthyroidism, and medications (Table 58.2).

DRUG-INDUCED NAIL ABNORMALITIES	
Nail Abnormality	**Responsible Agents**
Beau's lines and onychomadesis	Chemotherapeutic agents
True leukonychia	Chemotherapeutic agents
Nail thinning and brittleness	Chemotherapeutic agents Retinoids
Onycholysis/photo-onycholysis (see Fig. 58.2)	Chemotherapeutic agents, in particular taxanes Tetracyclines Psoralens NSAIDs
Apparent leukonychia (e.g. Muehrcke's nails)	Chemotherapeutic agents, in particular polychemotherapy including anthracyclines, vincristine
Melanonychia	Chemotherapeutic agents Psoralens Zidovudine (AZT)

Table 58.2 Drug-induced nail abnormalities.

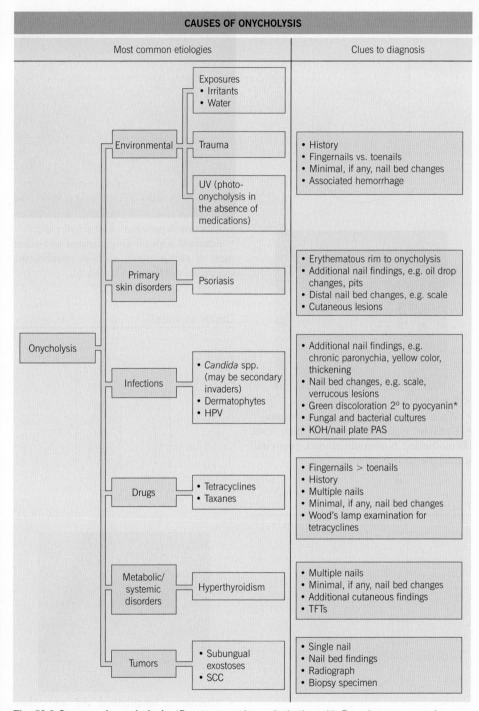

Fig. 58.2 Causes of onycholysis. *Due to secondary colonization with *Pseudomonas aeruginosa*. SCC, squamous cell carcinoma; TFTs, thyroid function tests.

Onychomadesis

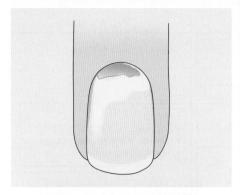

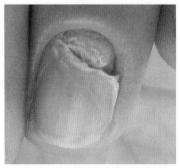

- Proximal detachment of nail plate.
- When single digit, often due to trauma.
- Consider systemic cause (e.g. high fever, chemotherapy, post-erythroderma, post-viral) if multiple nails involved.

Pitting in Psoriasis

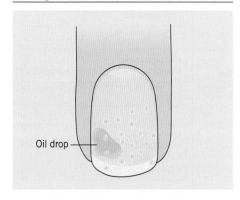

Oil drop

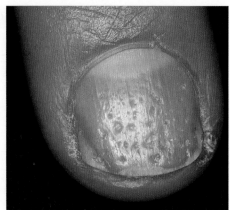

- Punctate depressions in the nail plate.
- Admixed with oil drop changes and other signs of nail psoriasis such as onycholysis, subungual debris (see Chapter 6).

Darier Disease

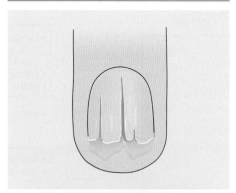

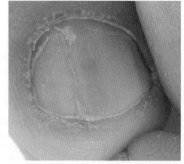

- Alternating longitudinal red and white streaks (i.e. erythronychia and leukonychia).
- Distal fissuring (notches).

Trachyonychia

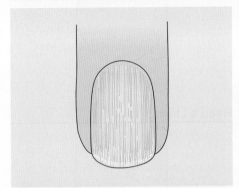

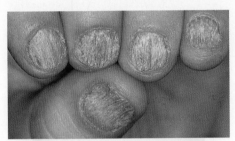

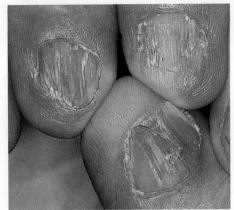

- Nail thinning/atrophy, especially laterally.
- Sometimes dorsal pterygium (see below).
- See Chapter 9.

- Rough, 'sandpaper' nails, often thin.
- Associated with alopecia areata or lichen planus >> psoriasis.
- May affect most or all nails, especially in children; often termed '20-nail dystrophy'.

Lichen Planus

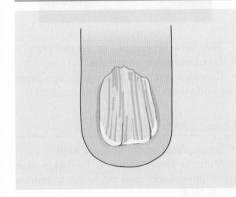

True Leukonychia

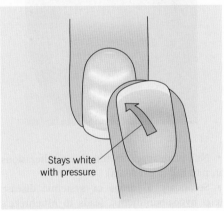

Stays white
with pressure

- White discoloration of nail.
- Punctate most common.
- Punctate > linear > diffuse.
- Linear bands may be transverse or longitudinal (see Darier disease).
- Punctate or transverse linear forms often due to trauma.

Apparent Leukonychia

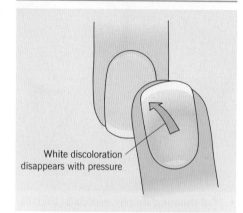

White discoloration disappears with pressure

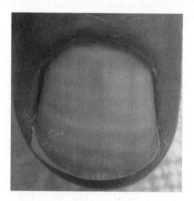

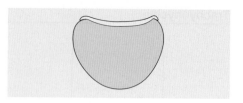

Beau's Lines

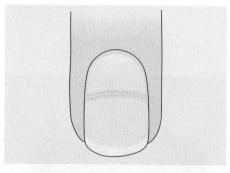

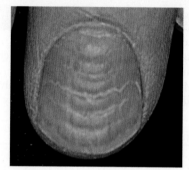

• Nail plate appears white due to alterations in nail bed (e.g. edema).

• Secondary to drugs or systemic disease (e.g. hypoalbuminemia leads to Muehrcke's lines).

• Terry's nails: only distal several millimeters of nail plate unaffected; associated with liver disease.

• Lindsay's nails: proximal half of nail is white and distal nail is red; associated with renal disease.

Koilonychia

• Spoon-shaped nails.

• Physiologic in children, associated with iron deficiency in adults.

• Transverse depressions in the nail plate.

• Often secondary to trauma.

• Consider systemic insult (e.g. high fever, chemotherapy) if multiple nails involved.

Longitudinal Melanonychia

• Longitudinal brown-to-black band.

• Multiple bands common in darker skin types (physiologic); also can be due to trauma (Table 58.3).

• Single band may be a sign of nail melanoma (Table 58.4).

• When melanoma is suspected, the nail matrix must be biopsied (see Fig. 58.1).

CAUSES OF LONGITUDINAL MELANONYCHIA	
Melanocyte activation	Racial Trauma • Manicures • Nail biting/onychotillomania • Frictional, primarily in toenails
	Drugs • Cancer chemotherapeutic agents, e.g. doxorubicin, 5-fluorouracil • Zidovudine (AZT) • Psoralens
	Pregnancy Laugier–Hunziker syndrome/Peutz–Jegher syndrome Addison's disease HIV infection Post-inflammatory • Lichen planus • Pustular psoriasis • Onychomycosis (*T. rubrum* and *Scytalidium* spp.) • Chronic radiodermatitis
Non-melanocytic tumors and proliferations	Bowen's disease Verrucae Basal cell carcinoma Subungual keratosis Myxoid cyst
Melanocyte hyperplasia	
Nail matrix nevus	
Nail matrix melanoma	

Table 58.3 Causes of longitudinal melanonychia.

ABCDEF RULE FOR CLINICAL SUSPICION OF NAIL MELANOMA	
A	• Age (peak incidence – 5th to 7th decades of life) • African-Americans, Asians, and Native Americans ($\frac{1}{3}$ of all nail melanoma cases)
B	• Brown to black • Breadth (3 mm or wider) • Borders (variegated)
C	• Change in the nail band (color/size) • Lack of change in the nail morphology despite presumed adequate treatment
D	• Digit most commonly involved (thumb and big toe)
E	• Extension of the pigment into the proximal and/or lateral nail fold (Hutchinson's sign)
F	• Family or personal history of melanoma

Adapted from Levit EK, et al. The ABC rule for clinical detection of subungual melanoma. J. Am. Acad. Dermatol. 2000;42:269–274.

Table 58.4 ABCDEF rule for clinical suspicion of nail melanoma.

Longitudinal Melanonychia, continued

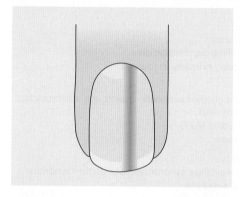

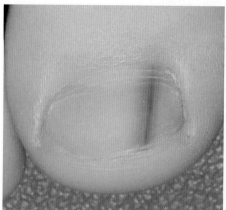

Onychorrhexis

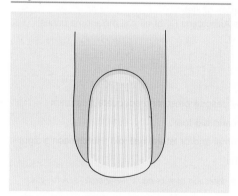

- Thinning and longitudinal ridging.
- May develop fissuring or notching.
- Less pronounced than trachyonychia.
- Normal finding with aging.
- Sometimes secondary to trauma.

Onychoschizia

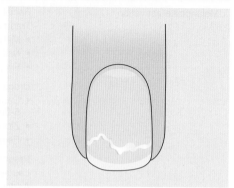

- Lamellar splitting of distal nail into multiple layers.
- Associated with the use of soap and irritants.
- Normal finding with aging.

Pitting in Alopecia Areata

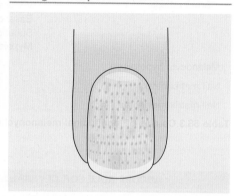

- Punctate depressions in nail plate; geometric or 'scotch-plaid' pattern.
- Compared to psoriasis, pits are smaller and more numerous.

Dorsal Pterygium

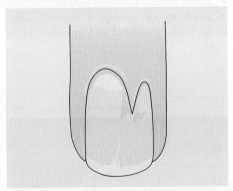

- Triangular extension of the proximal nail fold into the nail bed.
- Local loss of nail plate.
- Associated with lichen planus.

Proximal Nail Fold Telangiectasias

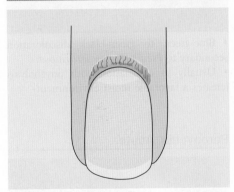

- Capillary prominence ± cuticular hemorrhages.
- Associated with lupus erythematosus and Osler–Weber–Rendu syndrome.
- Also associated with dermatomyositis and scleroderma, with a slightly different appearance (see below).

Proximal Nail Fold Telangiectasias with Capillary Dropout

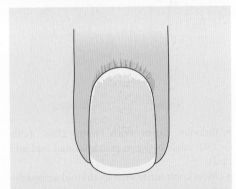

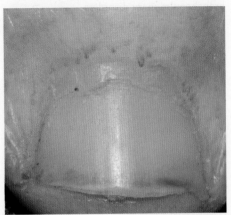

- Capillary dropout alternating with dilated capillary loops.
- Associated with dermatomyositis and scleroderma.
- In dermatomyositis, ragged cuticles may also be present.
- In scleroderma, ventral pterygium (loss of distal subungual space) may be seen.

Clubbing

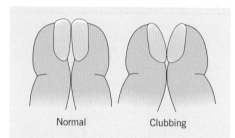

Normal   Clubbing

• Bulbous digits with watch-glass nails (> 180° angle between proximal nail fold and nail).

• Most commonly seen in thyroid acropachy and in association with cardiovascular and bronchopulmonary disorders.

Splinter Hemorrhages

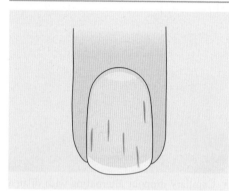

• Thin, longitudinal, dark-red subungual lines.
• Usually secondary to trauma.
• Can be seen in psoriasis, endocarditis.
• Pattern due to topography of nail bed.

Subungual Hematoma

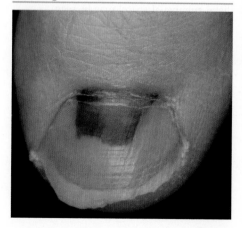

• Purple-red to black color beneath nail plate.
• Moves distally with nail growth.
• Secondary to trauma; if cuticle pushed back, band of normal nail growth may be seen.

Green Nail

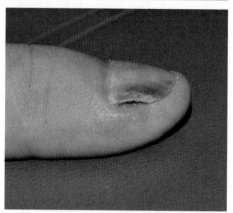

• Blue-green to green-black discoloration secondary to *Pseudomonas aeruginosa*.
• Usually in association with onycholysis (creates a favorable moist environment).

Paronychia, Acute

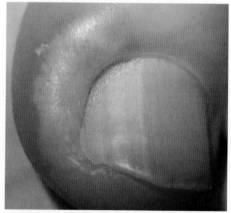

• Swollen nail fold with erythema and pain, sometimes with pustular drainage.
• Caused by bacteria (especially staphylococci).
• Recurrent episodes may be caused by herpes simplex virus infection (herpetic whitlow).

Paronychia, Chronic

- Chronic proximal nail fold inflammation with loss of cuticle (natural sealant).
- Exacerbated by exposure to water and irritants or overaggressive nail grooming.
- May have secondary *Candida* colonization.

Pustular Psoriasis

- Pustules can form under the nail.
- May have lesions of psoriasis on the tips of the digits.

Median Nail Dystrophy (Tic Deformity)

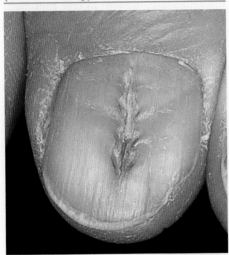

- Thumbnail(s).
- Multiple transverse grooves with central longitudinal depression.
- Due to manipulation of skin overlying matrix.

Malalignment

- Most commonly 1st toe(s).
- Lateral deviation of nail plate, often bilateral and congenital.

Nail Patella Syndrome

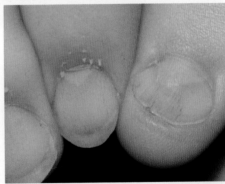

- Hypoplasia of fingernails, greatest on the thumb, least on the fifth digit, triangular lunulae.
- Absent or hypoplastic patella and renal disease.

Ingrown Toenails

- Painful inflammation of lateral fold with growth of granulation tissue.
- Can be side effect of drugs.
- **Rx:** see Table 58.1.

Onychomycosis

- See Chapter 64.

Onychogryphosis

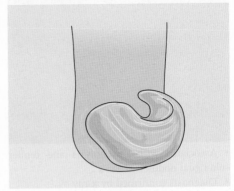

- Most commonly nail(s) of 1st toe(s).
- Curling of nail plate leads to ram's horn appearance.
- Affects elderly patients.

Subungual Exostosis

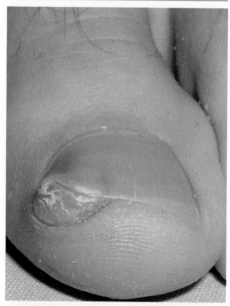

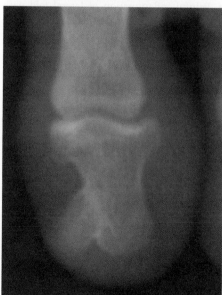

• Associated with onycholysis and tender subungual nodule
• Diagnosis confirmed by x-ray

Yellow Nail Syndrome

• Yellow coloration of all or most fingernails > toenails.
• Loss of cuticle, onychomadesis, overcurvature of nail plate.
• Associated with lymphedema and bronchopulmonary disease.

Tumors

• Various cysts, hyperplasias, and tumors may be seen on the distal digits, including fibromas (Fig. 58.3), myxoid cysts (Fig. 58.4), pyogenic granuloma (Fig. 58.5), glomus tumor (associated with paroxysmal pain) (see Chapter 94), Bowen's disease (Fig. 58.6), keratoacanthoma (symptoms include pain, rapid growth), melanoma (signs include longitudinal melanonychia [Fig. 58.7], Hutchinson's sign = pigmentation of proximal cuticle).

Additional details: onycholysis due to psoriasis; onychomadesis after an episode of acute paronychia; apparent leukonychia represents Muehrcke's lines; multiple Beau's lines were due to repeated cycles of systemic chemotherapy; proximal nail fold telangiectasias and ragged cuticles due to dermatomyositis.

Additional courtesies: Antonella Tosti, Julie V Schaffer, and Jean L Bolognia.

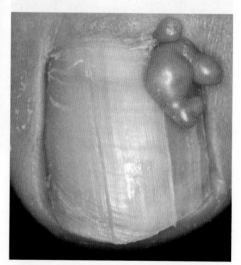

Fig. 58.3 Periungual fibroma producing a longitudinal groove due to matrix compression. *Courtesy, Antonella Tosti, MD.*

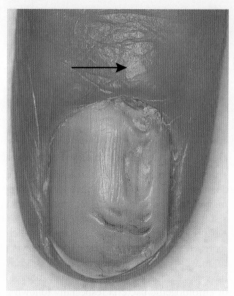

Fig. 58.4 Myxoid cyst. The longitudinal nail groove is a result of the compression of the nail matrix by the cyst (arrow). *Courtesy, Antonella Tosti, MD.*

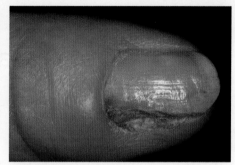

Fig. 58.6 Bowen's disease. The lateral portion of the nail plate is absent. The nail bed shows hyperkeratosis with scaling and fissuring of the epithelium. *Courtesy, Antonella Tosti, MD.*

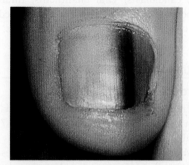

Fig. 58.7 Melanoma *in situ* of the nail. Darkly pigmented band in the nail bed and matrix. *Courtesy, Frank O Nestle, MD.*

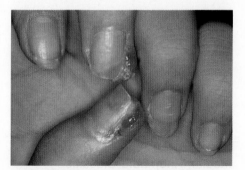

Fig. 58.5 Multiple periungual pyogenic granulomas in a patient taking indinavir. Similar lesions can be seen in patients receiving systemic retinoids or epidermal growth factor receptor inhibitors. *Courtesy, Antonella Tosti, MD.*

For further information see Ch. 71. From *Dermatology, Third Edition*.

59 | Oral Diseases

- In addition to common benign lesions such as bite fibromas and mucoceles, oral findings often represent clues to the diagnosis of skin disorders (e.g. lichen planus, early pemphigus vulgaris) or cutaneous signs of systemic disease (Table 59.1).
- Oral manifestations of infectious diseases (e.g. candidiasis, viral enanthems, findings associated with HIV infection) are covered in the chapters focused on these conditions.

Common Oral Mucosal Findings

Fordyce Granules
- 'Free' sebaceous glands (i.e. not associated with hair follicles) evident in as many as 75% of adults.
- Multiple 1- to 2-mm yellowish papules on the vermilion lips (upper > lower) and oral mucosa (especially buccal).

Geographic Tongue (Migratory Glossitis)
- Incidental finding on the dorsum of the tongue in ~2–3% of the population; may occasionally be associated with psoriasis, especially pustular variants.
- Well-demarcated areas of erythema and atrophy of the filiform papillae, surrounded by a whitish, hyperkeratotic serpiginous border (Fig. 59.1); lesions tend to migrate over time, may affect other oral sites, and are occasionally associated with a burning sensation.

Scrotal (Fissured) Tongue
- Asymptomatic finding that is occasionally associated with conditions such as granulomatous cheilitis (see below) and Down syndrome.
- Multiple grooves or furrows are present on the dorsal tongue, especially centrally (Fig. 59.2).

Hairy Tongue (Black Hairy Tongue)
- Reflects accumulation of keratin on the dorsum of the tongue; contributing factors may include poor oral hygiene, smoking, and a soft diet.
- Confluence of hairlike projections, which represent elongated papillae, with yellowish to brown-black discoloration (Fig. 59.3); may have exogenous staining from food, tobacco, or chromogenic bacteria (especially following antibiotic therapy); some patients report an unpleasant odor or taste.
- **DDx:** pigmented papillae of the tongue (in individuals with darkly pigmented skin).
- **Rx:** scraping or brushing the tongue.

Leukoedema
- Normal variant that is more often evident in smokers and individuals with darkly pigmented skin.
- Grayish-white, opalescent, sometimes 'moth-eaten' appearance of the buccal > labial mucosa; typically becomes less evident upon stretching.

Median Rhomboid Glossitis
- Found in ~1% of adults, often associated with local overgrowth of *Candida*.
- Well-demarcated diamond- or oval-shaped area of erythema and atrophy on the dorsum of the tongue (Fig. 59.4).
- **Rx:** clotrimazole troches or oral fluconazole (for dosage, see Table 64.5).

Periodontal and Dental Conditions with Dermatologic Relevance

Desquamative Gingivitis
- Clinical finding that can occur in several immune-mediated vesicular and erosive disorders (Fig. 59.5); favors women over 40 years of age.

SYSTEMIC DISEASES WITH ORAL MANIFESTATIONS	
Disorder	**Oral Findings**
Primary systemic amyloidosis (see Chapter 39)	• Macroglossia, often with scalloped edges (due to dental impressions) or hemorrhagic papulonodules (see Fig. 39.3); xerostomia
Nutritional deficiencies (see Chapter 43)	• Atrophic glossitis (see text), stomatitis • *Scurvy*: gingival enlargement, hemorrhage and erosions (see Fig. 43.6)
Inflammatory bowel disease	• *Crohn's disease*: oral cobblestoning and ulcers (aphthous or linear; Fig. 59.15), angular cheilitis, orofacial granulomatosis (see text) • *Pyostomatitis vegetans* (ulcerative colitis > Crohn's): oral pustules and erosions in a 'snail track-like' arrangement
Behçet's disease (see Chapter 21)	• Aphthae (see text)
Sarcoidosis (see Chapter 78)	• Orofacial granulomatosis (see text), xerostomia, salivary gland enlargement
Sjögren's syndrome (see Chapter 37)	• Xerostomia
Wegener's granulomatosis (see Chapter 19)	• Gingival hemorrhage with a friable micropapular surface ('strawberry gums'; Fig. 59.16)
Leukemia	• Hemorrhage due to thrombocytopenia, infections (viral, fungal, bacterial), gingival enlargement due to leukemic infiltration (especially in [myelo]monocytic forms)
Genodermatoses	• *Tuberous sclerosis*: oral fibromas, dental enamel pits • *Cowden disease*: oral papillomas favoring lips and tongue • *Multiple endocrine neoplasia type 2B*: mucosal neuromas – papulonodules favoring lips and anterior tongue • *Darier disease*: whitish papules and rugose plaques favoring palate and gingivae • *Lipoid proteinosis*: diffuse infiltration or cobblestoned papules favoring lips and tongue/frenulum, xerostomia • *Chronic mucocutaneous candidiasis* • *Classic hyper-IgE syndrome*: retention of primary teeth, candidiasis • *Ectodermal dysplasias*: hypodontia, cone-shaped teeth • *Nevoid BCC syndrome*: odontogenic keratocysts of mandible > maxilla • *Gardner syndrome*: osteomas of maxilla and mandible

Table 59.1 Systemic diseases with oral manifestations.

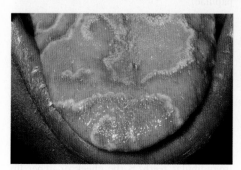

Fig. 59.1 Geographic tongue. A florid example, demonstrating well-delineated areas of erythema partially surrounded by white serpiginous borders. *Courtesy, Carl M. Allen, MD, and Charles Camisa, MD.*

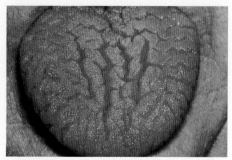

Fig. 59.2 Fissured tongue. Numerous asymptomatic furrows and grooves on the dorsal tongue. *Courtesy, Carl M. Allen, MD, and Charles Camisa, MD.*

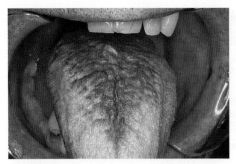

Fig. 59.3 Hairy tongue. The dorsum of the tongue exhibits marked accumulation of keratin and brown discoloration. *Courtesy, Carl M. Allen, MD, and Charles Camisa, MD.*

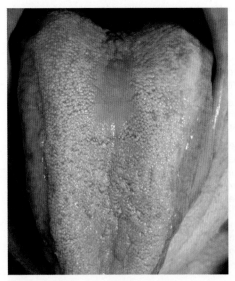

Fig. 59.4 Median rhomboid glossitis. On the dorsum of the tongue (anterior to the circumvallate papillae), there is a well-demarcated, smooth area with loss of the filiform papillae.

• Diffuse gingival erythema with varying degrees of sloughing and erosion; frequently painful.

• Because desquamative gingivitis is often a manifestation of mucous membrane (cicatricial) pemphigoid and other autoimmune bullous disorders, evaluation should include routine histology plus direct and indirect immunofluorescence studies (see Chapter 23).

• **Rx:** treatment of underlying condition plus meticulous oral hygiene.

CAUSES OF GINGIVAL ENLARGEMENT
Systemic medications
• Phenytoin (~50%) > other anticonvulsants • Cyclosporine (~25%)* • Nifedipine (~25%) > other calcium channel blockers • Others – e.g. amphetamines, estrogens
Other etiologies
• Poor oral hygiene,** periodontal disease • Hormone-related – pregnancy, acromegaly • Orofacial granulomatosis (see text) • Wegener's granulomatosis (friable 'strawberry' gums) • Scurvy • Genetic disorders – e.g. tuberous sclerosis, Cowden disease, hereditary gingival fibromatosis • Malignancies – e.g. leukemia, Kaposi's sarcoma • Deposition – e.g. primary systemic amyloidosis
*Consider substitution with oral tacrolimus. **Often contributes to gingival enlargement related to drugs and other factors.

Table 59.2 Causes of gingival enlargement. Another term for Wegener's granulomatosis is granulomatosis with polyangiitis (Wegener's).

Gingival Enlargement (Hyperplasia, Overgrowth)

• Systemic medications and other causes of gingival enlargement are listed in Table 59.2.

• Drug-related gingival enlargement typically develops during the first year of administration and is first evident in the interdental papillae.

Dental Sinus

• Occurs in the setting of a chronic periapical abscess in a carious tooth.

• *Intraoral ('parulis')*: soft, nontender, erythematous papule on the alveolar process in the region of the affected tooth.

• *Cutaneous*: erythematous papule, often with an umbilicated or ulcerated center; found on the chin or submandibular region (mandibular teeth) > the cheek or upper lip (maxillary teeth) (Fig. 59.6).

DIFFERENTIAL DIAGNOSIS OF DESQUAMATIVE GINGIVITIS

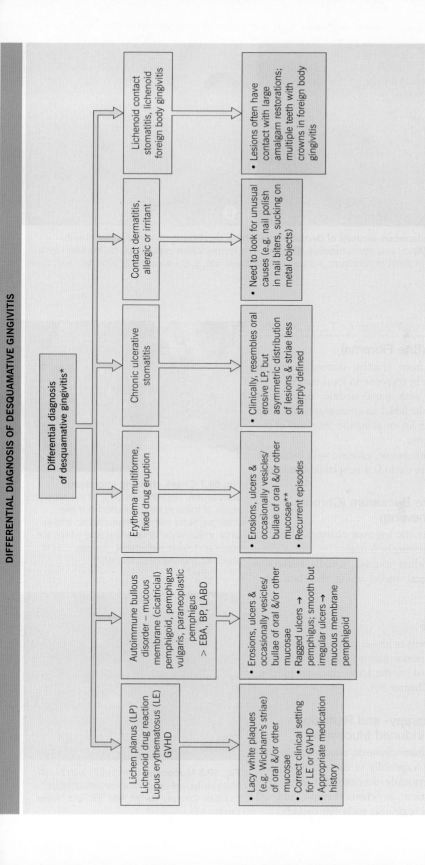

Fig. 59.5 Differential diagnosis of desquamative gingivitis. If the gingivae are painful, hemorrhagic, and necrotic with punched-out interdental papillae, then necrotizing ulcerative gingivitis (trench mouth) should also be considered. *No cutaneous lesions present. **Erythema multiforme is more likely to affect other mucosal sites. BP, bullous pemphigoid; EBA, epidermolysis bullosa acquisita; LABD, linear IgA bullous dermatosis. *Courtesy, Carl M. Allen, MD, and Charles Camisa, MD.*

ORAL DISEASES

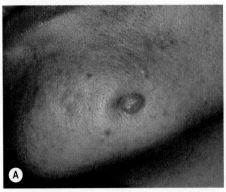
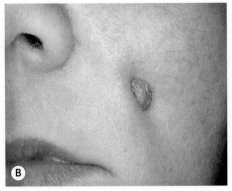

Fig. 59.6 Cutaneous sinuses of dental origin. These skin lesions can be associated with mandibular **(A)** or, less often, maxillary **(B)** teeth. The erythematous papule may be mistaken for a pyogenic granuloma or neoplasm. *A, Courtesy, Judit Stenn, MD; B, Courtesy, Carl M. Allen, MD, and Charles Camisa, MD.*

Sequelae of Trauma or Toxic Insults

Fibroma (Bite Fibroma)

- Results from reactive connective tissue hyperplasia in response to local trauma.
- Smooth pink papulonodule; most often located on the labial mucosa, especially of the lateral lower lip, or along the 'bite line' of the buccal mucosa.
- **Rx:** if bothersome, excision with histologic evaluation to exclude a neoplastic condition.

Morsicatio Buccarum (Chronic Cheek Chewing)

- Characteristic mucosal changes related to habitual chewing or biting.
- Shaggy white mucosa, usually bilaterally in the buccal region along the 'bite line' (Fig. 59.7).

Mucocele

- Translucent to bluish papule due to disruption of a minor salivary gland duct, most often located on the lower mucosal lip (Fig. 59.8; see Chapter 90).

Chemotherapy- and Radiation Therapy-Induced Mucositis

- Results from cytotoxic effects on the oral epithelium, especially in the setting of neutropenia; typically develops 4–7 days after administration of chemotherapy and ≥2 weeks after beginning radiation therapy.

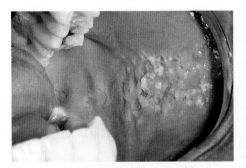

Fig. 59.7 Cheek chewing (morsicatio buccarum). Repetitive nibbling of the superficial layers of the epithelium resulted in these changes. Note that the characteristic shaggy, white lesion approximates the area where the upper and lower teeth meet. *Courtesy, Carl M. Allen, MD, and Charles Camisa, MD.*

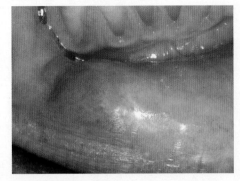

Fig. 59.8 Mucocele. Soft nodule with bluish hue in a typical location: lower lateral labial mucosa. *Courtesy, Carl M. Allen, MD, and Charles Camisa, MD.*

- Multiple erosions and/or ulcerations favor the gingivae, lateral tongue, and buccal mucosa; self-limited.
- **DDx:** herpetic or candidal infections (may be concomitant).
- **Rx:** topical anesthetics, analgesics, maintenance of oral hygiene; palifermin (recombinant human keratinocyte growth factor) can reduce severity but produces whitish discoloration of the dorsum of the tongue due to hyperkeratosis.

Cheilitis

- The differential diagnosis of cheilitis and clues to determining the etiology are outlined in Fig. 13.5; granulomatous cheilitis is discussed below.
- *Cheilitis glandularis*, seen primarily in men with a history of chronic sun exposure and/or lip irritation, is characterized by inflammatory hyperplasia of the lower labial salivary glands; this results in tiny erythematous macules (at sites of salivary ducts) and variable hypertrophy of the lower lip (Fig. 59.9).

Other Inflammatory Conditions

Aphthae (Aphthous Stomatitis; Canker Sores)

- Common condition characterized by recurrent oral ulcers, with a peak prevalence during the second and third decades of life; outbreaks may be triggered by trauma, psychological stress, or hormonal fluctuations.

- *Minor aphthae* (most frequent form): painful, round to ovoid, shallow ulcers that are usually <5 mm in diameter; feature a yellowish-white to gray pseudomembranous base, well-defined border, and prominent erythematous rim (Fig. 59.10); favor the buccal or labial mucosa and typically heal in 1–2 weeks without scarring.
- *Major aphthae*: larger (>1 cm), deeper ulcers that persist for up to 6 weeks; occasionally affect keratinized mucosa (e.g. dorsum of tongue, hard palate, attached gingiva) as well as nonkeratinized mucosa, may heal with scarring, and are more common in HIV-infected individuals.
- *Herpetiform aphthae*: simultaneous development of numerous small lesions that tend to coalesce; tends to favor nonkeratinized mucosa, unlike recurrent oral HSV, which favors keratinized mucosa.
- *Complex aphthosis*: frequent outbreaks of multiple (≥3) oral aphthae, or recurrent genital as well as oral aphthae, in the absence of Behçet's disease (see Chapter 21).
- Recurrent aphthae can occur in the setting of systemic disorders such as inflammatory bowel disease, SLE, and Behçet's disease (see Table 59.1).
- **DDx:** in addition to associated systemic conditions, may include HSV infection, trauma, and the disorders listed in Fig. 59.5.
- **Rx:** superpotent topical CS gel, topical analgesics; if severe or frequent recurrences:

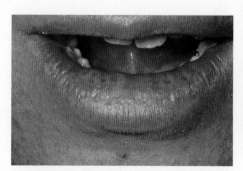

Fig. 59.9 Cheilitis glandularis. Erythematous macules on the mucosal lower lip at sites of inflamed salivary gland ducts. There is also evidence of actinic cheilitis. *Courtesy, Carl M. Allen, MD, and Charles Camisa, MD.*

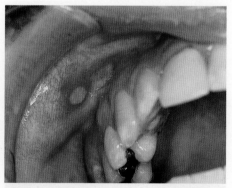

Fig. 59.10 Recurrent aphthous stomatitis. Shallow, creamy-white ulceration surrounded by an intensely red halo and located on nonkeratinized mucosa, representing a classic presentation. *Courtesy, Carl M. Allen, MD, and Charles Camisa, MD.*

vitamin B_{12}, colchicine, dapsone, thalidomide (the latter is especially helpful for major aphthae).

Granulomatous Cheilitis and Other Forms of Orofacial Granulomatosis

• The term *orofacial granulomatosis* refers to non-infectious, non-necrotizing granulomatous inflammation of the lips, face, and/or oral cavity; this term includes isolated granulomatous cheilitis as well as manifestations of Crohn's disease and sarcoidosis (see Table 59.1); usually develops during the second or third decade of life.

• *Granulomatous cheilitis* presents as diffuse swelling of the lip(s) (lower > upper or both) that can initially be intermittent (raising the possibility of angioedema) but is eventually persistent (Fig. 59.11); patients may have oral cobblestoning, recurrent aphthae, and gingival enlargement, and the less frequent association with a scrotal tongue and/or facial nerve palsy is referred to as *Melkersson–Rosenthal syndrome*.

• **Rx:** intralesional CS, topical calcineurin inhibitors, dapsone, tetracyclines (given for several months), thalidomide or TNF inhibitors (for severe disease); patients should be evaluated for signs of Crohn's disease and sarcoidosis.

Contact Stomatitis

• Irritant or allergic contact stomatitis can result from a variety of foods, food additives, and materials used in dentistry; in particular, cinnamon flavoring and dental amalgam ('silver' fillings) can lead to a lichenoid mucositis histologically.

• Shaggy white or erythematous areas, most often on the buccal mucosa or lateral tongue; lacy white streaks (resembling lichen planus) or erosions may be seen (Fig. 59.12).

• **Rx:** evaluation with patch testing and avoidance of offending agents, sometimes requiring replacement of amalgam with other materials.

Nicotine Stomatitis

• Presents as gray-white discoloration of the palate, often with umbilicated papules that represent inflamed salivary ducts (Fig. 59.13).

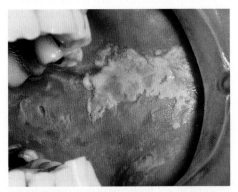

Fig. 59.12 Contact stomatitis from artificial cinnamon flavoring. Use of artificial cinnamon-flavored gum caused this shaggy, white keratotic lesion of the buccal mucosa. *Courtesy, Carl M. Allen, MD, and Charles Camisa, MD.*

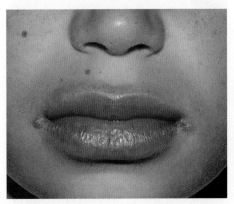

Fig. 59.11 Orofacial granulomatosis. Note the swelling of the lips (lower > upper) and angular cheilitis in this 10-year-old boy with Crohn's disease. *Courtesy, Julie V. Schaffer, MD.*

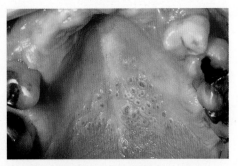

Fig. 59.13 Nicotine stomatitis. Gray-white palatal mucosa with numerous umbilicated papules representing inflamed palatal mucous glands. *Courtesy, Carl M. Allen, MD, and Charles Camisa, MD.*

Atrophic Glossitis

• Manifestation of several nutritional deficiencies (e.g. vitamin B_{12} [pernicious anemia], folate, iron, niacin [pellagra], riboflavin; see Chapter 43) and candidiasis.

• Presents with a smooth, 'beefy red' tongue (Fig. 59.14); involvement may initially be patchy but is eventually diffuse and may be associated with a burning sensation or sore mouth.

Oral Signs of Systemic Disease

• Systemic diseases that can present with oral findings are listed in Table 59.1 (Figs. 59.15 and 59.16).

Premalignant and Malignant Conditions

Leukoplakia and Erythroplakia

• *Leukoplakia* refers to a white patch or plaque on the oral mucosa that cannot be clinicopathologically characterized as a specific disease process; typically occurs in middle-aged and older adults (men > women), especially those who use tobacco ± alcohol, and is regarded as a premalignant condition for SCC.

- Often a homogeneous white patch or plaque, but may be nonhomogeneous and 'speckled' (e.g. white flecks on a red base); usually has sharply demarcated borders (Fig. 59.17).

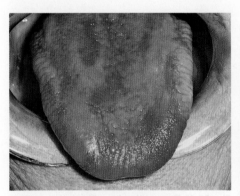

Fig. 59.14 Atrophic glossitis due to pernicious anemia plus candidiasis. Erythematous, atrophic tongue as a manifestation of pernicious anemia with a superimposed candidal infection. *Courtesy, Carl M. Allen, MD, and Charles Camisa, MD.*

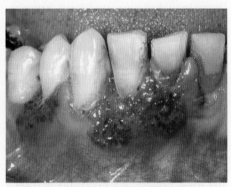

Fig. 59.16 Wegener's granulomatosis – strawberry gums. The affected areas of the gingiva are red-purple, micropapular, and friable, with a resemblance to ripe strawberries. *Courtesy, Carl M. Allen, MD, and Charles Camisa, MD.*

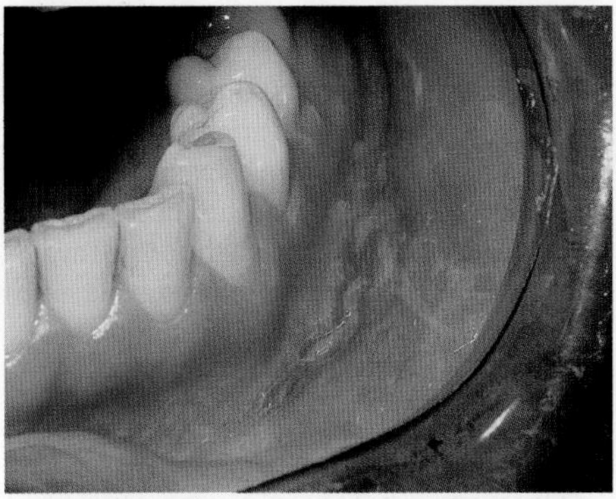

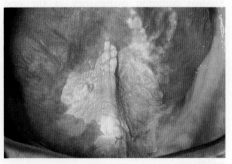

Fig. 59.15 Crohn's disease. Linear ulceration of the mandibular vestibule is the classic oral manifestation of this disease. *Courtesy, Carl M. Allen, MD, and Charles Camisa, MD.*

Fig. 59.17 Leukoplakia. Sharply demarcated, white plaque involving the ventral surface of the tongue and floor of the mouth. *Courtesy, Carl M. Allen, MD, and Charles Camisa, MD.*

• Similarly, *erythroplakia* is defined as a red intraoral patch or slightly elevated, velvety plaque that cannot be diagnosed as a particular disease; biopsies usually show more severe epithelial dysplasia than leukoplakia.

• Often affects the buccal mucosa, lower inner lip, floor of the mouth, and lateral or ventral tongue.

• The degree of histologic epithelial dysplasia influences the risk of transformation to SCC; nonhomogeneous leukoplakia, erythroplakia, and lesions located on the floor of the mouth or lateral/ventral tongue also have higher malignant potential.

• **DDx** of leukoplakia: may include SCC, lichen planus, candidiasis, morsicatio buccarum (see above), and nicotine or contact stomatitis.

• After elimination of possible causative factors (e.g. tobacco use, candidiasis, irritation/trauma) for 2–6 weeks, persistent lesions should be biopsied.

• **Rx:** for leukoplakia with moderate to severe dysplasia or in high-risk sites and for erythroplakia – excision, cryosurgery, or laser ablation; all patients need longitudinal evaluation and should avoid carcinogenic habits.

• *Proliferative verrucous leukoplakia*, which tends to occur in women without traditional risk factors, is characterized by multifocal red and white patches that eventually develop a verrucous surface; difficult to treat and associated with high risk of transformation to SCC.

Squamous Cell Carcinoma

• Most common malignancy of the oral cavity, favoring middle-aged and older men; risk factors include tobacco and alcohol use, HPV infection (see Chapter 66), and betel nut chewing.

• May present as an ulcer, exophytic mass, or area of induration; most often on the lateral or ventral tongue and floor of the mouth (Fig. 59.18).

• **DDx:** leukoplakia, traumatic ulcer (Fig. 59.19), salivary gland tumor, amelanotic melanoma.

• **Rx:** combinations of surgery, radiation therapy (especially if HPV-associated), and chemotherapy.

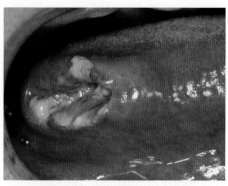

Fig. 59.18 Squamous cell carcinoma. Ulcerated, indurated, exophytic mass involving the right lateral border of the tongue, a typical presentation and site for this tumor. *Courtesy, Carl M. Allen, MD, and Charles Camisa, MD.*

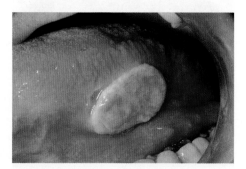

Fig. 59.19 Traumatic ulcer. This lesion on the lateral tongue has a yellow fibrinopurulent membrane and white hyperkeratotic border. Compare this to the oral SCC depicted in Fig. 59.18, which presented as an ulcerated, indurated mass. *Courtesy, Carl M. Allen, MD, and Charles Camisa, MD.*

• *Verrucous carcinoma (oral florid papillomatosis)* is a low-grade variant of SCC that presents as slowly growing, exophytic papillomatous masses that favor the buccal mucosa and gingiva; **Rx:** excision, traditionally avoiding radiation therapy due to a possible association with anaplastic transformation.

Melanoma

• Uncommon oral malignancy that favors middle-aged and older men; often diagnosed at a locally advanced stage.

• Pigmented (with findings similar to cutaneous melanoma; see Chapter 93) >

amelanotic, with a predilection for the hard palate and maxillary gingivae.

• **DDx:** for pigmented lesions – foreign body tattoo (Fig. 59.20), blue nevus, oral melanotic macule, physiologic pigmentation.

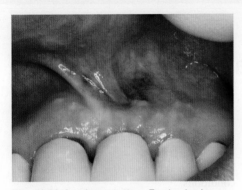

Fig. 59.20 Amalgam tattoo. Foreign body tattoos are the most common cause of acquired oral pigmentation, and most of them are due to implantation of dental amalgam. In this patient, the amalgam was used to seal the apices of endodontically treated teeth, resulting in tattooing of the maxillary vestibule. *Courtesy, Carl M. Allen, MD, and Charles Camisa, MD.*

For further information see Ch. 72. From *Dermatology, Third Edition.*

60 | Anogenital Diseases

Introduction

• The anatomy (Fig. 60.1), normal cutaneous findings, and benign lesions of the anogenital area (Table 60.1) should be appreciated before addressing diseases in this area.

• A number of systemic diseases affect the anogenital area (Table 60.2).

• Cutaneous disorders of the anogenital area may be more difficult to diagnose than those involving other cutaneous sites, as typical features may not be present.

• A number of dermatologic conditions affect the anogenital region, including inflammatory (Table 60.3; Figs. 60.2–60.6), bullous (Table 60.4; Fig. 60.7), infectious (Table 60.5; see Chapter 69), and premalignant and malignant (Table 60.6; Figs. 60.8–60.11) conditions.

• Pain and pruritus can be the presenting symptoms in a wide variety of anogenital diseases (Figs. 60.12 and 60.13).

• Patients with anogenital disease should use soap substitutes and bland emollient ointments; irritants and potential allergens (e.g. flushable moist wipes, previous topical medications) should be avoided.

• Ointments are preferred over creams in this area because of less irritation and burning with application, as well as providing a better barrier to urine and feces.

• The anogenital region is an area of occlusion and more prone to adverse side effects from and increased absorption of topical agents (e.g. CS).

THE NORMAL VULVA

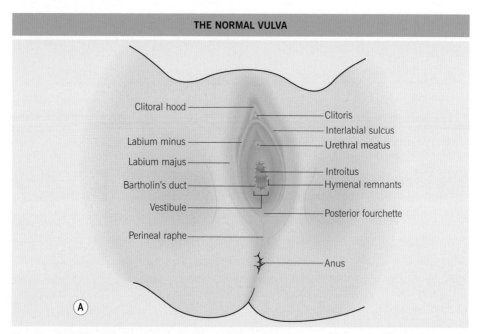

Clitoral hood
Clitoris
Interlabial sulcus
Labium minus
Urethral meatus
Labium majus
Introitus
Bartholin's duct
Hymenal remnants
Vestibule
Posterior fourchette
Perineal raphe
Anus

(A)

Fig. 60.1 Genital anatomy. A The normal vulva. *Continued*

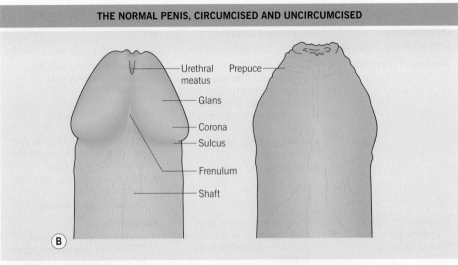

Urethral meatus
Prepuce
Glans
Corona
Sulcus
Frenulum
Shaft

Ⓑ

Fig. 60.1 *Continued* **B** The normal penis, circumcised and uncircumcised.

NORMAL FINDINGS AND BENIGN LESIONS OF THE ANOGENITAL REGION

Common	Less Common
Epidermoid cysts	Fox-Fordyce disease
Open comedones	Syringomas
Pearly penile papules (see Fig. 95.7)	Idiopathic calcinosis of the scrotum
Vestibular papillomatosis	Urethral caruncle
Angiokeratomas (see Fig. 87.11)	Hidradenoma papilliferum
Seborrheic keratoses and acrochordons	
Melanocytic nevi and genital lentigines	
Free sebaceous glands	

Table 60.1 Normal findings and benign lesions of the anogenital region. Papules in the anogenital region can also result from HPV infection, in particular condylomata acuminata and common warts (see Ch. 66).

SYSTEMIC DISEASES WITH ASSOCIATED ANOGENITAL CUTANEOUS FINDINGS

- Inflammatory bowel disease, especially Crohn's disease (see Chapter 45)
- Nutritional dermatoses, e.g. acrodermatitis enteropathica, necrolytic migratory erythema, cystic fibrosis (see Chapter 43)
- Langerhans cell histiocytosis (see Chapter 76)
- Kawasaki disease (see Chapter 3)
- Behçet's disease – ulcers (see Chapter 45)
- Infections (nonvenereal), e.g. recurrent toxin-mediated perineal erythema, Fournier's gangrene
- Infections (venereal) (see Chapter 69)
- Drug reactions (see Chapters 16 & 17), e.g. EM major, SJS, TEN; fixed drug eruption; toxic erythema of chemotherapy

EM, erythema multiforme; SJS, Stevens–Johnson syndrome; TEN, toxic epidermal necrolysis.

Table 60.2 Systemic diseases with associated anogenital cutaneous findings. *Courtesy, Susan M. Cooper, MD, and Fenella Wojnarowska, MD.*

INFLAMMATORY DERMATOLOGIC DISORDERS WITH ANOGENITAL FEATURES

Inflammatory Dermatologic Disorder	Anogenital Features	Rx
Anogenital dermatitis	• Female > male • Varied presentations, from mild erythema to significant lichenification (Fig. 60.2) • Unremitting itch/scratch cycle **Female:** perianal, labia majora, mons pubis **Male:** crura and scrotum	• Examine entire body for clues to etiology (e.g. seborrheic or atopic dermatitis) • Eliminate irritants and allergens • Break itch/scratch cycle with potent topical CS for several weeks and then taper • Oral antihistamines may help control pruritus • Consider patch testing
Psoriasis (including inverse psoriasis) (See Chapter 6)	• Perianal and intergluteal cleft fissuring; erythematous, smooth, well-demarcated plaques **Female:** labia majora and mons pubis **Male:** glans and shaft of penis (Fig. 60.3)	**Mild–Moderate** • Moderate potency topical CS for 2–3 weeks with taper to less potent topical CS plus antifungal • Topical calcineurin inhibitors and vitamin D analogs (may sting) **Severe** (see Chapter 6)
Lichen sclerosus (LS)	See Fig. 60.4 and Chapter 36	See Chapter 36
Classic lichen planus (LP) (See Chapter 9)	**Female:** mons pubis and labia **Male:** glans and shaft of penis; often annular (Fig. 60.5A)	• Moderate to high-potency topical CS as needed to control pruritus
Erosive lichen planus (oro-vaginal-vulvar LP) (See Chapter 9)	• Female > male • Erosions surrounded by white lacy pattern; prominent scarring and adhesions (Fig. 60.5B) • Desquamative vaginitis with discharge; significant pain and dyspareunia • Usually severe oral involvement/desquamative gingivitis • Increased risk for SCC	**Mild** • Topical potent CS with taper/maintenance • For vaginal disease use CS foams, enemas, suppositories **Severe** • Longer-term potent topical CS • Topical calcineurin inhibitors • Oral antimalarials • Systemic immunosuppressants
Zoon's balanitis/vulvitis (plasma cell balanitis/vulvitis)	• Male (uncircumcised) > female • Pruritus and pain **Male:** glans penis (Fig. 60.6) • Erythematous discrete moist plaques with speckled appearance and orange hue • Involvement of adjacent surfaces produce 'kissing lesions' **Female:** similar lesions involving vulva	• Circumcision curative • Topical CS if symptoms

The DDx of these disorders includes the other entities listed in this table; consider infections, either primary or superimposed (see Table 60.5); less commonly bullous disorders (see Table 60.4); if nonhealing consider malignancy, most commonly SCC (see Table 60.6).

Table 60.3 Inflammatory dermatologic disorders with anogenital features. Porokeratosis ptychotropica is a rare disorder and can mimic anogenital dermatitis or inverse psoriasis.

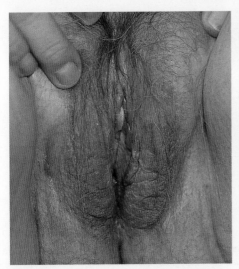

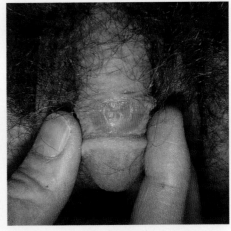

Fig. 60.3 Psoriasis of the penile shaft. Well-demarcated erythematous plaque with slight scale. Similar lesions can be seen in patients with reactive arthritis (formerly Reiter's disease). *Courtesy, Jean L. Bolognia, MD.*

Fig. 60.2 Vulvar dermatitis. Lichenification is prominent. The underlying diagnosis was atopic dermatitis. *Courtesy, Susan M. Cooper, MD, and Fenella Wojnarowska, MD.*

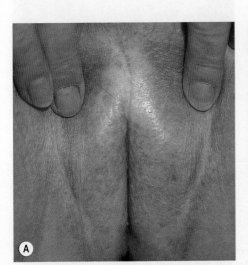

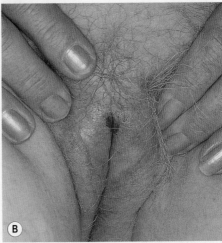

Fig. 60.4 Lichen sclerosus (LS). Typical involvement of the vulva demonstrating marked architectural change with the loss of the labia minora and midline fusion **(A)** and purpura **(B).** *A, Courtesy, Susan M. Cooper, MD, and Fenella Wojnarowska, MD; B, Courtesy, Kalman Watsky, MD. Continued*

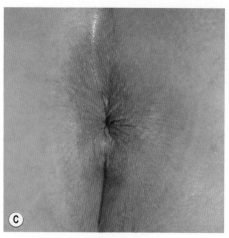

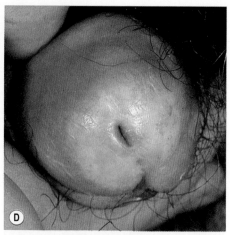

Fig. 60.4 *Continued* Perianal LS **(C)** and involvement of the penis **(D)** with an erythematous and hypopigmented plaque on the glans. *C, Courtesy, Susan M. Cooper, MD, and Fenella Wojnarowska, MD; D, Courtesy, Ronald P. Rapini, MD.*

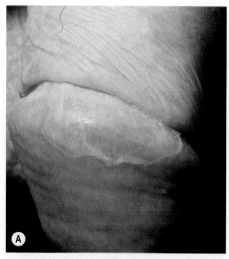

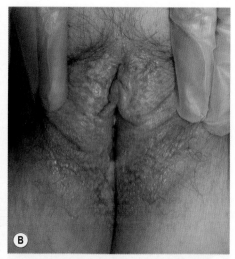

Fig. 60.5 Anogenital lichen planus. A Involvement of the penis with an annular band on the glans, a typical finding. **B** Erosive lichen planus of the vulva with fissures and an extensive white lacy pattern. *A, Courtesy, R. Turner, MD; B, Courtesy, Susan M. Cooper, MD, and Fenella Wojnarowska, MD.*

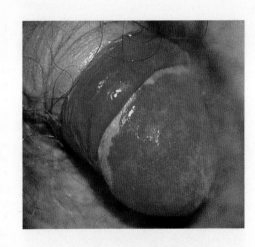

Fig. 60.6 Zoon's balanitis. There are moist 'kissing lesions' on adjacent surfaces of the glans and prepuce. *Courtesy, Susan M. Cooper, MD, and Fenella Wojnarowska, MD.*

BULLOUS DERMATOLOGIC DISORDERS WITH ANOGENITAL FEATURES		
Bullous Disorder	**Anogenital Features**	**Rx**
Hailey–Hailey disease	See Chapter 48	See Chapter 48
Bullous pemphigoid (BP) (See Chapter 24)	• Mostly affects the elderly, but a localized vulvar variant is occasionally seen in children • A vegetans form favors flexural sites • Less likely than PV to involve mucosal sites	**Mild** • Potent topical/ intralesional CS **Severe** • Systemic CS • Other systemic immunosuppressants
Mucous membrane (cicatricial) pemphigoid (MMP) (See Chapter 24)	• External genitalia and anus **Early:** erosions, ulcerations, blisters (Fig. 60.7) • Pain, pruritus, dysuria **Late:** scarring prominent with related disability • Phimosis, narrowing of vaginal introitus, anal stricture	• Methotrexate (BP) • Dapsone, cyclophosphamide (MMP) • Dapsone or sulfapyridine (LABD) • Mycophenolate mofetil, azathioprine (PV)
Pemphigus vulgaris (PV) (See Chapter 23)	• Vagina, labia, anus, penis • Widespread erosions; vegetative and papillomatous nodulo-plaques may develop (pemphigus vegetans)	See Chapter 23

Acquired autoimmune bullous diseases are clinically difficult to differentiate from one another and require biopsies for H&E and DIF, as well as serum for IIF and/or ELISA.
MMP can be clinically indistinguishable from erosive lichen planus in the anogenital area.
The DDx (especially of PV) may include other causes of erosions (Table 60.7).
Other blistering disorders, including LABD (linear IgA bullous dermatosis), can occur in the genital area.
H&E, hematoxylin and eosin; DIF, direct immunofluorescence; IIF, indirect immunofluorescence.

Table 60.4 Bullous dermatologic disorders with anogenital features.

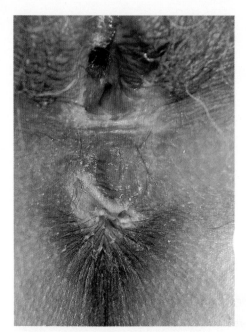

Fig. 60.7 Mucous membrane pemphigoid of the vulva. Ulcerations and scarring of the perianal area and perineum. Positive direct immunofluorescence with linear deposition of immunoreactants distinguished this from erosive lichen planus. *Courtesy, Susan M. Cooper, MD, and Fenella Wojnarowska, MD.*

• High-potency topical CS are generally avoided because of the increased risk for atrophy and striae, but they are used with confidence in certain situations (e.g. lichen sclerosus, erosive lichen planus) for periods of up to 12 weeks once to twice yearly.
• Because of increased moisture, warmth, and occlusion, anogenital diseases have an increased risk of superimposed bacterial and fungal infections.
• Diseases that result in scarring of the anogenital region (e.g. lichen sclerosus, erosive lichen planus) carry an increased long-term risk of developing invasive squamous cell carcinoma (SCC).

Intraepithelial Neoplasia

• The term *intraepithelial neoplasia* (*IN*) refers to a change within the anogenital epithelium that is premalignant, and as such has the potential to become an invasive SCC.

• IN has replaced older synonymous terms, such as genital Bowen's disease, erythroplasia of Queyrat, and genital SCC *in situ*; use of the term leukoplakia with atypia is also not recommended.
• IN is further subdivided based on location: vulvar IN (VIN), penile IN (PIN), perianal IN (PaIN), and anal IN (AIN) (see Table 60.6), as well as the degree of atypia: 1, mild; 2, moderate; 3, severe.
• Recently recommended terminology that can replace or qualify IN: high-grade and low-grade intraepithelial lesion.
• Bowenoid papulosis (BP) is a distinct clinical variant of IN that occurs in a younger (more sexually active) age group, is caused by the human papillomavirus (HPV subtypes 16 and 18), has a better prognosis, and sometimes spontaneously regresses (see Chapter 66).

Condyloma Acuminata

• See Chapter 66.

Dysesthetic Genital Pain Syndromes

• Includes several regional pain syndromes in which clinical appearance of the involved anogenital region is normal despite the patient's experience of debilitating pain (Fig. 60.14); associated depression is common.
• *Localized vulvodynia* (vestibulodynia) occurs in young, sexually active females and is characterized by superficial dyspareunia and tenderness upon localized pressure within the vulvar vestibule.
• *Generalized* (dysesthetic) *vulvodynia/scrotodynia* is characterized by persistent burning pain that involves the entire vulva, scrotum, or penis, and may extend down the thighs.
• *Cyclical vulvovaginitis* is a recurrent vulvovaginitis, with or without a typical candidal discharge, that most often occurs premenstrually and is associated with superficial dyspareunia; often responds to prolonged course of oral antifungals.
• *Anodynia* is an anal/perianal regional pain syndrome in males and females that shares many features of the previously described entities.

INFECTIOUS (NONVENEREAL) DERMATOLOGIC DISORDERS WITH ANOGENITAL FEATURES

Infectious (Nonvenereal) Dermatologic Disorder	Anogenital Features	Dx and DDx	Rx
Candidiasis (See Chapter 64 and Figs. 13.2 and 13.4)	• Favors the perianal area and inguinal crease, with sheet-like erythema, fissuring, erosions, and satellite pustules **Female** • Vulvar erythema, small fissures • Severe pruritus • Creamy-white vaginal discharge **Male** • Uncircumcised > circumcised • Balanitis or balanoposthitis • In the inguinal/scrotal folds, see erythema and focal white areas	• Many anogenital diseases may be misdiagnosed as a 'yeast' infection or develop superimposed candidiasis • Confirm by microscopy (KOH preparation) and/or culture • If pustules, consider impetigo	• Address precipitating factors (e.g. diabetes mellitus, systemic antibiotics) **Mild** • Topical antifungal/anti-yeast agents • Vaginal anti-yeast suppositories • Single, oral dose of fluconazole 150 mg (vaginal candidiasis) **Severe** • Fluconazole 50–100 mg daily for 14 days **Recurrent (>3 episodes/year)** • Treat sexual partners • Oral fluconazole 100 mg weekly for 6 months • Clotrimazole vaginal 500 mg tablets weekly for 6 months • Oral itraconazole 200 mg, twice a day, once per month, for 6 months
Dermatophytosis (tinea cruris) (See Chapter 64 and Fig. 13.2)	• Chronic, slowly advancing, scaly, erythematous patches and thin plaques; ± pustules • Favors the groin (but scrotum often spared) with extension onto upper, medial thighs; medial buttocks • Tinea pedis and toenail onychomycosis often present	• Confirm with microscopy (KOH preparation)	**Mild** • Topical antifungals **Severe** • Oral terbinafine 250 mg daily for 2 weeks

Table 60.5 Infectious (nonvenereal) dermatologic disorders with anogenital features. Condylomata acuminata and venereal diseases are covered in Chapters 66 and 69, respectively. *Continued*

Table 60.5 *Continued* **Infectious (nonvenereal) dermatologic disorders with anogenital features.** Condylomata acuminata and venereal diseases are covered in Chapters 66 and 69, respectively.

Infectious (Nonvenereal) Dermatologic Disorder	Anogenital Features	Dx and DDx	Rx
Erythrasma (See Chapter 61 and Fig. 13.2)	• Well-defined, pink to red-brown, pigmented patches or thin plaques with fine diffuse scale and wrinkling • Favors flexural areas, such as groin and intergluteal cleft • Caused by *Corynebacterium minutissimum*	• Wood's lamp examination (coral pink fluorescence)	**Mild** • Antibacterial soaps • Topical 10–20% aluminum chloride • Topical 2% clindamycin • Topical erythromycin **Severe** • Oral erythromycin for 5 days
Perianal streptococcal disease (See Chapter 61 and Fig. 13.4)	• Children >> adults • Sharply demarcated, bright perianal erythema, extending 2–3 cm around the anal verge • Painful defecation • Blood-streaked stools • Irritation or pruritus • Caused by group A β-hemolytic *Streptococcus* • May also involve the inguinal region, especially in children (streptococcal intertrigo) • May be preceded or accompanied by pharyngitis	• Diagnosis made with bacterial culture • Also consider: pinworm infection, child abuse, and early Kawasaki disease	• Oral cephalosporin, penicillin or erythromycin for 10–14 days • Follow with re-culture to exclude recurrence

The DDx of these disorders includes the other entities listed in this table; they may be confused with the disorders listed in Tables 60.2 and 60.3 as well as superimposed upon them; topical medications can also lead to a superimposed contact dermatitis. KOH, potassium hydroxide.

PREMALIGNANT AND MALIGNANT DERMATOLOGIC DISORDERS WITH ANOGENITAL FEATURES

Premalignant and Malignant Dermatologic Disorders	Anogenital Features	Other	Rx
Premalignant Lesions			
• Vulvar intraepithelial neoplasia (VIN) • Penile intraepithelial neoplasia (PIN) • Perianal intraepithelial neoplasia (PaIN) • Anal intraepithelial neoplasia (AIN)	Varied presentations • Erythematous or pigmented, well-demarcated plaque (genital Bowen's disease variant) • Verrucous white-gray plaque • Erosions • Nonhealing ulcer • Erythematous, shiny, velvety patch or plaque (erythroplasia of Queyrat variant) (Fig. 60.8)	Several etiologies/predisposing factors • Oncogenic HPV (e.g. subtypes 16, 18, 31, 33) • Inflammatory, scarring conditions (e.g. lichen sclerosus, erosive lichen planus) • Uncircumcised male • Immunosuppression • HIV infection	• In conjunction with gynecologic or urologic oncologist • Long-term evaluation necessary, including anal and cervical cytology • Examine sexual partners • Varies from topical agents (e.g. imiquimod, 5-fluorouracil) to surgical excision, including Mohs surgery • Prevention: HPV vaccination
• Bowenoid papulosis	See Fig. 60.9 and Chapter 66	See Chapter 66	See Chapter 66
Malignant Lesions			
• Invasive SCC	Varied presentations • Nonhealing ulcer or fissure • Erythematous plaque with heaped-up edges (Fig. 60.10) • Verrucous plaque • Nodule	• Most common anogenital tumor, but overall rare • Etiologies are similar to those listed for premalignant lesions	• Consult with gynecologic or urologic oncologist • First-line: surgical excision, including Mohs surgery • Second-line: RT
• Extramammary Paget's disease	• Slowly expanding erythematous plaque with demarcation between normal and involved skin; erosions and scale present (Fig. 60.11) • Favors vulva and perianal regions • Pruritus, burning, or asymptomatic	• Rare intraepithelial adenocarcinoma • More common in older females and Japanese males • May be primary or secondary to an underlying malignancy • Associated underlying visceral malignancy in 10–20% • Associated underlying adnexal adenocarcinoma in <5%	• Initial and periodic systemic evaluations for internal malignancy are necessary • Surgical excision vs. Mohs surgery • Combination therapy, e.g. topicals (see above), RT, photodynamic therapy

Multiple biopsies may be necessary to make a diagnosis.

The DDx of these disorders includes the other entities listed in this table and Table 60.2, as well as seborrheic keratosis, condyloma acuminata, NMSC, and amelanotic melanoma.

HPV, human papilloma virus; HIV, human immunodeficiency virus; RT, radiotherapy.

Table 60.6 Premalignant and malignant dermatologic disorders with anogenital features.

ANOGENITAL DISEASES

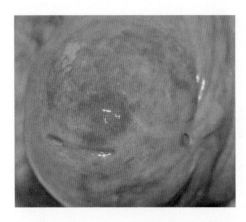

Fig. 60.8 Penile intraepithelial neoplasia (PIN). Persistent erythema not responding to topical steroids. *Courtesy, R. Turner, MD.*

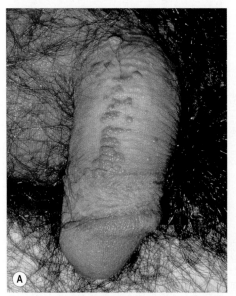

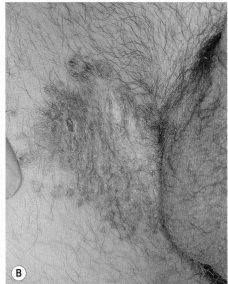

Fig. 60.9 Bowenoid papulosis variant of intraepithelial neoplasia. A Multiple red-brown to brown papules on the shaft of the penis. **B** Coalescence of red-brown to brown papules on the upper inner thigh. *B, Courtesy, Robert Hartman, MD.*

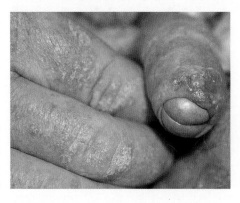

Fig. 60.10 Invasive squamous cell carcinoma of the foreskin. This patient with psoriasis had received PUVA therapy without genital protection. *Courtesy, Susan M. Cooper, MD, and Fenella Wojnarowska, MD.*

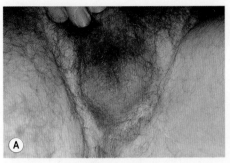
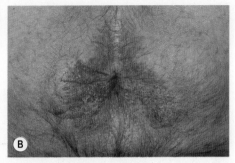

Fig. 60.11 Extramammary Paget's disease. A Erythematous plaque with hydrated scale at the base of the scrotum. **B** Well-demarcated perianal plaque with both erosions and scale, giving rise to a 'strawberries and cream' appearance. *B, Courtesy, Kalman Watsky, MD.*

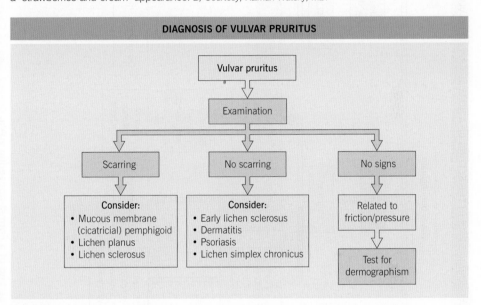

DIAGNOSIS OF VULVAR PRURITUS

Vulvar pruritus

Examination

Scarring → No scarring → No signs

Consider:
- Mucous membrane (cicatricial) pemphigoid
- Lichen planus
- Lichen sclerosus

Consider:
- Early lichen sclerosus
- Dermatitis
- Psoriasis
- Lichen simplex chronicus

Related to friction/pressure

Test for dermographism

Fig. 60.12 The diagnosis of vulvar pruritus. *Courtesy, Susan M. Cooper, MD, and Fenella Wojnarowska, MD.*

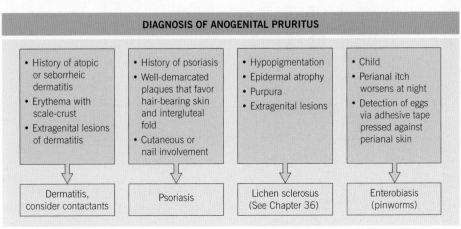

DIAGNOSIS OF ANOGENITAL PRURITUS

- History of atopic or seborrheic dermatitis
- Erythema with scale-crust
- Extragenital lesions of dermatitis

- History of psoriasis
- Well-demarcated plaques that favor hair-bearing skin and intergluteal fold
- Cutaneous or nail involvement

- Hypopigmentation
- Epidermal atrophy
- Purpura
- Extragenital lesions

- Child
- Perianal itch worsens at night
- Detection of eggs via adhesive tape pressed against perianal skin

Dermatitis, consider contactants

Psoriasis

Lichen sclerosus (See Chapter 36)

Enterobiasis (pinworms)

Fig. 60.13 The diagnosis of anogenital pruritus. Histologic evaluation may be required to confirm the clinical diagnosis (e.g. lichen sclerosus) or to exclude more unusual etiologies (e.g. extramammary Paget's disease). Systemic contact dermatitis reactions in this region may also be very pruritic.
Courtesy, Susan M. Cooper, MD, and Fenella Wojnarowska, MD.

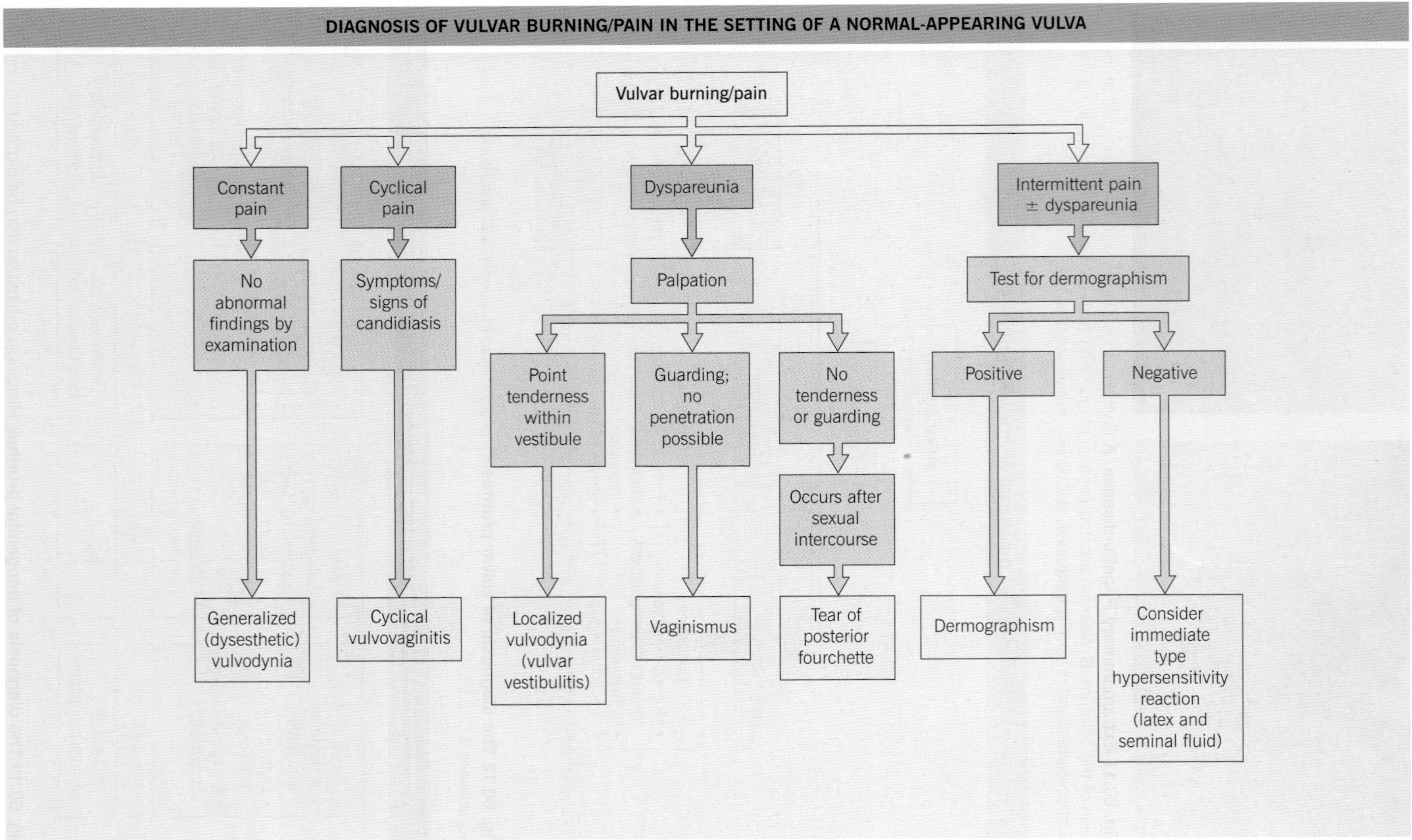

DIAGNOSIS OF VULVAR BURNING/PAIN IN THE SETTING OF A NORMAL-APPEARING VULVA

Fig. 60.14 The diagnosis of vulvar burning/pain in the setting of a normal-appearing vulva. *Courtesy, Susan M. Cooper, MD, and Fenella Wojnarowska, MD.*

CAUSES OF GENITAL EROSIONS

- Lichen sclerosus
- Erosive lichen planus
- Genital aphthae

- Infection
  - Candidiasis
  - Impetigo (*Staphylococcus/Streptococcus*)
  - Herpes simplex viral infection or herpes zoster
  - Primary syphilis, chancroid
  - Cytomegalovirus, Epstein–Barr virus,* *Mycoplasma*
  - Tuberculosis

- Squamous cell carcinoma and other malignancies
- Intraepithelial neoplasia

- Zoon's plasma cell balanitis/vulvitis

- Acquired bullous diseases
  - Pemphigus vulgaris
  - Bullous pemphigoid
  - Mucous membrane (cicatricial) pemphigoid
  - Linear IgA bullous dermatosis
  - Epidermolysis bullosa acquisita
  - Erythema multiforme, Stevens–Johnson syndrome
  - Fixed drug eruption
- Inherited bullous disease
  - Hailey–Hailey disease
  - Epidermolysis bullosa

- Complex aphthosis due to Behçet's disease or inflammatory bowel disease
- Crohn's disease
- Extramammary Paget's disease
- Langerhans cell histiocytosis
- Necrolytic migratory erythema, acrodermatitis enteropathica
- Papular acantholytic dyskeratosis
- Toxic erythema of chemotherapy

Diagnosed via EBV IgM antibodies or PCR; favors female children and adolescents.

Table 60.7 Causes of genital erosions.

- **Rx:** individualized and may include topical local anesthetics, oral tricyclic antidepressants, oral gabapentin, referral to a neurologist or specialized pain clinic (to exclude underlying neurologic disorder; see Chapter 4), acupuncture, or biofeedback.

For further information see Ch. 73. From *Dermatology, Third Edition.*

61 | Bacterial Diseases

Skin infection with bacteria may be a primary problem (e.g. impetigo) or a complication of another skin disease (e.g. atopic dermatitis). Nomenclature of these diseases often reflects the site and the depth of infection – that is, from the stratum corneum to the subcutaneous tissue (Fig. 61.1) – as well as the suspected causative organism.

Gram-Positive Cocci

Staphylococcal and Streptococcal Skin Infections

Streptococcal infections may be complicated by acute post-streptococcal glomerulonephritis; this occurs in <1% of patients in high-income countries, but it remains a significant problem in low-income countries.

IMPETIGO

• Major organisms are *Staphylococcus aureus* and *Streptococcus pyogenes* (group A streptococci [GAS]).
• A very common, highly contagious bacterial infection, most commonly seen on the face or extremities of children; usually the skin is eroded with overlying 'honey-colored' crusts, but there is a bullous variant (Fig. 61.2).
• Interestingly, bullae formation due to *S. aureus* can be explained by local release of an exfoliative toxin that binds to desmoglein 1 and leads to dissolution (i.e. acantholysis) of the upper epidermis (see Chapter 23).
• Risk factors for infection: nasal carriage of *S. aureus* and breaks in the epidermal barrier, e.g. atopic dermatitis, arthropod bites, trauma, scabies.
• **DDx** of eroded lesions: insect bites, prurigo simplex, dermatitis (e.g. atopic, nummular), herpes simplex viral infection.
• **DDx** of bullae: bullous insect bites, thermal burns, herpes simplex viral infection,

and occasionally autoimmune bullous dermatoses.
• **Rx:** local wound care (including soap), removal of crusts by soaking; for mild cases, topical mupirocin or retapamulin; for moderate to severe infections, oral antibiotics, the choice of which is dependent on prevalence of methicillin-resistant *S. aureus* (MRSA) in the local community (Table 61.1).

ECTHYMA

• Most commonly secondary to *Streptococcus pyogenes*.
• Ulceration with hemorrhagic crust that extends into the superficial dermis, i.e. is deeper than impetigo (Fig. 61.3); can heal with scarring.
• Often on the lower extremities, and risk factors include an edematous limb, arthropod bites, and a pre-existing ulceration.
• **Rx:** see Table 61.1.

BACTERIAL FOLLICULITIS

• *Staphylococcus aureus* is the most common cause, followed by gram-negative bacteria; the latter can occur in patients with acne vulgaris on long-term antibiotic therapy; see Chapter 31 for *Pseudomonas* folliculitis.
• Usually superficial, but occasionally deep, infection centered on hair follicles (see Fig. 61.1).
  – Superficial – 1- to 4-mm pustules on an erythematous base (see Fig. 31.2); centrally, a hair shaft may be noted.
  – Deep – also referred to as sycosis – tender, erythematous papulonodules, often with a central pustule.
• Commonly in the beard area, on the upper trunk, or on the buttocks and thighs; shaving can be an exacerbating factor.
• **DDx:** culture-negative (normal flora) folliculitis, acne vulgaris, folliculitis due to fungi

CATEGORIZATION OF BACTERIAL INFECTIONS BY DEPTH AND EXTENT OF SKIN INVOLVEMENT

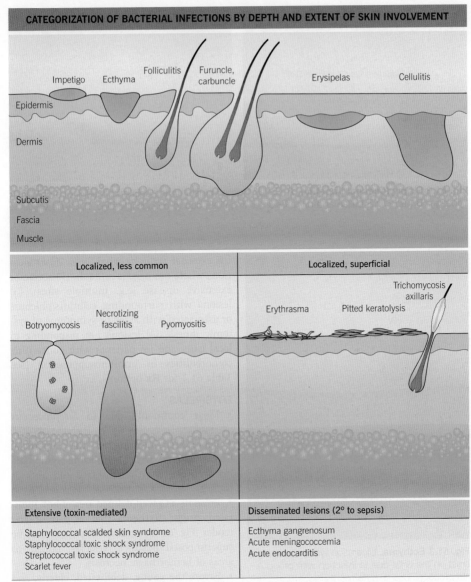

Fig. 61.1 Categorization of bacterial infections by depth and extent of skin involvement. More common, localized infections are depicted first; these infections are often secondary to *Staphylococcus aureus* or group A streptococci. *Adapted from 'Common bacterial infections of the skin,' American Academy of Dermatology.*

(e.g. *Pityrosporum*) or viruses (e.g. herpes simplex virus), rosacea, and pseudofolliculitis barbae (see Chapter 31).

• **Rx:** for superficial form – antibacterial washes (e.g. benzoyl peroxide, chlorhexidine) or topical gels (e.g. combination clindamycin/ benzoyl peroxide); widespread staphylococcal folliculitis – oral antibiotics (see Table 61.1).

ABSCESSES, FURUNCLES, AND CARBUNCLES

• By definition, a furuncle involves a hair follicle; involvement of multiple, adjacent follicles is termed a carbuncle (see Fig. 61.1).

• Most common organism is *S. aureus*, and this is the most frequent presentation for community-acquired MRSA (CA-MRSA).

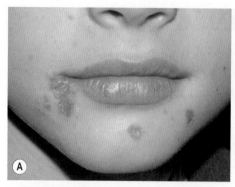
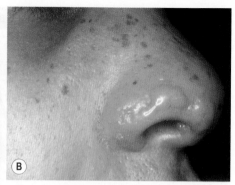

Fig. 61.2 Staphylococcal impetigo. A Honey-colored crusts on the chin and cheeks of a child with impetigo. **B** Superficial bullae and dry erosion on the nose due to bullous impetigo. *A, Courtesy, Julie V. Schaffer, MD.*

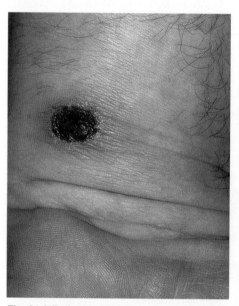

Fig. 61.3 Ecthyma. Ulceration with hemorrhagic crust on the wrist due to infection with group A streptococci. *Courtesy, Kalman Watsky, MD.*

• Clinically, furuncles appear as firm, tender, red nodules; carbuncles begin similarly but become larger in size and can develop multiple draining sinus tracts.

• Common locations are the face, neck, axillae, buttocks, perineum, and thighs.

• **DDx:** ruptured epidermoid inclusion cyst, hidradenitis suppurativa, and cystic acne.

• **Rx:** fluctuant lesions should be incised and drained; systemic antibiotics are generally reserved for: (1) furuncles around the nose, in

the external auditory canal, or in other locations where drainage is difficult; (2) severe or extensive disease (e.g. multiple sites); (3) lesions with surrounding cellulitis/phlebitis or associated with signs or symptoms of systemic illness; (4) lesions not responding to local care; and (5) patients with concerning comorbidities or immunosuppression (see Table 61.1 for **Rx** options).

ERYSIPELAS

• Most commonly due to *Streptococcus pyogenes*.

• Represents infection of the superficial dermis along with significant lymphatic involvement; often on the face and neck or the leg.

• Presents as a well-defined area of hot, indurated, bright erythema that is painful and tender (Fig. 61.4); occasionally, there may be superimposed pustules, vesicles, bullae, or areas of hemorrhagic necrosis.

• Favors the young, debilitated, elderly, and limbs with edema or lymphedema.

• **DDx:** cellulitis, erysipeloid breast cancer, irritant contact dermatitis, early necrotizing fasciitis or herpes zoster, erysipeloid, Sweet's syndrome, and if it involves the ear, chondritis.

• **Rx:** 10- to 14-day course of penicillin if due to *Streptococcus pyogenes*, with route depending on the severity and risk factors.

STREPTOCOCCAL INTERTRIGO/ PERIANAL DISEASE

• Presents as patches of erythema, especially in children (see Fig. 61.4 and Table 60.5).

EMPIRIC TREATMENT OF CUTANEOUS STAPHYLOCOCCAL AND STREPTOCOCCAL INFECTIONS IN ADULTS	
Organism/Situation	**Suggested Antibiotics**
Streptococci	• Dicloxacillin 500 mg PO four times a day • Nafcillin or oxacillin 1–2 g IV four times a day, if severe
Suspected MSSA	• First-generation cephalosporin, e.g. cephalexin 250–500 mg PO three or four times a day • Dicloxacillin 250–500 mg PO four times a day
Suspected CA-MRSA • Risk factors include participation in contact sports, contact with a person with HA-MRSA	• Doxycycline 100 mg PO two times a day* • Trimethoprim-sulfamethoxazole 1 or 2 double-strength tablets PO twice a day* • Clindamycin 300–450 mg PO four times a day
Suspected hospital-acquired MRSA (HA-MRSA) • Risk factors include recent contact with hospitals or health care facilities such as nursing homes or dialysis units	• See Suspected CA-MRSA
Penicillin-allergic patients	• Clindamycin (see above) • Clarithromycin 250 mg PO two times a day

Additional special considerations	• Furuncle/abscess: incision and drainage (without packing) is a key component of successful Rx
	• If recurrent infections, address carrier state:
	  – Mupirocin 2% nasal ointment twice a day for 5 days
	  – Mupirocin 2% cream to major body folds, e.g. axillae, groin, inframammary, as well as umbilicus
	  – Wash body with chlorhexidine, bathe in dilute Clorox® (Fig. 10.14A) once or twice a week, or use spray bottle with dilute Clorox®
	• Address fomites including sports equipment
	• Consider close human contacts or pets as source of infection

*Does not provide coverage of group A streptococci; if coverage of the latter is desired, a β-lactam is also prescribed.
MSSA, methicillin-sensitive Staphylococcus aureus.

Table 61.1 Empiric treatment of cutaneous staphylococcal and streptococcal infections in adults. Treatment duration is usually 7–10 days, depending on the severity and clinical response. Initial choice of antibiotic is dependent on known resistance patterns in a given community. The contents of pustules or exudate (e.g. underlying a crust) should be sent for culture and sensitivities prior to beginning therapy. Quinolones and macrolides are not optimal for treatment of community-acquired methicillin-resistant *Staphylococcus aureus* (CA-MRSA) because resistance is common and may develop rapidly.

- **DDx:** outlined in Fig. 13.4 and Table 60.5.
- **Rx:** 7- to 10-day course of a first-generation cephalosporin (see Table 61.1) or penicillin.

CELLULITIS

- Most commonly due to *Streptococcus pyogenes* or *S. aureus*; in diabetics and immunocompromised hosts, other organisms (e.g. gram-negative bacilli) may be the cause.
- In children, *Haemophilus influenzae* can be a cause of cellulitis, but its incidence has decreased since introduction of the *H. influenzae* vaccine.
- Infection of the deep dermis and sometimes the subcutaneous fat (see Fig. 61.1).

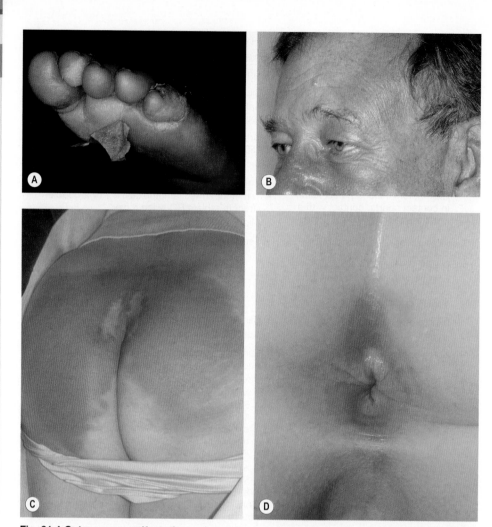

Fig. 61.4 Cutaneous manifestations of streptococcal infections. Prominent desquamation of the feet **(A)** following scarlet fever. Sharply demarcated erythema of the face, most obvious on the forehead **(B)**, and of the buttocks **(C)** in two patients with erysipelas. Bright red erythema extending from the anal verge in a young boy with streptococcal perianal disease **(D)**. *A, Courtesy, Eugene Mirrer, MD; B, Courtesy, Kalman Watsky, MD; C, Courtesy, Mary Stone, MD; D, Courtesy, Julie V. Schaffer, MD.*

• Skin rubor (redness), calor (warmth), dolor (pain), and tumor (swelling) are present; more ill-defined borders than erysipelas and may have skip areas; can become bullous or necrotic (Figs. 61.5 and 75.8).

• Systemic symptoms include fever, chills, and malaise; CBC usually shows leukocytosis and bandemia.

• Risk factors for cellulitis of the lower extremity include previous DVT, previous cellulitis with lymphangiitis, chronic edema, and tinea pedis (especially in patients who have undergone saphenous venectomy).

• **DDx:** on the lower extremity, lipodermatosclerosis and stasis dermatitis (see Fig. 11.5); elsewhere, erysipelas and the early stage of necrotizing fasciitis, as well as causes of pseudocellulitis (Table 61.2).

• **Rx:** see Table 61.1.

BLISTERING DISTAL DACTYLITIS

• Most commonly secondary to GAS or *S. aureus*.

• Localized infection of the volar fat pad of a finger or, less often, a toe; occurs most commonly in children.

- Initially erythema and swelling of the skin, followed by development of one or more vesicles or bullae.
- **Rx:** drainage of blisters and systemic antibiotics (see Table 61.1).

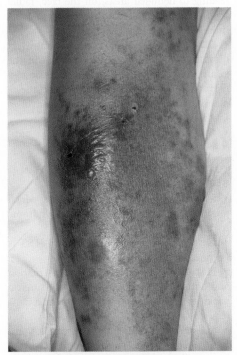

Fig. 61.5 Bullous cellulitis. Extensive soft tissue infection of the lower extremity due to group A streptococcal infection.

BOTRYOMYCOSIS

- Most commonly caused by *S. aureus*, followed by *Pseudomonas* spp.
- Cutaneous and subcutaneous nodules that may have superimposed pustules, purulent discharge, or become ulcerative or verrucous; often in immunosuppressed hosts.
- Grains, representing macroscopic colonies of bacteria, are seen in biopsy specimens as well as the pustular discharge; grains are also seen in eumycotic and actinomycotic mycetoma (see Chapter 64) and actinomycosis (see below).
- Often develops at sites of trauma.
- **DDx:** ruptured epidermoid cyst, abscess, mycetoma, actinomycosis, and atypical mycobacterial or dimorphic fungal infection.

NECROTIZING FASCIITIS

- Usually represents polymicrobial infection with both anaerobes and aerobes; ~10% secondary to GAS.
- Rapidly progressive necrosis of subcutaneous fat and fascia that leads to undermining and ulceration; may have a foul discharge.
- Risk factors include older age, diabetes mellitus, alcoholism, peripheral vascular disease, and immunosuppression.
- Initially may resemble cellulitis, but associated pain is often out of proportion to the clinical findings; additional clues include tense edema and a violaceous or gray color

CAUSES OF 'PSEUDOCELLULITIS'	
Infections and bites • Arthropod bite reactions (e.g. insect, spider) • Erythema migrans • Herpes zoster • Toxin-mediated erythema (e.g. recurrent toxin-mediated perineal erythema) Neutrophilic dermatoses • Sweet's syndrome, neutrophilic panniculitis • Familial Mediterranean fever, other periodic fever syndromes Drug reactions • Fixed drug eruptions (especially nonpigmenting) • Vaccine/injection site reactions • Toxic erythema of chemotherapy (e.g. due to gemcitabine)	Other inflammatory disorders • Allergic contact dermatitis (including airborne and dermal) • Phytophotodermatitis • Well's syndrome • Panniculitis, e.g. lipodermatosclerosis, erythema nodosum • Thrombophlebitis • Angioedema • Interstitial granulomatous dermatitis, inflammatory granuloma annulare • Inflammatory morphea Metabolic disorders • Gout Malignancy • Erysipeloid skin metastases (especially breast carcinoma)

Table 61.2 Causes of 'pseudocellulitis'.

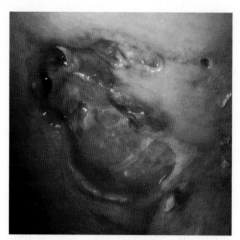

Fig. 61.6 Necrotizing fasciitis. Necrosis of the subcutaneous fat and fascia of the inner aspect of the upper arm in an elderly patient with diabetes mellitus. Note the watery discharge. *Courtesy, Jean L. Bolognia, MD.*

reflecting impending necrosis (Figs. 61.6 and 75.9).

• Diagnosis requires a high index of suspicion; when anogenital, it is referred to as Fournier's gangrene.

• Patients may have fever, chills, malaise, and leukocytosis.

• Dx: outlined in Fig. 61.7.

• **Rx:** surgical debridement is the mainstay of therapy; broad-spectrum IV antibiotics.

PYOMYOSITIS

• Primary bacterial infection of skeletal muscle, most commonly with *S. aureus* (see Fig. 61.1); associated with immunosuppression, including HIV infection.

STAPHYLOCOCCAL SCALDED SKIN SYNDROME (SSSS)

• Secondary to *S. aureus*, phage group II strains, which produce exfoliative toxins that bind to desmoglein 1 and lead to dissolution (i.e. acantholysis) of the upper epidermis.

• More commonly seen in infants and children; occasionally, adults with chronic renal insufficiency can develop SSSS.

• Prodrome of malaise, fever, irritability, sore throat, and tender skin; purulent rhinorrhea or conjunctivitis may be present because the initial site of staphylococcal infection is usually extracutaneous.

• Tender erythema on the face and in intertriginous zones that generalizes to the remainder of the body over 1 or 2 days; due to the split in the upper epidermis, the skin becomes 'wrinkled' and then sloughs over 3–5 days, leading to denuded areas; on the face, radial fissures with scale-crust develop around the mouth and eyes (see Fig. 3.11).

• **DDx:** sunburn, drug reaction, Kawasaki disease (erythema often first appears in the groin), Stevens–Johnson syndrome/toxic epidermal necrolysis (SJS/TEN; usually affects older children and adults, has mucosal involvement, and nearly always drug-induced).

• **Rx:** hospitalization and IV anti-staphylococcal antibiotics (see Table 61.1).

TOXIC SHOCK SYNDROME (OTHER THAN STREPTOCOCCAL) (TSS)

• Secondary to *Staphylococcus aureus*, which produces an exotoxin, toxic shock syndrome toxin-1.

• Case definition of staphylococcal TSS is outlined in Table 61.3.

• Historically associated with menstruation and tampon use, but nowadays with surgical packing, meshes, and cutaneous infections (e.g. abscesses).

• Sudden onset of high fever, myalgias, vomiting, diarrhea, headache, and pharyngitis; hypotension is a key finding.

• Clinically, scarlatiniform changes initially appear on the trunk and then spread centrifugally; erythema and edema of the palms and soles can be followed by desquamation 1–3 weeks later.

• Mucous membrane findings: erythema, strawberry tongue, hyperemia of the conjunctivae (Fig. 61.8).

• **DDx:** streptococcal TSS, drug reaction plus hypotension from sepsis; in children, Kawasaki disease and scarlet fever.

• **Rx:** hospitalization and IV antibiotics (see Table 61.1).

STREPTOCOCCAL TOXIC SHOCK SYNDROME (STREPTOCOCCAL TSS)

• Secondary to GAS (especially M types 1 and 3), which produce exotoxins A and/or B.

• Case definition of streptococcal TSS is outlined in Table 61.3.

• Most common site of the associated streptococcal infection is the skin, e.g. cellulitis or necrotizing fasciitis.

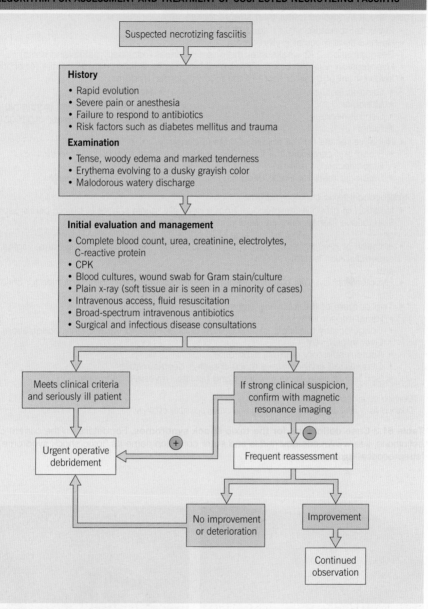

Fig. 61.7 Algorithm for assessment and treatment of suspected necrotizing fasciitis.

- **Rx:** hospitalization and IV antibiotics (see Table 61.1).

SCARLET FEVER

- Secondary to GAS, which produce erythrogenic toxins types A, B, and C.
- Seen in children (ages 1–10 years), usually following streptococcal tonsillitis or pharyngitis.

- Sore throat, headache, malaise, chills, anorexia, nausea, and high fevers precede erythema of the neck, chest, and axillae that becomes generalized over 4–6 hours.
- The erythema blanches with pressure and is studded with tiny papules ('sunburn with goose pimples'); the cheeks are also flushed with circumoral pallor.

CASE DEFINITIONS FOR THE TOXIC SHOCK SYNDROMES

Toxic shock syndrome (other than streptococcal)
- Fever: temperature >102°F (or >38.9°C)
- Rash: diffuse macular erythroderma
- Desquamation: 1–2 weeks after the onset of illness (especially palms and soles)
- Hypotension: systolic blood pressure <90 mmHg for adults (<5th percentile for children)
- Involvement of three or more of the following organ systems:
  - Gastrointestinal
  - Muscular
  - Central nervous
  - Renal
  - Hepatic
  - Mucous membranes (erythema)
  - Hematologic (platelets <100 000/mm^3)
- Negative results for the following tests (if done):
  - Blood and cerebrospinal fluid cultures (blood culture may be positive for *Staphylococcus aureus*)
  - Serologic tests for Rocky Mountain spotted fever, leptospirosis, measles

Streptococcal toxic shock syndrome
- Isolation of group A streptococci from a normally sterile site* (e.g. blood, cerebrospinal fluid, tissue biopsy, surgical wound)
  or
- Isolation of group A streptococci from a nonsterile site† (e.g. throat, sputum, vagina, superficial skin lesion)
  and
- Hypotension: systolic blood pressure <90 mmHg for adults (<5th percentile for children)
  and
- Two or more of the following signs:
  - Renal impairment
  - Coagulopathy (platelets ≤100 000/mm^3 or disseminated intravascular coagulation)
  - Liver impairment
  - Acute respiratory distress syndrome
  - Generalized erythematous macular rash ± desquamation
  - Soft tissue necrosis (e.g. necrotizing fasciitis, myositis, gangrene)

Defined as a definite case.
†*Defined as a probable case, excluding any other possible etiology.*

Table 61.3 Case definitions for the toxic shock syndromes. For details on the current case definitions, see www.cdc.gov/nndss and enter condition name as 'toxic shock syndrome' or 'streptococcal toxic shock syndrome'.

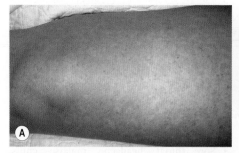
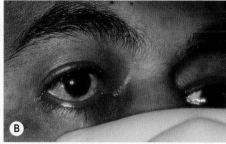

Fig. 61.8 Toxic shock syndrome due to *Staphylococcus aureus* infection. A Blotchy erythema is evident on the thigh. **B** Hyperemia of the conjunctiva is seen.

- Pastia lines (linear petechial streaks) are seen in major body folds, e.g. axillary, inguinal, antecubital.
- Desquamation of distal digits occurs after 7–10 days.
- Postinfectious sequelae include acute glomerulonephritis and rheumatic fever.
- **DDx** of palmoplantar desquamation: Kawasaki disease, TSS, and any preceding infection (including viral) with a high fever.
- **DDx** of exanthem: drug eruption, viral exanthem, early SSSS; a scarlatiniform eruption is also seen in TSS and Kawasaki disease.
- **Rx:** 10- to 14-day course of penicillin or amoxicillin.

BACTEREMIA/SEPTICEMIA

- Septic emboli can present as petechiae and purpura that may develop central pustules or hemorrhagic bullae; subcutaneous abscesses can also be seen.
- Endocarditis can be acute or subacute and caused by organisms including *S. aureus* and *Streptococcus* spp., respectively; cutaneous signs of endocarditis include splinter hemorrhages (see Chapter 58), Osler nodes, and Janeway lesions (see Table 18.2).

Gram-Positive Bacilli

Clostridial Skin Infections

- *Clostridia* spp. are gram-positive bacilli that live on dead organic matter and can cause anaerobic cellulitis or myonecrosis (gas gangrene).
- Anaerobic cellulitis.
  - Risk factors: trauma, diabetes mellitus, peripheral vascular disease, and injection drug use.
  - Generally due to *Clostridium perfringens* > other anaerobic bacteria (e.g. *Bacteroides*); incubation period >3 days with a rapid course.
  - Minimal visible skin changes; signs include crepitus and a thin, dark graybrown, foul-smelling ('dirty dishwater') exudate; pain often absent or mild without symptoms of toxemia (e.g. tachycardia).
- Myonecrosis, in contrast to anaerobic cellulitis, has a shorter incubation period with a very rapid course; overlying skin has a dark yellow to bronze discoloration,

sometimes with bullae or necrosis, and severe swelling; toxemia (e.g. hypotension) is generally present.
- **Rx:** early surgical debridement and empirical antibiotics (e.g. clindamycin plus a third-generation cephalosporin) until culture and sensitivities obtained.

Corynebacterium (And Kytococcus) Skin Infections

ERYTHRASMA

- Superficial, localized infection due to *Corynebacterium minutissimum*.
- Three major clinical variants.
  - Interdigital – the most common variant, characterized by chronic maceration with fissuring or scaling; needs to be distinguished from interdigital tinea pedis.
  - Intertriginous – thin red-brown plaques in the axillae and groin/upper inner thigh that may be misdiagnosed as tinea cruris (see Table 60.5; Fig. 61.9).
  - 'Disciform' – often on the trunk and diabetes mellitus is a risk factor (Fig. 61.7D).
- Bright, coral-red fluorescence with Wood's lamp examination (see Figs. 61.9B and 13.2).
- **Rx:** topical clindamycin or erythromycin; prevent moisture accumulation with topical aluminum chloride 6–20% (axillae).

PITTED KERATOLYSIS

- Secondary to *Kytococcus sedentarius* (*Micrococcus sedentarius*) and *Corynebacterium* spp.
- Hyperhidrosis, prolonged occlusion, and increased surface pH are contributing factors; the latter plus bacterial infection lead to 1- to 3-mm crater-like depressions in the stratum corneum that may coalesce, with involvement of soles >> palms (Fig. 61.10).
- Often accompanied by a distinctive malodor.
- **Rx:** topical clindamycin or erythromycin; decrease eccrine sweat production with topical aluminum chloride 20%.

TRICHOMYCOSIS AXILLARIS

- Common disorder that may be clinically subtle; often accompanied by malodor.
- Hair shafts are ensheathed with adherent yellow > red or black concretions composed

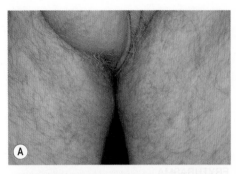
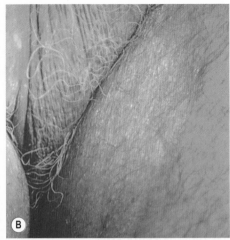
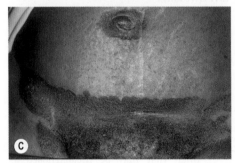
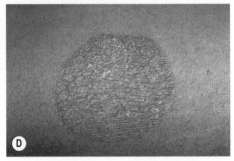

Fig. 61.9 Erythrasma. A Pink to brown scaly patches on the upper inner thighs. **B** Coral-red fluorescence upon illumination with a Wood's lamp. **C** Hyperpigmented plaques in the inguinal and periumbilical areas (intertriginous zones). **D** Well-demarcated, scaly, hyperpigmented plaque of disciform erythrasma. *A, B, Courtesy, Louis A. Fragola, MD.*

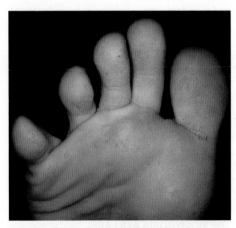

Fig. 61.10 Pitted keratolysis of the plantar surface of the foot. Multiple small craters with decreased stratum corneum that favor pressure points on the plantar surface. *Courtesy, Kalman Watsky, MD.*

of organisms (Fig. 61.11); most common in the axillae and a cause of chromhidrosis (see Chapter 32).

- **DDx:** other causes of nodules on hair shafts (see Fig. 64.3).
- **Rx:** shaving of hair; topical antimicrobials (e.g. benzoyl peroxide, erythromycin) can help prevent recurrence.

Other Gram-Positive Skin Infections
ANTHRAX

- *Bacillus anthracis* causes inhalational, gastrointestinal, and cutaneous disease.
- Occurs most commonly in farmers and ranchers exposed to animals such as sheep, cows, horses, and goats; also secondary to exposure to hides from these animals (e.g. skins used for drums).

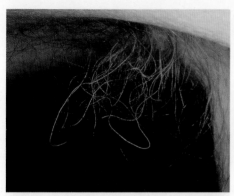

Fig. 61.11 Trichomycosis axillaris. Cylindrical sheaths and beading of the axillary hairs. A yellow color is seen most commonly.

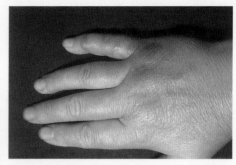

Fig. 61.12 Erysipeloid. Erythema and edema with vesicle formation on the hand and fifth digit.

ERYSIPELOID

• Due to *Erysipelothrix rhusiopathiae*.
• Variants.
  – Localized cellulitis – infection due to traumatic inoculation; seen in individuals who prepare fish and meat; the hand is a frequent site of involvement and the color is characteristically red-violet (Fig. 61.12).
  – Generalized – uncommon form; multiple pink plaques, usually in the setting of immunosuppression, with associated fever and arthralgias; blood cultures are generally negative.
• **DDx** of localized form: cellulitis due to more common infectious agents (see above), atypical mycobacterial infection, early *Vibrio* infection.
• **Rx** for localized form: penicillin 500 mg PO four times a day for 7–10 days.

Gram-Negative Cocci

ACUTE MENINGOCOCCEMIA

• Systemic infection due to *Neisseria meningitides*.
• Primarily seen in young children (6 months to 1 year of age) and young adults in close quarters (e.g. dormitories, barracks).
• In most individuals, infection results in an asymptomatic carrier state.
• In acute meningococcemia, one-third to one-half of patients have skin lesions due to septic emboli, initially subtle petechiae that evolve into irregularly shaped purpura with a central gunmetal gray color that reflects necrosis (Fig. 61.13); gram-negative cocci may be seen on Gram staining of lesional tissue.

CUTANEOUS ANTHRAX – CLINICAL CHARACTERISTICS

• Incubation period averages 7 days (range 1–12 days)
• A purpuric macule or papule develops in an exposed area (e.g. forearm, neck, chest, finger); the papule may resemble an insect bite and can be pruritic
• Within 48 hours of the lesion's appearance, a vesicle (1–3 mm) forms with surrounding nonpitting edema
• The central vesicle ulcerates and small vesicles may form around the ulcer
• The lesion becomes hemorrhagic and depressed, and a *painless*, black, necrotic eschar forms centrally with an increase in the surrounding erythema and edema
• The eschar dries, loosens, and sloughs over the next 1–2 weeks, with no permanent scar

Table 61.4 Cutaneous anthrax – clinical characteristics. *Adapted from Carucci JA, McGovern TW, Norton SA, et al. Cutaneous anthrax management algorithm. J. Am. Acad. Dermatol. 2002;47:766–769.*

• Emerged as an agent of biological terrorism.
• Clinical characteristics of cutaneous disease are outlined in Table 61.4.
• **Rx** for cutaneous disease: fluoroquinolone (e.g. ciprofloxacin 500 mg PO twice daily) for 60 days.

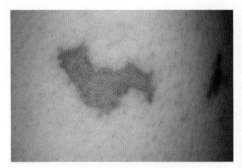

Fig. 61.13 Acute meningococcemia. Purpura with irregular outline and central gunmetal gray color. *Courtesy, Kalman Watsky, MD.*

• The septic lesions are to be distinguished from those due to disseminated intravascular coagulation (see Table 18.1).

• Additional systemic manifestations include fever, chills, hypotension, meningoencephalitis, pneumonia, pericarditis, and myocarditis.

• **Rx:** IV penicillin or ceftriaxone; vaccination is important for prevention.

CHRONIC MENINGOCOCCEMIA

• An indolent infection due to *Neisseria meningitides*.

• Recurrent episodes of fever, chills, night sweats, and arthralgias; skin lesions are polymorphous, e.g. pink macules and papules, nodules, petechiae/purpura; the skin lesions represent small vessel vasculitis without visible organisms by light microscopy, but PCR may be used to detect organisms.

GONORRHEA & DISSEMINATED GONOCOCCAL INFECTION
See Chapter 69.

Gram-Negative Bacilli

Pseudomonal Infections

Green nail syndrome is discussed in Chapter 58.

GRAM-NEGATIVE TOE-WEB INFECTION

• Although *Pseudomonas aeruginosa* is the most common cause, other gram-negative bacilli can be implicated (e.g. *Escherichia coli*, *Proteus mirabilis*).

• Risk factors are pre-existing tinea pedis and occlusion (e.g. tight-fitting shoes).

• Symptoms of burning and pain; signs include a malodorous exudate with a

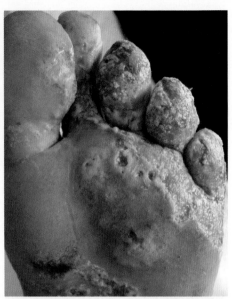

Fig. 61.14 Severe superficial infection of the skin with *Pseudomonas.* Note the macerated border, the erosions, and the moth-eaten appearance of the skin. *Courtesy, Kalman Watsky, MD.*

blue-green tinge, a grape-juice odor, and a moth-eaten appearance of skin due to maceration and erosions (Fig. 61.14).

• In severe cases, there can be cellulitis.

OTITIS EXTERNA ('SWIMMER'S EAR')

• Swollen auditory ear canal with greenish purulent discharge.

• Extreme pain with manipulation of the pinna.

• **Rx:** antimicrobial drops (e.g. ofloxacin) with or without an ear wick, oral analgesics (e.g. NSAIDs).

PSEUDOMONAL FOLLICULITIS (HOT TUB FOLLICULITIS)
See Table 31.2.

PSEUDOMONAS HOT-FOOT SYNDROME

• Develops acutely on the soles of children and adolescents who are otherwise healthy after swimming in water with high concentrations of *Pseudomonas aeruginosa*.

• Painful and tender, red-purple, 1- or 2-cm nodules appear on the weight-bearing aspects of the feet (Fig. 61.15).

• Self-limiting and **DDx** is primarily idiopathic palmoplantar hidradenitis (Chapter 32).

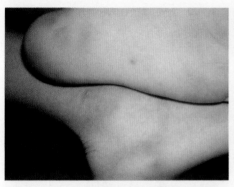

Fig. 61.15 Pseudomonas hot-foot syndrome. Tender erythematous nodules on the heel. *Courtesy, Justin J. Green, MD.*

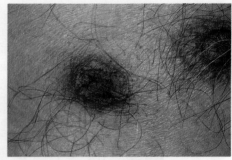

Fig. 61.16 Ecthyma gangrenosum. Embolic lesion of *Pseudomonas aeruginosa* on the chest. Note the necrotic center and inflammatory border.

CELLULITIS

• Clinical features are similar to those of cellulitis due to *S. aureus* (see above); can occur on the lower extremity in the setting of gram-negative toe-web infection or on the external ear postoperatively.

• Sometimes, it can be difficult to distinguish soft tissue infection from colonization with *Pseudomonas*, particularly in chronic ulcers.

ECTHYMA GANGRENOSUM

• A sign of bacteremia or septicemia.

• Most commonly due to gram-negative bacilli, including *Pseudomonas*, but can also be due to opportunistic fungi; primarily seen in immunocompromised hosts, especially those with prolonged neutropenia.

• A red-purple macule or patch that develops central necrosis; sometimes the necrosis is preceded by a hemorrhagic bulla; the number can vary from one to a dozen or more (Fig. 61.16).

• The most common location for ecthyma gangrenosum due to *Pseudomonas* is the groin.

• To establish the diagnosis, culture of tissue, obtained via sterile biopsy technique (see Fig. 2.10), is performed in combination with histopathology.

TREATMENT OF PSEUDOMONAL INFECTIONS

• For superficial infection (e.g. gram-negative toe-web infection): 5% acetic acid soaks followed by application of a topical antibiotic (e.g.

gentamicin, silver sulfadiazine); if minimal improvement or severe, oral fluoroquinolone.

• For severe or systemic infections: piperacillin/tazobactam or doripenem if penicillin-allergic; may be combined with an aminoglycoside antibiotic.

Diseases Caused by *Bartonella* Species

See Table 61.5.

Other Gram-Negative Skin Infections with Fever and Skin Findings

See Table 61.6.

Spirochetes

LYME DISEASE

See Chapter 15.

SYPHILIS

See Chapter 69.

OTHER TREPONEMAL DISEASES

• Like syphilis, other treponemal diseases may have primary, secondary, and tertiary stages.

• Endemic syphilis.

  – Due to *Treponema pallidum endemicum*.

  – Seen most commonly in Africa, the Arabian peninsula, and Southeast Asia.

  – Children younger than the age of 15 years are most often affected.

  – Primary lesion often missed.

  – Secondary stage: macerated patches on lips, tongue, and pharynx; angular

MAJOR HUMAN DISEASES CAUSED BY *BARTONELLA* SPECIES

Species	Disease	Vector	Epidemiology	Clinical Features
B. henselae	Cat-scratch disease	Cat flea (*Ctenocephalides felis*)*	Young people, <18 years of age	• Lymphadenopathy • Systemic symptoms (e.g. fever, malaise)
	Bacillary angiomatosis		Immunocompromised patients	• Bright red papules that can resemble pyogenic granulomas; lichenoid papules/plaques; subcutaneous nodules • Hepatic involvement (peliosis)
B. bacilliformis	Bartonellosis (Carrion disease, Oroya fever, verruga peruana)	Sand fly (*Lutzomyia verrucarum*)	Peru, Ecuador, and southwestern Colombia	• Oroya fever – fever, hemolytic anemia, secondary bacterial infections, e.g. *Salmonella* • Verruga peruana – erythematous patches with overlying bright red papules and nodules
B. quintana	Trench fever/'urban' trench fever	Human body louse (*Pediculus humanus corporis*)	Originally seen in World War I troops; today, associated with homelessness and poor hygiene	Relapsing fever
	Bacillary angiomatosis		See above	See above

Table 61.5 Major human diseases caused by *Bartonella* species. *More commonly by a cat scratch or bite.

SELECTED GRAM-NEGATIVE INFECTIONS THAT PRESENT WITH NONSPECIFIC SYSTEMIC SYMPTOMS (E.G. FEVER) AND SKIN FINDINGS

Infection	Common Organism(s)	Transmission/Other Factors	Unique/Characteristic Findings	Skin Findings
Infection with Vibrio vulnificus	Vibrio vulnificus	Raw seafood or exposure of cutaneous wounds to infected sea water, primarily in warmer climates; patients at risk are middle-aged men with chronic liver disease or diabetes		Hemorrhagic bullae with cellulitis
Tularemia	Francisella tularensis	Infected rabbits; deerfly or tick (e.g. Amblyomma americanum) as vector	May show sporotrichoid pattern	Ulcers, lymphadenopathy
Glanders	Burkholderia mallei	Direct contact with infected animals (horses, mules, donkeys)	Sporotrichoid (lymphocutaneous) pattern	Nodule, pustule, or vesicle surrounded by erythema
Plague	Yersinia pestis	Contaminated food, water, or raw milk; fleas can be the vector	Bubonic form can have a sporotrichoid pattern	• Bubonic form due to inoculation: wound becomes a pustule or ulcer with painful regional lymphadenopathy • Septicemic form: emboli present as vesicles, carbuncles, petechiae, or purpura
Melioidosis	Burkholderia pseudomallei	Contact with contaminated soil or water; ingestion or inhalation; sexual intercourse; fleas can be the vector		Abscesses, granulomatous lesions, purpura, pustules, urticaria, ecthyma gangrenosum

Table 61.6 Selected gram-negative infections that present with nonspecific systemic symptoms (e.g. fever) and skin findings. *Continued*

BACTERIAL DISEASES

Table 61.6 *Continued* **Selected gram-negative infections that present with nonspecific systemic symptoms (e.g. fever) and skin findings.**

Infection	Common Organism(s)	Transmission/Other Factors	Unique/Characteristic Findings	Skin Findings
Rat-bite fever (Haverhill fever)	*Streptobacillus moniliformis*	Close contact with infected rodents or contaminated food, water, or raw milk (Haverhill fever)	Migratory polyarthritis in 50% of patients that mimics rheumatoid arthritis	Acral palmoplantar eruption of macules, papules, petechiae, vesicles, pustules, with secondary crusts
Brucellosis	*Brucella abortus*	Consumption of unpasteurized milk products	Malodorous perspiration	• Erythema nodosum • Vasculitis
Typhoid fever	*Salmonella typhi*	Contact with infected persons	Rose spots	• Rose spots – 2–8 mm pink, blanching papules, often in clusters of 5–15 on the anterior trunk • Erythema multiforme, Sweet's syndrome, hemorrhagic bullae, pustules
Malacoplakia (malakoplakia)	*Escherichia coli* (less commonly *Pseudomonas* or other bacteria)	Immunocompromised hosts	Michaelis–Gutmann bodies: intracytoplasmic concretions within large histiocytes	Most commonly perianal abscesses or ulcers
Rhinoscleroma	*Klebsiella rhinoscleromatis*	Endemic to Central Europe, India, Egypt, other countries (e.g. Indonesia)	Intracellular bacteria within large histiocytes (Mikulicz cells)	Rhinitis that progresses to granulomatous nodules and scarring of nose and upper respiratory tract

stomatitis; condyloma lata; generalized lymphadenopathy.
– Tertiary stage: gummas that can lead to destruction of the palate and nasal septum.
• Pinta.
– Due to *T. carateum*.
– Seen primarily in Central and South America.
– Primary stage: minute macules or papules with erythematous haloes, most commonly on the lower extremities, that develop into infiltrated plaques over several months.
– Secondary stage: smaller, variably pigmented (red, blue, black, or hypopigmented), scaly macules and papules that may coalesce; clustered near the initial primary lesion or generalized.
– Tertiary stage: symmetric, depigmented, vitiligo-like lesions that are atrophic or keratotic.
• Yaws.
– Due to *T. pallidum pertenue*.
– Seen in warm, humid, tropical climates.
– Children younger than the age of 15 years are most often affected.
– Primary: erythematous, infiltrated, painful papule, usually on the extremities; enlarges to become up to 5 cm in diameter and ulcerates; heals spontaneously over 3–6 months.
– Secondary: smaller lesions adjacent to orifices or adjacent to site of initial primary lesion (Fig. 61.17).
– Tertiary: destructive skin lesions, palmoplantar thickening that can lead to difficulty with ambulation, chronic osteitis (sabre tibia).

Filamentous Bacteria
ACTINOMYCOSIS
• Most commonly due to *Actinomyces israelii*.

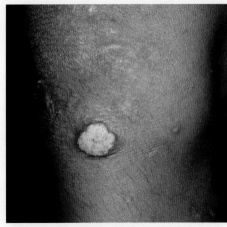

Fig. 61.17 Cutaneous yaws on the knee of an adolescent from Indonesia. *Courtesy, Peter Ehrnstrom, MD.*

• Three major sites of involvement – cervical, pulmonary, and gastrointestinal.
• Skin involvement is most common with the cervical variant and is sometimes referred to as 'lumpy jaw' due to irregular subcutaneous nodules; the latter can drain and the exudate contains grains (Fig. 61.18).
• **Rx:** penicillin.

ACTINOMYCOTIC MYCETOMA
• Most commonly due to *Nocardia* as well as *Actinomadura madurae*, *Actinomadura pelletieri*, and *Streptomyces somaliensis*; organisms are found in soil and on plant material (Table 61.7).
• **DDx:** distinguishing this entity from eumycotic mycetoma requires culture of grains or tissue; prior to the return of tissue or grain culture results, a presumptive diagnosis can be made based on the diameter of the filaments or hyphae composing the grains in biopsy specimens.

NOCARDIOSIS
See Table 61.7.

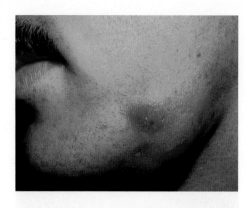

Fig. 61.18 Cervicofacial actinomycosis or 'lumpy jaw' with soft tissue swelling and draining ulcerated nodules. The discharge contained sulfur granules, a term used when the grains are yellow in color. *Courtesy, M. Joyce Rico, MD.*

FOUR MAJOR CLINICAL FORMS OF CUTANEOUS NOCARDIOSIS	
Primary	
Actinomycotic mycetoma	• Half of all cases of actinomycotic mycetoma are due to *Nocardia* species*
	• Traumatic inoculation causes a painless nodule that enlarges, suppurates, and drains via sinus tracts
	• Purulent discharge contains grains
	• The foot is the usual site of involvement
	• May involve underlying muscle and bone
Lymphocutaneous	• Occurs days to weeks after trauma
	• Appears as a persistent crusted pustule or abscess, often resistant to shorter courses of antibiotics
	• Ascending lymphatic streaks, a sporotrichoid pattern of papulonodules, and tender palpable lymph nodes may be seen
Superficial cutaneous	• Traumatic implantation of foreign objects (including soil and gravel) into the skin
	• The diagnosis is based on a high index of suspicion, lack of response to routine antibiotic treatment, and laboratory results
Secondary	
Pulmonary/systemic	• Subcutaneous abscesses of the chest wall
	• Pustules, nodules, cutaneous fistulae
	• Almost universally fatal if left untreated
	• Most commonly caused by *Nocardia asteroides*

In Mexico and Central and South America, N. brasiliensis is the etiologic agent of 90% of actinomycotic mycetomas, whereas in the United States, most mycetomas are caused by true fungi.

Table 61.7 Four major clinical forms of cutaneous nocardiosis. Rx: Sulfonamides are the drugs of choice for primary cutaneous nocardiosis, with minocycline being an alternative for sulfonamide-allergic patients. Duration of treatment is at least 6-12 weeks for localized disease in immunocompetent hosts. Surgical excision may be required for deep abscesses.

For further information see Ch. 74. From *Dermatology, Third Edition.*

Mycobacterial Diseases | 62

Key Points

- Mycobacteria are the etiologic agents of three major types of infection:
  - Leprosy – *Mycobacterium leprae*.
  - Tuberculosis – *Mycobacterium tuberculosis*.
  - Atypical or nontuberculous infections – e.g. *Mycobacterium marinum*, *Mycobacterium chelonae* (Tables 62.1 and 62.2).

Leprosy

- Slowly progressive disease characterized by granuloma formation in nerves and the skin.
- Affects all ages, but bimodal peak distribution – ages 10–15 years and 30–60 years.

- Currently, the highest incidence is in Brazil (Fig. 62.1).
- Spread of leprosy is dependent on: (1) a contagious person (predominantly through nasal/oral droplets); (2) a susceptible person; and (3) close/intimate contact.
- Incubation period averages 4–10 years.
- Degree of immunity is reflected in clinical findings (Table 62.3; Figs. 62.2 and 62.3) and histopathologic features; the latter range from macrophages containing numerous bacilli (globi) in lepromatous leprosy to granulomas without organisms in tuberculoid leprosy.
- Nerves are often affected, particularly ones close to the surface of the skin (Figs. 62.4 and 62.5); sensations of pain, temperature, and/or touch should be evaluated within skin lesions.
- Sequelae of leprosy can be disfiguring (Figs. 62.6 and 62.7).

MYCOBACTERIA THAT CAUSE CUTANEOUS DISEASE		
Group and Pigment	**Rate of Growth**	**Examples of Pathogens**
Slow growers		
Photochromogens*	2–3 weeks	*M. kansasii, M. marinum, M. simiae*
Scotochromogens†	2–3 weeks	*M. scrofulaceum, M. szulgai, M. gordonae, M. xenopi*
Nonchromogens‡	2–3 weeks	*M. tuberculosis, M. avium, M. intracellulare, M. ulcerans, M. haemophilum, M. bovis*§
Rapid growers	3–5 days	*M. fortuitum, M. chelonae, M. abscessus*
Noncultured (to date)		*M. leprae*

*Capable of yellow pigment formation upon exposure to light.
†Capable of yellow pigment production without light exposure.
‡Incapable of pigment production.
§Including bacillus Calmette–Guérin.

Table 62.1 Mycobacteria that cause cutaneous disease. *Modified classification of Runyon from Hautmann G, Lotti T. Atypical mycobacterial infections of the skin. Dermatol. Clin. 1994;12:657–668; Yates VM, Rook GAW. Mycobacterial infections. In: Burns T, Breathnach S, Cox N, Griffiths C (eds). Rook's Textbook of Dermatology, 7 edn. London: Blackwell Science, 2004;28.1–39; Neves RG, Pradinaud R. Micobacterioses atípicas. In: Neves RG, Talhari S (eds). Dermatologia Tropical. Rio de Janeiro: Medsi, 1995:283–290.*

IMPORTANT FEATURES OF ATYPICAL MYCOBACTERIA		
Mycobacteria	**Clinical Features**	**Clinical Setting**
M. marinum	• See text	Found in the environment
M. fortuitum, *M. chelonae,* *M. abscessus*	• Infected tattoos and post-pedicure lower extremity furuncles • Infected surgical sites	Can occur in immunocompetent hosts
M. ulcerans	• Often infects children • Can form large ulcers • May require surgical Rx as responds poorly to antibiotic therapy	
M. avium intracellulare *M. kansasii*	• Skin lesions rare	Found in the environment
M. scrofulaceum	• Classically causes lymphadenopathy	Often develops in immunocompromised hosts

Table 62.2 Important features of atypical mycobacteria. Disseminated skin lesions are an HIV-defining criterion, most commonly due to *M. avium intracellulare* or *M. kansasii*.

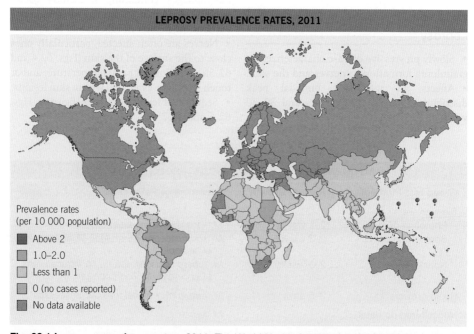

LEPROSY PREVALENCE RATES, 2011

Prevalence rates
(per 10 000 population)

■ Above 2
□ 1.0–2.0
□ Less than 1
□ 0 (no cases reported)
■ No data available

Fig. 62.1 Leprosy prevalence rates, 2011. The World Health Organization (WHO) has achieved its goal of a prevalence rate of less than 1 case per 10 000 persons in all but a few countries. *Reproduced from the World Health Organization, http://www.who.int/lep/situation/prevalence/en.*

CLASSIFICATION OF LEPROSY: RIDLEY–JOPLING AND OPERATIONAL

Operational	Multibacillary, >5 skin lesions		Paucibacillary, 1–5 skin lesions	
Ridley–Jopling*	Lepromatous leprosy (LL)	Borderline leprosy (BL)	Tuberculoid leprosy (TT)	Indeterminate (I)
Clinical findings				
Cellular immunity	Least (Th2 CD4$^+$ T-cell response)		Greatest (Th1 CD4$^+$ T-cell response)	
Type of lesions	Macules, papules, and plaques and sometimes diffuse infiltration of the skin	Macules, papules, and plaques with variable induration	Infiltrated thin plaques with raised edges, often hypopigmented	Macules, often hypopigmented
Distribution	Symmetric; favors face, buttocks, lower extremities	Tendency to symmetry	Localized, asymmetric	Variable
Definition	Vague, difficult to distinguish normal versus affected skin	Less well-defined borders	Well-defined, sharp borders	Not always defined
Sensation	Not affected	Diminished	Absent	Impaired
Bacilli in skin lesions				Usually none detected

*Disease states intermediate between LL and TT include borderline LL, mid-borderline leprosy, borderline TT, and indeterminate.

Table 62.3 Classification of leprosy: Ridley–Jopling and operational. *Adapted from A Guide to Leprosy Control, 2nd ed. Geneva: World Health Organization, 1988;27–28.*

MYCOBACTERIAL DISEASES

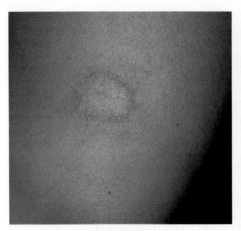

Fig. 62.2 Tuberculoid leprosy. Note the elevated border and central hypopigmentation. *Courtesy, Robert Hartman, MD.*

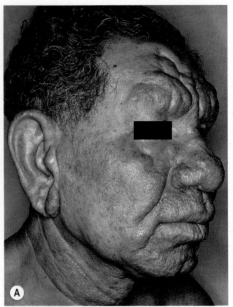

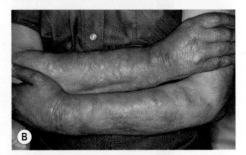

Fig. 62.3 Lepromatous leprosy. A Note the diffuse infiltration with leonine facies and madarosis. **B** Numerous nodules and thick plaques on the forearms. *A, B, Courtesy, Louis A. Fragola, Jr., MD.*

- Reactive states that can involve the skin may develop, especially following institution of antimicrobial treatment.
  - Type 1 (reversal reaction) – acute inflammation of cutaneous lesions (Fig. 62.8A) and nerves; appears rapidly due to a change in the immunologic state of the patient; in the case of upgrading, subclinical lesions can become clinically apparent.
  - Type 2 (vasculitis) – formation of immune complexes in the setting of an excessive humoral immune reaction, leading to the appearance of cutaneous lesions, particularly erythema nodosum leprosum (Fig. 62.8B).
- **DDx:** outlined in Table 62.4.
- **Rx** for adults: multibacillary leprosy – rifampin 600 mg PO once a month, dapsone 100 mg PO daily, and clofazimine 300 mg PO once a month plus 50 mg PO daily for 12 months; paucibacillary leprosy – rifampin 600 mg PO once a month and dapsone 100 mg PO daily for 6 months; single lesion – one-time dose of rifampin 600 mg, ofloxacin 400 mg, and minocycline 100 mg; prednisone for type 1 (reversal) reactions; thalidomide for type 2 reactions.

Cutaneous Tuberculosis (TB)

- Cutaneous lesions reflect mode of exposure and the degree of immunity.

- Exogenous exposure (inoculation).
  - Tuberculous chancre – seen in previously uninfected persons; 2–4 weeks after inoculation, a painless, firm, red-brown papulonodule appears that ulcerates centrally; generally heals within 3–12 months.
  - TB verrucosa cutis – secondary to inoculation in persons with moderate to high immunity to *M. tuberculosis*; asymptomatic, wart-like papule that gradually enlarges (Fig. 62.9); may heal spontaneously after several years.

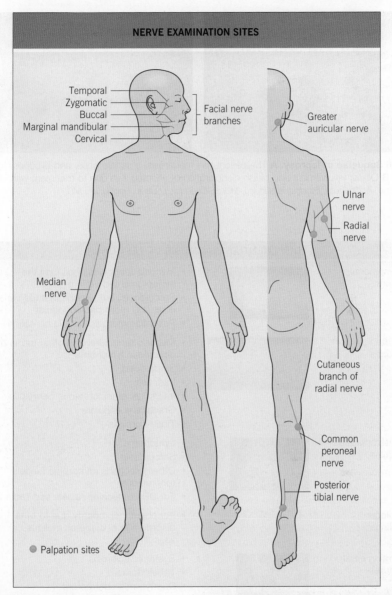

NERVE EXAMINATION SITES

Temporal
Zygomatic
Buccal
Marginal mandibular
Cervical

Facial nerve
branches

Greater
auricular nerve

Ulnar
nerve

Radial
nerve

Median
nerve

Cutaneous
branch of
radial nerve

Common
peroneal
nerve

Posterior
tibial nerve

● Palpation sites

Fig. 62.4 Nerve examination sites.

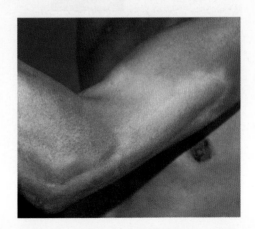

Fig. 62.5 Leprosy. Enlargement of the radial
nerve with a circumscribed area of
hypopigmentation. *Courtesy, Regional Dermatology
Training Centre, Moshi, Tanzania.*

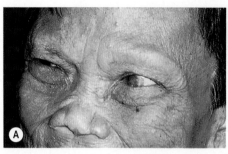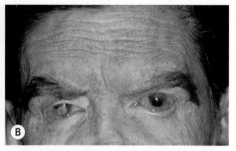

Fig. 62.6 Sequelae of leprosy. A The patient has madarosis, a saddle nose, and blindness in the left eye. **B** Ocular involvement and bluish discoloration of affected skin due to treatment with clofazimine. *A, Courtesy, Evangeline Handog, MD; B, Courtesy, Louis A. Fragola, Jr., MD.*

DIFFERENTIAL DIAGNOSIS OF LEPROSY		
Hypopigmented lesions		• Mycosis fungoides, including the hypopigmented variant • Sarcoidosis, but hypopigmented variant is usually more papulonodular • Postinflammatory hypopigmentation
Circinate (annular) plaques		• Mycosis fungoides and other forms of cutaneous lymphoma • Sarcoidosis • Psoriasis • Interstitial granulomatous dermatitis • Granuloma annulare • Tinea corporis
Infiltrated plaques/ nodules		• Lymphoma • Sarcoidosis • Other infections (dimorphic fungal, tuberculous) • For DDx of leonine facies, see Table 38.1
Neurologic findings		• Peripheral neuropathy due to other disorders (e.g. diabetes mellitus, vasculitis)
Deforming acral features		• Systemic sclerosis • Tabes dorsalis • Dupuytren's contracture
Type 1 reaction		• Acute lupus erythematosus • Cellulitis • Drug reactions • Misdiagnosed as worsening of disease as subclinical lesions may become apparent
Type 2 reaction		• Sweet's syndrome • Medium-vessel vasculitis • Panniculitides, e.g. erythema nodosum • Infections, including other mycobacterial, bacterial, dimorphic fungal, and other opportunistic fungal

Table 62.4 Differential diagnosis of leprosy.

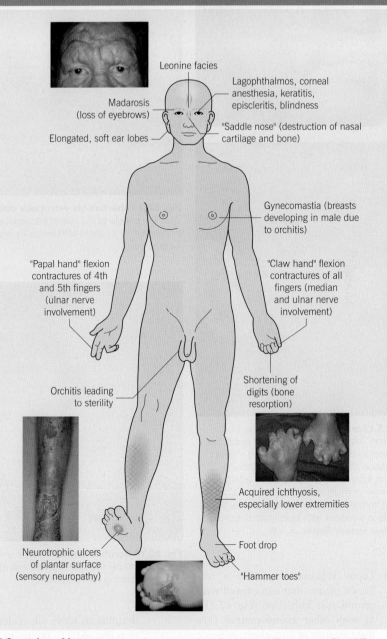

Leonine facies

Lagophthalmos, corneal
anesthesia, keratitis,
episcleritis, blindness

Madarosis
(loss of eyebrows)

"Saddle nose" (destruction of nasal
cartilage and bone)

Elongated, soft ear lobes

Gynecomastia (breasts
developing in male due
to orchitis)

"Papal hand" flexion
contractures of 4th
and 5th fingers
(ulnar nerve
involvement)

"Claw hand" flexion
contractures of all
fingers (median
and ulnar nerve
involvement)

Orchitis leading
to sterility

Shortening of
digits (bone
resorption)

Acquired ichthyosis,
especially lower extremities

Neurotrophic ulcers
of plantar surface
(sensory neuropathy)

Foot drop

"Hammer toes"

Fig. 62.7 Sequelae of leprosy. *Inserts, Courtesy, Louis A. Fragola, Jr., MD, and Joyce Rico, MD.*

- Endogenous spread of infection.
  - Some degree of cellular immunity (TST/PPD [tuberculin skin test] usually positive).
    • Scrofuloderma – firm, subcutaneous nodules that become fluctuant; may ulcerate or drain via sinus tracts that heal as tethered scars; represents spread of infection from underlying disease (e.g. in bones and lymph nodes, often cervical; Fig. 62.10).

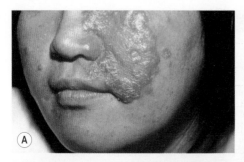

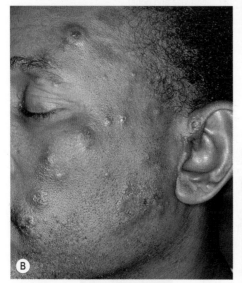

Fig. 62.8 Leprosy reactions. A Type 1 'upgrading' reaction in a patient with borderline lepromatous disease characterized by marked inflammation of a facial plaque. **B** Erythema nodosum leprosum (type 2 reaction) with the appearance of multiple red papulonodules as a result of immune complex-mediated small vessel vasculitis in a patient with lepromatous leprosy. *B, Courtesy, Louis A. Fragola, Jr., MD.*

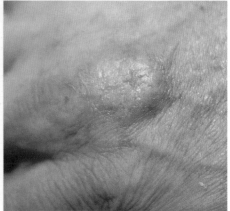

Fig. 62.9 Tuberculosis verrucosa cutis. A wart-like papule at the site of exogenous inoculation in a patient with immunity against *M. tuberculosis.*

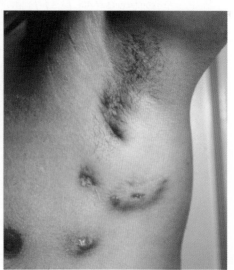

Fig. 62.10 Scrofuloderma. Plaques and nodules with central ulceration as well as resultant scarring with retraction.

- Lupus vulgaris – typically a red-brown plaque that can expand with central scar formation (Fig. 62.11); as with other granulomatous skin diseases such as sarcoidosis, pressure (diascopy) results in a yellow-brown color; represents direct extension or hematogenous/lymphatic spread of infection.
  - Impaired cellular immunity (TST/PPD usually negative).
    - Orificial TB – autoinoculation of skin or mucosa adjacent to an orifice draining an active tuberculous infection (Fig. 62.12); occurs in patients with advanced internal TB.
    - Miliary TB – small erythematous papules that develop central crusting and may resemble a viral exanthem or pityriasis lichenoides et varioliformis acuta (PLEVA); secondary to hematogenous spread from a primary lung focus.

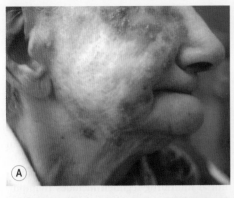

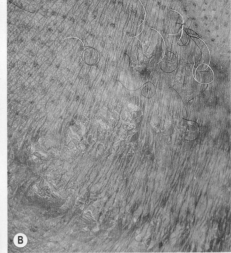

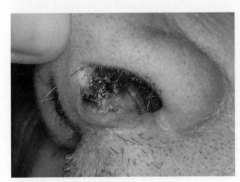

Fig. 62.11 Lupus vulgaris. A Annular granulomatous plaque with central scarring. **B** Two dull red-brown plaques with papular borders, scale and central clearing. **C** Violet-brown plaque on the neck. *A, Courtesy, Marcia Ramos-e-Silva, MD; C, Courtesy, Eugene Mirrer, MD.*

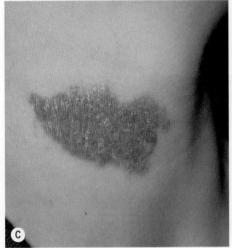

Fig. 62.12 Orificial tuberculosis. A nonhealing ulcer of the nasal mucosa. *Courtesy, Louis A. Fragola, Jr., MD.*

- Tuberculous gumma – firm subcutaneous nodule or fluctuant swelling that often ulcerates; seen in the setting of hematogenous dissemination.
- Tuberculids (cutaneous immune reactions to *M. tuberculosis*).
  - Papulonecrotic tuberculid – widely distributed, dusky red papules or papulopustules, sometimes with central crusts; favors the extremities and may resemble PLEVA (Fig. 62.13).
  - Lichen scrofulosorum – small pink to yellow-brown perifollicular papules with scale, often in clusters on the trunk.

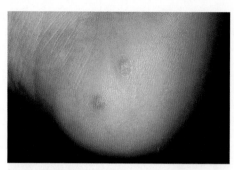

Fig. 62.13 Papulonecrotic tuberculid.
Erythematous papules and papulopustules on the heel.

– Erythema induratum, a form of panniculitis – subcutaneous nodules that may ulcerate; favors the posterior calves (see Chapter 83).

• Confirmation of diagnosis: tuberculin skin test (TST/PPD) or IFN-γ release assays (e.g. QuantiFERON-TB Gold [In-Tube]) or testing of tissue with polymerase chain reaction for *M. tuberculosis* DNA; advantages and disadvantages of the first two tests are outlined in Table 62.5.

• **Rx:** pending sensitivities, an example of an initial multidrug regimen includes rifampin, isoniazid, pyrazinamide, and ethambutol.

ADVANTAGES AND DISADVANTAGES OF INTERFERON-γ (IFN-γ) RELEASE ASSAYS AND TUBERCULIN SKIN TESTING		
	Tuberculin Skin Test	**IFN-γ Release Assays**
Advantages	Does not require a laboratory Relatively low cost	Requires a single patient visit Results can be available within 24 hours Prior BCG vaccination does not cause a false-positive result Does not boost responses measured by subsequent tests
Disadvantages	Requires two patient visits Results not available for 48 hours Prior BCG vaccination can cause a false-positive result May boost responses in subsequent tests Infections with nontuberculous mycobacteria may lead to a false-positive result	Requires laboratory processing within 16 hours (for QuantiFERON®-TB Gold [In-Tube]) or 8 hours (for T-SPOT®.TB; time limit of 30 hours if use T-cell Xtend®) Relatively high cost Infections with some nontuberculous mycobacteria (e.g. *M. kansasii*, *M. szulgai*, and *M. marinum*) may lead to a false-positive result
Situations where preferable	Children <5 years of age	Patient groups that historically have low rates of returning for a second visit (e.g. homeless persons, drug users) Individuals who have received BCG

BCG, bacille Calmette–Guérin.

Table 62.5 Advantages and disadvantages of interferon-γ (IFN-γ) release assays and tuberculin skin testing. Both types of tests may be negative in patients with early active tuberculosis. Indeterminate IFN-γ release assay results due to failure of the internal positive control (i.e. a 'low mitogen' response) are more common in immunocompromised individuals and young children. Indeterminate results due to inappropriately high IFN-γ levels in the negative control ('high nil') can also occur. Testing with a second method after an initial negative test may be useful when the risk of infection/progression is high or when there is clinical suspicion of active tuberculosis. The QuantiFERON®-TB Gold (In-Tube) test directly measures IFN-γ levels, whereas the T-SPOT®.TB test determines the number of IFN-γ-producing T cells; both use a peripheral blood sample.

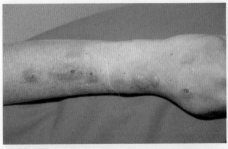

Fig. 62.14 Complication of injection of methanol extraction residue (MER) of bacille Calmette–Guérin (BCG), an attenuated strain of *Mycobacterium bovis.* Nodules, some of which have ulcerated, are arranged in a linear 'lymphatic' pattern in a patient with a high-risk extremity melanoma who had received an injection of MER of BCG as adjuvant immunotherapy.

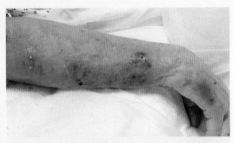

Fig. 62.15 *Mycobacterium avium* complex cellulitis in a patient on chronic CS for rheumatoid arthritis. Note the sporotrichoid (lymphocutaneous) pattern of the coalescing nodules with abscess formation.

Atypical Mycobacteria

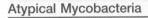

• Found in the natural environment (water, wet soil, vegetation, cold-blooded animals [e.g. fish], dairy products, human feces).

• Skin infections most commonly arise via traumatic inoculation; other routes include surgical or cosmetic procedures (e.g. liposuction, tattooing) and exposure to contaminated water (e.g. soaking distal lower extremities prior to pedicure; see Table 62.2).

• Clinically, pustules, plaques, or nodules develop that may become keratotic or centrally ulcerated.

• A sporotrichoid or lymphocutaneous pattern (linear arrangement of lesions along draining lymphatics) may be seen (Figs. 62.14 and 62.15).

• Disseminated infection can occur in immunocompromised hosts.

• *Mycobacterium marinum* infection is seen most frequently in the United States.

– Found in aquatic environments, including fish tanks and swimming pools.

– Bluish-red inflammatory nodule or pustule that may ulcerate; over time, can develop additional lesions in a sporotrichoid pattern (Fig. 62.16).

• **DDx:** other infections with sporotrichoid spread (e.g. sporotrichosis, nocardiosis) (see Table 64.7).

• **Rx:** pending sensitivities, empiric treatment of infection with *M. marinum* is clarithromycin, and additional antibiotics include minocycline and rifampin; localized infection with *M. ulcerans* or *M. scrofulaceum* can be excised; more disseminated disease usually requires a multidrug regimen for at least 3–6 months.

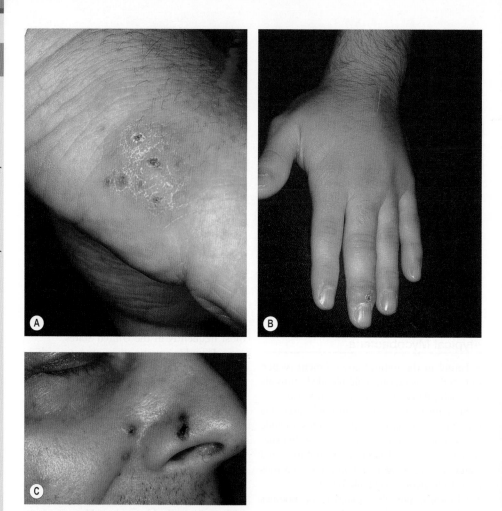

Fig. 62.16 *Mycobacterium marinum* infections. A range of presentations, including an erythematous plaque with scale-crust at the inoculation site on the lateral hand **(A),** a sporotrichoid pattern with the inoculation site on the distal third finger **(B),** and disseminated necrotic lesions on the face of an immunocompromised patient **(C).**

For further information see Ch. 75. From *Dermatology, Third Edition.*

Rickettsial Diseases | 63

Rickettsial infections often have cutaneous manifestations that can vary from nonspecific maculopapular eruptions to an eschar at the site of inoculation (by the vector) to petechiae and retiform purpura (Table 63.1). These gram-negative bacteria reside within an arthropod – tick, flea, mite, or louse – during a portion of their life cycle and are transmitted to humans while feeding, either via saliva or via feces (Table 63.2). As a result, rickettsial diseases exhibit both seasonality and geographic diversity.

DERMATOLOGIC MANIFESTATIONS OF RICKETTSIAL INFECTIONS				
Disease	Rash Incidence (%)	Appearance of Rash after Onset of Illness	Characteristics	Eschar (%)
Rocky Mountain spotted fever	90	3–5 days	Early macules, later papules; petechiae in 50% of cases; retiform purpura	<1
Rickettsialpox	100	2–3 days	Early macules and papules; later papulovesicles and crusts	90
Boutonneuse fever	97	3–5 days	Early macules, later papules	50
North Asian tick typhus	100	4–5 days	Macules and papules	75
Queensland tick typhus	90	2–6 days	Macules, papules, and vesicles	75
Flinders Island spotted fever	85	A few days	Early macules and papules, later (in some patients) petechiae	50
Japanese spotted fever	100	A few days	Early macules, later (in some patients) petechiae	90
Flea-borne spotted fever	83	A few days	Macules and papules; occasionally pustules	17
African tick bite fever	50	3–5 days	Generally relatively few lesions; macules, often vesicles	90, often multiple
Maculatum disease (American tick bite fever)	80	2–4 days	Macules, papules, often vesicles	100

Table 63.1 Dermatologic manifestations of rickettsial infections. *Courtesy, David H. Walker, MD.*
Continued

Table 63.1 *Continued* **Dermatologic manifestations of rickettsial infections.** *Courtesy, David H. Walker, MD.*

Disease	Rash Incidence (%)	Appearance of Rash after Onset of Illness	Characteristics	Eschar (%)
R. aeschlimannii infection	50	Not known	Macules, papules	100
Tick-borne lymphadenopathy	5	Not reported	Macules, papules	100
Epidemic louse-borne typhus	50–100	4–5 days	Early macules, later papules; petechiae	None
Brill–Zinsser disease	50	4–6 days	Macules, papules	None
Flying squirrel typhus	66	2–8 days	Macules, papules	None
Murine (endemic) typhus	80	5 days	Early macules, later papules	None
Scrub typhus	50	4–6 days	Early macules, later papules	60–90
Human monocytotropic ehrlichiosis	40	Median, 5 days	Macules, papules, occasionally petechiae	None
Ehrlichiosis ewingii infection	None	NA	NA	None
Human granulocytotropic anaplasmosis	Rare	NA	NA	None
Q fever	Rare	Associated with chronic infection	Macules, papules, palpable purpura; rarely erythema nodosum	None

NA, not applicable.

EPIDEMIOLOGY OF RICKETTSIAL INFECTIONS			
Agent	Disease	Transmission	Geographic Distribution
Rickettsia rickettsii	Rocky Mountain spotted fever	Bite of tick: *Dermacentor variabilis* (Fig. 63.1)	Eastern two-thirds and Pacific Coast of US
		D. andersoni	Rocky Mountain states
		Rhipicephalus sanguineus	Southwestern US; northern Mexico
		Amblyomma cajennense, A. aureolatum	Central and South America
Rickettsia akari	Rickettsialpox	Bite of mouse mite: *Liponyssoides sanguineus*	North America; Eurasia

Table 63.2 Epidemiology of rickettsial infections. A new *Ehrlichia* species transmitted by *Ixodes scapularis*, provisionally called *E. muris*-like, was recently found to cause a febrile illness in the upper midwestern United States. *Continued*

Table 63.2 *Continued* **Epidemiology of rickettsial infections.**

Agent	Disease	Transmission	Geographic Distribution
Rickettsia conorii	Boutonneuse fever (Mediterranean spotted fever)	Bite of tick: *Rhipicephalus sanguineus*	Southern Europe; Africa; western and southern Asia
		Rh. pumilio	Southern Russia
Rickettsia sibirica	North Asia tick typhus, lymphangitis-associated rickettsiosis	Bite of tick: *Dermacentor nuttallii, D. silvarum, Haemaphysalis concinna, Hyalomma asiaticum,* other species	Eurasia and Africa
Rickettsia australis	Queensland tick typhus	Bite of tick: *Ixodes holocyclus*	Eastern Australia
Rickettsia honei	Flinders Island spotted fever	Bite of tick: *Bothriocroton hydrosauri,* other species	Australia and southeastern Asia (Flinders Island is located between Tasmania and Australia)
Rickettsia japonica	Japanese spotted fever	Bite of tick: Vector status not established for ticks that carry the agent (*Haemaphysalis flava, H. longicornis, Ixodes ovatus, Dermacentor taiwanensis*)	Japan; eastern Asia
Rickettsia felis	Flea-borne spotted fever	By flea: e.g. *Ctenocephalides felis*	Worldwide
Rickettsia africae	African tick bite fever	Bite of tick: *Amblyomma hebraeum*	Southern Africa
		A. variegatum	Central, eastern, and western Africa; Caribbean islands
Rickettsia parkeri	Maculatum disease (American tick bite fever)	Bite of tick: *Amblyomma maculatum, A. americanum*	North America
		A. triste	South America

Table 63.2 *Continued* **Epidemiology of rickettsial infections.**

Agent	Disease	Transmission	Geographic Distribution
Rickettsia aeschlimannii	Unnamed disease	Bite of tick: *Hyalomma marginatum*	Africa
Rickettsia slovaca	Tick-borne lymphadenopathy*	Bite of tick: *Dermacentor marginatus, D. reticularis*	Europe
Rickettsia prowazekii	Epidemic louse-borne typhus	Feces of human body louse (*Pediculus humanus* var. *corporis*)	South America; Africa; Eurasia
	Brill–Zinsser disease	None (recrudescence of latent infection)	
	Flying squirrel typhus	Contact with flying squirrel (*Glaucomys volans*) and its fleas and lice	North America
Rickettsia typhi	Murine (endemic) typhus	Feces of fleas: *Xenopsylla cheopis Ctenocephalides felis*	Worldwide North America
Orientia tsutsugamushi	Scrub typhus	Bite of larval trombiculid mites: *L. deliense, L. fletcheri, L. scutellare, L. arenicola*	Southern and eastern Asia; islands of the southwestern Pacific and Indian Oceans; northern Australia
		e.g. *L. pallidum*	Japan; Korea; Russian Far East
		e.g. *L. scutellare*	China; Malaysia
		e.g. *L. deliense, L. fletcheri, L. arenicola*	Tropical regions
Ehrlichia chaffeensis	Human monocytotropic ehrlichiosis	Bite of tick: *Amblyomma americanum* (Fig. 63.1), *Dermacentor variabilis*	Southeastern and south central US
Ehrlichia ewingii	*Ehrlichia ewingii* infection	Bite of tick: *Amblyomma americanum*	Southeastern and south central US

Table 63.2 *Continued* **Epidemiology of rickettsial infections.** 63

Agent	Disease	Transmission	Geographic Distribution
Anaplasma phagocytophilum	Human granulocytotropic anaplasmosis	**Bite of tick:** *Ixodes scapularis* (Fig. 63.1) *I. pacificus* *I. ricinus,* *I. persulcatus*	Northern US Far western US Eurasia
Coxiella burnetii	Q fever	**Aerosol** of infected products of parturition of ruminants and other animals**	Worldwide

*Also reported to be caused by Rickettsia raoultii.
**Less common means of transmission include ingestion of contaminated dairy products and tick bites (e.g. Dermacentor spp.).
Courtesy, David H. Walker, MD.

Rickettsia and *Orientia* spp. target endothelial cells of multiple organs, including the skin, whereas *Ehrlichia*, *Anaplasma*, and *Coxiella* spp. target monocytes or neutrophils, neutrophils, and macrophages, respectively.

Rocky Mountain Spotted Fever (RMSF)

• Due to transmission of *Rickettsia rickettsia* by the bite of a tick, most commonly *Dermacentor* spp. (Fig. 63.1); the incubation period is 2–14 days (mean, 7 days) following the bite.
• Highest incidence in the South Atlantic and South Central states (Fig. 63.2), not the Rocky Mountain states, with peak incidence from late spring to the end of summer (tick season).
• Begins as a subtle cutaneous eruption with pink to erythematous macules then papules, initially in acral sites (e.g. wrists, ankles); over time central petechiae develop and lesions become more widespread (Figs. 63.3–63.6).
• In the majority of patients, the skin findings are preceded by a fever (for 3–5 days), myalgias, and severe headache; some patients also develop nausea and vomiting and a change in mental status; if not treated appropriately, acute renal failure, hypotension, and coma can ensue, with a mortality rate of up to 25%.

• Dx: biopsy of petechial papule or eschar followed by PCR and/or immunohistochemistry (Table 63.3); serologic results are not helpful in the acute setting.
• **DDx:** viral exanthem (e.g. enterovirus, EBV, measles, parvovirus B19, dengue virus; see Fig. 68.1), other rickettsial spotted fevers (similar eruption but more likely to have an inoculation eschar; see Table 63.1), typhus (several forms), ehrlichiosis, morbilliform drug reaction; when severe and purpuric, meningococcemia, vasculitis, hemorrhagic fevers.
• **Rx:** begun empirically; doxycycline or tetracycline represents first-line therapy, even in children (Table 63.4).

Typhus – Epidemic and Endemic (Murine)

• While the vector differs for epidemic (human body louse) versus endemic (flea) typhus, spread of the infection involves deposition of feces onto the skin followed by scratching into the skin, rubbing into mucous membranes, or inhalation.
• The eruption often begins in the axillae and then becomes more widespread, with relative sparing of the face; individual lesions are similar to those seen in RMSF.
• **DDx** and **Rx:** see section on RMSF.

COMPARISON OF *IXODES SCAPULARIS*, *AMBLYOMMA AMERICANUM*, AND *DERMACENTOR VARIABILIS*, BY LIFE STAGE

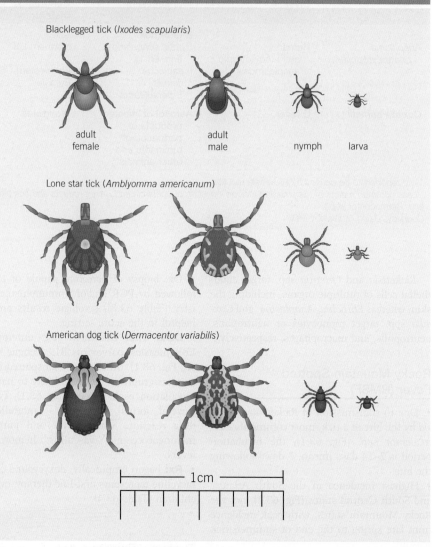

Blacklegged tick (*Ixodes scapularis*)

adult female   adult male   nymph   larva

Lone star tick (*Amblyomma americanum*)

American dog tick (*Dermacentor variabilis*)

├───── 1cm ─────┤

Fig. 63.1 Comparison of *Ixodes scapularis* (blacklegged tick), *Amblyomma americanum* (lone star tick), and *Dermacentor variabilis* (American dog tick), by life stage. *From Chapman, A. S., et al. MMWR Recomm. Rep. 2006;55:1–27.*

Rickettsialpox

• Most often occurs in urban areas.
• Within 48 hours, a papulovesicle (then eschar) develops at the site of the bite of the mouse mite (Fig. 63.7A); fever, myalgias, and headache appear 1–2 weeks later followed soon thereafter by a cutaneous eruption.
• The eruption has a widespread distribution that includes the face, but the number of lesions is usually limited, i.e. ~20–40; the individual macules and papules develop central vesicles and hemorrhagic crusts (Fig. 63.7B).
• **DDx:** varicella, other vesicular viral exanthems (e.g. Coxsackie), pityriasis lichenoides et varioliformis acuta (PLEVA), bullous insect bite reactions, scabies.
• **Rx:** tetracycline or doxycycline (dosages in Table 63.4).

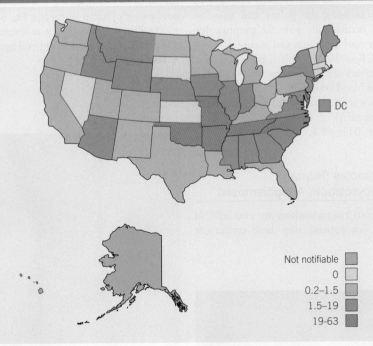

ANNUAL REPORTED INCIDENCE (PER MILLION POPULATION)
FOR ROCKY MOUNTAIN SPOTTED FEVER IN THE UNITED STATES FOR 2010

DC

Not notifiable
0
0.2–1.5
1.5–19
19-63

Fig. 63.2 Annual reported incidence (per million population) for Rocky Mountain spotted fever in the United States for 2010. Five states account for >60% of cases. *From* www.cdc.gov/rmsf/stats/#reportsurv.

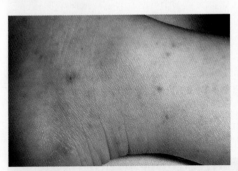

Fig. 63.3 Rocky Mountain spotted fever. The cutaneous lesions often first appear on the ankles and wrists. These are nonblanching due to hemorrhage within the skin. *Courtesy, Philippe Berbis, MD.*

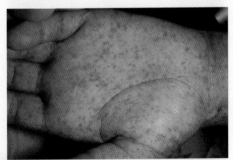

Fig. 63.4 Rocky Mountain spotted fever. Petechiae on the palms and soles often develop relatively later in the disease course. *Courtesy, Ronald Rapini, MD.*

Ehrlichiosis

• The primary vector for ehrlichiosis is the lone star tick *Amblyomma americanum* (Figs. 63.1 and 63.8), with the white-tailed deer serving as a major reservoir.

• In addition to fever, headache, and myalgias, patients with human monocytotropic ehrlichiosis (HME) can develop meningoencephalitis and acute respiratory distress syndrome, with overwhelming disease in immunocompromised hosts.

• Mucocutaneous lesions appear an average of 5 days into the illness of HME and vary from a widespread morbilliform eruption to petechiae favoring the palms and soles to vesicular; occasionally palpable purpura due to small vessel vasculitis can occur.

• Dx: PCR of blood, with intracytoplasmic macrocolonies of bacteria sometimes noted in peripheral blood smears.

• **DDx:** see sections on RMSF and rickettsialpox (if vesicular).

• **Rx:** see Table 63.4.

Anaplasmosis (Human Granulocytotropic Anaplasmosis)

• Cutaneous manifestations are rare (<5% of patients), but patients may have concurrent

signs and symptoms of Lyme borreliosis and/or babesiosis because all three infections are transmitted by *Ixodes* ticks, e.g. *I. scapularis* in the northeastern United States (see Fig. 63.8).

• The illness is usually not as severe as HME and patients may have peripheral neuropathy.

• **Rx:** see Table 63.4.

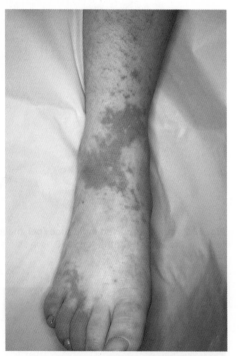

Fig. 63.6 Rocky Mountain spotted fever. Retiform purpura on the distal lower extremity in a patient with more severe disease.

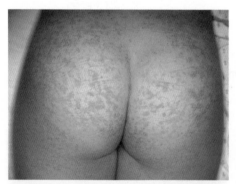

Fig. 63.5 Rocky Mountain spotted fever. Petechiae are present within erythematous papules and plaques on the buttocks. Some of the lesions have a retiform pattern.

EVALUATION OF SUSPECTED CUTANEOUS LESION(S) OF A SPOTTED FEVER, INCLUDING ROCKY MOUNTAIN SPOTTED FEVER (RMSF), VIA REAL-TIME PCR
• Contact the state health department to assist (required if utilizing the CDC) • 3- to 5-mm skin biopsy of a fresh but developed lesion, i.e. in the case of a spotted fever, a maculopapular lesion with pinpoint hemorrhage • Appropriate treatment for <24 hours does not appear to alter sensitivity • Appropriate treatment for ≥72 hours often results in a negative test • Fresh tissue preferred with placement of skin biopsy inside sterile urine container on gauze moistened with sterile saline (transport overnight with ice packs) (see Fig. 2.10B) • PCR can be done on frozen tissue (transport overnight with dry ice)

Table 63.3 Evaluation of suspected cutaneous lesion(s) of a spotted fever, including Rocky Mountain spotted fever (RMSF), via real-time PCR. As recommended by the Centers for Disease Control and Prevention (CDC). www.cdc.gov/rmsf/resources/SkinBiopsyInformation.docx.

TREATMENT OF RICKETTSIAL DISEASES

	Medication	Adult Dose	Pediatric Dose	Treatment Duration
• First choice for virtually all rickettsial infections in children and adults*	Doxycycline	100 mg PO or iv twice daily	2.2 mg/kg (max. 100 mg) PO or iv twice daily	Until ≥3 days after defervescence, for a minimum total course of 5–7 days[†]
• First choice for non-life-threatening RMSF in pregnant women	Chloramphenicol[‡]	500 mg iv every 6 hours	Not recommended	Until ≥3 days after defervescence, for a minimum total course of 5–7 days[†]
• First choice for non-life-threatening HME or HGA in pregnant women • Alternative for resistant scrub typhus	Rifampin	300 mg PO twice daily	10 mg/kg (max. 300 mg) twice daily	Until ≥3 days after defervescence, for a minimum total course of 7–10 days
• First choice for scrub typhus in pregnant women and potentially in children • Alternative for mild rickettsioses (e.g. early boutonneuse fever) during pregnancy or in children	Azithromycin[§]	500 mg PO daily	10 mg/kg PO daily	3 days

*With the exception of infections in pregnant women, although doxycycline administration during pregnancy can be considered in life-threatening situations when the suspicion of RMSF or other severe rickettsioses is high; other tetracyclines are also effective for rickettsial infections.
[†]Recommended by the CDC; others recommend a 10-day course.
[‡]May be associated with gray baby syndrome when administered late in the third trimester of pregnancy.
[§]Clarithromycin may also be considered.

Table 63.4 Treatment of rickettsial diseases. Empiric treatment with an appropriate agent should be initiated immediately when a diagnosis of Rocky Mountain spotted fever (RMSF), human monocytotropic ehrlichiosis (HME), human granulocytotropic anaplasmosis (HGA), or another potentially severe rickettsiosis is suspected clinically.

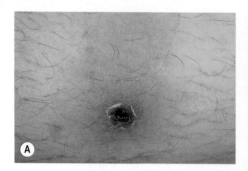

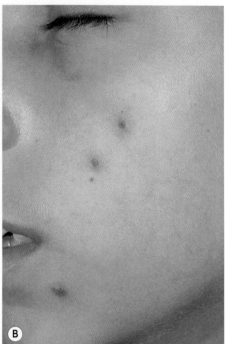

Fig. 63.7 Rickettsialpox. A Eschar at the site of the mite bite. **B** Scattered papules with central hemorrhagic crusts.

APPROXIMATE DISTRIBUTION IN THE US OF VECTOR TICK SPECIES FOR HUMAN MONOCYTOTROPIC EHRLICHIOSIS, HUMAN GRANULOCYTOTROPIC ANAPLASMOSIS, MACULATUM DISEASE AND LYME BORRELIOSIS

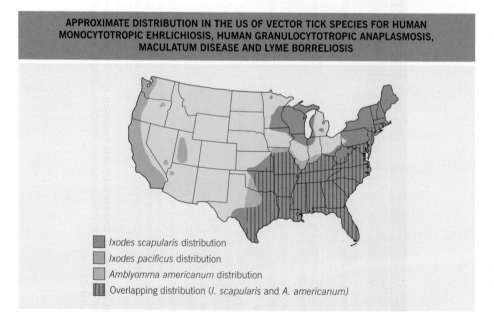

Ixodes scapularis distribution
Ixodes pacificus distribution
Amblyomma americanum distribution
Overlapping distribution (*I. scapularis* and *A. americanum*)

Fig. 63.8 Approximate distribution in the United States of vector tick species for human monocytotropic ehrlichiosis, human granulocytotropic anaplasmosis, maculatum disease, and Lyme borreliosis. It has been postulated that *Amblyomma maculatum*, which is classically found primarily along the Atlantic and Gulf coasts, has a range as broad as that of *Amblyomma americanum*. *From Chapman, A. S., et al. MMWR Recomm. Rep. 2006;55:1–27.*

For further information see Ch. 76. From *Dermatology, Third Edition*.

Fungal Diseases

64

Key Points

- Cutaneous fungal diseases can be broadly divided into two groups:
  - Superficial – limited to the stratum corneum, hair, and/or nails.
  - Deep – dermal and/or subcutaneous.
- Superficial fungal infections can be further subdivided into:
  - Noninflammatory – most commonly tinea versicolor, but includes tinea nigra and piedra.
  - Inflammatory – primarily infections due to dermatophytes (*Trichophyton*, *Microsporum*, *Epidermophyton*; e.g. tinea corporis, tinea cruris) or *Candida* spp. (e.g. cutaneous candidiasis of the groin).
- Deep fungal infections are often secondary to implantation (e.g. sporotrichosis, chromoblastomycosis, eumycetoma) or hematogenous spread of an underlying systemic infection (e.g. cryptococcosis, coccidioidomycosis).
- Opportunistic pathogens (e.g. *Aspergillus*, *Mucor*) can lead to systemic infection in immunosuppressed hosts.

Superficial Fungal Infections

Tinea (Pityriasis) Versicolor

- Secondary to transformation of *Malassezia* spp., especially *M. furfur*, from the yeast form to the hyphal form (see Fig. 2.1A).
- *Malassezia* spp. are part of the normal flora.
- Multiple, brown (hyperpigmented), tan (hypopigmented), or pink, oval to round macules, patches, or thin plaques; there is often coalescence of lesions centrally with scattered lesions at the periphery.
- Associated scale may be subtle but becomes more obvious with gentle scratching or stretching of the skin.

- Most commonly develops on the upper trunk and shoulders, but can also involve flexural sites such as the antecubital fossae, submammary folds, and groin (Fig. 64.1); in children more frequently than adults, there can also be facial involvement.
- Often first noticed in the summer, and a suntan accentuates the hypopigmented variant.
- **DDx:** postinflammatory hypopigmentation and idiopathic macular hypomelanosis (if hypopigmented); confluent and reticulated papillomatosis of Gougerot and Carteaud (if hyperpigmented; see Chapter 89).
- **Rx:** outlined in Table 64.1.
- Following appropriate **Rx**, the associated hypopigmentation may persist for months until there is repigmentation or fading of the suntan.

Tinea Nigra, Black Piedra, and White Piedra

- Typically seen in tropical areas.
- Tinea nigra.
  - Most commonly due to infection with *Hortaea werneckii*, a pigmented fungus found in soil.
  - Brown, sharply marginated macule or patch; most commonly on the palms (Fig. 64.2).
  - **Rx:** keratolytic agents (e.g. salicylic acid 6% cream) and topical antifungals (e.g. terbinafine 1% cream).
- Black piedra and white piedra are characterized by the formation of nodules on hair shafts (Table 64.2; Fig. 64.3).

Dermatophytoses (Tinea Infections)

- The names of dermatophyte infections consist of the word 'tinea' followed by the Latin name for the involved body site;

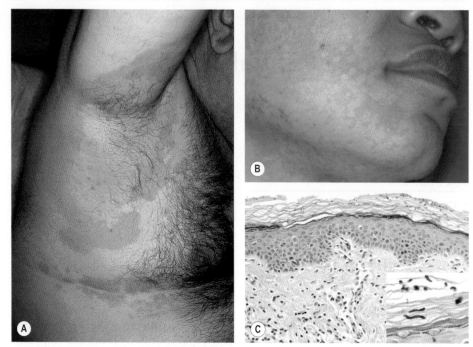

Fig. 64.1 Tinea (pityriasis) versicolor. A Hyperpigmented variant. **B** Hypopigmented variant on the face. **C** Yeast and short hyphae in the stratum corneum highlighted by a PAS stain (*insert*).
A, B, Courtesy, Kalman Watsky, MD; C, Courtesy, Lorenzo Cerroni, MD.

TREATMENT OF TINEA (PITYRIASIS) VERSICOLOR	

Initial therapy (often combination)	Topical
	• Application of antifungal shampoo for 10 minutes to 1 hour weekly to twice weekly for 2–4 weeks
	  • Selenium sulfide shampoo, 1% (OTC) or 2.5%
	  • Ketoconazole shampoo, 1% (OTC) or 2%
	• Imidazoles, e.g. ketoconazole 2% cream daily to BID × 2 weeks
	• Apply several hand-widths beyond clinically visible lesions
	Oral
	• Fluconazole 200–400 mg PO once weekly × 2–3 doses

Maintenance therapy (tinea versicolor commonly recurs)	Examples of topical regimens • Treat previously affected sites with topical imidazole daily for 2 weeks prior to anticipated sun exposure (temperate climates) • Apply antifungal shampoo (see above) 1–2 times every month (tropical climates)

Table 64.1 Treatment of tinea (pityriasis) versicolor.

examples are tinea pedis (foot) and tinea cruris (groin) (Fig. 64.4).

• Due to fungi of three genera – *Trichophyton*, *Microsporum*, and *Epidermophyton* – that invade only keratinized tissue (stratum corneum, hair, and nails).

– With the exception of tinea capitis, *Trichophyton rubrum* and *T. mentagrophytes* are the most common pathogens.

– *Trichophyton mentagrophytes* has two major variants that infect the skin, which can lead to confusion; *T. mentagrophytes* var. *interdigitale* is spread human-to-human, whereas *T. mentagrophytes* var. *mentagrophytes* is acquired from animals; these variants are also known as *T. interdigitale* [anthropophilic] and [zoophilic], respectively.

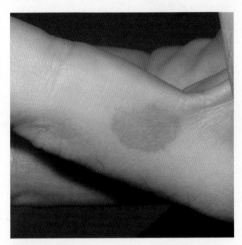

Fig. 64.2 Tinea nigra. Single, sharply demarcated brown macule on the finger. *Courtesy, Frank Samarin, MD.*

• Transmission occurs via close contact with infected humans or domestic animals, occupational or recreational exposure (e.g. locker rooms), and contact with contaminated clothing, furniture, or brushes; the latter inanimate objects serve as fomites.

• More commonly seen in adults, with the exception of tinea capitis, which occurs more often in children.

• The classic presentation is an erythematous, annular lesion with an active, scaly border; superficial pustules may also be present (Fig. 64.5).

• Occasionally, vesicles may develop, especially in tinea pedis or manuum due to *T. mentagrophytes*.

• Dx: KOH ± fungal culture of skin scrapings (see Fig. 2.1) as well as hairs and nails, in the case of tinea capitis and tinea unguium, respectively.

• Important variants:

  – *Tinea incognito* refers to atypical clinical presentations, often due to inappropriate treatment with potent topical CS or combination topical therapies that contain CS; lesions may lack scale or be minimally inflamed (Fig. 64.6; see Fig. 64.5E).

COMPARISON OF BLACK AND WHITE PIEDRA		
	White Piedra	**Black Piedra**
Nodule color	White (occasionally red, green, or light brown)	Brown to black
Nodule firmness	Soft	Hard
Nodule adherence to the hair shaft	Loose	Firm
Typical anatomic location	Face, axillae, and pubic region (occasionally scalp)	Scalp and face (occasionally pubic region)
Favored climate	Tropical	Tropical
Causative organism	*Trichosporon beigelii*	*Piedraia hortae*
KOH examination of 'crush prep' of cut hair shafts	Nondematiaceous hyphae with blastoconidia and arthroconidia (see Fig. 2.17A)	Dematiaceous hyphae with asci and ascospores (sexual reproduction)
Culture on Sabouraud's agar	Moist, cream-colored, yeast-like colonies*	Slow-growing, dark green to dark brown-black colonies
Treatment	Clip affected hairs, wash affected hairs with antifungal shampoo	Clip affected hairs, wash affected hairs with antifungal shampoo

Growth inhibited by cycloheximide.

Table 64.2 Comparison of black and white piedra.

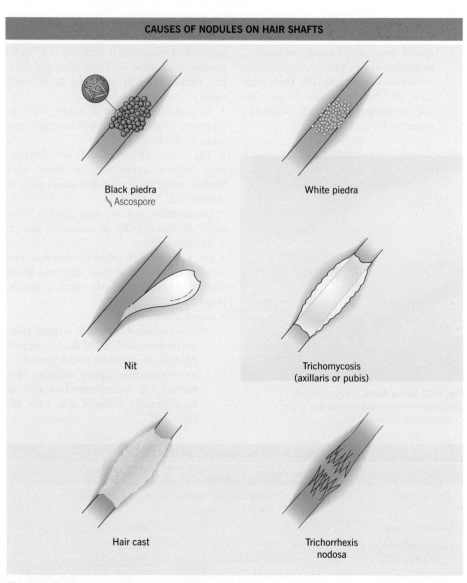

Black piedra
Ascospore

White piedra

Nit

Trichomycosis
(axillaris or pubis)

Hair cast

Trichorrhexis
nodosa

Fig. 64.3 Causes of nodules on hair shafts.

– *Majocchi's granuloma* is characterized by erythematous papules or pustules within an area of tinea corporis; the papules represent sites of hair shaft invasion, usually due to *T. rubrum*; often seen in women with tinea pedis who shave their legs or in immunosuppressed patients (see Fig. 31.4A; Fig. 64.7).

Examples of Specific Types of Dermatophytoses

• Tinea pedis (Fig. 64.8).
  – Most commonly due to *T. rubrum* or *T. mentagrophytes* var. *interdigitale* > *Epidermophyton floccosum*.
  – Three major types: (1) interdigital – erythema, scaling, and maceration in the web spaces, especially the two

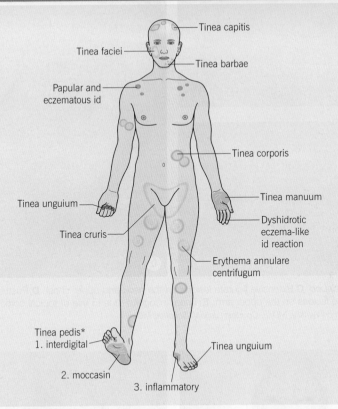

Tinea capitis

Tinea faciei

Tinea barbae

Papular and eczematous id

Tinea corporis

Tinea unguium

Tinea manuum

Tinea cruris

Dyshidrotic eczema-like id reaction

Erythema annulare centrifugum

Tinea pedis*
1. interdigital

Tinea unguium

2. moccasin

3. inflammatory

Fig. 64.4 Dermatophyte infections of the skin and potential associated reactions. *Often associated with an id reaction, particularly dyshidrotic eczema-like findings on the palms and lateral digits; papular and eczematous id may also be seen, especially in association with tinea capitis. Erythema annulare centrifugum is a reaction pattern that can be idiopathic or associated with tinea infections (see Chapter 15).

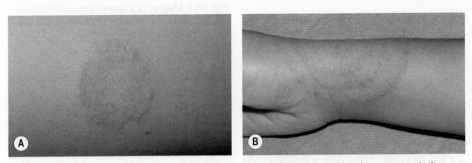

Fig. 64.5 Tinea corporis. A Lesions with subtle annular configuration and border composed of individual, slightly scaly papules. **B** Scaly concentric rings on the arm. *A, B, Courtesy, Julie V. Schaffer, MD.* *Continued*

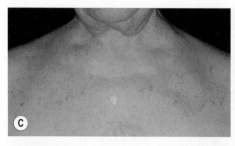

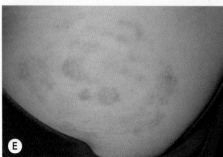

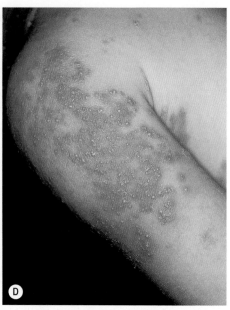

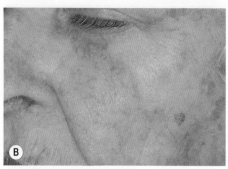

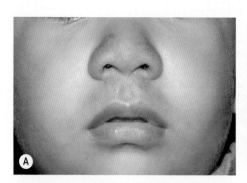

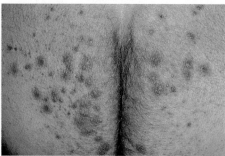

Fig. 64.5 *Continued* **C** Extensive figurate lesions on the neck and upper chest. **D** Pustules within multiple figurate lesions on the upper arm. **E** Tinea 'incognito' due to use of topical corticosteroids. *C, Courtesy, Kalman Watsky, MD; E, Courtesy, Julie V. Schaffer, MD.*

Fig. 64.7 Majocchi's granuloma. Perifollicular inflammation and pustules on the buttocks due to *Trichophyton rubrum.*

Fig. 64.6 Tinea faciei. A Area of erythema and scale on the nose and philtrum of a young child. **B** Serpiginous lesion with minimal scale on the upper cheek of an older woman. *A, Courtesy, Julie V. Schaffer, MD; B, Courtesy, Jean L. Bolognia, MD.*

lateral web spaces, which have the most occlusion; can be accompanied by fissures as well as superimposed bacterial infection; (2) moccasin – diffuse scaling and erythema that extends onto the lateral aspect of the feet; and (3) inflammatory (vesicular) – vesicles and bullae, especially on the medial aspect of the plantar surface.

– Occasionally, especially in immunocompromised and diabetic patients, a more severe ulcerative toe-web

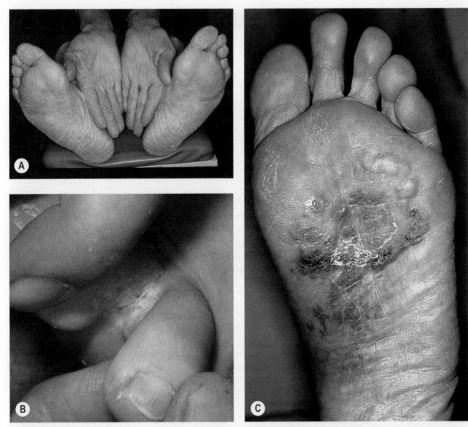

Fig. 64.8 Tinea pedis. Diffuse scaling in the moccasin type **(A)**, maceration between the third and fourth toes in the interdigital form **(B)**, and erythema, scale-crust, and bullae in the inflammatory form **(C)**. The patient in **(A)** also has involvement of the right hand (i.e. one hand–two feet tinea). *B, Courtesy, Jean L. Bolognia, MD.*

infection can occur where there is both a dermatophyte and a bacterial (e.g. pseudomonal) infection; see discussion of gram-negative toe-web infection in Chapter 61.

– Consider use of oral antifungal medications if the tinea pedis fails to respond to topical agents or is severe (Table 64.3).

• Tinea unguium (Fig. 64.9).

– Dx: KOH preparation and/or fungal culture of nail plate and subungual scale, PAS-staining of nail clippings.

– Of note, *onychomycosis* is a more general term that includes nail infections due to dermatophytes, *Candida* spp., and saprophytes (up to 10% of toenail infections; Table 64.4).

• Tinea cruris (Fig. 64.10).

– Favors the upper inner thighs and can extend to the lower abdomen and buttocks; associated with tinea pedis.

– Most commonly due to *T. rubrum* > *Epidermophyton floccosum* > *T. mentagrophytes* var. *interdigitale*.

• Tinea manuum (Fig. 64.11).

• Often due to same dermatophyte as associated tinea pedis.

• Can be unilateral ('one hand, two feet syndrome'; see Fig. 64.8A).

• Tinea unguium of the involved hand is a clinical clue.

• Tinea faciei (see Fig. 64.6).

– Misdiagnosis is common and application of topical CS is a typical history, often leading to tinea incognito.

THERAPEUTIC REGIMENS FOR DERMATOPHYTOSES

Topical Medications

Twice daily for 2–4 weeks
- Allylamines (e.g. terbinafine 1% cream, naftifine 1% gel)
- Imidazoles (e.g. econazole 1% cream, sulconazole 1% solution)
- Hydroxypyridinones (e.g. ciclopirox 0.77% cream or gel)

Oral Medications

	Fluconazole	Griseofulvin	Itraconazole*	Terbinafine
Tinea corporis and pedis (moccasin type)/tinea manuum (*adults*)**	150–200 mg/week × 2–6 weeks	500–1000 mg/day (microsize) or 375–750 mg/day (ultra-microsize) × 2–4 weeks	200–400 mg/day × 1 week	250 mg/day × 1–2 weeks
Tinea corporis and pedis (moccasin type)/tinea manuum (*children*)**	6 mg/kg/week × 2–6 weeks	15–20 mg/kg/day (microsize suspension) × 2–4 weeks	3–5 mg/kg/day (maximum 400 mg) × 1 week	Daily dosing as for tinea capitis (see below) × 1–2 weeks
Tinea unguium (*adults*)	Toenail ± fingernail involvement			
	150–200 mg/week × 9 months	1–2 g/day (microsize) or 750 mg/day (ultra-microsize) until nails are normal†	200 mg/day × 12 weeks or 200 mg BID × 1 week per month for 3–4 consecutive months	250 mg/day × 12 weeks
	Fingernail involvement only			
	150–200 mg/week × 6 months	1–2 g/day (microsize) or 750 mg/day (ultra-microsize) until nails are normal†	200 mg/day × 6 weeks or 200 mg BID × 1 week per month for 2 consecutive months	250 mg/day × 6 weeks
Tinea capitis (*adults*)‡	6 mg/kg/day × 3–6 weeks	10–15 mg/kg/day (ultra-microsize; usually maximum 750 mg/day) × 6–8 weeks	5 mg/kg/day (maximum 400 mg) × 4–8 weeks	250 mg/day × 3–4 weeks§
Tinea capitis (*children*)‡	6 mg/kg/day × 3–6 weeks	20–25 mg/kg/day (microsize suspension) × 6–8 weeks	5 mg/kg/day (maximum 400 mg) × 4–8 weeks	Granules 125 mg (<25 kg), 187.5 mg (25–35 kg), or 250 mg (>35 kg) × 3–4 weeks§

*Not approved in the United States for use in children.
**In general, the shorter courses and lower doses tend to be used for tinea corporis.
†No longer commonly used for this indication.
‡Combined with 2.5% selenium sulfide shampoo or ketoconazole 2% shampoo; 'id' reaction should not be confused with a medication allergy.
§Not recommended for Microsporum canis, unless given at double-dose.

Table 64.3 Therapeutic regimens for dermatophytoses.

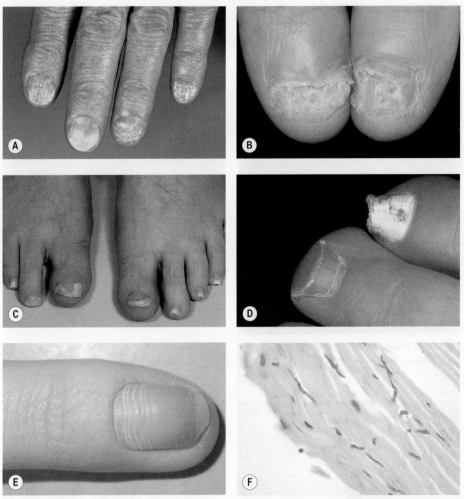

Fig. 64.9 Tinea unguium. Onycholysis, yellowing, crumbling, and thickening of the fingernails **(A)**, thumb nails **(B)**, and toenails **(C)** in the distal/lateral subungual variant. Diffuse **(D)** and striate **(E)** white discoloration of the toenail in the superficial white variant. Hyphae within a formalin-fixed, PAS-stained nail plate **(F)**. *A, C, D, Courtesy, Jean L. Bolognia, MD; B, Courtesy, Louis A. Fragola, Jr., MD; E, Courtesy, Boni Elewski, MD; F, Courtesy, Mary Stone, MD.*

– An arciform shape with pustules in the border points to the diagnosis.

• Tinea barbae (Fig. 64.12; see Fig. 31.7).
  – Often secondary to a zoophilic dermatophyte – i.e. acquired from an animal, e.g. *T. mentagrophytes* var. *mentagrophytes* (small mammals) and *T. verrucosum* (cattle).
  – Favors postpubertal males.
  – Invasion of hair shafts and intense inflammation with follicular pustules and abscess formation; can resemble a kerion.

• Tinea capitis (Fig. 64.13).
  – Occurs more frequently in children.
  – In the United States as well as other regions such as the United Kingdom, *T. tonsurans* is the most common pathogen; for example, in the United States, it causes >95% of tinea capitis; *T. tonsurans* primarily affects those with afrocentric hair.
  – Tinea capitis due to *T. tonsurans* can be more difficult to diagnose because the clinical findings may be subtle with only seborrheic dermatitis-like scaling

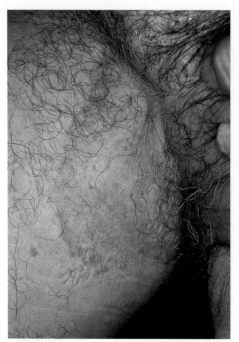

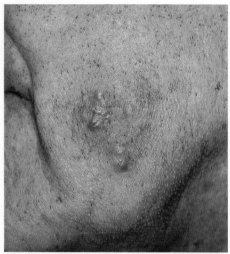

Fig. 64.12 Tinea barbae. More superficial form due to *Trichophyton rubrum*. Several follicular pustules are seen. *Courtesy, Jean L. Bolognia, MD.*

Fig. 64.10 Tinea cruris. Note the arciform erythematous border on the upper inner thigh.

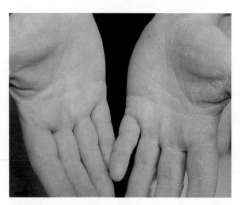

Fig. 64.11 Tinea manuum. Diffuse scaling of the palm of one hand, with accentuation in the creases.

of the scalp, minimal alopecia, and no fluorescence by Wood's lamp examination (in contrast to ectothrix infection due to *M. canis*).

– Multiple spores (conidia) within or surrounding hair shafts, referred to as endothrix or ectothrix tinea capitis, respectively, cause fragility and breakage

of hair, leading to areas of alopecia (see Figs. 2.2 and 2.3).

– In addition to alopecia, clinical clues include pustules, scale, and crusting; occasionally, there is formation of a kerion (see Fig. 64.13E) or development of posterior cervical and posterior auricular lymphadenopathy.

– A type of tinea capitis seen in the Mediterranean basin and Middle East is favus, in which there are keratotic masses that contain hyphae and keratin (Fig. 64.14).

– **Rx:** oral treatment is required; for children, an adequate dose of griseofulvin is 20–25 mg/kg/day (microsized suspension) × 6–8 weeks; combination therapy with 2.5% selenium sulfide or 2% ketoconazole shampoo is recommended to kill spores and reduce transmission; see Table 64.3 for additional oral therapies.

• Id reactions (see Chapter 11) can occur in the setting of dermatophyte infections; two of the more common examples are as follows (see Fig. 64.4):

– Dyshidrotic eczema-like papules and vesicles of the palms and fingers seen in association with tinea pedis.

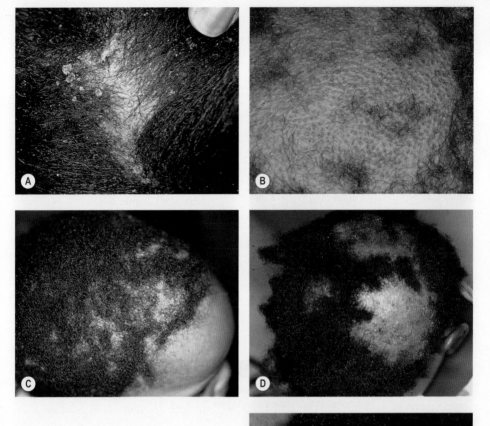

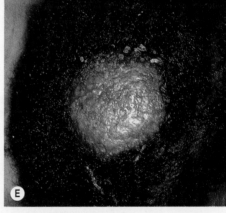

Fig. 64.13 Tinea capitis. The range of clinical presentations of tinea capitis due to *Trichophyton tonsurans*, from mild scalp scaling **(A)** to patchy alopecia with black dots **(B)** or scale **(C)** to large areas of alopecia with pustules and scale-crust **(D). E** Kerion formation due to *T. tonsurans*. There is a boggy plaque that can be misdiagnosed as a bacterial abscess. *B, Courtesy, Louis A. Fragola, Jr., MD.*

- Pruritic papules favoring the upper trunk in the setting of tinea capitis, often following the initiation of appropriate therapy.
• Erythema annulare centrifugum may also be present in association with tinea pedis (see Chapter 15 and Fig. 64.4).
• **DDx:** outlined in Table 64.4.
• **Rx:** outlined in Table 64.3.

Superficial Mucocutaneous *Candida* Infections

• Most commonly due to *Candida albicans* or *C. tropicalis*.
• Wide spectrum of clinical presentations, from diaper dermatitis in infants (see Fig. 13.4) to intertrigo (see Table 60.5 and Fig. 13.2) to chronic mucocutaneous candidiasis (see Chapter 49).

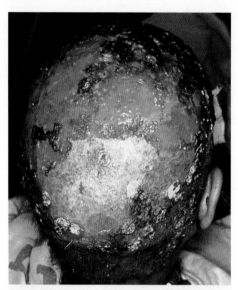

Fig. 64.14 Favus due to *Trichophyton schoenleinii*. Scarring alopecia with erosions and several scutula on the occipital scalp. The latter represent masses of keratin plus fungi. *Courtesy, Israel Dvoretzky, MD.*

- Mucosal.
  - Oral candidiasis (thrush) presents as a white exudate resembling cottage cheese; risk factors include diabetes mellitus, treatment with broad-spectrum antibiotics, use of inhaled CS, dentures, and immunosuppression; common in otherwise healthy neonates and infants.
  - Additional forms: intraoral erythematous patches and adherent white plaques, glossitis, angular cheilitis (see Fig. 13.5), and vulvovaginitis and balanitis (see Chapter 60).
- Cutaneous.
  - Most common presentation is an erosive, erythematous patch with satellite pustules in an intertriginous zone (inframammary, axillary, inguinal, beneath a pannus; Fig. 64.15), on the scrotum, or in the diaper area of infants (see Fig. 13.4).

DIFFERENTIAL DIAGNOSIS OF DERMATOPHYTE INFECTIONS	
Tinea corporis	• Dermatitis (atopic, nummular, contact, stasis) • Erythema annulare centrifugum • Annular psoriasis • Parapsoriasis • Granuloma annulare (lacks scale)
Tinea capitis	• Alopecia areata • Seborrheic dermatitis (unusual in prepubertal populations) • Psoriasis • Tinea amiantacea
Tinea unguium	• Onychomycosis due to saprophytes (e.g. *Fusarium*); primarily toenails • Candidal onychomycosis (primarily fingernails; often there is concurrent paronychia) • Psoriasis • Chronic trauma
Tinea faciei	• Dermatitis (seborrheic, contact, atopic) • Rosacea • Lupus erythematosus • Acne vulgaris • Annular psoriasis (children)
Tinea pedis	• Dermatitis (dyshidrotic, contact) • Psoriasis • Juvenile plantar dermatosis • Palmoplantar pustulosis If interdigital: • Erythrasma • Gram-negative toe-web infection

Table 64.4 Differential diagnosis of dermatophyte infections.

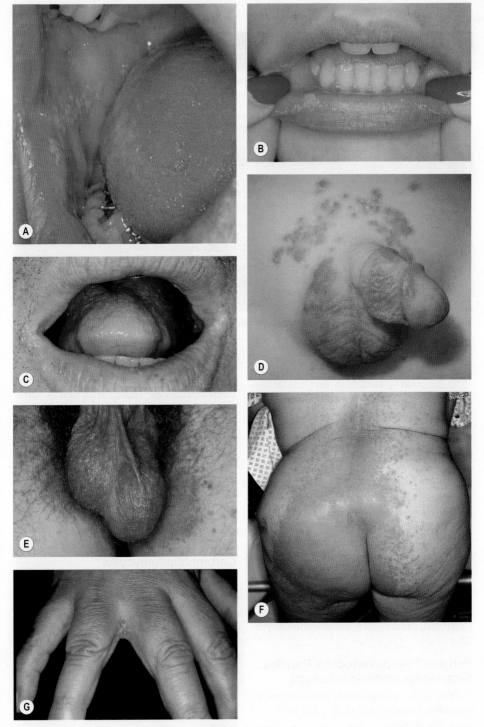

Fig. 64.15 Mucocutaneous candidiasis. A Thrush with 'cottage cheese'-like exudate on the buccal mucosa. **B** Candidal cheilitis with white plaques of the vermilion lip. **C** Angular cheilitis (perlèche). **D** Candidiasis of the suprapubic area, scrotum and penis in a young boy. Note the collarettes of scale on the coalescing, brightly erythematous papules. **E** Candidiasis of the scrotum and medial thighs with beefy red erythema, scale, and satellite papules. **F** This infection occurred in a hospitalized patient with diabetes mellitus who was receiving broad-spectrum antibiotics. Note the multiple satellite lesions. **G** Erosio interdigitalis blastomycetica in the classic location between the third and fourth fingers. *A, Courtesy, Judit Stenn, MD; B, Courtesy, Kalman Watsky, MD; C, Courtesy, Louis A. Fragola, Jr., MD; E, G, Courtesy, Eugene Mirrer, MD.*

TREATMENT OF MUCOCUTANEOUS CANDIDIASIS	
Candidiasis	**Treatment**
Mucosal (continue treatment for 7–14 days after clinical resolution)	Immunocompetent patient • Clotrimazole 10 mg troche five times daily • Nystatin 100 000 units/ml suspension: 4–6 ml swish and swallow four times daily (adults); 1 ml in each cheek four times daily (infants)
	Immunocompromised patient OR failure to respond to topical **Rx** • Oral fluconazole 200 mg PO on day 1, then 100–200 mg PO daily
Cutaneous	If mild, topical treatment • Imidazoles (e.g. ketoconazole 2% cream twice daily for 2 weeks or until resolved)
	If moderate to severe OR fails to respond to topical **Rx** • Fluconazole 50–100 mg daily for 14 days OR • Fluconazole 150 mg PO weekly for 2–4 weeks
	Chronic mucocutaneous candidiasis • Fluconazole 400–800 mg PO daily for 4–6 months • May require lifelong suppressive treatment with fluconazole 200 mg PO daily

Table 64.5 Treatment of mucocutaneous candidiasis.

– Predisposing factors for cutaneous infection – similar to oral candidiasis plus hyperhidrosis with occlusion.
• **DDx** of candidal intertrigo: see Chapter 13.
• **Rx:** outlined in Table 64.5.
• **Rx** of candidal intertrigo or balanitis: outlined in Table 60.5.

Systemic Candidiasis

• Generally affects immunosuppressed hosts in the setting of neutropenia.
• Clinical features are outlined in Table 64.6.
• Although the skin lesions represent septic emboli, blood cultures may be negative; as a result, skin biopsy for tissue culture and histology can play a critical role.

Congenital Candidiasis

Congenital candidiasis is discussed in Chapter 28.

Perianal Pseudoverrucous Papules (Granuloma Gluteale Infantum)

• Etiology is multifactorial, including moist occlusion, irritation from urine and stool, and candidal infection.
• Seen primarily in infants but also in older individuals with urinary and fecal incontinence.
• Erythematous papules and nodules, as well as erosions, develop in the anogenital region.
• **DDx:** outlined in Fig. 13.4.

Deep Fungal Infections

Deep mycoses are treated with oral or intravenous antifungal medications, often for an extended period of time (e.g. 6 months). Culture results direct therapy, but initial empiric treatment is often started based on the clinical presentation plus histologic findings (e.g. itraconazole 200–400 mg/day for chromoblastomycosis).

Dermal/Subcutaneous

Chromoblastomycosis

• Commonly due to several species of dematiaceous fungi – *Fonsecaea pedrosoi*, *F. compacta*, *F. monophora*, *Phialophora verrucosa*, *Cladosporium carrionii*, and *Rhinocladiella aquaspersa* – that are found in soil and decaying wood.
• Follows trauma and implantation of the fungus into the skin.
• Expanding, verrucous plaque, usually on an extremity (Fig. 64.16); central scarring can occur.
• More common in tropical and subtropical regions.
• Diagnostic histologic finding – round, pigmented bodies with internal septations that are said to resemble copper pennies, also referred to sclerotic bodies or Medlar bodies.

CUTANEOUS FEATURES OF COMMON OPPORTUNISTIC MYCOSES	
Mycosis	**Common Cutaneous Presentations**
Systemic candidiasis* • *Candida albicans* • *C. tropicalis* • Other *Candida* spp.	• Firm erythematous papules and nodules, often with a pale center • Lesions can be hemorrhagic, especially in the setting of thrombocytopenia • Ecthyma gangrenosum-like lesions • Occasionally, the lesions are nonspecific, i.e. purpuric macules

Aspergillosis*
• *Aspergillus flavus*
• *A. fumigatus*
Serum assays to screen high-risk patients
• galactomannan (more specific, lower sensitivity)
• 1,3-D-glucan (less specificity)
	• Primary cutaneous
	  – Necrotic papulonodules
	  – May be associated with an intravenous catheter site, burns, trauma, or surgical wounds
	• Secondary cutaneous (septic emboli from disseminated infection)
	  – Necrotic papulonodules and ecthyma gangrenosum-like lesions
	  – Associated with the final stages of AIDS

Zygomycosis* • *Mucor* • *Rhizopus* • *Absidia*	• Ecthyma gangrenosum-like lesions, cellulitis, facial edema (commonly unilateral due to contiguous spread of sino-orbital disease), necrotic papulonodules, plaques, large hemorrhagic crusts on the face • May be associated with an intravenous catheter site (primary cutaneous) • Also associated with poorly controlled diabetes mellitus
Cryptococcosis† • *Cryptococcus neoformans*	• Molluscum contagiosum-like lesions, ulceration, cellulitis
Phaeohyphomycosis*,‡ • *Alternaria* • *Exophiala* • *Phialophora*	• Subcutaneous cysts, ulcerated plaques, necrotic papulonodules
Hyalohyphomycosis*,‡ • *Fusarium* • *Penicillium* • *Paecilomyces*	• Umbilicated or necrotic papules, pustules, abscesses, cellulitis, subcutaneous nodules • *Fusarium* infection can begin with a periungual focus

*With use of prophylactic fluconazole and (more recently) voriconazole in high-risk oncology patients, incidences of systemic candidiasis and (with voriconazole use) aspergillosis have decreased, but incidences of zygomycosis and (with fluconazole use) fusariosis have increased as well as other hyalohyphomycoses.
†Especially in the setting of AIDS; also histoplasmosis, coccidioidomycosis, penicilliosis, and sporotrichosis.
‡Less common infections.

Table 64.6 Cutaneous features of common opportunistic mycoses.

Mycetoma (Madura Foot)

• Two subtypes: (1) actinomycotic mycetoma – secondary to filamentous bacteria, especially *Nocardia* and *Actinomyces* (see Chapter 61); and (2) eumycotic mycetoma – caused by true fungi, e.g. *Madurella mycetomatis*, *Pseudallescheria boydii*.

• Contracted from trauma and implantation of fungus into the skin (Fig. 64.17A).

• Most common site is the distal lower extremity but can also be seen in other sites, such as the distal upper extremity, trunk, and scalp.

• Clinical triad of draining sinuses, grains (macroscopic colonies of organisms; see Chapter 61), and edema (Fig. 64.18).

• **Rx:** excision of more localized lesions; for larger areas of involvement as well as pre- and

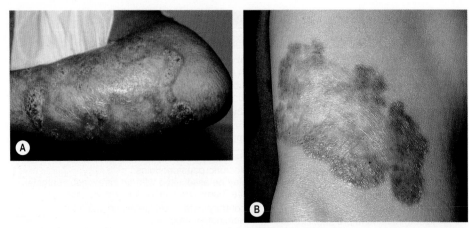

Fig. 64.16 Chromoblastomycosis. Annular and figurate plaques due to central clearing and scarring with a verrucous surface on the arm **(A)** and a more granulomatous appearance on the leg **(B).**

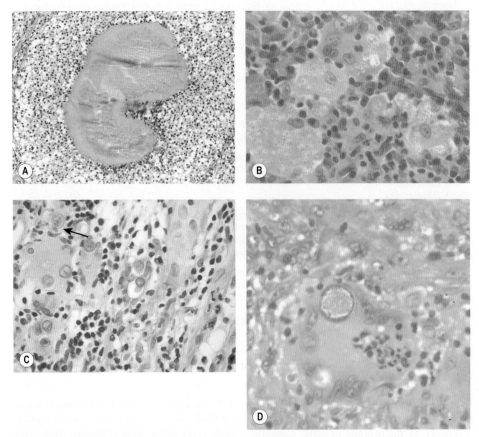

Fig. 64.17 Histologic features of selected deep fungal infections. A Eumycetoma with formation of a grain, which represents tightly packed colonies of fungal organisms. **B** Histoplasmosis – *Histoplasma capsulatum* yeast forms are present within macrophages. **C** Blastomycosis – budding yeast forms within the dermis, several of which are within a giant cell (PAS stain). Note the single, broad-based budding (*arrow*). **D** Coccidioidomycosis – an endospore-containing spherule within a giant cell. *A, Courtesy, Lorenzo Cerroni, MD; B, D, Courtesy Jennifer McNiff, MD; C, Courtesy, Mary Stone, MD.*

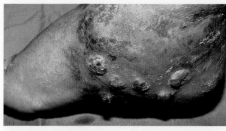

Fig. 64.18 Madura foot. Note the soft tissue swelling of the foot as well as multiple nodules with pustular discharge.

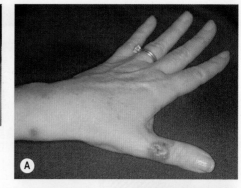

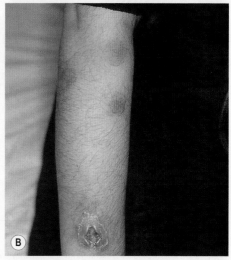

INFECTIOUS CAUSES OF A LYMPHOCUTANEOUS ('SPOROTRICHOID') PATTERN

Most common
- Atypical mycobacteria, especially *Mycobacterium marinum*, but also other species (e.g. *M. chelonae, M. kansasii*)
- Sporotrichosis

Unusual
- Nocardiosis
- Pyogenic bacteria (e.g. *Staphylococcus aureus, Streptococcus pyogenes*)
- *Pseudallescheria boydii*

Rare (in high-income countries)
- Leishmaniasis
- Tularemia*
- Tuberculosis*
- Dimorphic fungi (other than *Sporothrix schenckii*)
- Opportunistic fungi in immunocompromised hosts (e.g. *Fusarium, Alternaria* spp.)
- Glanders (*Burkholderia mallei*)*
- Cat scratch disease*
- Anthrax

Often ulceroglandular.

Table 64.7 Infectious causes of a lymphocutaneous ('sporotrichoid') pattern. There are also noninfectious causes, such as lymphoma, Langerhans cell histiocytosis, and in-transit metastases. In addition, perineural spread of leprosy can mimic a lymphocutaneous pattern.

Fig. 64.19 Lymphocutaneous (sporotrichoid) pattern. A An eroded nodule on the thumb, representing the primary lesion, with a secondary lesion along the lymphatics due to sporotrichosis. **B** Ulcerated nodule on the extensor forearm with multiple more proximal nodules due to nocardiosis in a patient with lymphoma who was receiving systemic corticosteroids. *B, Courtesy, Jean L. Bolognia, MD.*

postoperatively, long-term course (i.e. 6 months or longer) of oral antifungal medication (e.g. itraconazole 400 mg PO daily × 3 months followed by 200 mg PO daily for 9 months).

Sporotrichosis

- Secondary to *Sporothrix schenkii*, a dimorphic fungus, i.e. a yeast at 37°C (human body) and a mold at 25°C (soil).
- Worldwide distribution; present in soil and sphagnum moss.
- Most common presentation is a lymphocutaneous or 'sporotrichoid' pattern (~75% of patients) that initially presents as a papule or nodule at the site of inoculation; this is followed by the appearance of papulonodules along the draining lymphatics (Fig. 64.19; Table 64.7).

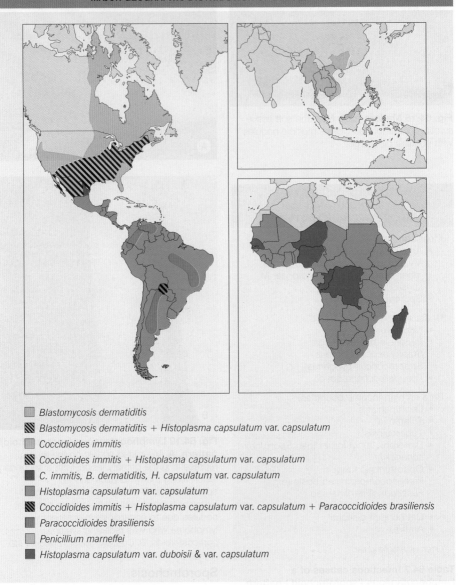

MAJOR GEOGRAPHIC DISTRIBUTION OF DIMORPHIC FUNGI

- *Blastomycosis dermatiditis*
- *Blastomycosis dermatiditis* + *Histoplasma capsulatum* var. *capsulatum*
- *Coccidioides immitis*
- *Coccidioides immitis* + *Histoplasma capsulatum* var. *capsulatum*
- *C. immitis, B. dermatiditis, H. capsulatum* var. *capsulatum*
- *Histoplasma capsulatum* var. *capsulatum*
- *Coccidioides immitis* + *Histoplasma capsulatum* var. *capsulatum* + *Paracoccidioides brasiliensis*
- *Paracoccidioides brasiliensis*
- *Penicillium marneffei*
- *Histoplasma capsulatum* var. *duboisii* & var. *capsulatum*

Fig. 64.20 Major geographic distribution of dimorphic fungi. *Courtesy, Braden A. Perry, MD.*

- Less common variants: (1) a fixed, ulcerated plaque on the face in someone with prior exposure, a form prevalent in Brazil due to transmission by infected cats; and (2) cutaneous dissemination from a systemic infection.

Systemic (Unless Primary Inoculation into Skin)

Blastomycosis

- Due to *Blastomyces dermatitidis*, a dimorphic fungus; yeast form displays broad-based budding (see Fig. 64.17C).

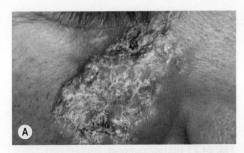

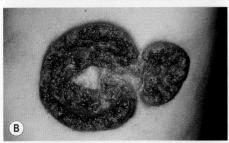

Fig. 64.21 Blastomycosis. A Facial plaque with scale-crust and a border with a granulomatous appearance. **B** Well-demarcated plaques with erosions, central scarring, and black crusting. *A, Courtesy, Louis A. Fragola, Jr., MD; B, Courtesy, Paul Lucky, MD.*

• Endemic to the southeastern United States and other areas of North America (Fig. 64.20).
• Contracted via inhalation, with the skin, bones, and genitourinary tract being the most common sites of secondary infection.
• Cutaneous lesions can vary from papulo-pustules to verrucous plaques with crusted borders (Fig. 64.21).

Coccidioidomycosis

• Due to *Coccidioides immitis*, a dimorphic fungus that forms arthrospores in the soil and spherules within the skin (see Fig. 64.17D).
• Endemic to the southwestern United States (see Fig. 64.20).
• Contracted via inhalation, with dis-seminated disease more common in African-Americans, Mexicans, and immuno-compromised hosts.
• Cutaneous manifestations: lesions vary from papules to pustules, abscesses, and plaques with sinus tracts (Fig. 64.22).

• Noninfectious hypersensitivity reactions include toxic erythema, erythema multi-forme, and erythema nodosum.
• Molluscum contagiosum-like lesions may be seen in HIV-infected persons.

Cryptococcosis

• Molluscum contagiosum-like lesions may be seen in HIV-infected patients and other immunocompromised hosts (see Fig. 64.25G), in addition to ulcers and cellulitis (see Fig. 64.25F).

Histoplasmosis

• Due to *Histoplasma capsulatum* var. *cap-sulatum*, a dimorphic fungus (see Fig. 64.17B).
• Endemic to the southeastern and central United States and many other countries with reservoirs in birds, including fowl, and bats (see Fig. 64.20).
• Disease contracted through inhalation or, rarely, implantation.
• Immunocompetent hosts: oral ulcers in up to 75% of patients; occasionally cutaneous papulonodules.
• Immunosuppressed hosts: oral ulcers and multiple papules or plaques (Fig. 64.23), including ones that resemble molluscum contagiosum.

Paracoccidioidomycosis

• Due to *Paracoccidioides brasiliensis*, a dimorphic fungus that displays multiple narrow-based buds in tissue, including the skin.
• Endemic to South America.
• Disease contracted via inhalation, with dissemination primarily to lymph nodes > oropharynx > adrenal glands > spleen and gastrointestinal tract, in addition to the skin.
• Cutaneous lesions are primarily periorifi-cial and associated with involvement of the oral mucosa; verrucous and ulcerative plaques are seen (Fig. 64.24).

Opportunistic Pathogens

See Table 64.6 and Fig. 64.25.

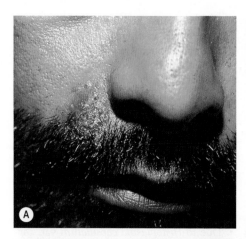

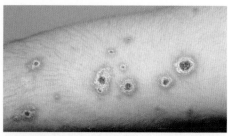

Fig. 64.23 Histoplasmosis. Papules and nodules with scale-crust in a patient with AIDS.

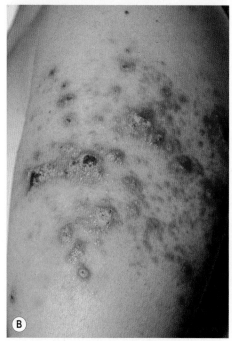

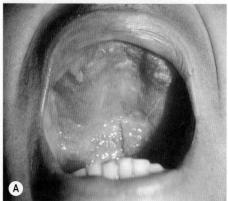

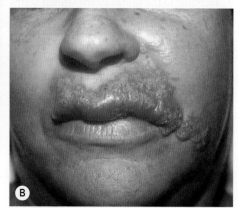

Fig. 64.22 Coccidioidomycosis. Moist erythematous plaque on the face **(A)** and multiple papules and suppurative nodules on the arm **(B)** in two patients living in the southwestern United States.

Fig. 64.24 Paracoccidioidomycosis. Ulcerated plaques on the palate **(A)** and verrucous granulomatous red-brown plaques with crusting involving the perioral region and upper lip **(B).**
A, B, Courtesy, Marcia Ramos-e-Silva, MD, PhD.

For further information see Ch. 77. From *Dermatology, Third Edition.*

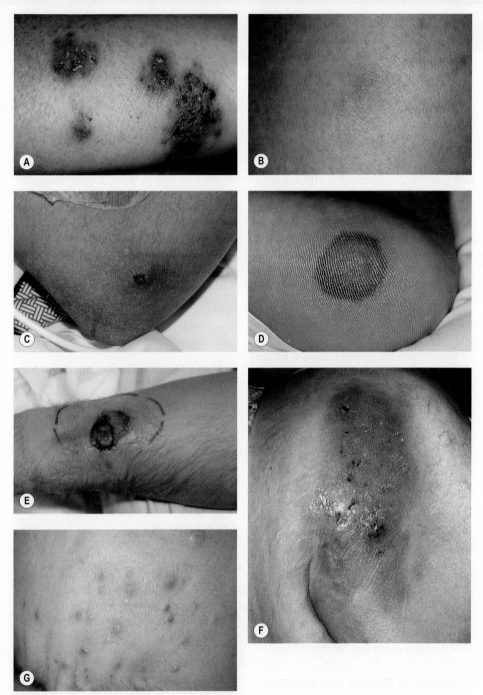

Fig. 64.25 Clinical findings of opportunistic fungal infections in immunocompromised hosts.
Primary cutaneous aspergillosis characterized by hyperpigmented plaques with brown-black
scale-crusts at the site of intravenous catheters on the arm **(A);** firm pink papulonodule due to
disseminated candidiasis **(B);** erythematous papulonodule with central necrosis due to embolus of
Mucor circinelloides **(C);** necrotic hemorrhagic bulla due to embolus of *Aspergillus flavus* **(D);** cellulitis
with area(s) of necrosis due to *Rhizopus* **(E)** and *Cryptococcus neoformans* **(F);** and crusted
molluscum contagiosum-like lesions due to disseminated cryptococcosis **(G).** *C, Courtesy,
Julie V. Schaffer, MD; F, Courtesy, Kalman Watsky, MD; G, Courtesy, Athanasia Syrengelas, MD, PhD.*

65 | Cutaneous Manifestations of HIV Infection

There are a number of cutaneous disorders that point to the diagnosis of HIV infection. For some, it is the mere presence of the skin disease, whereas for others, the disease is extensive or proves recalcitrant to therapy (Table 65.1; Figs. 65.1–65.12). As HIV infection is associated with immunosuppression, the clinical presentation of various infectious diseases is often reminiscent of that observed in individuals whose immunocompromised state is due to medications (e.g. CS plus chemotherapy) or underlying diseases (e.g. acute leukemia).

In HIV-infected patients, several cutaneous diseases (e.g. disseminated coccidioidomycosis, Kaposi's sarcoma) are AIDS-defining conditions (see http://www.cdc.gov/mmwr), whereas others such as oral hairy leukoplakia and seborrheic dermatitis can serve as early clues to the infection, i.e. when there are >500 CD4+ cells/mm^3.

Epidemiology

• With the advent of antiretroviral therapy (ART), HIV infection/AIDS has become a chronic disease.
• High-risk groups still include commercial sex workers, men who have sex with men (MSM), and intravenous drug users, but heterosexual transmission has become a significant mode of transmission.
• Nearly two-thirds of individuals living with HIV infection are in sub-Saharan Africa.

Exanthem of Primary HIV Infection (Acute Retroviral Syndrome)

• Follows an incubation period of 3–6 weeks, but the latter may be shorter if infection acquired hematogenously.
• Morbilliform eruption (40–80% of patients) appears in the setting of peak viremia; accompanied by orogenital ulcerations (5–20%) as well as fever, fatigue, headache, pharyngitis, arthralgia, myalgia and GI symptoms and a decrease in circulating CD4+ T cells.
• While the cutaneous eruption usually lasts 4–5 days, the constitutional symptoms can last from a few days to a few months.
• Dx: detection of viral RNA by PCR and/or p24 antigen in the plasma; assays for anti-HIV-1 antibodies are less reliable as they may be negative.

Immune Reconstitution Inflammatory Syndrome (IRIS)

• Those disorders that can 'flare' or 'worsen' due to an increase in the ability to mount an inflammatory response following the institution of ART are outlined in Table 65.2 (Fig. 65.13).
• It is noteworthy that depending on the patient, some of these disorders improve rather than 'worsen' in the setting of ART, e.g. Kaposi's sarcoma.

Antiretroviral Therapy (ART)

• For naive patients, initial combination ART currently consists of one of the following: (1) efavirenz/tenofovir/emtricitabine; (2) ritonavir-boosted atazanavir + tenofovir/emtricitabine; (3) ritonavir-boosted darunavir + tenofovir/emtricitabine; or (4) raltegravir + tenofovir/emtricitabine (see http://aidsinfo.nih.gov/contentfiles/lvguidelines/adultandadolescentgl.pdf).
• Table 65.3 (Figs. 65.14 and 65.15) outlines the mucocutaneous side effects of these antiretroviral drugs (Fig. 65.16); such reactions can lead to the discontinuation of the incriminated medication.

MUCOCUTANEOUS DISORDERS ASSOCIATED WITH HIV INFECTION

Inflammatory Disorders

When severe, recalcitrant, or of sudden onset, consider HIV infection

- Seborrheic dermatitis (e.g. face, scalp)
- Psoriasis vulgaris (Fig. 65.1)
- Reactive arthritis (previously referred to as Reiter's disease)

Alone raises the possibility of HIV infection

- Eosinophilic folliculitis (Fig. 65.2; Chapter 31)*
- Pityriasis rubra pilaris (type VI with follicular spines & acne conglobata)

Infectious Diseases and Infestations*

When severe and/or recalcitrant, consider HIV infection

- Human papilloma virus infections (warts), including acquired epidermodysplasia verruciformis-like lesions (Chapter 66)
- Molluscum contagiosum, numerous, coalescent, and/or giant-sized, especially in adults (Fig. 65.3)
- Dermatophyte infections (Chapter 64)

Alone raises the possibility of HIV infection

- Syphilis and other sexually transmitted infections (e.g. chancroid; Chapter 69)
- Bacillary angiomatosis (Fig. 65.4)
- Botryomycosis ("grains" within the dermis composed of *Staphylococcus*, *Pseudomonas*)
- Disseminated mycobacterial infections (tuberculous and nontuberculous)

- Chronic oral and anogenital herpes simplex (Fig. 65.5) or disseminated HSV
- Herpes zoster, especially if multi-dermatomal, disseminated, verrucous or chronic, but can have classic presentation (Fig. 67.11A)
- Oral hairy leukoplakia due to EBV infection (Fig. 65.6)
- Anogenital and oral ulcers, verrucous plaques or morbilliform eruption due to CMV (Chapter 67)
- Kaposi's sarcoma due to HHV-8 infection (Fig. 65.7; Chapters 67 and 94)

- Oropharyngeal candidiasis (thrush; Fig. 65.8; Chapter 64)
- Proximal subungual onychomycosis (Chapter 64)
- Disseminated cryptococcosis (Fig. 65.9; Chapter 64)
- Disseminated dimorphic fungal infections (e.g. coccidioidomycosis, histoplasmosis, penicilliosis; Fig. 65.10)

- Crusted scabies (Norwegian scabies; Fig. 65.11)

- Disseminated or necrotic cutaneous leishmaniasis

Other

- Papular pruritic eruption of HIV
- Xerosis and acquired ichthyosis
- Major aphthae (Fig. 65.12); acute necrotizing ulcerative stomatitis with gingivitis
- Porphyria cutanea tarda, often in association with hepatitis C
- Facial hyperpigmentation, idiopathic or due to photolichenoid drug eruption
- Linear telangiectasias of the chest
- Trichomegaly of the eyelashes and change in texture of scalp hair (e.g. curly -> fine and straight)
- *Demodex* folliculitis
- Cutaneous lesions of non-Hodgkin's lymphoma
- Anal intraepithelial neoplasia/anal carcinoma
- Acral persistent papular mucinosis; atypical variants of granuloma annulare

In particular when there is no known cause of immunosuppression.

Table 65.1 Mucocutaneous disorders associated with HIV infection.

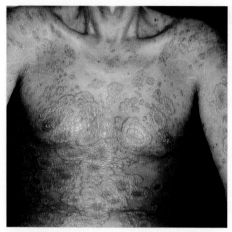

Fig. 65.1 Severe psoriasis in a patient with AIDS. Both sudden acute exacerbations and treatment resistance can be observed.

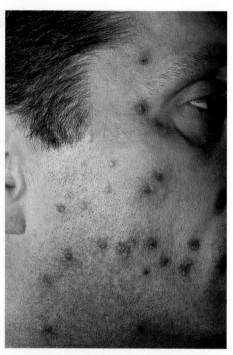

Fig. 65.2 Eosinophilic folliculitis. Due to associated pruritus, follicular papules are often excoriated; lesions favor the head and upper trunk. *Courtesy, Clay J. Cockerell, MD.*

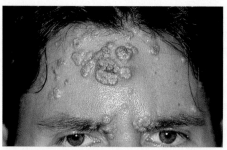

Fig. 65.3 Molluscum contagiosum in the setting of HIV infection. Large lesions due to coalescence of individual papules. The face is a common location.

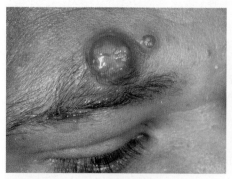

Fig. 65.4 Bacillary angiomatosis. Lesions can resemble vascular tumors or pyogenic granulomas and are a reflection of infection with *Bartonella henselae* or *B. quintana*.

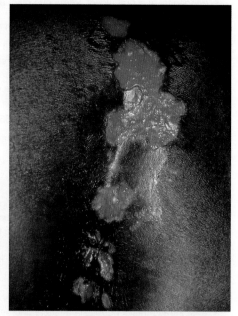

Fig. 65.5 Chronic ulcerative herpes simplex viral infection in an HIV-infected patient. These slowly enlarging ulcers of the buttocks and perianal area have a characteristic scalloped border.

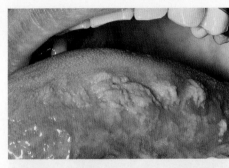

Fig. 65.6 Oral hairy leukoplakia. Shaggy white keratotic plaques along the lateral aspect of the tongue. A corrugated pattern is often seen. *Courtesy, Charles Camisa, MD.*

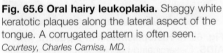

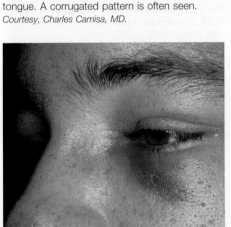

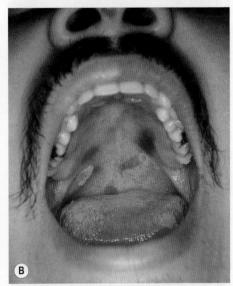

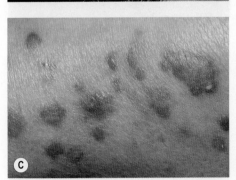

Fig. 65.7 Kaposi's sarcoma in the setting of AIDS. Violaceous papules and plaques involving the face **(A)**, palate **(B)**, and an extremity **(C)**. The patient also has oral candidiasis. *C, Courtesy, Thomas Horn, MD.*

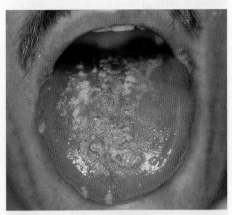

Fig. 65.8 Both oral candidiasis and oral herpes viral infection involving the tongue. The white plaques represent the former, whereas the circular and scalloped areas of detached epithelium represent the latter. Either of these infections, and especially their combination, points to immunosuppression and the possibility of HIV infection.

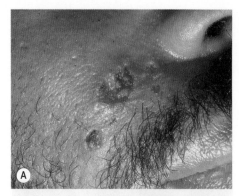

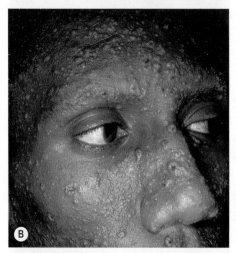

Fig. 65.9 Disseminated cryptococcosis in the setting of AIDS. A Several ulcers with rolled borders. **B** Numerous molloscum contagiosum-like lesions. Microscopic examination and culture of either dermal scrapings or a biopsy specimen confirm the diagnosis.

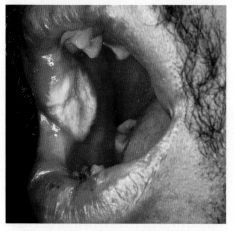

Fig. 65.12 Major aphthae in a patient with AIDS. Resolution of these oral ulcers may require thalidomide.

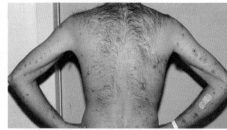

Fig. 65.10 Histoplasmosis in a patient with AIDS. Disseminated papules and nodules, some with central scale-crust.

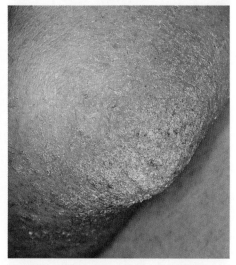

Fig. 65.11 Crusted scabies in the setting of HIV infection. Crusted scabies is often misdiagnosed as dermatitis, but these scale-crusts are teeming with mites. This form of the disease was previously referred to as Norwegian scabies.

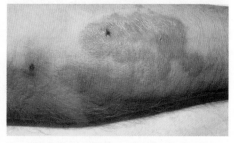

Fig. 65.13 Exacerbation of leprosy due to immune reconstitution inflammatory syndrome (IRIS) following institution of ART. *Courtesy, Beatriz Trope, MD, PhD.*

CUTANEOUS DISEASES THAT CAN 'FLARE' DUE TO THE IMMUNE RECONSTITUTION INFLAMMATORY SYNDROME (IRIS)

Infections

- *Mycobacterium tuberculosis*
- *Mycobacterium leprae* (Fig. 65.13)
- *Mycobacterium avium* complex and other species
- Herpes simplex virus 1 and 2
- Varicella–zoster virus
- Epstein-Barr virus (e.g. oral hairy leukoplakia)
- Cytomegalovirus
- Human papillomavirus
- Molluscum contagiosum virus
- *Candida* spp.
- Dermatophytes
- *Cryptococcus* spp.
- *Histoplasma capsulatum*, *Penicillium marneffei*
- *Demodex*, *Malassezia* spp. (e.g. folliculitis)
- *Leishmania* spp.

Inflammatory Disorders

- Psoriasis, seborrheic dermatitis
- Sarcoidosis
- Foreign body reactions (granulomatous)
- Eosinophilic folliculitis
- Acne vulgaris, rosacea
- Papular pruritic eruption
- Lupus erythematosus (systemic, discoid, tumid), relapsing polychondritis
- Alopecia areata
- Dyshidrotic eczema

Neoplasms

- Kaposi's sarcoma
- Non-Hodgkin lymphoma
- Multiple eruptive dermatofibromas

Table 65.2 Cutaneous diseases that can 'flare' due to the immune reconstitution inflammatory syndrome (IRIS). IRIS can also occur in other settings of immunosuppression (e.g. solid organ transplants, TNF administration).

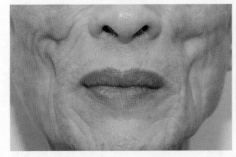

Fig. 65.14 HIV/ART-associated lipodystrophy. Marked indentation of the medial cheeks due to lipoatrophy is a characteristic finding, as is a decrease in subcutaneous fat of the extremities and an increase in abdominal fat (central obesity). *Courtesy, Priya Sen, MD.*

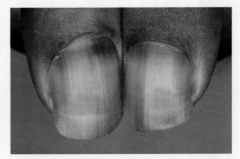

Fig. 65.15 Zidovudine-associated melanonychia. Patients receiving zidovudine (AZT) may develop longitudinal streaks, horizontal bands, or diffuse hyperpigmentation as well as oral and cutaneous hyperpigmentation.

CUTANEOUS MANIFESTATIONS OF HIV INFECTION

For further information see Ch. 78. From *Dermatology, Third Edition.*

CUTANEOUS SIDE EFFECTS OF ANTIRETROVIRAL THERAPY (ART)

Type of Skin Reaction	NRTIs/NtRTIs	NNRTIs	Protease Inhibitors	Integrase Inhibitors	CCR5 Inhibitors	Fusion Inhibitors
Injection site reaction						
Morbilliform eruption	Emtricitabine*, Abacavir**	Nevirapine > etravirine, efavirenz	Atazanavir, fosamprenavir^ > darunavir^, tipranavir^ > lopinavir			
DRESS [DIHS]	Abacavir**	Etravirine, efavirenz, Nevirapine	Atazanavir, darunavir^, fosamprenavir^, tipranavir^, lopinavir	Rare	Rare	Rare
SJS/TEN	Rare	Rare, Nevirapine > efavirenz, etravirine	Rare	Rare		
Lipodystrophy (also insulin resistance and elevated TTGs)	Stavudine	Efavirenz	Fig. 65.14			
Paronychia, excessive periungual granulation tissue	Lamivudine		Indinavir			
Xerosis			Indinavir			
Hyperpigmentation of skin and nails	AZT (Fig. 65.15), emtricitabine (palmoplantar)					

*Palmoplantar eruption.

**Associated with HLA-B*5701 allele.

^Sulfonamide-like structure and should be used cautiously in patients with sulfonamide allergy.

AZT, zidovudine; CCR5, CC-chemokine receptor 5; DIHS, drug-induced hypersensitivity syndrome; DRESS, drug reaction with eosinophilia and systemic symptoms; NNRTIs, non-nucleoside reverse transcriptase inhibitors; NRTIs/NtRTIs, nucleoside/nucleotide reverse transcriptase inhibitors; SJS, Stevens–Johnson syndrome; TEN, toxic epidermal necrolysis; TTGs, triglycerides.

Table 65.3 Cutaneous side effects of antiretroviral therapy (ART). In general, patients with HIV infection have an increased risk of developing drug-induced morbilliform eruptions and toxic epidermal necrolysis, e.g. to sulfonamides. Dark-colored cells = common; light-colored cells = less common. A whole cell that lacks specific drug names refers to that class of drugs, whereas in subdivided cells, it refers to the remainder of that class of drugs.

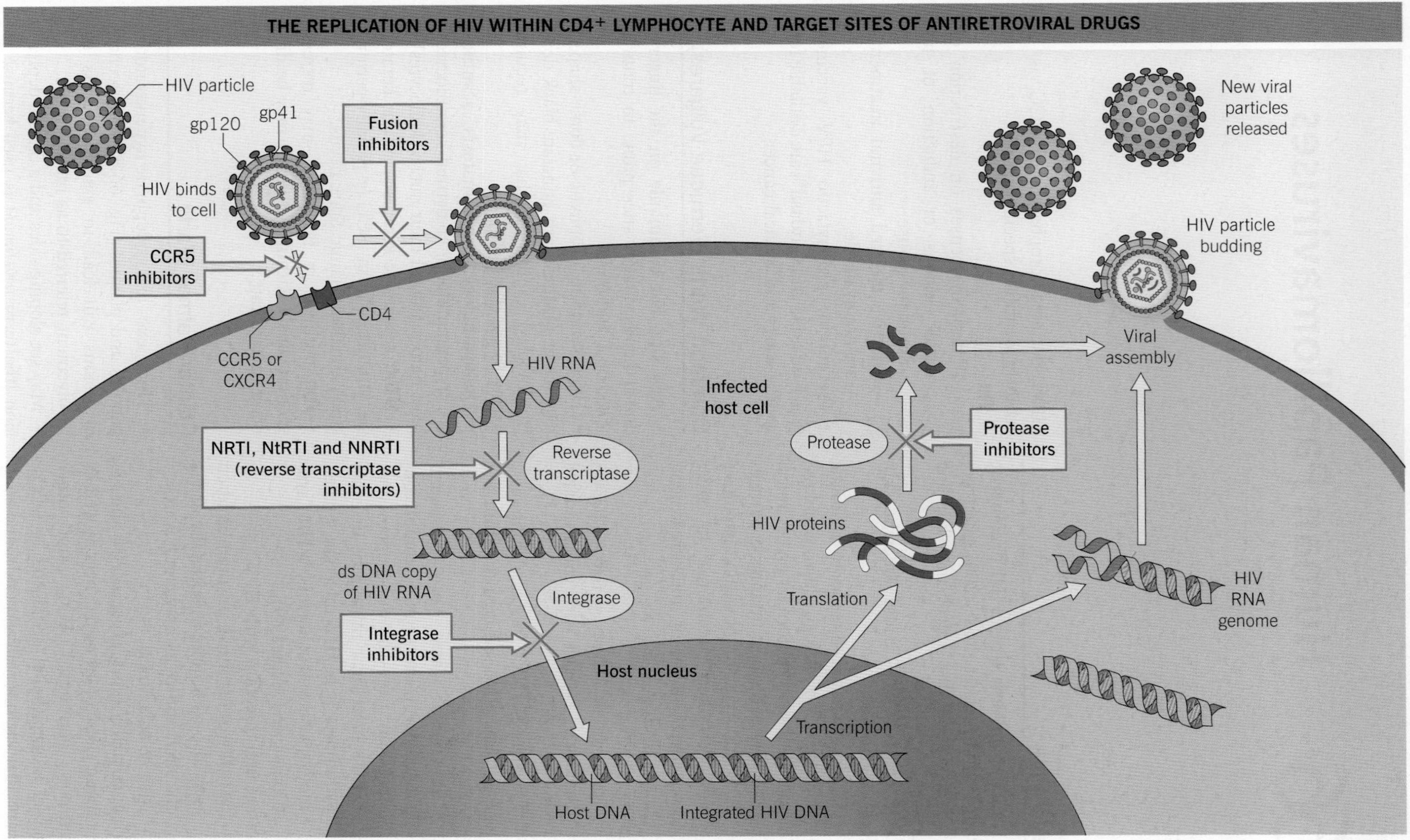

Fig. 65.16 Replication of HIV within CD4+ lymphocyte and target sites of antiretroviral drugs. CCR5, CC-chemokine receptor 5; NRTI, nucleoside reverse transcriptase inhibitor; NtRTI, nucleotide reverse transcriptase inhibitor; NNRTI, non-nucleoside reverse transcriptase inhibitor.

CUTANEOUS MANIFESTATIONS OF HIV INFECTION

66 | Human Papillomaviruses

Key Points

• Human papilloma viruses (HPV) comprise a large group of at least 200 genotypes of DNA viruses that infect the skin and mucosa.
• Different genotypes cause different skin lesions (Table 66.1).
  – Clinical variants differ as to anatomic location, morphology, histopathology, and HPV subtype; correlation of clinical and histopathologic findings is particularly important for bowenoid papulosis and verrucous carcinoma in order to prevent over- or undertreatment, respectively.
• Nongenital warts.
  – Transmitted via person-to-person contact or contact with contaminated surfaces/objects.
  – Prevalence of 20% in schoolchildren.
  – A third or more self-regress within 1–2 years.
  – Numerous warts or persistent/progressive warts should prompt consideration of immunosuppression, defects in cellular immunity, or other syndromes [e.g. HIV infection, epidermodysplasia verruciformis, WHIM syndrome (see Chapter 49)].
• Anogenital infection with HPV.
  – Sexually transmitted; in young children may also be acquired perinatally or via the same routes as nongenital warts.
  – May be subclinical.
• High-risk HPV types, especially 16 and 18, are a major cause of cervical cancer as well as cutaneous (periungual SCC) and other mucosal intraepithelial neoplasias or SCCs, in particular vaginal, vulvar, penile, and anal;

HPV-associated oropharyngeal SCC is a recently identified specific subtype.
• **Rx**.
  – If desired, focuses on destruction of visible lesions or induction of an immune response.
  – Effective targeted antiviral treatments are not available.
• Prevention: prophylactic HPV vaccines (e.g. Cervarix® and Gardasil®) are available for genital warts and cervical cancer.

Common Warts (Verrucae Vulgares)

• Any site, but commonly on the fingers, dorsal hands, and/or sites prone to trauma (Figs. 66.1 and 66.2).
• Hyperkeratotic, exophytic or dome-shaped papules or plaques with punctate black dots (thrombosed capillaries) that may require paring to see (Fig. 66.3).
• Histopathology: papillomatosis, acanthosis, hypergranulosis; epidermal keratinocytes have haloes around their nuclei (koilocytes).
• **DDx:** seborrheic keratosis, actinic keratosis, cutaneous horn, SCC (especially periungual), trichilemmoma, Spitz nevus.
• **Rx:** outlined in Fig. 66.4; may regress spontaneously within 1–2 years; may be difficult to eradicate.

Plantar/Palmar Warts

• Thick, exo- and endophytic hyperkeratotic papules and plaques (Fig. 66.5); coalescence of lesions can lead to extensive areas of involvement referred to as mosaic warts.
• May see sloping sides and a central depression (the term *myrmecia* is used because it

CLINICAL MANIFESTATIONS OF COMMON HUMAN PAPILLOMAVIRUS (HPV) TYPES	
Skin Lesions	**Frequently Detected HPV Type**
Common, palmar, plantar, myrmecial warts	1, 2, 4
Flat warts	3, 10
Epidermodysplasia verruciformis	5, 8* > others (e.g. 9, 20)
Condylomata acuminata (anogenital warts)	6, 11
High-grade squamous intraepithelial neoplasia (cervical lesions, bowenoid papulosis, erythroplasia of Queyrat)	16, 18, 31, 33 > others (e.g. 35)
Cervical cancer	16, 18

*Oncogenic, like HPV types 16, 18.

Table 66.1 Clinical manifestations of common human papillomavirus (HPV) types. In clinical practice, subtyping is generally only performed routinely on Papanicolaou smears. Subtyping does not usually change management of cutaneous lesions.

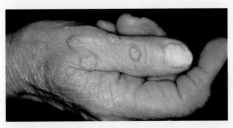

Fig. 66.1 Verrucae vulgares (common warts).
Courtesy, A. Geusau, MD.

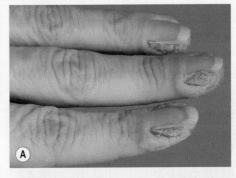

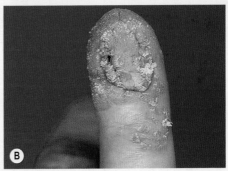

Fig. 66.2 Periungual common warts.
Destruction of the nail matrix and bed can lead to partial **(A)** or complete **(B)** absence of the nail plate. Bowen's disease may be considered in the differential diagnosis, especially for a single, recalcitrant digital wart. *A, B, Courtesy, Reinhard Kirnbauer, MD, and Petra Lenz, MD.*

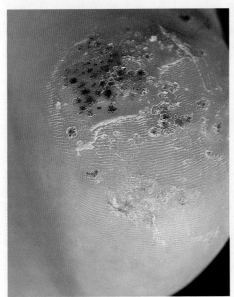

Fig. 66.3 Verrucae plantares (plantar warts).
The photo was taken after shaving of the hyperkeratotic surface; the black dots represent thrombosed capillaries. *Courtesy, Reinhard Kirnbauer, MD, and Petra Lenz, MD.*

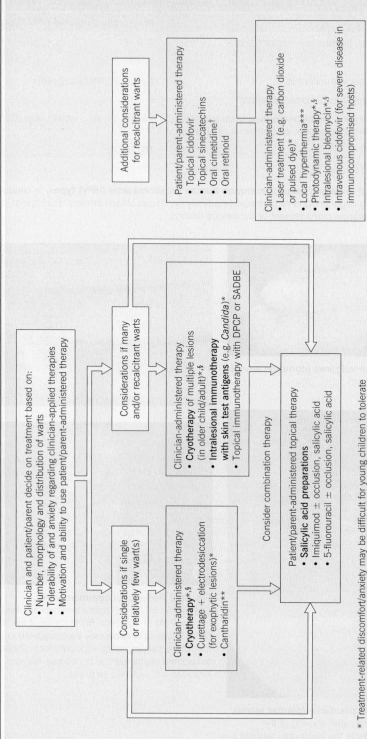

Fig. 66.4 Treatment of common warts. Therapies found to be effective in controlled trials are in bold. DPCP, diphenylcyclopropenone; SADBE, squaric acid dibutyl ester.

TREATMENT OF COMMON WARTS

Clinician and patient/parent decide on treatment based on:
- Number, morphology and distribution of warts
- Tolerability of and anxiety regarding clinician-applied therapies
- Motivation and ability to use patient/parent-administered therapy

Considerations if single or relatively few wart(s)

Clinician-administered therapy
- **Cryotherapy***,§
- Curettage + electrodesiccation (for exophytic lesions)*
- Cantharidin**

Considerations if many and/or recalcitrant warts

Clinician-administered therapy
- **Cryotherapy** of multiple lesions (in older child/adult)*,§
- **Intralesional immunotherapy with skin test antigens** (e.g. *Candida*)*
- Topical immunotherapy with DPCP or SADBE

Consider combination therapy

Patient/parent-administered topical therapy
- **Salicylic acid preparations**
- Imiquimod ± occlusion, salicylic acid
- 5-fluorouracil ± occlusion, salicylic acid

Additional considerations for recalcitrant warts

Patient/parent-administered therapy
- Topical cidofovir
- Topical sinecatechins
- Oral cimetidine†
- Oral retinoid

Clinician-administered therapy
- Laser treatment (e.g. carbon dioxide or pulsed dye)*
- Local hyperthermia***
- Photodynamic therapy*,§
- Intralesional bleomycin*,§
- Intravenous cidofovir (for severe disease in immunocompromised hosts)

* Treatment-related discomfort/anxiety may be difficult for young children to tolerate
** Higher likelihood of "doughnut" wart formation; may be combined with podophyllotoxin and salicylic acid
§ Results in controlled trials have been inconsistent
† Randomized controlled trials did not demonstrate efficacy
*** 44°C/111°F for 30 minutes on days 1, 2, 3, 17 and 18

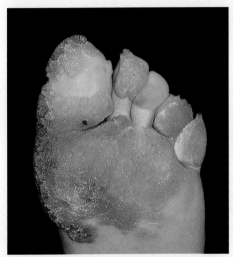

Fig. 66.5 Extensive and chronic verrucosis of the sole causing pain when walking. HPV-2a was isolated from the lesion of this otherwise immunocompetent and healthy patient. *Courtesy, Reinhard Kirnbauer, MD, and Petra Lenz, MD.*

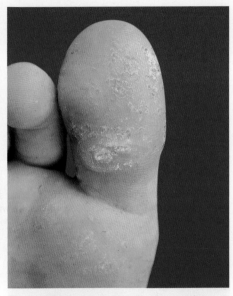

Fig. 66.6 Myrmecial wart. The wart at the base of the distal phalanx of the hallux is painful due to deep endophytic growth; in addition, there are confluent plaques of superficial warts (mosaic warts). *Courtesy, Reinhard Kirnbauer, MD, and Petra Lenz, MD.*

can resemble an anthill); tender with pressure (Fig. 66.6).
• **DDx:** corns (clavi; see Chapter 74), punctate palmoplantar keratoderma (see Table 47.1), arsenical keratoses, SCC, amelanotic melanoma.
• **Rx:** overlaps with Rx of common warts (see Fig. 66.4).

Flat Warts (Verrucae Planae)

• Commonly on the dorsal hands, arms, and face, as well as the legs (exacerbated by shaving).
• Skin-colored to pink or brown (sometimes hypopigmented in darker skin), minimally elevated papules; the surface is smooth and often flat-topped (Fig. 66.7).
• **DDx:** small seborrheic keratoses, common warts, Gottron's papules of dermatomyositis, lichen nitidus, lichen planus, acrokeratosis verruciformis (see Chapter 48), epidermodysplasia verruciformis (see below).
• **Rx**.
  – If a few lesions, destructive or ablative therapies (e.g. cryosurgery, trichloroacetic acid; see Fig. 66.4).

  – If numerous, topical application of irritants (e.g. retinoids), immunotherapy (see Fig. 66.4), topical 5-fluorouracil.

Oral Warts

• Buccal, gingival, and labial mucosae as well as tongue and hard palate (Fig. 66.8).
• Small, soft, mucosal-colored to white, slightly elevated papillomatous papules.
• **DDx:** Heck's disease (focal epithelial hyperplasia; multiple white to pink sessile papules; secondary to HPV types 13 and 32), early SCC, verrucous proliferative leukoplakia, bite fibroma.

Condylomata Acuminata

• Involve primarily the anogenital region.
• Range from discrete, sessile, smooth-surfaced papillomas to large cauliflower-like lesions (Figs. 66.9 and 66.10).
• Skin-colored to pink to brown.
• If present in children, especially those >3 years of age, the possibility of sexual abuse should be considered (see Chapter 75).

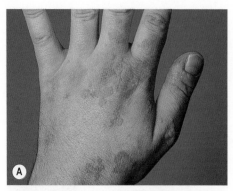

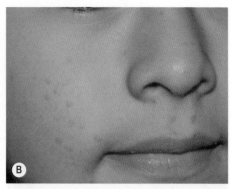

Fig. 66.7 Verrucae planae (flat warts). Multiple skin-colored or pink **(A)** to brown **(B)** smooth-surfaced, flat-topped papules. These lesions are typically caused by HPV-3 or -10. *A, Courtesy, Reinhard Kirnbauer, MD, and Petra Lenz, MD; B, Courtesy, Julie V. Schaffer, MD.*

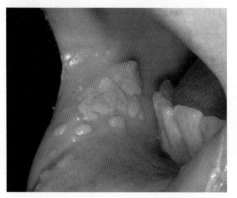

Fig. 66.8 Oral warts. Papillomas of the labial mucosa in a 6-year-old child. *Courtesy, Reinhard Kirnbauer, MD, and Petra Lenz, MD.*

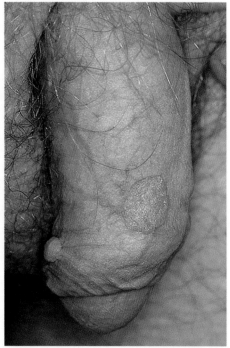

Fig. 66.9 Penile condylomata acuminata (genital warts). Both sessile and exophytic warts are present. *Courtesy, Reinhard Kirnbauer, MD, and Petra Lenz, MD.*

- **DDx:** seborrheic keratosis, skin tag, molluscum contagiosum, Bowenoid papulosis, SCC, pearly penile papules (see Chapter 95), free sebaceous glands, condyloma lata of secondary syphilis.
- **Rx:** outlined in Fig. 66.11.

Bowenoid Papulosis (Intraepithelial Neoplasia-3; High-Grade Squamous Intraepithelial Lesion)

- Similar to condylomata acuminata, primarily in the anogenital region.
- Multiple pink to red-brown smooth to warty papules or plaques (Fig. 66.12; see Fig. 60.9).

- Histopathology: numerous mitoses scattered throughout the epidermis (which distinguishes it from condyloma acuminatum); keratinocytes may show less atypia than in an SCC.
- **Rx:** outlined in Fig. 66.11.

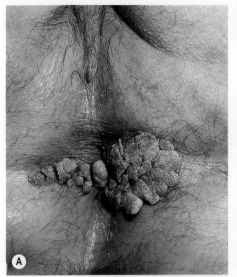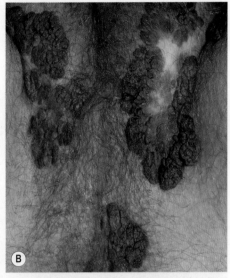

Fig. 66.10 Condylomata acuminata. A Perianal papillomas that are macerated due to moisture from occlusion. **B** Confluent lesions forming hyperpigmented plaques in the perineal region and along the inguinal fold. A depigmented scar is seen at the site of treatment with liquid nitrogen. *A, B, Courtesy, Reinhard Kirnbauer, MD, and Petra Lenz, MD.*

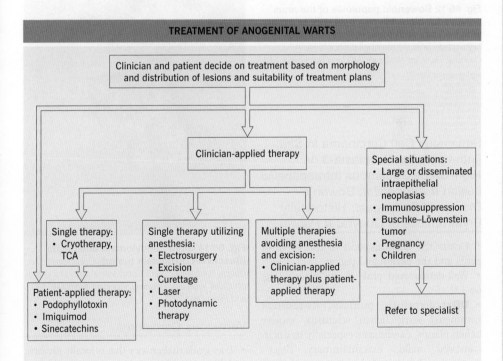

Fig. 66.11 Treatment of anogenital warts. TCA, trichloroacetic acid. *Courtesy, Reinhard Kirnbauer, MD, and Petra Lenz, MD.*

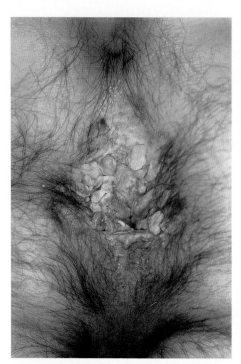

Fig. 66.12 Bowenoid papulosis of the anus positive for high-risk mucosal HPV in a man who had sex with men. Histology revealed high-grade anal intraepithelial neoplasia (AIN). *Courtesy, Reinhard Kirnbauer, MD, and Petra Lenz, MD.*

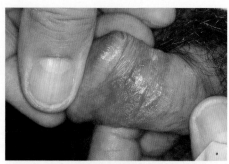

Fig. 66.13 Erythroplasia of Queyrat. A well-demarcated velvety plaque of the prepuce positive for high-risk HPV; histology detected a high-grade penile intraepithelial neoplasia (PIN). *Courtesy, Reinhard Kirnbauer, MD, and Petra Lenz, MD.*

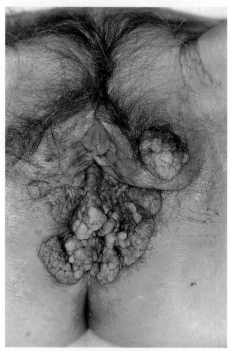

Fig. 66.14 Giant condylomata acuminata (Buschke–Löwenstein tumor). Cauliflower-like, deeply infiltrating giant condylomata acuminata in an older woman. *Courtesy, Reinhard Kirnbauer, MD, and Petra Lenz, MD.*

Squamous Cell Carcinoma *In Situ* (Intraepithelial Neoplasia-3 or High-Grade Squamous Intraepithelial Lesion *If Anogenital*; Bowen's Disease *If Periungual*; Historically Erythroplasia of Queyrat *If Penile*)

- Favors the glabrous skin of the vulva or penis and the periungual region.
- Well-demarcated pink to red plaque (Fig. 66.13).
- **DDx:** dermatitis, psoriasis, Rx-resistant periungual wart, lichen sclerosus, erosive lichen planus, candidiasis especially in uncircumcised male, extramammary Paget's disease, Zoon's balantis, amelanotic melanoma.
- **Rx:** excision, Mohs surgery, or other destructive modalities depending on patient/lesion characteristics; imiquimod with careful re-evaluation.

Verrucous Carcinoma

- Low-grade malignancy that is locally invasive and destructive, but rarely metastasizes; lesions can attain a large size when left untreated.
- Major types.
  - Buschke–Löwenstein tumor (Fig. 66.14) – anogenital region; fistulas and/or abscesses may be present.

– Oral florid papillomatosis – oral mucosa or perinasal sinuses – pebbly confluence of whitish papillomas.

– Epithelioma cuniculatum – plantar surface – irregularly shaped, well-demarcated, verrucous nodule, often several centimeters in diameter.

• **Rx:** excision.

Epidermodysplasia Verruciformis (EDV)

• Cutaneous infection with particular HPV types in patients with an inherited predisposition [mutations in *TMC6* (*EVER1*), *TMC8* (*EVER2*)] or acquired immunosuppression (e.g. HIV infection); see Table 66.1.

• Widespread lesions that begin to appear during childhood (inherited form), with a predisposition for sun-exposed areas.

• Lesions vary in color from white to pink to brown and can resemble flat warts or tinea versicolor (Fig. 66.15).

• Distinctive histopathology with expanded gray-blue cytoplasm within the keratinocytes of the upper stratum spinosum.

• Increased risk of SCC, especially in sun-exposed areas.

• **Rx:** difficult (similar to that for flat warts), sun protective measures, address immunosuppression in acquired cases.

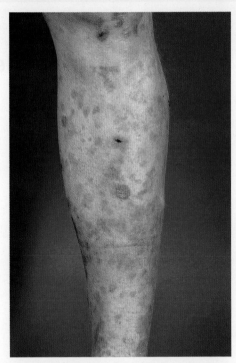

Fig. 66.15 Epidermodysplasia verruciformis. Generalized erythematous macules and plaques are seen. Lesions tested positive for HPV-8 and -36. *Courtesy, Reinhard Kirnbauer, MD, and Petra Lenz, MD.*

For further information see Ch. 79. From *Dermatology, Third Edition.*

67 | Human Herpesviruses

General

• Human herpesviruses (HHV) are a family of double-stranded DNA viruses (8 members) with a lipid envelope.

• All share the ability to establish lifelong latency in their host following primary infection.

• Basic pathogenesis of HHV infections involves a sequence of primary infection, establishment of latency, reactivation, and recurrent (secondary) infection.

• Clinical presentations depend on the host's age, anatomic location, immune status, and ethnicity (e.g. EBV).

• Spread of infection is usually the result of contact with bodily secretions containing the virus.

• Asymptomatic shedding of virus is common.

Herpes Simplex Viruses (HSV-1/ HHV-1 and HSV-2/HHV-2)

• Ubiquitous pathogens that produce primarily orolabial (HSV-1 > HSV-2) and genital infections (HSV-2 > HSV-1) characterized by recurrent vesicular eruptions (Table 67.1).

• *Transmission* can occur during both symptomatic and asymptomatic periods of viral shedding.

• *Reactivation* can occur either spontaneously or due to an appropriate stimulus (e.g. stress, UVR, fever, tissue trauma, or immunosuppression).

• A wide range of clinical presentations exist, with asymptomatic infection being the most common.

• In *primary infection*.
  – Onset is usually 3–7 days after exposure.
  – *Generalized prodrome* (before the onset of mucocutaneous lesions) of tender lymphadenopathy, fever, and malaise; localized pain, burning, and tenderness.

– Initial lesions: small round vesicles on an erythematous base; often painful or burning; the grouping of these vesicles is a clue to the diagnosis; vesicles may become umbilicated or pustular, followed by erosions or ulcerations with hemorrhagic crusts, often with a scalloped border; lesions resolve over 2–6 weeks (Fig. 67.1).

• In *reactivation infection*.
  – *Localized prodrome* of dysesthesia (e.g. burning/tingling, pain, pruritus) and tenderness.
  – Mucocutaneous lesions similar as in primary but fewer in number, less severe, and shorter duration (Fig. 67.2).

• In addition to the classic orolabial and genital infections, HSV can cause other infections (Table 67.2; Figs. 67.3–67.7).

• **DDx** and Dx: see Table 67.1 and Fig. 67.8.

• **Rx:** outlined in Table 67.3.

Varicella–Zoster Virus (VZV or HHV-3)

• **Primary varicella infection (chickenpox)**.
  – Usually self-limited in otherwise healthy children but more severe with more numerous lesions and a greater risk for complications in adults (including pregnant women) and immunocompromised individuals (Table 67.4; Fig. 67.9).

• **Herpes zoster (shingles) – reactivation of VZV**.
  – Incidence, severity, and risk of complications increase significantly with age and immunosuppression due to a decline in specific cell-mediated immune response to VZV.
  – Reactivation results in a sensory neuritis and painful neuralgia, followed by a

MAJOR CLINICAL FEATURES OF CLASSIC HERPES SIMPLEX VIRUS (HSV) OROLABIAL AND GENITAL INFECTIONS

Mucocutaneous HSV Infection	Primary Infection*	Reactivation Infection*	DDx
Orolabial HSV (HSV1 > HSV2) Latency is established in the neuronal cells of dorsal root ganglia, especially trigeminal	• Asymptomatic infection most common • Gingivostomatitis primarily in children <10 years of age (Fig. 67.1A) • Pharyngitis and mononucleosis-like syndrome in young adults • Dysphagia and drooling may occur	• Favors vermilion border of lips (Fig. 67.2A) and occurs less commonly in the perioral region and cheek, nasal mucosa, and hard mucosa (i.e. mucosa overlying bone) such as the hard palate and gingivae (Fig. 67.2B) • In immunocompromised hosts, can see on the soft mucosa, e.g. buccal mucosa and soft palate	**Vermilion lips/perioral** • Impetigo • Coxsackie infection (also intraoral) • EM major or SJS (also intraoral) **Intraoral** • Aphthous stomatitis • Pharyngitis (e.g. EBV)/herpangina • Drug-induced mucositis
Genital HSV (HSV2 > HSV1) Latency is established in the neuronal cells of dorsal root ganglia, especially sacral	• Seropositive persons often report no history of primary genital infection • Frequently presents with excruciatingly painful erosive balanitis, vulvitis, or vaginitis • In males typically involves the glans or shaft of the penis • In **females** can also involve cervix, buttocks, and perineum with associated dysuria, urinary retention, and inguinal lymphadenopathy (Fig. 67.1C)	• Usually a subclinical presentation • Typically a limited number of grouped vesicles* occur on the genitalia or buttocks (especially in females) (Fig. 67.2B,C) • Frequency of recurrence correlates with the severity of the primary infection	• Trauma • EBV infection • Aphthae • Syphilitic chancre • Chancroid • Lymphogranuloma venereum

Diagnosis is made at the bedside by either (1) performance of a Tzanck smear (see Fig. 2.7; results in minutes); DFA or PCR (Fig. 67.8; results in hours); or viral culture (results in days) or (2) performing a skin biopsy for H&E staining (see Fig. 2.6; results in days). *~90% of U.S. adults are seropositive for HSV-1 and ~25–30% are seropositive for HSV-2, with an increasing seroprevalence for the latter. Treatment is outlined in Table 67.3.*

*For the description of typical lesions, see text; occasionally, intact vesicles are not seen but rather grouped ulcerations with hemorrhagic crusts predominate. In immunocompromised hosts it is prudent to request testing for HSV-1, HSV-2, and VZV, as clinical presentations are often atypical.

EM, erythema multiforme; SJS, Stevens–Johnson syndrome; DFA, direct fluorescent antibody; H&E, hematoxylin and eosin.

Table 67.1 Major clinical features of classic herpes simplex virus (HSV) orolabial and genital infections. ~90% of U.S. adults are seropositive for HSV-1 and ~25–30% are seropositive for HSV-2, with an increasing seroprevalence for the latter. Treatment is outlined in Table 67.3.

HUMAN HERPESVIRUSES

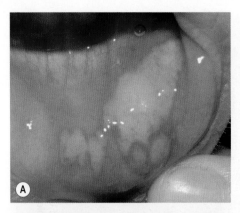

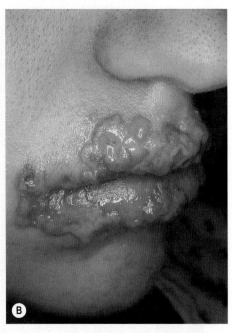

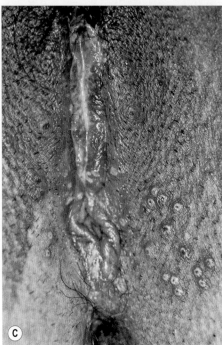

Fig. 67.1 Primary herpes simplex virus (HSV) infections. A Primary herpes gingivostomatitis due to HSV-1 in a child. Note the coalescing lesions with scalloped borders. **B** HSV-2 infection in a teenager (primary vs. non-primary initial infection). Note the scalloped borders. **C** Primary genital HSV infection. In addition to 1- to 2-mm hemorrhagic crusts, there are perifollicular vesicopustules. *A, Courtesy, Julie V. Schaffer, MD; B, Courtesy, Jean L. Bolognia, MD; C, Courtesy, Stephen K. Tyring, MD.*

dermatomal vesicular eruption; clinical course is outlined in Table 67.4 (Figs. 67.10–67.12).

– Exposure of a susceptible person to an individual with chickenpox or zoster can lead to primary varicella but not zoster.

– **Rx:** early antiviral treatment (within 72 hours of the onset of the first vesicle) is ideal, but initiation after 72 hours but within 7 days may also be helpful (see Table 67.3).

– **Selected complications of herpes zoster:**

1. **Disseminated zoster.**
   • Defined as >20 vesicles outside the area of the primary or adjacent dermatomes.

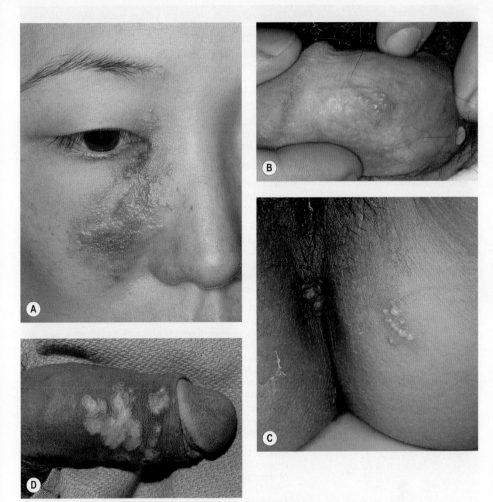

Fig. 67.2 Reactivation of herpes simplex virus (HSV) infections. A Recurrent HSV-1 infection on the cheek. Occasionally such lesions are misdiagnosed as cellulitis or bullous impetigo. **B** Intact grouped vesicles on the penis. Note the genital wart at the base of the penis. **C** Grouped vesiculopustules on the buttock, a common location in women. **D** Healing ulcerations with scalloped borders on the penis. *A, Courtesy, Kalman Watsky, MD; B, C, Courtesy, Louis A. Fragola, Jr., MD; D, Courtesy, Joseph L. Jorizzo, MD.*

- Implies viremia and an increased risk for visceral or CNS involvement (see Table 67.4).
- Requires intravenous acyclovir.
2. **Post-herpetic neuralgia (PHN) and post-herpetic itch (PHI)**.
    - Affects 10–15% of patients; incidence and severity increase with age.
    - Characterized by persistent pain, dysesthesia (PHN) or pruritus (PHI) along the affected dermatome for weeks to years after the resolution of the eruption.
    - **Rx:** gabapentin, tricyclic antidepressants (e.g. amitriptyline, nortriptyline); topical agents (e.g. lidocaine patch, capsaicin); oral analgesics (e.g. ibuprofen, opioids).
    - Note that opioids are typically ineffective or even aggravating in patients with PHI.

MAJOR CLINICAL FEATURES OF OTHER HERPES SIMPLEX VIRUS (HSV) INFECTIONS

HSV Infection	Major Clinical Features
Eczema herpeticum (Kaposi's varicelliform eruption [KVE])	• Widespread eruption of HSV, usually occurring in association with skin conditions that disrupt the epidermal barrier (e.g. atopic dermatitis, burns, Darier disease) (Fig. 67.3); DDx includes infections with coxsackievirus or *Streptococcus*
Herpetic whitlow	• HSV infection of the digit(s) (Fig. 67.4); most often seen in children; in the past was common in healthcare workers who did not wear gloves
Herpes gladiatorum	• Occurs in contact sports (e.g. wrestling) (Fig. 67.5)
HSV folliculitis	• Uncommon; most often seen in patients who shave with a blade razor (e.g. herpes sycosis in the beard region) or in immunocompromised hosts
HSV in immunocompromised hosts (e.g. HIV (+), solid organ and hematopoietic stem cell transplant recipients, leukemia and lymphoma patients)	• May present with chronic or atypical mucocutaneous presentations (e.g. multiple sites; disseminated lesions; verrucous, exophytic or pustular lesions; Fig. 67.6) • Most common presentation is a chronic, enlarging ulceration; in the buttock area may be misdiagnosed as a pressure ulcer (Fig. 67.6D)
Ocular HSV	• Most often acquired in newborns during the vaginal birthing process • *Primary infection:* typically presents as unilateral or bilateral keratoconjunctivitis, eyelid edema, tearing, photophobia, chemosis, and preauricular lymphadenopathy; with *recurrent infection* usually unilateral and may be confused with a contact dermatitis or periocular cellulitis • Potential complications: corneal ulceration, scarring • Pathognomonic finding: branching, dendritic lesions of the corneal epithelium
Neonatal HSV	• Greatest risk of transmission (30–50%) from infected mother to neonate is among women with first episode of genital HSV near the time of delivery; lowest risk (<3%) is among women with recurrent genital HSV • Significant morbidity and mortality in affected infants, especially if disseminated disease • Clinical presentations vary (Fig. 67.7 and see Chapter 28)
Herpes encephalitis	• *No* cutaneous manifestations • Most common cause of sporadic, fatal viral encephalitis in the U.S.

Table 67.2 Major clinical features of other herpes simplex virus (HSV) infections. Treatment is outlined in Table 67.3.

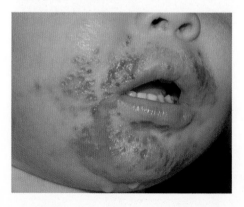

Fig. 67.3 Eczema herpeticum. Monomorphic, punched-out erosions with a scalloped border in this infant with a history of facial atopic dermatitis. *Courtesy, Julie V. Schaffer, MD.*

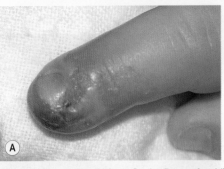
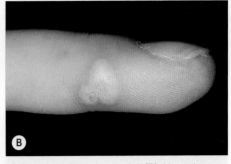

Fig. 67.4 Herpetic whitlow. On the finger of a child **(A)** and on the finger in an adult **(B).** Herpetic whitlow is sometimes misdiagnosed as cellulitis or blistering dactylitis, or, depending on the distribution, paronychia. *B, Courtesy, Eugene Mirrer, MD.*

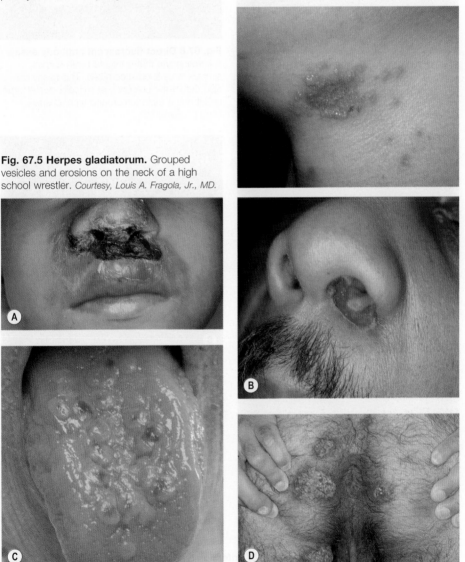

Fig. 67.5 Herpes gladiatorum. Grouped vesicles and erosions on the neck of a high school wrestler. *Courtesy, Louis A. Fragola, Jr., MD.*

Fig. 67.6 Herpes simplex viral infections in immunocompromised hosts. A Enlarging ulcerations in a child with acute lymphocytic leukemia who was presumed to have a *Rhizopus* infection, and **(B)** in a young man with AIDS. **C** Coalescence of eroded, yellow-white papules and plaques on the tongue. **D** Chronic perianal ulcerations in an HIV-infected male. *D, From Callen JP, Jorizzo JL, et al. Dermatological Signs of Internal Disease, 4th edn.; Saunders/Elsevier, 2009.*

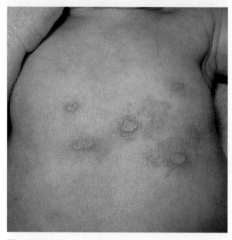

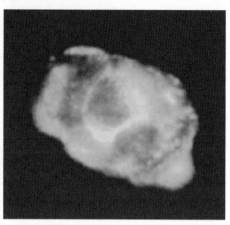

Fig. 67.7 Neonatal herpes. Grouped papulovesicles with an erythematous base on the chest. Note the scalloped borders in areas of coalescence. *Courtesy, Frank Samarin, MD.*

Fig. 67.8 Direct fluorescent antibody assay. A keratinocyte that is infected with herpes simplex virus fluoresces green. This assay can also detect the presence of varicella–zoster virus and it has a rapid turnaround time. *Courtesy, Marie L. Landry, MD.*

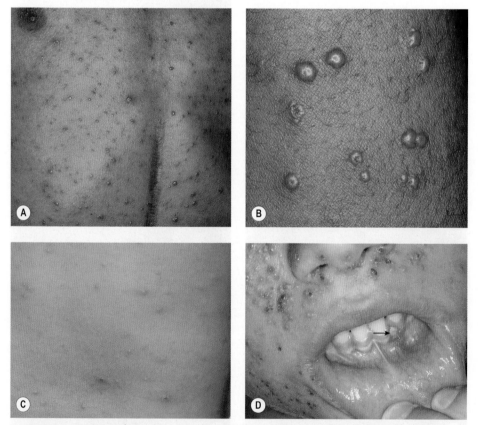

Fig. 67.9 Primary varicella–zoster virus (VZV) infection (varicella or chickenpox). Widespread lesions in different stages of evolution **(A).** Vesicles often develop central umbilication **(B)** and some lesions become pustular **(C).** Note the dermatographism related to scratching **(C).** Oral lesions can also occur **(D).** *A, B, Courtesy, Robert Hartman, MD; C, Courtesy, Julie V. Schaffer, MD; D, Courtesy, Judit Stenn, MD.*

3. **Ocular involvement** (see Fig. 67.10F).
   - Occurs in ~10% of patients, with 20–70% developing ocular disease (occasionally blindness).
   - Due to VZV reactivation in the first division of the trigeminal nerve (V1).
   - Clues to its diagnosis include lesions in the V1 distribution (see Fig. 67.11), which may be accompanied by unilateral eye pain or conjunctivitis.
   - *Hutchinson's sign* is the presence of vesicles at the tip, side, or bridge of the nose, indicating involvement of the nasociliary branch of the trigeminal nerve, which also innervates the cornea.
   - Initial and longitudinal evaluation by ophthalmology is required.

4. **Ramsay–Hunt syndrome (herpes zoster oticus)**.
   - Due to VZV reactivation in the geniculate ganglion.
   - Clues to its diagnosis: vesicles in the ear canal, tongue, and/or hard palate.

- Patients may have severe ear pain, acute facial nerve paralysis, and/or taste loss of the anterior two-thirds of the tongue.
- If the vestibulocochlear nerve is also affected, may have tinnitus, hearing loss, or vertigo.
- Consider referral to otolaryngology.

Epstein–Barr Virus (EBV or HHV-4)

- Table 67.5 and Figs. 67.13 and 67.14.

Cytomegalovirus (CMV or HHV-5)

- Table 67.6 and Fig. 67.15.

Human Herpesvirus 6 and 7 (HHV-6 and HHV-7)

- Table 67.7 and Fig. 67.16.

Human Herpesvirus 8 (Kaposi's Sarcoma-Associated Herpesvirus [KSHV])

- Table 67.8 and Fig. 67.17.

For further information see Ch. 80. From *Dermatology, Third Edition*.

ANTIVIRAL THERAPY FOR HERPES SIMPLEX VIRUS AND VARICELLA–ZOSTER VIRUS INFECTIONS	
Disease Context	**Drug and Dosage**
Herpes Simplex Infections	
Orolabial herpes* (recurrence)	Penciclovir: 1% cream applied q2h × 4 days Acyclovir + hydrocortisone: 5%/1% cream applied 5×/day × 5 days Famciclovir: 1.5 g PO × 1 dose Valacyclovir: 2 g PO BID × 1 day
Genital herpes (first episode)	Acyclovir: 200 mg PO 5×/day × 10 days or 400 mg PO TID × 10 days Famciclovir: 250 mg PO TID × 10 days Valacyclovir: 1 g PO BID × 10 days
Genital herpes (recurrence)	Acyclovir: 400 mg PO TID × 5 days or 800 mg PO BID × 5 days or 800 mg PO TID × 2 days Famciclovir: 1 g PO BID × 1 day or 500 mg PO × 1 dose then 250 mg PO BID × 2 days or 125 mg PO BID × 5 days Valacyclovir: 500 mg PO BID × 3 days or 1 g PO daily × 5 days

Table 67.3 Antiviral therapy for herpes simplex virus and varicella–zoster virus infections. *Continued*

Table 67.3 *Continued* **Antiviral therapy for herpes simplex virus and varicella–zoster virus infections.**

Disease Context	Drug and Dosage
Chronic suppression	Acyclovir: 400 mg PO BID Famciclovir: 250 mg PO BID Valacyclovir: 500 mg PO daily for <10 outbreaks/year or 1 g PO daily for ≥10 outbreaks/year
Neonatal	Acyclovir: 20 mg/kg iv q8 h × 14–21 days
Immunocompromised	Recommend use until all mucocutaneous lesions are healed Acyclovir: 400 mg PO 5×/day or 5 mg/kg (if age ≥12 years) to 10 mg/kg (if age <12 years) iv q8h Famciclovir: 500 mg PO BID Valacyclovir: 1 g PO BID
Eczema herpeticum/ Kaposi's varicelliform eruption	Recommend use for 10–14 days or (especially if immunocompromised) until all mucocutaneous lesions are healed Acyclovir: 15 mg/kg (400 mg max) PO 3–5×/day or, if severe, 5 mg/kg (if age ≥12 years) to 10 mg/kg (if age <12 years) iv q8h Famciclovir: 500 mg PO BID Valacyclovir: 1 g PO BID
Genital herpes, recurrent in the setting of HIV infection	Recommend use until all mucocutaneous lesions are healed Acyclovir: 400 mg PO TID Famciclovir: 500 mg PO BID Valacyclovir: 1 g PO BID
Chronic suppression in the setting of HIV infection	Acyclovir: 400–800 mg PO BID–TID Famciclovir: 500 mg PO BID Valacyclovir: 500 mg PO BID
Acyclovir-resistant HSV in immunocompromised patients	Foscarnet: 40 mg/kg iv q8–12h × 2–3 weeks (or until all lesions are healed) Cidofovir: 1% cream or gel daily × 2–3 weeks or (for severe disease) 5 mg/kg iv weekly × 2 weeks then every other week (together with probenecid)
Varicella–Zoster Virus Infections	
Varicella	Acyclovir: 20 mg/kg (800 mg max) PO QID × 5 days Valacyclovir[†]: 20 mg/kg (1 g max) PO TID × 5 days
Zoster	Acyclovir: 800 mg PO 5×/day × 7–10 days Famciclovir: 500 mg PO TID × 7 days Valacyclovir: 1 g PO TID × 7 days
Immunocompromised	Acyclovir: 10 mg/kg (500 mg/m^2) iv q8h × 7–10 days *or until cropping has ceased* (depending on the setting, consider continuing until lesions are healed)

Indications for and efficacy of antiviral treatment for initial episodes of orolabial herpes in immunocompetent adults have not been defined, but the regimens used for initial genital episodes can be considered in individuals with severe disease; acyclovir 15 mg/kg (200 mg max) PO 5×/day × 7 days (initiated within 3 days of disease onset) has been shown to be beneficial in young children with primary herpes gingivostomatitis.

†*FDA-approved for ages 2–17 years; pharmacies can compound valacyclovir tablets into an oral suspension (25 or 50 mg/ml).*

BID, twice daily; iv, intravenously; PO, orally; q2h, every 2 hours; daily, once a day; qid, four times a day; TID, three times a day.

MAJOR CLINICAL FEATURES OF VARICELLA–ZOSTER VIRUS (VZV) INFECTIONS

VZV Infection	Major Clinical Features	Complications (Also See Text)	DDx
Primary infection*: Varicella (chickenpox) Latency is established in the neuronal cells of dorsal root ganglia ~98% of adults worldwide are seropositive	• 11- to 20-day incubation period • *Generalized prodrome* of mild fever, malaise, and myalgia, followed by an eruption of erythematous, pruritic macules and papules that develop central vesicles ('dew drops on a rose petal') and then evolve into pustules and crusts (Fig. 67.9); lesions heal over 7–10 days • Favors scalp and face first, with progression to trunk, extremities, and sometimes oral mucosa (Fig. 67.9D) • **Hallmark**: lesions in all stages of development (Fig. 67.9A) • Affected individual is contagious via airborne droplets and contact with vesicular fluid (until all lesions have crusted over) • *Breakthrough varicella*: seen in previously immunized persons; characterized by a much milder course and often an atypical presentation, e.g. only a few papules or papulovesicles	***Immunocompetent host*** **Most common**: secondary bacterial infection (especially staphylococcal and streptococcal), scarring **Less common**: pneumonia **Rare**: CNS (e.g. Reye's syndrome, encephalitis); glomerulonephritis; optic neuritis; hepatitis **Congenital varicella**: associated with multiple fetal abnormalities as well as cutaneous scarring ***Immunocompromised host*** • Significant morbidity and mortality with more extensive, atypical eruptions (e.g. hemorrhagic, purpuric) and an increased likelihood of CNS and visceral involvement (lung, liver)	• Vesicular viral exanthems (e.g. coxsackievirus, ECHO) • PLEVA • Disseminated HSV*** • Rickettsialpox • Drug eruption • Scabies • Insect bites
Reactivation infection**: Zoster (shingles)	• *Localized (dermatomal) prodrome* of intense pain and dysesthesia, with subsequent development of cutaneous lesions • Painful grouped vesicles on erythematous bases, developing within a sensory dermatome (Figs. 67.10 and 67.11) • Most often on the trunk > face, neck, scalp, extremity • Typically self-limited in children and young adults • Occasionally localized dysesthesia but no cutaneous eruption ('zoster sine herpete')	***Immunocompetent host*** • Post-herpetic neuralgia (~10–15%) • Local: secondary bacterial infection; scarring; motor paralysis • Systemic (see below); occasionally pneumonitis • Ophthalmic zoster (Fig. 67.10F) • Ramsay–Hunt syndrome ***Immunocompromised host*** (Fig. 67.12) • More severe and unusual presentations (e.g. persistent and verrucous lesions or post-herpetic hyperhidrosis) • Disseminated disease • Visceral involvement: pneumonitis; meningoencephalitis; hepatitis	• Zosteriform HSV • Localized contact dermatitis • Bacterial skin infection (e.g. bullous impetigo, cellulitis)

Diagnosis is outlined in Table 67.1.

*Prevention is now a major focus: In the United States, all eligible children are recommended to receive the two-dose, live-attenuated VZV vaccine. Varicella IgG (VIG) given to immunocompromised hosts with first-time exposure; VIG given to neonates whose mothers became infected shortly before birth.

**Prevention is now a major focus in the United States and United Kingdom; The FDA has approved a one-time live-attenuated VZV vaccine for eligible persons older than 50 years (efficacy is ~50%).

***Especially in immunocompromised hosts.

HSV, herpes simplex virus; ECHO, enteric cytopathic human orphan; PLEVA, pityriasis lichenoides et varioliformis acuta; DFA, direct fluorescent antibody; H&E, hematoxylin and eosin.

Table 67.4 Major clinical features of varicella–zoster virus (VZV) infections. Treatment is outlined in Table 67.3.

HUMAN HERPESVIRUSES

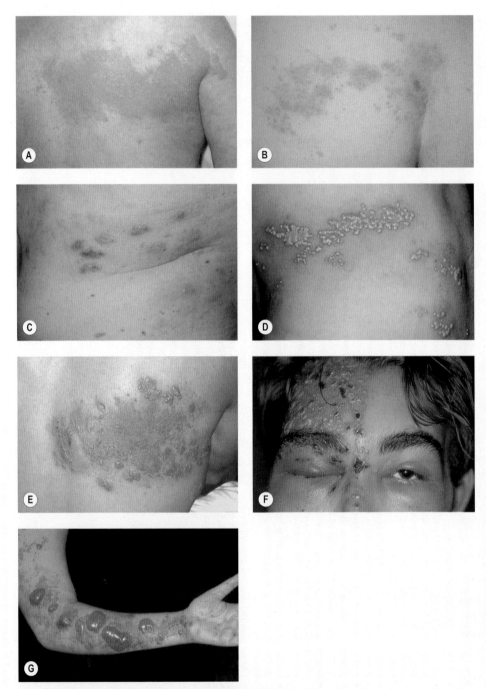

Fig. 67.10 Herpes zoster (shingles) infection. A–C Erythematous, edematous plaques with early vesicle formation. Note the perifollicular accentuation **(B)**. **D** and **E** Later stages of evolution with prominent pustule formation **(D)** and a dusky purple color associated with older vesicles **(E)**. **F** Ophthalmic zoster (V1) with sharp midline demarcation of erythema and crusts on the forehead as well as contralateral periorbital edema. **G** Bullous variant on the flexor arm. *B, Courtesy, Jean L. Bolognia, MD; D, Courtesy, Louis A. Fragola, Jr., MD.*

DISTRIBUTION OF DERMATOMES

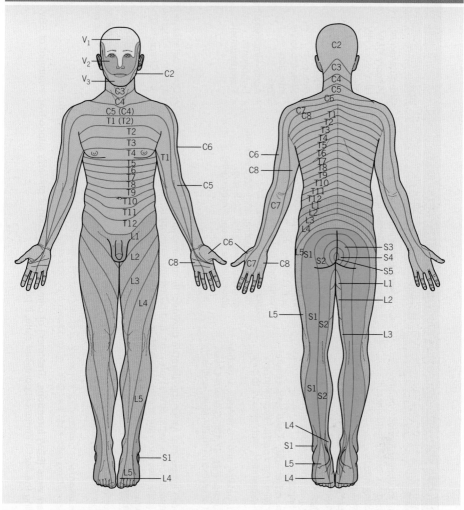

Fig. 67.11 Distribution of dermatomes.

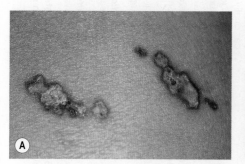

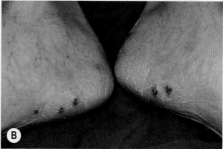

Fig. 67.12 Herpes zoster (shingles) in immunocompromised hosts. A Chronic verrucous zoster in an HIV-infected patient. **B** Disseminated cutaneous zoster with multiple violet-black papules on the feet. Patients with disseminated cutaneous skin lesions should be evaluated for possible CNS or visceral involvement, e.g. hepatic, pulmonary, especially if they are immunocompromised.

MAJOR CLINICAL FEATURES OF EPSTEIN-BARR VIRUS (EBV) INFECTIONS

EBV Infection	Major Clinical Features	Complications	DDx
Primary infection*: Infectious mononucleosis (IM) Latency is established in B lymphocytes ~95% of adults worldwide are seropositive	• Long, 30- to 50-day incubation period; usually asymptomatic in children, but symptomatic in adolescents and young adults • *Generalized prodrome* of headache, malaise, fatigue • *Classically*, ~80% present with triad of fever, pharyngitis, and lymphadenopathy • *Other clinical findings:* exudative tonsillitis, splenomegaly (50%), lymphocytosis with atypical lymphocytes, mild hepatitis • *Cutaneous eruption:* onset ~day 4 and lasts several days; most often a faint, nonspecific exanthem on trunk and proximal extremities, with spread to face and forearms • Occasionally eyelid, palatal, and cutaneous petechiae • Less often genital ulcers (Fig. 67.13), Gianotti–Crosti syndrome, urticaria > erythema multiforme, erythema nodosum	**Common, *not* serious:** antibiotic-induced hypersensitivity reaction (most often with penicillins or cephalosporins); this is not a true allergic reaction and typically safe for that patient to take the antibiotic in the future (Fig. 67.14) **Rare, but serious:** splenic rupture, especially post-traumatic; airway and oral compromise from oropharyngeal lymphoid tissue swelling **Other:** severe hepatitis; thrombocytopenia; hemolytic anemia; glomerulonephritis; CNS (e.g. encephalitis, aseptic meningitis)	**Oro-cutaneous** • Primary CMV, HHV-6, or HIV infections • Drug eruption (e.g. DRESS/DIHS) **Pharyngitis** • Group A *Streptococcus* infection **Other** • Acute viral hepatitis • Lymphoma • Toxoplasmosis
Reactivation infection**: EBV lymphoproliferative disorders	***In United States***: B-cell lymphoma; lymphoproliferative disorders in immunocompromised hosts (e.g. solid organ transplant recipients; HIV (+) infection; and taking immunosuppressive medications, classically methotrexate and/or infliximab in the setting of rheumatoid arthritis) ***Worldwide:*** Hydroa vacciniforme, necrotic hypersensitivity to mosquito bites, African (endemic) Burkitt's lymphoma, nasopharyngeal carcinoma		• Other cutaneous and systemic lymphomas (see Chapters 97–99)

*Diagnosis of suspected *primary EBV infection* is confirmed by a positive heterophile antibody test ('Monospot' test); if the heterophile antibody test is still suspected (e.g. early in the course of disease (≤6 weeks)) or in younger children (<2-years), then consider: repeat heterophile antibody testing, EBV-specific serologies, and/or EBV DNA levels.

Diagnosis of a suspected **EBV lymphoproliferative disorder is confirmed by the presence of elevated circulating EBV DNA levels.

DRESS, drug reaction with eosinophilia and systemic symptoms (also known as DIHS, drug-induced hypersensitivity syndrome); CMV, cytomegalovirus.

Table 67.5 Major clinical features of Epstein–Barr virus (EBV) infections. Treatment of primary EBV infection is primarily supportive; treatment of EBV lymphoproliferative disorders is focused on reversing the host's immunosuppressed state, if possible.

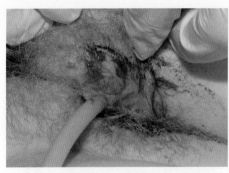

Fig. 67.13 Genital ulcers associated with primary EBV infection. Extreme pain with urination required placement of a Foley catheter in this 13-year-old girl. EBV-related genital ulcers are often misdiagnosed as a genital herpes simplex virus infection. *Courtesy, Julie V. Schaffer, MD.*

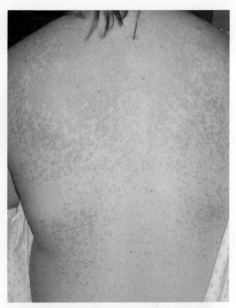

Fig. 67.14 Ampicillin-induced eruption in a patient with infectious mononucleosis due to Epstein–Barr virus infection. Erythematous macules and papules have become confluent on the upper trunk.

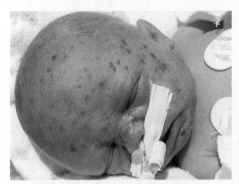

Fig. 67.15 TORCH syndrome due to cytomegalovirus. Multiple firm, red-violet papules of dermal erythropoiesis. *Courtesy, Mary S. Stone, MD.*

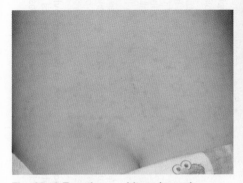

Fig. 67.16 Exanthem subitum (roseola infantum). Small pink-red macules and papules developed on the trunk and neck of this 9-month-old boy during defervescence of a high fever that lasted 5 days. *Courtesy, Julie V. Schaffer, MD.*

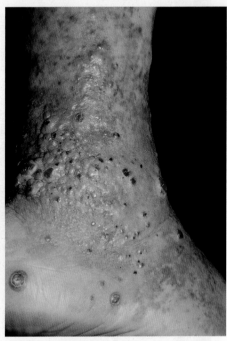

Fig. 67.17 Classic Kaposi's sarcoma. Multiple red-violet nodules with hemorrhagic crusting and plaques on the ankle and foot. *Courtesy, Joyce Rico, MD.*

MAJOR CLINICAL FEATURES OF CYTOMEGALOVIRUS (CMV) INFECTIONS

CMV Infection*	Major Clinical Features	Complications	DDx of Skin Lesions
Primary infection Latency is established primarily in monocytes and macrophages ~40–100% of adults are seropositive	• 4–8 week incubation period **Immunocompetent hosts** • >90% are subclinical and in children > adults • Occasionally (adults > children) presents as a mononucleosis-like syndrome; usually less severe, no exudative tonsillitis, and heterophile antibody (–); in those patients, ~33% have a morbilliform or petechial eruption **Congenital and neonates** • ~5–10% of infected neonates present with jaundice, IUGR, thrombocytopenia, chorioretinitis, and petechiae or the papules of extramedullary hematopoiesis ('blueberry muffin' lesions) (Fig. 67.15) **AIDS patients** • Chorioretinitis, esophagitis, colitis, pneumonitis • Rarely, chronic perineal and lower extremity ulcerations **Organ transplant recipients** • Gastrointestinal involvement and pneumonitis	**Immunocompetent hosts:** rarely colitis, encephalitis, myocarditis, and anterior uveitis **Congenital and neonates:** congenital deafness; mental retardation **AIDS patients:** blindness	**Immunocompetent hosts** • Other mononucleosis-like syndromes (e.g. EBV, HHV-6, toxoplasmosis) • Morbilliform drug eruption • Other causes of petechiae (see Chapter 18) **Congenital and neonates** • Other causes of TORCH
Reactivation infection	• May result from reactivation of latent CMV (greatest risk in immunosuppressed hosts) or from reinfection with a novel exogenous strain of CMV • Overall rare in immunocompetent hosts • Clinical presentations are similar to those described in primary CMV infections		

*Diagnosis is made via various techniques: (1) serologies (e.g. IgM and IgG antibodies); (2) various molecular amplification techniques (e.g. PCR); (3) cultures (helpful to determine if drug resistance is present); (4) CMV antigenemia assays (helpful in immunosuppressed hosts); (5) biopsy of cutaneous lesions (e.g. ulcerations) may show characteristic findings of enlarged endothelial cells with prominent intranuclear inclusions ('owl's eyes')
EBV, Epstein–Barr virus; IUGR, intrauterine growth retardation; TORCH, toxoplasmosis, other agents, rubella, cytomegalovirus, herpes simplex virus.

Table 67.6 Major clinical features of cytomegalovirus (CMV) infections. Treatment of uncomplicated CMV infection in immunocompetent hosts is primarily supportive; treatment in immunocompromised hosts or in those with complicated infections involves systemic therapy (e.g. intravenous ganciclovir, oral valganciclovir, cidofovir, foscarnet). Prevention is possible by matching CMV serologies between donor and transplant recipients.

	MAJOR CLINICAL FEATURES OF HUMAN HERPESVIRUS 6 AND 7 (HHV-6 AND HHV-7) INFECTIONS		
Infection	Primary Infection	Reactivation Infection	DDx
HHV-6* Latency is established in T lymphocytes ~70–90% of adults are seropositive	• Usually acquired between 6 months and 2 years of age • ~30% of children develop observable clinical manifestations • Febrile seizures may occur in infants **Clinical presentations** ***Exanthem subitum (roseola, sixth disease)*** • 3–5 days of high fever followed by cutaneous eruption as fever fades (Fig. 67.16) • Discrete circular 'rose red,' 2- to 5-mm macules or maculopapules, often surrounded by a white halo • Enanthem of red papules on soft palate (Nagayama's spots) • Late, may see palpebral edema ***Febrile syndrome without a cutaneous eruption*** ***Mononucleosis-like syndrome in adults***	• Seen primarily in immunosuppressed hosts • Fever, cutaneous eruption, hepatitis, pneumonitis, bone marrow suppression, encephalitis, colitis • Also implicated in DRESS/DIHS syndrome and possibly pityriasis rosea	***Exanthem subitum*** • Other viral exanthems (see Chapter 68); Kawasaki disease (if fever persists after appearance of eruption) **Mononucleosis-like syndrome** • EBV, CMV, toxoplasmosis
HHV-7** Latency is established in T lymphocytes ~85% of U.S. adults are seropositive	• Usually acquired in the first 5 years of life, peaking at about age 3 years • Usually asymptomatic • Can cause *exanthem subitum*, but is less common than HHV-6 • Potential complications include febrile seizures and acute hemiplegia	• Implicated in DRESS/DIHS syndrome and possibly pityriasis rosea	• See above, under *exanthem subitum*

*Diagnosis of HHV-6 is clinical in most cases of classic exanthema subitum in children; laboratory investigation with serologies and seroconversion data (e.g. IgM and IgG antibodies and titers) or detection of HHV-6 DNA in clinical/tissue specimens is reserved for atypical presentations and complications or in immunosuppressed hosts.
**Serologic tests and quantitative PCR may be useful for immunosuppressed hosts.
DRESS, drug reaction with eosinophilia and systemic symptoms (also known as DIHS, drug-induced hypersensitivity syndrome); EBV, Epstein–Barr virus; CMV, cytomegalovirus.

Table 67.7 Major clinical features of human herpesvirus 6 and 7 (HHV-6 and HHV-7) infections. No definitive treatment is available.

MAJOR CLINICAL FEATURES OF HUMAN HERPESVIRUS 8 (HHV-8) INFECTIONS		
HHV-8 Infection	**Major Clinical Features**	**DDx**
Primary infection Latency is established in B lymphocytes and vascular endothelial cells	**Children** • Fever and morbilliform eruption **Men who have sex with men (MSM)** • New-onset lymphadenopathy, fatigue, diarrhea, and a localized cutaneous eruption **Immunosuppressed hosts (e.g. solid organ transplant recipients, HIV (+) infection)** • Fever, splenomegaly, lymphoid hyperplasia, pancytopenia • Occasionally rapid-onset KS	

Reactivation infection	**Kaposi's Sarcoma (KS) (Four Subtypes)**
	• Cutaneous lesions progress through stages as red, brown, or violaceous papules, plaques, and nodules
	1. *Classic KS* (Fig. 67.17)
	  • Indolent; primarily seen in elderly males of Mediterranean and Jewish descent; favors the lower extremities
	2. *Endemic or African KS*
	  • Seen in equatorial Africa; primarily in children and young adults; more aggressive than classic KS; may disseminate to lymph nodes, bone, or skin
	3. *Iatrogenic or organ transplant-associated KS*
	  • Similar to AIDS-related KS; may be acquired from the donor or transplanted tissue; typically regresses with reduction of immunosuppression medications or a change to sirolimus
	4. *Epidemic or AIDS-related KS*
	  • Most common tumor in HIV (+) persons; can improve with ART treatment, but can also flare as part of IRIS
	
	Primary Effusion Lymphoma
	• B-cell lymphoma
	
	Multicentric Castleman's Disease
	• Lymphoproliferative disorder characterized by fever, hepatosplenomegaly, and massive lymphadenopathy
		KS (Lower Extremity)
		• Acroangiodermatitis (pseudo-KS)
		• Lymphoma
		• Ecchymoses
		
		KS (More Widespread Distribution)
		• Bacillary angiomatosis
		• Ecchymoses
		• Other vascular tumors and hyperplasias (see Chapter 94)
		• Lymphoma

The optimal serologic assay for diagnosis of HHV-8 is not known; when cutaneous lesions are present, a skin biopsy for histochemical analysis for LNA-1 can be diagnostic.

ART, antiretroviral therapy; IRIS, immune reconstitution inflammatory syndrome.

Table 67.8 Major clinical features of human herpesvirus 8 (HHV-8) infections. HHV-8 is also known as Kaposi's sarcoma (KS)-associated herpesvirus. Treatment of KS involves reconstitution of the host's immune system (e.g. decrease immunosuppressive therapy, ART, change to sirolimus); systemic and intralesional chemotherapy; radiation therapy; cryotherapy.

Other Viral Diseases | 68

Viral infections frequently have cutaneous manifestations, especially in children. This chapter covers classic childhood exanthems, poxvirus infections, and several other viral infections with characteristic skin findings. *Nonspecific viral exanthems*, typically presenting with blanchable erythematous macules and papules in a widespread distribution, are also common in children infected with enteroviruses (see below) and a variety of respiratory viruses, generally resolving spontaneously within a week. Fig. 68.1 outlines clinical features to consider when evaluating a patient with a morbilliform ('maculopapular') exanthem, and Chapter 3 addresses considerations in patients with fever and a rash. HIV, human papillomavirus, and herpesvirus (including infectious mononucleosis and roseola infantum) infections are discussed in Chapters 65–67.

Enterovirus Infections

• Non-polio enteroviruses (e.g. coxsackieviruses, echoviruses) are single-stranded RNA picornaviruses with a worldwide distribution; they cause a variety of exanthems, enanthems, and systemic manifestations.

• Spread via fecal–oral (e.g. swimming pools, ingestion of oysters) and respiratory routes, with an incubation period of 3–6 days; most common in the summer and fall in temperate climates, favoring young children.

• *Hand, foot, and, mouth disease* (HFMD; in the United States, coxsackievirus A16 > others) features oval vesicles on the hands and feet (palms/soles > dorsally) and buttocks plus an erosive stomatitis (e.g. tongue, buccal mucosa, palate, tonsils), often associated with fever and malaise (Fig. 68.2A–D); onychomadesis occasionally occurs 1–2 months later.

• Recently, coxsackievirus A6 infection has been associated with a more widespread

vesiculobullous exanthem favoring the perioral area, extremities > trunk, and areas of previous dermatitis ('eczema coxsackium') or injury as well as the classic sites of HFMD (Fig. 68.2B, D, E; see Fig. 3.5B, C).

• *Herpangina* presents with fever and oropharyngeal erosions, but usually no exanthem.

• The diverse spectrum of enteroviral exanthems also includes morbilliform, scarlatiniform, Gianotti–Crosti syndrome-like, petechial, and pustular eruptions (see Fig. 3.5A); eruptive pseudoangiomatosis is an uncommon manifestation.

• Organ systems that can be affected by enteroviral infections include the respiratory (upper > lower) and gastrointestinal tracts, liver, CNS (meningitis > encephalitis; especially with enterovirus 71), eyes (hemorrhagic conjunctivitis), joints, muscles, and heart.

• Spontaneous resolution typically occurs within 1–2 weeks.

Measles (Rubeola)

• Incidence has decreased dramatically since introduction of a live vaccine for this single-stranded RNA paramyxovirus in 1963; however, measles outbreaks still occur in both low- and high-income countries, often because of unfounded fears of vaccination.

• Highly contagious and spread by respiratory droplets, with an incubation period of 10–14 days.

• Prodrome of fever, cough, coryza, and conjunctivitis (the 3 C's), followed in 2–4 days by the appearance of pathognomonic Koplik spots (gray-white papules on the buccal mucosa).

• An exanthem develops 3–5 days after the onset of symptoms, with erythematous macules and papules spreading cephalocaudally from the forehead, hairline, and behind

APPROACH TO THE PATIENT WITH A PRESUMED MORBILLIFORM OR MACULAR/PAPULAR VIRAL EXANTHEM

1. Exclude other causes → Drug reaction, Kawasaki disease. Bacterial (e.g. Group A β-hemolytic *Streptococcus* or *Arcanobacterium haemolyticum**, meningococcemia if petechiae, ehrlichiosis, leptospirosis, rickettsioses, syphilis). HIV seroconversion exanthem (see Chapter 78), dengue, Chikungunya fever, Barmah Forest/Ross River virus infections (depending on geographic region/travel history)

2. Specific features

Clinical signs and symptoms		Measles (rubeola)	Rubella	Parvovirus B19	Human herpesvirus 6 or 7	Epstein–Barr virus	Adenovirus	Enterovirus	Cytomegalovirus†	West Nile virus
Exanthem	Cephalocaudad spread	✓	✓							
	Rose-pink macules		✓							
	Red cheeks; reticulate or lacy			✓						✓
	Punctate lesions on extremities				✓					
	Starts as fever subsides				✓					
	Most prominent following antibiotics					✓			✓	
	Petechiae	✓		✓					✓	
Enanthem	Gray-white papules, buccal mucosa (Koplik's)	✓								
	Red macules, soft palate (Forscheimer's)		✓							
	Red papules, soft palate/uvula (Nagayama's)				✓					
	Uvulo-palatoglossal junctional ulcers				✓					
	Painful erosions, esp. of posterior pharynx			✓				✓		
	Pharyngitis					✓		✓		
Lymphadenopathy	Generalized					✓		✓	✓	
	Localized: occipital, posterior auricular		✓							
	Localized: cervical					✓	✓	✓	✓	
Musculoskeletal	Arthralgias/arthritis	✓		✓		✓				✓
	Muscle weakness									✓
Eye	Conjunctivitis	✓	✓				✓			✓
Liver/spleen	Hepatosplenomegaly	✓	✓			✓		✓	✓	✓
CNS	Encephalitis (E) ± Meningitis (M)	✓(E)	✓(E)		✓(E**)		✓(E,M)	✓(E,M)	✓(E)	✓(E,M)
Lungs	Pneumonia	✓					✓	✓		✓
Heart	Myocarditis	✓	✓					✓		

3. Laboratory tests

(Laboratory test row, by agent)
- Measles (rubeola): virus isolation NP; PCR xxxxx
- Rubella: serology; virus isolation NP/U/CSF; PCR xxxxx
- Parvovirus B19: serology; PCR xxxxx
- Human herpesvirus 6 or 7: serology; PCR xxxxx
- Epstein–Barr virus: serology; heterophile antibody; atypical lymphocytosis; PCR xxxxx
- Adenovirus: antigen detection T/S, NP; virus isolation; PCR xxxxx
- Enterovirus: virus isolation T/S/V; PCR xxxxx
- Cytomegalovirus: antigen detection Blood[a,b]; virus isolation U[b]; serology ✓(E); PCR xxxxx
- West Nile virus: serology (also CSF); PCR xxxxx

Legend

- (serology) Serology
- (virus isolation icon) Virus isolation
- xxxxx Polymerase chain reaction assay
- Antigen detection
- Heterophile antibody
- Atypical lymphocytosis

- CSF = Cerebrospinal fluid
- NP = Nasopharyngeal
- V = Vesicle fluid
- U = Urine
- T = Throat
- S = Stool

Notes: [a] Immunocompromised host [b] Immunocompetent host

Fig. 68.1 Approach to the patient with a presumed morbilliform or macular/papular viral exanthem. *Gram-positive rod; may result in severe pharyngitis and scarlatiniform exanthem in adolescents and young adults. †Intracellular inclusions in endothelial cells are another finding. **Usually febrile seizures.

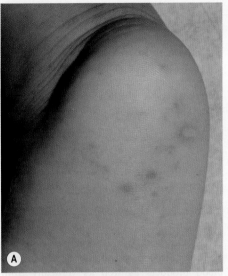

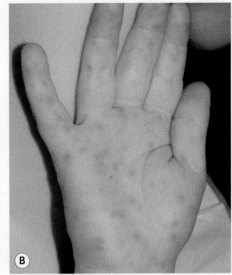

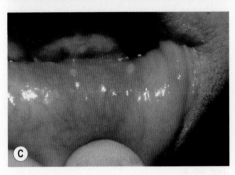

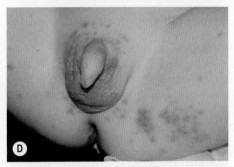

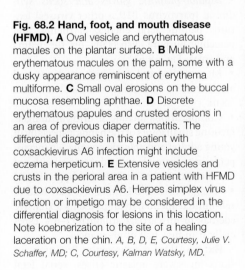

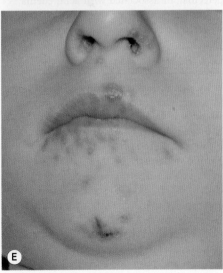

Fig. 68.2 Hand, foot, and mouth disease (HFMD). A Oval vesicle and erythematous macules on the plantar surface. **B** Multiple erythematous macules on the palm, some with a dusky appearance reminiscent of erythema multiforme. **C** Small oval erosions on the buccal mucosa resembling aphthae. **D** Discrete erythematous papules and crusted erosions in an area of previous diaper dermatitis. The differential diagnosis in this patient with coxsackievirus A6 infection might include eczema herpeticum. **E** Extensive vesicles and crusts in the perioral area in a patient with HFMD due to coxsackievirus A6. Herpes simplex virus infection or impetigo may be considered in the differential diagnosis for lesions in this location. Note koebnerization to the site of a healing laceration on the chin. *A, B, D, E, Courtesy, Julie V. Schaffer, MD; C, Courtesy, Kalman Watsky, MD.*

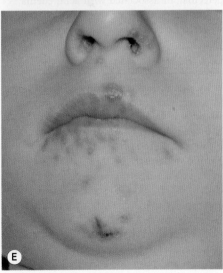

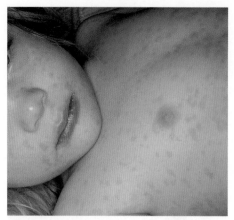

Fig. 68.3 Measles. Pink macules and minimally elevated papules. *Courtesy, Louis Fragola, MD.*

the ears to the trunk and extremities (Fig. 68.3); after 5 days, the eruption fades in the order it appeared.

• Complications include otitis media, pneumonia, and encephalitis; subacute sclerosing panencephalitis occasionally develops 5–10 years later.

• *Atypical measles* in the setting of partial immunity features high fevers, cough, and a variable exanthem that may be vesicular, petechial, or associated with acral edema.

• **Rx:** vitamin A administration for children with acute disease; prevention via vaccination.

Rubella (German Measles)

• Incidence has markedly declined since introduction of a live vaccine for this single-stranded RNA togavirus in 1969.

• Spread via respiratory droplets, with an incubation period of 16–18 days.

• Mild prodrome of fever, headache, and upper respiratory symptoms, followed in 1–5 days by an eruption of erythematous macules and papules that spreads downward from the face and lasts ~3 days; Forchheimer's spots (red or petechial macules on the soft palate) and tender lymphadenopathy (especially occipital and posterior auricular) are characteristic findings.

• Although usually self-limited, complications include arthralgias/arthritis (especially

in adolescent girls and women), thrombocytopenia, and encephalitis.

• *Congenital rubella syndrome*, most common with maternal infection in the first 16 weeks of pregnancy; can result in cataracts, deafness, congenital heart defects, and microcephaly; a 'blueberry muffin baby' presentation occasionally occurs (see Fig. 67.15).

Parvovirus B19 Infection (Erythema Infectiosum, Fifth Disease, 'Slapped Cheek Disease')

• Single-stranded DNA virus with tropism for erythroid progenitor cells; found worldwide.

• Transmitted via respiratory secretions and blood products as well as vertically from mother to fetus, with an incubation period of 4–14 days; peak incidence in the winter and spring, favoring children 4–10 years of age.

• A mild prodrome (e.g. low-grade fever, myalgias, headache) is followed in 7–10 days by bright red, macular erythema on the cheeks; a few days later, a lacy, reticulated pattern of erythematous macules and papules may appear on the extremities > trunk, lasting 1–3 weeks and fluctuating in intensity (with flares upon sun exposure and overheating) (Fig. 68.4).

• *Papular–purpuric gloves and socks syndrome* (parvovirus B19 > other viruses) features painful acral edema, erythema, and petechiae/purpura (especially on the palms and soles; Fig. 68.5).

• More widespread petechial eruptions and an enanthem (petechiae, erosions) can also occur.

• Complications include arthritis/arthralgias favoring small joints of the hands (especially in young adults) and aplastic anemia > pancytopenia in susceptible individuals (e.g. with red blood cell disorders or immunosuppression).

• *Fetal parvovirus B19 infection* may lead to self-limited anemia, hydrops fetalis (extensive edema), or miscarriage/stillbirth (2–6%, especially if in first half of pregnancy).

• **Rx:** NSAIDs for arthropathy, RBC transfusions for severe aplastic crises, serial fetal ultrasonography for infections during the first two trimesters of pregnancy.

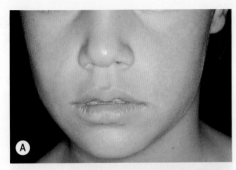

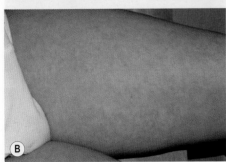

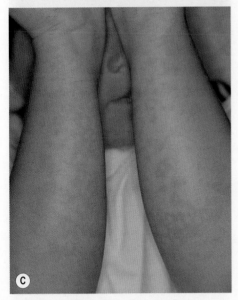

Fig. 68.4 Erythema infectiosum. Bright macular erythema on the cheeks, with characteristic sparing of periorificial areas **(A)**. Lacy, reticulated erythematous eruption on the thigh **(B)** and arms **(C)** during the second stage of the exanthem. *A, Courtesy, Louis Fragola, MD; B, Courtesy, Julie V. Schaffer, MD; C, Courtesy, Kalman Watsky, MD.*

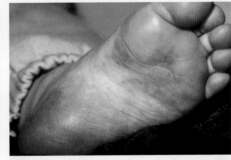

Fig. 68.5 Papular–purpuric gloves and socks syndrome. Erythematous patches with petechiae on the plantar surface. *Courtesy, Anthony Mancini, MD.*

Unilateral Laterothoracic Exanthem (Asymmetric Periflexural Exanthem of Childhood)

• A consistent causative infectious agent has not been identified.
• Most often occurs in the spring and favors preschool-aged children.
• Morbilliform or eczematous eruption that begins unilaterally (axilla > trunk or thigh) and then spreads to contralateral sites (Fig. 68.6).
• Often pruritic and may be preceded by upper respiratory or gastrointestinal symptoms.
• **DDx:** allergic contact dermatitis, eczematous reaction to molluscum contagiosium, pityriasis rosea, scabies; eruptions with a more widespread distribution may overlap with Gianotti–Crosti syndrome.
• Resolves spontaneously, usually within 3–8 weeks.
• **Rx:** topical CS are often of limited benefit.

Gianotti–Crosti Syndrome (Papular Acrodermatitis of Childhood)

• Associated with a variety of infectious triggers, most often Epstein–Barr virus, hepatitis B virus (outside the United States), and vaccines.
• Most common in the spring and early summer, favoring young children.
• Often preceded by a low-grade fever and/or upper respiratory symptoms.

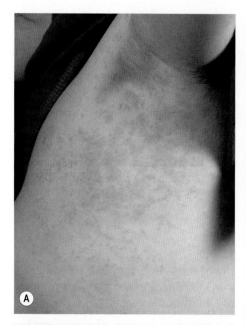

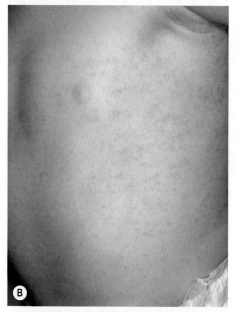

Fig. 68.6 Unilateral laterothoracic exanthem. Erythematous macules and papules involving the left axilla and upper flank **(A)** and a slightly more extensive distribution on the left lateral trunk **(B)**.

• Rapid onset of monomorphic, skin-colored to pink-red, edematous papules > papulovesicles in a symmetric distribution on the extensor surfaces of the extremities, buttocks, and face (Fig. 68.7); pruritus, purpuric lesions, and extension to the trunk occasionally occur.

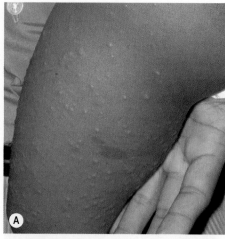

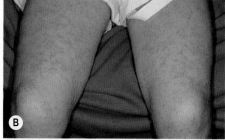

Fig. 68.7 Gianotti–Crosti syndrome.
A Monomorphic erythematous papules on the thigh. **B** A more exuberant eruption of multiple edematous, erythematous papules on the thighs and knees. *B, Courtesy, Anthony Mancini, MD.*

• **DDx:** inflammatory response to molluscum contagiosum, id reaction (e.g. due to allergic contact dermatitis to nickel), papular urticaria, another viral exanthem (e.g. coxsackievirus A6), drug eruption, scabies.
• Resolves spontaneously, usually within 3–8 weeks (longer than a classic viral exanthem); laboratory evaluation for specific viral agents can be performed if indicated by clinical findings and geographic region.
• **Rx:** topical CS are often of limited benefit.

Molluscum Contagiosum (MC)

• Common cutaneous infection caused by a poxvirus.
• Spread by skin-to-skin contact > fomites (e.g. towels), favoring young children but also

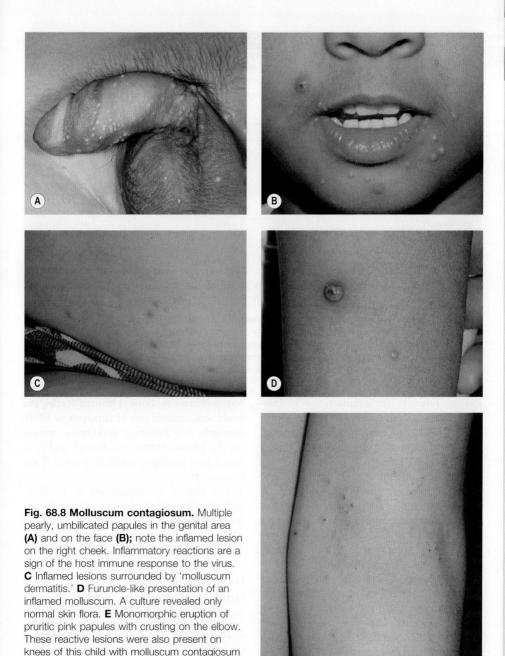

Fig. 68.8 Molluscum contagiosum. Multiple pearly, umbilicated papules in the genital area **(A)** and on the face **(B)**; note the inflamed lesion on the right cheek. Inflammatory reactions are a sign of the host immune response to the virus. **C** Inflamed lesions surrounded by 'molluscum dermatitis.' **D** Furuncle-like presentation of an inflamed molluscum. A culture revealed only normal skin flora. **E** Monomorphic eruption of pruritic pink papules with crusting on the elbow. These reactive lesions were also present on knees of this child with molluscum contagiosum on the trunk. *A, C, Courtesy, Anthony Mancini, MD; B, D, E, Courtesy, Julie V. Schaffer, MD.*

occurring via sexual contact in adults; larger and more numerous lesions may be seen in immunocompromised hosts, especially those with HIV infection.

• Firm, skin-colored to pink papules or papulonodules with a waxy surface and central umbilication; predilection for the skin folds (e.g. axillae, neck, groin), lateral trunk, thighs, buttocks, genitals, and face (Fig. 68.8).

• Inflammatory reactions frequently occur, including eczematous dermatitis (diffuse or nummular) in the skin surrounding MC

TREATMENT OF MOLLUSCUM CONTAGIOSUM
No Direct Therapy
Eventual spontaneous involution in immunocompetent patients
Treatment of associated dermatitis with a topical CS can prevent autoinoculation from scratching
Physical Modalities
Curettage* (1) or manual extraction (3)
Cryotherapy (2)
Electrodesiccation* (3)
Topical Therapy
Cantharidin (2)
Imiquimod** (1)
Podophyllotoxin (1)
Retinoids (3)
Trichloroacetic acid (1)

*Discomfort can be minimized by prior application of a topical anesthetic (e.g. lidocaine 4–5% cream).
**Based on publications, but ineffective in 2 unpublished randomized controlled trials.

Table 68.1 Treatment of molluscum contagiosum. Other options include topical sinecatechins, intralesional immunotherapy with *Candida* antigen, pulsed dye laser, and (for extensive lesions) systemic medications (e.g. oral cimetidine or [in immunosuppressed patients] intravenous cidofovir). Key to evidence-based support: (1) prospective controlled trial; (2) retrospective study or large case series; (3) small case series or individual case reports.

lesions, furuncle-like inflammation of individual MC lesions, and a Gianotti–Crosti syndrome-like eruption of pruritic erythematous papules favoring the elbows and knees (see Fig. 68.8B–E).

• **DDx** (in addition to above): *multiple lesions* – verrucae, condyloma acuminata, papular eczema; *solitary to few lesions* – juvenile xanthogranuloma or Spitz nevus in a child, BCC in an adult; *in immunocompromised hosts* – cryptococcosis, histoplasmosis, other dimorphic fungal infections.

• Microscopic evaluation following curettage of lesional contents or biopsy shows large, round intracytoplasmic inclusion bodies (see Chapter 2); dermoscopy can identify a characteristic yellow-white, lobular central structure surrounded by a 'crown' of blood vessels.

• Resolves spontaneously over months to several years in immunocompetent children, with larger numbers of lesions often developing in those with atopic dermatitis.

• **Rx:** options are listed in Table 68.1.

Other Poxvirus Infections

• The most historically significant poxvirus infection was smallpox, which has been responsible for millions of human deaths; the world was declared free of smallpox in 1980, although two reference collections remain (in the United States and Russia) and it is feared that smallpox could be exploited for bioterrorism.

• The clinical manifestations of smallpox and varicella are compared in Table 68.2, and selected poxvirus infections and complications of smallpox vaccination are presented in Figs. 68.9, 68.10 and Table 68.3.

Hemorrhagic Fevers and Other Viral Infections with Cutaneous Manifestations

• *Hemorrhagic fevers*: group of zoonotic viral infections with nonspecific cutaneous manifestations that include petechiae, purpura, and mucosal hemorrhage; although overall most common in Africa and South America (e.g. Ebola, Marburg, and yellow fever viruses), some have a worldwide distribution (e.g. hantavirus).

• Cutaneous manifestations of hepatitis A, B, and C infections are listed in Table 68.4.

• Major features of other viral infections with cutaneous findings are presented in Table 68.5.

COMPARISON OF VARICELLA/DISSEMINATED ZOSTER TO SMALLPOX		
	Varicella/Disseminated Zoster	**Smallpox**
Prodrome	None or mild fever and malaise	Fever ≥101°F/38.3°C for 1–4 days prior to rash onset, plus malaise, headache, backache and/or abdominal pain
Distribution of lesions	Initially on face/scalp; trunk > distal extremities May have an enanthem	Concentrated on face and limbs; can progress to involve entire body surface Oropharyngeal lesions often precede cutaneous eruption
Stage of lesions	Different stages occur simultaneously in any one area of the skin (nonsynchronous)	Adjacent lesions are all at same stage of development (synchronous)
Types of lesions	Superficial papules, vesicles, and pustules	Papulovesicles → firm, deep-seated pustules with a tendency to confluence
Course	Lesions appear in crops over a 3-day period	Lesions spread over 1–2 weeks Crusting develops over 1 week
Scarring	Rare in uncomplicated cases	Common and marked

Table 68.2 Comparison of varicella/disseminated zoster to smallpox.

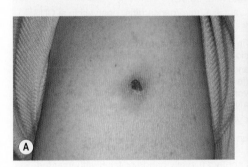

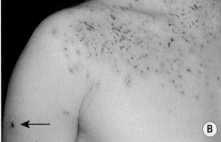

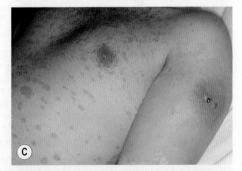

Fig. 68.9 Smallpox vaccine. A Crusted papule at the site of vaccination, 14 days following administration. **B** Eczema vaccinatum in a patient with atopic dermatitis. Spread from the vaccination site (arrow) to areas of eczema. **C** Erythema multiforme-like reaction associated with marked erythema and edema at the vaccination site. *B, C, Courtesy, Louis Fragola, MD.*

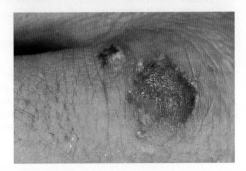

Fig. 68.10 Orf. Vesiculopustule and ulceration on the finger. *Courtesy, Anthony Mancini, MD.*

SELECTED POXVIRUS INFECTIONS	
Disease/Virus (Genus; Host)	**Major Features**
Smallpox/variola (*Orthopoxvirus*; only humans)	• Theoretically eradicated; respiratory transmission, 7- to 17-day incubation period • See Table 68.2 for clinical findings* • Complications: panophthalmitis, arthritis, encephalitis

Vaccinia (*Orthopoxvirus*; used as vaccine in humans)	• Currently used for smallpox vaccination in the military and first responders
	• Papule at vaccination site (e.g. deltoid or thigh) → vesiculopustules → crust (Fig. 68.9A) → scar, occasionally with satellite lesions; fever and LAN are common, and urticarial or exanthematous eruptions may develop 1–3 weeks postvaccination
	• Possible adverse events*
	   – Superinfection of the vaccination site or lymph nodes
	   – Inadvertent autoinoculation or contact transmission
	   – Generalized or progressive vaccinia (especially in immunocompromised hosts)
	   – Eczema vaccinatum (e.g. in patients with atopic dermatitis) (Fig. 68.9B)
	   – Postvaccination nonviral pustulosis or erythema multiforme (Fig. 68.9C)
	   – Ocular vaccinia, myo/pericarditis, postvaccinial CNS disease

Monkeypox (*Orthopoxvirus*; monkeys, rodents)	• Primarily in Africa; cutaneous inoculation or respiratory transmission, 10- to 12-day incubation period • Malaise and fever, then nonsynchronous eruption of papules (few to >100) → vesiculopustules → crusts → scars, favoring face and extremities (often on palms/soles); LAN and respiratory symptoms • Smallpox vaccination protective
Cowpox (*Orthopoxvirus*; cats > rodents > cattle)	• Primarily in Europe and Central Asia; 7-day incubation period • At site of contact (usually hands or face) with infected animal: papule → vesicle → pustule → crusted eschar → scar; often fever and LAN • Occasionally generalized in patients with atopic dermatitis
Orf (*Parapoxvirus*; sheep, goats, reindeer)	• At-risk occupations: shepherds, veterinarians, butchers • On hands (Fig. 68.10) following contact with infected animal (especially perioral area and udder of ewes): papule (1 to few) → targetoid lesion → nodule (weeping then dry with black dots then papillomatous) → regression without scar; ± fever and LAN, and erythema multiforme may occur 10–14 days later • Diagnosis often made histologically
Milker's nodules (bovine papular stomatitis)/paravaccinia (*Parapoxvirus*; cattle)	• At-risk occupations: dairy farmers, ranchers, butchers, veterinarians • Lesions on hands virtually identical to orf (see above)

*Additional information (e.g. diagnostic criteria, algorithms, case definitions) is available at http://www.bt.cdc.gov/agent/smallpox.
LAN, lymphadenopathy.

Table 68.3 Selected poxvirus infections. Real-time PCR is currently the diagnostic method of choice. Other poxviruses that occasionally lead to skin lesions (single or few) in humans include *deer-associated parapoxvirus* (eastern United States; reported in deer hunters) and *tanapox* (equatorial Africa; endemic in nonhuman primates, likely arthropod vector).

CUTANEOUS MANIFESTATIONS OF HEPATITIS A, B, AND C INFECTIONS	
Acute urticaria (A, B, C)	Necrolytic acral erythema (C)
Serum sickness-like reaction (B, C)	Porphyria cutanea tarda (B, C)
Gianotti–Crosti syndrome (B > A, C)	Pruritus (B, C > A)
Small vessel vasculitis (B, C > A)	Lichen planus – especially erosive oral disease (C)
Cryoglobulinemic vasculitis (C > B > A)	
Urticarial vasculitis (B, C)	Sarcoidosis (with interferon and/or ribavirin therapy; C > B)
Polyarteritis nodosa (classic – B, cutaneous – C)	
Livedo reticularis (C)	Erythema multiforme (B, C)
	Erythema nodosum (B > C)

Table 68.4 Cutaneous manifestations of hepatitis A, B, and C infections.

ADDITIONAL VIRAL INFECTIONS WITH CUTANEOUS FINDINGS		
Viral Infection (Family)	Geography/Source of Infection	Major Features
Dengue (Flaviviridae)	Caribbean, Mexico, Central and South America, Africa, Asia (especially tropics)/ mosquitoes	• 3- to 14-day incubation period → variable fever, headache (especially retro-orbital), myalgias, vomiting* • ~50% of patients: macular erythema of head, neck, and upper trunk, followed by morbilliform eruption with islands of sparing and often petechiae*
West Nile (Flaviviridae)	Africa, Europe, Asia, North > South America, Australia/ mosquitoes that feed on infected birds	• 5- to 14-day incubation period → fever, headache, myalgias > meningoencephalitis, flaccid paralysis • ~25% of patients: exanthem with erythematous macules/papules, often punctate and favoring extremities
Chikungunya (Togaviridae)	India, Indian Ocean islands, Southeast Asia, Africa, Italy/ mosquitoes	• 1- to 14-day incubation period → fever, headache, myalgias/ arthralgias • ~50% of patients: acrofacial erythema/edema, morbilliform eruption; occasionally ulcers (genital, intertriginous, oral), vesiculobullae, and postinflammatory hyperpigmentation (freckle-like, flagellate or diffuse)
Viral-associated trichodysplasia of immunosuppression (Polyomaviridae)	Worldwide**	• Numerous erythematous to skin-colored, spiny papules favoring the mid face and ears; ± alopecia or leonine facies

*In the hemorrhagic form (often representing a repeat infection with a second serotype) marked thrombocytopenia with bleeding into skin and other organs.
**In solid organ transplant recipients or patients receiving chemotherapy for a hematologic malignancy.

Table 68.5 Additional viral infections with cutaneous findings. Other viruses with limited geographic distributions have prominent skin findings, e.g. Barmah Forest virus in Australia.

For further information see Ch. 81. From *Dermatology, Third Edition.*

69 Sexually Transmitted Diseases

In this chapter, five sexually transmitted diseases (STDs) are covered – syphilis, gonorrhea, chancroid, lymphogranuloma venereum (LGV), and granuloma inguinale. Additional more common STDs including herpes simplex infections, molluscum contagiosum, condyloma acuminata, crab lice, and HIV infection are discussed in Chapters 67, 68, 66, 71, and 65, respectively. When one STD is present, a search for others is indicated.

Syphilis (Lues)

• Etiologic agent is the spirochete *Treponema pallidum*; the infection is divided into four phases: primary, secondary, latent, and tertiary (Fig. 69.1), in addition to a congenital form.

• Syphilis is 7–8 times more common in men than in women in the United States, and the highest rates are in black and Hispanic individuals and in men who have sex with men (MSM); there is an increased risk of transmission of HIV infection in those with ulcers due to syphilis as well as chancroid or herpes simplex viral infection.

• One or more ulcers, usually anogenital, characterize *primary syphilis* and are referred to as chancres (Fig. 69.2); the ulcers are painless (unless secondarily infected) and upon palpation the base is firm; regional lymphadenopathy may be present (Fig. 69.3).

• *Secondary syphilis* reflects hematogenous dissemination and the skin lesions vary from macular to papulosquamous and from annular to granulomatous (Figs. 69.4 and 69.5); mucosal involvement is common and includes mucous patches, split papules at the angles of the mouth and condyloma lata (Fig. 69.6);

usually accompanied by constitutional symptoms (Table 69.1).

• *Tertiary syphilis* is preceded by a latent phase that can last for years (Fig. 69.7); the skin and mucous membranes, as well as the bones, develop gummas (Fig. 69.8), with cardiovascular syphilis and neurosyphilis representing the major causes of death in those who remain untreated.

• *In utero* infection of a fetus can occur, primarily during the secondary or latent phases, leading to congenital syphilis or stigmata (Tables 69.2 and 69.3); the cutaneous lesions of early congenital syphilis are similar to those of secondary syphilis (Fig. 69.9), but they may be bullous; additional findings include a bloody or purulent nasal discharge ('snuffles'), perioral and perianal fissures, and osteochondritis.

• Dx: darkfield microscopic examination (serous exudate from primary or secondary lesions); anti-cardiolipin antibodies (rapid plasma reagin [RPR], Venereal Disease Research Laboratory [VDRL] assay), ~80%+ in primary and 99%+ in secondary; anti-*T. pallidum* (TP) antibodies (microhemagglutination assay [MHA-TP], fluorescent treponemal antibody absorption [FTA-ABS], ~90%+ in primary and 99%+ in secondary.

• A false-positive VDRL can occur in pregnant women and in association with a number of disorders including antiphospholipid antibody syndrome, lupus erythematosus (LE), lymphoma, and drug abuse as well as infections (e.g. endemic treponematoses, borreliosis, malaria), while a false-positive FTA-ABS can occur in patients with LE, HIV infection, hypergammaglobulinemia, endemic treponematoses, and borreliosis.

• **DDx:** see Table 69.4.

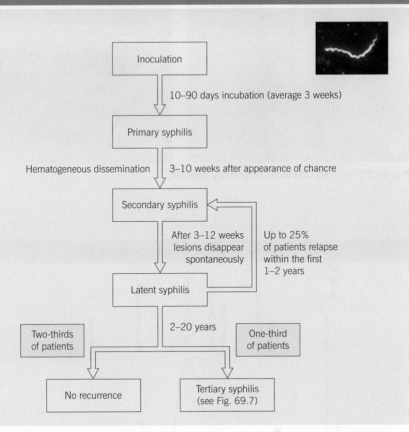

Inoculation

↓ 10–90 days incubation (average 3 weeks)

Primary syphilis

Hematogeneous dissemination ↓ 3–10 weeks after appearance of chancre

Secondary syphilis

After 3–12 weeks lesions disappear spontaneously

Up to 25% of patients relapse within the first 1–2 years

Latent syphilis

2–20 years

Two-thirds of patients

One-third of patients

No recurrence

Tertiary syphilis (see Fig. 69.7)

Fig. 69.1 Natural history of untreated syphilis. Chancres spontaneously resolve after a few weeks (see Fig. 69.3). In the group of patients with no recurrence, the rapid plasma reagin (RPR) becomes negative in 50% and remains positive in 50%. *Adapted from Rein MF, Musher DM. Late syphilis. In: Rein MF (Ed.), Atlas of Infectious Diseases, Vol. V: Sexually Transmitted Diseases. New York: Current Medicine, 1995:10.1–10.13. Inset figure: Adapted from Morse SA, et al. Atlas of Sexually Transmitted Diseases and AIDS, 3rd ed. London: Mosby; 2003.*

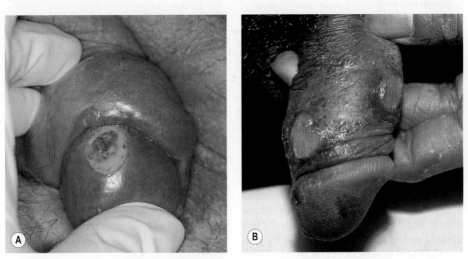

Fig. 69.2 Chancres of primary syphilis. The lesions are firm to palpation and are occasionally multiple. Sites of chancres include the penis **(A, B),** perianal area **(C),** and lip **(D),** as well as the fingers, cervix, and breast. *A, C, D, Courtesy, Angelika Stary, MD. Continued*

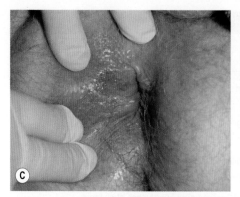
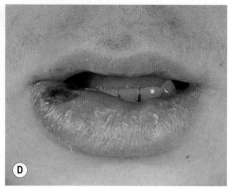

Fig. 69.2 *Continued* **Chancres of primary syphilis.**

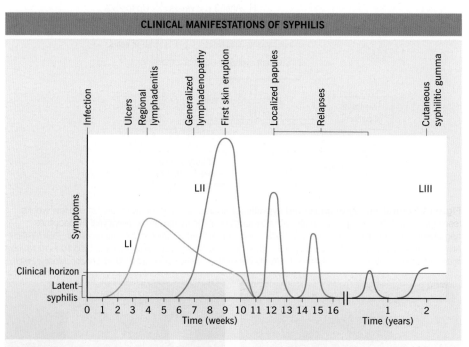

CLINICAL MANIFESTATIONS OF SYPHILIS

Fig. 69.3 Clinical manifestations of syphilis. LI, primary syphilis (lues); LII, secondary syphilis (lues); LIII, tertiary syphilis (lues). *Adapted from Fritsch P, Zangerle R, Stary A. Venerologie. In: Fritsch P (Ed.), Dermatologie und Venerologie. Berlin: Springer, 1998:865–886.*

- **Rx:** see Table 69.5 for treatment of primary, secondary, and early latent syphilis; patients with symptoms or signs suggesting neurologic disease should have CSF analysis and HIV-infected patients are at increased risk for neurosyphilis; for treatment of late latent, ocular, tertiary, and congenital syphilis as well as neurosyphilis, see www.cdc.gov/std/treatment or download the CDC STD Tx Guide App; a fourfold decrease in the antibody titer based on the RPR or VDRL assay is indicative of successful treatment.

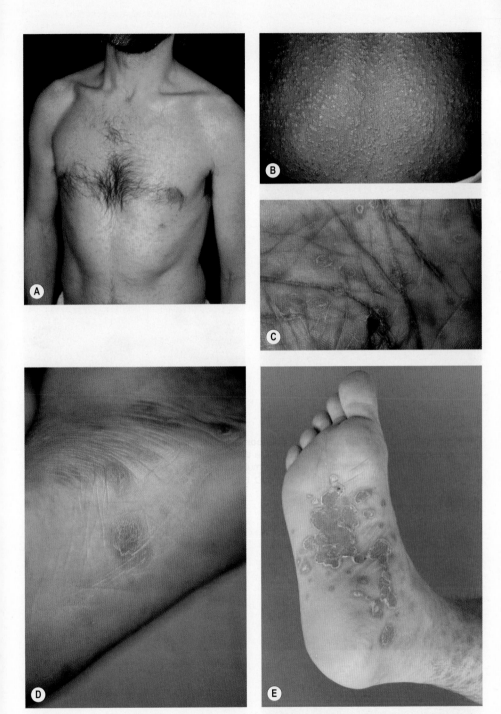

Fig. 69.4 Secondary syphilis – cutaneous manifestations. Widespread exanthem of pink papules **(A)** and generalized papulosquamous lesions **(B)**. Lesions on the palms **(C)** and soles **(D, E)** can have a collarette of scale; in patients with more darkly pigmented skin, these lesions may have a copper color. *E, Courtesy, Angelika Stary, MD.*

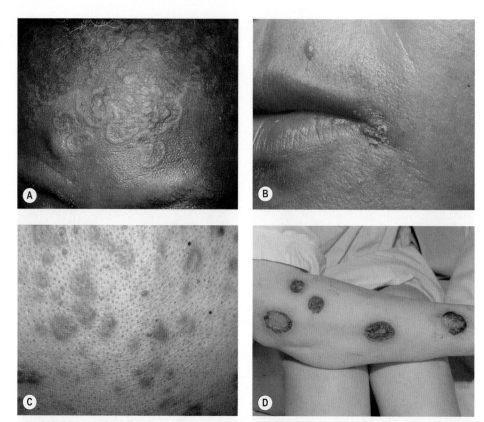

Fig. 69.5 Less common manifestations of secondary syphilis. A Annular plaques with central hyperpigmentation on the forehead. **B** Split papule at the oral commissure. **C** Granulomatous nodules and plaques. **D** 'Malignant' syphilis with multiple necrotic, ulcerated, and crusted lesions associated with severe constitutional symptoms. *D, Courtesy, Angelika Stary, MD.*

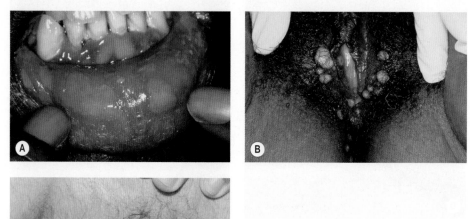

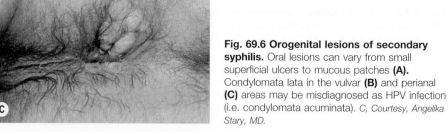

Fig. 69.6 Orogenital lesions of secondary syphilis. Oral lesions can vary from small superficial ulcers to mucous patches **(A)**. Condylomata lata in the vulvar **(B)** and perianal **(C)** areas may be misdiagnosed as HPV infection (i.e. condylomata acuminata). *C, Courtesy, Angelika Stary, MD.*

CLINICAL FEATURES OF SECONDARY SYPHILIS

- Prodromal symptoms and signs
    - Weight loss
    - Low-grade fever
    - Malaise
    - Headache (meningeal irritation)
    - Sore throat
    - Conjunctivitis (iridocyclitis)
    - Arthralgia (periostitis)
    - Myalgias, bone pain
    - Hepatosplenomegaly (mild hepatitis)

- Generalized lymphadenopathy with indolent enlargement of lymph nodes (50–85%)

- Skin manifestations
    - Early (10%): generalized eruption; non-pruritic, roseola-like, discrete macules, initially distributed on the flanks and shoulders
    - Late (70%): generalized maculopapular and papulosquamous eruptions; more infiltrated lesions, often copper-colored; annular plaques on the face; corymbose arrangement (satellite papules around a larger central lesion); occurs in successive waves and is polymorphic
    - Localized syphilids (specific infiltrations of treponemes; positive darkfield examination):
        - palms and soles: symmetric papules and plaques with a collarette of scale (collarette of Biett)
        - anogenital area: condylomata lata
        - seborrheic area: 'corona veneris' along the hairline
    - Hypopigmented macules, mainly on the neck (postinflammatory; 'necklace of Venus')

- Manifestations involving mucous membranes (30%)
    - Syphilitic perlèche, split papules
    - Mucous patches: 'plaques muqueuses' in the oropharynx (equivalent to condylomata lata in the genital area)
    - Syphilitic sore throat: inflammation of the whole pharynx

- Patchy alopecia (7%): 'moth-eaten' localized areas of hair loss; toxic telogen effluvium

Table 69.1 Clinical features of secondary syphilis. *Courtesy, Angelika Stary, MD.*

CLINICAL MANIFESTATIONS OF LATE SYPHILIS

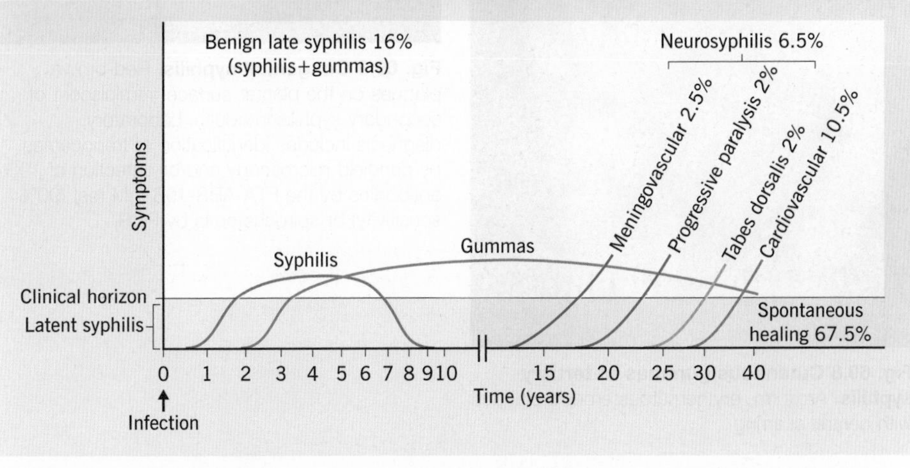

Fig. 69.7 Clinical manifestations of late syphilis. Gummas occur most commonly in the skin (70%) and less often in the bones (10%) or mucous membranes (10%). In neurosyphilis, both endarteritis and direct invasion of the brain parenchyma can occur. Tabes dorsalis presents with painful paresthesias of the limbs, ataxia, and Argyll Robertson pupils. *Adapted from Fritsch P, Zangerle R, Stary A. Venerologie. In: Fritsch P (Ed.), Dermatologie und Venerologie. Berlin: Springer, 1998:865–886.*

MOTHER-TO-CHILD TRANSMISSION OF UNTREATED SYPHILIS AND ITS CONSEQUENCES
Risk
• Infection of the mother from conception to 7th month of pregnancy: transmission in nearly 100% (often fetal demise or severe congenital syphilis) • Infection at least 2 years before pregnancy: reduced risk of transmission to 50% • Infection during 7th, 8th, or early 9th month: reduced risk of transmission • Infection 3–6 weeks before labor: no placental transmission; risk of perinatal transmission
Consequences of infection
• Spontaneous abortion (second or third trimester) (10%) • Stillbirth (10%) • Infant death (20%) • Congenital syphilis (20%) • Healthy child (40%)

Table 69.2 Mother-to-child transmission of untreated syphilis and its consequences. *Courtesy, Angelika Stary, MD.*

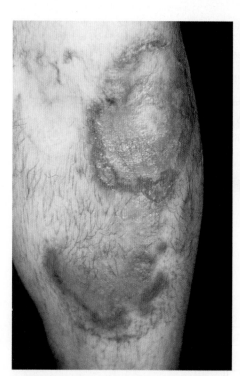

Fig. 69.8 Cutaneous gummas of tertiary syphilis. Arciform, erythematous eroded plaques with central scarring.

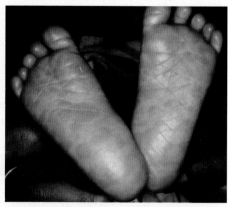

Fig. 69.9 Congenital syphilis. Red-brown plaques on the plantar surface, reminiscent of secondary syphilis in adults. Laboratory diagnosis includes identification of treponemes by darkfield microscopy and/or detection of 19S antibodies by the FTA-ABS-19S-IgM test (90% sensitivity) or spirochetemia by PCR.

STIGMATA OF CONGENITAL SYPHILIS

Cutaneous
- Rhagades (radial periorificial [mouth, nose, eyes, anus] scars at sites of previous fissures)

Dental
- Hutchinson's teeth (peg-shaped, notched permanent incisors)*
- Mulberry molars (multiple rounded rudimentary cusps on the permanent first molars)
- Caries due to defective enamel

Skeletal
- Saddle nose (depression of the nasal root due to destruction of cartilage/bone)
- Frontal bossing of Parrot ('Olympian brow')
- Hypoplastic maxilla, relatively prominent mandible
- High palatal arch ± perforation
- Higouménakis' sign (thickening of the medial clavicle)
- Scaphoid scapulae
- Saber shins (anterior tibial bowing)
- Clutton's joints (painless synovitis and effusions of the knees)

Other
- Eighth nerve deafness*
- Interstitial keratitis (leading to corneal ulcers and opacities)*

*Components of Hutchinson's triad.

Table 69.3 Stigmata of congenital syphilis. These findings represent the delayed consequences of inflammation at the sites of infection. *Courtesy, Angelika Stary, MD.*

DIFFERENTIAL DIAGNOSES FOR SYPHILIS

Primary syphilis
  Other causes of genital ulcers should be considered:
- Genital trauma
- Fixed drug eruption
- Ulcerative genital carcinoma (e.g. squamous cell carcinoma)
- Primary EBV infection
- Behçet's disease
- See Table 69.8

Secondary syphilis
- Cutaneous: pityriasis rosea, guttate psoriasis, viral exanthems, lichen planus, pityriasis lichenoides chronica, primary HIV infection, drug eruption, nummular eczema, folliculitis
- Mucous membranes: lichen planus; chronic aphthae; hand, foot, and mouth disease; herpangina; perlèche
- Condylomata lata: warts due to HPV, bowenoid papulosis, squamous cell carcinoma

Tertiary syphilis
- Cutaneous: lupus vulgaris, chromoblastomycosis, dimorphic fungal infections, leishmaniasis, lupus erythematosus, mycosis fungoides, sarcoidosis, tumors, venous ulcer

Table 69.4 Differential diagnoses for syphilis. *Courtesy, Angelika Stary, MD.*

TREATMENT RECOMMENDATIONS FOR EARLY SYPHILIS (PRIMARY, SECONDARY, AND EARLY LATENT [ACQUIRED <1 YEAR PREVIOUSLY])

Recommended
- Benzathine penicillin, 2.4 million units* im as a single dose

Alternative regimens for penicillin-allergic patients‡
- Doxycycline, 200 mg daily (100 mg PO BID preferred over a single 200-mg dose) for 14 days *or*
- Tetracycline, 500 mg PO qid for 14 days *or*
- Ceftriaxone, 1 g im or iv daily for 10–14 days *or*
- Azithromycin, 2 g PO as a single dose§

Pregnancy

Recommended
- Benzathine penicillin, 2.4 million units im weekly for two doses

In the case of penicillin allergy
- Desensitization to penicillin *or*
- Alternative regimens**
  - Azithromycin, 500 mg daily for 10 days *or*
  - Ceftriaxone, 1 g im or iv daily for 10–14 days

In children, 50 000 U/kg up to the adult dose.
‡*Limited data; desensitization to penicillin is recommended when compliance is an issue.*
§*Resistance reported; not recommended in men who have sex with men and pregnant women.*
***Limited data; not recommended by the CDC but included in the European Branch of the International Union against Sexually Transmitted Infections (IUSTI) guidelines.*
BID, twice daily; h, hours; im, intramuscularly; iv, intravenously; PO, orally; qid, four times daily.

Table 69.5 Treatment recommendations for early syphilis (primary, secondary, and early latent [acquired <1 year previously]). A Jarisch–Herxheimer reaction characterized by the acute onset of fever, headache, and myalgias can occur upon treatment of early syphilis. See the Centers for Disease Control and Prevention (CDC) guidelines (http://www.cdc.gov/std/treatment) or download the CDC STD Tx Guide App.

Gonorrhea

- The etiologic agent is *Neisseria gonorrhoeae* and the primary infection is usually genital but can be anal, rectal, or oral; gonorrhea is acquired primarily via sexual contact and the incubation period is 2–5 days.
- While acute urethritis in men accompanied by a purulent discharge is the most common clinical presentation, the manifestations of gonorrhea are varied (Table 69.6); asymptomatic infections are common in women and when the rectum or pharynx is the site of infection.
- In disseminated gonococcal infection, often referred to as the arthritis–dermatosis syndrome, a limited number of acral inflammatory pustules appear due to septic vasculitis, along with fever, arthralgia, and tenosynovitis (Fig. 69.10); risk factors include menstruation

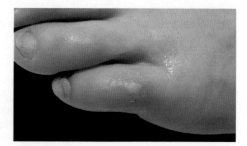

Fig. 69.10 Gonococcemia (arthritis–dermatosis syndrome). Pustule with surrounding erythema on the toe. *Courtesy, Angelika Stary, MD.*

and deficiencies of the late components of complement (C5–C9; see Chapter 49).
- Dx: stained smears of urethral and cervical exudates or cutaneous pustules; culture, PCR, or DNA hybridization of samples from any site of infection.

CLINICAL MANIFESTATIONS OF GONORRHEA	
Disseminated infection • Arthritis • Fever • Tenosynovitis • Acral cutaneous pustules • Scalp abscesses* • Endocarditis • Meningitis	**Local extension** • Prostatitis • Vesiculitis • Epididymitis • Salpingitis • Oophoritis • Pelvic inflammatory disease
Direct mucosal infection • Urethritis • Cervicitis • Proctitis • Pharyngitis • Vulvovaginitis (children) • Ophthalmia neonatorum	
*In neonates at sites of fetal scalp monitor electrodes.	

Table 69.6 Clinical manifestations of gonorrhea. Both urethritis and cervicitis lead to a purulent discharge. *Courtesy, Angelika Stary, MD.*

• **DDx:** for the urethral or cervical discharge, other infections, in particular due to *Chlamydia trachomatis*; for the cutaneous lesions due to gonococcemia, other infectious emboli, small vessel vasculitis, and neutrophilic dermatoses.
• **Rx:** see Table 69.7.

Chancroid

• The etiologic agent is *Haemophilus ducreyi*; this infection occurs more commonly in Africa and South Asia (Fig. 69.11), and it has a male:female ratio of 10:1.
• After an incubation period of 3–10 days, painful genital ulcers, usually multiple, develop in conjunction with tender inguinal lymphadenitis (usually unilateral; Fig. 69.12); the base of the ulcer is purulent and soft, as opposed to the induration of syphilitic chancres.
• Dx: stained smears and culture (on special media) of ulcer exudate; PCR.
• **DDx:** see Table 69.8.
• **Rx:** see Table 69.9.

Lymphogranuloma Venereum (LGV)

• The etiologic agent is *Chlamydia trachomatis* serovars L1–L3; endemic in regions of Africa, Asia, and South America; elsewhere, e.g. in the United States and Western Europe, primarily MSM are affected.
• Infection is acquired via the anogenital or rectal mucosa with subsequent lymphatic spread, leading to lymphadenopathy which is usually unilateral (Fig. 69.13); ~50% of patients develop a herpetiform lesion at the initial site of infection that heals spontaneously, following an incubation period of 3–12 days; the subsequent clinical manifestations are outlined in Table 69.10.
• Dx: detection of *Chlamydia*-specific DNA by PCR from affected tissues.
• **DDx:** see Table 69.8.
• **Rx:** see Table 69.9.

Granuloma Inguinale (Donovanosis)

• The etiologic agent is *Klebsiella granulomatis* (previously named *Calymmatobacterium granulomatis*), and the majority of infections occur in southern Africa, Southeast Asia, and northern Australia; histologically, 'parasitized' macrophages with intracellular organisms (Donovan bodies) are seen.
• Clinically, an initial small papulonodule in the anogenital region ulcerates and then enlarges following an incubation period of up to 1 year (usually ~15–20 days); the base of

TREATMENT RECOMMENDATIONS FOR GONOCOCCAL INFECTIONS

Uncomplicated gonococcal infections of the urethra, cervix or rectum
Recommended regimens
- Ceftriaxone, 250 mg im as single dose* *versus*
- Ceftriaxone, 500 mg im as a single dose plus azithromycin 2 g as a single dose (IUSTI)
Alternative regimens (plus test-of-cure in one week)
- Cefixime, 400 mg PO as single dose*
- Cefixime, 400 mg PO as single dose plus azithromycin 2 g as a single dose (IUSTI)
Alternative regimen if severe cephalosporin allergy (plus test-of-cure in one week)
- Azithromycin, 2 g im as single dose

Uncomplicated gonococcal infections of the pharynx*
- Ceftriaxone, 250 mg im as single dose

Gonococcal conjunctivitis*
- Ceftriaxone, 1 g im as single dose

Disseminated gonococcal infection*
Recommended regimen
- Ceftriaxone, 1 g im or iv q24h until 24–48 hours after improvement begins, *then* cefixime, 400 mg PO BID to complete at least 1 week of therapy
Alternative regimens
- Cefotaxime or ceftizoxime, 1 g iv q8h until 24–48 hours after improvement begins, then cefixime as above

Additional treatment with azithromycin 1 g as single dose or doxycycline 100 mg BID for 7 days is recommended for all patients being treated for gonococcal infections; use of azithromycin is preferred. BID, twice daily; h, hours; im, intramuscularly; iv, intravenously; PO, orally; q, every; IUSTI, European Branch of the International Union against Sexually Transmitted Infections guidelines.

Table 69.7 Treatment recommendations for gonococcal infections. Examination and treatment of sexual partners is also indicated. See the Centers for Disease Control and Prevention (CDC) guidelines (http://www.cdc.gov/std/treatment) or download the CDC STD Tx Guide App.

ESTIMATED WORLDWIDE PREVALENCE OF CHANCROID

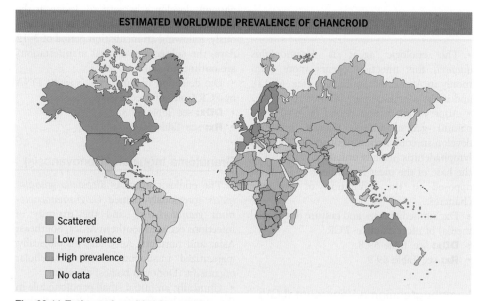

- Scattered
- Low prevalence
- High prevalence
- No data

Fig. 69.11 Estimated worldwide prevalence of chancroid. *Adapted from Ronald A. Chancroid. In: Mandell GL (Ed.-in-Chief), Rein MF (Ed.),* Atlas of Infectious Diseases: Vol. 5. Sexually Transmitted Diseases. *New York: Current Medicine, 1995:16.1–10.*

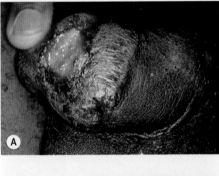

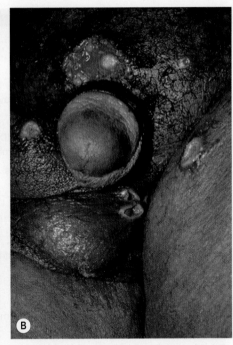

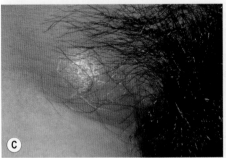

Fig. 69.12 Chancroid. A Well-demarcated painful ulcers on the penis. **B** Multiple purulent ulcers with undermined borders. **C** Unilateral lymphadenitis with overlying erythema. *B, Courtesy, Joyce Rico, MD.*

INFECTIOUS CAUSES OF GENITAL ULCER DISEASE				
Disease	**Incubation Time**	**Clinical Lesion**	**Diagnosis**	**Organism**
Genital herpes	3–7 days	Vesicles, erosions, ulcers; history of herpes infection; painful	DFA, Tzanck (if vesicles), culture, PCR	HSV 2 > 1
Primary syphilis	10–90 days, average 3 weeks	Nonpurulent; usually single ulcer; indurated; relatively painless	Darkfield microscopy, serology	*Treponema pallidum*
Chancroid	3–10 days	Purulent; often multiple ulcers; soft, undermined edges; painful	Smear, culture, PCR	*Haemophilus ducreyi*
LGV	3–12 days	Transient ulcer; indurated; painless	PCR, serology, culture	*Chlamydia trachomatis* serovars L1–L3
Donovanosis	2–12 weeks	Chronic ulcer; indurated, beefy red, friable	Smears, histology	*Klebsiella* (*Calymmatobacterium*) *granulomatis*

DFA, direct fluorescent assay; HSV, herpes simplex virus; LGV, lymphogranuloma venereum; PCR, polymerase chain reaction.
Courtesy, Angelika Stary, MD.

Table 69.8 Infectious causes of genital ulcer disease.

TREATMENT REGIMENS FOR CHANCROID, LGV, AND GRANULOMA INGUINALE

Chancroid

- Azithromycin, 1 g PO, single dose
- Ceftriaxone, 250 mg im, single dose
- Ciprofloxacin, 500 mg PO BID for 3 days*,†
- Erythromycin base, 500 mg PO QID for 7 days†

LGV

- Recommended: doxycycline, 100 mg PO BID
- Alternative and in case of pregnancy: erythromycin base, 500 mg PO QID

Duration for both regimens: at least 3 weeks

Granuloma Inguinale

Recommended**
- Doxycycline, 100 mg PO BID

Alternative**
- Trimethoprim–sulfamethoxazole, 1 double-strength (160 mg/800 mg) tablet PO BID *or*
- Ciprofloxacin, 750 mg PO BID *or*
- Erythromycin base, 500 mg PO QID *or*
- Azithromycin 1 g PO once weekly

Duration for all regimens: until all lesions completely healed (at least 3 weeks)

Contraindicated for pregnant or lactating women.
†Worldwide, isolates with intermediate resistance.
**For any of the regimens, the addition of an aminoglycoside (e.g. gentamicin 1 mg/kg iv q8h) should be considered if lesions do not respond within the first few days of therapy.
BID, twice daily; im, intramuscularly; LGV, lymphogranuloma venereum; PO, orally; QID, four times daily.

Table 69.9 Treatment regimens for chancroid, LGV, and granuloma inguinale. Examination and treatment of sexual partners is also indicated. *Courtesy, Angelika Stary, MD.*

CLINICAL MANIFESTATIONS OF LYMPHOGRANULOMA VENEREUM

Initial manifestations: 3–12 days
- Papule
- Erosion or ulcer
- Herpetiform vesicle
- Nonspecific urethritis or cervicitis

Inguinal syndrome: 10–30 days up to 6 months
- Regional lymphadenopathy (mostly inguinal and femoral; also perirectal, deep iliac)
- Overlying erythema
- Constitutional symptoms
- Eruption of buboes
- Pelvic inflammatory disease (PID), back pain

Ano-genito-rectal syndrome: months to years
- Proctocolitis
- Hyperplasia of intestinal and perirectal lymphatic tissue
- Perirectal abscesses
- Ischiorectal and rectovaginal fistulas
- Anal fistulas
- Rectal strictures and stenoses

Table 69.10 Clinical manifestations of lymphogranuloma venereum. *Courtesy, Angelika Stary, MD.*
Continued

Table 69.10 *Continued* **Clinical manifestations of lymphogranuloma venereum.** *Courtesy, Angelika Stary, MD.*

Other manifestations
• Urethro-genito-perineal syndrome
• Peno-scrotal elephantiasis
• Erythema nodosum
• Submaxillary or cervical lymphadenopathy associated with oropharyngeal lesions

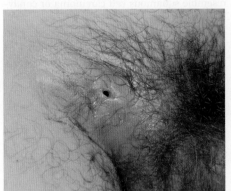

Fig. 69.13 Lymphogranuloma venereum.
Inguinal bubo that has ruptured and drained.
Courtesy, Angelika Stary, MD.

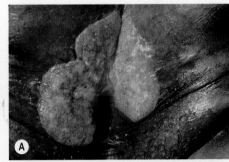

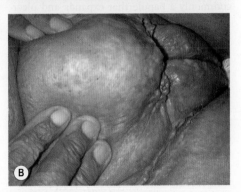

the ulcer is often quite vascular with a foul-smelling drainage (Fig. 69.14).
• Dx: Detection of Donovan bodies in smears of tissue scrapings or touch preps of biopsy specimens (see Chapter 2).
• **DDx:** see Table 69.8.
• **Rx:** see Table 69.9.

Fig. 69.14 Granuloma inguinale (donovanosis). A Large ulcers with a characteristic 'beefy' appearance. **B** The vulva is the most common site of involvement in women with granulomatous plaques as well as ulcerations. *A, Courtesy, Joyce Rico, MD; B, Courtesy, Francisco Bravo, MD.*

For further information see Ch. 82. From *Dermatology, Third Edition.*

70 | Protozoa and Worms

Leishmaniasis

• Three major forms: (1) cutaneous (Fig. 70.1); (2) mucocutaneous (Fig. 70.2); and (3) visceral (e.g. liver, spleen).

• Caused by more than 15 different species of *Leishmania* (Table 70.1).

• Vector = sandfly (*Phlebotomus* and *Lutzomyia* spp.) (Fig. 70.3).

• Disease seen worldwide but endemic in areas of Asia, Africa, Latin America, and the Mediterranean basin (Fig. 70.4).

• Cutaneous disease affects skin only and is commonly a papule that expands and ulcerates (Fig. 70.5); pattern may be sporotrichoid (Fig. 70.6); lesion(s) may heal spontaneously (Fig. 70.7).

• Mucocutaneous form, often due to *Leishmania brasiliensis*, involves mucosal (e.g. nose, lips, oropharynx) sites as well as the skin.

• Visceral leishmaniasis (kala-azar) affects the bone marrow, spleen, and liver and is commonly due to *Leishmania donovani*; symptoms include fever, cough, lymphadenopathy, and hepatosplenomegaly; post-kala-azar dermal leishmaniasis may follow treatment.

• **Rx:** for an isolated lesion, conservative therapy (e.g. observation, heat, cryotherapy) or topical paromycin can be used; for more extensive disease, IV or IM pentavalent antimony (sodium stibogluconate, meglumine antimonate), oral miltefosine.

• For assistance in diagnosis and treatment, helpful sources of information include the Centers for Disease Control and World Health Organization.

Amebiasis

• Protozoan infection (*Entamoeba histolytica*) that most commonly causes colitis; fecal–oral spread.

• Occasionally presents in the skin with necrotic ulcers that can resemble pyoderma gangrenosum or verrucous plaques that resemble squamous cell carcinoma or condyloma acuminatum.

• Skin involvement generally secondary to extension of rectal amebiasis to perianal or perigenital skin or extension of a liver abscess to skin of abdominal wall.

• **Rx:** for *Entamoeba histolytica*, metronidazole; other treatments include diloxanide, tinidazole.

Free-Living Ameba

• *Balamuthia mandrillaris* can infect immunocompetent (especially children) and immunocompromised patients; the typical cutaneous lesion is a slow-growing indurated plaque on the central face with eventual hematogenous spread to the central nervous system.

• *Acanthamoeba* spp. can cause cutaneous papulonodules and encephalitis in immunocompromised patients.

Trypanosomiasis – American

• *Trypanosoma cruzi* carried by reduviid (kissing) bugs.

• Endemic in areas of Central and South America.

• Systemic disease that can affect the autonomic nervous system, gastrointestinal tract, and heart.

• Primary acute phase: local erythema and edema at inoculation site ± regional lymphadenopathy; when periorbital, termed Romaña sign (Fig. 70.8).

• Chronic phase seen after years to decades: congestive heart failure, arrhythmias, including heart block, megacolon, megaesophagus.

Trypanosomiasis – African

• Vector = tsetse fly.

• Found in both West (*Trypanosoma brucei gambiense*) and East (*Trypanosoma brucei rhodesiense*) Africa.

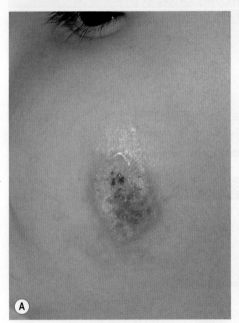

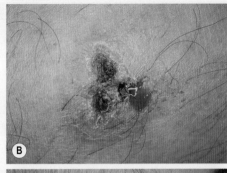

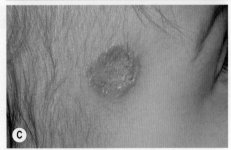

Fig. 70.1 Variable presentations of cutaneous leishmaniasis. Ulcerated plaques with rolled border **(A)** and central crusting **(A, B)**. Plaque with translucent borders containing telangiectasias and central scarring **(C)**. Cutaneous leishmaniasis is sometimes mistaken for a basal cell carcinoma in adults. *A, C, Courtesy, Julie V. Schaffer, MD.*

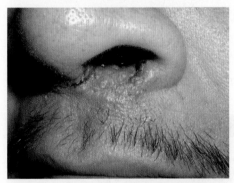

Fig. 70.2 Mucocutaneous leishmaniasis. Ulceration and induration of the nasal vestibule extending onto the cutaneous lip due to *Leishmania braziliensis. Courtesy, Kalman Watsky, MD.*

• Skin findings: trypanosomal chancre (localized bite reaction; Fig. 70.9) and annular erythematous eruption with fever.

• Winterbottom's sign – enlargement of nodes of posterior cervical triangle – classic finding in West African form.

Toxoplasmosis

• Worldwide infection secondary to *Toxoplasma gondii*; oocytes present in cat feces or infected meat.

• Rare skin involvement; congenital infections present with necrotic or hemorrhagic papules on the trunk ('T' in TORCH complex).

• Common presentations include cervical lymphadenitis or chorioretinitis.

• Tissue cysts may lead to recrudescence in immunosuppressed individuals.

Cutaneous Larva Migrans

• Secondary to larvae of *animal* (e.g. usually wild/domestic dogs/cats) hookworms (intestinal nematodes), e.g. *Ancylostoma braziliense*.

• Worldwide, but especially common in tropical/subtropical areas and the southwestern United States.

• Larvae in infected soil, including sand, penetrate the skin.

• Pruritic, inflamed, serpiginous tracks are produced by migrating organisms (Fig. 70.10); migration averages 1–2 cm/day.

FOUR MAJOR SPECIES OF *LEISHMANIA* THAT CAUSE CUTANEOUS DISEASE		
Complex	**Species**	**Major Geographic Distribution**
Leishmania tropica	*L. major*	Arid areas of Africa (north and south of the Sahara), Arabia and Central Asia
	L. tropica	Towns in Eastern Mediterranean countries, Middle East and Central Asia
Leishmania mexicana	*L. mexicana*	Mexico and Central America
Leishmania braziliensis	*L. braziliensis**	South and Central America

*Can also cause mucosal leishmaniasis or visceral leishmaniasis in immunocompromised individuals.

Table 70.1 Four major species of *Leishmania* that cause cutaneous disease.

LIFE CYCLE OF *LEISHMANIA* SPECIES

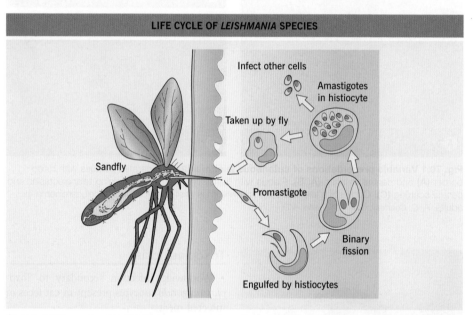

Fig. 70.3 Life cycle of *Leishmania* species. Promastigotes develop within the gut of the sandfly and then migrate to the proboscis.

DISTRIBUTION OF CUTANEOUS LEISHMANIASIS

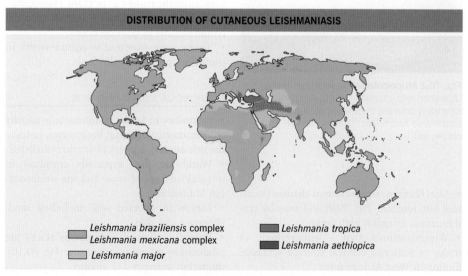

Fig. 70.4 Distribution of cutaneous leishmaniasis. *Adapted with permission from Davidson RN, Leishmaniasis. In Cohen J, Powderly WG (Eds.), Infectious Diseases. Edinburgh, UK: Mosby, 2004.*

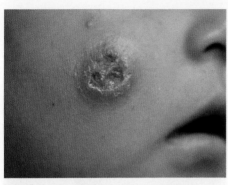

Fig. 70.5 Ulcerated nodule with rolled border. *Courtesy, Omar P. Sangüeza, MD.*

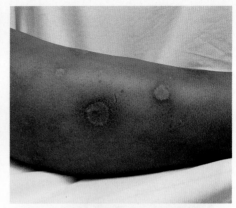

Fig. 70.7 Scars secondary to previous cutaneous leishmaniasis. Circular scars at previous sites of cutaneous leishmaniasis are often the only sign of a prior infection. *Courtesy, Omar P. Sangüeza, MD.*

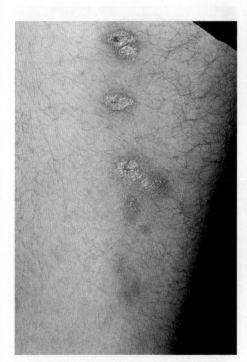

Fig. 70.6 Sporotrichoid form of cutaneous leishmaniasis. *With permission from Tyring S, Lupi O, Hengge U (Eds.),* Tropical Dermatology. *Oxford: Churchill Livingstone, 2005.*

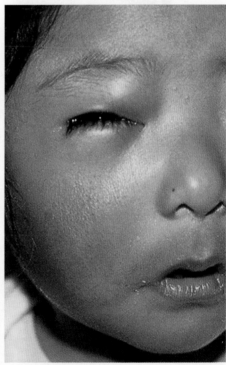

Fig. 70.8 Chagas disease. Young child with unilateral periorbital edema characteristic of this disease (Romaña sign) when the conjunctiva is the portal of entry. *Courtesy, Omar P. Sangüeza, MD.*

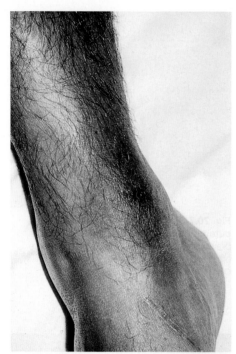

Fig. 70.9 Trypanosomal chancre. The bite reaction, the earliest clinical lesion, is known as a 'trypanosomal chancre.' It resembles a boil but is usually painless. Fluid aspirated from the nodule contains actively dividing trypanosomes. This reaction is seen more commonly in *T. b. rhodesiense* than in *T. b. gambiense* infection. *With permission from Peters W, Pasvol G, Tropical Medicine and Parasitology, 6th ed. London: Mosby, 2007.*

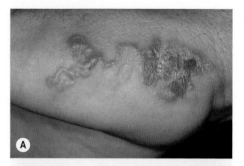

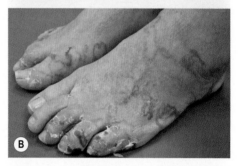

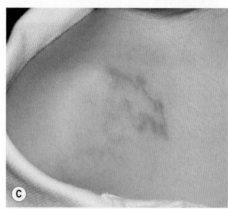

• Most common locations are the lower extremities, especially the feet, and buttocks, due to walking and sitting at the beach.

• **DDx:** not to be confused with larva currens (secondary to *Strongyloides*; see Table 70.2).

• Disease is self-limited but treatment can include oral albendazole or ivermectin; topical thiabendazole for localized disease.

Onchocerciasis

• Secondary to *Onchocerca volvulus*, a tissue-dwelling nematode.

• Vector = black fly (*Simulium*).

• Endemic in Africa, Yemen, and some areas of Central and South America; near fast-flowing rivers.

Fig. 70.10 Cutaneous larva migrans. Note the characteristic serpiginous erythematous tracks on the lateral foot **(A)**, both feet **(B)**, and the shoulder **(C)**. Vesiculation and crusting **(B)** are sometimes seen. *B, Courtesy, Peter Klein, MD; C, Courtesy, Julie V. Schaffer, MD.*

• Skin findings: subcutaneous nodules containing adult worms (onchocercomas), pruritic papular dermatitis, depigmented, lichenified skin, especially over the shins (sowda) (Fig. 70.11).

• Chronic ocular involvement leads to sclerosing keratitis, iridocyclitis, and ultimately blindness, hence the name river blindness.

• **Rx:** oral ivermectin.

OTHER MAJOR PARASITIC WORMS THAT CAUSE CUTANEOUS MANIFESTATIONS IN HUMANS					
Disease	Organism	Distribution	Mode of Spread	Skin Findings	Systemic Findings
Enterobiasis (pinworms), intestinal nematode	*Enterobius vermicularis*	Widespread and high prevalence, especially in countries within temperate zones	Ingestion of eggs	Perianal and perineal pruritus	Restlessness Asymptomatic in most patients
Ancylostomiasis (human hookworms), intestinal nematode	*Ancylostoma duodenale, Necator americanus*	Tropical and subtropical distribution	Percutaneous via contact with infective larvae in soil	Dermatitis ('ground itch') at the site of larval entry	Iron deficiency anemia, GI symptoms, Loeffler's syndrome, eosinophilia
Strongyloidiasis, intestinal nematode	*Strongyloides stercoralis*	Occurs worldwide, especially in tropical areas; in cooler climates found in warm humid deep mines	Percutaneous via contact with infective larvae; occasionally ingestion of larvae Autoinfection via penetration of perianal skin Hyperinfection in immunocompromised patients, due to penetration of intestinal mucosa	Generalized or localized urticarial eruption beginning perianally and extending to the buttocks, thighs, and abdomen (larva currens) 'Thumbprint' purpura in hyperinfection (Fig. 70.13)	Diarrhea, eosinophilia, pulmonary symptoms Symptoms more severe in immuno-compromised patients
Loiasis, tissue nematode	*Loa loa*	West and central Africa	Transmitted by bite of tabanid flies of the genus *Chrysops* (mango flies) carrying infective larvae Mature in connective tissue	Transient localized subcutaneous edema (Calabar swellings), often of the hands, wrists and forearms; represent tracts of migrating adult worms; associated with pruritus and pain	Conjunctivitis (due to movement of adult worms under conjunctiva), eosinophilia, renal disease

Table 70.2 Other major parasitic worms that cause cutaneous manifestations in humans. *Continued*

Table 70.2 *Continued* **Other major parasitic worms that cause cutaneous manifestations in humans.**

Disease	Organism	Distribution	Mode of Spread	Skin Findings	Systemic Findings
Dirofilariasis, tissue nematodes of animals	*Dirofilaria immitis* (dog heartworms); *D. tunuis* (filaria of raccoons); *D. repens* (filaria of dogs and cats); *D. ursi* (filaria of bears)	*D. immitis* occurs worldwide; *D. tunuis* in southeast US; *D. repens* in Europe and Asia; *D. ursi* in North America and Japan	Transmitted by mosquitoes carrying infective larvae Do not mature in humans	*D. tunuis*, *D. repens*, and *D. ursi* cause small painful subcutaneous nodules with or without inflammation	*D. immitis* causes nodules in the lungs
Dracunculiasis, guinea worm, tissue nematode	*Dracunculus medinensis*	Africa, particularly Ghana and the Sudan	Ingestion of infected water fleas of the genus *Cyclops* in drinking water Migrate from intestine to subcutaneous tissue, usually of the legs	Papulonodule then blister and/or ulceration, usually of the lower extremity; calcified nodules	Anaphylactic shock, rheumatic symptoms
Trichinosis, tissue nematode	*Trichinella spiralis*	Widespread in temperate zones	Ingestion of encysted larvae from raw/ undercooked animal meat, usually pork	Periorbital edema in severe infection, splinter hemorrhages	Most infections are subclinical Heavy infection also leads to fever, enteritis, myositis, and eosinophilia; occasionally myocarditis and encephalitis
Sparganosis, larval stage of tapeworms of dogs and cats, cestode	*Spirometra* spp.	Sporadic in most countries, seen most frequently in the Far East	Ingestion of larvae in intermediate hosts (e.g. snakes, frogs, fish) Occasionally following application of frogs to eyes as poultice	Painless small subcutaneous nodules at sites of larval proliferation Edema if periorbital involvement	Rarely, pulmonary or CNS involvement

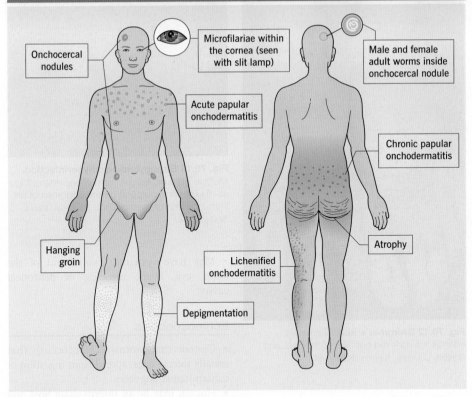

Fig. 70.11 Cutaneous findings in onchocerciasis.

Filariasis

• Tissue nematodes (*Wuchereria bancrofti* or *Brugia malayi/B. timori*) infect the lymphatic system.
• Vector = mosquito (*Culex*, *Anopheles*, *Aedes* spp.).
• Endemic in tropical and subtropical regions of India, the Americas, and Africa.
• Acute form: lymphangitis and orchitis.
• Chronic form: lymphedema, elephantiasis (the enlarged limb becomes indurated with skin folds and overlying verrucous changes), hydrocele, chyluria.
• Complicated by recurrent cellulitis.

Schistosomiasis

• Trematode (fluke) infection secondary to three major species with specific geographic distributions (Africa – *Schistosoma hematobium*, Asia – *S. japonicum*, South America – *S. mansoni*); intermediate host is the freshwater snail; organisms penetrate skin.
• Variants of cutaneous disease – cercarial dermatitis (transient erythema, urticaria, or pruritic papules), Katayama fever (systemic allergic reaction with urticaria, fever, chills, sweats, headache, peripheral eosinophilia).
• Chronic fibro-occlusive disease in the liver (*S. japonicum*), intestine (*S. mansoni*), or urinary tract (*S. hematobium*).

Swimmer's Itch

• Cercariae of >20 species of *animal* schistosomes (e.g. *Ornithobilharzia*) can penetrate skin and cause swimmer's itch.
• Worldwide; endemic to the Great Lakes.
• Erythematous papules on exposed skin (Fig. 70.12).

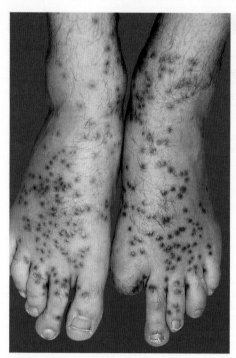

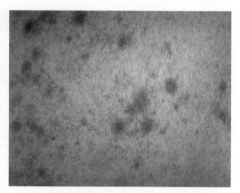

Fig. 70.13 Strongyloidiasis hyperinfection. Multiple purpuric lesions (sometimes referred to as 'thumbprint' purpura) on the abdomen of an immunocompromised patient. *Courtesy, Jean L. Bolognia, MD.*

• May have systemic involvement of the brain, eye, heart, muscles, or peritoneal cavity.

Echinococcosis

• Cestode (tapeworm *Echinococcus*) that usually infects dogs; spread from ingestion of contaminated dog feces.
• Human may be an intermediate host and develop liver or lung hydatid cysts.
• Rarely leads to urticaria, asthma, or anaphylaxis.

Gnathostomiasis

• Due to ingestion of raw or poorly cooked fresh water fish (e.g. ceviche) and eels or frogs that contain larvae of *Gnathostoma* spp. (nematodes).
• Transient subcutaneous swellings that may be pruritic are due to migration of the larvae.

See Table 70.2 for a summary of other major parasitic worms that cause skin findings.

Fig. 70.12 Swimmer's itch. Numerous edematous dark red papules on the feet and ankles. *Courtesy, Kalman Watsky, MD.*

• Self-limited (7–10 days).
• Not to be confused with seabather's eruption (secondary to *Linuche, Edwardsiella* spp.), which affects areas under the swimsuit (see Chapter 72).

Cysticercosis

• Cestodes (tapeworms; e.g. *Taenia solium*) that more commonly infect animals may infect humans; spread from ingestion of contaminated meat or fecal–oral spread.
• Skin findings: small, asymptomatic papulonodules.

For further information see Ch. 83. From *Dermatology, Third Edition*.

Infestations | 71

Scabies

• Infestation by *Sarcoptes scabiei* var. *hominis*, a mite that lives within the stratum corneum of human skin (Fig. 71.1).

• Transmission is primarily by direct contact with an infested person and occasionally by fomites (e.g. clothing); incubation period may be up to 6 weeks; in some tropical regions, scabies can infest the majority of individuals in a community.

• Asymptomatic infestation by scabies is not uncommon ('carriers' of scabies).

• In symptomatic cases, pruritus is severe, often worse at night or after a hot shower; secondary bacterial infections (e.g. staphylococcal, streptococcal) may occur.

• Skin lesions are variable and include erythematous papules with scale-crust, small patches of eczema, excoriations, vesicles (especially acrally in infants), and nodules; the classic burrow – a thread-like, grayish-white, wavy, 1- to 10-mm linear structure – favors acral sites (Figs. 71.2 and 71.3).

• Clinical confirmation is by mineral oil examination of skin scrapings (see Chapter 2) or dermoscopy (see Fig. 71.2D).

• Usually <100 mites, but often no more than 10–15, living on an infested individual (Fig. 71.4); there may be thousands of mites in crusted scabies (thick scale, especially acrally, with minimal inflammation), which affects immunocompromised hosts, those with altered skin sensation, and sometimes the elderly (Fig. 71.5).

• In general, the mites live off the body ≤3 days; if accompanied by sloughed skin, as in crusted scabies, the duration may be longer.

• **DDx:** arthropod bites, including bites of animal mites (e.g. *Cheyletiella*); diseases associated with generalized pruritus (e.g. atopic dermatitis; see Table 4.1); in infants, infantile acropustulosis, which may also occur following successful treatment of scabies.

• **Rx:** see Table 71.1.

  – Two overnight applications of a topical antiscabetic medication, 1 week apart, to the entire body surface from the neck down to the toes; in infants, the elderly, and the immunocompromised, need to include the face and scalp.

  – Permethrin 5% cream is the preferred topical agent.

  – Oral ivermectin (200–400 microg/kg given on days 1 and 8) is increasingly replacing topical medications, especially when large groups of individuals are affected as in a nursing home.

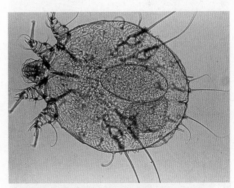

Fig. 71.1 Female scabies mite with egg. The female scabies mite in a potassium hydroxide wet mount obtained from skin scrapings, revealing a flattened, oval body with wrinkle-like corrugations, eight short legs, and an egg ready for deposition (40×). *With permission from Taplin D, Meinking TL. Infestations. In: Schachner LA, Hansen RC (Eds.), Pediatric Dermatology, 4th edn. Edinburgh, UK: Mosby, 2011:1141–1180.*

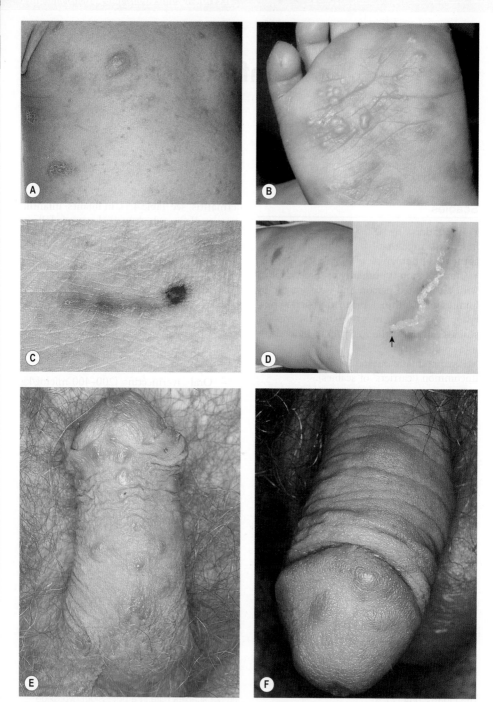

Fig. 71.2 Scabies. A, B Erythematous papules, linear burrows, areas of crusting and acral vesiculopustules in two infants with scabies. **C** Close-up of a linear burrow post scraping for examination under mineral oil. **D** By dermoscopy, a characteristic 'jet with contrail' structure can be identified corresponding to the anterior part of the mite (arrow) and the burrow behind it. **E, F** Penile involvement with erythematous papules and nodules. *D, Courtesy, Iris Zalaudek, MD; F, Courtesy, Robert Hartman, MD. Continued*

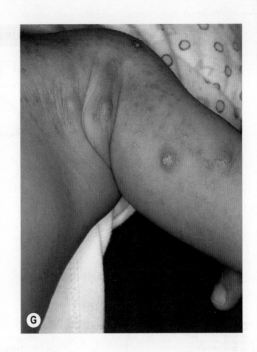

Fig. 71.2 *Continued* **G** Nodular scabies in an infant. *G, Courtesy, Kalman Watsky, MD.*

RANGE OF CUTANEOUS LESIONS IN SCABIES

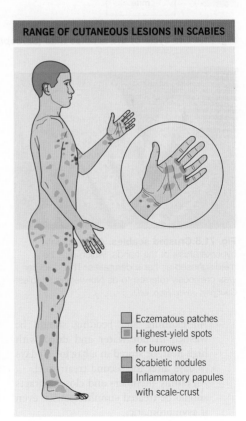

Eczematous patches
Highest-yield spots for burrows
Scabietic nodules
Inflammatory papules with scale-crust

Fig. 71.3 Range of cutaneous lesions in scabies. Typical sites affected by scabies are highlighted. In infants and the elderly or immunocompromised, all surfaces can be involved, including the scalp and face.

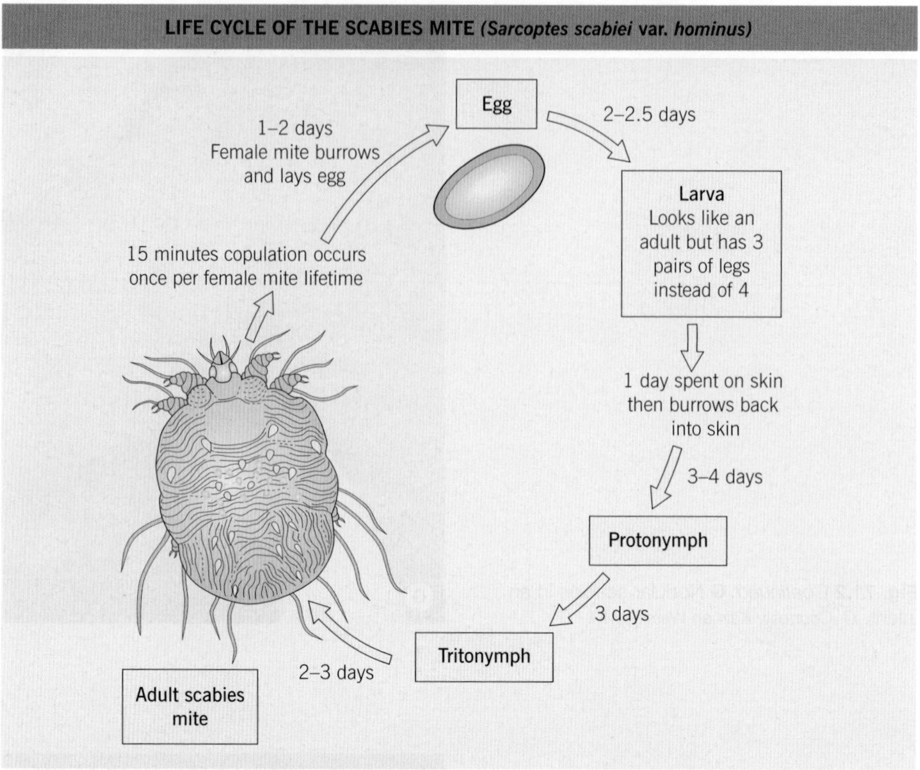

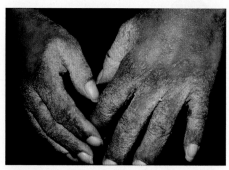

LIFE CYCLE OF THE SCABIES MITE *(Sarcoptes scabiei var. hominus)*

Egg

1–2 days
Female mite burrows
and lays egg

2–2.5 days

15 minutes copulation occurs
once per female mite lifetime

Larva
Looks like an
adult but has 3
pairs of legs
instead of 4

1 day spent on skin
then burrows back
into skin

3–4 days

Protonymph

3 days

Tritonymph

2–3 days

**Adult scabies
mite**

Fig. 71.4 Life cycle of the scabies mite (*Sarcoptes scabiei* var. *hominus*).

Fig. 71.5 Crusted scabies. Asymptomatic hyperkeratosis of the hands, which may be misdiagnosed as hand dermatitis. This disorder was previously referred to as Norwegian scabies. *Courtesy, Joyce Rico, MD.*

– All clothing and bedding should be washed in hot water and dried with high heat, or stored in a bag for 10 days (3 days after the second treatment).
– All family members and close contacts should be treated simultaneously, even if asymptomatic.

– Pruritus and cutaneous lesions often last 2–4 weeks after successful treatment, but patients may feel relief within 3 days.
– Once the diagnosis is established and initial treatment has been administered, topical corticosteroids (mild to moderate strength) can be used for symptomatic relief.
– In crusted scabies, additional measures are necessary (e.g. combined and/or repeated treatments, cutting of nails, longer storage of clothing, vacuuming upholstery).

Head Lice (Pediculosis Capitis)

• Secondary to *Pediculus capitis*, a blood-sucking, six-legged insect that lays its eggs near the base of the hairs on the scalp (Fig. 71.6); the casing remains after the egg hatches and migrates outward with growth of the hair shaft.

TOPICAL AND ORAL TREATMENTS FOR SCABIES

Treatment	Administration on Days 1 and 8	Concerns	Efficacy and Resistance	Use in Infants	FDA Pregnancy Category
Permethrin cream (5%)	Topically overnight	Allergic contact dermatitis in individuals with sensitivity to formaldehyde	Good, but some signs of resistance developing	FDA approved for infants ≥2 months of age	B
Ivermectin (available as 3 mg tablets)	Oral dose of 200–400 microg/kg	Potential CNS toxicity in infants and young children	Excellent	Safety not established for children weighing <33 pounds (15 kg) or breast-feeding mothers	C (but generally not recommended for scabies in pregnant women)

Table 71.1 Topical and oral treatments for scabies. All treatments should be given on two separate occasions, 1 week apart. Other topical therapies are sometimes utilized, based on availability, but suffer from inferior efficacy and toxicities, e.g. lindane (CNS toxicity), sulfur 5–10%, and crotamiton.

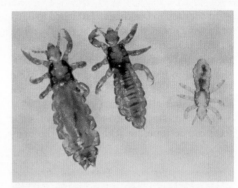

Fig. 71.6 Head louse family. From left to right: female, male, and nymph. *With permission from Taplin D, Meinking TL. Infestations. In: Schachner LA, Hansen RC (Eds.), Pediatric Dermatology, 4th edn. Edinburgh, UK: Mosby, 2011:1141–1180.*

- Transmission is by direct contact with an infested person or fomites (e.g. hats, brushes).
- Pruritus is variable.
- In addition to the presence of lice and eggs, there may be erythema, scaling, and excoriations of the head and neck region; occasionally there is a secondary pyoderma.
- Diagnosis is generally made by visual examination, followed by microscopic inspection and the detection of 0.8 mm eggs or their casings attached to scalp hairs ('nits'); high-yield locations include hairs above the ears and the lower occipital scalp (Fig. 71.7).
- **DDx** of scalp pruritus: seborrheic dermatitis, psoriasis, atopic dermatitis.
- **DDx** of nits: hair casts, dandruff, hair gel, and other causes of hair shaft nodules (see Fig. 64.3).
- **Rx:** outlined in Table 71.2.

Crab Lice (Pediculosis Pubis)

- Secondary to *Phthirus pubis*, a bloodsucking, six-legged insect that lives on the terminal hairs of the pubic region, beard, eyelashes, axillae, and perianal region.
- While body and head lice are similar in appearance, crab lice are shorter and broader, thus actually resembling crabs (Fig. 71.8).
- Transmission is by direct contact (may be sexual) or occasionally via contaminated clothing, towels, or bedding.
- May coexist with other STDs; pruritus is common.

- In addition to lice that are attached to hairs or moving about the surface of the skin (Fig. 71.9A), hemorrhagic crusts, perifollicular erythema, and macula caerulea (asymptomatic slate-gray to blue macules on the trunk and thighs) may be seen; secondary bacterial infection may also occur.
- If the infestation involves the eyelashes, feces can accumulate at the base of the hairs and at the inferior margin of the lower eyelid (Fig. 71.9B).
- **DDx:** other causes of genital pruritus; nits must be distinguished from other causes of hair nodules (see Fig. 64.3).
- **Rx:** see Table 71.3.

Body Lice (Pediculosis Corporis)

- Secondary to infestation of clothing and humans by *Pediculus humanus* var. *corporis*, a bloodsucking six-legged insect.
- Associated with overcrowding, poor hygiene, poverty, wars, and natural disasters.
- Body lice can transmit epidemic typhus (*Rickettsia prowazekii*), trench fever (*Bartonella quintana*), and relapsing fever (*Borrelia recurrentis*).

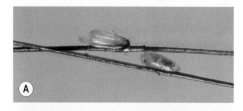

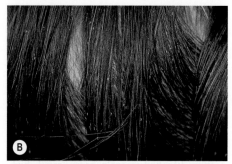

Fig. 71.7 Head lice. A The head louse egg or nit is 0.8 mm in length. **B** Head lice nits on hair. *With permission from Taplin D, Meinking TL. Infestations. In: Schachner LA, Hansen RC (Eds.), Pediatric Dermatology, 4th edn. Edinburgh, UK: Mosby, 2011:1141–1180.*

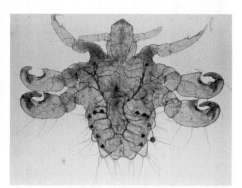

Fig. 71.8 Adult crab louse. The shape is shorter and broader than that of head and body lice. *Courtesy, Tony Burns, MD.*

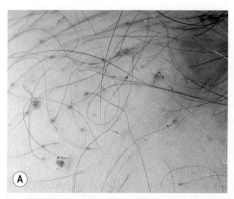

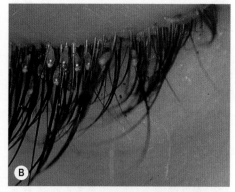

Fig. 71.9 Crab lice. A Both adult crab lice and nits are evident on pubic hairs. **B** Crab lice nits and feces on the eyelashes. *A, Courtesy, Louis A. Fragola, Jr., MD; B, With permission from Taplin D, Meinking TL. Infestations. In: Schachner LA, Hansen RC (Eds.), Pediatric Dermatology, 4th edn. Edinburgh, UK: Mosby, 2011:1141–1180.*

TOPICAL AND ORAL TREATMENTS FOR HEAD LICE

Treatment	Administration on Days 1 and 8	Concerns	Efficacy and Resistance
Permethrin cream rinse or lotion (1%)*	Topical application for 10 minutes to clean, dry hair	None	Poor–fair; resistance common
Pyrethrins (0.33%) synergized with piperonyl butoxide (4%), various formulations*	Topical application for 10 minutes to dry hair	Allergic reactions in individuals with sensitivity to chrysanthemums, ragweed, and related plants	Poor–fair; resistance common
Malathion lotion or gel (0.5%)**	Topical application for 8–12 hours to dry hair (Ovide® and gel products with isopropyl alcohol base are effective at 20 minutes)	Flammable isopropyl alcohol base; burning or stinging at sites of eroded skin	Excellent (in United States); resistance noted in United Kingdom and France, but to date not in United States
Benzyl alcohol lotion (5%)^	Topical application for 10 minutes to dry hair	Potential skin irritation	Fair–good; no resistance noted to date
Spinosad cream rinse (0.9%)+	Topical application for 10 minutes to dry hair	None	Good; no resistance noted to date
Ivermectin lotion (0.5%)^	Topical application for 10 minutes to dry hair	Ocular irritation	Good; no resistance noted to date
Ivermectin (available as 3 mg tablets)	Oral dose of 200–400 microg/kg	Potential CNS toxicity; not recommended for children weighing <33 pounds (15 kg), breast-feeding mothers, or pregnant women (category C)	Excellent; no resistance noted to date

*Over-the-counter products.
**Approved for individuals ≥6 years of age; pregnancy category B.
+Approved for individuals ≥4 years of age; avoid in infants <6 months of age; pregnancy category B.
^Approved for individuals ≥6 months of age; pregnancy category B.

Table 71.2 Topical and oral treatments for head lice. All treatments should be given on two separate occasions, 1 week apart, with the exception of a single application for ivermectin lotion. Carbaryl shampoo (0.5%), lindane shampoo (1%), and permethrin cream (5%) are sometimes used, but generally have inferior efficacy.

TOPICAL AND ORAL TREATMENTS FOR CRAB LICE

Treatment	Administration on Days 1 and 8	Efficacy
Permethrin (1%) cream rinse or synergized pyrethrin shampoo*	Topical application for 10 minutes to clean, dry hair	Fair
Permethrin cream (5%)	Topical application for 8–12 hours	Good
Ivermectin (available as 3 mg tablets)	Oral dose of 250 microg/kg	Excellent

*Over-the-counter product.

Table 71.3 Topical and oral treatments for crab lice. All crab lice treatments should be given on two separate occasions, 1 week apart. Lindane shampoo (1%) is occasionally used but has inferior efficacy.

- Severe pruritus common, especially on the back, waist, shoulders, and neck.
- Body lice and nits are primarily found in clothing seams (Fig. 71.10).
- **DDx:** bites from other arthropods and other causes of generalized pruritus (see Table 4.1).
- **Rx:** incinerate clothing and bedding if possible; otherwise wash and dry with high heat; in epidemics, mass delousing with dusting powders (e.g. DDT).

Tungiasis

- Secondary to the burrowing flea, *Tunga penetrans*.
- Endemic in Central and South America, Caribbean Islands, Africa, Pakistan, and India.
- Pregnant female flea burrows into the skin, especially on the feet of individuals who do not wear shoes or wear only flip-flops (Fig. 71.11).

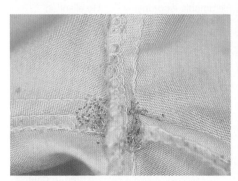

Fig. 71.10 Body lice eggs in the seams of clothing.

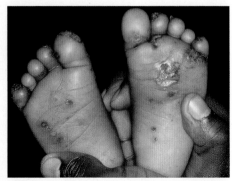

Fig. 71.11 Tungiasis in a child. *Courtesy, Terri L. Meinking, MD, Craig N. Burkhart, MD, and Craig G. Burkhart, MD.*

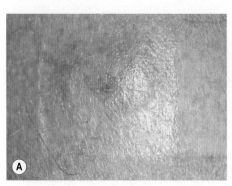

(A)

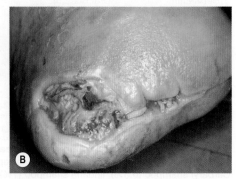

(B)

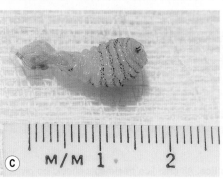

(C)

Fig. 71.12 Cutaneous myiasis. A Furuncular myiasis presenting as a papulonodule with a central punctum on the leg. **B** Wound myiasis in an amputation stump. **C** Botfly larva. *B, Courtesy, Louis A. Fragola, Jr., MD.*

- Commonly, a 1- or 2-cm nodule with surrounding erythema develops; there may be multiple lesions.
- Rarely, tetanus, gangrene, or autoamputation may result.
- **DDx:** myiasis, persistent arthropod bite reaction, cercarial dermatitis, pyoderma, wart, squamous cell carcinoma.
- **Rx:** removal of the flea; tetanus prophylaxis should be considered.
- Prevention: wear shoes and avoid sitting on sandy beaches in endemic areas.

Cutaneous Myiasis

- Infestation of skin by fly larvae; furuncular myiasis presents as a boil-like lesion, most commonly secondary to *Dermatobia hominis* (human botfly) and *Cordylobia anthropophaga* (tumbu fly); wound myiasis is most often due to *Cochliomyia hominivorax* or *Chrysomya bezziana* (Fig. 71.12).
- Complications may occur, especially when the sinuses, nasal cavity, or scalp are involved.
- **DDx** for furuncular myiasis: ruptured cyst, abscess, furunculosis, and foreign body reaction.
- **Rx:** excision or removal of larvae for furuncular myiasis; debridement and irrigation for wound myiasis; consider oral ivermectin if oral/ocular involvement.
- Prevention: insect repellent, including on the scalp; ironing all line-dried items will kill eggs of the tumbu fly.

For further information see Ch. 84. From *Dermatology, Third Edition*.

72 | Bites and Stings

Insects

• The bite of any insect can lead to a local cutaneous reaction whose intensity can vary depending on the individual's level of sensitivity; the typical presentation is a 2 to 8 mm, erythematous urticarial papule in an exposed area (Fig. 72.1); lesions are often multiple and can be grouped.

• Secondary changes consisting of excoriations may be present; less often, vesicles or bullae develop at the site of bites (Fig. 72.2).

• Bite reactions typically resolve over 5–10 days; occasionally, patients develop persistent bite reactions that on biopsy may be diagnosed as pseudolymphoma (see Chapter 99).

• Postinflammatory hyperpigmentation is common, especially in patients with darkly pigmented skin.

• Secondary infection is a potential complication, most commonly from staphylococci or streptococci.

• Exaggerated bite reactions can be seen in patients with chronic lymphocytic leukemia; rarely, hypersensitivity reactions to mosquito bites that become necrotic can be associated with EBV infection (see Chapter 67).

• Anaphylaxis with urticaria and angioedema is generally due to stings from hymenopterids (bees, wasps, hornets, and fire ants) (Fig. 72.3).

• Insects may be vectors of infectious diseases (Table 72.1).

• Bites can trigger papular urticaria, especially in children, in which edematous papules are more widespread and longer-lasting; some of the lesions can represent reactivation.

• Prevention: insect repellents (e.g. DEET), mosquito netting, and protective or permethrin-treated clothing.

• **Rx:** anti-pruritic topical agents (e.g. pramoxine, calamine), topical CS ± occlusion; for persistent lesions, intralesional CS (e.g. triamcinolone 5 mg/ml).

Arachnids

Hard Ticks

• Site of the tick bite can become papular, nodular, bullous, or plaque-like; expanding lesion suggests possible erythema migrans.

• Attached ticks may go unnoticed (e.g. scalp, groin); occasionally the attached tick is misinterpreted as a 'new mole'.

• Ticks are important disease vectors, especially in the nymphal stage (Table 72.2; see Fig. 63.1); tick control measures are important for public health (see Fig. 63.8 for geographic distribution of vector tick species).

• Removal of ticks should be performed carefully by grasping the protruding end of the tick as close to the skin surface as possible and firmly pulling away from the attachment site with fine-tipped tweezers.

• Prevention: permethrin repellent can be sprayed on clothing or other fabrics; protective clothing.

• **Rx** of persistent tick bite reactions: potent topical CS, intralesional CS, or even excision in severe cases; doxycycline is recommended in suspected cases of Rocky Mountain spotted fever (10-day course; see Chapter 63) or Lyme disease (14- to 21-day course).

Mites

• Thousands of species; parasitize humans as well as animals and plants.

• Human mites include *Demodex folliculorum* and *D. brevis* (may lead to folliculitis and exacerbate rosacea) and *Sarcoptes scabiei*, which causes scabies (see Chapter 71); these mites complete their life cycle on humans.

• *Cheyletiella* mites ('walking dandruff') are found on small mammals (e.g. cats, dogs) and may cause papulovesicular lesions in humans (Fig. 72.4).

• Chigger mites in Asia are vectors for scrub typhus.

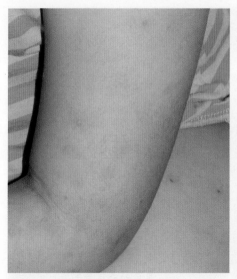

Fig. 72.1 Insect bite reactions. In this patient, there are papulovesicles as well as excoriated papules with hemorrhagic crusting. In more darkly pigmented individuals, residual hyperpigmentation is common and can persist for months. *Courtesy, Julie V. Schaffer, MD.*

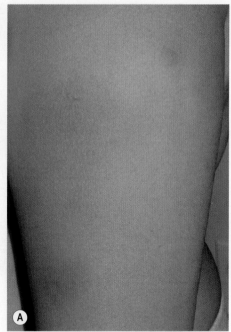

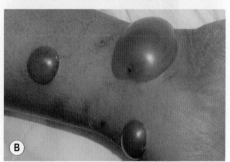

Fig. 72.2 Insect bite reactions. Sometimes patients develop large, erythematous, edematous plaques **(A)** or frank bullae **(B).** *Courtesy, Julie V. Schaffer, MD.*

• House mouse mites are vectors for rickettsialpox.

Spiders

• Black widow spider (*Latrodectus mactans* is the primary species in the United States).
  – Bites lead to acute pain and edema.
  – Systemic symptoms may include an acute abdomen or rhabdomyolysis.
  – **Rx:** if severe reaction, emergency medical treatment.

• Brown recluse spider (*Loxosceles reclusa* is the predominant species in the United States) (Fig. 72.5).
  – Bites can cause dermonecrosis (sphingomyelinase D is the major toxin) which begins with erythema and/or vesiculation that becomes dusky, sometimes with bullae formation and eventual necrosis (Fig. 72.6).
  – Rarely, systemic findings of shock, hemolysis, renal insufficiency, and disseminated intravascular coagulation.
  – **Rx:** rest, ice, and elevation are the mainstay of treatment.

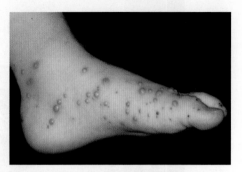

Fig. 72.3 Fire ant bites presenting as clusters of sterile pustules on the foot.
Courtesy, Dirk M. Elston, MD.

MAJOR INSECTS OF DERMATOLOGIC SIGNIFICANCE

Insect		Size of an Adult (Length)	Example(s)	Lesional Clues	Vector of:	Rx/Prevention
Bedbugs		~5–8 mm	*Cimex lectularius*, species most commonly found in the United States	• Lesions noted upon awakening • Bites often in groups of 2 or 3		• Extermination
Triatome reduviids		~1–3 cm	*Triatoma dimidiata*, *Rhodnius prolixus*	• Painless bites with delayed erythema, edema, and pruritus • Unilateral eyelid swelling (Romaña sign), a conjunctival reaction to infected feces	American trypanosomiasis (bugs defecate as they eat and infectious feces are rubbed into the wound)	• Elimination of hiding spots/breeding grounds (e.g. cracked stone walls) • Extermination

Fleas*		~2-10 mm	• *Pulex irritans* (human flea; shown here) • *Ctenocephalides felis* (often found on dogs) • *Xenopsylla cheopsis* (oriental rat flea)	• Lesions often limited to lower extremities as fleas jump but cannot fly • Wider distribution if an infested pet is held, groomed, or shares bed	• Endemic (murine) typhus, primarily oriental rat flea • Flea-borne spotted fever and plague, primarily oriental rat flea	• Treat infested animals (e.g. firponil, methoprene) • Treat house with insecticide
Fire ants		2–6 mm	*Solenopsis invicta*	Clusters of sterile pustules (Fig. 72.3), sometimes in rosettes		• Eradication of fire ant mounds
Blister beetles		~1–2.5 cm	*Paederus eximium,* found primarily in Kenya	Vesicles/bullae result from secreted cantharidin		

See Chapter 71 for information on Tunga penetrans, a burrowing flea. Photographs courtesy, Dirk M. Elston, MD.

Table 72.1 Major insects of dermatologic significance.

BITES AND STINGS

MAJOR TICKS OF DERMATOLOGIC SIGNIFICANCE

Tick	Example/Distribution	Vector of:
Ixodes 	• *Ixodes scapularis* (black-legged tick; shown here), United States: eastern and mid-Atlantic states, Great Lakes region • *Ixodes pacificus* (western black-legged tick), western United States • *Ixodes ricinus*, Europe • *Ixodes persulcatus*, Eurasia	• Lyme disease • Babesiosis • Human granulocytotropic anaplasmosis
Amblyomma 	• *Amblyomma americanum* (lone star tick; shown here), United States: from Texas to Iowa and Connecticut • *Amblyomma maculatum*, U.S. Gulf Coast	• Human monocytotropic ehrlichiosis • *Ehrlichia ewingii* infection • Southern tick-associated rash illness (STARI) • Occasionally, rickettsial diseases are transmitted by *Amblyomma* species • Tularemia

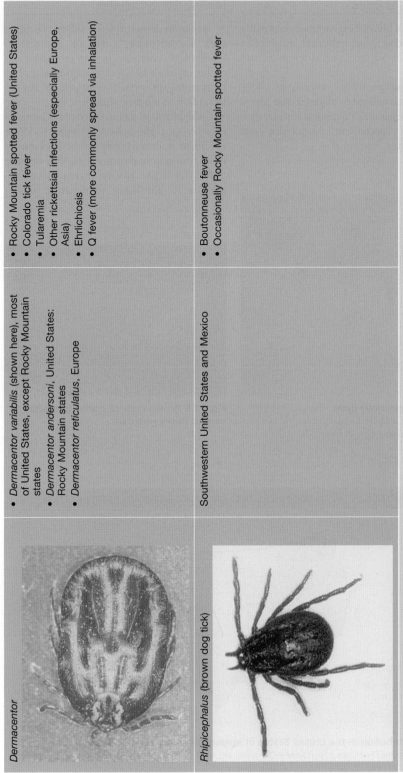

| Dermacentor | • Dermacentor variabilis (shown here), most of United States, except Rocky Mountain states
• Dermacentor andersoni, United States: Rocky Mountain states
• Dermacentor reticulatus, Europe | • Rocky Mountain spotted fever (United States)
• Colorado tick fever
• Tularemia
• Other rickettsial infections (especially Europe, Asia)
• Ehrlichiosis
• Q fever (more commonly spread via inhalation) |
| Rhipicephalus (brown dog tick) | Southwestern United States and Mexico | • Boutonneuse fever
• Occasionally Rocky Mountain spotted fever |

Photographs courtesy, Dirk M. Elston, MD.

Table 72.2 Major ticks of dermatologic significance. *Dermacentor* ticks primarily attach to the head and neck region; *Amblyomma* ticks prefer the lower legs and buttocks; *Ixodes* ticks may be found at any site, but the trunk is common.

BITES AND STINGS

Dog and Cat Bites

- Infection of bite sites is common, especially with streptococci, staphylococci, *Pasteurella multocida*, *Capnocytophaga canimorsus*, and anaerobes.
- **Rx:** broad-spectrum antibiotics (e.g. amoxicillin–clavulanate) to cover the above organisms; depending on clinical setting, consider rabies vaccine/immunoglobulin and tetanus booster.

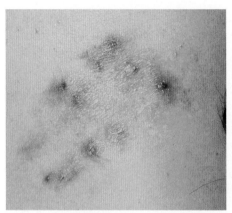

Fig. 72.4 *Cheyletiella* bites. These mites are nonburrowing and are found on cats, rabbits, and dogs. *Courtesy, Dirk M. Elston, MD.*

Marine Stings/Injuries

- Vary from dermatitis (secondary to contact with sea anemone, coral, or sponges) to foreign body reactions (e.g. to embedded sea urchin spines) to acute reactions (e.g. erythematous, urticarial or hemorrhagic streaks secondary to jellyfish stings).
- Complications include secondary bacterial infection (e.g. *Staphylococcus aureus*); *Vibrio vulnificus* infections with hemorrhagic bullae more common in patients with liver disease.
- **Rx:** for acute marine envenomations – soaking in hot water to denature venom

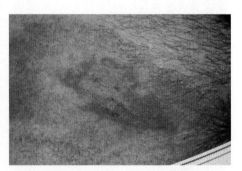

Fig. 72.6 Brown recluse spider bite with central dusky necrosis.

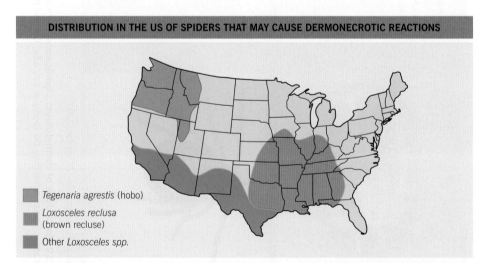

DISTRIBUTION IN THE US OF SPIDERS THAT MAY CAUSE DERMONECROTIC REACTIONS

- *Tegenaria agrestis* (hobo)
- *Loxosceles reclusa* (brown recluse)
- Other *Loxosceles spp.*

Fig. 72.5 Distribution in the United States of spiders that may cause dermonecrotic reactions. *Adapted from Sams HH, Dunnick CA, Smith ML, et al. Necrotic arachnidism. J. Am. Acad. Dermatol. 2001;44:561–573.*

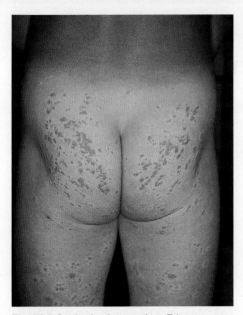

Fig. 72.7 Seabather's eruption. Edematous pink papules in the same distribution as the bathing trunks. *Courtesy, Kalman Watsky, MD.*

proteins; for symptoms of delayed reactions or dermatitis – topical CS; for foreign body reactions – removal of foreign material.

- Seabather's eruption.
  - Pruritic papules, localized to the bathing suit area and intertriginous areas (Fig. 72.7).
  - Secondary to a variety of stinging larvae, e.g. *Linuche unguiculata* (jellyfish), *Edwardsiella lineata* (sea anemone).

For further information see Ch. 85. From *Dermatology, Third Edition.*

73 | Photodermatoses

Photo Facts

• The UV radiation (UVR) emitted by the sun is arbitrarily subdivided based on wavelength into UVA (400–320 nm), UVB (320–290 nm), and UVC (290–200 nm).
• More than 95% of UVR that reaches the earth's surface is UVA.
• UVA, but not UVB, can penetrate through glass windows.
• The penetration of UVR into the skin is wavelength-dependent (Fig. 73.1).
• Principles and formulations of sunscreens are discussed in the Appendix.

Cutaneous Effects of UVR Exposure: Acute

• The visible short-term effects of UVR include sunburn and tanning; in addition, it leads to vitamin D synthesis, epidermal hyperplasia, proinflammatory responses, and immunosuppression.
• **Sunburn** = inflammation + erythema; UVC (absorbed by ozone) > UVB > UVA in potential to cause sunburn.
• **MED** = 'minimal erythema dose' = the lowest dose of UVR capable of inducing erythema (sunburn) in a given individual.

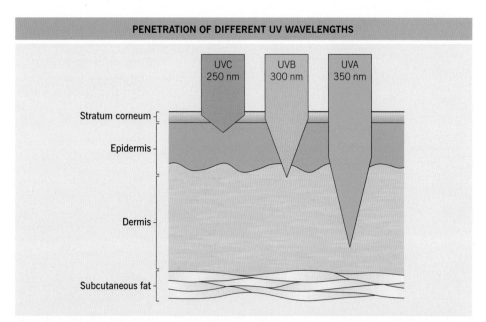

PENETRATION OF DIFFERENT UV WAVELENGTHS

Fig. 73.1 Depth of penetration of different wavelengths of UV light into human skin. Depth of penetration varies greatly with the thickness of the different skin layers and their composition (e.g. melanin content). The beginning of the wedge-shaped portion of the penetration symbol represents a decrease to approximately one-third of the incident energy density, and the tip of the symbol represents a decrease to approximately 1%. Figure not drawn to scale.

Typically, a UVB-induced sunburn appears within 30 minutes to 8 hours of sufficient exposure, peaks at 12–24 hours, and diminishes over hours to days with desquamation.

- **Tanning** occurs as a biphasic response to UVR and is wavelength-dependent.
  - **'Immediate pigment darkening'** occurs during and immediately after exposure and is most prominent with UVA.
  - **'Delayed tanning'** usually results from UVB exposure and peaks about 3 days after sun exposure.
- A 'UVA-induced tan,' such as from the use of tanning beds, provides 5–10 times less protection from subsequent UVR exposure than does a 'UVB-induced tan,' most likely because UVB also induces epidermal hyperplasia.

Cutaneous Effects of UVR Exposure: Chronic

- The visible long-term effects of UVR include **photoaging** and **photocarcinogenesis**.
- Cutaneous signs of photoaging are pictured in Fig. 73.2 and also include solar lentigines, sunburn lentigines, and ephelides; in more darkly pigmented skin, small seborrheic keratoses, melasma, and dyspigmentation may be seen.

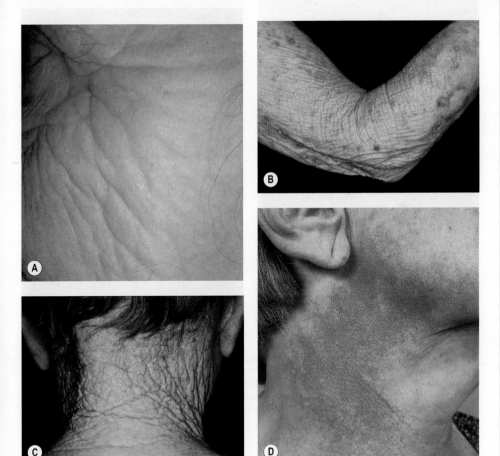

Fig. 73.2 Cutaneous signs of significant photoaging. A, B Solar elastosis of the cheek and arm with the characteristic yellow discoloration and thickening of the skin. **C** Cutis rhomboidalis nuchae with deep furrowing of the posterior neck. **D** Poikiloderma of Civatte with sparing of the anterior neck. *A, Courtesy, Henry Lim, MD; B, Courtesy, Jean L. Bolognia, MD. Continued*

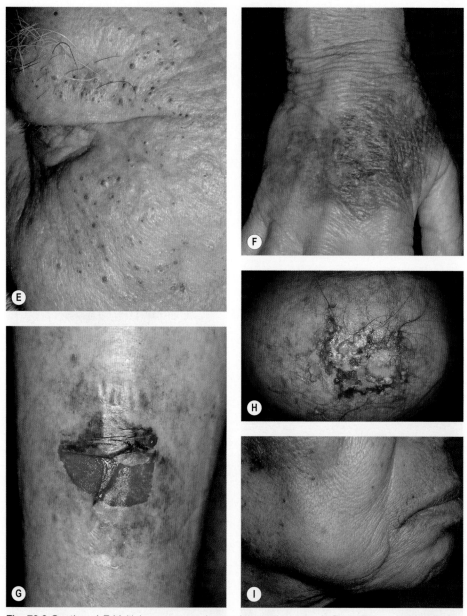

Fig. 73.2 *Continued* **E** Multiple open comedones of the malar region in Favre–Racouchot syndrome. **F** Brown discoloration of the dorsal hand due to hemosiderin deposits from recurrent solar purpura. **G** Fragility of atrophic photodamaged skin of the shin. **H** Erosive pustular dermatosis of the bald scalp. **I** Photoaging in a 93-year-old African-American woman, demonstrating fine wrinkling and numerous tiny seborrheic keratoses. *E, I, Courtesy, Henry Lim, MD; F, G, Courtesy, Jean L. Bolognia, MD.*

CLASSIFICATION OF THE MORE COMMON PHOTODERMATOSES
Idiopathic, probably immunologically based photodermatoses (Table 73.2)
• Polymorphic light eruption (PMLE) • Actinic prurigo • Hydroa vacciniforme • Chronic actinic dermatitis (CAD) • Solar urticaria
Photoaggravated dermatoses (Table 73.2)
• Atopic dermatitis • Seborrheic dermatitis > psoriasis • Lupus erythematosus, dermatomyositis • Rosacea • Grover's disease (transient acantholytic dermatosis) • Other: erythema multiforme, bullous pemphigoid, pityriasis rubra pilaris, Darier disease
Chemical- and drug-induced photosensitivity (Table 73.3)
Inherited disorders characterized by defective DNA repair or chromosomal instability (Table 73.5)

Table 73.1 Classification of the more common photodermatoses.

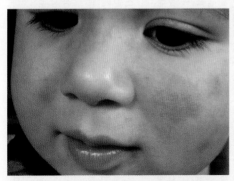

Fig. 73.3 Polymorphic light eruption (PMLE) of the face. Edematous erythematous plaques on the cheeks of a young child.

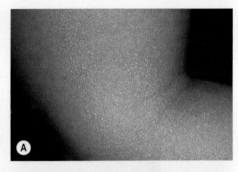

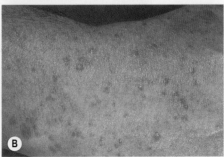

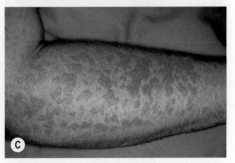

Fig. 73.4 Polymorphic light eruption (PMLE) of the upper extremity. Small papules **(A),** papulovesicles **(B),** and larger edematous papules and plaques **(C).**

• Chronic UVR is responsible for development of actinic keratoses, squamous cell carcinoma, basal cell carcinoma, and cutaneous melanoma (see Chapters 88 and 93).

Photodermatoses

• The photodermatoses are classified into four broad categories (Table 73.1) and are discussed in Tables 73.2 (Figs. 73.3–73.10), Table 73.3 (Fig. 73.11), and Table 73.5 (Fig. 73.12).

• Of all the photodermatoses, polymorphic light eruption (PMLE) is the most common, followed by photoaggravated dermatoses; drug-induced photosensitivity is also a common disorder.

• *Phototoxicity* results from direct tissue and cellular injury following UVR-induced activation of a phototoxic agent; resembles a sunburn (Table 73.4).

CLINICAL FEATURES OF THE IDIOPATHIC, PROBABLY IMMUNOLOGICALLY BASED, PHOTODERMATOSES AND PHOTOAGGRAVATED DERMATOSES

Photodermatosis (Action Spectrum)	Clinical Features	DDx	Rx
Polymorphic light eruption (PMLE) See Figs. 73.3–73.5 (UVB and UVA; rarely visible light)	• **Onset:** one to several hours after sun exposure; appears primarily in spring and early summer, but initial episode may follow intense sun exposure (e.g. trip to the tropics in the winter) • **Duration:** lesions last days; tends to diminish or cease with repeated sun = 'hardening' phenomenon • **Clinical:** lesions seen on sun-exposed skin (extensor forearms > dorsal hands > face and neck > other areas); typically, recurrences have a similar appearance in a given individual • Symmetric, pruritic, skin-colored to red, various-sized papules and/or papulovesicles that often coalesce into larger plaques • Confluent erythema or edema may be seen on the face • 'Juvenile spring eruption' is a clinical variant seen most often in boys, presenting as papulovesicles on the helices of the ears	• LE (lasts weeks to months, nonpruritic) • Solar urticaria (more rapid onset and resolution) • Photoaggravated atopic or seborrheic dermatitis (eczematous) • Erythema multiforme • EPP (painful) • In children also consider rare entities in Table 73.5	**Mild:** photoprotection,* topical CS **Severe** • Short course of antimalarials • 'Hardening' via phototherapy (may lead to flare requiring oral CS)
Actinic prurigo See Fig. 73.6 (UVR: UVA + UVB)	• **Onset:** childhood; flares within hours of sun exposure • **Duration:** lesions are chronic and persistent throughout childhood, but often fade in adolescence • **Clinical:** seen most commonly in Native Americans; females > males • Typically involves sun-exposed skin (e.g. face/nose, distal limbs), but with time can involve nonexposed skin • Pruritic, erythematous papules and nodules with hemorrhagic crusts and lichenification • Cheilitis, conjunctivitis	• Photoaggravated atopic dermatitis • Photoallergic contact dermatitis • PMLE (resolves more quickly) • Scabies, arthropod bites • Prurigo nodularis	**Mild:** photoprotection,* topical CS or CIs **Moderate–severe** • Antimalarials • 'Hardening' phototherapy as for PMLE **Recalcitrant:** thalidomide, azathioprine, cyclosporine

Hydroa vacciniforme (HV) See Figs. 73.7 and 73.8 (Primarily UVA)	• **Onset:** childhood; flares within hours of sun exposure • **Duration:** active lesions last weeks; may resolve during adolescence or early adulthood • **Clinical:** males > females • Typically presents on sun-exposed skin (e.g. face, dorsal hands) as symmetric, pruritic or painful, erythematous macules and papules that progress to vesicles/bullae with central umbilication and hemorrhagic crusts • Resolves with varioliform scarring • Severe form features ulcerated nodules, a more widespread distribution, systemic findings (e.g. fever, hepatosplenomegaly, high circulating EBV DNA load and NK cells), and a high risk of hemophagocytic syndrome/lymphoma	• Overlaps with EBV-related necrotic hypersensitivity to mosquito bites • HSV, VZV • LE, dermatomyositis • Cutaneous porphyrias • Lymphoma	• Often refractory to therapy, as no effective medication is available for underlying EBV infection **Mild:** photoprotection,* beta-carotene, fish oil, antimalarials **Severe:** thalidomide, hematopoietic stem cell transplant (if progression to lymphoma)
Chronic actinic dermatitis (CAD) See Fig. 73.9 (UVB > UVA; occasionally visible light)	• **Onset:** older age at onset (>50 years) • **Duration:** persistent for years; typically ~10% of cases resolve within 5 years, ~20% by 10 years, and 50% by 15 years • **Clinical:** males > females; darker phototypes • Presents on sun-exposed skin (initially with sharp cut-off at lines of clothing) as pruritic, eczematous papules and plaques with lichenification • Occasionally pseudolymphomatous papules, plaques, and erythroderma are seen • There is often a coexisting allergic contact dermatitis to plants (e.g. daisies)	• Photoaggravated dermatoses (e.g. atopic dermatitis) • Photoallergic contact dermatitis • Photoallergic drug • LE • Mycosis fungoides	**Mild:** photoprotection,* topical CS and CIs, and avoid relevant contact allergens and drugs **Severe/recalcitrant:** cyclosporine, azathioprine, mycophenolate mofetil, low-dose PUVA

Table 73.2 Clinical features of the idiopathic, probably immunologically based, photodermatoses and photoaggravated dermatoses. *Continued*

Table 73.2 *Continued* Clinical features of the idiopathic, probably immunologically based, photodermatoses and photoaggravated dermatoses.

Photodermatosis (Action Spectrum)	Clinical Features	DDx	Rx
Solar urticaria See Fig. 73.10 (UVA, UVB, visible light; this action spectrum may change over the years)	• **Onset:** within minutes of sun exposure; often older age at onset (40s–50s) • **Duration:** lesions last <24 hours; ~15% of cases resolve within 5 years and ~25% by 10 years • **Clinical:** females > males • Seen on sun-exposed skin only, favoring the upper chest and outer arms • Individual lesions look like typical urticaria and cause pruritus > burning or pain • 20–50% of affected individuals also have atopic dermatitis • Several clinical variants exist, e.g. severe, anaphylactoid attacks; fixed; delayed; and drug-induced	• Other urticarias (not solely photodistributed) • EPP (childhood, pain) • PMLE (more delayed onset and lasts longer) • LE	Mild: photoprotection* is recommended but often not helpful because of visible light induction; oral antihistamines **Moderate–severe** • Graduated exposure to UVA, PUVA Recalcitrant: antimalarials, cyclosporine, plasmapheresis, IVIg
Photoaggravated dermatoses See Table 73.1 for list of disorders (UVA, UVB)	• **Onset:** usually flares within hours of sun exposure, but sometimes delayed a day or more • **Duration:** days to months • **Clinical:** exacerbation of underlying skin condition in sun-exposed and sometimes non-sun-exposed areas	• Sweat-aggravated dermatoses • PMLE • CAD	• Photoprotection* and treat the underlying dermatosis

*Photoprotection generally includes avoidance of sun, sun-protective clothing, broad-spectrum sunscreens, hats, sunglasses; for UVA-sensitive disorders, must also caution about protection from UVR received while driving or through glass windows; zinc- and titanium dioxide-based sunscreens are best for visible light-sensitive disorders. UVA, ultraviolet A; UVB, ultraviolet B; LE, lupus erythematosus; EPP, erythropoietic protoporphyria; CI, calcineurin inhibitor; PUVA, psoralens plus ultraviolet A; UVR, ultraviolet radiation, including both UVA and UVB; HSV, herpes simplex virus; VZV, varicella–zoster virus; EBV, Epstein–Barr virus; PMLE, polymorphic light eruption; CAD, chronic actinic dermatitis.

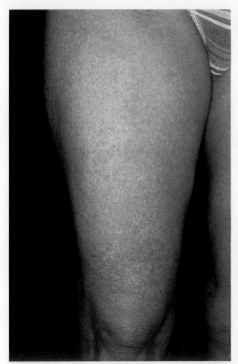

Fig. 73.5 Polymorphic light eruption (PMLE) of the thigh. Edematous papules becoming confluent into plaques. *Courtesy, Jean L. Bolognia, MD.*

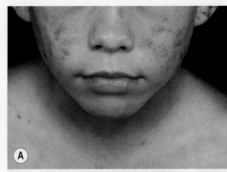

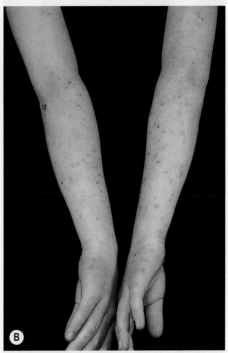

Fig. 73.6 Actinic prurigo. A The clinical features, including a photodistribution and worsening in the summer, are somewhat suggestive of polymorphic light eruption, but the lesions were persistent and the HLA type was that seen in association with actinic prurigo. Note the involvement of the ears. **B** The crusted papules are more dense on the distal arms. *Continued*

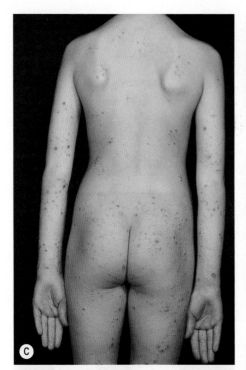

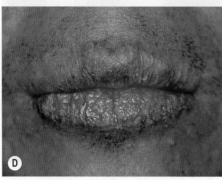

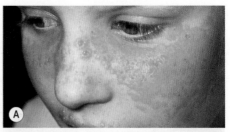

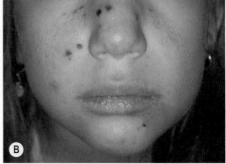

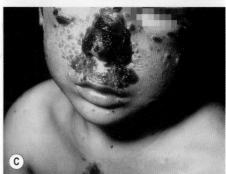

Fig. 73.6 *Continued* **C** This patient with severe actinic prurigo has involvement of the buttocks. **D** Significant cheilitis that is more severe on the lower lip in a Peruvian man with Native American (as well as European) ancestry. *A–C, Courtesy, John L. M. Hawk, MD; D, Courtesy, Jean L. Bolognia, MD.*

Fig. 73.7 Hydroa vacciniforme. A There is an early, polymorphic light eruption-like appearance, but with vesicles around the mouth and umbilicated lesions on the nose. **B** Hemorrhagic crusts are admixed with varioliform scars; the latter are the sequelae of repeated acute attacks. Note the telangiectasias on the nasal tip. **C** More severe crusting and scarring. *A, C, Courtesy, John L. M. Hawk, MD; B, Courtesy, Jean L. Bolognia, MD.*

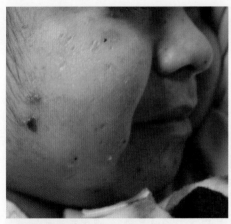

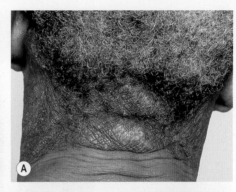

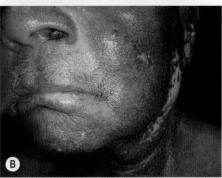

Fig. 73.8 EBV-associated hydroa vacciniforme-like eruption. This Hispanic child had >50000 copies of EBV DNA/100000 WBCs as well as EBV RNA within skin lesions by *in situ* hybridization; he subsequently died of lymphoma. Note the facial edema, erythema, papulovesicles, hemorrhagic crusts, and varioliform scars. *Courtesy, Richard Antaya, MD.*

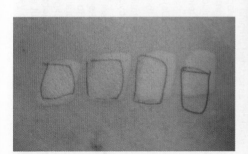

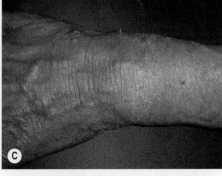

Fig. 73.10 Solar urticaria. Wheal and flare responses within minutes of exposure to UVB irradiation in a patient undergoing phototesting. *Courtesy, John L. M. Hawk, MD.*

Fig. 73.9 Chronic actinic dermatitis (CAD).
A Chronic eczematous changes of the posterior neck with lichenification and a sharp cut-off at the collar in a patient with phototype V skin.
B Lichenification and hyperpigmentation in sun-exposed sites with areas of depigmentation. Note the sparing of sun-protected areas (i.e. nasolabial fold and shoulder). **C** Chronic eczematous changes of the dorsal hand and wrist with associated hyperpigmentation and scaling. Note the sharp cut-off at the distal forearm. *Courtesy, Henry Lim, MD.*

CHEMICAL- AND DRUG-INDUCED PHOTOSENSITIVITY

Disorder and Etiology	Clinical Features	DDx/Evaluation
Exogenous		
Phototoxicity • Phototoxic drug reaction to systemic medication > phototoxic contact dermatitis to topical medication or chemical (Table 73.4) • Requires exposure to drug or chemical plus exposure to UVR (UVA > UVB)	• **Onset:** hours after sun exposure • **Clinical:** Typically presents as an exaggerated sunburn reaction; associated burning or stinging; when severe, vesicles and/or bullae develop; resolves with desquamation and hyperpigmentation • Other skin findings may include 1. Photo-onycholysis (e.g. tetracyclines, psoralens; Chapter 58) 2. Pseudo-PCT (e.g. NSAIDs) (Chapter 41) 3. Lichenoid eruption (e.g. thiazide diuretics, quinidine)* 4. Slate-gray hyperpigmentation (e.g. amiodarone, diltiazem [Fig. 73.11], tricyclic antidepressants)	• Sunburn • LE • Photoallergy (see below) • Airborne contact dermatitis • EPP • Solar urticaria **Evaluation** • If persistent despite discontinuation of suspected drug or chemical, consider phototesting and photopatch testing (Fig. 73.13)
Phytophotodermatitis (Chapter 12) • Photoactive reaction due to exposure to plants ('phyto') that contain a phototoxin plus exposure to UVA • Most commonly due to furocoumarins found in limes, celery, and false Bishop's weed	• **Inflammatory reaction** (onset usually within 1 day): initially erythematous streaks, often with vesicles or bullae, reflecting exposure to the plant or its juice; painful, nonpruritic; configuration may be unusual, depending on the type of exposure • **Delayed pigmentary reaction:** hyperpigmented streaks (occasionally appear without a preceding inflammatory phase); may last months to years	• Allergic contact dermatitis to plants, e.g. poison ivy or poison oak; distribution includes sites that are exposed to the environment but not the sun, e.g. inner arms • May be confused with child abuse

Photoallergy

- Photoallergic contact dermatitis to topical medication or chemical > photoallergic drug reaction to systemic medication
- Requires exposure to drug or chemical plus UVR (Table 73.4)

- **Onset:** first exposure: 7–10 days; subsequent: minutes to hours
- **Clinical:** pruritic, eczematous eruption; occasionally vesicles and bullae

- Allergic contact dermatitis
- Photoaggravated dermatosis (e.g. atopic dermatitis)
- Airborne contact dermatitis
- Phototoxicity

Evaluation

- If persistent despite discontinuation of suspected topical medication or systemic drug, consider phototesting and photopatch testing; photopatch testing is positive, whereas phototoxicity is negative (Fig. 73.13)

Endogenous

Erythropoietic protoporphyria (EPP) (Chapter 41)

Porphyria cutanea tarda (PCT) (Chapter 41)

*Lichenoid drug eruptions, including photolichenoid drug eruptions, are discussed in Chapter 9.
UVR, ultraviolet radiation, including both UVA and UVB; UVA, ultraviolet A; UVB, ultraviolet B; PCT, porphyria cutanea tarda; NSAIDs, nonsteroidal anti-inflammatory drugs; EPP, erythropoietic protoporphyria; LE, lupus erythematosus.

Table 73.3 Chemical- and drug-induced photosensitivity. Treatment of phototoxic and photoallergic reactions includes discontinuation of the offending agent or medication, photoprotection, symptomatic care, and occasionally topical or oral CS if severe. Photoprotection generally includes avoidance of sun, sun-protective clothing, broad-spectrum sunscreens, hats, and sunglasses; for UVA-sensitive disorders, must also caution about protection from UVR received while driving or through glass windows; zinc- and titanium dioxide-based sunscreens are best for visible light-sensitive disorders.

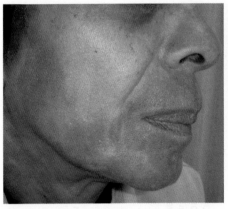

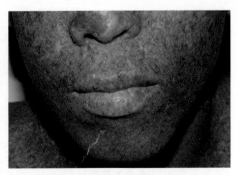

Fig. 73.12 Xeroderma pigmentosum. A 17-year-old boy with skin phototype V who has hyper- and hypopigmentation admixed with scarring, lentigines, and seborrheic as well as actinic keratoses. Note the squamous cell carcinoma *in situ* of the lower lip in association with severe actinic cheilitis. *Courtesy, Julie V. Schaffer, MD.*

Fig. 73.11 Drug-induced photosensitivity and hyperpigmentation. Gray-brown patches involving the sun-exposed skin of a patient receiving diltiazem. *Courtesy, Henry Lim, MD.*

COMMON PHOTOTOXIC AND PHOTOALLERGIC AGENTS

Common Phototoxic Agents	Common Photoallergic Agents

• Antiarrhythmics
  – Amiodarone
  – Quinidine
• Triazole antifungals
  – Voriconazole
• Diuretics
  – Furosemide
  – Thiazides
• Nonsteroidal anti-inflammatory drugs
  – Nabumetone
  – Naproxen
  – Piroxicam
• Phenothiazines
  – Chlorpromazine
  – Prochlorperazine
• Psoralens
  – 5-Methoxypsoralen
  – 8-Methoxypsoralen
  – 4,5′,8-Trimethylpsoralen
• Quinolones
  – Ciprofloxacin
  – Lomefloxacin
  – Nalidixic acid
  – Sparfloxacin
• St. John's wort
  – Hypericin
• Sulfonamides
• Sulfonylureas
• Tar (topical)
• Tetracyclines
  – Doxycycline
  – Demeclocycline
	Topical agents
	• Sunscreens (e.g. oxybenzone [benzophenone-3])
	• Fragrances
	  – 6-Methylcoumarin
	  – Musk ambrette
	  – Sandalwood oil
	• Antimicrobial agents
	  – Bithionol
	  – Chlorhexidine
	  – Fenticlor
	  – Hexachlorophene
	• Nonsteroidal anti-inflammatory drugs
	  – Diclofenac
	  – Ketoprofen
	• Phenothiazines
	  – Chlorpromazine
	  – Promethazine
	Systemic agents
	• Antiarrhythmics
	  – Quinidine
	• Antimalarials
	  – Quinine
	• Antifungals
	  – Griseofulvin
	• Antimicrobials
	  – Quinolones (e.g. enoxacin, lomefloxacin)
	  – Sulfonamides
	• Nonsteroidal anti-inflammatory drugs
	  – Ketoprofen
	  – Piroxicam*
	• Diuretics
	  – Furosemide
	• Thiazides

Often have positive patch test to thimerosol.

Table 73.4 Common phototoxic and photoallergic agents.

CLINICAL FEATURES OF SELECTED INHERITED PHOTOSENSITIVITY DISORDERS ASSOCIATED WITH DEFECTIVE DNA NUCLEOTIDE EXCISION REPAIR OR CHROMOSOMAL INSTABILITY

Inherited Disorder	Clinical Features
Defective DNA Nucleotide Excision Repair	
Xeroderma pigmentosum (XP) See Fig. 73.12	• Photosensitivity • Early onset lentigines (about age 2 years) and dyspigmentation • Xerotic skin • BCCs, SCCs, cutaneous melanomas in sun-exposed areas; median age of NMSC onset is 8 years • Photophobia, keratitis, corneal opacification • Increased incidence of intraoral and ocular malignancies as well as CNS tumors
Cockayne syndrome (CS)	• Photosensitivity without pigmentary changes • Progressive signs of premature aging • Cachectic dwarfism • No increase in malignancies
Chromosomal Instability	
Bloom syndrome	• More common in Ashkenazi Jews • Presents in first few weeks of life with malar erythema and telangiectasias, exacerbated by sun exposure • Café-au-lait macules with adjacent hypopigmented macules • Growth delay, short stature • Increased incidence of internal malignancies (e.g. leukemia)
Rothmund–Thomson syndrome	• Presents in first few months of life with photodistributed erythema, edema, and vesicles on cheeks and face • Later develop poikiloderma on extremities and buttocks • Acral keratoses and radial ray defects • Increased risk of SCC and osteosarcoma • DDx: consider poikiloderma with neutropenia (Clericuzio type; 'Navajo poikiloderma')

BCC, basal cell carcinoma; SCC, squamous cell carcinoma.

Table 73.5 Clinical features of selected inherited photosensitivity disorders associated with defective DNA nucleotide excision repair or chromosomal instability. All four listed diseases are rare and inherited in an autosomal recessive fashion, but they are the more common of these disorders.

• *Photoallergy* is a delayed-type hypersensitivity response that requires both a photoallergen (usually topical) and UVR exposure; resembles eczema (Table 73.4).

• Photosensitivity to some medications (e.g. methotrexate, 5-fluorouracil, retinoids) does not require UVR activation of the drug.

• It is important to recognize photodistributed versus photoprotected areas on the body; sparing of certain sites, including behind the ears, under the chin, the upper eyelids, and the nasolabial folds, is a clue to a photodistributed eruption (Fig. 73.14).

• Some patients may have no cutaneous findings at the time of the visit and the diagnosis is based on historical information, in particular those with PMLE and solar urticaria.

• Clues to the diagnosis of various photodermatoses are outlined in Fig. 73.15.

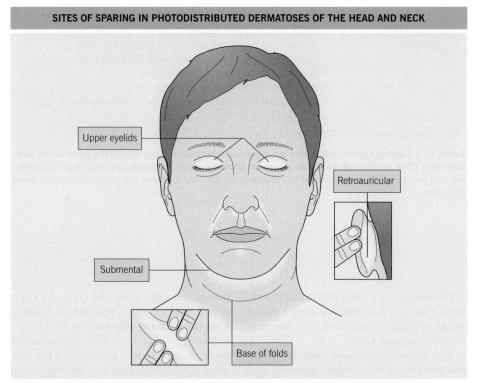

EXOGENOUS CHEMICAL-INDUCED PHOTOSENSITIVITY: INTERPRETATION OF PHOTOPATCH TESTS

UVA

Unirradiated

○   ○ + ──────→ Photoallergy

○ +   ○ + + ──────→ Contact allergy + photoallergy

○ +   ○ + ──────→ Contact allergy

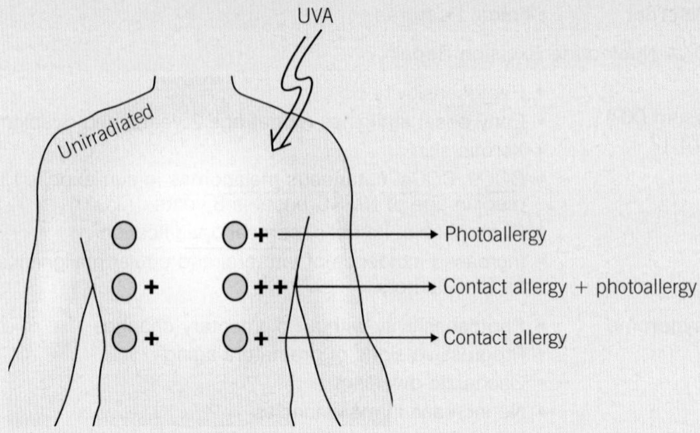

Fig. 73.13 Exogenous chemical-induced photosensitivity: Interpretation of photopatch tests. This schematic demonstrates the interpretation of photopatch tests. The UVA dose is usually the lower of 5 J/cm^2, or 50% of the MED to UVA.

SITES OF SPARING IN PHOTODISTRIBUTED DERMATOSES OF THE HEAD AND NECK

Upper eyelids

Retroauricular

Submental

Base of folds

Fig. 73.14 Sites of sparing in photodistributed dermatoses of the head and neck (e.g. chronic actinic dermatitis and photoallergic dermatitis). Relatively sun-protected sites include the upper eyelids, nasolabial folds, retroauricular areas, submental region, and deepest portion of skin furrows. In airborne contact dermatitis, these areas may be involved.

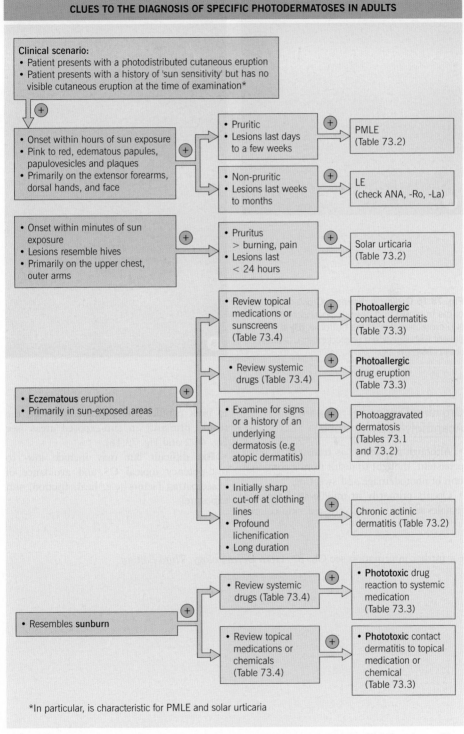

Fig. 73.15 Clues to the diagnosis of specific photodermatoses in adults. PMLE, polymorphic light eruption; LE, lupus erythematosus; ANA, antinuclear antibody.

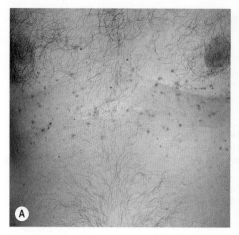

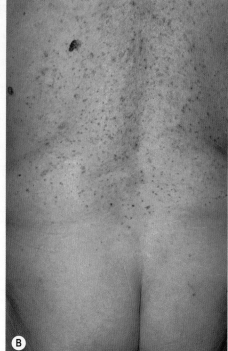

Fig. 73.16 Grover's disease. Crusted papules of the trunk **(A)** and obvious sparing of the sun-protected skin of the buttocks **(B)** in this patient with significant photodamage. *Courtesy, Jean L. Bolognia, MD.*

Grover's Disease (Transient Acantholytic Dermatosis)

- Although referred to as transient, is often persistent; thought to result from a combination of photodamage and sweating.
- Occurs primarily in middle-aged males > females as pruritic, often crusted, skin-colored to pink papules and papulovesicles on the trunk, primarily in sun-exposed areas (see Fig. 48.2 and Fig. 73.16).
- **Rx:** difficult but may include low- to mid-potency topical CS and avoidance of exacerbating factors (e.g. heat, friction, sun exposure).

For further information see Ch. 87. From *Dermatology, Third Edition*.

Environmental and Sports-Related Skin Diseases

74

Cutaneous Injury Due to Heat Exposure

Thermal Burns

• Traumatic injury to the skin caused by an external heat source.

• The depth of the burn injury depends on the temperature of and the amount of contact time with the heat source as well as the thickness of the affected skin.

• The *burn depth* determines the severity and classification of the injury, its potential for healing and need for surgical intervention (Table 74.1).

• In 2009, the American Burn Association replaced the traditional classification of burn wounds (i.e. first-, second-, third-degree) with a system that reflects the need for surgical intervention (see Table 74.1; Fig. 74.1).

• An exact classification of the burn injury may not be possible upon initial presentation and may take up to 3 weeks to determine; burns may be deeper than initially suspected when occurring on thinner skin (e.g. in pediatric and elderly patients; on ears, volar forearms, medial thighs, and perineum).

• The *extent of burn injury* is expressed as a percentage of the body surface area (BSA) involved and is essential for guiding therapy and determining a patient's disposition (e.g. hospital admission for a partial-thickness burn involving >10% BSA in an individual 10–50 years of age).

• The most accurate method for estimating BSA involvement in adults and children is the Lund–Browder chart (http://www.tg.org.au/etg_demo/phone/etg-lund-and-browder.pdf); the 'rule of nines' method is perhaps more expeditious in adults, but it cannot be used for children (Fig. 74.2).

• General principles of treatment are outlined in Table 74.1.

Erythema Ab Igne

• Localized areas of reticulated erythema and hyperpigmentation due to chronic exposure to heat that is below the threshold for a thermal burn.

• Multiple heat sources have been implicated (Table 74.2).

• Most commonly seen in the lumbosacral region (due to heating pads applied to relieve pain from degenerative spinal disease); more recently seen on the anterior thighs from heated batteries in laptop computers.

• In long-standing erythema ab igne (latency period ≥30 years) there is an associated risk of malignant degeneration, resulting in thermal keratoses and SCC.

• *Early lesions*: asymptomatic, initially transient, blanchable macular erythema in a broad, reticulated pattern that corresponds to the venous plexus; size and shape approximates that of the heat source (Fig. 74.3A).

• *Later lesions*: dusky reticulated hyperpigmentation; lesions are fixed and no longer blanchable (Fig. 74.3B).

• *End stage*: may become keratotic and bullae may appear.

• **DDx:** livedo reticularis, cutis marmorata, poikiloderma (e.g. due to CTCL, dermatomyositis, several genodermatoses); the latter has a tighter net-like pattern.

• **Rx:** remove the heat source; if applicable, identify and treat the underlying source of pain.

Burns Associated with MRI and Fluoroscopy

MRI

• MRI may produce first-, second-, or third-degree burns due to metal or wire contact with skin, creating a closed-loop conduction system.

CLASSIFICATION AND TREATMENT OF THERMAL BURNS

Type	Depth	Clinical Features Treatment*
Superficial (first-degree)	Epidermis only	– Pain, tenderness – Dry, erythema, no blistering – Blanches with pressure – Heals without scar in 3–6 days
		– No specific treatment needed – Aloe vera,** sun protection
Superficial partial-thickness (second-degree, partial) (Figure 74.1)	Epidermis and superficial dermis	– Severe pain and tenderness – Serous or hemorrhagic bullae, deep rubor, erosion and exudation – Blanches with pressure – Heals in 7–21 days with mild but variable scarring

		– Daily dressing changes with topical antibiotic
		  (e.g. silver sulfadiazine,¶ silver nitrate,¶¶
		  mafenide acetate, mupirocin) and gauze until
		  re-epithelialization occurs***
		– Sun protection

Deep partial-
thickness
(second-degree,
deep)
	Epidermis and
	most of dermis
	destroyed,
	including deep
	follicular
	structures
		– Intense pain but reduced sensation (pressure
		  only)
		– Deep red to pale and speckled in color
		– Does not blanch with pressure
		– Serosanguinous bullae (easily unroofed), erosions
		– May appear devitalized initially
		– Prolonged healing time (> 21 days)
		– Hypertrophic scars and marked wound
		  contracture

		– Surgical intervention¶¶¶
Full-thickness (third-degree)	Full-thickness epidermal and dermal destruction	– Sensation to deep pressure only – Dry, hard, waxy white to gray or charred black in color – Does not blanch with pressure – Small lesions heal with significant scarring – Most require surgical correction
		– Surgical intervention¶¶¶
Fourth degree	Extends through the skin into fascia, muscle, bone, and/or joints	– Sensation to deep pressure only – Does not heal unless surgical intervention – Potentially life-threatening
		– Surgical intervention¶¶¶

*General principles of treatment include removal of the heat source; assessment and treatment of cardiopulmonary issues; cool compresses; pain control; cleaning of the wound (soap and water) and removal of foreign material; prevention of infection; tetanus prophylaxis; and creation of a proper wound healing environment.

**May act as an anti-inflammatory agent and decrease levels of thromboxane, but can cause allergic contact dermatitis.

***A basic dressing may include a first layer of a nonadherent gauze (e.g. Adaptic or Xeroform), a second layer of dry gauze, and an outer layer of wrapped gauze.

¶Extensive use/percutaneous absorption may cause leukopenia, pseudoeschar, and argyria.

¶¶Potential for argyria.

¶¶¶Serial excisions; skin substitutes.

Table 74.1 Classification and treatment of thermal burns. *Based on the 2009 American Burn Association revised classification system for burns. http://www.ameriburn.org/Chapter14.pdf*

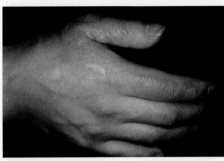

Fig. 74.1 Thermal burn. This superficial partial-thickness burn is characterized by bullae that contain serous fluid. *Courtesy, Kalman Watsky, MD.*

ASSESSING THE EXTENT OF BODY SURFACE AREA INVOLVEMENT IN BURN INJURIES

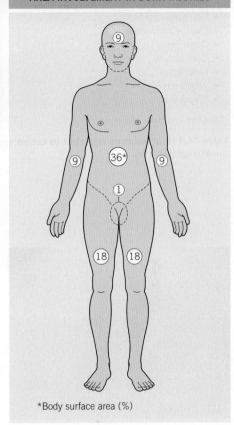

*Body surface area (%)

Fig. 74.2 Assessing the extent of body surface area involvement in burn injuries: Rule of nines. In adults, an estimate of burn extent is often based on this surface area distribution chart. Infants and children have a relatively increased head : trunk surface area ratio and this chart is ineffective for them. These estimates are also used for primary cutaneous disorders. The most accurate method of estimating the BSA involvement of burn injury in adults and children is with the Lund–Browder chart (http://www.tg.org.au/etg_demo/phone/etg-lund-and-browder.pdf).

ENVIRONMENTAL AND SPORTS-RELATED SKIN DISEASES

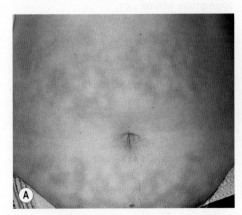

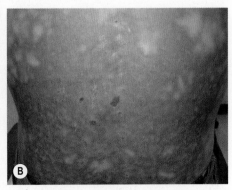

Fig. 74.3 Erythema ab igne. A Early phase with pink reticulated patches predominating over reticulated hyperpigmentation. **B** Later phase with large area of reticulated hyperpigmentation and superimposed pink keratotic plaques centrally. *A, Courtesy, Jeffrey Callen, MD; B, Courtesy, Peter Klein, MD.*

HEAT SOURCES REPORTED TO CAUSE ERYTHEMA AB IGNE	
• Heating pads • Hot water bottles • Electric stove/heater • Open fires • Coal stoves • Peat fires • Wood stoves • Sauna belt	• Steam radiators • Heated car seats • Heated reclining chairs • Heating blanket • Hot bricks • Infrared lamps • Microwave popcorn • Laptop computer*

*Anterior thighs >> abdomen.

Table 74.2 Heat sources reported to cause erythema ab igne. *Courtesy, Mary Beth Cole, MD, and Michael Smith, MD.*

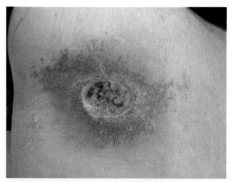

Fig. 74.4 Fluoroscopy-induced radiation dermatitis. The left upper back is a characteristic location for patients who have undergone attempts at coronary artery revascularization (e.g. angioplasty, stent placement). *Courtesy, Jeffrey Callen, MD.*

• The shape and size of the burns are determined by the conductor causing the injury (e.g. circular burns under ECG electrodes).

FLUOROSCOPY

• Fluoroscopy, especially when performed repeatedly in patients with cardiovascular disease, may result in radiation-induced injury (radiodermatitis).

• This radiodermatitis may be acute, but with time continued changes can develop, e.g. hair loss, desquamation, permanent erythema, and ulceration (Fig. 74.4).

Cutaneous Injury Due to Cold Exposure

Frostbite

• Can occur when the skin temperature drops below about −2°C (28°F).

• Tissue freezing, vasoconstriction, and inflammatory mediator release are key features of its pathophysiology.

• There are four categories of severity based on depth of tissue injury; these are only recognizable upon rewarming (Fig. 74.5).

• Symptomatically, early erythema, edema, and numbness are replaced by marked hyperemia and pain.

• **Rx:** rapid rewarming in a warm water bath is the cornerstone of treatment, followed by appropriate wound care.

Pernio (Chilblains)

• An abnormal inflammatory response to cold, damp, nonfreezing conditions.

• Classically presents with single or multiple erythematous to blue-violet macules, papules, or nodules distributed symmetrically on distal toes (Fig. 74.6) and fingers, and less often on the remainder of the foot or hand, nose and ears.

• In severe cases, blistering and ulceration may be seen.

• Patients describe pruritus, burning, or pain; histology demonstrates a perivascular and perieccrine lymphohistiocytic infiltrate.

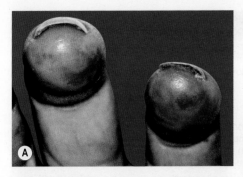

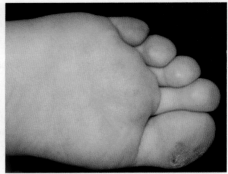

Fig. 74.6 Pernio. Violaceous macules and patches, primarily on the toes but also on the plantar surface of the foot; note the associated scaling. *Courtesy, Jean L. Bolognia, MD.*

Cutaneous Injury Due to Chemical Exposure

Chemical Hair Discoloration

• May be a voluntary cosmetic change or the result of chemical or metal exposure (Table 74.4).

• Most hair discoloration normalizes over time upon discontinuation of the offending exposure.

• Numerous anecdotal treatment remedies have been described, e.g. hot oil, hydrogen peroxide, and various shampoos (e.g. alkaline or EDTA-based).

Chronic Arsenical Dermatoses

• Chronic arsenic exposure most often occurs via contaminated drinking water or occupational exposure; long latency period (up to 40 years).

• Chronic arsenicism is characterized by mottled hyperpigmentation with areas of hypopigmentation (Fig. 74.7A); arsenical keratoses on the palms and soles (Fig. 74.7B–C); multiple non-melanoma skin cancers (particularly Bowen's disease); peripheral neuropathy and internal malignancies (e.g. bladder, lung, liver).

Cutaneous Findings Resulting from Toxic and Heavy Metal Exposure

• Various toxic and heavy metals are known to cause irritant and/or allergic contact dermatitis, including the following (Table 74.5):

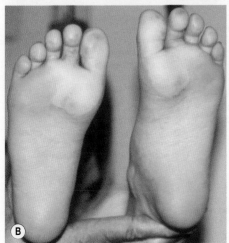

Fig. 74.5 Frostbite. A Erythema, edema, and hemorrhage are seen on the fingertips in a *first-degree frostbite (frostnip)*; full recovery is expected, with only mild desquamation. **B** Bullae filled with clear fluid on the distal plantar surfaces in a **second-degree frostbite**; many such patients develop long-term sensory neuropathies. In **third-degree frostbite** there is full-thickness dermal loss with hemorrhagic bullae or waxy, dry, mummified skin. In *fourth-degree frostbite* there is full-thickness loss of the entire part, with skin, muscle, tendon, and bone damage; amputation may occur. *A, Courtesy, Michael L. Smith, MD; B, Courtesy, Timothy Givens, MD.*

• Lesions typically resolve in 1–3 weeks but can take much longer or become chronic in elderly patients with venous insufficiency.

• **DDx:** chilblain lupus; frostbite; lupus pernio (a variant of sarcoidosis involving mainly the nose and ears) (Table 74.3).

• **Rx:** adequate clothing; avoidance of cold, damp conditions; keeping feet dry; avoidance of smoking; and use of nifedipine in recalcitrant cases.

DIFFERENTIAL DIAGNOSIS AND EVALUATION OF SKIN LESIONS INDUCED BY NONFREEZING COLD EXPOSURE		
Disorder	**Features**	**Possible Associated Conditions**
Acrocyanosis	Red to purple discoloration Hands and feet Painless	Erythromelalgia Cryoproteins Anorexia nervosa
Pernio (chilblains) (see Fig. 74.6)	Erythrocyanotic Symmetric distribution of painful macules and papules, mostly on digits; scaling develops as lesions heal	
Raynaud's phenomenon (see Chapter 35)	Well-demarcated pallor, followed by blue, then red discoloration; painful Idiopathic form (common) – no nailfold capillary changes; pulp ulcerations rare	AI-CTD (especially systemic sclerosis) Blood dyscrasias (e.g. polycythemia vera) Drugs (e.g. beta-blockers, bleomycin) Trauma
Livedo reticularis (see Chapter 87)	Bluish, broad reticulated patches corresponding to venous plexus May be idiopathic	Vascular occlusive diseases (e.g. severe atherosclerosis) AI-CTD (e.g. lupus erythematosus) Hematologic disorders (e.g. antiphospholipid syndrome) Infections (e.g. hepatitis C infection) Medications (e.g. amantadine)
Cold panniculitis (see Chapter 83)	Erythematous indurated plaques, most often on cheeks of children or thighs in equestrians	
Cold urticaria (see Chapter 14)	Cold-induced wheals	Cryoproteins Familial cold autoinflammatory syndrome
Chilblain lupus (see Chapter 33)	Cold-induced acral lesions, similar to pernio Histopathologic features of LE Coexistent LE	
Retiform purpura due to cryoproteins* • Cryoglobulins	Favors acral sites (see Fig. 18.3) Cold serum protein precipitate	Type I (monoclonal) cryoglobulinemia due to plasma cell dyscrasias Lymphoproliferative disorders (e.g. Waldenström macroglobulinemia)
• Cryofibrinogen**	Cold plasma protein precipitate	Infections (e.g. hepatitis C infection) Malignancies (e.g. non-Hodgkin lymphoma)
• Cold agglutinins or hemolysins**	RBCs agglutinate or lyse in cold Paroxysmal hemoglobinuria if RBC lysis	Infections (e.g. with *Mycoplasma*, EBV, CMV) Lymphoproliferative disorders

Table 74.3 Differential diagnosis and evaluation of skin lesions induced by nonfreezing cold exposure. *Courtesy, Michael L. Smith, MD. Continued*

Table 74.3 *Continued* **Differential diagnosis and evaluation of skin lesions induced by nonfreezing cold exposure.** *Courtesy, Michael L. Smith, MD.*

Evaluation Considerations
• CBC with platelets and differential • ANA with profile • Hypercoagulable evaluation (see Table 18.5) • Cryoprotein analysis • Serum protein electrophoresis and immunofixation electrophoresis • Lesional biopsy

Acrocyanosis, Raynaud's phenomenon, livedo reticularis, and cold urticaria can also be observed in association with cryoproteins.
**Rarely cause cold-related occlusion syndromes.*
AI-CTD, autoimmune connective tissue disease; CMV, cytomegalovirus; EBV, Epstein–Barr virus; RBC, red blood cell; CBC, complete blood count; ANA, anti-nuclear antibody.

CAUSES OF UNINTENTIONAL HAIR DISCOLORATION		
Green (Chlorotrichosis)	**Yellow, Orange, or Golden**	**Purple**
Copper (swimming pools) Selenium sulfide Tar shampoo Cobalt Chromium Nickel Yellow mercuric oxide	Tar shampoo Anthralin Minoxidil Copper (cosmetic plant extracts, metallic eyeglass frames)	Alkalinized anthralin

Table 74.4 Causes of unintentional hair discoloration. *Courtesy, Michael L. Smith, MD.*

– *Beryllium* is a metal known to cause dermatitis and sarcoidosis-like granulomas of the skin and lung.
– *Gold*, as an elemental salt, can cause a variety of cutaneous eruptions (Table 74.6).
– *Mercury*, in elemental, inorganic, or organic forms, may cause acrodynia, tattoo reaction (cinnabar), granulomas, exanthems, cutaneous hyperpigmentation, allergic and irritant contact dermatitis, baboon syndrome.
– Cutaneous contact with *silver* may result in argyria, irritant contact dermatitis, or skin ulceration.
– *Thallium*, in its soluble form, may cause alopecia, acneiform papules, hyperkeratotic plaques on hands and feet, and Mee's lines in nails.
• For most cutaneous exposures to these toxic and heavy metals, effective treatment requires prompt soap and/or water washing;

an exception is lithium, in which washing is contraindicated and gentle brushing off is preferred.

Cutaneous Findings of Frictional and Traumatic Injury to the Skin

Corns and Calluses

• Keratotic lesions resulting from repeated trauma and the subsequent cycle of friction, pressure, and thickening (Fig. 74.8).
• Contributing factors include ill-fitting footwear, bony protuberances, abnormal biomechanical foot function, and specific activities that involve repetitive activity.
• *Hard corns* are usually located on the dorsal aspects of the toes, while *soft corns* are typically found in the interdigital web spaces.
• Corns and calluses can often be mistaken for verrucae; gentle paring of the lesions with a blade and noticing the lesion's effect on

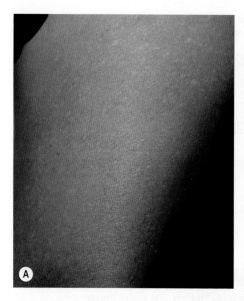

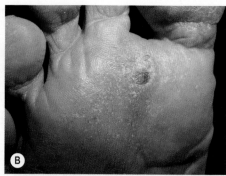

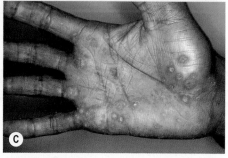

Fig. 74.7 Cutaneous manifestations of chronic arsenicism. A Guttate hypopigmentation superimposed on hyperpigmentation resembles 'raindrops on a dusty road.' **B, C** Arsenical keratoses on the plantar and palmar surface. *A, Courtesy, John Steinbaugh, MD; C, Courtesy, Jeffrey Callen, MD.*

SELECTED TOXIC AND HEAVY METALS KNOWN TO CAUSE CONTACT DERMATITIS	
Irritant Contact Dermatitis	**Allergic Contact Dermatitis**
• Cobalt salts • Copper salts • Lithium • Mercury, organic and inorganic • Selenium	• Chromium • Cobalt • Gold • Mercury, organic • Nickel

Table 74.5 Selected toxic and heavy metals known to cause contact dermatitis.

CUTANEOUS ERUPTIONS ASSOCIATED WITH GOLD EXPOSURE (AS AN ELEMENTAL SALT)	
Most Common	**Less Common**
• Lichen planus, lichenoid drug eruption • Allergic contact dermatitis • Pityriasis rosea-like eruptions • Erosive stomatitis	• Chrysiasis • Erythema nodosum • Erythema multiforme, toxic epidermal necrolysis • Exfoliative dermatitis

Table 74.6 Cutaneous eruptions associated with gold exposure (as an elemental salt).

dermatoglyphics can help distinguish between these three entities (Table 74.7).

• Treatment involves both symptomatic relief and correction of the underlying biomechanical problem:

    – *Symptomatic relief.*

       1. Paring of the callosity with removal of the corn's central core may bring

immediate relief of discomfort, followed by periodic foot filing.

    2. Application of keratolytic agents (e.g. 40% salicylic acid pads; 6% salicylic acid, 10–40% urea, or 12% ammonium lactate creams), from daily to twice weekly, depending on strength.

DISTINGUISHING FEATURES OF VERRUCAE, CORNS, AND CALLUSES		
Lesion	**Paring Revelations**	**Effect on Dermatoglyphics**
Verruca	Thrombosed capillaries, multiple bleeding points	Interrupted
Corn	Central translucent, whitish-yellow core	Interrupted
Callus	Layers of yellowish keratin	Accentuated

Table 74.7 Distinguishing features of verrucae, corns, and calluses.

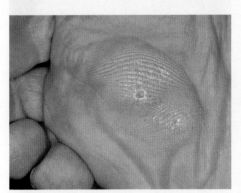

Fig. 74.8 Callus plus hard corns. Calluses are broad based and have increased skin markings while corns are round, more sharply defined papules with a central translucency and an interruption in dermatoglyphics. The skin overlying the second and third metatarsal heads is a common location for such lesions. *Courtesy, Jean L. Bolognia, MD.*

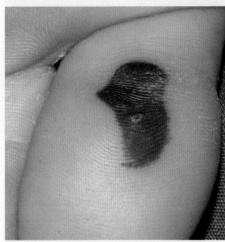

Fig. 74.9 Black heel (talon noir) and palm. This black color is due to hemoglobin within the thickened stratum corneum of plantar skin. *Courtesy, Julie V. Schaffer, MD.*

3. Soft cushions (e.g. silicone sheet, sheep skin) and donut-shaped corn pads.
 – *Biomechanical* correction – properly-fitted footwear and use of appropriate orthotics.
 – *Recalcitrant* lesions – consider x-ray to look for exostoses and referral to orthopedic or podiatric surgeon.

Black Heel (Talon Noir)

• Black macules on the palms or soles due to hemoglobin within the thickened stratum corneum (Fig. 74.9).
• Secondary to impact trauma and resolves with paring or spontaneously with time.
• Harmless, but because of its dark color must be differentiated from acral cutaneous melanoma (does not resolve with gentle paring).

Chondrodermatitis Nodularis Helicis (CNH)

• A tender, inflammatory process of the ear that primarily affects patients older than 50 years of age; initiated by ischemia-related inflammation of the cartilage.
• Presents with a skin-colored to erythematous, dome-shaped papule or nodule with a central crust or keratin-filled crater; often exquisitely tender (Fig. 74.10).
• Most often a unilateral process affecting the most protuberant portion of the ear, primarily the upper helical rim or the middle to lower antihelical rim.
• **DDx:** SCC, KA, BCC, AK, cutaneous horn, weathering nodule, verruca, calcinosis cutis, gouty tophus; often distinguished via biopsy.
• **Rx:** mostly anecdotal and not standardized (e.g. intralesional CS, topical antibiotics, specially designed CNH pillows for sleeping,

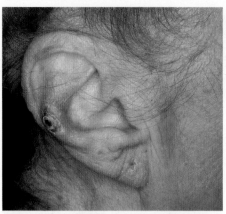

Fig. 74.10 Chondrodermatitis nodularis helicis (CNH). Tender, erythematous papulonodule with central scale-crust on the mid antihelix of an older woman. This represented the site most susceptible to pressure-induced ischemia. *Courtesy, Kalman Watsky, MD.*

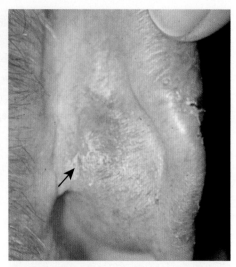

Fig. 74.11 Acanthoma fissuratum. Thin pink plaque with scale of the postauricular sulcus. Note the linear fissure (arrow). *Courtesy, Mary Beth Cole, MD, and Michael L. Smith, MD.*

cryosurgery, electrodesiccation and curettage, CO$_2$ laser ablation); full-thickness excision is the most definitive and favored treatment for particularly bothersome lesions.

Acanthoma Fissuratum

• Results from ill-fitting eyeglass frames that create a frictional injury to the postauricular sulcus or the upper lateral nose (Fig. 74.11).

• Presents as a firm or sometimes soft, skin-colored to erythematous nodule or plaque with a central vertical groove or fissure; occasionally tenderness, serous discharge, or slight hyperkeratosis.

• **DDx:** BCC, SCC, chronic dermatitis or benign acanthoma; biopsy is occasionally necessary to exclude a non-melanoma skin cancer.

• **Rx:** adjust or replace the offending eyeglasses.

Weathering Nodules of the Ears

• Multiple, bilateral, firm (feels like cartilage), asymptomatic, whitish, 2- to 3-mm papules located along the inner rim of the helices in older males >> females (Fig. 74.12).

• Associated consistently with a history of significant sun exposure and actinic damage.

• **DDx:** CNH, gouty tophi, calcinosis cutis, elastotic nodules, granuloma annulare.

• **Rx:** not necessary.

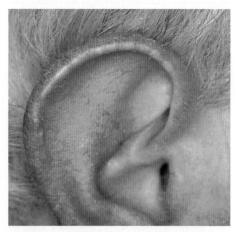

Fig. 74.12 Weathering nodules. Multiple asymptomatic, small, whitish papules along the helix of an older man with photodamage. *Courtesy, Jean L. Bolognia, MD.*

Sports-Related Dermatoses

• Participation in sports is often associated with a number of cutaneous injuries, dermatoses, or infections, related to acute and chronic mechanical trauma (Tables 74.8 and 74.9; Fig. 74.13 and 74.14).

SELECTED FRICTIONAL AND MECHANICAL DERMATOSES IN ATHLETES

Condition	Clinical Features	Sports	Etiology/Pathogenesis
			Prevention/Treatment
Subungual hematoma	Red/maroon, purple or black discoloration beneath all or part of the nail (see Chapter 58 and Figure 74.13)	Running Tennis	Sudden impact of toe tip with end of shoe
			Enlarged shoe toe box with proper arch and metatarsal support; drainage of hematoma may be necessary
Jogger's nipple	Pain, erythema, fissuring, occasional bleeding	Running	Repeated friction of rough shirt fabric
			Woman: jogging bra Man: taping, lubrication, semisynthetic or silk shirt
Tennis toe	Toe tip callus, nail thickening, subungual hyperkeratosis (see Figure 74.14)	Tennis Running	Repeated trauma of longest toe against inside of toe box
			Proper shoe fit, enlarged toe box, improved arch support
Fibrotic knots (e.g. surfer's nodules)	Thick fibrotic nodules on knees, knuckles, dorsal feet, and anterior lower ribs (surfers)	Surfing, boxing, football, marbles, yoga, video game playing	Chronic pressure over bony prominences
			Position change, padding

Table 74.8 Selected frictional and mechanical dermatoses in athletes. *Courtesy, Michael L. Smith, MD.*

CUTANEOUS INFECTIONS IN ATHLETES

Bacterial

- Impetigo (see Fig. 61.2)
- Folliculitis (see Chapter 31)
- Hot tub folliculitis (see Fig. 31.3)
- *Pseudomonas* hot-foot syndrome (see Fig. 61.15)
- Furuncles (boils)
- Erythrasma (see Fig.13.2 and/or Fig. 61.9)
- Pitted keratolysis (toxic sock syndrome) (see Fig. 61.10)
- Otitis externa (swimmer's ear)

Mycobacterial

- Swimming pool granuloma (see Fig. 62.16)

Viral

- Verruca vulgaris (warts) (see Chapter 66)
- Herpes simplex viral infection (herpes gladiatorum) (see Fig. 67.5)
- Molluscum contagiosum (see Fig. 68.8)

Fungal (see Chapter 64)

- Tinea pedis (athlete's foot)
- Tinea cruris (jock itch)
- Tinea corporis (tinea gladiatorum)

Other

- Seabather's eruption (sea lice) (see Fig. 72.7)
- Swimmer's itch (see Fig. 70.12)

Table 74.9 Cutaneous infections in athletes. *Courtesy, Michael L. Smith, MD.*

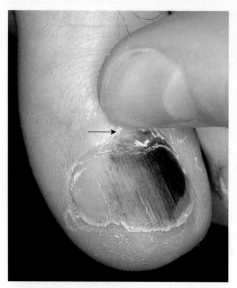

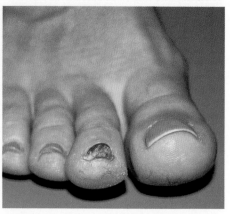

Fig. 74.14 Chronic 'tennis toe.' Chronic and repeated trauma of the longer second toe against the end of the tennis shoe toe box during sudden stops creates the distal callus formation and nail plate thickening known as 'tennis toe.' *Courtesy, Michael L. Smith, MD.*

Fig. 74.13 Subungual hematoma. A common sports-related (e.g. tennis, running, basketball) injury due to the sudden impact of the toe tip with the end of the shoe. Note the subungual dark purplish discoloration, which may be misdiagnosed as melanoma. Clues to the diagnosis of subungual hematoma include: a normal-appearing proximal nail plate upon gentle retraction of the cuticle (arrow); characteristic dermoscopic features (e.g. red-brown to purplish-black round globules); and determination that the discoloration grows out distally. *Courtesy, Jean L. Bolognia, MD.*

For further information see Ch. 88. From *Dermatology, Third Edition.*

Cutaneous Signs of Drug, Child, and Elder Abuse

75

Drug Abuse

- The skin often displays evidence of injection and inhalation drug abuse.
- A broad spectrum of cutaneous findings can result from local and systemic effects of the drug itself, adulterants, or associated infectious agents (Tables 75.1 and 75.2; Figs. 75.1–75.9).
- Skin and soft tissue infections as well as thrombophlebitis are the most common conditions for which drug addicts seek medical care and are hospitalized.

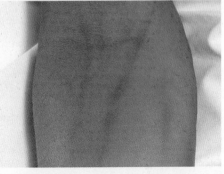

Fig. 75.1 Injection sites ('skin tracks') in an intravenous drug user. There is overlying hyperpigmentation and scarring of veins due to inflammation from repeated nonsterile injections as well as injections of irritating drugs and adulterants. *Courtesy, Mark Pittelkow, MD.*

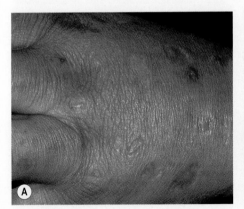

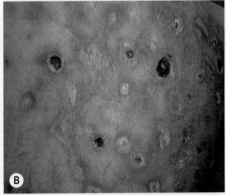

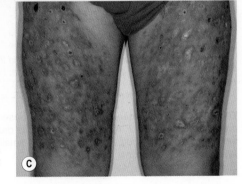

Fig. 75.2 'Skin popping' scars. A–C Multiple circular depressed scars, some with rims of post-inflammatory hyperpigmentation, admixed with circular hemorrhagic crusts overlying ulcerations. Cocaine was injected into the thighs. *A, Courtesy Miguel Sanchez, MD; B, C, Courtesy, Mark Pittelkow, MD.*

MUCOCUTANEOUS SIGNS OF DRUG ABUSE

Finding	Route(s) and Example Drugs
Sequelae of Tissue Injury	
Skin tracks (Fig. 75.1) and skin popping scars (Fig. 75.2)	IV and SC/intradermal, respectively
Lymphedema	IV, SC
Ulcers	IV – cocaine, propoxyphene* SC – barbiturates, pentazocine Intra-arterial injection leading to ischemia
Retiform purpura (Fig. 75.3) with ulceration (associated with neutropenia)	Snorting/IV cocaine or smoking crack cocaine adulterated with levamisole
Sclerosis	SC – pentazocine (Fig. 75.4), barbiturates, cocaine
Hyperkeratosis ± linear or circular black plaques on palms/fingers; erosions or blisters on lips; madarosis	Smoking crack cocaine
Circumferential pigmented bands due to tourniquet	IV
Pseudoaneurysm (tender pulsatile mass with bruit) associated with petechiae/purpura ± reduced pulses	Intra-arterial injection in groin > an extremity
Pressure erythema, bullae (Fig. 75.7), and ulcers	Overdose with barbiturates or other sedatives
Sequelae of CNS Effects	
Pruritus ± excoriations	Methamphetamine (dry, leathery skin), heroin (associated with flushing), cocaine (with chronic use)
Formication/delusions of parasitosis leading to skin picking (Fig. 75.6) and self-induced ulcers	Cocaine, methamphetamine
Other Skin Findings	
Granulomas (Fig. 75.5; onset may be delayed)	Injection of talc (e.g. in narcotic tablets) or starch
Hyperhidrosis	Amphetamines, LSD
Acne vulgaris	Anabolic steroids,† methamphetamine (especially acne excoriée), marijuana
Perinasal or perioral irritant dermatitis	Sniffing volatile solvents/inhalants
Oral Findings	
Xerostomia	Amphetamines, heroin
Dental caries, gingivitis, tooth loss	Methamphetamine, heroin

*Withdrawn from prescription drug market in 2010 in the United States and Europe.
†May also be associated with androgenetic alopecia, hirsutism, clitoral enlargement, testicular atrophy, and gynecomastia.
IV, intravenous; LSD, lysergic acid diethylamide; SC, subcutaneous.

Table 75.1 Mucocutaneous signs of drug abuse. Infections associated with drug abuse are presented in Table 75.2. A variety of cutaneous drug reactions can also develop, such as morbilliform or fixed drug eruptions, urticaria, small vessel vasculitis, and Stevens–Johnson syndrome/toxic epidermal necrolysis.

INFECTIOUS COMPLICATIONS OF DRUG ABUSE

Finding	Route(s) and Example Drugs
Abscesses and cellulitis (Fig. 75.8): *Staphylococcus aureus* > *Streptococcus* spp. > GNRs, anaerobes; often polymicrobial and associated with lymphangitis*	IV, SC, intradermal • Adulterated (e.g. 'black tar') heroin: *Clostridium* (including wound botulism from *C. botulinum*) • Heroin or pentazocine: *Pseudomonas*
Necrotizing fasciitis (Fig. 75.9; severe, disproportionate pain): usually polymicrobial, may include anaerobes	IV, SC
Disseminated candidiasis with pustular folliculitis	Injection of heroin (e.g. brown heroin in 1980s)
Zygomycosis (necrotic cellulitic plaque or abscess)	IV
Nasal verrucae in setting of nasal irritation	Snorting cocaine or heroin
Hepatitis C > B viral infection leading to cryoglobulinemic vasculitis (e.g. palpable purpura)	Needle/syringe sharing

May also be associated with osteomyelitis, septic arthritis, bacteremia, septic thrombophlebitis, and endocarditis (often tricuspid valve).
GNRs, gram-negative rods; IV, intravenous; SC, subcutaneous.

Table 75.2 Infectious complications of drug abuse.

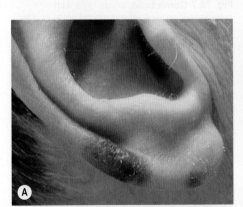
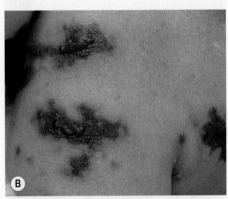

Fig. 75.3 Retiform purpura due to levamisole-adulterated cocaine. A, B The earlobe is a common site of involvement and purpuric lesions of the earlobe had been described previously as a side effect of levamisole. At the time of writing, up to 70% of the cocaine in the United States contained levamisole, compared to <3% of the heroin. *Courtesy, Jeffrey Callen, MD.*

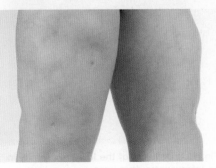
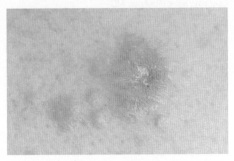

Fig. 75.4 Atrophic depressions on the thighs and extensive calcification from multiple pentazocine injections. The calcified areas are firm upon palpation. *Courtesy, Mark Pittelkow, MD.*

Fig. 75.5 Foreign body granuloma formation leading to papules at the sites of injection of adulterated heroin. *Courtesy, Mark Pittelkow, MD.*

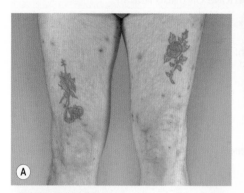

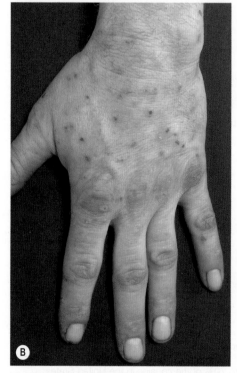

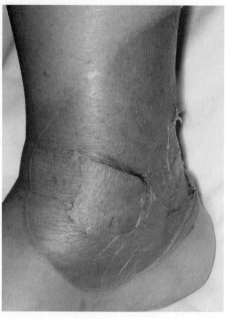

Fig. 75.7 Coma bulla. Large bulla with subsequent erosion on the medial ankle due to a prolonged coma from barbiturate overdose. *Courtesy, Mark Pittelkow, MD.*

Fig. 75.6 Multiple excoriations in a cocaine addict. The patient felt 'crawling' in his skin. *Courtesy, Mark Pittelkow, MD.*

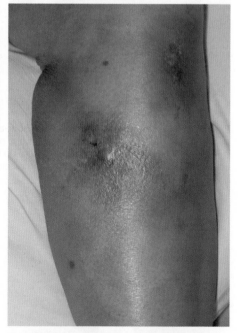

Fig. 75.8 Cellulitis of the lower extremity in an intravenous drug user. *Courtesy, Mark Pittelkow, MD.*

- Children with disabilities, behavioral problems, and stressful home situations (e.g. parental unemployment or substance use) are at increased risk of abuse, and serious injury is more frequent in boys.
- Cutaneous signs of physical abuse.
  - Unexplained bruises (Fig. 75.10), curvilinear or binding marks (e.g. produced by belts, ropes, or cords), buckle imprints, and burns (e.g. from cigarettes or scalding; Fig. 75.11).
  - Skin injuries in areas less prone to accidental trauma (e.g. trunk, buttocks, genitals, chin, ears, neck) or in infants who are not independently mobile.
  - Delay between the injury and seeking medical care.
- Physical signs of sexual abuse include tears, attenuation, or scars of the hymen and extension of the anal margin onto perianal skin.
- Anogenital warts in children may be perinatally acquired, transmitted during routine child care, autoinoculated from other sites, or acquired from sexual abuse; the latter is an uncommon etiology of anogenital warts in children <3 years of age.
- **DDx:** conditions that can mimic physical and sexual abuse in children are listed in Tables 75.3 and 75.4 (Fig. 75.12).
- **Rx:** guidelines for evaluation of suspected child abuse are available at http://pediatrics .aappublications.org/content/119/6/1232.full .pdf (physical abuse) and http://pediatrics .aappublications.org/content/116/2/506.full .pdf (sexual abuse).

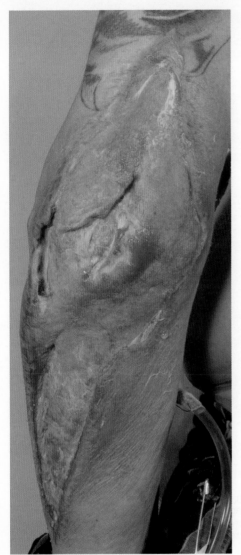

Fig. 75.9 Necrotizing fasciitis of the upper extremity with extensive tissue necrosis in an intravenous drug user. Surgical debridement has been performed. *Courtesy, Mark Pittelkow, MD.*

Child Abuse

- Child abuse encompasses a broad spectrum of nonaccidental maltreatment of children, including physical, emotional, and sexual abuse as well as neglect.

Elder Abuse

- Elder abuse may involve intentional actions that cause harm (physical, psychological, sexual, or financial) as well as failure by a caretaker to satisfy the basic needs of an elder or to protect him or her from harm.
- Risk factors include dementia and social isolation.
- The National Center on Elder Abuse (http://www.ncea.aoa.gov) provides resources to assist in the recognition and management of elder abuse.

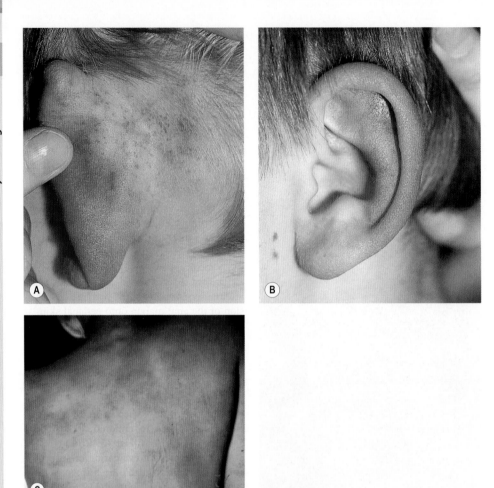

Fig. 75.10 Bruising and petechiae. A, B Bruising and petechiae of the pinna and post-auricular area in a 6-year-old boy, consistent with a hand slap by an adult. **C** Bruising from a belt and belt buckle on the back of an 8-year-old boy. *A, B, From Hobbs CJ, Wynne JM. Physical Signs of Child Abuse. © 2001 WB Saunders; C, Courtesy, Sharon Ann Raimer, MD.*

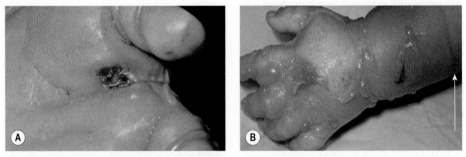

Fig. 75.11 Injuries produced by burns. A Cigarette burn. **B** Bullae and erosions due to dunking in hot water, with a sharp line of demarcation on the arm (arrow; 'glove/stocking' distribution). 'Donut-type sparing' on the child's buttocks may be seen when the buttocks are held against the cooler tub while water scalds the surrounding immersed skin. *Courtesy, Sharon Ann Raimer, MD.*

CONDITIONS THAT CAN MIMIC CHILD ABUSE

Bleeding into the skin (ecchymoses, purpura)

- Multiple bruises due to platelet/clotting disorders or Ehlers–Danlos syndrome (especially on shins, knees)
- Bruising due to 'cupping' or cao gio (coin rubbing)
- Vasculitis, particularly Henoch–Schönlein purpura (HSP; favors lower extremities) and acute hemorrhagic edema of infancy (favors face)

Blue discoloration of skin mistaken as bruising

- Dermal melanocytosis (favors sacral area and back; color does not progress to green/yellow)
- Infantile hemangioma (deep) or vascular malformation

Linear hyperpigmentation

- Phytophotodermatitis (Fig. 75.12A)
- Sock-line or mitten-line hyperpigmentation

Vesicles, bullae, or erosions mistaken as nonaccidental burns or other intentional injuries

- Impetigo, ecthyma, blistering distal dactylitis
- Erythema multiforme, fixed drug eruption
- Bullous mastocytosis
- Irritant contact dermatitis (e.g. from laxative and mimicking immersion burn)
- Arthropod bite reaction
- Moxibustion
- Burn from a hot car seat or seat belt buckle
- Genetic disorders of skin fragility, e.g. epidermolysis bullosa or porphyria

Other

- Osteogenesis imperfecta
- Hair tourniquet
- Self-inflicted injury

Table 75.3 Conditions that can mimic child abuse.

CONDITIONS OCCASIONALLY MISDIAGNOSED AS SEXUAL ABUSE IN CHILDREN

- Congenital anomalies or normal variants (e.g. white line in the posterior vestibule)
- Accidental injury
- Perianal streptococcal infection
- Lichen sclerosus (Fig. 75.12B; may be associated with purpura or hemorrhagic bullae)
- Genital vitiligo
- Localized vulvar bullous pemphigoid or other bullous diseases
- Crohn's disease (Fig. 75.12C)
- Entities misdiagnosed as genital or perianal warts
  - Perianal pyramidal protrusion (Fig. 75.12D)
  - Molluscum contagiosum
  - Pseudoverrucous papules and nodules due to encopresis or urinary incontinence

Table 75.4 Conditions occasionally misdiagnosed as sexual abuse in children.

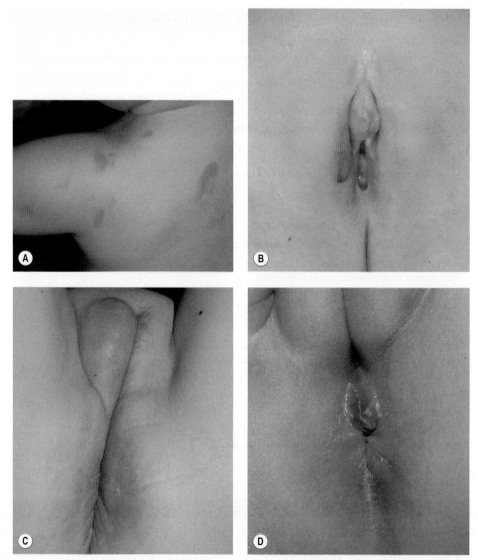

Fig. 75.12 Cutaneous disorders that may be misdiagnosed as physical or sexual abuse.
A Linear hyperpigmented streaks due to phytophotodermatitis on the back of a 2-year-old girl; the mother had lime juice on her hand when she touched the child. **B** Genital lichen sclerosus may have associated purpura or hemorrhagic bullae. **C** Cutaneous Crohn's disease can present with vulvar erythema and swelling as well as perianal ulcers. **D** A perianal pyramidal protrusion in the typical location, just anterior to the anus in the midline. This finding is most common in infant girls. *A, Courtesy, Anthony J. Mancini, MD; B, Courtesy, Sharon Ann Raimer, MD; C, D, Courtesy, Julie V. Schaffer, MD.*

For further information see Chs. 89 and 90. From *Dermatology, Third Edition.*

Histiocytoses

76

- Group of disorders in which the predominant cell type is a Langerhans cell, a mononuclear cell/macrophage, or a dermal dendrocyte.
- Two major groups: Langerhans cell histiocytoses and non-Langerhans cell histiocytoses.
- Within these two main groups, the disorders overlap and form a clinicopathologic spectrum.

Langerhans Cell Histiocytoses

- Langerhans cells, which represent the major antigen-presenting cells of the epidermis, are CD1a-positive, S-100 protein-positive, langerin (CD207)-positive.
- Langerhans cells have Birbeck granules by electron microscopy.
- Common in children ages 1–3 years, but can occur at any age.
- Traditionally classified into the following categories but they exist along a clinical spectrum.

Letterer–Siwe Disease (Multifocal, Multisystem)

- Acute, diffuse form.
- Multisystem involvement (skin, lung, liver, lymph nodes, bone, bone marrow).
- Classically in those <1–2 year(s) of age.
- Small, 2- to 3-mm, skin-colored to pink papules, which can coalesce; sometimes admixed with pustules or vesicles.
- Favors scalp, flexural neck, axilla, perineum, trunk (Fig. 76.1).
- Secondary changes include scale, crusts, petechiae/purpura.
- **DDx** includes seborrheic dermatitis, intertrigo, scabies, impetigo, atopic dermatitis, contact dermatitis.

Hand–Schüller–Christian Disease

- Triad of diabetes insipidus (in 30%), exophthalmos, osteolytic bone lesions (especially in cranium).
- Chronic, progressive course.
- Classically in children ages 2–6 years.
- 30% with skin lesions, sometimes resembling those of Letterer–Siwe disease; older lesions often more xanthomatous (i.e. yellow in color due to accumulations of lipid within macrophages) and occasionally lesions are ulcerated.
- Premature loss of teeth can occur.

Eosinophilic Granuloma (Unifocal)

- Localized variant (Fig. 76.2).
- Classically in children, ages 7–12 years.
- Skin and mucous membrane involvement rare.
- Often presents as a single, asymptomatic bony lesion (cranium > ribs > vertebrae > pelvis > scapulae > long bones).

Hashimoto–Pritzker Disease (Congenital Self-Healing Reticulohistiocytosis)

- Limited to skin, rapidly self-healing.
- At birth or during first few days of life.
- Variable presentation from a single nodule to widespread red-brown papules/nodules that crust and involute after several weeks (Fig. 76.3).
- Longitudinal follow-up is recommended because a small percentage of patients can develop systemic disease.

Non-Langerhans Cell Histiocytoses

Juvenile Xanthogranuloma

- Most common of the non-Langerhans cell histiocytoses.

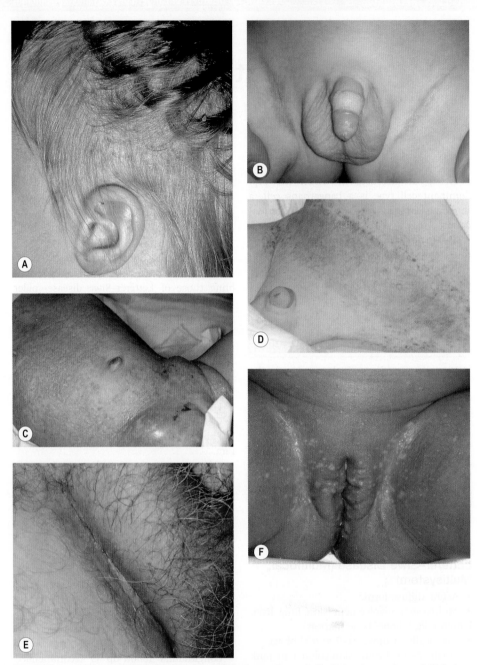

Fig. 76.1 Langerhans cell histiocytosis – clinical spectrum. A Scalp involvement may initially be diagnosed as seborrheic dermatitis; however, there are usually more discrete papules and crusting. **B** Pink, thin plaques with fissuring along the inguinal crease can also resemble seborrheic dermatitis. **C** Advanced disease with coalescence of papules into large plaques and prominent inguinal lymphadenopathy. **D** The presence of petechiae and purpuric papules is a clue to the diagnosis. **E** In an adult, the clinical presentation of inguinal involvement is similar to that of infants. **F** In patients with darkly pigmented skin, the papules can be hypopigmented. *B, Courtesy, Richard Antaya, MD; D, F, Courtesy, Julie V. Schaffer, MD.*

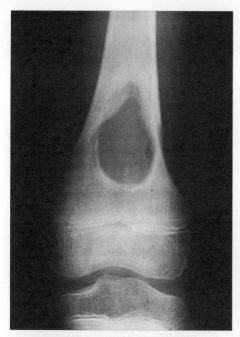

Fig. 76.2 Langerhans cell histiocytosis (eosinophilic granuloma of the bone). Radiography of the femur shows a large well-circumscribed osteolytic lesion. *Courtesy, Edward McCarthy, MD.*

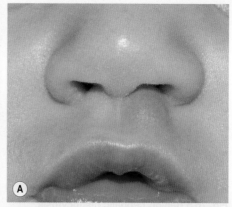

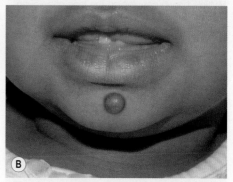

Fig. 76.4 Juvenile xanthogranuloma. A Pink nodule with a few telangiectasias representing an early lesion. **B** Well-developed yellow-brown papulonodule on the chin, with the color reflecting the accumulation of lipid within histiocytes. *Courtesy, Julie V. Schaffer, MD.*

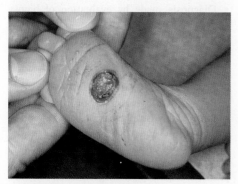

Fig. 76.3 Congenital self-healing reticulohistiocytosis (Hashimoto–Pritzker disease). Solitary eroded nodule on the plantar surface of a neonate. *Courtesy, Richard Antaya, MD.*

- Appears primarily in infants and children (75% present during the first year of life).
- Usually a single papule or nodule (Fig. 76.4).
- The color is initially pink to red-brown, but over time a yellow hue develops due to accumulation of intracellular lipid.

- Head/neck > trunk > upper extremities > lower extremities.
- Self-limiting; no treatment necessary.
- If multiple lesions, consider ophthalmologic examination for ocular involvement.
- If multiple café-au-lait macules are present, then consider the rare triple association with neurofibromatosis type I and an increased risk of developing juvenile myelomonocytic leukemia.
- **DDx:** molluscum contagiosum, Spitz nevus.

Benign Cephalic Histiocytosis

- Rare, generally in infants <1 year old.
- 2- to 5-mm red-brown macules or papules on the face and neck, rarely elsewhere (Fig. 76.5).

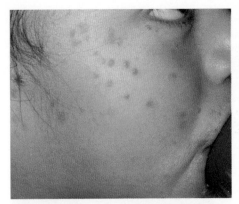

Fig. 76.5 Benign cephalic histiocytosis. Multiple brown papules on the face of a young child.

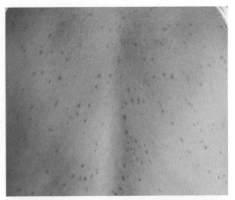

Fig. 76.7 Generalized eruptive histiocytoma. Multiple firm pink to red-brown papules on the trunk. The arms and legs were extensively involved. *Courtesy, Ingo Haase, MD, and Iliana Tantcheva-Poor, MD.*

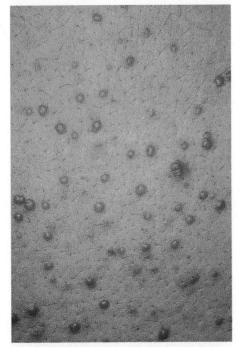

Fig. 76.6 Generalized eruptive histiocytoma. Multiple firm red papules on the trunk.

• Self-limiting after months to years; no treatment necessary.

Generalized Eruptive Histiocytoma

• Rare, generally in adults.
• Recurrent crops of tens to hundreds of small red-brown, firm papules (Figs. 76.6 and 76.7).

• Widespread on trunk.
• Self-limiting; no treatment necessary.

Indeterminate Cell Histiocytosis

• Rare, all ages affected.
• Clinically indistinguishable from generalized eruptive histiocytoma.
• Diagnosis made by evaluation of biopsy specimen, with cells expressing CD1a, S100-protein, and CD68 (a marker of macrophages); lack of Birbeck granules ultrastructurally.

Necrobiotic Xanthogranuloma

• Rare, generally in adults >50 years of age.
• Firm, yellowish plaques or papulonodules; sometimes ulcerated.
• Classically periorbital (Fig. 76.8).
• IgG monoclonal gammopathy in 80% of patients; hepatosplenomegaly, increased ESR, leukopenia, hypocomplementemia.
• Underlying plasma cell dyscrasia common; also increased risk of lymphoproliferative disorders.

Multicentric Reticulohistiocytosis/ Giant Cell Reticulohistiocytoma

• Generally in adults.
• When single:
  – A skin-colored to pink papulonodule often on the head.
  – Cutaneous disease only.

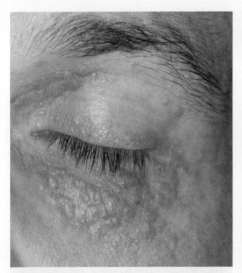

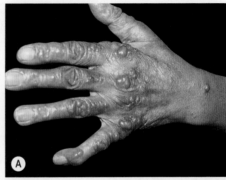

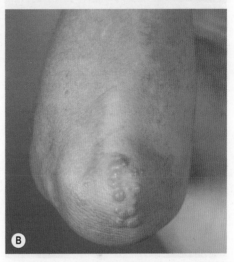

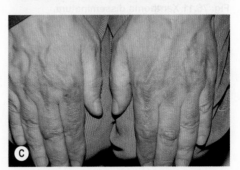

Fig. 76.8 Necrobiotic xanthogranuloma.
Yellow-brown papules and plaques in a periorbital distribution in a patient with chronic lymphocytic leukemia. Such lesions may initially be mistaken for xanthelasma. *Courtesy, Kalman Watsky, MD.*

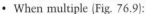

- When multiple (Fig. 76.9):
  - Pink to red-brown papulonodules that favor the hands (especially periungual) and elbows; occasionally photodistributed.
  - 50% with mucous membrane involvement.
  - Associated with destructive arthritis that can clinically resemble rheumatoid arthritis; in up to 50%, arthritis is preceded by skin disease.
  - Up to one third of affected patients can have an associated malignancy.

Rosai–Dorfman Disease (Sinus Histiocytosis with Massive Lymphadenopathy)

- Generally in children and young adults.
- Nonspecific red, red-brown, or yellow papulonodule(s) (Fig. 76.10).
- Favor eyelids and malar area.
- Skin-limited form being increasingly recognized.
- Often self-limited, but there may be a protracted course.
- Systemic disease presents as massive bilateral cervical lymphadenopathy; fever and IgG polyclonal hypergammaglobulinimia may be present.

Fig. 76.9 Multicentric reticulohistiocytosis.
A Grouped firm pink papules on the dorsal surface of the fingers, hand, and wrist of a 73-year-old African-American woman.
B Grouped pink papulonodules on the elbow in a second patient. **C** A more subtle presentation in a third patient, with small pink papules and thin plaques that favor the skin overlying the small joints of the hands; this is the form that can initially be confused with dermatomyositis.
A, Courtesy, Susan D. Laman, MD; B, Courtesy, Jean L. Bolognia, MD; C, Courtesy, Kalman Watsky, MD.

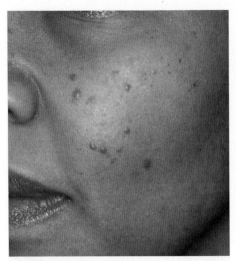

Fig. 76.10 Cutaneous Rosai–Dorfman disease. Discrete, dome-shaped, brown papules.

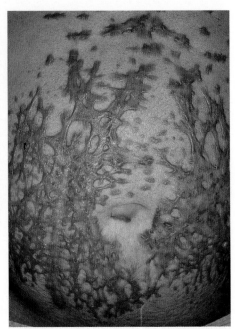

Fig. 76.12 Xanthoma disseminatum. Sclerotic form of xanthoma disseminatum in a patient who developed multiple myeloma.

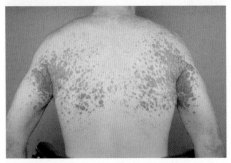

Fig. 76.11 Xanthoma disseminatum. Symmetric involvement of the major flexures is a characteristic finding. Note the yellow discoloration of some of the coalescing papulonodules. *Courtesy, David Wetter, MD.*

Xanthoma Disseminatum

- Rare, generally before age 25 years.
- Triad of cutaneous xanthomas, mucous membrane xanthomas (in 40–60%), and diabetes insipidus (in 40%).
- Symmetric eruption of tens to hundreds of yellow, red, or brown papules and plaques.
- Favors face and flexural areas, including major folds (Fig. 76.11).
- Rarely sclerosis (Fig. 76.12).
- Mucous membrane involvement: oral, upper airway, ocular (may threaten vision).
- Can be associated with a monoclonal gammopathy.
- May self-resolve, be persistent, or progressive.

Papular Xanthoma

- Any age.
- Generalized yellow papulonodules, sparing flexures.

Progressive Nodular Histiocytoma

- Any age.
- Generalized yellow papulonodules with prominent facial involvement.

Although we have made all these distinctions in the non-Langerhans cell histiocytoses, patients may have overlapping clinical and histopathologic features (including immunohistochemical staining). As a result, the evaluation of a patient with a non-Langerhans cell histiocytosis should include a total body skin examination and general physical examination, inclusive of eyes, mucosae, and lymph nodes. In addition, laboratory testing should include serum protein electrophoresis, immunofixation electrophoresis, and evaluation for diabetes insipidus.

For further information see Ch. 91. From *Dermatology, Third Edition.*

Xanthomas | 77

Key Points

- Cutaneous xanthomas are due to an accumulation of lipid, primarily within dermal macrophages (foam cells), and they have a characteristic yellow-orange hue.
- Four major types of xanthomas: eruptive, tuberous, tendinous, and plane.

- They may be a sign of hyperlipidemia, either primary or secondary, or an underlying monoclonal gammopathy.
- The type of xanthoma and its anatomic location are clues to the specific lipid abnormality or associated disorder (Table 77.1; Figs. 77.1 and 77.2).

MAJOR TYPES OF HYPERLIPIDEMIA			
Type	**Laboratory Findings**	**Clinical Findings**	
		Skin (Types of Xanthoma)	**Systemic**
Type I (familial LPL deficiency, familial hyperchylomicronemia)	Slow chylomicron clearance Reduced LDL and HDL levels Hypertriglyceridemia	Eruptive	No increased risk of coronary artery disease
Type II (familial hypercholesterolemia or familial defective apo B-100)	Reduced LDL clearance Hypercholesterolemia	Tendinous, tuberoeruptive, tuberous, plane (xanthelasma, intertriginous areas, interdigital web spaces*)	Atherosclerosis of peripheral and coronary arteries
Type III (familial dysbetalipoproteinemia, remnant removal disease, broad beta disease, apo E deficiency)	Elevated levels of chylomicron remnants and IDLs Hypercholesterolemia Hypertriglyceridemia	Tuberoeruptive, tuberous Plane (palmar creases) – most characteristic Tendinous	Atherosclerosis of peripheral and coronary arteries
Type IV (endogenous familial hypertriglyceridemia)	Increased VLDLs Hypertriglyceridemia	Eruptive	Frequently associated with type 2 non-insulin-dependent diabetes mellitus, obesity, alcoholism
Type V	Decreased LDLs and HDLs Hypertriglyeridemia	Eruptive	Diabetes mellitus

*Plane xanthomas in the interdigital web space are said to be pathognomonic for the homozygous state.

Table 77.1 Major types of hyperlipidemia. apo, apolipoprotein; HDL, high-density lipoprotein; LDL, low-density lipoprotein; LPL, lipoprotein lipase; VLDL, very-low-density lipoprotein.

DISTRIBUTION OF DIFFERENT TYPES OF XANTHOMAS

Eruptive
Tuberous
Tuberoeruptive
Tendinous
Plane
Xanthelasma
Normolipemic plane
Verruciform xanthoma

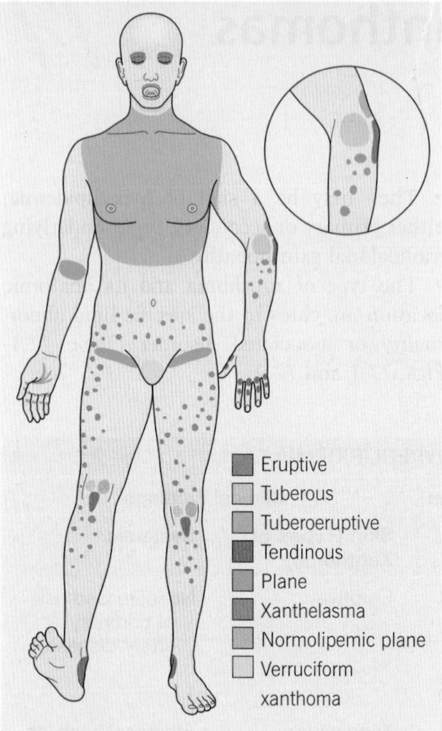

Fig. 77.1 Distribution of different types of xanthomas.

DIFFERENTIAL DIAGNOSIS OF XANTHOMAS

Eruptive Xanthomas

Disseminated granuloma annulare
Non-Langerhans cell histiocytosis
Xanthomatous lesions of Langerhans cell histiocytosis

Tuberous/Tuberoeruptive Xanthomas

Rheumatoid nodules
Erythema elevatum diutinum
Multicentric reticulohistiocytosis

Tendinous Xanthomas

Rheumatoid nodules
Erythema elevatum diutinum
Subcutaneous granuloma annulare
Giant cell tumor of the tendon sheath

Xanthelasma

Syringomas
Necrobiotic xanthogranuloma
Periocular xanthogranuloma and adult-onset asthma

Table 77.2 Differential diagnosis of xanthomas.

• **DDx** depends on the type of xanthoma (Table 77.2).
• In general, **Rx** is focused on correcting any underlying hyperlipidemia.

Xanthomas Associated with Hyperlipidemia

Eruptive Xanthomas

• Yellow-pink papules, 1–5 mm in diameter.
• May be widespread, but favor the extensor surfaces of the extremities and buttocks (Figs. 77.3 and 77.4).
• An inflammatory halo, tenderness, and/or pruritus may be present.
• Associated with hypertriglyceridemia (often >3000–4000 mg/dl) (see Fig. 77.2).
• Seen in the setting of type I, IV, or V hyperlipidemia and most commonly when associated diabetes mellitus is under poor control.

• Lesions often resolve within weeks of aggressive **Rx:** insulin; triglyceride-lowering agents, e.g. fenofibrate.

Tuberous/Tuberoeruptive Xanthomas

• Pink-yellow to yellow-brown papules (tuberoeruptive) or nodules (tuberous) on extensor surfaces, especially the elbows and knees (Figs. 77.5 and 77.6); tuberous xanthomas can be >3 cm in diameter.
• Associated with hypercholesterolemia (type II or III hyperlipidemia).
• May be slow to regress with cholesterol-lowering agents (e.g. 'statins').

Tendinous Xanthomas

• Firm, smooth, skin-colored nodules due to lipid deposits within the Achilles tendons and the extensor tendons of the hands, knees, and/or elbows (Figs. 77.7 and 77.8).
• Can serve as an early clue to the presence of type II hyperlipidemia.

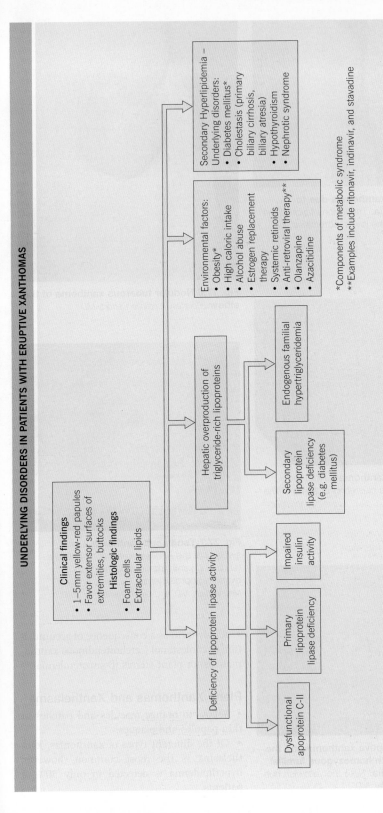

UNDERLYING DISORDERS IN PATIENTS WITH ERUPTIVE XANTHOMAS

Clinical findings
- 1–5mm yellow-red papules
- Favor extensor surfaces of extremities, buttocks

Histologic findings
- Foam cells
- Extracellular lipids

Deficiency of lipoprotein lipase activity

Dysfunctional apoprotein C-II

Primary lipoprotein lipase deficiency

Impaired insulin activity

Hepatic overproduction of triglyceride-rich lipoproteins

Secondary lipoprotein lipase deficiency (e.g. diabetes mellitus)

Endogenous familial hypertriglyceridemia

Environmental factors:
- Obesity*
- High caloric intake
- Alcohol abuse
- Estrogen replacement therapy
- Systemic retinoids
- Anti-retroviral therapy**
- Olanzapine
- Azacitidine

Secondary Hyperlipidemia – Underlying disorders:
- Diabetes mellitus*
- Cholestasis (primary biliary cirrhosis, biliary atresia)
- Hypothyroidism
- Nephrotic syndrome

*Components of metabolic syndrome
**Examples include ritonavir, indinavir, and stavadine

Fig. 77.2 Underlying disorders in patients with eruptive xanthomas.

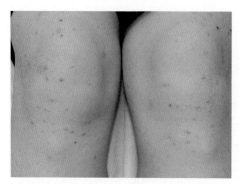

Fig. 77.3 Eruptive xanthomas due to hypertriglyceridemia. The lesions favored the extensor surface of the lower extremities, in particular the knees.

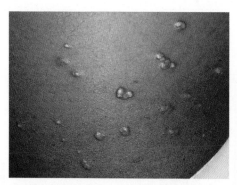

Fig. 77.4 Eruptive xanthomas. Note the yellowish hue and the clustering of some of the lesions.

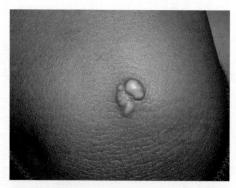

Fig. 77.5 Tuberoeruptive xanthomas on the elbow of a child with homozygous familial hypercholesterolemia. Note the yellowish hue. *Courtesy, Julie V. Schaffer, MD.*

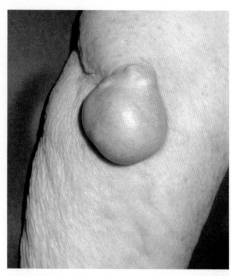

Fig. 77.6 Nodular tuberous xanthoma of the elbow. *Courtesy, Lorenzo Cerroni, MD.*

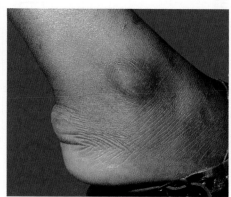

Fig. 77.7 Tendinous xanthoma. Linear swelling of the Achilles area, representing a tendinous xanthoma in a patient with dysbetalipoproteinemia. *Courtesy, W. Trent Massengale, MD, and Lee T. Nesbitt, Jr., MD.*

• Rarely form as a consequence of accumulation of cholestanol (cerebrotendinous xanthomatosis) or plant sterols (β-sitosterolemia).

Plane Xanthomas and Xanthelasma
• Yellow to orange macules and patches or thin papules and plaques.
• Of the different types of xanthomas, xanthelasma is the most common; however, hyperlipidemia is detected in only 50% of patients.

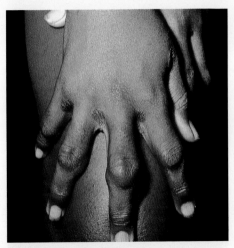

Fig. 77.8 Tendinous xanthomas of the fingers in a patient with homozygous familial hypercholesterolemia. Note interdigital plane xanthomas of the web spaces. *Courtesy, W. Trent Massengale, MD, and Lee T. Nesbitt, Jr., MD.*

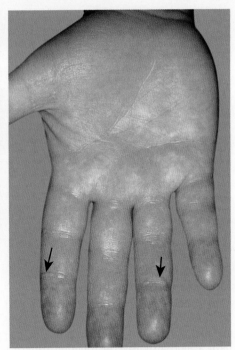

Fig. 77.10 Plane xanthomas of the palmar creases (arrows) in a patient with dysbetalipoproteinemia. They are seen in approximately two-thirds of patients with this disorder. Plane xanthomas are also seen in the setting of cholestasis, e.g. biliary atresia or primary biliary cirrhosis. *Courtesy, W. Trent Massengale, MD, and Lee T. Nesbitt, Jr., MD.*

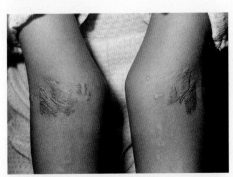

Fig. 77.9 Plane xanthomas of the antecubital fossae. This young patient had dysbetalipoproteinemia. *Courtesy, W. Trent Massengale, MD, and Lee T. Nesbitt, Jr., MD.*

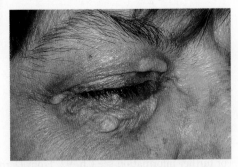

Fig. 77.11 Xanthelasma palpebrarum with typical yellowish hue.

- Site:
  - Intertriginous – antecubital fossae, finger web spaces, and palmar creases (Figs. 77.9 and 77.10).
  - Eyelids (xanthelasma), especially the medial aspect of the upper eyelid (Fig. 77.11).
- Intertriginous plane xanthomas can be seen in primary hyperlipidemia (type II or III) as well as secondary hyperlipidemia (e.g. biliary atresia, primary biliary cirrhosis).

- **Rx** of xanthelasma: destructive methods (e.g. trichloroacetic acid application, laser ablation), surgical excision.

Laboratory evaluation for suspected hyperlipidemia is outlined in Table 77.3.

- Fasting lipid panel*
- Fasting glucose level
- Liver function tests**
- Thyroid-stimulating hormone (TSH) level
- Serum albumin

*If elevated serum lipids, evaluate for systemic disease (see Table 77.1).
**If elevated serum alkaline phosphatase and bilirubin, evaluate for biliary disease.

Table 77.3 Laboratory evaluation of suspected hyperlipidemia.

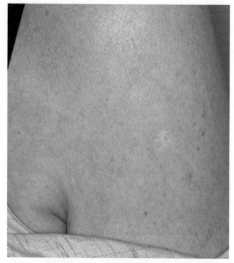

Fig. 77.12 Plane xanthoma. The large thin plaques have a yellow-orange color. On longitudinal evaluation, the patient was found to have a monoclonal gammopathy. *Courtesy, Whitney High, MD, JD.*

Normolipemic Xanthomas

Plane Xanthomas Associated with Monoclonal Gammopathy

- In contrast to plane xanthomas due to hyperlipidemia, these yellow-orange patches and thin plaques are usually larger in size and have a more extensive distribution pattern; the latter often includes the trunk (Fig. 77.12).
- In addition to the trunk, lesions may be seen on the neck, in flexural folds, and in the periorbital region.
- The monoclonal gammopathy is most commonly due to a plasma cell dyscrasia, and occasionally due to a lymphoproliferative disorder.

Verruciform Xanthoma

- Asymptomatic verrucous plaque, 1 to 2 cm in diameter (Fig. 77.13).
- Oral mucosa or anogenital region.
- May be seen in association with lymphedema, epidermolysis bullosa, and CHILD (congenital hemidysplasia with ichthyosiform erythroderma and limb defects) syndrome.

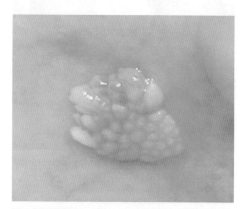

Fig. 77.13 Verruciform xanthoma of the oral mucosa. *Courtesy, Kishore Shetty, DDS.*

For further information see Ch. 92. From *Dermatology, Third Edition.*

Non-infectious Granulomatous Disorders, Including Foreign Body Reactions

78

When histiocytes form granulomas within the skin, the cutaneous disorders are referred to as granulomatous. This group of disorders is further divided into infectious (e.g. mycobacterial infections, dimorphic fungal infections) and non-infectious (e.g. sarcoidosis, granuloma annulare). This chapter focuses on the latter category.

Sarcoidosis

- Disorder of unknown etiology in which granulomas develop in one or more organs, most commonly the lung, skin, liver, and spleen.
- Cutaneous manifestations occur in >30% of patients and may be the first and/or only sign of the disease (Table 78.1).
- The classic lesion is a red-brown papule or plaque with a yellowish color on compression (diascopy), most commonly on the face (Figs. 78.1 and 78.2).
- Variants.
  - Lupus pernio – purple to red-brown papules and plaques of the nose, ears, and cheeks; may be beaded along the nasal rim (Fig. 78.2C); associated with chronic pulmonary sarcoidosis (75% of patients) or upper respiratory tract sarcoidosis (50%) and cysts within the distal phalanges.
  - Darier–Roussy sarcoidosis (subcutaneous variant) – painless, firm, mobile nodules or plaques.
  - Löfgren's syndrome – hilar adenopathy, fever, migrating polyarthritis, and acute iritis; erythema nodosum is the primary skin finding (see Table 83.2); often spontaneously remits.
  - Heerfordt's syndrome – parotid gland enlargement, uveitis, fever, cranial nerve palsies.

- **DDx of classic papule/plaque**: other entities in this chapter, cutaneous tuberculosis, dimorphic fungal infections, granulomatous rosacea.
- **Rx of cutaneous lesions**: CS (topical, intralesional); oral medications include minocycline, antimalarials, methotrexate, tacrolimus, TNF-α inhibitors, and thalidomide.

Granuloma Annulare

- May be a delayed-type hypersensitivity reaction to an unknown antigen; by history can follow an arthropod bite, trauma.
- Common clinical variants (see Table 78.1) – localized, often acral (Fig. 78.3); subcutaneous on hands, shins, and scalp in children; generalized (Fig. 78.4).
- Less common variants are perforating, often on the hands (Fig. 78.5), patch type on the trunk, and micropapular (Fig. 78.6).
- Generalized granuloma annulare is more likely to be associated with diabetes mellitus or lipid abnormalities (e.g. hypercholesterolemia) compared to other variants; atypical presentations seen in HIV-infected patients (Fig. 78.7).
- **DDx:** other entities in this chapter, tinea, interstitial granulomatous dermatitis, inflammatory morphea.
- **Rx:** spontaneous resolution may occur; first-line – CS (topical including under occlusion, intralesional); second-line – cryosurgery, tetracycline + niacinamide, antimalarials, retinoids, PUVA/UVA1/excimer laser.

Necrobiosis Lipoidica

- Formerly referred to as 'necrobiosis lipoidica diabeticorum,' a term abandoned given that the minority (~10%) of patients with this disorder have diabetes mellitus.

CLINICAL FEATURES OF THE MAJOR GRANULOMATOUS DERMATITIDES

	Sarcoidosis*	Classic Granuloma Annulare	Necrobiosis Lipoidica	AEGCG	Cutaneous Crohn's Disease	Rheumatoid Nodule
Average age (years)	25–35, 45–65	<30	30	50–70	35	40–50
Sex predilection	Female	Female	Female	None	Female	Male†
Racial/ethnic predilection in United States	African-American	None	None	Caucasian	Ashkenazi Jews	None
Sites	Symmetric on face, neck, upper trunk, extremities	Hands, feet, extensor aspects of extremities	Anterior and lateral aspects of distal lower extremities	Face, neck, forearms (sites of chronic sun exposure)	Oral/perioral, genital areas, lower > upper extremities	Juxta-articular areas, especially elbows, hands, ankles, feet
Appearance	Red to red-brown papules and plaques; occasionally violaceous or annular	Papules coalescing into annular plaques	Plaques with elevated borders, telangiectasias centrally	Annular plaques	Dusky erythema and swelling, ulceration	Skin-colored, firm, mobile subcutaneous nodules
Size of lesions	0.2 to >5 cm	1- to 3-mm papules, annular plaques usually <6 cm	3 to >10 cm	1–6 cm	Variable	1–3 cm
No. of lesions	Variable	1–10	1–10	1–10	1–5	1–10
Associations	Systemic manifestations of sarcoidosis; interferon-α therapy for hepatitis C viral infection >> melanoma	Rare diabetes mellitus, HIV infection, malignancy	Diabetes mellitus	Actinic damage	Intestinal Crohn's disease	Rheumatoid arthritis
Special clinical characteristics	Occasional central atrophy and hypopigmentation; development within scars	Central hyperpigmentation	Yellow-brown atrophic centers, ulceration	Central atrophy and hypopigmentation	Draining sinuses and fistulas	Occasional ulceration, especially at sites of trauma

*Clinical variants include lupus pernio and subcutaneous (Darier–Roussy), psoriasiform, ichthyosiform, angiolupoid, and ulcerative sarcoidosis.
†Although rheumatoid arthritis has a female:male ratio of 2–3:1.
AEGCG, annular elastolytic giant cell granuloma.

Table 78.1 Clinical features of the major granulomatous dermatitides.

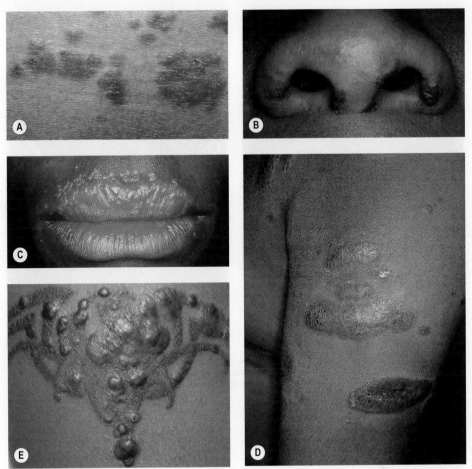

Fig. 78.1 Sarcoidosis. A Cutaneous sarcoidosis usually consists of papules and plaques with a typical reddish-brown color. **B, C** Lesions often favor the nose, lips, and perioral region. **D** Hyperpigmented plaques, some of which have scale. **E** Papules of cutaneous sarcoidosis arising within a tattoo; the differential diagnosis includes foreign body reaction. *B, Courtesy, Louis A. Fragola, Jr., MD.*

- Typically red-brown plaques on the shins with central clearing that may become yellow and atrophic over time; occasionally, lesions involve the upper extremities, face, and scalp (Fig. 78.8; see Table 78.1).
- **DDx:** granuloma annulare, sarcoidosis, and non-X histiocytoses, in particular necrobiotic xanthogranuloma.
- **Rx:** CS (topical, intralesional, rarely systemic) are the mainstay; for intralesional CS, test sites are recommended.

Annular Elastolytic Giant Cell Granuloma

- Clinically most closely resembles granuloma annulare but lesions have an atrophic,

hypopigmented center and sites of predilection are sun-exposed sites including the face, neck, and forearms (Fig. 78.9; see Table 78.1).
- Biopsy needs to be elliptical and involve the center, the border, and uninvolved skin with longitudinal sectioning.
- **Rx:** often ineffective, can try topical and intralesional CS.

Cutaneous Crohn's Disease

- Skin lesions may be the presenting sign of Crohn's disease in up to 20% of patients and they may be specific or nonspecific; examples of the latter include pyoderma gangrenosum and erythema nodosum.

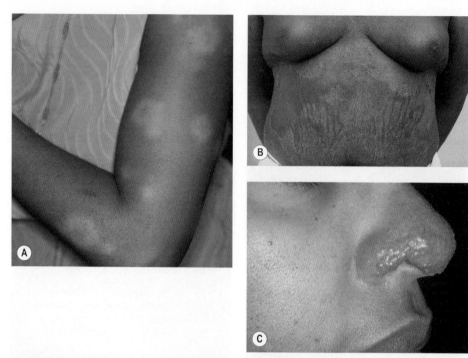

Fig. 78.2 Sarcoidosis – clinical variants. A The hypopigmented variant is more noticeable in individuals with dark skin. **B** Ichthyosiform presentation with obvious scale. **C** Coalescing violaceous papules on the nose in lupus pernio; note the notching of the nasal rim. *A, Courtesy, Louis A. Fragola, Jr., MD; B, Courtesy, Jean L. Bolognia, MD.*

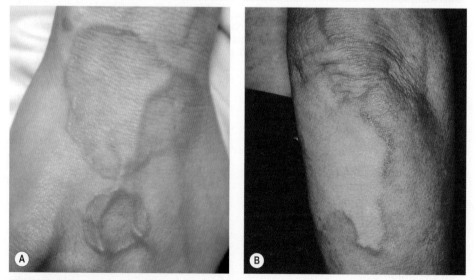

Fig. 78.3 Granuloma annulare. A Annular plaques on the dorsal aspect of the hand, a common location. **B** Larger lesion on the arm with a figurate border composed of coalescing papules. Note the red-brown color of previously involved skin.

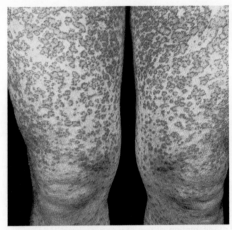

Fig. 78.4 Generalized granuloma annulare. Numerous papules and small annular plaques.

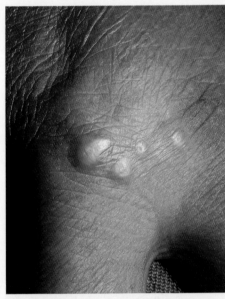

Fig. 78.5 Perforating granuloma annulare. Papules can have a central keratotic plug or umbilication. *Courtesy, Ronald P. Rapini, MD.*

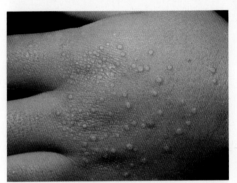

Fig. 78.6 Papular granuloma annulare of the dorsal hand. Several of the lesions have a central dell. *Courtesy, Joyce Rico, MD.*

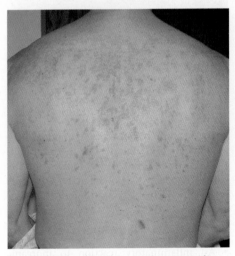

Fig. 78.7 Disseminated granuloma annulare in an HIV-infected patient. *From Callen, JP, et al. Dermatological Signs of Internal Disease, 4th edn. 2009. Saunders: Philadelphia. Courtesy, Kalman Watsky, MD.*

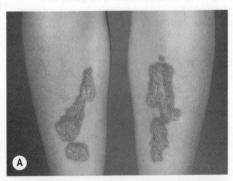

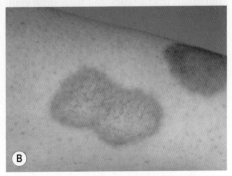

Fig. 78.8 Necrobiosis lipoidica. A Pink-brown atrophic plaques on the shins. **B** Annular plaques with central telangiectasias.

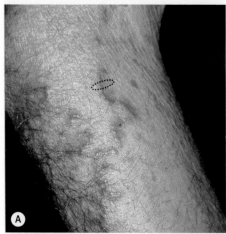

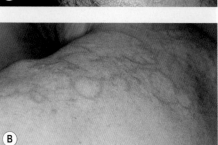

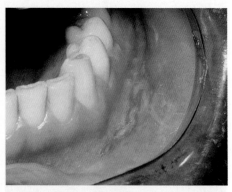

Fig. 78.10 Crohn's disease. Linear ulceration of the mandibular vestibule: the classic oral manifestation of this disease. *Courtesy, Charles Camisa, MD.*

Fig. 78.9 Annular elastolytic giant cell granuloma. The border resembles granuloma annulare but the central portion is hypopigmented and/or atrophic **(A, B)**. A biopsy specimen that includes the area outlined in **A** would contain the three characteristic histologic zones: absence of elastic fibers, granulomatous inflammation, and normal skin. Longitudinal sectioning of the surgical specimen is preferred. *B, Courtesy, Kalman Watsky, MD.*

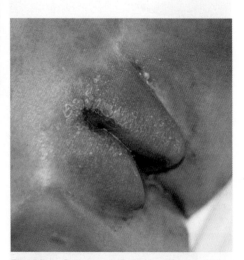

Fig. 78.11 Cutaneous Crohn's disease. Note the swelling and violaceous discoloration of the labia majora in this prepubescent girl. *Courtesy, Joseph L. Jorizzo, MD.*

- Specific lesions can be contiguous or non-contiguous (metastatic), and both show granulomas on biopsy.
  - Contiguous lesions are seen in the mouth, perioral, anogenital region, and peristomal areas with clinical presentations varying from fissures to cobblestoning to swelling (Figs. 78.10 and 78.11).
  - Metastatic lesions present as vegetating plaques or nodules, most commonly on the lower extremities (see Table 78.1).
  - Sinuses from GI disease may extend to the skin, particularly in the anogenital region or surgical sites on the abdomen.

- **Rx of skin lesions**: often improve with systemic Rx of GI disease; oral metronidazole (250 mg three times daily); topical, intralesional, and oral CS; other systemic agents (e.g. sulfasalazine, TNF-α inhibitors).

Foreign Body Granulomas

- An inflammatory reaction to inorganic (e.g. suture) or organic (e.g. keratin) materials implanted into the skin.

- The most common foreign body is keratin due to ruptured cysts or hair follicles (Table 78.2; Figs. 78.12–78.18).
- The clinical presentation is usually a red to red-brown papule, nodule, or plaque that may be ulcerated or extruding the foreign material.

- History and histologic findings including polarization can aid in identifying the foreign material; occasionally other procedures (e.g. energy dispersive x-ray analysis) are necessary.

FEATURES OF SELECTED FOREIGN BODY REACTIONS		
Foreign Body	**Clinical Presentations**	**Cause/Common Site(s)**
Endogenous Material		
Keratin	• Erythema, induration, papules, nodules • Pseudofolliculitis/acne keloidalis nuchae • Pyogenic granuloma-like lesions • Pilonidal disease	• Ruptured follicle/cyst • Ingrown hair/nail • Beard area • Sacral area
Generally Exogenous Material		
Tattoo pigment	• Erythema, induration, papules, nodules (Fig. 78.12) • Lichenoid papules and plaques • Eczematous dermatitis (including photoallergic reactions)	• Decorative/cosmetic • Accidental (Fig. 78.13) • Iatrogenic
Silica (silicon dioxide)	• Nodules, indurated plaques within scar (Fig. 78.14) • Disseminated papules (blast injury) • Prolonged incubation period (sometimes decades)	• Wound contamination • Blast injury
Zirconium	• Persistent, brown, soft papules • Involvement of axillary skin	• Topical application of deodorants, antipruritic medications
Beryllium	• Nodule, ulcer • Widely scattered papules (systemic reaction)	• Laceration by broken fluorescent lamps • Inhalation
Cactus	• Dome-shaped, skin-colored papules with a central black dot	• Accidental • Occupational
Jellyfish, corals, sea urchin spines	• Pruritic lichenoid papules and plaques (onset 2–3 weeks after exposure) • Linear, zigzag, and whip-like (flagellate) patterns of erythema/edema (early), hyperpigmentation or lichenoid papules (late) (Fig. 78.15)	• Accidental • Swimming or diving
Implanted/Injected Material During Procedures (Fig. 78.16)		
Suture	• Wound/scar appears inflamed, red, edematous (or develops papules or nodules) and opens to form a fistula	
Intralesional corticosteroids	• Skin-colored to yellow-white papules or nodules develop at the site of a previous intralesional injection of corticosteroid • Incubation period varies from weeks to months	

Table 78.2 Features of selected foreign body reactions. *Continued*

Table 78.2 *Continued* **Features of selected foreign body reactions.**

Foreign Body	Clinical Presentations	Cause/Common Site(s)
Talc	• Sarcoid-like papules • Thickening and erythema of an old scar • Involvement of intertriginous zones, IV injection sites (e.g. self-prepared drugs) • Umbilical stumps • Pyogenic granuloma-like	
Starch	• Papules and nodules	
Aluminum	• Persistent subcutaneous nodule at vaccine injection site	
Zinc	• Furuncles at insulin injection sites	
Injected Material for Tissue Augmentation		
Paraffin	• Firm nodules, indurated plaques on genitalia or breasts • Ulceration or abscess formation (Fig. 78.17) • Occasionally periorbital (due to topical paraffin-containing preparations)	
Silicone	• Erythema, induration, nodules, ulcers on breasts • Often appears after years • Sometimes injected into the face for HIV-associated lipodystrophy (see Chapter 84)	
Bovine collagen,* hyaluronic acid,* fillers containing synthetic particles	• Generally used on the face • Induration and erythema • Papules and nodules (Fig. 78.18) • Abscesses	

*Often resorbable.

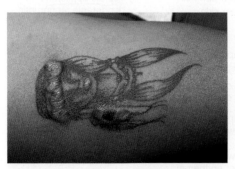

Fig. 78.12 Granulomatous reaction to the red (cinnabar) portions of a tattoo. During the past several years, cinnabar (mercuric sulfide) has been gradually replaced by cadmium selenide (cadmium red), ferric hydrate (sienna), and organic compounds. *Courtesy, Ronald P. Rapini, MD.*

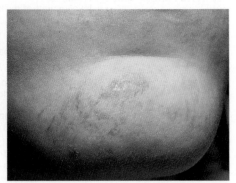

Fig. 78.13 Traumatic tattoo of the chin. Bluish discoloration and slight erythema, predominantly due to silica. *Courtesy, Ronald P. Rapini, MD.*

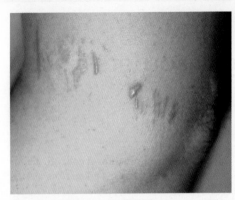

Fig. 78.14 Silica granulomas. *Courtesy, Kenneth Greer, MD.*

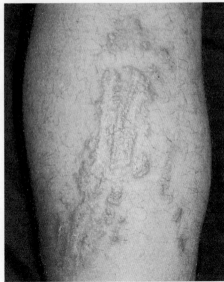

Fig. 78.15 Coral envenomation. Delayed lichenoid reaction on the calf. The patient accidentally came into contact with a coral reef and developed acute dermatitis that resolved, to be followed 3 weeks later by this severely itchy eruption that responded favorably to intralesional triamcinolone injection. *Courtesy, M. A. Abdallah, MD.*

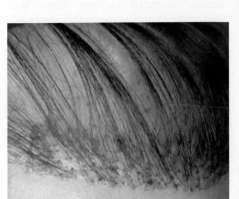

Fig. 78.16 Foreign body reactions to polyamide synthetic 'hair' implantation. In addition to multiple perifollicular granulomas, there is evidence of chronic folliculitis. *Courtesy, Marwa Abdallah, MD.*

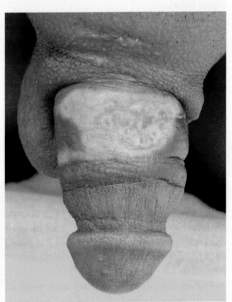

Fig. 78.17 Sclerosing lipogranuloma of the penis. The penis was injected in order to relieve urinary retention following a motorbike accident, and an ulcerated, indurated yellow plaque with telangiectasias developed at the site. *Courtesy, Glen Foxton, MD, and Clare Tait, MD.*

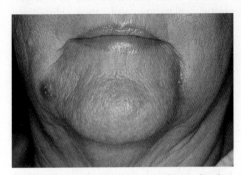

Fig. 78.18 Granulomatous reaction to bovine collagen injection.

For further information see Chs. 93 and 94. From *Dermatology, Third Edition.*

79 | Perforating Disorders

Classically, a group of disorders in which there is transepidermal elimination ('perforation') of components of the dermis, in particular collagen and/or elastic fibers (Table 79.1). Etiologies are multiple, including inheritance as an isolated cutaneous disease or in association with genetic disorders that affect connective tissue (e.g. Ehlers–Danlos syndrome). Most commonly, however, the perforating disorder is acquired and is related to the cutaneous trauma that results from scratching pruritic skin, especially in the setting of chronic kidney disease. A number of other cutaneous diseases occasionally undergo perforation, e.g. granuloma annulare, calcinosis cutis, chondrodermatitis nodularis helicis.

Acquired Perforating Dermatosis (APD)

• The most commonly observed perforating disorder (see Table 79.1); it is an acquired disease that affects primarily adults; the term APD encompasses several overlapping entities including *acquired* reactive perforating collagenosis (RPC), Kyrle's disease, and perforating folliculitis.
• In general, affected individuals have pruritic skin that has been scratched; the vast majority of patients have chronic kidney disease and/or diabetes mellitus, with most of the latter individuals having diabetic nephropathy; it affects up to 10% of patients receiving chronic hemodialysis.
• Occurs less often in patients with pruritus due to other causes, e.g. biliary cirrhosis, Hodgkin's disease.
• Erythematous, skin-colored or hyperpigmented papules and papulonodules with a central keratotic core that favor the extensor surfaces of the extremities (Figs. 79.1 and 79.2); the central core is a reflection of the transepidermal elimination of collagen and/or elastic fibers as well as hyperkeratosis associated with epidermal hyperplasia.
• **DDx:** see Table 79.2.
• **Rx:** difficult; topical antipruritics (e.g. pramoxine), sedating antihistamines, CS-impregnated tape, intralesional CS, cryotherapy, tangential excision, Unna boot (impregnated gauze wrapping that serves as a physical barrier against scratching), NB- or BB-UVB, topical or oral retinoids.

Elastosis Perforans Serpiginosa (EPS)

• Annular or serpiginous plaques composed of keratotic papules that are usually skin-colored (Fig. 79.3); lesions favor flexural sites, in particular the neck and antecubital fossae, and can be several centimeters in diameter.
• Occurs in patients with inherited disorders that affect connective tissue (~40% of cases of EPS; Fig. 79.4) or as a consequence of medications that disrupt elastin formation, e.g. penicillamine; in the former group, the onset is during childhood or early adulthood; there is also a skin-limited childhood form that may be inherited.
• Elastic fibers are surrounded by a hyperplastic epidermis and then eliminated transepidermally.
• **DDx:** see Table 79.2.
• **Rx:** lesions may spontaneously resolve over a period of years; cryotherapy, tangential excision, nonaggressive electrosurgical or laser therapy (to avoid scarring).

Familial Reactive Perforating Collagenosis (RPC)

• Rare inherited disorder with an onset during childhood; affects sites of trauma, especially the arms and hands.

MAJOR PERFORATING DISORDERS

Disease	Incidence	Time of Onset	Most Common Location	Perforating Substance	Associations
Acquired perforating dermatosis (APD)	Common	Adulthood	Extensor extremities (legs > arms); occasionally generalized	Necrotic material +/or collagen >> elastic fibers	Pruritus, usually in the setting of chronic kidney disease +/or diabetes mellitus*; affects 10% of patients on chronic hemodialysis
Elastosis perforans serpiginosa (EPS)	Rare	Childhood, early adulthood; variable if drug-induced	Flexures, especially neck, antecubital fossae; face	Elastic fibers	Genetic disorders (see Fig. 79.4); penicillamine
Familial reactive perforating collagenosis (RPC)	Rare	Childhood	Arms, hands, sites of trauma	Collagen	None
Perforating calcific elastosis	Rare, but more common in African-American women	Adulthood	Periumbilical, abdomen > breast	Calcified elastic tissue	Primarily multiparity, obesity; occasionally chronic kidney disease
Perforating folliculitis	Common	Early adulthood	Extremities, trunk	Necrotic tissue	May represent rupture of ordinary folliculitis

*Occasionally affects patients with pruritus due to other disorders, e.g. Hodgkin disease, biliary cirrhosis.

Table 79.1 Major perforating disorders. *Courtesy, Ronald Rapini, MD.*

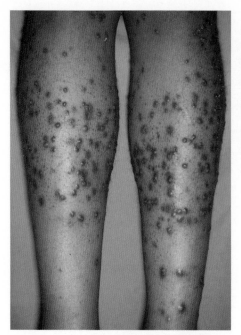

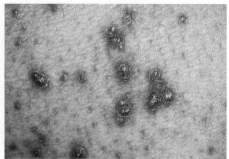

Fig. 79.2 Acquired perforating dermatosis. Keratotic papules on the arm of a diabetic woman on hemodialysis. Note the central keratotic core which is sometimes dislodged by the patient.

Fig. 79.1 Acquired perforating dermatosis. Numerous papules and papulonodules on the legs in a patient with diabetes mellitus and chronic kidney disease. *Courtesy, Ronald Rapini, MD.*

DIFFERENTIAL DIAGNOSIS OF PERFORATING DISEASES
Acquired Perforating Dermatosis and Reactive Perforating Collagenosis
• Excoriations from a variety of causes (prurigo simplex) • Prurigo nodularis • Folliculitis • Arthropod bites • Perforation of exogenous foreign material • Perforation of endogenous substances (e.g. calcium) • Multiple keratoacanthomas • Dermatofibromas • If Koebner phenomenon, verrucae, lichen planus
Elastosis Perforans Serpiginosa (see Chapter 15 for **DDx** of annular lesions)
• Granuloma annulare ⎱ Common annular diseases • Tinea ⎰ • Sarcoidosis • Actinic granuloma (annular elastolytic giant cell granuloma) • Perforating calcific elastosis • Perforating pseudoxanthoma elasticum

Table 79.2 Differential diagnosis of perforating diseases.

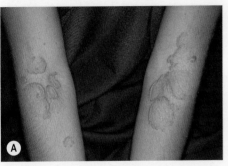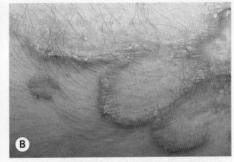

Fig. 79.3 Elastosis perforans serpiginosa. A Multiple annular plaques favoring the antecubital fossae, a flexural site. **B** Closer view with foci of hyperkeratosis at sites of transepidermal elimination. The patient had received penicillamine.

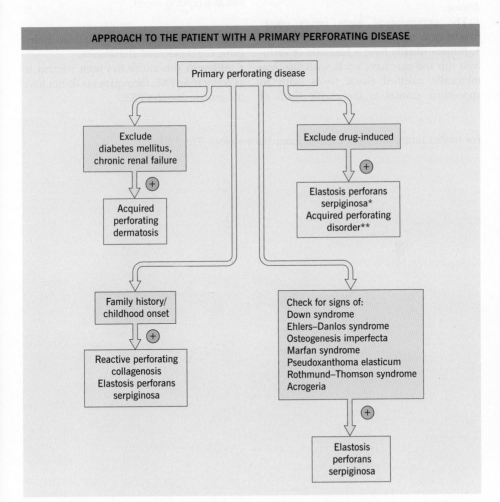

APPROACH TO THE PATIENT WITH A PRIMARY PERFORATING DISEASE

Primary perforating disease

Exclude diabetes mellitus, chronic renal failure
(+)
Acquired perforating dermatosis

Exclude drug-induced
(+)
Elastosis perforans serpiginosa*
Acquired perforating disorder**

Family history/ childhood onset
(+)
Reactive perforating collagenosis
Elastosis perforans serpiginosa

Check for signs of:
Down syndrome
Ehlers–Danlos syndrome
Osteogenesis imperfecta
Marfan syndrome
Pseudoxanthoma elasticum
Rothmund–Thomson syndrome
Acrogeria
(+)
Elastosis perforans serpiginosa

Fig. 79.4 Approach to the patient with a primary perforating disease. *Penicillamine. **Tumor necrosis factor-alpha inhibitors, bevacizumab, sirolimus, indinavir.

- Skin-colored papules with a central core composed of 'perforating' collagen fibers; a linear array due to Koebner phenomenon may be seen.
- **DDx:** other perforating disorders, perforating GA.
- **Rx:** lesions spontaneously resolve over a period of a few months.

Perforating Calcific Elastosis

- Most common site of involvement is periumbilical (Fig. 79.5); may be seen on the breast in the setting of chronic kidney disease.
- The periumbilical form favors obese, middle-aged, multiparous black women.
- Plaques usually have a keratotic or verrucous rim and may have a yellowish hue; histologically, calcified elastic fibers (with an appearance similar to the elastic fibers of

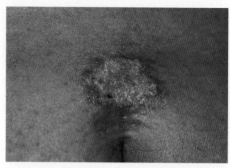

Fig. 79.5 Perforating calcific elastosis. When a biopsy was performed from the elevated edge of this supraumbilical plaque in a multiparous African-American woman, resistance was felt, as well as a grinding sound.

pseudoxanthoma elasticum [PXE]) are undergoing transepidermal elimination.
- Although this entity has been referred to as perforating PXE, these patients do not have the genetic disorder PXE.

For further information see Ch. 96. From *Dermatology, Third Edition.*

Heritable Connective Tissue Disorders

80

Heritable connective tissue disorders present with a broad range of cutaneous and extracutaneous manifestations. Recognition of characteristic skin findings is often critical to establishing the diagnosis and identifying associated internal involvement, which may include life-threatening cardiovascular disease (e.g. in the vascular type of Ehlers–Danlos syndrome [EDS] and pseudoxanthoma elasticum [PXE]).

Ehlers–Danlos Syndrome

• Clinically and genetically heterogeneous group of connective tissue disorders caused by defective function of various collagens, collagen-processing enzymes, and associated proteins.
• The cardinal physical findings of hyperextensible, fragile skin, and hypermobile joints (Fig. 80.1) are present to varying degrees in different subtypes of EDS (Table 80.1).
• Manifestations of cutaneous fragility include easy bruising (sometimes leading to suspicion of a bleeding disorder; see Fig. 80.1D) and gaping, 'fish-mouth' wounds from minor trauma that heal with widened, atrophic scars (see Fig. 80.1C); additional findings may include smooth velvety skin, molluscoid pseudotumors (fleshy nodules in sites of repetitive trauma), subcutaneous spheroids over bony prominences (small, hard nodules that represent calcified fat lobules), piezogenic papules (see Chapter 82), and elastosis perforans serpiginosa (see Chapter 79).
• **Rx:** prevention of trauma; patients with the vascular type of EDS require close monitoring (especially during pregnancy) to avoid serious complications.

Pseudoxanthoma Elasticum

• Uncommon autosomal recessive disorder characterized by distorted and calcified elastic fibers in the skin, eyes, and cardiovascular system; caused by mutations in the *ABCC6* gene, which encodes an ABC-cassette transporter (expressed primarily in the liver) that exports anti-mineralization factors into the circulation.
• Skin changes and asymptomatic ocular findings usually appear during the first two decades of life, with ocular and cardiovascular complications typically developing in the third and fourth decades.
• Thin yellowish papules coalesce to form cobblestoned plaques (resembling 'plucked chicken skin') on the lateral neck and in other flexural sites (e.g. antecubital and popliteal fossae, axillae, groin) (Fig. 80.2); decreased elasticity leads to sagging skin in affected areas (see Fig. 80.2D), and yellow papules on the oral mucosa may be evident (see Fig. 80.2E).
• Early ocular findings include angioid streaks, which reflect breaks in the calcified elastic lamina of Bruch's membrane (also seen in other metabolic/genetic disorders, e.g. sickle cell anemia), and mottling of the retinal pigment epithelium; choroidal neovascularization and hemorrhage can result in progressive loss of vision.
• Calcification of elastic fibers in the walls of medium-sized arteries leads to luminal narrowing and clinical sequelae such as intermittent claudication, renovascular hypertension, angina, myocardial infarction, and stroke; GI hemorrhage may also occur.
• **DDx:** PXE-like cutaneous and extracutaneous findings can be seen in generalized arterial calcification of infancy (*ENPP1* mutations), PXE-like disorder with coagulation factor deficiency (*GGCX* mutations), β-thalassemia, and sickle cell anemia; other conditions featuring PXE-like skin lesions are outlined in Table 80.2.
• **Rx:** an approach to management of PXE is presented in Table 80.3.

MAJOR TYPES OF EHLERS–DANLOS SYNDROME			
EDS Type	Cutaneous Findings	Extracutaneous Manifestations	Inheritance, Mutated Protein
Classic (I/II)*	Hyperextensible and fragile skin, with easy bruising and atrophic scars	Joint hypermobility, absence of inferior labial and lingual frenula, ability to touch nose with tongue (Gorlin's sign)	AD, type V collagen AR, tenascin-X**
Hypermobility (III)	Hyperextensible skin	Joint hypermobility, pain and dislocations; absence of inferior labial and lingual frenula	AD, tenascin-X (F > M)
Vascular (IV)†	Thin, translucent skin with excessive bruising; decreased facial fat	Distal joint hypermobility; arterial, gastrointestinal, and uterine rupture	AD, type III collagen
Kyphoscoliosis (VIA)	Hyperextensible and fragile skin	Joint hypermobility, congenital scoliosis, osteopenia; neonatal hypotonia; ocular fragility	AR, lysyl hydroxylase
Musculocontractural (VIB)	Hyperextensible and fragile skin; wrinkled palms	Joint hypermobility, contractures, scoliosis, craniofacial anomalies; ocular fragility	AR, dermatan-4-sulfotransferase
Arthrochalasia (VIIA/B)	Hyperextensible and fragile skin	Severe joint hypermobility with congenital bilateral hip dislocation	AD, type I collagen
Dermatosparaxis (VIIC)	Sagging, doughy and extremely fragile skin, with easy bruising and tearing	Hernias; PROM; delayed closure of fontanelles, puffy eyelids, micrognathia	AR, procollagen N-peptidase

*Most common form of Ehlers–Danlos syndrome.
**May be associated with congenital adrenal hyperplasia due to a contiguous gene syndrome.
†Loeys–Dietz syndrome type II (see Table 80.5) can have a similar clinical presentation.
AD, autosomal dominant; AR, autosomal recessive; PROM, premature rupture of fetal membranes.

Table 80.1 Major types of Ehlers–Danlos syndrome.

Cutis Laxa

• Heterogeneous group of heritable and acquired disorders (Table 80.4) characterized by loose, sagging skin due to sparse and fragmented elastic fibers.

• Skin involvement is often generalized, giving patients a prematurely aged appearance

(Fig. 80.3), but it may be localized to acral or periorbital sites; cutaneous findings are present at birth in most heritable forms of cutis laxa, developing later in acquired cutis laxa and some autosomal dominant variants.

• Extracutaneous manifestations can include emphysema, hernias (e.g. umbilical, inguinal), diverticula (e.g. GI, genitourinary),

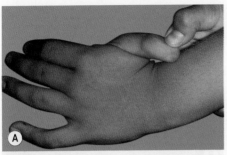
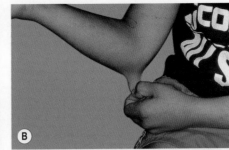
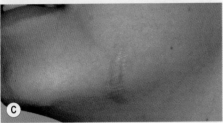
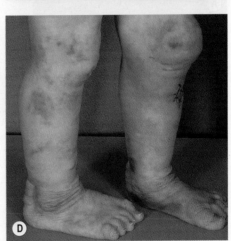
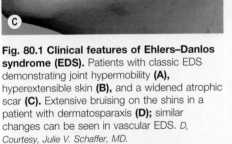

Fig. 80.1 Clinical features of Ehlers–Danlos syndrome (EDS). Patients with classic EDS demonstrating joint hypermobility **(A),** hyperextensible skin **(B),** and a widened atrophic scar **(C).** Extensive bruising on the shins in a patient with dermatosparaxis **(D);** similar changes can be seen in vascular EDS. *D, Courtesy, Julie V. Schaffer, MD.*

DIFFERENTIAL DIAGNOSIS OF PSEUDOXANTHOMA ELASTICUM (PXE)-LIKE SKIN FINDINGS		
Disorder	**Patient Characteristics**	**Clinical Features**
Actinic elastosis	Middle-aged and older adults with lightly pigmented skin and a history of chronic sun exposure	Yellow to gray, thickened, lax, finely to coarsely wrinkled skin; photodistribution on the lateral forehead, neck, dorsal aspect of the forearms
Perforating calcific elastosis*	5th–8th decades; primarily multiparous black women**	Plaque composed of coalescing keratotic papules (most apparent at the periphery); periumbilical area >> breasts
PXE-like papillary dermal elastolysis (PPDE)[†] and white fibrous papulosis of the neck (WFPN)[†]	5th–9th decades; primarily Caucasian women and (for WFPN) Japanese men	Multiple 2- to 3-mm yellow, skin-colored, or (in WFPN) whitish papules; in PPDE, coalesce to form plaques with a cobblestone appearance; neck > upper trunk, axillae, flexor forearms, lower abdomen

*Also referred to as periumbilical perforating PXE.
**Occasionally associated with an increased calcium-phosphate product in chronic kidney disease.
[†]Related conditions within the spectrum of fibroelastolytic papulosis; late-onset focal dermal elastosis has a similar clinical presentation.

Table 80.2 Differential diagnosis of pseudoxanthoma elasticum (PXE)-like skin findings. Additional considerations may include PXE-like skin lesions in patients receiving D-penicillamine, exposed to saltpeter, or with chronic kidney disease, β-thalassemia, or sickle cell anemia.

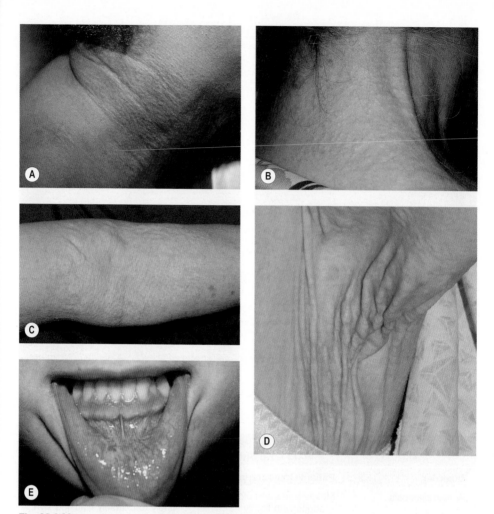

Fig. 80.2 Mucocutaneous findings in pseudoxanthoma elasticum. Yellowish papules and 'cobblestoned' plaques on the neck **(A, B)** and in the antecubital fossa **(C).** Thickened, yellowish, sagging skin in the axilla **(D).** Yellow papules on the inner aspect of the lower lip **(E).** *C, D, Courtesy, Julie V. Schaffer, MD.*

cardiovascular defects, musculoskeletal or craniofacial anomalies, and developmental delay; these findings are most common in autosomal recessive variants and occasionally occur in acquired forms.

- **DDx:** PXE and related conditions, mid-dermal elastolysis (see Chapter 82), aneto-derma (see Chapter 82; smaller, circumscribed lesions), hereditary gelsolin amyloidosis.

- **Rx:** reconstructive surgery for cutaneous disease; multidisciplinary approach for internal involvement.

Other Disorders

- Additional heritable connective tissue disorders with cutaneous manifestations are summarized in Table 80.5.

A MULTIDISCIPLINARY APPROACH TO THE MANAGEMENT OF PSEUDOXANTHOMA ELASTICUM

General

- Antioxidant and magnesium supplementation, moderate calcium intake
- Regular exercise, weight control, avoidance of smoking or excessive alcohol intake

Skin

- Surgical intervention for excessive skin folds

Eyes

- Biannual funduscopic examination, use of Amsler grid to assess for central visual field defects
- Use of sunglasses; avoidance of head trauma or heavy straining
- Laser photocoagulation or photodynamic therapy for choroidal neovascularization if visual symptoms
- Intravitreal injections of VEGF antagonists

Cardiovascular System

- Baseline electrocardiogram and echocardiogram, annual cardiac examination
- Low-dose acetylsalicylic acid (if not contraindicated), correction of hyperlipidemia and hypertension
- Pentoxyfylline, cilostazol or clopidogrel for intermittent claudication

VEGF, vascular endothelial growth factor.

Table 80.3 A multidisciplinary approach to the management of pseudoxanthoma elasticum.

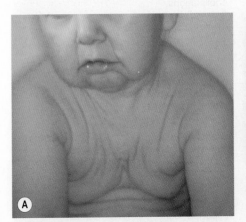 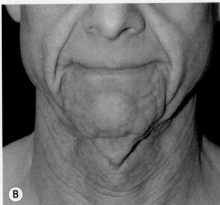

Fig. 80.3 Clinical features in cutis laxa. A Loose skin and drooping jowls in an infant with heritable cutis laxa. **B** Sagging folds of skin giving a prematurely aged appearance to a man with acquired cutis laxa associated with multiple myeloma. *A, Courtesy, Thomas Schwarz, MD. B, Courtesy, Jeffrey P Callen, MD.*

ETIOLOGIES OF CUTIS LAXA

Hereditary Cutis Laxa

Defects in elastic fiber components, e.g. elastin, fibulin-4/5 or latent TGF-β binding protein-4
Defective vesicular trafficking of elastic fiber components
Defective mitochondrial proline biosynthetic enzymes

Acquired Cutis Laxa*

Skin disorders, e.g. Sweet syndrome-like eruptions (Marshall syndrome),* urticaria/angioedema, drug eruptions, cutaneous lymphoma
Monoclonal gammopathies with various underlying plasma cell dyscrasias; cutis laxa may be acral or (especially with heavy chain disease) generalized
Direct effects of drug intake, particularly penicillamine

*Sometimes in the setting of α_1-antitrypsin deficiency.
TGF-β, transforming growth factor-β.

Table 80.4 Etiologies of cutis laxa.

ADDITIONAL HERITABLE CONNECTIVE TISSUE DISORDERS WITH CUTANEOUS FINDINGS			
Disease	Cutaneous Findings	Extracutaneous Manifestations	Inheritance, Mutated Protein
Marfan syndrome	Striae, elastosis perforans serpiginosa, decreased fat in extremities	Tall stature with long limbs, arachnodactyly, scoliosis; lens subluxations (upward), myopia; dilation/dissection of ascending aorta*	AD, fibrillin-1
Loeys–Dietz syndrome types I and II	In type II: translucent skin, easy bruising, atrophic scarring	Marfanoid habitus, joint hypermobility; aortic aneurysms, arterial tortuosity; in type I: craniofacial anomalies	AD, TGF-β receptors 1 and 2
Homocystinuria	Malar flush, livedo reticularis, diffuse pigmentary dilution, tissue paper-like scars	Marfanoid habitus, lens subluxations (downward), thrombosis, mental retardation	AR, cystathionine synthase > other enzymes
Buschke–Ollendorff syndrome	Connective tissue nevi (dermatofibrosis lenticularis disseminata); occasionally cutaneous sclerosis associated with melorheostosis	Osteopoikilosis ('spotted' bones); occasionally melorheostosis (sclerotic bone resembling 'dripping candle wax' on radiographs)	AD, LEM domain-containing 3 (antagonist of TGF-β signaling)

***Rx:** β-blockers and angiotensin II receptor blockers, which antagonize pathogenic TGF-β signaling.
AD, autosomal dominant; AR, autosomal recessive; TGF-β, transforming growth factor-β.

Table 80.5 Additional heritable connective tissue disorders with cutaneous findings.

For further information see Chs. 95 and 97. From *Dermatology, Third Edition.*

Dermal Hypertrophies | 81

Hypertrophic Scar

• Firm, initially pink to purple in color then becomes skin-colored to hypopigmented, occasionally hyperpigmented; papule or plaque limited to an excision site or wound (Figs. 81.1 and 81.2).

• Most commonly seen on the trunk/shoulders.

• Sometimes pruritic.

• With treatment, can reduce pruritus and height but not width of scar.

• Treatment options include silicone gel sheets, intralesional triamcinolone, re-excision (but may recur), laser (to improve color), massage/pressure, postoperative radiotherapy.

Keloid

• More common in patients with darkly pigmented skin who have a familial predisposition.

• Rarely associated with syndromes (e.g. Rubinstein–Taybi or Goeminne syndromes).

• Raised, often skin-colored firm plaque(s) that, in contrast to hypertrophic scars, extend beyond the wound margin (Fig. 81.3; Table 81.1); color may vary as in hypertrophic scars.

• Follow trauma from surgical procedures (including ear piercing) and inflammatory disorders, especially acne (see Fig. 81.2), but can occur spontaneously (Fig. 81.4).

• Poor response to treatment.

• Treatment options include silicone gel sheets; intralesional injections of triamcinolone, interferon-α-2b, or 5-fluorouracil; pressure; laser (to improve color); excision followed by other modalities such as low-dose radiation or topical imiquimod.

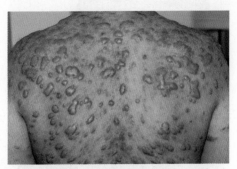

Fig. 81.2 Multiple hypertrophic scars due to acne vulgaris. The posterior trunk is a common location for hypertrophic scars. *Courtesy, Julie V. Schaffer, MD.*

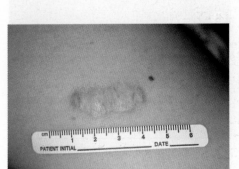

Fig. 81.1 Hypertrophic scar at the site of an excision of an atypical melanocytic nevus. The deltoid region is a common location for hypertrophic scars. *Courtesy, Jean L. Bologna, MD.*

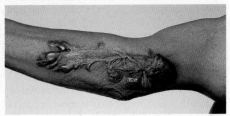

Fig. 81.3 Keloid of the flexor arm in an African-American man. Note the extension of the keloid into the normal surrounding skin in a claw-like manner and the central involution. *Courtesy, Claude Burton, MD.*

KEY FEATURES OF NORMAL, HYPERTROPHIC, AND KELOID SCARS			
	Normal Scar	**Hypertrophic Scar**	**Keloid Scar**
Preceded by injury	Yes	Yes	Not always
Onset	Immediate	Immediate	Delayed (sometimes months)
Erythema	Temporary	Prominent	Varies
Profile	Flat	Raised	Raised
Symptomatic	No	Yes	Yes
Confined to wound margin	Yes	Yes	No
Increased mast cells	No	Yes	Yes
Contains myofibroblasts within nodules	N/A	Yes	No
Spontaneous resolution	N/A	Sometimes, gradual	Rare
Treatment response	N/A	Good	Poor

N/A, not applicable.

Table 81.1 Key features of normal, hypertrophic, and keloid scars.

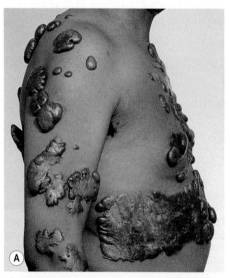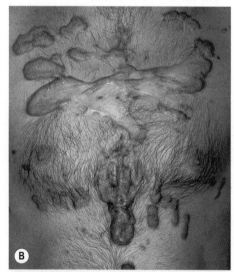

Fig. 81.4 Spontaneous generalized keloids. Extensive spontaneous keloids in a patient with darkly pigmented skin **(A)** and a patient with lightly pigmented skin **(B)**. *A, Courtesy, Claude Burton, MD.*

Dupuytren's Contracture

• Fibromatosis of the fascia of the ventral aspect of the digit and the palm.
• Starts as a linear thickening proximal to the fourth > fifth finger that is most apparent with extension of the digits.
• May gradually progress to flexion contractures (Fig. 81.5).
• Associated with other fibromatoses (e.g. plantar, penile), alcoholism, and diabetes mellitus.
• Surgical correction usually helpful; injection of collagenase also sometimes effective.

Cutis Verticis Gyrata

• Hypertrophy and linear folding of the scalp only (Fig. 81.6).
• Idiopathic in most cases.
• Primary form may be associated with systemic findings (neurologic, ophthalmologic).
• Secondary form associated with acromegaly, myxedema, and Turner syndrome.

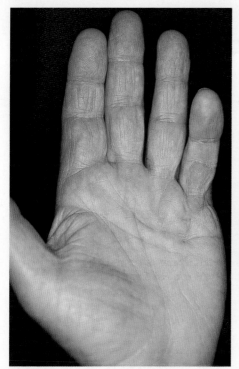

Fig. 81.5 Dupuytren's contracture. There is greater involvement of the fifth finger than the fourth finger. Fibrotic cords can be felt and are accentuated by extension of the digits. Eventually, flexion contractures develop. *Courtesy, Jean L. Bolognia, MD.*

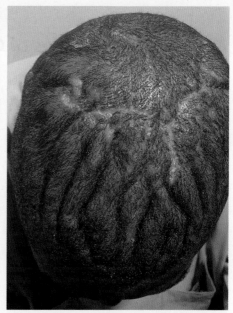

Fig. 81.6 Cutis verticis gyrata. Cerebriform folding of the skin of the scalp. Erythema in the posterior grooves is related to a previous superinfection.

• Differential diagnosis includes several disorders, including pachydermoperiostitis (involves the face and acral sites as well as the scalp), dissecting cellulitis (scalp is boggy and painful), and plexiform neurofibroma.

Hyaline Fibromatosis Syndrome (Juvenile Hyaline Fibromatosis and Infantile Systemic Hyalinosis)

• Autosomal recessive spectrum of disorders due to *ANTXR2* mutations.
• Presents during infancy or early childhood with papulonodules on the ears, hands, and periorificial areas (Fig. 81.7), in addition to gingival hypertrophy and flexion contractures.
• Severe form (infantile systemic hyalinosis) has internal organ involvement.

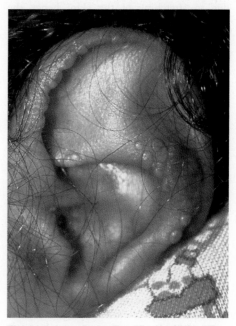

Fig. 81.7 Juvenile hyaline fibromatosis. Firm pearly papules favor the ears.

For further information see Ch. 98. From *Dermatology, Third Edition.*

82 | Atrophies of Connective Tissue

This chapter focuses primarily on entities in which there is a reduction in collagen and/or elastic tissue within the dermis. They vary from very common skin disorders such as striae to cutaneous manifestations of rare genetic syndromes. Loss of subcutaneous fat, i.e. lipoatrophy, is covered in Chapter 84, while acrodermatitis chronica atrophicans is covered in Chapter 61 and Ehlers–Danlos syndrome and cutis laxa are covered in Chapter 80.

Striae (Distensae)

• Linear atrophic lesions that reflect dermal damage ('breaks') at sites of mechanical stress due to stretching of the skin, hence the popular term 'stretch marks'; most commonly observed in adolescents undergoing growth spurts or weight gain and on the abdomen in up to 75% of pregnant women.

• Striae are multiple, symmetric, and arranged along the lines of cleavage, with the typical sites of involvement and characteristic patterns shown in Fig. 82.1; early lesions may be red-purple in color (striae rubra) but with time, most striae become skin-colored to white with fine wrinkling (striae alba) (Fig. 82.2).

• Additional causes include hypercortisolism (e.g. Cushing's syndrome), application of potent topical CS (especially in areas of occlusion such as major body folds), and heredity; in weightlifters, mechanical stress and muscle enlargement can lead to striae.

• **DDx:** linear focal elastosis, in particular when lesions are present on the lower mid-back.

• **Rx:** difficult and striae often become less noticeable over a period of years; possible modest improvement with topical tretinoin 0.1% cream; lasers (e.g. pulsed dye for striae rubra, 308 nm excimer for striae alba) reportedly lead to improvement.

Pizogenic Pedal Papules (Piezogenic Papules)

• Herniations of fat in the heel region where there is reduced dermal connective tissue; the skin-colored papules appear with the pressure of weight-bearing and disappear when the leg is raised (Fig. 82.3A); occasionally occur on the wrist.

• In an infantile variant, larger nodules occur on the medial aspect of the heel and their appearance does not require weight-bearing (Fig. 82.3B).

Anetoderma

• Well-circumscribed, skin-colored, flaccid lesions that result from a marked focal decrease in elastic tissue within the dermis (Fig. 82.4).

• Often arises *de novo* (primary form), with lesions usually measuring 1–2 cm in diameter; there are also secondary forms of anetoderma that can follow inflammation or infection of the skin (e.g. acute cutaneous lupus, varicella, lepromatous leprosy) or are seen in association with cutaneous tumors (e.g. involuted infantile hemangiomas) or the antiphospholipid antibody syndrome.

• Anetoderma of prematurity presents as atrophic lesions resulting from minor iatrogenic trauma to immature skin in the setting of neonatal intensive care.

• Although the individual lesions of the primary form are often elevated, they can be even with the skin surface or depressed (Fig. 82.4C); however, all lesions are soft to palpation and the focal reduction in elastic tissue results in a feel similar to

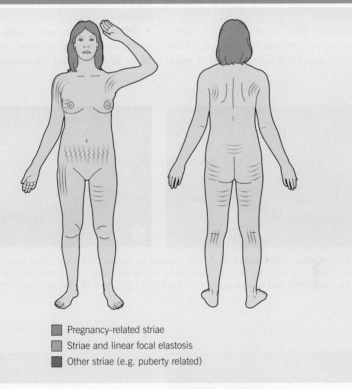

Pregnancy-related striae
Striae and linear focal elastosis
Other striae (e.g. puberty related)

Fig. 82.1 Common anatomic sites of striae and linear focal elastosis.

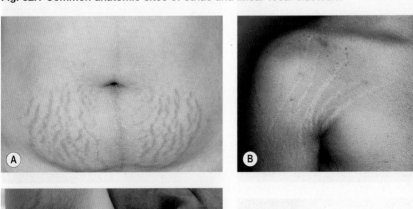

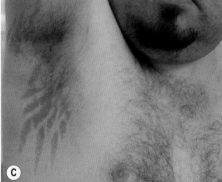

Fig. 82.2 Striae. A Linear erythematous lesions on the abdomen (striae rubra). **B** Multiple linear atrophic streaks of striae alba in a teenager. **C** Large axillary striae in a patient receiving chronic, high-dose systemic corticosteroids.
B, Courtesy, Kalman Watsky, MD.

that of an abdominal hernia (referred to as a 'buttonhole' sign which is also seen in neurofibromas).

• The primary form favors the neck, upper trunk, and upper extremities of young adults, with lesions appearing over a period of years, while the distribution pattern of the secondary form reflects that of the preceding inflammatory disorder.

• **DDx:** post-traumatic scars, papular elastorrhexis (similar clinical appearance but firm to palpation), anetoderma-like scars

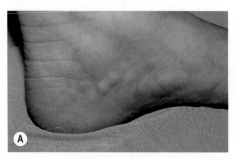 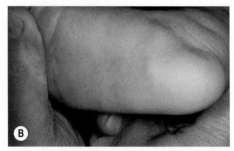

Fig. 82.3 Pizogenic pedal papules. A Skin-colored to yellowish outpouchings on the heel represent herniation of subcutaneous fat through the plantar fascia and they are sometimes painful. **B** Soft nodules on the medial and plantar surface of the foot in an infant. *B, Courtesy, Julie V. Schaffer, MD.*

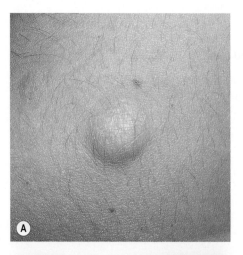 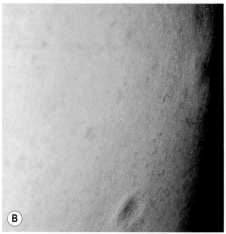

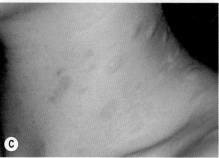

Fig. 82.4 Anetoderma – primary and secondary. Lesions can range from soft, skin-colored papules that herniate upon palpation **(A)** to flaccid papules that have a central depression **(B).** The upper trunk and neck is a common location for primary anetoderma; an admixture of elevated, macular and depressed lesions is seen **(C).** *A, Courtesy, Ronald Rapini, MD; B, Courtesy, Catherine Maari, MD, and Julie Powell, MD; C, Courtesy, Thomas Schwarz, MD. Continued*

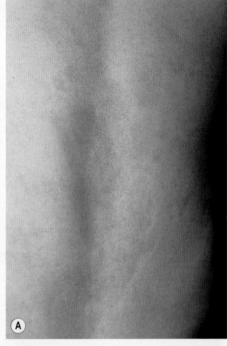

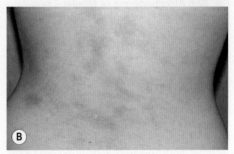

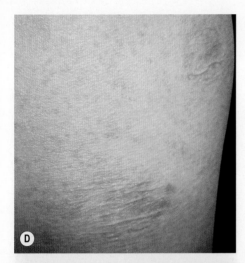

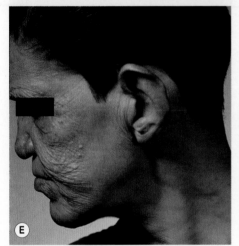

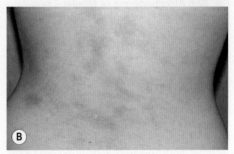

Fig. 82.4 *Continued* Wrinkling of the skin from secondary anetoderma due to sarcoidosis **(D)** and lepromatous leprosy **(E).** *D, Courtesy, Catherine Maari, MD, and Julie Powell, MD; E, Courtesy, Louis A. Fragola, Jr., MD.*

Fig. 82.5 Atrophoderma of Pasini and Pierini. A, B Multiple light brown patches on the back; note the subtle depression of the lesions with a 'cliff-drop' edge. In **(B)**, dermal blood vessels are seen within a few patches; the white papule is a healed biopsy site. *A, Courtesy, Catherine C. McCuaig, MD; B, Courtesy, Julie V. Schaffer, MD.*

(perifollicular elastolysis) due to acne vulgaris, pseudoxanthoma elasticum-like papillary dermal elastolysis (flexural areas).

• **Rx:** difficult; for secondary form, treatment of underlying disease may prevent new lesions; surgical excision can lead to scars.

Atrophoderma of Pasini and Pierini

• Minimally depressed hyperpigmented patches, primarily of the posterior trunk (Fig. 82.5); the characteristic 'cliff-drop' sign at the peripheral edge may be subtle; significant overlap with 'burnt-out' plaque-type morphea, and notably a minority of patients have both disorders.

• Onset typically during adolescence or young adulthood; the patches are often oval in shape, 2–8 cm in diameter, number from one to several, and persist for decades; rarely, lesions are present at birth or arise along the

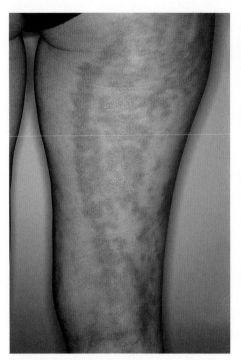

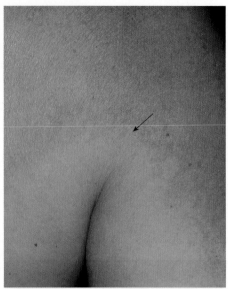

Fig. 82.7 Mid-dermal elastolysis. Large patch with fine wrinkling and a slightly reticulated border on the upper back and shoulder. The junction of involved and uninvolved skin is marked with an arrow. *Courtesy, Judit Stenn, MD.*

Fig. 82.6 Atrophoderma of Moulin. Linear hyperpigmented streaks along the lines of Blaschko. Note the subtle depression of the lesions on the upper lateral thigh. *Courtesy, Jean L. Bolognia, MD.*

lines of Blaschko (atrophoderma of Moulin; Fig. 82.6).

• Because the reduction in the thickness of the dermis is subtle, an elliptical biopsy that includes both involved and uninvolved skin and is sectioned longitudinally is usually required for diagnosis.

• **DDx:** morphea, but in contrast to atrophoderma, induration and/or an inflammatory rim is observed; post-inflammatory hyperpigmentation; if a limited number of lesions, dermatofibrosarcoma protuberans (primarily in children).

• **Rx:** difficult; modest improvement in hyperpigmentation reported with pigment-specific laser therapy.

Mid-Dermal Elastolysis

• Idiopathic disorder characterized by large, skin-colored patches with fine wrinkling and occasionally follicular papules with central delling; the lesions are often clinically subtle

(Fig. 82.7) and histologically, there is a selective loss of elastic tissue in the mid dermis best demonstrated by special elastic stains.

• Most commonly affects the trunk, neck, and arms of middle-aged Caucasian women.

• **DDx:** the major entity is generalized acquired cutis laxa.

• **Rx:** none currently available.

Follicular Atrophoderma

• Small depressions at the sites of hair follicles.

• Clinical presentations include.

  – As atrophoderma vermiculatum of the cheeks (Fig. 82.8), which can be sporadic, inherited in an autosomal dominant manner, or be a component of the keratosis pilaris atrophicans spectrum in which there is also follicular hyperkeratosis (Table 82.1; Fig. 82.9).

  – As patulous follicles on the dorsal aspect of the hands and feet in the X-linked dominant Bazex–Dupré–Christol syndrome in which patients also develop BCCs and alopecia.

THE SPECTRUM OF KERATOSIS PILARIS ATROPHICANS						
Disorder	Mode of Inheritance	Age of Onset	Distribution	Cutaneous Features	KP*	Other Findings and Associations
Keratosis pilaris atrophicans faciei (ulerythema ophryogenes)	AD	Infancy	Eyebrows, particularly the lateral third (Fig. 82.9) > temples, cheeks, forehead	• Erythematous follicular papules with central keratotic plugs, eventuating in follicular atrophy • Scarring alopecia of the lateral eyebrows distinguishes it from KP rubra	+	Associated with Noonan syndrome
Atrophoderma vermiculata	See text and Fig. 82.8				–	
Keratosis follicularis spinulosa decalvans	XR (*MBTPS2* mutations)	Childhood	Face, scalp, limbs, trunk	• Erythematous follicular papules with central keratotic plugs, eventuating in follicular atrophy • Scarring alopecia of the scalp, eyebrows, and eyelashes	++	• Palmoplantar keratoderma, facial erythema • Keratitis, photophobia

*Associated keratosis pilaris (KP) on the extremities and trunk, which does not typically eventuate in atrophy.
AD, autosomal dominant; MBTPS2, membrane-bound transcription factor peptidase, site 2 (involved in sterol regulation); XR, X-linked recessive; +, mild to moderate; ++, severe.

Table 82.1 The spectrum of keratosis pilaris atrophicans.

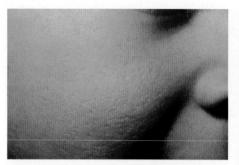

Fig. 82.8 Atrophoderma vermiculatum.
Multiple small pitted scars on the cheek of a young girl. Note the honeycomb pattern on the lower inner cheek; the skin is said to appear 'worm-eaten.' The atrophic lesions may be preceded by inflammatory papules. *Courtesy, Robert Hartmann, MD.*

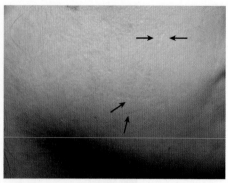

Fig. 82.10 Atrophia macularis varicelliformis cutis. Multiple linear scar-like depressions (between and above arrows) with no history of trauma. *Courtesy, Jean L. Bolognia, MD.*

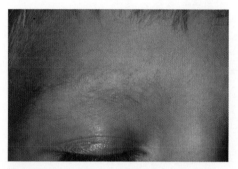

Fig. 82.9 Ulerythema ophryogenes. Alopecia of the eyebrows admixed with tiny follicular papules with a thin erythematous rim. *Courtesy, Jean L. Bolognia, MD.*

– As follicular pits within streaks along the lines of Blaschko in the X-linked dominant disorder Conradi–Hünermann–Happle syndrome (form of chondrodysplasia punctata).

Atrophia Macularis Varicelliformis Cutis (AMVC)

• Acquired thin linear depressions on the face that measure 2–10 mm in length and can be admixed with small circular depressions; there is no history of preceding inflammation, acne, or trauma (Fig. 82.10).

For further information see Ch. 99. From *Dermatology, Third Edition*.

Panniculitis | 83

Introduction

• Adipose tissue plays many active roles in the body beyond insulation, e.g. storing and releasing lipids, mediating inflammation, and modulating endocrinologic and reproductive systems.

• Panniculitis = inflammation of adipose tissue.

• Clinically and histopathologically, the adipose tissue has a limited repertoire of responses to insults and inflammation.

• Most often clinically presents as tender, inflamed, subcutaneous nodules or plaques; with the exception of erythema nodosum, ulceration with drainage may develop.

• There are various etiologies, and a clinical classification system is presented in Table 83.1.

CLINICAL CLASSIFICATION OF THE PANNICULITIDES
Reactive Panniculitis
• Erythema nodosum (EN) • Subacute nodular migratory panniculitis • Erythema induratum (EI)
Predominantly Childhood Panniculitis (see Table 83.3)
Metabolic Panniculitis
• α_1-Antitrypsin deficiency panniculitis • Pancreatic panniculitis
Connective Tissue Disease Panniculitis
• Lupus erythematosus panniculitis • Dermatomyositis-associated panniculitis • Morphea/systemic sclerosis (see Chapters 35 and 36)
Physical/Traumatic Panniculitis
• Cold panniculitis • Facticial panniculitis • Blunt trauma panniculitis • Injection-related panniculitis • Sclerosing lipogranuloma
Infection-Induced Panniculitis (see Table 83.2)
Panniculitis-like T-Cell Lymphomas (see Table 83.4 and Chapter 98)
Other
• Lipodermatosclerosis (LDS) • Idiopathic neutrophilic lobular panniculitis (overlapping with subcutaneous Sweet's syndrome) • Cytophagic hemophagocytic panniculitis (CHP)*

*The majority represent an underlying subcutaneous lymphoma.

Table 83.1 Clinical classification of the panniculitides.

- Diagnosis is challenging and involves consideration of (1) patient characteristics such as age, immune status, underlying diseases; (2) location of the lesions (Fig. 83.1); (3) the presence or absence of ulceration and/or drainage; and (4) histopathological findings.
- A biopsy is usually necessary to establish the diagnosis, and it is critical that the specimen include a generous portion of the subcutaneous (SC) fat.
- Excisional biopsies or narrow incisional biopsies that incorporate a broad expanse of SC fat are preferable to punch biopsies.

- Once the diagnosis of panniculitis is made, further evaluation for underlying etiology or associated conditions is necessary (Tables 83.2–83.4).
- **DDx:** Primarily differentiating among the various forms of panniculitis, superficial thrombophlebitis.
- **Rx:** involves specific treatment of the panniculitis and often treatment of an underlying disorder (see Tables 83.2–83.4).

MOST COMMON LOCATIONS FOR SEVERAL FORMS OF PANNICULITIS

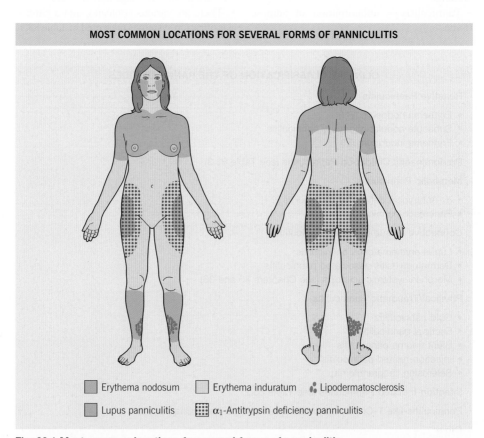

Erythema nodosum   Erythema induratum   Lipodermatosclerosis

Lupus panniculitis α_1-Antitrypsin deficiency panniculitis

Fig. 83.1 Most common locations for several forms of panniculitis.

83

THE MORE COMMON PANNICULITIDES

Panniculitis	Classic Clinical and Histopathologic Features	Systemic Findings and Further Evaluation	Treatment
Most Common			
Erythema nodosum (EN)	• Females > males; 2nd–4th decade • Acute eruption of inflamed, tender SC nodules, favoring the pretibial area bilaterally (Fig. 83.2), but may occur elsewhere • No ulceration or drainage • May last days to weeks • Late lesions can have a bruise-like appearance • Histopathology: prototypical septal panniculitis	• ± fevers, arthralgias, malaise • Other findings may be related to underlying etiology (see Table 83.5)	• Address and treat underlying etiology • See Table 83.6
Lipodermatosclerosis (LDS)	• Typically middle-aged to older individuals with chronic venous disorders (CVD) **ACUTE** • Painful, warm, red-purple, poorly defined plaques with variable induration (Fig. 83.3A) • Favors the lower extremities, usually initially involves the skin above the medial malleolus • Sometimes involves lower abdominal pannus **CHRONIC** • Induration and hyperpigmentation of the lower legs (Fig. 83.3B), with an 'inverted champagne bottle' appearance **ACUTE on CHRONIC** • Occasionally acute onset of pain in the region of chronic LDS • Histopathology: lipomembranous change	• Strong association with obesity, venous insufficiency, systemic hypertension • Consider Doppler studies to evaluate venous system and to look for valvular or vein incompetence • Consider ABI before instituting compression therapy	**ACUTE** • Compression therapy (consider the Velcro strip variant) • If too painful for compression therapy alone, add fibrinolytic agent (e.g., anabolic steroids such as oxandrolone 10 mg BID) plus pentoxifylline (400–800 TID) **CHRONIC** • Compression stockings (≥20–30 mmHg) • Consider endovenous laser or radiofrequency ablation of incompetent veins
Less Common			
Erythema induratum (Nodular vasculitis)	• Females >> males; young to middle-aged • Tender, inflamed nodules or plaques on posterior lower legs (Fig. 83.4) • Ulceration and drainage can occur • Heal with scarring; recurrent • Histopathology: neutrophilic vasculitis	• Other findings may be related to underlying etiology (see Table 83.5)	• Address and treat underlying etiology • See Table 83.6

Table 83.2 The more common panniculitides. *Continued*

Table 83.2 *Continued* **The more common panniculitides.**

Panniculitis	Classic Clinical and Histopathologic Features	Systemic Findings and Further Evaluation	Treatment
α_1-Antitrypsin deficiency panniculitis	• Autosomal co-dominant inheritance • Panniculitis may be initial presentation of disease or develop well into its course • Painful red or purpuric SC nodules or plaques favoring the lower trunk or proximal extremities (Fig. 83.5) • May spontaneously ulcerate and drain an oily material • Histopathology: liquefactive necrosis of dermis and SC septa	• COPD • Chronic liver disease • Autosomal recessive inheritance • Dx made by demonstrating low plasma concentrations of α_1-antitrypsin (AAT) and either observation of a deficient variant of the protein AAT by protease inhibitor typing (PI ZZ variant most common) or by molecular genetic testing for *SERPINA1* gene mutations	• **MILD disease** – Doxycycline, dapsone • **SEVERE disease** – Intravenous α_1-antitrypsin replacement • **REFRACTORY disease** – Plasma exchange, liver transplant
Lupus erythematosus panniculitis	• Uncommon form of chronic cutaneous LE • Associated with SLE in at least 10% of cases • Associated with discoid LE (DLE) in at least one-third of cases, but may be an isolated finding • Painful SC nodules or plaques in a characteristic pattern – on face, shoulders, upper arms, breasts, hips, and buttocks (Fig. 83.6), notably sparing lower extremities • Chronic remitting course; can be elicited by trauma • Overlying skin may be normal, depressed, bound down, or have changes of DLE ('lupus profundus') • Histopathology: hyaline necrosis and lymphoplasmacytic infiltrate	• May have other findings of SLE (see Chapter 33) • If associated with SLE often portends a good prognosis • ANA often (+) but in low titers • Hematologic abnormalities may be the only other abnormality	• Intralesional CS • Systemic medications most effective • **First-line** – Antimalarials • **Second-line** – Methotrexate, mycophenolate mofetil, azathioprine, thalidomide
Infection-induced panniculitis • Bacterial • Mycobacterial • Fungal • Viral • Parasitic	• Most often seen in immunocompromised patients, but not exclusively • Three typical clinical scenarios: – Direct inoculation of infectious organisms into the SC fat (may see sporotrichoid pattern) – Hematogenous spread to SC fat, as in septicemia (disseminated lesions) – Extension to the SC fat from underlying infection • Typically presents with ≥1 fluctuant nodules that ulcerate and drain • Favors lower extremities • Histopathology: necrosis and neutrophils; special stains can highlight organisms, but tissue culture ± PCR also recommended	• May be profoundly ill (e.g. septicemia) or appear well (e.g. normal host with isolated lesion) • Dx requires a high index of suspicion, *pre*-biopsy, so that a sterile, deep biopsy specimen can be sent to microbiology for tissue culture ± PCR, in addition to pathology	• Empirical, broad-spectrum coverage in severely ill host • Otherwise tailored to identified organism

SC, subcutaneous; ABI, ankle brachial index; COPD, chronic obstructive pulmonary disease; ANA, antinuclear antibody; BID, twice daily; TID, three times a day.

PREDOMINANTLY CHILDHOOD PANNICULITIDES

Panniculitis	Classic features*	Systemic Findings and Further Evaluation	Treatment
Subcutaneous fat necrosis of the newborn[†]	• Seen in full-term, usually healthy neonates • Onset during the first 2–3 weeks of life • Mobile, firm SC nodules or plaques, favoring the cheeks, shoulders, back, buttocks, and thighs (Fig. 83.7)	• Thrombocytopenia, hypertriglyceridemia, hypercalcemia (can occur months later) • May be precipitated by hypothermia, hypoglycemia, birth trauma	• Spontaneous resolution common • Favorable prognosis • Supportive care
Post-steroid panniculitis[†]	• Onset usually within 10 days after the rapid withdrawal of systemic CS • Firm red plaques on the cheeks, arms, trunk	• May be related to the condition that required the systemic CS	• May resolve spontaneously • Consider readministration and slower tapering of systemic CS
Cold panniculitis	• Favors the cheeks of infants and children due to popsicles or ice cubes and the medial thighs of equestrians due to riding in cold temperatures plus tight-fitting clothing (Fig. 83.8)	• Possibly other signs of hypothermia	• Remove cold exposure and re-warm
Sclerema neonatorum[†]	• Seen in premature, extremely ill neonates • Onset during the first week of life • Diffusely cold, rigid, board-like skin	• Death common due to septicemia • May be precipitated by hypothermia, dehydration, perinatal asphyxia	• No good treatment • Supportive care

*All entities, except for cold panniculitis, will demonstrate needle-shaped clefts on histopathology.
[†]Seen exclusively in infants or children.
SC, subcutaneous.

Table 83.3 Predominantly childhood panniculitides.

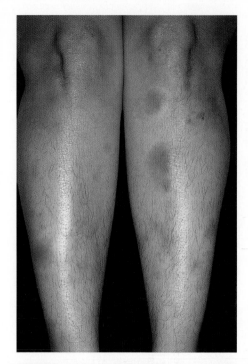

Fig. 83.2 Erythema nodosum. Erythematous, tender nodules located bilaterally on the shins. *Courtesy, Kenneth E. Greer, MD.*

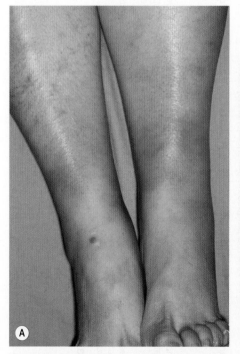

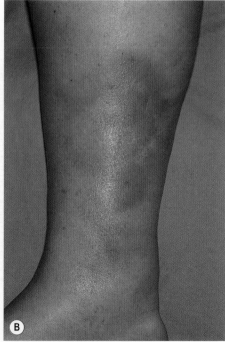

Fig. 83.3 Lipodermatosclerosis. A Acute phase with tender erythematous plaques on both lower extremities. This condition is often misdiagnosed as 'bilateral recurrent cellulitis.' **B** Chronic phase with sclerotic red-brown plaque on the lower medial leg. *A, Courtesy, James Patterson, MD; B, Courtesy, Kenneth E. Greer, MD.*

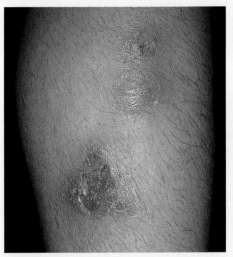

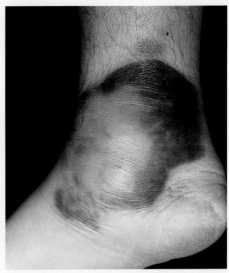

Fig. 83.4 Erythema induratum. Nodular lesions on the lower leg, with evidence of ulceration. *Courtesy, Kenneth E. Greer, MD.*

Fig. 83.5 α₁-Antitrypsin deficiency panniculitis. Purpuric nodules on the ankles. *Courtesy, Kenneth E. Greer, MD.*

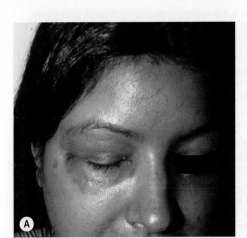

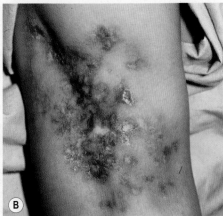

Fig. 83.6 Lupus panniculitis. A Erythematous plaque involving the orbital area. **B** Red-brown plaques on the upper outer arm. Note the significant subcutaneous atrophy and overlying lesions of discoid lupus erythematosus. *A, Courtesy, James Patterson, MD; B, Courtesy, Kenneth E. Greer, MD.*

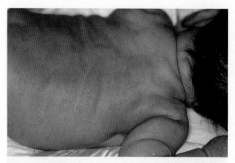

Fig. 83.7 Subcutaneous fat necrosis of the newborn. Indurated plaques on the trunk.

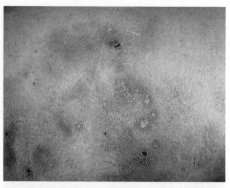

Fig. 83.8 Cold panniculitis. Erythematous to violaceous plaques on the thighs of a young woman with equestrian cold panniculitis. *Courtesy, Kenneth E. Greer, MD.*

THE LESS COMMON PANNICULITIDES	
Panniculitis	**Classic Features**
Subacute nodular migratory panniculitis (chronic EN)	• Resembles EN but is typically chronic, unilateral, and tends to migrate and/or form annular lesions • May be associated with streptococcal infections or thyroid disease
Pancreatic panniculitis	• May be the initial presentation of pancreatic disease (pancreatitis > cancer) or develop during its course • Favors lower legs (Fig. 83.9), but also arms, chest, abdomen • May become fluctuant, ulcerate, and drain an oily substance • Eosinophilia and polyarthritis are associated findings
Dermatomyositis-associated panniculitis	• More common in juvenile dermatomyositis • Tender SC nodules or plaques on thighs, arms, buttocks, and abdomen; calcify with time
Panniculitis-like T-cell lymphomas (see Chapter 98)	• Dx is often suggested after a biopsy is performed in a patient whose lesions fail to improve or worsen, e.g. in a patient with a clinical Dx of EN • Two major types, requiring histopathologic differentiation: subcutaneous panniculitis-like T-cell lymphoma ($\alpha\beta$ type) and $\gamma\delta$ T-cell lymphoma • Evaluation for systemic involvement is necessary • DDx includes lupus panniculitis
Cytophagic histiocytic panniculitis (CHP)	• Dx is usually made after histopathologic examination of SC nodules or plaques (Fig. 83.10) when the finding of hematophagocytosis is identified • The majority of patients have subcutaneous involvement with an aggressive lymphoma, e.g. $\gamma\delta$ T-cell lymphoma; may have a fatal course due to a hemophagocytic syndrome

EN, erythema nodosum; SC, subcutaneous.

Table 83.4 The less common panniculitides.

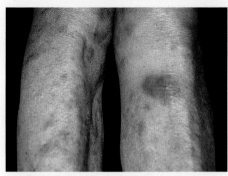

Fig. 83.9 Pancreatic panniculitis. Multiple nodules on the legs. *Courtesy, Kenneth E. Greer, MD.*

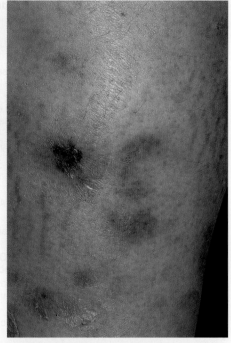

Fig. 83.10 Cytophagic histiocytic panniculitis. Subcutaneous nodules with purpura. The majority of these patients have an underlying subcutaneous lymphoma. *Courtesy, Kenneth E. Greer, MD.*

CAUSES OF ERYTHEMA NODOSUM AND ERYTHEMA INDURATUM AND SUGGESTED EVALUATIONS		
	Erythema Nodosum	**Erythema Induratum**

Most Common Causes	• Idiopathic
	• Streptococcal infections, especially of the upper respiratory tract
	• Other infectious associations:
	  – Bacterial gastroenteritis – *Yersinia* > *Salmonella*, *Campylobacter*
	  – Viral upper respiratory tract infections
	  – Coccidioidomycosis
	• Sarcoidosis*
	• Inflammatory bowel disease
	• Drugs:
	  – Estrogens/oral contraceptives
	  – Sulfonamides
	  – Penicillins
		• Tuberculosis
		• Idiopathic

Table 83.5 Causes of erythema nodosum and erythema induratum and suggested evaluations. *Continued*

Table 83.5 *Continued* **Causes of erythema nodosum and erythema induratum and suggested evaluations.**

	Erythema Nodosum	Erythema Induratum
Uncommon Causes	• Less common infectious associations (e.g. brucellosis, tuberculosis, hepatitis B†) • Neutrophilic dermatoses (e.g. Sweet's syndrome, Behçet's disease) • Pregnancy • Malignancy (e.g. acute myelogenous leukemia)	• Less common infectious associations (e.g. *Nocardia*, *Pseudomonas*, viral hepatitis) • Non-infectious associations (e.g. superficial thrombophlebitis, hypothyroidism, RA, Crohn's disease) • Drugs (e.g. propylthiouracil)
Suggested Workup**	• Chest x-ray • Tuberculin skin test or IGRA • Viral hepatitis panel • Anti-streptolysin O and/or anti-DNase B titers • If diarrhea check fecal WBC and stool culture for bacteria, ova and parasites • Consider GI referral if bloody diarrhea, fecal WBC, and negative cultures • β-HCG in women • Malignancy workup as indicated by history and physical exam	• Chest x-ray • Tuberculin skin test or IGRA • Consider PCR of skin biopsy for *M. tuberculosis* • Viral hepatitis panel • TSH • CBC, ESR • Rheumatoid factor • Consider GI referral if diarrhea

*Lofgren's syndrome is an acute, spontaneously resolving form of sarcoidosis characterized by erythema nodosum, fever, hilar lymphadenopathy, polyarthritis, and uveitis.
†Erythema nodosum secondary to hepatitis B vaccine has also been reported.
**Basic workup in patients with erythema nodosum and erythema induratum with no obvious etiology.
WBC, white blood cell count; GI, gastrointestinal; RA, rheumatoid arthritis; TSH, thyroid-stimulating hormone; CBC, complete blood count; ESR, erythrocyte sedimentation rate; IGRA, interferon-γ release assay.*

TREATMENT RECOMMENDATIONS FOR ERYTHEMA NODOSUM AND ERYTHEMA INDURATUM		
Treatment	**Erythema Nodosum**	**Erythema Induratum**
In all patients	• Discontinue possible causative medications • Diagnose and treat underlying cause/infection • Bed rest and leg elevation • Compression	
First-line	• Nonsteroidal anti-inflammatory medications • Salicylates • Potassium iodide	
Second-line$	• Colchicine* • Infliximab** • Hydroxychloroquine***	• Systemic CS • Mycophenolate mofetil
Third-line$	• Systemic CS • Thalidomide** • Cyclosporine*	

*Helpful for erythema nodosum occurring in the setting of Behçet's disease.
**Helpful for erythema nodosum occurring in the setting of inflammatory bowel disease.
***Helpful for chronic erythema nodosum.
$Immunosuppressives to be used only if underlying infection has been excluded and/or treated.*

Table 83.6 Treatment recommendations for erythema nodosum and erythema induratum.

For further information see Ch. 100. From *Dermatology, Third Edition.*

Lipodystrophies

84

Key Points

- Lipodystrophy is characterized by areas of fat loss/absence (lipoatrophy), and/or fat accumulation (lipohypertrophy), with both often coexisting in the same patient; lipoatrophy can lead to the appearance of muscular hypertrophy (Fig. 84.1).

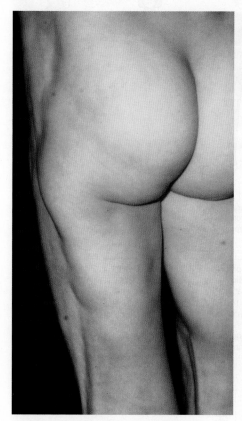

Fig. 84.1 Lipoatrophy of the lower extremities, leading to the appearance of muscular hypertrophy. *Courtesy, William D. James, MD.*

- Lipoatrophy may be classified as.
  - Generalized, partial, or localized (Fig. 84.2).
  - Inherited (often appears during childhood) or acquired.
  - Stable or progressive.
- Localized lipo*atrophy* may be idiopathic or secondary to various causes, e.g. injection of medications (in particular CS), pressure (Fig. 84.3), trauma, autoimmune connective tissue disease (e.g. lupus panniculitis; Fig. 84.4), and other panniculitides due to inflammation or lymphoma.
- Localized lipo*hypertrophy* is most commonly seen in the setting of multiple insulin injections.
- Human immunodeficiency virus/ antiretroviral therapy (HIV/ART) causes a distinct syndrome of central lipohypertrophy and peripheral lipoatrophy (Figs. 84.5 and 84.6).
- Extensive lipodystrophy syndromes have characteristic distributions of fat atrophy and hypertrophy (Figs. 84.2 and 84.7–84.9).
- Fat is a metabolically active tissue with important endocrine functions; therefore, nonlocalized lipodystrophy is often seen in conjunction with the metabolic syndrome (insulin resistance, diabetes mellitus, hyperinsulinemia, hypertriglyceridemia, cardiovascular disease, and fatty liver).
- Other associations include hormonal abnormalities, anabolic syndrome, glomerulonephritis.
- **Rx:** depends in part on underlying etiology (see Fig. 84.2); (1) remove inciting cause (e.g. relieve pressure or rotate sites of injections); (2) address the metabolic syndrome if present; (3) improve cosmetic appearance (e.g. injection of poly-L-lactic acid or autologous fat transfer into the cheeks).

SECTION 16: Disorders of Subcutaneous Fat

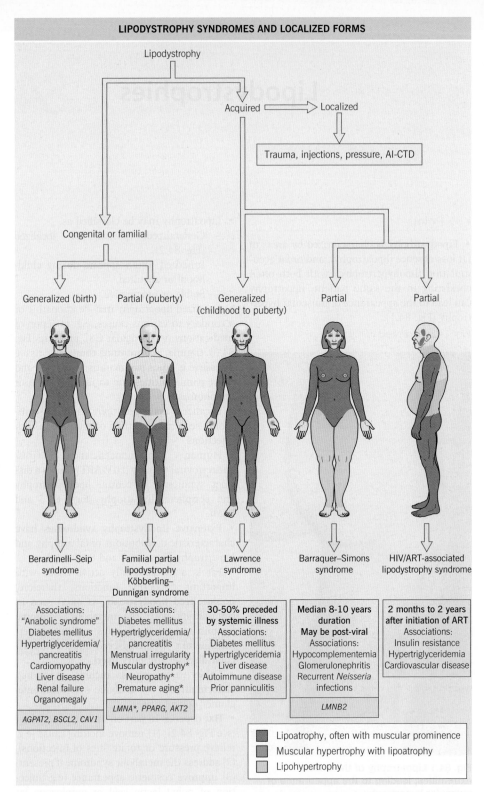

LIPODYSTROPHY SYNDROMES AND LOCALIZED FORMS

Lipodystrophy

Acquired ⟹ Localized

Trauma, injections, pressure, AI-CTD

Congenital or familial

Generalized (birth) Partial (puberty) Generalized (childhood to puberty) Partial Partial

Berardinelli–Seip syndrome

Familial partial lipodystrophy Köbberling–Dunnigan syndrome

Lawrence syndrome

Barraquer–Simons syndrome

HIV/ART-associated lipodystrophy syndrome

Associations:
"Anabolic syndrome"
Diabetes mellitus
Hypertriglyceridemia/ pancreatitis
Cardiomyopathy
Liver disease
Renal failure
Organomegaly

AGPAT2, BSCL2, CAV1

Associations:
Diabetes mellitus
Hypertriglyceridemia/ pancreatitis
Menstrual irregularity
Muscular dystrophy*
Neuropathy*
Premature aging*

LMNA*, PPARG, AKT2

30-50% preceded by systemic illness
Associations:
Diabetes mellitus
Hypertriglyceridemia
Liver disease
Autoimmune disease
Prior panniculitis

Median 8-10 years duration
May be post-viral
Associations:
Hypocomplementemia
Glomerulonephritis
Recurrent *Neisseria* infections

LMNB2

2 months to 2 years after initiation of ART
Associations:
Insulin resistance
Hypertriglyceridemia
Cardiovascular disease

Lipoatrophy, often with muscular prominence
Muscular hypertrophy with lipoatrophy
Lipohypertrophy

Fig. 84.2 Lipodystrophy syndromes and localized forms. Shaded boxes include best-described underlying genetic mutations. In familial partial lipodystrophy, *LMNA* mutations are associated with facial lipohypertrophy and abdominal lipoatrophy while *PPARG* mutations are associated with abdominal lipohypertrophy.

808

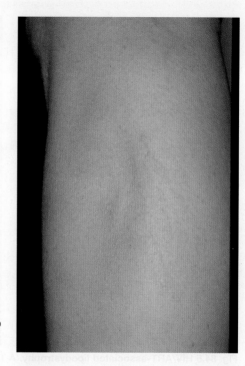

Fig. 84.3 Localized lipoatrophy of the upper lateral calf. A common finding in women due to crossing the legs while seated. *Courtesy, Jean L. Bolognia, MD.*

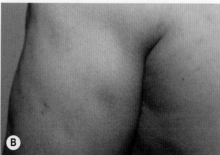

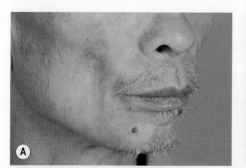

Fig. 84.4 Lipoatrophy secondary to lupus panniculitis. A An area of depression on the cheek due to burnt-out lupus panniculitis; note the dyspigmentation and scarring from an overlapping lesion of discoid lupus erythematosus. **B** Circular depressions on the upper arm, a common location for lupus panniculitis. Lipoatrophy can be seen with other connective tissue disorders, including dermatomyositis in children. *A, Courtesy National Skin Centre, Singapore.*

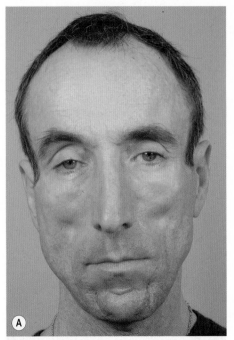
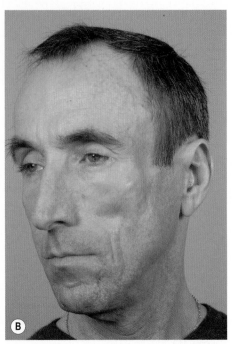

Fig. 84.5 HIV/ART-associated lipodystrophy. A There is symmetric loss of buccal, parotid, and preauricular (Bichat's) fat pads, resulting in prominent zygomata, sunken eyeballs, and a cachectic appearance. **B** The side view highlights the loss of temporal fat. In particular, stavudine and protease inhibitors are most strongly associated with lipoatrophy. *Courtesy, Ken Katz, MD.*

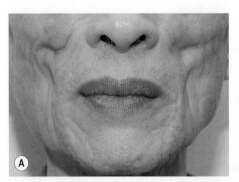
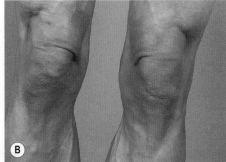

Fig. 84.6 HIV/ART-associated lipodystrophy. A Marked indentation of the medial cheeks in an older patient, with redundant melolabial folds. **B** Lower extremities with prominent veins and defined musculature. *A, Courtesy, Priya Sen, MD; B, Courtesy, Alison Sharpe Avram, MD and Matthew Avram, MD.*

For further information see Ch. 101. From *Dermatology, Third Edition.*

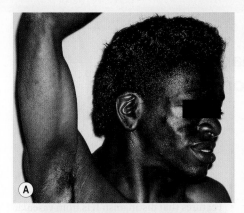

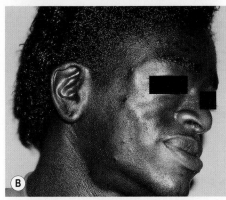

Fig. 84.7 Congenital generalized lipodystrophy. A Extensive acanthosis nigricans, facial and extremity lipodystrophy, and muscular habitus. **B** Close-up view demonstrating loss of Bichat's fat pad and buccal fat. *A, B, Courtesy, Kenneth E. Greer, MD.*

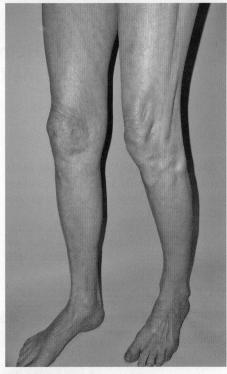

Fig. 84.8 Acquired generalized lipodystrophy. There is loss of subcutaneous fat, resulting in a muscular appearance of the legs and accentuation of the tendons. *Courtesy, Jacqueline Junkins-Hopkins, MD.*

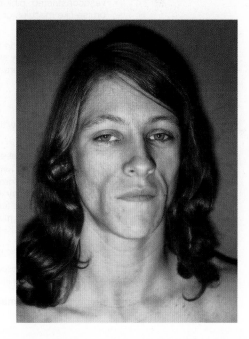

Fig. 84.9 Acquired partial lipodystrophy in a patient with nephritic factor and renal disease. Lipoatrophic features are most prominent on the face, with a marked loss of buccal fat. Axillary acanthosis nigricans was present. *Courtesy, Kenneth E. Greer, MD.*

85 | Infantile Hemangiomas and Vascular Malformations

- Vascular anomalies, which often present at birth or during early infancy, are classified into two groups based on their biologic and clinical behavior:
  - *Vascular tumors*, most commonly the infantile hemangioma (IH), that are characterized by endothelial cell proliferation.
  - *Vascular malformations* that result from defective vascular morphogenesis.
- Features that distinguish IHs from vascular malformations are presented in Table 85.1, and differences in their natural histories are depicted in Fig. 85.1.
- Additional vascular neoplasms are discussed in Chapter 94; other vascular ectasias,

COMPARISON OF INFANTILE HEMANGIOMAS WITH VASCULAR MALFORMATIONS		
Characteristic	**Infantile Hemangiomas**	**Vascular Malformations**
Epidemiology	More common in: • Girls (female : male ratio 3–5 : 1) • Premature and/or low-birth-weight infants • Infants whose mothers are older or underwent CVS	• Equal sex ratio • No predilection based on gestational history • Certain variants have autosomal dominant inheritance (see text)
Appearance at birth	• Often absent • ~50% with a subtle precursor lesion, e.g. telangiectatic, vasoconstricted, pink or bluish bruise-like macules or patches (Fig. 85.2)	• Typically present and already demonstrate characteristic clinical findings
Natural history	• *Postnatal proliferation* for 6–9 months, followed by *slow involution* over several years	• *Lifelong persistence*, with commensurate growth during childhood and often *gradual worsening* (e.g. thickening of capillary malformations) over time
Radiology	• Well-defined mass with high-flow vessels	• Varies depending on the type (see text)
Pathology	In the proliferative phase: • Dense lobules of hyperplastic endothelial cells forming capillaries with tiny lumens • Increased cellular turnover demonstrated by markers of proliferation (e.g. Ki-67)	• Ectatic or distorted vascular channels • Typically no increase in cellular turnover
Immunophenotype	• GLUT1-positive	• GLUT1-negative

CVS, chorionic villus sampling; GLUT1, glucose transporter protein-1 (expressed by the placenta as well as infantile hemangiomas, but no diffuse expression in other vascular tumors).

Table 85.1 Comparison of infantile hemangiomas with vascular malformations.

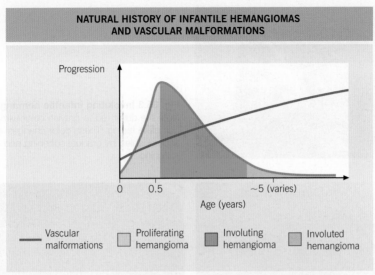

NATURAL HISTORY OF INFANTILE HEMANGIOMAS AND VASCULAR MALFORMATIONS

Fig. 85.1 **Natural history of infantile hemangiomas and vascular malformations.**

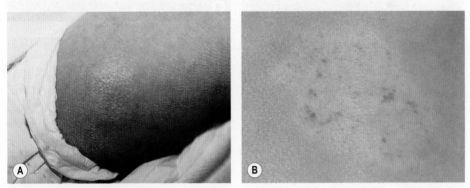

Fig. 85.2 **Hemangioma precursors.** These initial lesions can have a 'bruised' **(A)** or blanched **(B)** appearance. *A, Courtesy, Maria Garzon, MD; B, Courtesy, Julie V. Schaffer, MD.*

such as telangiectasias and angiokeratomas, are covered in Chapter 87.

Infantile Hemangioma (IH)

• Benign vascular neoplasm that represents the most common tumor of infancy.
  – Affects ~5% of infants, with a predilection for girls and premature neonates (see Table 85.1).
• IHs appear during the first few weeks of life, with a characteristic course:
  – *Proliferation* for 6–9 months, tending to 'mark out their territory' early on and

then grow primarily in volume; overall, ~80% of growth is in the first 5 months of life.
  – Subsequent *involution* gradually over several years (e.g. 30% completed by 3 years of age and 50% by 5 years), with softening and a duller or lighter color followed by flattening (Fig. 85.3).
  – Some IHs involute with little or no visible sequelae, whereas others (especially pedunculated or exophytic lesions) leave atrophic, fibrofatty, or telangiectatic residua in addition to scars at sites of previous ulceration (discussed later; Fig. 85.4).

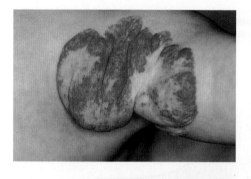

Fig. 85.3 Involuting infantile hemangioma.
Note the duller red to grayish color with areas of complete fading. These color changes were accompanied by gradual softening and flattening.

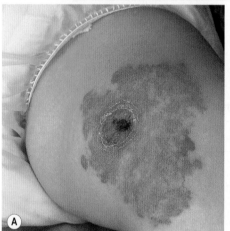

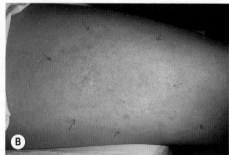

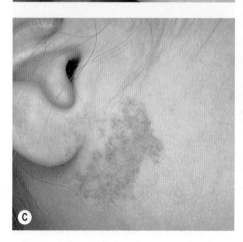

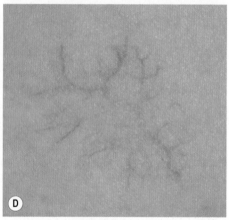

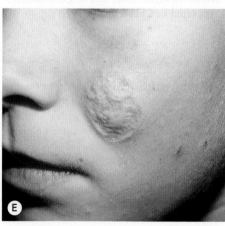

Fig. 85.4 Residua of infantile hemangiomas.
A Superficial hemangioma with a healing ulcer in an infant. **B** Hypopigmentation (*arrows*) and a circular scar at the site of the previous ulcer in the same patient 20 years later. **C, D** Residual telangiectasias. **E** Atrophy and fibrofatty changes. *A, B, E, Courtesy, Ronald P. Rapini, MD; D, Courtesy, Jean L. Bolognia, MD.*

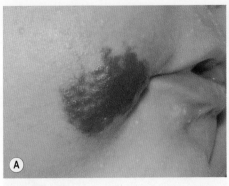

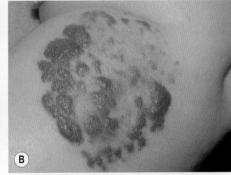

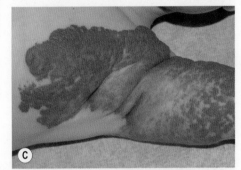

Fig. 85.5 Superficial infantile hemangiomas. Note the bright red color and finely lobulated surface. Involvement may be diffuse or broken up. *Courtesy, Julie V. Schaffer, MD.*

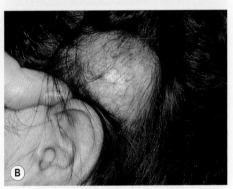

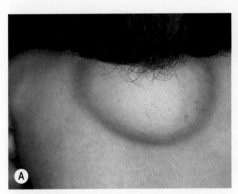

Fig. 85.6 Deep infantile hemangiomas. Note the skin-colored to bluish hue with scattered telangiectasias. *A, Courtesy, Anthony J. Mancini, MD.*

- Divided into three clinical subtypes based on the depth of cutaneous involvement:
  - *Superficial* lesions (~50%; upper dermis) are bright red with a finely lobulated surface ('strawberry' hemangiomas) during proliferation, changing to a mixture of purple-red and gray during involution (Fig. 85.5).
  - *Deep* lesions (~15%; lower dermis and subcutis) present as warm, ill-defined, light blue-purple, rubbery nodules or masses (Fig. 85.6); often become evident

later and proliferate ~1 month longer than superficial lesions.
  - *Mixed* lesions (~35%) have superficial and deep components – e.g. a well-defined red plaque overlying a poorly circumscribed bluish nodule.
- IHs have two major distribution patterns:
  - *Focal* lesions arise from a localized nidus (see Fig. 85.5A).
  - *Segmental* lesions cover a broader area or developmental unit and are more likely to be associated with regional

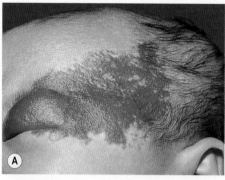
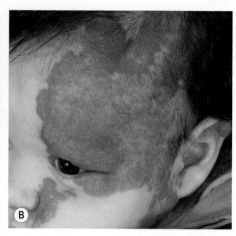
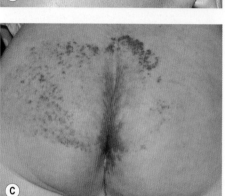

Fig. 85.7 Segmental infantile hemangiomas. A Segmental facial hemangioma mimicking a capillary malformation. **B** Thicker segmental facial hemangioma partially obstructing the visual axis. Both of these patients had PHACE(S) syndrome. **C** Segmental lumbosacral hemangioma. This child is at risk for LUMBAR syndrome. *A, Courtesy, Maria Garzon, MD; B, C, Courtesy, Julie V. Schaffer, MD.*

extracutaneous abnormalities – e.g. PHACE(S) and LUMBAR syndromes (discussed later) (Fig. 85.7).

- **DDx:** *precursors and early lesions*: capillary malformation, telangiectasias; *well-developed lesions*: pyogenic granuloma, other vascular tumors, venous/lymphatic malformation, and rare entities such as nasal glioma and soft tissue sarcomas (see Table 53.1); *multiple lesions*: glomuvenous malformations, blue rubber bleb nevus syndrome, multifocal lymphangioendotheliomatosis with thrombocytopenia, 'blueberry muffin baby' (see Chapter 99).
- When an atypical clinical appearance or natural history leads to consideration of entities in the DDx of an IH, additional evaluation may include ultrasonography, other imaging, and biopsy.

Complications of IHs

- *Ulceration*: occurs in ~10% of lesions, especially those on the lip and in the anogenital region or other skin folds, at a median age of 4 months (Fig. 85.8); whitish discoloration of an IH in an infant <3 months of age may signal impending ulceration; results in pain, a risk of infection (relatively uncommon), and eventual scarring (see Fig. 85.4A,B).
- *Disfigurement and interference with function due to the IH's location and/or large size.*
  - *Periocular IH* – risk of astigmatism if puts pressure on globe, amblyopia if obstructs the visual axis, and strabismus if affects orbital musculature (see Fig. 85.7A,B); requires ophthalmologic evaluation.
  - *IH on nasal tip, columella, or lip (especially if crosses the vermilion border)* – high risk of distortion of facial structures (as well as ulceration if on the lip) (Fig. 85.9).
  - *IH on breast* (in girls) – may affect underlying breast bud, so early surgery should be avoided.

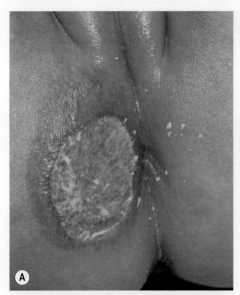

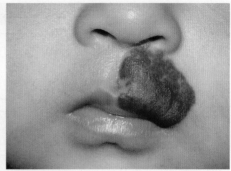

Fig. 85.9 Infantile hemangioma on the lip. This is a cosmetically sensitive site, especially when lesions cross the vermilion border, and hemangiomas in this location are prone to ulceration. *Courtesy, Julie V. Schaffer, MD.*

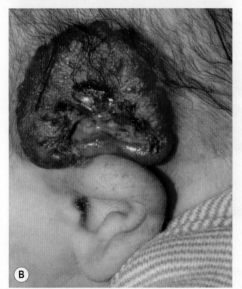

Fig. 85.8 Ulcerated infantile hemangiomas. A Ulcerated hemangioma on the buttock. Because the hemangioma component may not be obvious, this diagnosis should be considered when an infant presents with an ulcer in the diaper area. **B** Ulcerated superficial hemangioma above the ear. Note the distortion of the pinna. *Courtesy, Julie V. Schaffer, MD.*

- *Associated extracutaneous abnormalities.*
  - *IHs in 'beard' area of the lower face* – often associated with *airway IHs*, which may present with noisy breathing or biphasic stridor; otolaryngologic evaluation is needed for infants with symptoms or when the IH is likely to be actively proliferating (i.e. <4–5 months of age) (Fig. 85.10).
  - *Large facial IHs, particularly segmental lesions* – risk of *PHACE(S)* syndrome: P, posterior fossa malformations; H, hemangioma; A, arterial abnormalities (cervical, cerebral); C, cardiac defects, especially coarctation of the aorta; E, eye anomalies; S, sternal defects and supraumbilical raphe (Table 85.2; Figs. 85.11 and 85.12; see Fig. 85.7A,B).
  - *Large IHs on the lower body, particularly segmental lesions* – risk of *LUMBAR* syndrome: L, lower body/lumbosacral IH and lipomas; U, urogenital anomalies and ulceration; M, myelopathy (spinal dysraphism); B, bony deformities; A, anorectal and arterial anomalies; R, renal anomalies (see Figs. 85.7C and 85.12).
  - *Midline lumbosacral IHs* – risk of *spinal dysraphism* (see Chapter 53).
  - *Multiple (≥5) IHs* – may be associated with *visceral hemangiomatosis*, most often hepatic; the cutaneous IHs are usually relatively small and superficial, but hepatic involvement can be

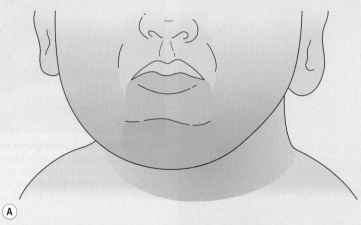

A
- Involvement of each of the five areas scores as 1 point
- In one study of 16 children with a score ≥ 4, 63% had some degree of symptomatic airway involvement

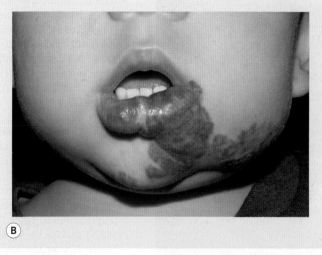

B

Fig. 85.10 Infantile hemangiomas in a 'beard' distribution. A Anatomic sites associated with risk of an airway hemangioma. **B** Infant with a laryngeal hemangioma in addition to cutaneous lesions in a 'beard' distribution. *A, Adapted with permission from Orlow SJ, Isakoff MS, Blei F. Increased risk of symptomatic hemangiomas of the airway in association with cutaneous hemangiomas in a 'beard' distribution. J. Pediatr. 1997;131:643–646; B, Courtesy, Julie V. Schaffer, MD.*

associated with complications such as high-output cardiac failure and hypothyroidism (due to iodothyronine diodinase production by the IH) (Fig. 85.13; see Fig. 85.12).

Treatment of IHs

- 'Active non-intervention,' including education of parents and observation with periodic photography, is sufficient for most small hemangiomas expected to have a good cosmetic outcome; frequent visits (e.g. at 2- or 3-week intervals) are helpful to monitor early lesions with the potential to become problematic.
- **Local Rx:** topical timolol (systemic absorption possible, especially if ulcerated or involving mucous membranes) or superpotent CS

DIAGNOSTIC CRITERIA FOR PHACE(S) SYNDROME		
Definite PHACE(S)		
• Facial hemangioma >5 cm in diameter plus 1 major criterion or 2 minor criteria		
Possible PHACE(S)		
• Facial hemangioma >5 cm plus 1 minor criterion; *or*		
• Hemangioma of the neck or upper torso plus 1 major criteria or 2 minor criteria; *or*		
• Two major criteria in the absence of a hemangioma		
Organ System	**Major Criteria**	**Minor Criteria**
Cerebrovascular	Anomalies of major cerebral arteries* (e.g. dysplasia, hypoplasia, stenosis, aneurysm, aberrant origin/course) Persistent trigeminal artery	Persistent embryonic arteries (other than trigeminal artery) Intracranial hemangioma
Structural brain	Posterior fossa anomalies (e.g. Dandy–Walker complex, cerebellar hypoplasia/dysplasia)	Midline anomalies Neuronal migration disorder
Cardiovascular	Aortic arch anomalies Anomalous origin of subclavian artery ± vascular ring	Ventricular septal defect Right aortic arch
Ocular	Posterior segment anomalies (e.g. retinal vascular anomalies, optic nerve hypoplasia)	Anterior segment anomalies (e.g. sclerocornea, cataract, coloboma)
Ventral or midline	Sternal defect Supraumbilical raphe	Hypopituitarism Ectopic thyroid

Major cerebral arteries include internal carotid artery; middle, anterior, or posterior cerebral artery; and vertebrobasilar system.

Table 85.2 Diagnostic criteria for PHACE(S) syndrome.

REASONS TO CONSIDER SYSTEMIC THERAPY FOR INFANTILE HEMANGIOMAS
Threatened vital functions
• Vision • Airway
Potential for disfigurement
• Nasal tip or columella • Lip, especially if crosses the vermilion border • Large or rapidly growing lesion, especially if on the face
Severe/recalcitrant ulceration
High-output cardiac failure

Table 85.3 Reasons to consider systemic therapy for infantile hemangiomas.

for thin superficial lesions; intralesional CS for thicker lesions (avoiding the periocular area); pulsed dye laser for residual telangiectasias and possibly for thin superficial lesions.
• **Systemic Rx:** indications are listed in Table 85.3; oral propranolol (Table 85.4) has replaced prednisolone as the first-line systemic therapy.
• Management of an ulcerated IH includes wound care (e.g. hydrocolloid dressings), monitoring for infection, pain management, and specific therapies directed at the ulcer (e.g. becaplermin gel, pulsed-dye laser) or IH (e.g. β-blockers).
• Surgical excision is useful to remove fibro-fatty tissue and redundant skin in involuted or partially involuted IHs; often done in preschool-aged children with cosmetically significant lesions (e.g. on the nasal tip or lip), and earlier resection may be considered when eventual surgery is inevitable (e.g. for some pedunculated lesions) and for small, persistently ulcerated IHs.

Hemangioma Variants

• *IHs with minimal or arrested growth* present with reticulated erythema, telangiectasias, and larger ectatic vessels, often on a vasoconstricted background; a proliferative

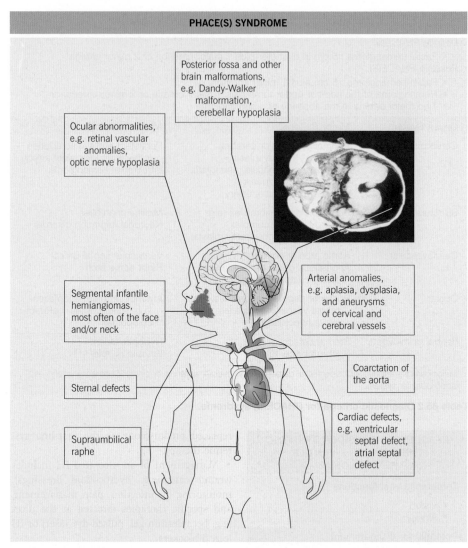

Posterior fossa and other brain malformations, e.g. Dandy-Walker malformation, cerebellar hypoplasia

Ocular abnormalities, e.g. retinal vascular anomalies, optic nerve hypoplasia

Segmental infantile hemangiomas, most often of the face and/or neck

Arterial anomalies, e.g. aplasia, dysplasia, and aneurysms of cervical and cerebral vessels

Sternal defects

Coarctation of the aorta

Supraumbilical raphe

Cardiac defects, e.g. ventricular septal defect, atrial septal defect

Fig. 85.11 PHACE(S) syndrome. Major clinical features are illustrated.

component is either absent or represents <25% of the surface area (often small red papules at the periphery) (Fig. 85.14); histologically, these lesions are GLUT1-positive like classic IHs (see Table 85.1).

• *Congenital hemangiomas* are fully developed at birth, typically presenting as a warm, pink to blue-violet mass or plaque with overlying coarse telangiectasias, surrounded by a vasoconstricted rim and/or radiating veins; unlike true IHs, congenital hemangiomas are GLUT1-negative.

– *Rapidly involuting congenital hemangioma (RICH)* – rapid involution during the first year of life (Fig. 85.15A,B).
– *Non-involuting congenital hemangioma (NICH)* – postnatal growth in proportion to the child, without involution (Fig. 85.15C).

Kasabach–Merritt Phenomenon (KMP)

• Life-threatening thrombocytopenic coagulopathy associated with a vascular tumor,

EVALUATION OF A CHILD WITH INFANTILE HEMANGIOMAS FOR POSSIBLE EXTRACUTANEOUS INVOLVEMENT

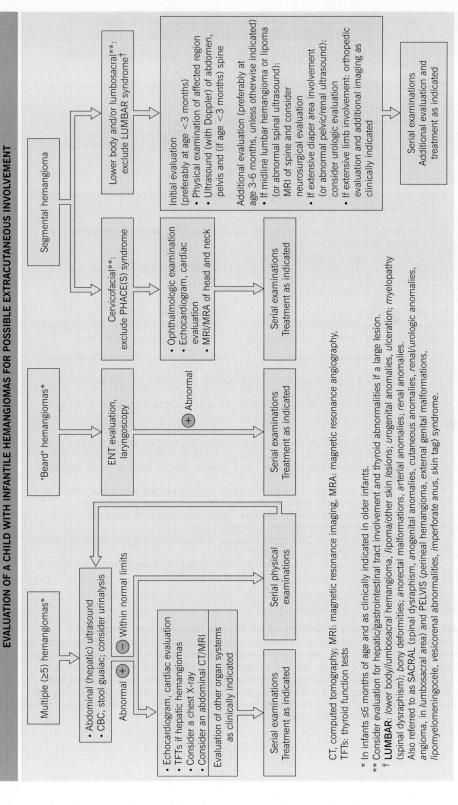

Fig. 85.12 Evaluation of a child with infantile hemangiomas for possible extracutaneous involvement. See Fig. 85.11 and Table 85.2 for additional information on PHACE(S) syndrome.

INFANTILE HEMANGIOMAS AND VASCULAR MALFORMATIONS

ADMINISTRATION OF PROPRANOLOL FOR INFANTILE HEMANGIOMAS: CONSENSUS RECOMMENDATIONS

Pretreatment evaluation (typically done in conjunction with a pediatrician or pediatric cardiologist)

- Cardiopulmonary history and examination; asthma/reactive airway disease is usually considered as a contraindication
- Heart rate and blood pressure
- Electrocardiogram, especially if low heart rate, history/evidence of arrhythmia, family history of heart conditions, or maternal autoimmune connective tissue disease
- If at risk for PHACE(S) (see Table 85.2): MRI/MRA of head/neck/aortic arch and echocardiogram

Dosing and course

- Use propranolol 20 mg/5 ml oral solution, divided into 3 daily doses at a minimum of 6-hour intervals
- *Initial* dose: 1 mg/kg/day (0.33 mg/kg/dose)
- *Target* dose: usually 2 mg/kg/day (0.66 mg/kg/dose), with range of 1–3 mg/kg/day
- Indications for initiation as inpatient:
  - ≤8 weeks of age (gestationally corrected); *or*
  - Comorbid cardiovascular or respiratory* disorders or problems with glucose regulation; *or*
  - Inadequate social support

If *inpatient* initiation:	If *outpatient* initiation:
• Increase from 0.33 to 0.66 mg/kg/dose *after 1–3 doses* (slower if not tolerated)	• Increase from 0.33 to 0.5 to 0.66 mg/kg/dose, each *after 3–7 days*

- Treatment is typically continued for 6–12+ months, depending on the clinical setting and course
  - Often longer if younger at initiation (e.g. until 9–15+ months of age) to prevent rebound
- Taper over ≥2 weeks before discontinuing (primarily to prevent rebound tachycardia)

Monitoring

- Risks of propranolol include symptomatic hypotension (<0.5%), bradycardia (<0.1%), hypoglycemia (<0.5%), sleep disturbances (up to 10%), and bronchospasm (~3%)
- Check heart rate and blood pressure 1 and 2 hours after an initial or newly increased dose is given
- Educate parents about signs of hypoglycemia (early[†]: sweating, rapid heart rate, shakiness, fussiness; late: lethargy, poor feeding, hypothermia, seizures) and hypotension/bradycardia (cold extremities, delayed capillary refill, lethargy)
- Infants should be fed in conjunction with each dose
  - Feed at least every 4 hours if age <6 weeks, every 5 hours if age 6 weeks–4 months, and every 6–8 hours if age >4 months
  - Suspend therapy during intercurrent illnesses, especially if decreased oral intake or vomiting

*Including symptomatic airway hemangiomas.
†May be masked with the β-adrenergic blockade.

Table 85.4 Administration of propranolol for infantile hemangiomas: consensus recommendations. Propranolol, a nonselective β-blocker, binds to β_2-adrenergic receptors on hemangioma endothelial cells, with effects including vasoconstriction (leading to softening and dulling of color within 24 hours), decreased expression of pro-angiogenic growth factors, and induction of apoptosis. Practices vary widely, and some pediatric dermatologists and cardiologists recommend more or less intensive evaluation and monitoring. The patient's age, hemangioma-related issues, and medical comorbidities also affect management. *Based on Drolet BA, Frommelt PC, Chamlin SL, et al. Pediatrics 2013;131:128–140.*

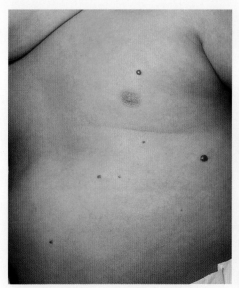

Fig. 85.13 Multiple cutaneous infantile hemangiomas in a child with hepatic involvement ('diffuse neonatal hemangiomatosis'). Many small, superficial skin lesions are present. *Courtesy, Ronald P. Rapini, MD.*

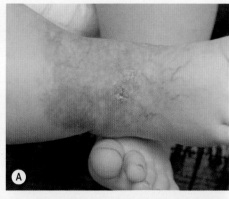

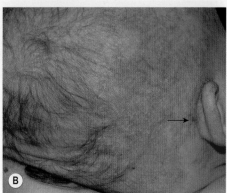

Fig. 85.14 Minimal/arrested growth infantile hemangiomas. Telangiectasias and larger ectatic vessels are evident. Note the focal crusting **(A)** and small bright red papules behind the ear (arrow) **(B)**. The presence of the latter (which may be subtle or absent), reticulated erythema, and characteristic telangiectasias (often both fine and coarse) help to distinguish these lesions from capillary–venous malformations. *A, Courtesy, Maria Garzon, MD, and Anita Haggstrom, MD; B, Courtesy, Julie V. Schaffer, MD.*

usually a kaposiform hemangioendothelioma or tufted angioma (see Chapter 94) in an infant (*not* an IH).

- Prior to onset of KMP, lesions may appear as thin red-violet plaques or deeper masses.

• Presents with a rapidly enlarging, indurated, ecchymotic mass associated with marked thrombocytopenia and a consumptive coagulopathy (Fig. 85.16).

• **Rx:** difficult; traditionally vincristine and prednisone, with sirolimus (rapamycin) showing promise in recent reports.

Vascular Malformations

• Categorized based on the predominant type(s) of vascular channels, which are divided into slow- and fast-flow groups:

- *Slow-flow*: capillary (port-wine stain), venous, microcystic lymphatic ('lymphangioma'), and macrocystic lymphatic ('cystic hygroma').
- *Fast-flow*: arteriovenous (arterial anomalies + arteriovenous shunting).

• Although they can affect any organ, vascular malformations are most easily identified in the skin and mucous membranes, where they may extend into deeper structures or be associated with other extracutaneous abnormalities.

Capillary Malformations (CMs) and Related Conditions

NEVUS SIMPLEX (SALMON PATCH)

• Common congenital capillary stain (*not* a true CM) on the mid face (forehead, glabella, nasal tip, and philtrum), eyelids, occiput, and

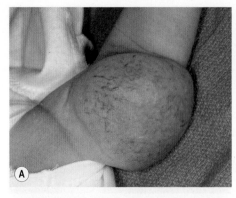

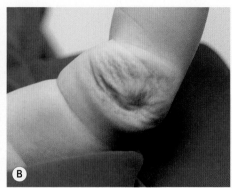

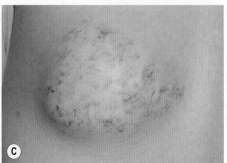

Fig. 85.15 Congenital hemangiomas. A Rapidly involuting congenital hemangioma (RICH) presenting as a violaceous tumor on the upper extremity with surface telangiectasias in a neonate. **B** Spontaneous involution of the RICH at 5 months of age, with fibrofatty residua. **C** Non-involuting congenital hemangioma (NICH) in a school-aged child. This lesion was fully formed at birth and is still warm and firm to palpation. Note the coarse telangiectasias and pallor. *A, B, Courtesy, Annette Wagner, MD; C, Courtesy, Julie V. Schaffer, MD.*

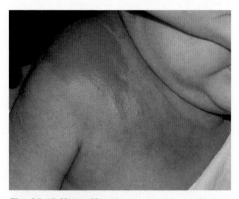

Fig. 85.16 Kaposiform hemangioendothelioma associated with Kasabach–Merritt phenomenon in a 5-week-old boy. Progressive induration and ecchymosis developed rapidly over a 24-hour period. An eczematous eruption is also evident. *Courtesy, Julie V. Schaffer, MD.*

nape ('stork bite') (Fig. 85.17A,B); multiple lesions may be present and can occur in the lumbar area.

- Facial lesions often fade by early childhood.

PORT-WINE STAIN (PWS)
- Mosaic activating mutations in the *GNAQ* gene, which encodes a G protein α subunit, underlie both nonsyndromic PWSs and Sturge–Weber syndrome.
- PWSs present at birth as pinkish-red macules and patches, often in a segmental pattern (Fig. 85.17C).
- Over time, may develop a deeper purplish-red color, and affected skin (especially on the face) often thickens and becomes nodular; overgrowth of underlying soft tissues and bones can also occur (Figs. 85.18 and 85.19).

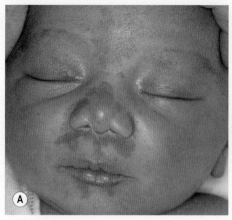

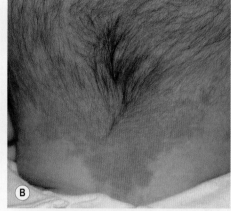

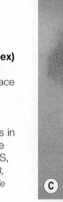

Fig. 85.17 Salmon patches (nevus simplex) versus port-wine stain (PWS) in a V2 distribution. A Involvement of the central face in a symmetrical pattern is common with a salmon patch; such lesions fade over the first few years of life but are sometimes misdiagnosed as a PWS. **B** Salmon patches in the nape area ('stork bites') tend to be more persistent. **C** In this young infant with a PWS, the skin is smooth. This lesion will persist. *B, Courtesy, Julie V. Schaffer, MD; C, Courtesy, Odile Enjolras, MD.*

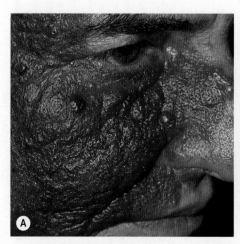

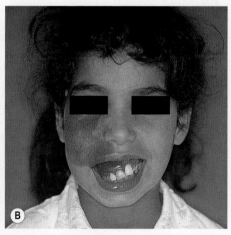

Fig. 85.18 Facial port-wine stains in a V2 distribution with hypertrophic changes. A Prominent skin thickening and nodularity. **B** Markedly enlarged gingiva and overgrowth of the right maxilla. *Courtesy, Odile Enjolras, MD.*

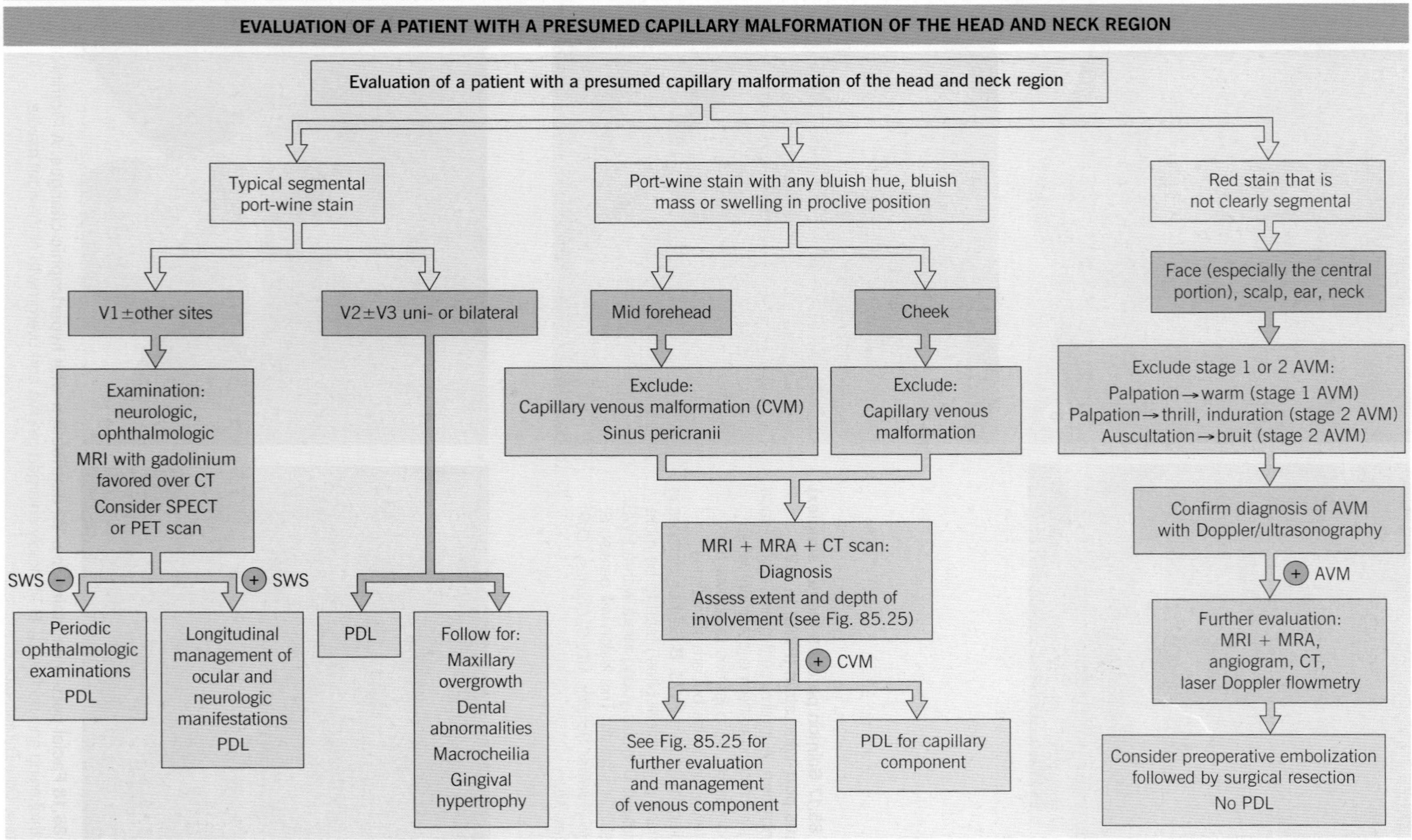

EVALUATION OF A PATIENT WITH A PRESUMED CAPILLARY MALFORMATION OF THE HEAD AND NECK REGION

Fig. 85.19 Evaluation of a patient with a presumed capillary malformation of the head and neck region. AVM, arteriovenous malformation; CT, computed tomography; CVM, capillary venous malformation; PDL, pulsed dye laser; MRA, magnetic resonance arteriography; MRI, magnetic resonance imaging; PET, positron emission computed tomography; SPECT, single photon emission computed tomography; SWS, Sturge–Weber syndrome.

- **DDx:** *in infant*: nevus simplex, early or arrested-growth IH; CMTC (especially if on an extremity), stage 1 arteriovenous malformation, *verrucous 'hemangioma'* (congenital red-purple hyperkeratotic plaques, often in a segmental pattern, composed of capillaries and with growth proportional to the child).
- **Rx:** pulsed dye laser therapy, preferably initiated during infancy for facial lesions to avoid psychosocial distress and lesional thickening.
- *Sturge–Weber syndrome:* association of a facial PWS, usually involving the trigeminal V1 dermatome (upper eyelid, forehead) ± other sites (Fig. 85.20), with ipsilateral ocular and leptomeningeal vascular malformations; the latter can lead to glaucoma and neurologic sequelae such as developmental delay and contralateral seizures or hemiparesis.
- *Phakomatosis pigmentovascularis (PPV)*: forms of 'twin spotting' in which a PWS coexists with aberrant Mongolian spots (dermal melanocytosis, also caused by mosaic *GNAQ* mutations; type 2 PPV) (Fig. 85.21) or a nevus spilus (type 3 PPV); a nevus anemicus may also be present.

- *Megalencephaly–capillary malformation* (previously *macrocephaly–CMTC*): reticulated PWS and persistent nevus simplex associated with asymmetric overgrowth, macrocephaly, and developmental delay; due to mosaic *PIK3CA* mutations (Fig. 85.22).

CUTIS MARMORATA TELANGIECTATICA CONGENITA (CMTC)

- Red-purple, broad reticulated vascular pattern intermingled with telangiectasias, ± prominent veins and atrophy; most often affects a limb, which may be hypoplastic; occasionally generalized (Fig. 85.23).
- *Adams–Oliver syndrome* features CMTC together with aplasia cutis congenita and limb defects (see Table 53.3).

Venous Malformations (VMs; Former Misnomer of 'Cavernous Hemangioma')

CLASSIC VMs

- Soft, compressible bluish nodules that fill with dependency; may be focal, segmental, or widespread, and often extend into underlying muscles and bones (Fig. 85.24).

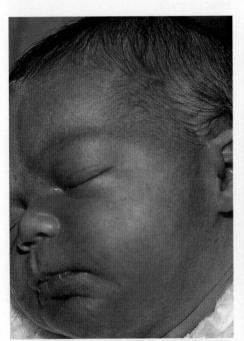

Fig. 85.20 Infant at risk for Sturge–Weber syndrome. Port-wine stain with involvement of V1 as well as V2 and V3. *Courtesy, Odile Enjolras, MD.*

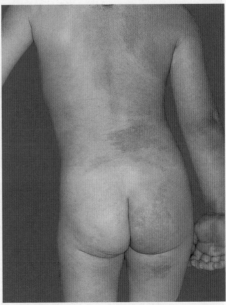

Fig. 85.21 Phakomatosis pigmentovascularis type 2. A large port-wine stain and extensive dermal melanocytosis are seen. *Courtesy, Odile Enjolras, MD.*

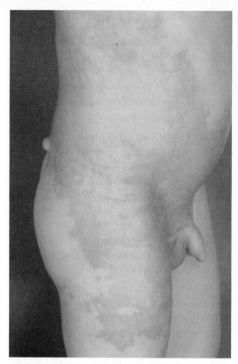

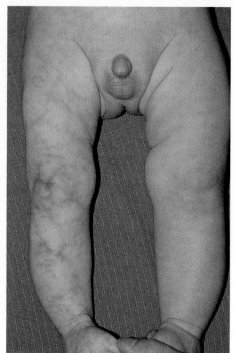

Fig. 85.22 Reticulated port-wine stain (PWS) in a patient with megalencephaly–capillary malformation syndrome. This boy has hemihypertrophy of the side of the body *opposite* to the PWS. *Courtesy, Julie V. Schaffer, MD.*

Fig. 85.23 Cutis marmorata telangiectatica congenita (CMTC) with atrophy of the affected limb. The color of the broad vascular network can be red-purple (as in this infant) to brownish-purple.

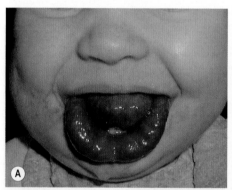

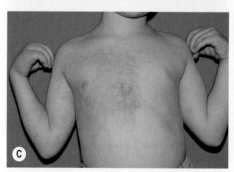

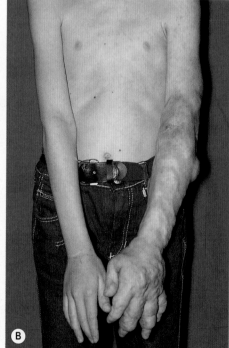

Fig. 85.24 Venous malformations (VMs). A Distortion of the tongue and lower lip has led to an open bite. **B** The skin and muscles of the entire arm are affected, with soft bluish nodules and obvious swelling in the dependent position. **C** This VM has a segmental distribution on the right trunk and involvement of the ipsilateral arm. *Courtesy, Odile Enjolras, MD.*

• Both *multiple cutaneous and mucosal VMs* with autosomal dominant inheritance and sporadic VMs can result from mutations in the *TEK* gene, which encodes an endothelial cell-specific tyrosine kinase.

• *Blue rubber bleb nevus (Bean) syndrome* also presents with multiple cutaneous and mucosal (e.g. GI) VMs.

• An approach to the evaluation and management of VMs at different sites is presented in Fig. 85.25.

GLOMUVENOUS MALFORMATIONS (GVMs; PREVIOUSLY KNOWN AS GLOMANGIOMATOSIS)

• Pink to blue-purple nodules and cobble-stoned plaques that resist full compression and are painful upon palpation; may be focal, segmental, or widespread and (unlike classic VMs) are typically limited to the skin and subcutis (Fig. 85.26).

• Autosomal dominant inheritance due to mutations in the glomulin gene (*GLMN*).

MAFFUCCI SYNDROME

• Association of VMs with enchondromas, most often of the extremities; skin lesions may also have features of a spindle cell hemangioma.

Lymphatic Anomalies

• *Lymphatic malformations (LMs)* are due to excessive aberrant lymphatic channels, whereas *lymphedema* results from hypoplasia or disruption of the lymphatics.

LYMPHATIC MALFORMATIONS

• *Microcystic LM ('lymphangioma circumscriptum')*: clusters of clear or hemorrhagic, vesicle-like papules favoring the proximal limbs and chest; intermittent hemorrhage and leakage of lymph can occur (Fig. 85.27A–D).

• *Macrocystic LM ('cystic hygroma')*: ballo-table subcutaneous masses representing larger lymphatic cysts; favor the neck, axilla, and lateral chest wall (Fig. 85.27E).

• Cellulitis-like inflammatory reactions can be triggered by trauma or infection and may result in expansion and worsening over time.

• Cervicofacial lesions often distort underlying bony structures, and oropharyngeal involvement can lead to airway compromise; rare complications include visceral 'lymphan-giomatosis' and massive osteolysis (*Gorham-Stout [disappearing bone] disease*).

• **DDx:** acquired cutaneous lymphangiectasia (e.g. due to Crohn's disease, recurrent cellulitis, or intralymphatic metastases).

• Radiologic evaluation: ultrasonography, MRI with gadolinium (lack enhancement).

• **Rx:** sclerotherapy, laser therapy (for microcystic lesions), surgical excision (but recurrences are common).

PRIMARY LYMPHEDEMA

• Most often affects the extremities (lower > upper), with occasional genital, cephalic, or generalized involvement; may be associated with pulmonary or GI lymphangiectasia.

• *Congenital lymphedema* is present at birth or develops during infancy; etiologies include *Milroy disease* (mutations in the gene encoding vascular endothelial growth factor receptor 3) and *Turner* and *Noonan syndromes*.

• *Lymphedema praecox* presents around puberty; etiologies include *Meige disease* and *lymphedema–distichiasis syndrome*.

• Secondary lymphedema is discussed in Chapter 86.

Arteriovenous Malformations (AVMs)

• Fast-flow malformations with potential for serious complications (e.g. amputation, deformity).

• Often involve the cephalic region, especially the central face, with approximately half of lesions evident at birth; may worsen with puberty, pregnancy, trauma, partial excision, or proximal embolization.

• Divided into four stages based on clinical severity:
  – *Stage 1 – dormant*: red, warm and macular (mimicking a PWS) or slightly infiltrated (Fig. 85.28A,B).
  – *Stage 2 – expansion*: warm mass with thrill/throbbing and dilated draining veins (Fig. 85.28C).
  – *Stage 3 – destruction*: pain, necrosis, and ulceration; ± lytic bone lesions (Fig. 85.28D).
  – *Stage 4 – cardiac decompensation*: high-output cardiac failure.

• Radiologic evaluation: ultrasonography, MRI/MRA, arteriography.

• **Rx:** complete excision after judicious preoperative embolization.

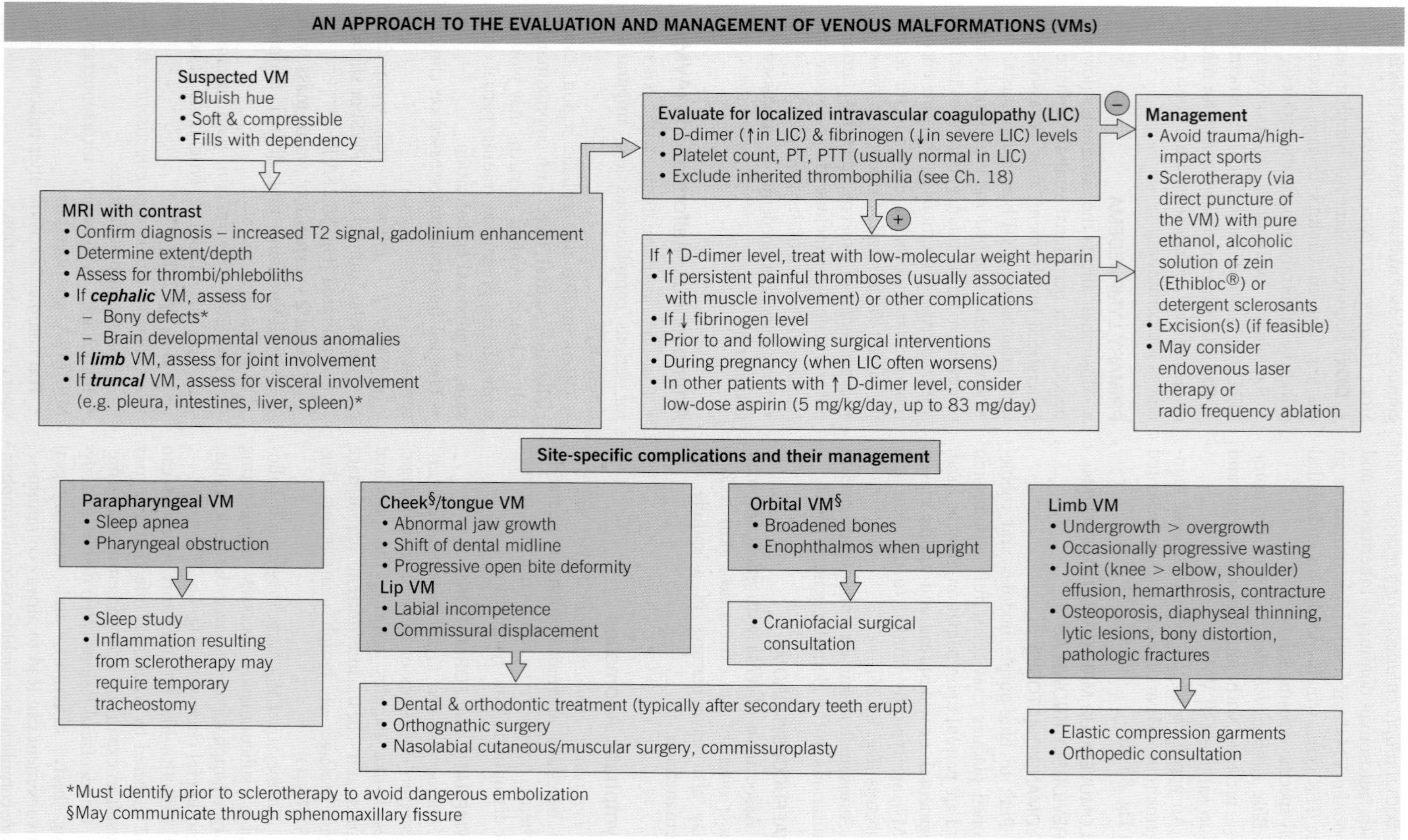

AN APPROACH TO THE EVALUATION AND MANAGEMENT OF VENOUS MALFORMATIONS (VMs)

Suspected VM
- Bluish hue
- Soft & compressible
- Fills with dependency

MRI with contrast
- Confirm diagnosis – increased T2 signal, gadolinium enhancement
- Determine extent/depth
- Assess for thrombi/pheboliths
- If *cephalic* VM, assess for
  - Bony defects*
  - Brain developmental venous anomalies
- If *limb* VM, assess for joint involvement
- If *truncal* VM, assess for visceral involvement (e.g. pleura, intestines, liver, spleen)*

Evaluate for localized intravascular coagulopathy (LIC)
- D-dimer (↑in LIC) & fibrinogen (↓in severe LIC) levels
- Platelet count, PT, PTT (usually normal in LIC)
- Exclude inherited thrombophilia (see Ch. 18)

If ↑ D-dimer level, treat with low-molecular weight heparin
- If persistent painful thromboses (usually associated with muscle involvement) or other complications
- If ↓ fibrinogen level
- Prior to and following surgical interventions
- During pregnancy (when LIC often worsens)
- In other patients with ↑ D-dimer level, consider low-dose aspirin (5 mg/kg/day, up to 83 mg/day)

Management
- Avoid trauma/high-impact sports
- Sclerotherapy (via direct puncture of the VM) with pure ethanol, alcoholic solution of zein (Ethibloc®) or detergent sclerosants
- Excision(s) (if feasible)
- May consider endovenous laser therapy or radio frequency ablation

Site-specific complications and their management

Parapharyngeal VM
- Sleep apnea
- Pharyngeal obstruction

- Sleep study
- Inflammation resulting from sclerotherapy may require temporary tracheostomy

Cheek§/tongue VM
- Abnormal jaw growth
- Shift of dental midline
- Progressive open bite deformity

Lip VM
- Labial incompetence
- Commissural displacement

- Dental & orthodontic treatment (typically after secondary teeth erupt)
- Orthognathic surgery
- Nasolabial cutaneous/muscular surgery, commissuroplasty

Orbital VM§
- Broadened bones
- Enophthalmos when upright

- Craniofacial surgical consultation

Limb VM
- Undergrowth > overgrowth
- Occasionally progressive wasting
- Joint (knee > elbow, shoulder) effusion, hemarthrosis, contracture
- Osteoporosis, diaphyseal thinning, lytic lesions, bony distortion, pathologic fractures

- Elastic compression garments
- Orthopedic consultation

*Must identify prior to sclerotherapy to avoid dangerous embolization
§May communicate through sphenomaxillary fissure

Fig. 85.25 An approach to the evaluation and management of venous malformations (VMs).

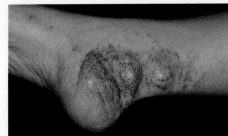

Fig. 85.26 Plaque-type glomuvenous malformation on the distal lower extremity.

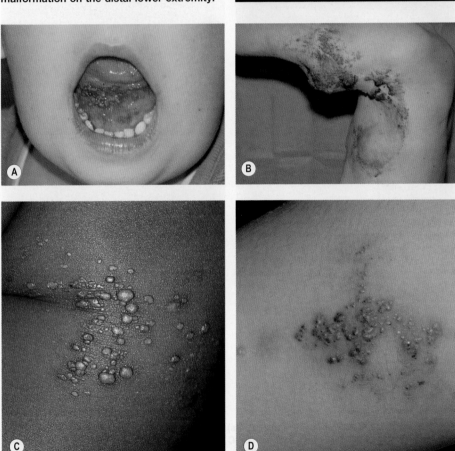

Fig. 85.27 Lymphatic malformations (LMs).
A–D Microcystic LMs presenting as clusters of clear or hemorrhagic vesicles, with active bleeding from lesions in the mouth. The crops of vesicles in **(B)** recurred years after surgical resection (utilizing grafting and linear closure) of a large microcystic LM affecting the skin and deeper structures of the arm and thorax. **E** Macrocystic LM on the lateral trunk. The mass was soft except for a focal firm area of hemorrhage associated with bruise-like discoloration of the overlying skin. *A, B, Courtesy, Odile Enjolras, MD; D, E, Courtesy, Julie V. Schaffer, MD.*

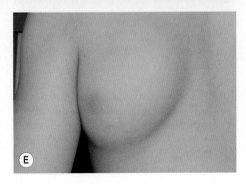

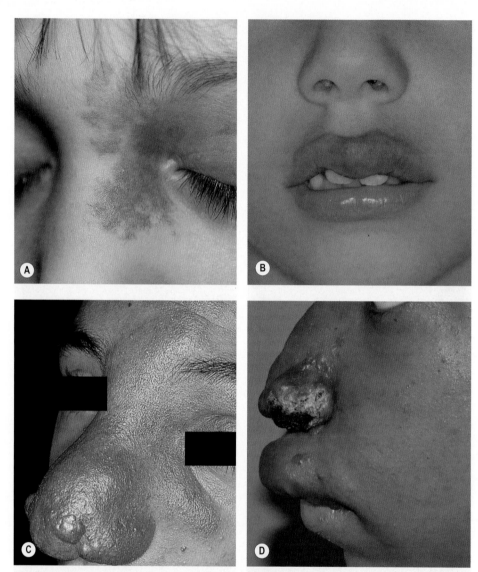

Fig. 85.28 Arteriovenous malformations (AVMs). A, B Dormant (stage 1) AVMs mimicking a port-wine stain **(A)** and infantile hemangioma **(B). C** Expanding (stage 2) centrofacial AVM associated with AVMs of the retina and brain in a boy with Bonnet–Dechaume–Blanc syndrome. **D** Destructive (stage 3) AVM that has led to cutaneous necrosis. *Courtesy, Odile Enjolras, MD.*

- *Acroangiodermatitis* (pseudo-Kaposi sarcoma; see Chapter 86) can occur in association with a lower extremity AVM.
- *Metameric AVMs.*
  - *Cobb syndrome*: cutaneous (may mimic a CM or angiokeratomas) in dermatomal distribution + intraspinal/vertebral.
  - *Bonnet–Dechaume–Blanc (Wyburn–Mason) syndrome*: cutaneous facial + orbit/eye and/or brain (see Fig. 85.28C).

Syndromes Associated with Complex–Combined or Multiple Types of Vascular Malformations

- *Klippel–Trenaunay syndrome*: CM + VM ± LM associated with progressive overgrowth of the affected extremity; well-demarcated geographic stains usually have a lymphatic component, which increases the likelihood of massive overgrowth and cellulitis; risk of deep venous thrombosis/pulmonary embolism (Fig. 85.29).

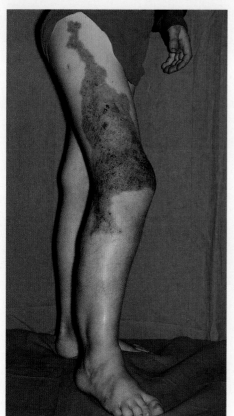

Fig. 85.29 Klippel–Trenaunay syndrome (KTS). Dilated incompetent veins and an enlarged lower limb are evident. The sharply demarcated *geographic* borders of this capillary stain and the superimposed purple papulovesicles (representing lymphangiectasias) are clues to the presence of a lymphatic malformation. In contrast, KTS without a lymphatic component often presents with an ill-defined *patchy* capillary stain in a segmental or haphazard distribution.

• *Proteus syndrome* (see Table 51.3): mosaic disorder due to *AKT1* mutations; can feature CM, VM, and/or LM.

• *CLOVES syndrome: c*ongenital *l*ipomatous *o*vergrowth, *v*ascular malformations (slow- or fast-flow), *e*pidermal nevi, and *s*keletal anomalies (e.g. scoliosis, splayed feet) due to mosaic *PIK3CA* mutations.

• *PTEN hamartoma–tumor syndrome* (see Chapter 52): often intramuscular fast-flow anomalies associated with ectopic fat and dilated draining veins; ± CM and LM components.

• *Cerebral CM and hyperkeratotic cutaneous CM-VM:* autosomal dominant disorder, usually due to *KRIT1* mutations; congenital red-purple plaques and red-brown macules with peripheral telangiectatic puncta.

• *CM-AVM syndrome*: autosomal dominant disorder due to *RASA1* mutations; presents with multiple small CMs ± AVM(s) and sometimes *Parkes–Weber syndrome* (limb overgrowth associated with an AVM).

For further information see Chs. 103 and 104. From *Dermatology, Third Edition*.

INFANTILE HEMANGIOMAS AND VASCULAR MALFORMATIONS

86 | Ulcers

- An ulcer is defined as a wound with loss of the entire epidermis plus dermal tissue, sometimes extending as deep as the subcutis.
- The most common types of leg ulcers – venous, arterial, and neuropathic – as well as pressure ulcers, lymphedema, and an approach to wound healing are reviewed (see below); additional physical, inflammatory, infectious, metabolic, and neoplastic causes of leg ulcers are outlined in Fig. 86.1.
- Features to consider in the history and physical examination of patients with a leg ulcer are presented in Table 86.1, and routine laboratory testing often includes a CBC, ESR, and blood glucose and serum albumin levels; microbial cultures, evaluation for hypercoagulability (see Table 18.5), and additional studies depend on the clinical setting.
- Ulcers with atypical features or a lack of response to appropriate therapy should be re-evaluated, with expansion of the DDx and

consideration of a skin biopsy (preferably including the ulcer margin and bed) to exclude less common etiologies, such as SCC, vasculitis, and fungal or mycobacterial infections (via tissue culture).

Venous Ulcers

- Venous hypertension and insufficiency represent the most common causes of chronic leg ulcers.
- Prevalence increases with age, and risk factors include female sex, obesity, pregnancy, prolonged standing, and family history of venous insufficiency; hypercoagulability can be a contributing factor, especially in patients with a history of deep vein thrombosis or livedoid vasculopathy (Fig. 86.3; see Chapter 18).
- Ulcers tend to have irregular borders and a yellow fibrinous base, with a predilection for the area above the medial malleolus

POINTS TO INCLUDE IN THE HISTORY AND PHYSICAL EXAMINATION OF PATIENTS WITH A LEG ULCER	
History	**Physical Examination**

• Onset and clinical course of ulcer
• Symptoms, including those of vascular disease or neuropathy
• Alleviating factors
• Exacerbating factors
• Past medical history, e.g. diabetes mellitus, atherosclerotic cardiovascular disease, AI-CTD
• Family history
• Medications, topical and systemic
• Personal habits (e.g. smoking, alcohol intake)
	General, emphasizing the following:
	• Ulcer characteristics
	  – Location and size
	  – Morphology, including depth, shape, border, and base
	  – Surrounding skin, e.g. edema, dermatitis, fibrosis, cellulitis, necrosis
	• Peripheral pulses
	• Capillary refill time
	• Evidence of peripheral neuropathy
	• Deep tendon reflexes

Table 86.1 Points to include in the history and physical examination of patients with a leg ulcer. *Adapted from Kanj LF, Phillips TJ. Management of leg ulcers. Fitpatrick's J. Clin. Dermatol. 1994;Sept/Oct:52–60.*

CAUSES OF LEG ULCERS

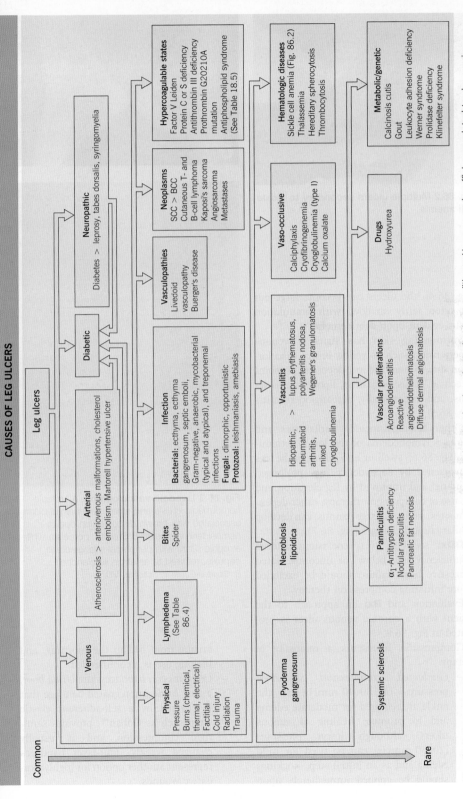

Fig. 86.1 Causes of leg ulcers. Patients with Behçet's disease can also develop leg ulcers due to vasculitis and/or venous insufficiency related to deep vein thromboses. Erosive pustular dermatosis is another occasional cause of leg ulcers. Hydroxyurea-induced leg ulcers are exceedingly painful, surrounded by atrophic skin, and often located on the malleolus or tibial crest.

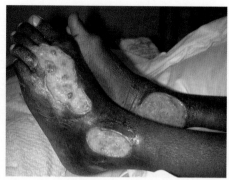

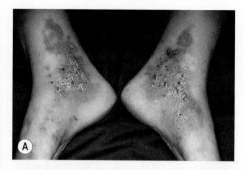

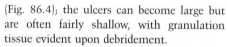

Fig. 86.2 Multiple ulcers secondary to sickle cell anemia.

(Fig. 86.4); the ulcers can become large but are often fairly shallow, with granulation tissue evident upon debridement.

• Surrounding skin has signs of venous hypertension such as yellow-brown discoloration due to hemosiderin deposits, pinpoint petechiae, stasis dermatitis, lipodermatosclerosis, and, occasionally, acroangiodermatitis (Fig. 86.5).

• Other findings include varicosities and edema > lymphedema of the lower extremities (Fig. 86.6); swelling and aching of the legs is worsened by dependency (e.g. prolonged standing) and improved by leg elevation and the use of compression therapy; other dependent sites, such as a large pannus, can develop similar clinical changes (Fig. 86.7).

• **DDx:** see Fig. 86.1; coexistent arterial insufficiency (see below) or uncompensated congestive heart failure should be excluded before initiating compression therapy.

• Evaluation and **Rx:** an approach to the patient with a chronic venous ulcer is presented in Fig. 86.8.

• Compression represents a mainstay of therapy.

  – *Graduated compression stockings*: pressures of 30–40 mmHg at the ankle are required for moderate edema and to promote healing of venous ulcers, although lower pressures (20–30 mmHg) can be used for mild edema and as an initial step; stockings should be applied immediately upon

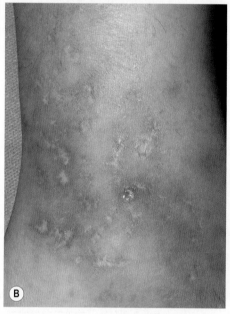

Fig. 86.3 Livedoid vasculopathy. **A** Multiple hemorrhagic crusts and small, very painful ulcers associated with brown discoloration due to hemosiderin deposits. **B** Stellate, porcelain-white atrophic scars with peripheral telangiectatic papules, referred to as atrophie blanche. *B, Courtesy, Julie V. Schaffer, MD.*

arising from bed in the morning, and lifelong use is recommended.

  – *Compression bandages*: the *Unna boot*, a zinc oxide-impregnated bandage that is covered by a self-adherent elastic wrap such as Coban™, provides semi-rigid compression and is usually changed weekly; four-layer bandages represent another option for highly exudative wounds.

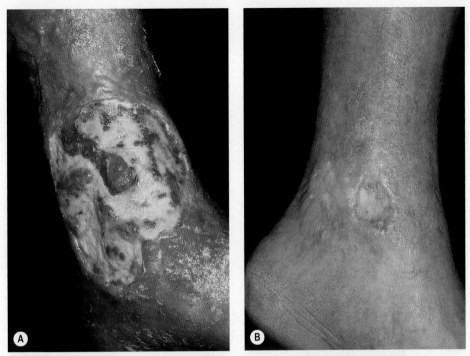

Fig. 86.4 Venous ulcers over the medial malleolus. A Granulation tissue is evident in ~15% of the ulcer bed. Note the surrounding stasis dermatitis with erythema, crusting, and scaling as well as scarring. **B** Induration due to lipodermatosclerosis, hemosiderin deposition, and atrophie blanche scars are present in the surrounding skin. *B, Courtesy, Jean L. Bolognia, MD.*

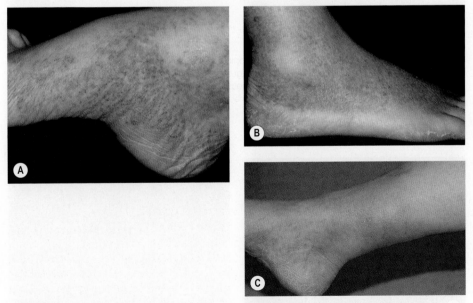

Fig. 86.5 Associated findings in patients with venous hypertension and insufficiency.
A Venulectasias of the instep. **B** Brown discoloration of the foot and ankle due to hemosiderin deposits within dermal macrophages in addition to hyperpigmentation. Note the cutoff at Wallace's line. **C** Lipodermatosclerosis with violet-brown discoloration, tenderness, and induration that typically begins above the medial malleolus. *A, B, Courtesy, Jean L. Bolognia, MD; C, Courtesy, Kalman Watsky, MD.*
Continued

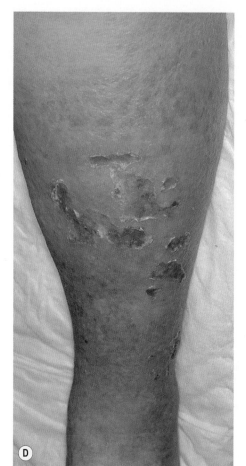

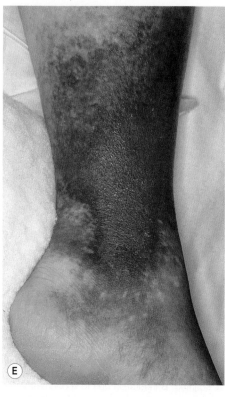

Fig. 86.5 *Continued* **D** Stasis dermatitis and chronic lipodermatosclerosis with serous crusts and the 'inverted champagne bottle' or 'bowling pin' configuration. **E** Acroangiodermatitis (pseudo-Kaposi's sarcoma). Violaceous plaque in a patient with venous hypertension. Histologically, these lesions can resemble Kaposi's sarcoma. *D, Courtesy, Ariela Hafner, MD, and Eli Sprecher, MD.*

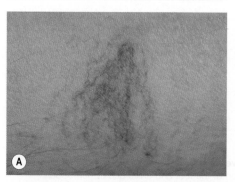

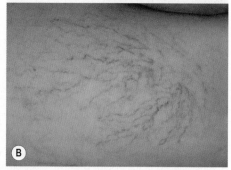

Fig. 86.6 Venous abnormalities of the lower extremity. A Venulectasias and a few reticular varicosities at the site of a perforator vein. **B** Reticular varicosities; note the blue-green color. *Courtesy, Jean L. Bolognia, MD. Continued*

838

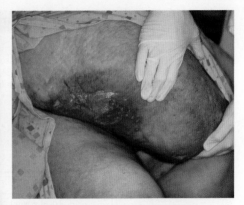

Fig. 86.7 Lymphedema, lipodermato-sclerosis, and chronic ulceration of the dependent portion of the pannus. The changes are similar to those that can be seen on the distal lower extremities.

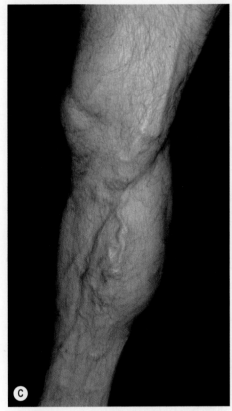

Fig. 86.6 *Continued* **C** Larger saphenous varicosities may also be evident. *Courtesy, Jean L. Bolognia, MD.*

Arterial Ulcers

• Peripheral arterial disease (PAD), a manifestation of atherosclerosis, is present in up to 25% of patients with leg ulcers; risk factors include cigarette smoking, diabetes mellitus, dyslipidemia, and hypertension; ulceration is often precipitated by trauma.

• Well-demarcated, round, 'punched out' ulcers with a dry necrotic base; occur primarily on the distal lower extremities, favoring the toes and sites of pressure.

• Surrounding skin is typically hairless, shiny, and atrophic (Fig. 86.9).

• Other findings include cool feet, weak or absent peripheral pulses, prolonged capillary refill time (>3–4 seconds), pallor ± pain upon leg elevation (45° for 1 minute), and dependent rubor; patients may report pain induced by ambulation and relieved by rest.

• **DDx:** other causes of ulcers in patients with PAD include cholesterol emboli (Fig.

86.10), diffuse dermal angiomatosis (painful violaceous plaques with central ulceration), and Buerger's disease (thrombangiitis obliterans; inflammatory and vaso-occlusive disorder in smokers affecting upper and lower extremities); patients with co-existing diabetes mellitus may have overlapping features (see below).

• Evaluation: the ankle–brachial index (ABI) is used to screen for PAD (Table 86.2); additional assessment may include duplex ultrasonography, CT angiography, and magnetic resonance angiography.

• **Rx:** surgical or endovascular restoration of blood flow; wound care (see below), but with avoidance of sharp debridement.

Neuropathic (Mal Perforans) and Diabetic Ulcers

• Diabetes mellitus confers a 15–25% lifetime risk of foot ulcers, ~15% of which eventuate in an amputation; diabetic neuropathy is the major cause of these ulcers, although ischemia, venous hypertension, and infection often contribute to pathogenesis.

• *Sensory* neuropathy leads to unrecognized foot trauma, *motor* neuropathy leads to altered biomechanics and structural deformities that increase mechanical stress, and *autonomic* neuropathy leads to both arteriovenous shunting that decreases perfusion and reduced sweating that predisposes to dryness and fissuring.

APPROACH TO THE TREATMENT OF CHRONIC VENOUS ULCERS

Confirm reflux – duplex ultrasound scan
Exclude arterial disease – ABI >0.8*
Screen for neuropathy – nylon monofilament testing

↓

Treatment

• Compression
• Leg elevation

+

Local wound care, including:
• Dressings
• Debridement (autolytic, chemical, and/or mechanical)
• Treat surrounding stasis dermatitis if present
• Antimicrobial therapy, as needed (topical or systemic)
Tetanus booster vaccination

Healing

Non-healing

Consider venous surgery if superficial reflux present

Consider skin constructs, pinch grafts

Reconsider the diagnosis, including possible biopsy (see Fig. 86.1)

*May be falsely high in diabetics
ABI, ankle brachial index

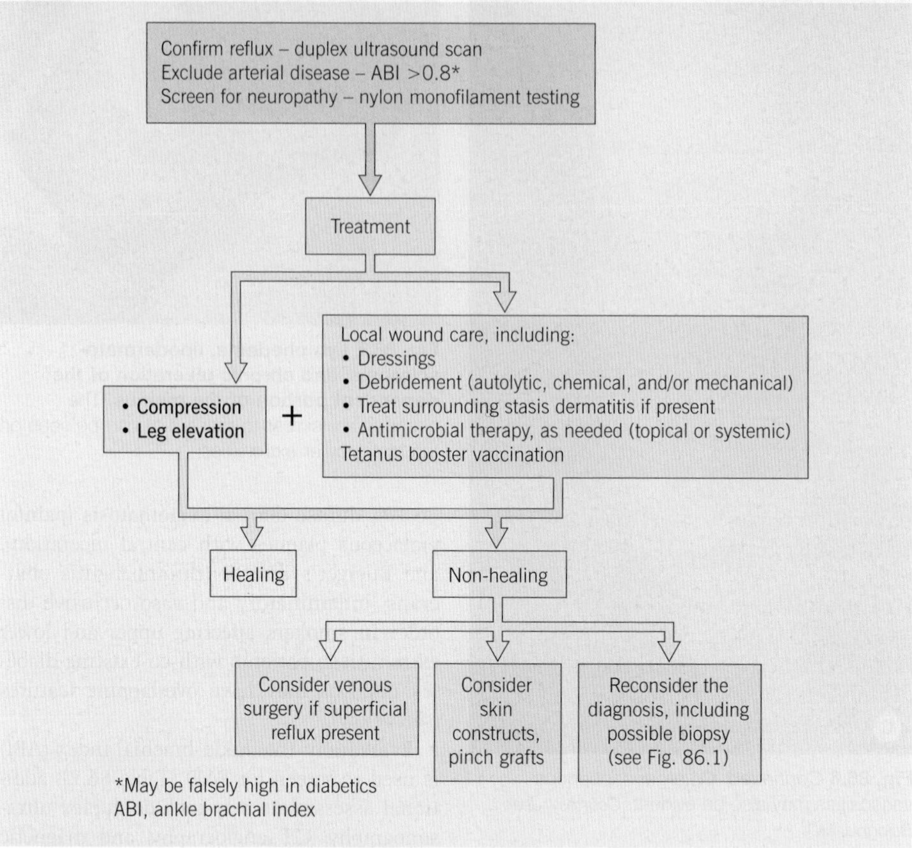

Fig. 86.8 Approach to the treatment of chronic venous ulcers. *Courtesy, Tania Phillips, MD.*

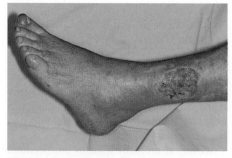

Fig. 86.9 Arterial ulcer. The punched-out appearance and surrounding smooth shiny skin are common features. *Courtesy, Ariela Hafner, MD, and Eli Sprecher, MD.*

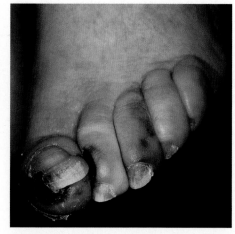

Fig. 86.10 Cholesterol emboli. Ischemia of the toes and necrosis with early ulcer formation.

DETERMINATION AND INTERPRETATION OF THE ANKLE–BRACHIAL INDEX (ABI)

- With the patient in a supine position, the systolic blood pressure is measured in the:
  - Brachial arteries (right and left)
  - Dorsalis pedis and posterior tibial arteries (right and left)
- The ABI is determined by:

$$\frac{\text{the highest of the systolic pressures from the dorsalis pedis or posterior tibial arteries}}{\text{the higher of the brachial artery systolic pressures}}$$

- Interpretation of the ABI:
  0.91–1.30 = normal range
  >1.30 = suggests incompressible tibial arteries due to medial calcification (diabetes mellitus, chronic renal insufficiency)
  <0.9 = indicative of peripheral artery disease (PAD)
      0.41–0.90 = mild to moderate PAD
      0.00–0.40 = severe PAD

Table 86.2 Determination and interpretation of the ankle–brachial index (ABI).

- Neuropathic ulcers are typically 'punched out' with a hyperkeratotic rim, arising in a background of callused skin; they are usually located on pressure points and over bony prominences (e.g. metatarsal heads, heels, great toes) (Fig. 86.11).
- Other findings include decreased sensation due to peripheral neuropathy and sometimes foot deformities (e.g. hammer toes, Charcot foot).
- Evaluation: neurologic examination using nylon monofilament to test sensation ± nerve conduction studies/electromyography and determination of the ABI (see Table 86.2); assessment for infection utilizing laboratory studies (e.g. CBC, ESR/C-reactive protein), wound cultures (tissue from biopsy is higher yield than swabs), and imaging to exclude osteomyelitis (e.g. radiographs [low sensitivity], MRI) as indicated by clinical suspicion.
- **Rx:** wound care with debridement of necrotic material and the hyperkeratotic rim, eradication of infection, and mechanical offloading (e.g. bed rest, wheelchair, crutches, total contact casting, felted foam, orthotic shoes); additional options include hyperbaric oxygen and becaplermin gel (recombinant platelet-derived growth factor [PDGF]); patient instructions are provided in Table 86.3.

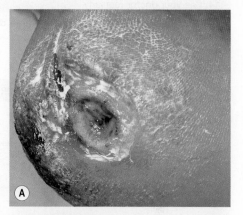

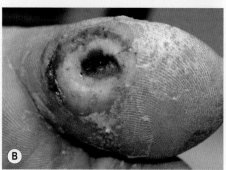

Fig. 86.11 Neuropathic ulcers in patients with diabetes mellitus and peripheral neuropathy. Common locations are the plantar surface of the heel **(A)** and the great toe **(B)**. Note the thick rim of callus. *A, Courtesy, Ariela Hafner, MD, and Eli Sprecher, MD.*

Pressure (Decubitis) Ulcers (Bed Sores)

- Occur as a consequence of prolonged immobility, affecting ~10% of hospitalized

INSTRUCTIONS FOR THE PATIENT WITH A DIABETIC OR NEUROPATHIC ULCER

1. Stop smoking, control blood sugar levels, and lose weight if overweight.
2. Inspect feet daily for blisters, scratches, and red areas. If your vision is impaired, get someone to do this for you.
3. Wash your feet daily in warm water. Dry carefully between the toes.
4. Apply petroleum jelly to dry areas of skin but not between the toes.
5. Always test water temperature before bathing.
6. Inspect the insides of your shoes before putting them on.
7. Do not remove corns or apply strong chemicals to your feet.
8. Cut nails straight across.
9. See your podiatrist regularly.
10. Wear properly fitting shoes. New shoes should be worn for 1–2 hours daily only. Check your feet for red spots afterwards.
11. Avoid open-toed sandals and shoes with pointed toes.
12. Never walk barefoot.
13. If you develop any breaks in the skin or blisters, inform your doctor.
14. See your doctor regularly.

Table 86.3 Instructions for the patient with a diabetic or neuropathic ulcer. *Adapted with permission from Levin M, O'Neal ME.* The Diabetic Foot. *St Louis: Mosby, 1988.*

COMMON SITES FOR PRESSURE ULCERS

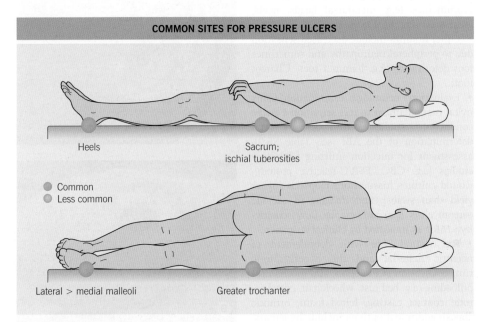

Heels

Sacrum; ischial tuberosities

● Common
◐ Less common

Lateral > medial malleoli

Greater trochanter

Fig. 86.12 Common sites for pressure ulcers.

patients and ~25% of nursing home residents; other risk factors include sensory deficits, older age, and poor nutrition.

• Soft tissues are compressed between a bony prominence (e.g. sacrum, ischial tuberosity; Figs. 86.12 and 86.13) and an external surface; pathogenic factors include continuous pressure, shearing forces/friction, and moisture (e.g. perspiration, urine, feces).

• Classified according to a four-stage system (Fig. 86.14); ulcers do not necessarily progress sequentially through these stages, and

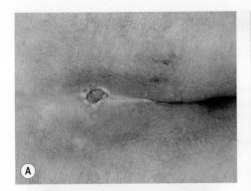

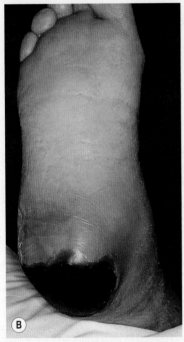

Fig. 86.13 Pressure ulcers. A Stage III ulcer over the sacrum. **B** Black eschar on the heel due to pressure necrosis. *A, Courtesy, Ariela Hafner, MD, and Eli Sprecher, MD.*

extensive deep tissue damage may initially have few superficial manifestations.

• Prevention: frequent position changes together with use of softer surfaces (e.g. containing foam, air, or liquid) and devices (e.g. pillows, foam wedges) to relieve pressure; optimize nutrition.

• **Rx:** relief of pressure and wound care – for example, utilizing an occlusive dressing (see below); stage IV ulcers may require surgical intervention.

CAUSES OF SECONDARY LYMPHEDEMA
Infections
• Recurrent cellulitis and lymphangitis • Parasitic infections (e.g. filariasis)
Cancer-Related, Including Iatrogenic
• Lymph node dissection (e.g. for melanoma or breast cancer) or other surgical excisions (e.g. mastectomy) • Radiation injury • Malignant obstruction (e.g. by lymphoma or Kaposi's sarcoma)
Inflammatory
• Acne vulgaris and rosacea (midfacial) • Granulomatous disorders (e.g. anogenital in Crohn's disease)
Other
• Obesity • Podoconiosis (exposure to mineral microparticles in volcanic soils)

Table 86.4 Causes of secondary lymphedema.

Lymphedema

• Lymphedema is the interstitial accumulation of lymphatic fluid due to reduced drainage by lymphatic vessels.

• Divided into *primary* forms due to abnormal lymphatic development (see Chapter 85) and *secondary* forms due to lymphatic damage or obstruction (Table 86.4).

• Usually presents as chronic, painless swelling and heaviness of an extremity (leg > arm), typically beginning distally (e.g. on the dorsal foot) and progressing proximally (Fig. 86.15); initially pitting, but becomes indurated and nonpitting as fibrosis develops; prone to ulceration and often worsens following secondary infections.

• *Elephantiasis nostras verrucosa* is a complication of severe lymphedema characterized by massive enlargement of the affected area, marked fibrosis, and verrucous epidermal changes with a mossy, cobblestoned appearance (Fig. 86.16).

• **DDx:** edema secondary to venous insufficiency, lipedema (bilateral lower extremity swelling that spares the feet, almost exclusively affecting women; Fig. 86.17), obesity-associated lymphedematous mucinosis.

NATIONAL PRESSURE ULCER ADVISORY PANEL CLASSIFICATION OF PRESSURE ULCERS

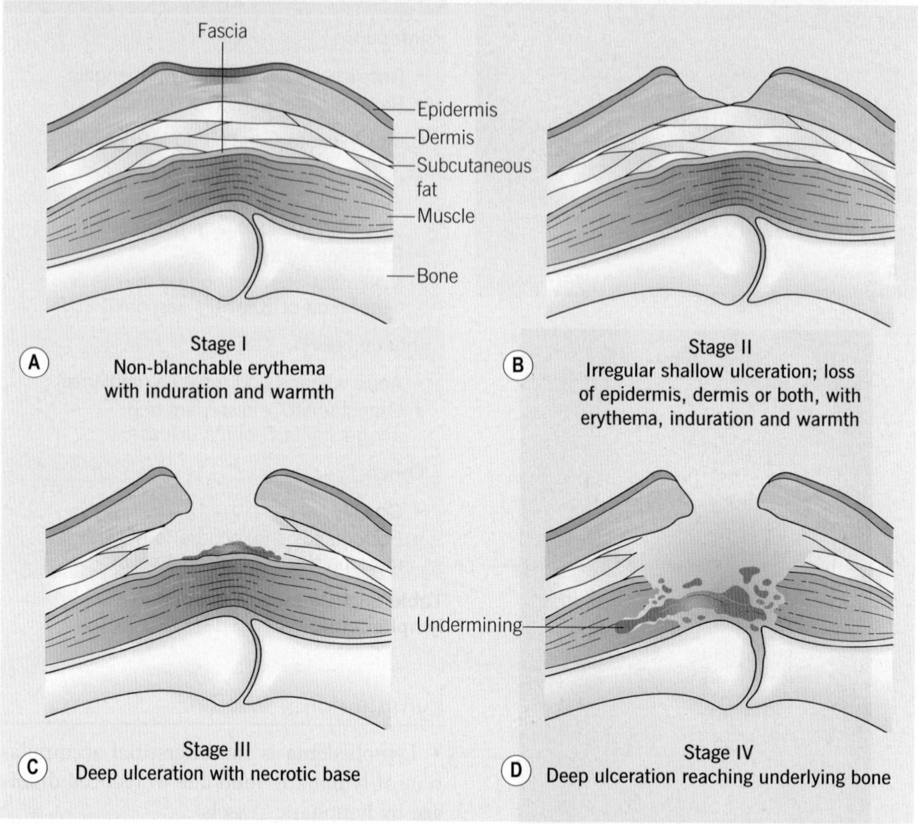

Fig. 86.14 National Pressure Ulcer Advisory Panel classification of pressure ulcers. A Stage I: nonblanchable erythema of intact skin. This lesion is the heralding sign of impending skin ulceration. For darker-skinned individuals, other signs may be indicators and include warmth, edema, discoloration of the skin, and induration. **B** Stage II: partial-thickness skin loss involving the epidermis, dermis, or both. This superficial lesion presents as an abrasion, blister, or shallow crater. **C** Stage III: full-thickness skin loss, in which subcutaneous tissue is damaged or necrotic and may extend down into, but not including, the underlying fascia. This deep lesion presents as a crater and sometimes involves adjacent tissue. **D** Stage IV: full-thickness skin loss and extensive tissue necrosis, destruction to muscle, bone, or supporting structures such as a tendon or joint capsule. Undermining or sinus tracts can be present.

• **Rx:** difficult; compression (e.g. garments, wrapping), pneumatic pumps and massage to decrease accumulation of lymph; treatment of secondary infections.

General Approach to Wound Healing

• In a patient with an ulcer, modifiable local and systemic factors that may impair wound healing should be addressed, including deleterious mechanical forces, inadequate perfusion, and poor nutritional or immune status.

• A moist wound environment such as that provided by a semipermeable 'occlusive' dressing enhances healing by stimulating collagen synthesis, promoting angiogenesis, encouraging re-epithelialization, and providing autolytic debridement.

• The choice of dressing depends on the wound type and amount of exudate (Table 86.5), and it may be helpful to protect the

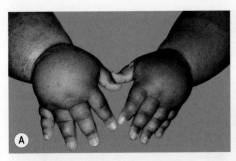

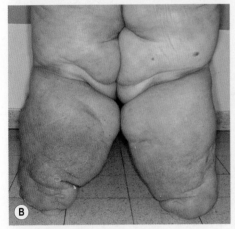

Fig. 86.15 Lymphedema. A Primary lymphedema of the upper extremities due to Milroy disease (see Chapter 85). **B** Lymphedema of the lower extremities secondary to morbid obesity and associated with myxedema. *B, Courtesy, Ariela Hafner, MD, and Eli Sprecher, MD.*

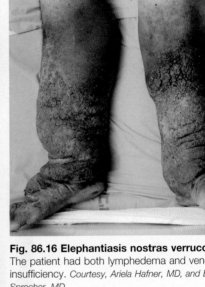

Fig. 86.16 Elephantiasis nostras verrucosa. The patient had both lymphedema and venous insufficiency. *Courtesy, Ariela Hafner, MD, and Eli Sprecher, MD.*

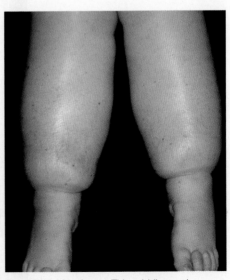

Fig. 86.17 Lipedema. This middle-aged woman has bilateral 'stovepipe' enlargement of the legs and minimal involvement of the feet. Note the sharp demarcation between normal and abnormal tissue at the ankle, referred to as the 'cuff sign.' *Courtesy, Jean L. Bolognia, MD.*

skin around the wound with a thin coat of ointment to prevent maceration; the frequency of dressing changes is based on their absorbency as well as the amount of exudate.

• Debridement of nonviable tissue from the wound bed also promotes healing.

– *Autolytic debridement* utilizing the body's own proteolytic enzymes is provided by moist retentive dressings; it is best suited for non-infected wounds with minimal debris.

– *Mechanical debridement* (e.g. 'sharp' with surgical instruments, wet-to-dry [can disrupt viable tissue]) may be helpful for wounds with large amounts of necrotic and/or infected tissue.

– *Enzymatic debridement* utilizes topical proteolytic enzyme preparations such as collagenase and papain-urea.

TYPES OF WOUND DRESSINGS

Dressing Type	Properties	Disadvantages	Indications

Gauzes	• Good absorption
	• Can be impregnated with:
	  – NaCl to become highly absorbent, discourage bacterial overgrowth, and prevent formation of excess granulation tissue
	  – Petrolatum so less drying and adherent, but then less absorbent
	  – Iodine or silver as an antiseptic
		• Adhere to wound bed and promote desiccation
		• Can cause pain and trauma, including disruption of epithelium, upon removal
			• Wet wounds with heavy exudate
			• As a secondary dressing

Films	• Thin polyurethane membranes • Maintain a moist environment • Semipermeable (only to vapors, not to liquids) • Transparency enables wound visualization	• Non-absorbent • Can cause maceration of surrounding skin if applied to wounds with heavy exudate	• Wounds with minimal exudate • As a secondary dressing
Hydrogels	• Maintain a moist environment • Promote autolytic debridement • Non-adhesive • Relieve pain	• Can cause maceration of surrounding skin if applied to wounds with heavy exudate	• Wounds with minimal exudate

Hydrocolloids	• Adhesive, occlusive dressings that absorb exudates with the formation of hydrophilic gel • Provide a moist environment	• Not suitable for wounds with heavy exudate or infected wounds • May produce a brown, malodorous gel • May lead to maceration of surrounding skin, and removal can be traumatic	• Wounds with mild to moderate exudate
Alginates	• Fibrous dressings derived from brown seaweed • Highly absorbent and require moisture to function • Ion exchange between calcium in the alginate and sodium in the wound fluid leads to the formation of a moist retentive gel • Hemostatic	• May adhere to dry wounds • May leave fibrous debris in the wound • Can lead to maceration around the wound unless cut to the size of the wound bed	• Wounds with moderate to heavy exudate • Undermined or tunneling wounds
Foams (polyurethane)	• Good absorbance capacity • Nontraumatic upon removal • Provide thermal and shear protection	• Not suitable for dry wounds • Maceration around wound possible	• Wounds with moderate to heavy exudate
Collagens	• Collagen matrix that physically entraps MMPs and facilitates growth factor activity	• Nonspecific inhibition of MMPs	• Clean, non-infected, recalcitrant chronic wounds

MMPs, matrix metalloproteinases.
Courtesy, Ariela Hafner, MD, and Eli Sprecher, MD.

Table 86.5 Types of wound dressings. A conventional layered dressing usually has three components: (1) a nonadherent, fluid-permeable material that directly contacts the wound; (2) an absorbent layer (e.g. cotton pad or gauze); and (3) an outer wrap. However, some dressings (e.g. hydrocolloids) that are waterproof and adhere directly do not require secondary layers.

- *Maggot debridement* can be considered for recalcitrant ulcers with excessive necrotic tissue.

• Bacterial colonization occurs in all chronic wounds and must be distinguished from true soft tissue infection; wounds with clinical evidence of infection (e.g. purulent discharge, surrounding cellulitis) should be cultured and treated with systemic antibiotics (initially broad-spectrum and then adjusted based on sensitivities); topical antimicrobial agents (e.g. dressings containing silver or cadexomer-iodine) can be considered for nonhealing wounds with 'critical colonization' ($>10^6$ colony-forming units of bacteria per gram of tissue).

• In addition to wound care, treatment of ulcers should be directed at the underlying cause (see above).

• Other adjuncts to wound care may include topical growth factors (e.g. PDGF), topical negative pressure therapy, and tissue-engineered skin equivalents.

For further information see Ch. 105. From *Dermatology, Third Edition*.

Other Vascular Disorders | 87

This chapter covers a range of vascular disorders from livedo reticularis to common vascular ectasias such as venous lakes and telangiectasias. Additional disorders characterized by proliferation of blood vessels are covered in Chapters 85 (infantile hemangiomas and vascular malformations) and 94 (vascular neoplasms).

Livedo Reticularis

• Blue-violet netlike pattern that reflects an increase in deoxygenated blood within the venous plexus of the skin (Fig. 87.1); this increase can be due to a number of causes, including vasospasm of arterioles supplying the skin and sluggish flow due to hypercoagulability or luminal pathology.

• A common physiologic vasospastic response to cold that resolves with rewarming, as well as a sign of a number of systemic diseases, from severe atherosclerosis to systemic lupus erythematosus (Table 87.1; Fig. 87.2).

• Most commonly observed on the legs but may be more widespread, especially in the setting of systemic diseases.

• **DDx:** early phase of erythema ab igne; viral exanthems (e.g. erythema infectiosum), retiform purpura and necrosis due to more

ANATOMICAL BASIS FOR THE DEVELOPMENT OF LIVEDO RETICULARIS

Zone of venous predominance | Zone of arterial predominance

Venous drainage

Arterial cone

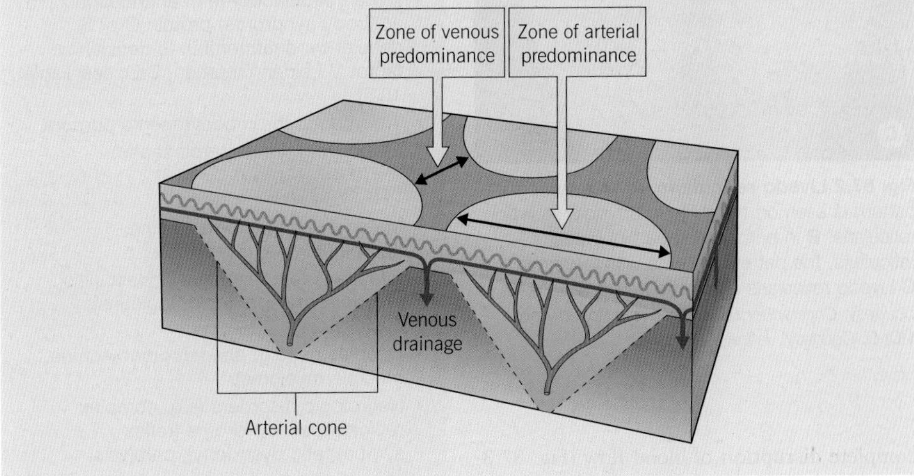

Fig. 87.1 Anatomic basis for the development of livedo reticularis. At the edges of arterial cones, the venous plexus is prominent. An increase in deoxygenated blood within this plexus (due to a decrease in blood flow into or through the skin or impeded drainage of blood) leads to livedo reticularis. If disease of the feeding arteriole is suspected, a wedge biopsy of the central cone can be performed.

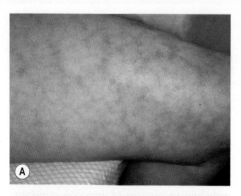

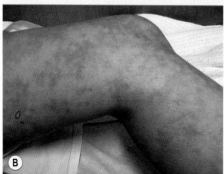

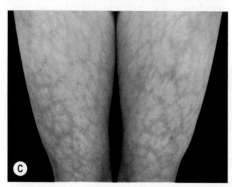

Fig. 87.2 Livedo reticularis. A An even, netlike pattern is seen on the thigh in physiologic livedo reticularis. **B** In primary (idiopathic) livedo reticularis, the pattern persists with rewarming. **C** Livedo reticularis in a patient with SLE. *A, B, Courtesy, Christopher Baker, MD, and Robert Kelly, MD; C, Courtesy, Jeffrey Callen, MD.*

complete disruption of blood flow (Fig. 87.3; see Chapter 18); underlying etiologies are outlined in Table 87.1.

• **Rx:** can improve with treatment of an underlying systemic disorder; no treatment currently available for the idiopathic form.

CAUSES OF LIVEDO RETICULARIS

Congenital Livedo Reticularis

Cutis marmorata telangiectatica congenita

Acquired Livedo Reticularis

Vasospasm

- Cutis marmorata/physiologic livedo reticularis (more common in young children)
- Primary (idiopathic) livedo reticularis
- Autoimmune connective tissue diseases (e.g. SLE)
- Raynaud's phenomenon/disease

Vessel Wall Pathology

- Vasculitis (medium-sized arterioles)
  - Cutaneous polyarteritis nodosa (nearly all patients)
  - Systemic polyarteritis nodosa
  - Cryoglobulinemic vasculitis
  - Autoimmune connective tissue-associated vasculitis (e.g. rheumatoid arthritis, SLE, Sjögren's syndrome)
- Calciphylaxis
- Sneddon syndrome
- Livedoid vasculopathy (also intraluminal obstruction)

Intraluminal Pathology

- Increased normal blood components (e.g. thrombocythemia, polycythemia vera)
- Abnormal proteins (e.g. cryoglobulinemia, paraproteinemia; see Chapter 18)
- Hypercoagulability (e.g. antiphospholipid antibody syndrome, protein C or S deficiency, antithrombin III deficiency, factor V Leiden mutation, DIC; see Table 18.5)
- Thrombotic thrombocytopenic purpura
- Emboli (e.g. cholesterol, septic)

Other

- Medications (e.g. amantadine, norepinephrine, interferon)
- Infections (e.g. hepatitis C [vasculitis], *Mycoplasma* spp. [cold agglutins], syphilis)
- Neoplasms (e.g. pheochromocytomas, multiple myeloma)
- Neurologic disorders (e.g. complex regional pain syndrome [reflex sympathetic dystrophy], paralysis)
- Moyamoya disease

DIC, disseminated intravascular coagulation; SLE, systemic lupus erythematosus.

Table 87.1 Causes of livedo reticularis.

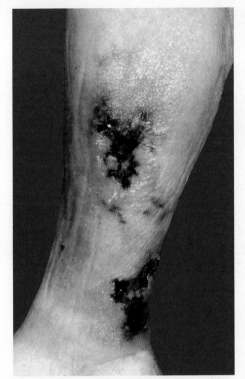

Fig. 87.3 Reticulated purpura and necrosis due to calciphylaxis. These patients can also have patchy areas of livedo reticularis. *Courtesy, Norbert Sepp, MD.*

CAUSES OF FLUSHING
• Physiologic
• Estrogen deficiency (e.g. menopause, tamoxifen)
• Rosacea (also triggered by exogenous agents)
• Exogenous agents
– Alcohol, especially poor metabolizers
– Drugs (e.g. nicotinic acid, nitrates, sildenafil, prostaglandins, disulfiram*, chlorpropamide*, methylphenidate, calcium channel blockers, calcitonin)
– Foods (e.g. spoiled scombroid fish)
– Food additives (e.g. monosodium glutamate, sodium nitrite, sulfites)
• Neurologic disorders
– Anxiety
– Autonomic dysfunction
– Tumors (e.g. hypogonadal pituitary tumors)
– Migraine
– Frey's syndrome (auriculotemporal syndrome)
• Systemic disease
– Carcinoid syndrome (also vascular rosacea-like changes, pellagra, facial edema)**
– Mastocytosis (also red-brown papules, plaques, or nodules)
– Pheochromocytoma (also macular amyloidosis if MEN 2a)
– Medullary carcinoma of the thyroid (also macular amyloidosis if MEN 2a)
– Thyrotoxicosis (also hyperhidrosis)
– POEMS syndrome
– Pancreatic tumors (e.g. VIPomas)

*With alcohol intake.
**Midgut tumors with liver metastases, type III gastric tumors, and bronchial tumors.
POEMS, polyneuropathy, organomegaly, endocrinopathy, M-protein (monoclonal gammopathy), skin changes; VIP, vasoactive intestinal polypeptide.

Table 87.2 Causes of flushing.

Flushing

• Exaggerated physiologic dilatation of superficial cutaneous blood vessels that can be triggered by a number of factors, including heat, spicy foods, hot drinks, and anxiety; the resultant erythema of the skin is episodic and transient and may be accompanied by sweating.

• Common etiologies are menopause, other causes of estrogen deficiency (e.g. tamoxifen), rosacea, and medications (e.g. nicotinic acid, nitrates); uncommon causes are carcinoid syndrome, mastocytosis, and pheochromocytoma (Table 87.2).

• Sites of involvement, primarily the face > ears, neck, and chest, are both visible and characterized by greater vasculature capacitance; an approach to the evaluation of a patient with flushing is outlined in Table 87.3.

• **Rx:** avoidance of exacerbating factors; addressing any underlying systemic disorder; for physiologic flushing – propranolol, nadolol, or clonidine; for menopausal 'hot flashes' – hormone replacement therapy, SSRIs, or clonidine; laser therapy can address telangiectasias that may result from repeated episodes of flushing.

CLINICAL APPROACH TO THE EVALUATION OF FLUSHING

1. Identify provocative factors
  • Direct questioning
  • Patient diary (food, medications, activities)

2. Check for associated symptoms
  • Sweating
  • Urticaria
  • Diarrhea
  • Bronchospasm

3. Investigation
Not required in all cases
Indicated if flushing:
  • Of sudden or recent onset
  • Severe
  • Associated with systemic symptoms
Investigations to consider:
  • Complete blood count with differential and platelets
  • Thyroid function tests
  • Serum tryptase, histamine, and/or chromogranin A levels; plasma free metanephrines
  • 24-hour urine collection for:
    – Serotonin metabolites such as 5-hydroxyindole acetic acid (5-HIAA)
    – Fractionated metanephrines
    – Histamine metabolites such as methylimidazole acetic acid (MIAA)
    – CT/MRI scans; somatostatin receptor scintigraphy (using radiolabeled analogue of somatostatin)

4. Elimination   • Exclude suspected drugs and food additives

Table 87.3 Clinical approach to the evaluation of flushing.

Erythromelalgia

• Erythema, warmth, and painful burning sensation of the distal extremities (lower > upper) that is usually episodic but may be constant (Fig. 87.4); relieved by cooling and precipitated by warming, with attacks often beginning in the evening.

• Three major forms: (1) associated with thrombocythemia, (2) primary or 'idiopathic' that can be familial, and (3) associated with underlying disorders other than thrombocythemia (e.g. myelodysplasia, SLE); in some families, gain-of-function mutations in *SCN9A*, which encodes a subunit of a voltage-gated sodium channel, have been identified

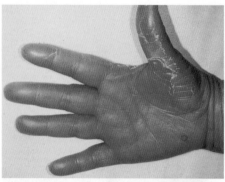

Fig. 87.4 Erythromelalgia. Red hot hand with painful burning sensation. *Courtesy, Agustin Aloma, MD.*

and are thought to lead to 'overexcitability' of pain-signaling sensory neurons.

• **DDx:** complex regional pain syndrome (reflex sympathetic dystrophy), peripheral neuropathy, autonomic dysfunction, acrodynia, thromboangiitis obliterans, calcium channel blockers.

• **Rx:** cooling techniques, leg elevation, oral analgesics, topical anesthetics, SSRIs, tricyclic antidepressants, gabapentin, carbamazepine; for those with thrombocythemia, aspirin; for those with *SCN9A* mutations, sodium channel blocking agents (e.g. mexiletine, flecainide).

Telangiectasias

• Permanently dilated superficial cutaneous blood vessels; fine (diameter 0.1–1mm), red to blue-violet in color, and usually fade with pressure (Fig. 87.5).

• Although most commonly seen on the face and on the lower extremities in the settings of photodamage and venous hypertension, respectively, telangiectasias are associated with a number of conditions (Table 87.4) and have several variants (see later).

• **Rx:** fine wire diathermy, injection sclerotherapy (legs), laser or intense pulsed light therapy.

Spider Telangiectasia (Spider Angioma)

• Characterized by a red papule with multiple radiating fine vessels ('legs'); the papular component is the site of the feeding arteriole; usually present as isolated lesions in children but are often multiple when associated with

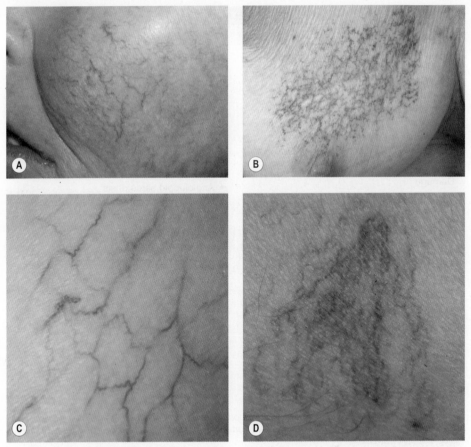

Fig. 87.5 Telangiectasias. A Sun-induced telangiectasias on the cheek. **B** Prominent telangiectasias on the breast following radiation therapy. Note the overall rectangular configuration. **C** Fine blue-violet telangiectasias of the leg. **D** Venulectasias of the leg, which have a larger diameter (1–2 mm). The latter are a reflection of venous hypertension. *A, B, Courtesy, Christopher Baker, MD, and Robert Kelly, MD. C, D, Courtesy, Jean L. Bolognia, MD.*

hyperestrogenemia, e.g. in the setting of pregnancy or hepatic cirrhosis in men.
• Usually develop in otherwise healthy women and children, with the most common locations being the face, neck, chest, and hands (Fig. 87.6).

Generalized Essential Telangiectasia

• Broad areas composed of multiple linear telangiectasias that vary in color from red to purple; involvement is often symmetrical and usually begins on the ankles, primarily of adult women; over time, there is typically proximal spread.
• Although these linear telangiectasias can become quite extensive, the disorder remains a cosmetic one, i.e. there are no associated systemic manifestations.
• **DDx:** cutaneous collagenous vasculopathy (similar clinical appearance but central distribution and perivascular deposits of type IV collagen histologically); initially, telangiectasias due to venous hypertension.

Hereditary Hemorrhagic Telangiectasia (Osler–Weber–Rendu Disease)

• Autosomal dominant disorder due to mutations in several genes, particularly the two that encode endoglin and ALK-1, both of which are TGF-β receptors expressed in the vascular endothelium.

CAUSES OF TELANGIECTASIAS

Primary

- Spider telangiectasias (also associated with estrogen excess) (Fig. 87.6)
- Hereditary benign telangiectasia*
- Costal fringe
- Angioma serpiginosum (Fig. 87.7)
- Unilateral nevoid telangiectasia (Fig. 87.8)
- Generalized essential telangiectasia
- Cutaneous collagenous vasculopathy

Secondary to Physical Changes or Damage

- Photodamage (Fig. 87.5A)
- Post radiation therapy (Fig. 87.5B)
- Traumatic
- Venous hypertension (Fig. 87.5C,D)

Skin Disease

- Telangiectatic rosacea (see Chapter 30)
- Incipient or involuted infantile hemangiomas (see Figs. 85.2 and 85.3)

Hormonal/Metabolic

- Estrogen-related
  - Liver disease
  - Pregnancy
  - Exogenous estrogens
- Corticosteroids

Systemic Conditions

- Carcinoid syndrome
- Mastocytosis (telangiectasia macularis eruptiva perstans) (see Fig. 96.6)
- Autoimmune connective tissue diseases
  - Lupus erythematosus
  - Dermatomyositis (see Fig. 34.3)
  - Systemic sclerosis (see Fig. 35.6)
- Mycosis fungoides, including poikilodermatous
- B-cell lymphomas
- Angiolupoid sarcoidosis
- GVHD (in the context of poikiloderma)
- HIV infection (anterior chest)

Congenital Malformations and Genodermatoses**

- Cutis marmorata telangiectatica congenita
- Hereditary hemorrhagic telangiectasia (Fig. 87.9)
- Ataxia–telangiectasia (see Fig. 49.1)
- Bloom syndrome (see Chapter 73)
- Goltz syndrome (in Blaschko's lines)

*Childhood onset of multiple punctate, linear, or arborizing telangiectasias favoring the sun-exposed areas of the face and upper extremities; the vermilion lips and palate are occasionally affected, but there is no visceral involvement.
**Not exhaustive list.

Table 87.4 Causes of telangiectasias.

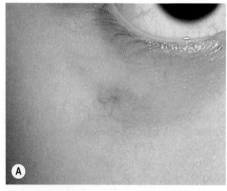 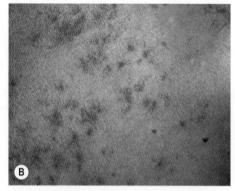

Fig. 87.6 Spider telangiectasias. A Central red papule representing the feeding arteriole with radiating telangiectatic 'legs' on the cheek of a young child. **B** Multiple lesions in a jaundiced patient with liver disease. *A, Courtesy, Phillip Bekhor, MD; B, Courtesy, Ronald Rapini, MD.*

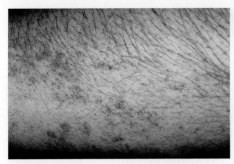

Fig. 87.7 Angioma serpiginosum. Clusters of dark red puncta on the arm in a serpiginous pattern. This disorder initially favors a single extremity, usually in a girl, and may be confused with a pigmented purpuric eruption.

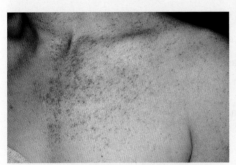

Fig. 87.8 Unilateral nevoid telangiectasia. Discrete telangiectasias in a unilateral, segmental distribution pattern. This is a common location. *Courtesy, Robert Hartman, MD.*

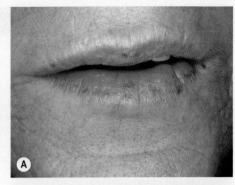

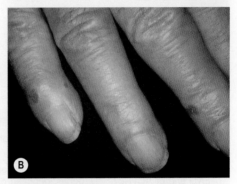

Fig. 87.9 Hereditary hemorrhagic telangiectasia (Osler–Weber–Rendu disease). The majority of lesions are papular, but occasionally they resemble the mat telangiectasias observed in systemic sclerosis. *Courtesy, Irwin Braverman, MD.*

• The vascular lesions are actually arteriovenous malformations and are found in the skin, mucous membranes, GI tract, CNS, and other visceral organs (e.g. lung, liver); the disorder most often initially presents as recurrent epistaxis due to involvement of the nasal mucosa, with hemorrhage at other sites usually occurring later in life.

• The oral mucosal lesions (tongue, lips) usually appear during adolescence and predate the cutaneous 'telangiectasias' (face, hands); there is an increase in the overall number of lesions with time (Fig. 87.9).

• Clinical criteria: (1) spontaneous recurrent epistaxis, (2) characteristic mucocutaneous telangiectasias/AVMs, (3) visceral telangiectasias/AVMs, and (4) HHT in a first-degree relative; definite diagnosis if ≥3 criteria and possible/suspected diagnosis if 1 or 2 criteria (especially in children and young adults).

• Evaluation is outlined in Table 87.5.

• **Rx:** laser therapy, diathermy, transcatheter embolotherapy (e.g. for lung AVMs so as to avoid right-to-left shunting and risk of paradoxical embolization), surgical intervention.

Ataxia–Telangiectasia
(See Chapter 49)

• Primary immunodeficiency syndrome inherited in an autosomal recessive manner in which telangiectasias appear on the bulbar conjunctivae during childhood as well as in the head and neck region (eyelids, malar, ears) and antecubital and popliteal fossae.

Venous Lake

• A blue, soft papule that is compressible and, with pressure, both its color and elevation are diminished (Fig. 87.10); represents dilation of superficial blood vessels.

STUDIES RECOMMENDED TO SCREEN FOR SYSTEMIC INVOLVEMENT AND ASSIST IN THE DIAGNOSIS OF HEREDITARY HEMORRHAGIC TELANGIECTASIA (HHT)

Study and Purpose	Frequency	Indication(s)	% of HHT Patients
Transthoracic contrast echocardiography (bubble study) to detect pulmonary AVMs	If initial screening negative, repeat every 5–10 years as well as prior to and following pregnancies	Suspected or confirmed HHT	15–50
Brain MRI with and without gadolinium to detect cerebral AVMs and other vascular malformations	If initial screening negative, repeat at age 18 years	Suspected or confirmed HHT	~25
Hemoglobin and hematocrit levels to detect GI bleeding due to GI AVMs	Yearly after age 35 years	HHT patients	~25
Doppler ultrasonography or triphasic spiral CT of liver to detect hepatic AVMs	If sign or symptoms of heart failure or hepatobiliary disease	HHT patients	30–80
	As a clinical criterion (see text)	Suspected or confirmed HHT	
Genetic analysis of *ENG* and/or *ACVRL1* (then *SMAD4* if negative) of index case	Once unless additional genes identified or improved methodology	Also performed in first-degree relatives of HHT patients or suspected HHT	~75 for *ENG* or *ACVRL1*; 1–3 for *SMAD4*

Table 87.5 Studies recommended to screen for systemic involvement and assist in the diagnosis of hereditary hemorrhagic telangiectasia (HHT).

• Most common sites are vermilion lip > face, ears.

• **Rx:** electrosurgery, vascular laser therapy.

Angiokeratomas

• Dark red to purple papules that represent vascular ectasias; the affected blood vessels are often located in the most superficial portion of the dermis.

• Most commonly occur as multiple lesions on the scrotum or vulva (Fig. 87. 11) or as an isolated lesion on the lower extremity (Fig. 87.12).

• Occasionally, angiokeratomas are grouped (circumscriptum and Mibelli forms) or rarely more widely distributed (diffusum form), especially within the girdle area; the latter form is a cutaneous manifestation of several lysosomal storage disorders (e.g. Fabry disease) (see Chapter 52).

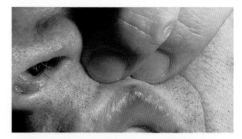

Fig. 87.10 Venous lake on the vermilion lip. This dark blue papule is soft and, with compression, can be emptied of most of its blood content. *Courtesy, Ronald Rapini, MD.*

Nevus anemicus

• Congenital circumscribed area of pale vasoconstriction, often 5–10 cm in diameter and occurs most commonly on the trunk (Fig. 87.13).

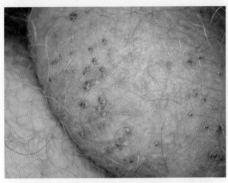

Fig. 87.11 Angiokeratomas of the scrotum. These lesions typically arise along superficial vessels, and similar lesions are seen on the vulva in women. *Courtesy, Christopher Baker, MD, and Robert Kelly, MD.*

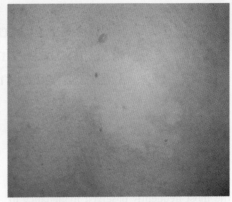

Fig. 87.13 Nevus anemicus. Pale area of vasoconstriction with irregular borders on the back.

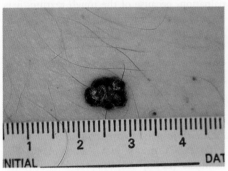

Fig. 87.12 Solitary angiokeratoma. Because of its dark color, this lesion may resemble cutaneous melanoma. Dermoscopy will readily distinguish between these two entities. *Courtesy, Jean L. Bolognia, MD.*

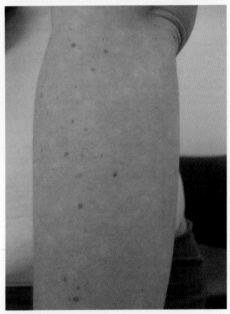

Fig. 87.14 Angiospastic macules (Bier spots). Multiple pale macules due to vasoconstriction within a background of erythema on the forearm.

• The edges are irregular and disappear via diascopy (pressure), allowing distinction from nevus depigmentosus or vitiligo; application of heat or an ice cube accentuates the border as a result of hyperemia of surrounding uninvolved skin.

Angiospastic Macules (Bier Spots)

• Pale macules due to relative vasoconstriction within areas of subtle vascular mottling (Fig. 87.14); as with nevus anemicus, the border disappears with diascopy (pressure); dependency leads to accentuation of lesions due to venous congestion.

• Most commonly observed in young healthy adults with lightly pigmented skin; no effective **Rx**.

For further information see Ch. 106. From *Dermatology, Third Edition.*

88 Actinic Keratosis, Basal Cell Carcinoma, and Squamous Cell Carcinoma

Introduction

• Non-melanoma skin cancer (NMSC) is the most frequently observed malignancy in Caucasians, affecting up to 20% of this population.
• NMSC typically refers to the keratinocyte carcinomas – i.e. basal cell carcinoma (BCC) and squamous cell carcinoma (SCC) – but can also include rare tumors such as Merkel cell carcinoma (see Chapter 95).
• ~75–80% of NMSCs are BCCs, and up to 25% are SCCs.
• The two most important risk factors for developing NMSC are skin phototype (see Appendix) and UV light exposure (Table 88.1).
• The presence of actinic keratoses (AKs) and/or NMSCs increases the likelihood of future NMSCs and cutaneous melanoma, particularly lentigo maligna; such persons require lifelong surveillance via total body skin examination (TBSE).

Actinic Keratoses (AKs)

• Also referred to as solar keratoses, AKs are considered "precancerous" lesions that have the potential to progress into invasive SCC; estimates of progression vary from a rate of 0.075–0.1% per lesion per year to ~10% over 10 years.
• The atypical keratinocytes are confined to the lower portion of the epidermis (Fig. 88.1).
• AKs are one of the most frequently encountered lesions in clinical practice.
• Occur primarily in sites that have received the greatest amount of cumulative sun exposure (e.g. scalp in bald individuals, face, ears, neck, dorsal forearms and hands, shins); seen primarily in middle-aged to older, fair-skinned individuals.
• Classic presentation is a gritty papule with an erythematous base; the associated scale is usually white to yellow in color and feels rough (Fig. 88.2).
• Common clinical variants: hypertrophic (referred to as HAK [Fig. 88.2C,D]), pigmented, lichenoid, and atrophic (Fig. 88.2B); in actinic cheilitis, there is scaling and roughness of the lower vermilion lip (see Fig. 13.5).
• Dx: usually made by visual inspection and palpation; because of the rough texture, it is sometimes easier to detect lesions via touch.
• AKs have the potential to persist, spontaneously regress, or progress to SCC, but clinically it is difficult to predict which course a given AK will take.
• Clinical clues to progression to invasive SCC and need for biopsy: tenderness, volume (particularly thickness), inflammation, and failure to respond to appropriate therapy.
• **DDx:** SCC *in situ*, BCC, lichen planus-like keratosis (LPLK; see Chapter 89), irritated seborrheic keratosis (SK) or verruca vulgaris, and amelanotic melanoma; for thicker lesions (e.g. HAK), invasive SCC; for lesions on extensor extremities, actinic porokeratosis; occasionally, isolated lesions of psoriasis or seborrheic dermatitis may resemble an AK.
• **Rx:** localized or lesion-targeted treatments are best for an isolated or limited number of lesions; field treatments are best for more numerous or larger lesions (Table 88.2).
• Prevention is possible with broad-spectrum sunscreens and sun avoidance measures.

SCC *In Situ* (Bowen's Disease)

• May arise *de novo* or from a pre-existing AK; sometimes caused by oncogenic strains of human papillomavirus (HPV, e.g. periungual [see Chapter 66]).
• Keratinocyte atypia is seen throughout the entire epidermis (full-thickness) (see Fig. 88.1) and has the potential to progress to

RISK FACTORS FOR THE DEVELOPMENT OF BASAL CELL CARCINOMAS (BCCs) AND SQUAMOUS CELL CARCINOMAS (SCCs)		
RISK FACTORS	**SCC**	**BCC**
Environmental Exposures		
Cumulative/occupational sun exposure	+	
Intermittent/recreational sun exposure		+
Other exposures to UV light (PUVA, tanning beds)	+	+
Ionizing radiation	+	+
Arsenic	+	(+)
Chemicals (e.g. coal tar, polycyclic aromatic hydrocarbons, polychlorinated biphenyls, psoralen [plus UVA], nitrogen mustard, 4,4′-bipyridyl)	+	(+)
HPV	+	
Cigarette smoking	+	
Pigmentary Phenotype		
Fair skin	+	+
Always burns, never tans	+	+
Freckling	+	+
Red hair	+	+
Genetic Syndromes		
Xeroderma pigmentosum	+	+
Oculocutaneous albinism	+	(+)
Epidermodysplasia verruciformis	+	
Dystrophic epidermolysis bullosa (primarily recessive)	+	
Ferguson–Smith syndrome	+	
Muir–Torre syndrome	+*	(+)*
Nevoid basal cell carcinoma syndrome		+
Bazex and Rombo syndromes		+
Predisposing Clinical Settings		
Chronic nonhealing wounds	+	
Long-standing discoid lupus erythematosus, lichen planus (erosive) or lichen sclerosus	+	
Porokeratosis (especially linear)	+	
Nevus sebaceus		+†
Immunosuppression		
Organ transplantation	+	(+)
Other (e.g. chronic lymphocytic leukemia treated with fludarabine, AIDS patients with HPV infection)	+	

*Both SCCs (keratoacanthoma type) and BCCs typically have sebaceous differentiation.
†More often trichoblastomas.
HPV, human papillomavirus.

Table 88.1 Risk factors for the development of basal cell carcinomas (BCCs) and squamous cell carcinomas (SCCs).

THE HISTOPATHOLOGIC SPECTRUM OF ACTINIC KERATOSIS (AK), SCC *IN SITU*, AND INVASIVE SCC

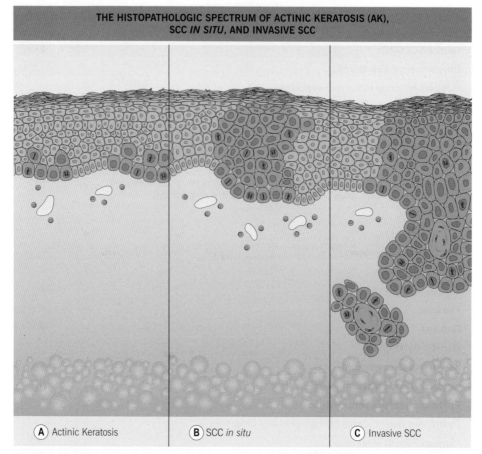

A Actinic Keratosis **B** SCC *in situ* **C** Invasive SCC

Fig. 88.1 The histopathologic spectrum of actinic keratosis (AK), SCC *in situ*, and invasive SCC. A An AK consists of a lower epidermal proliferation of cytologically abnormal keratinocytes; the adnexal epithelium is notably spared. **B** In SCC *in situ*, the atypical keratinocytes occupy the entire epidermis and intraepidermal portion of adnexal structures, without invasion into the dermis. **C** Invasive SCC is distinguished by the extension of the malignant keratinocytes into the dermis. If an invasive SCC is clinically suspected, the biopsy specimen should be deep enough to determine the extent of dermal invasion.

invasive SCC, with an estimated risk of ~3–5% if untreated.

• With the exception of HPV- or arsenic-related SCC *in situ*, the risk factors for and the locations of SCC *in situ* are similar to those for AKs (see above and Table 88.1).

• Clinically presents as an erythematous patch or thin plaque with scale (Fig. 88.3); occasionally, the lesions are pigmented.

• Less common sites (may be related to HPV infection): beard area, periungual (see Figs. 88.3B and 58.7) and subungual, anogenital (now referred to as intraepithelial neoplasia, further qualified by anatomic site [see Chapter

60 and Fig. 88.4]); SCC *in situ* in non-sun-exposed sites may also be related to arsenic exposure.

• Dx: biopsy; dermoscopy may assist in diagnosis (Fig. 88.3C).

• **DDx:** AK, invasive SCC, BCC, LPLK, irritated SK, amelanotic melanoma; occasionally may be misdiagnosed as an isolated lesion of psoriasis or nummular eczema, but a clue is its lack of response to appropriate therapy.

• **Rx:** tangential excision with curettage or electrodesiccation and curettage (especially for smaller lesions), excision, Mohs micrographic surgery (e.g. head and neck, acrogenital);

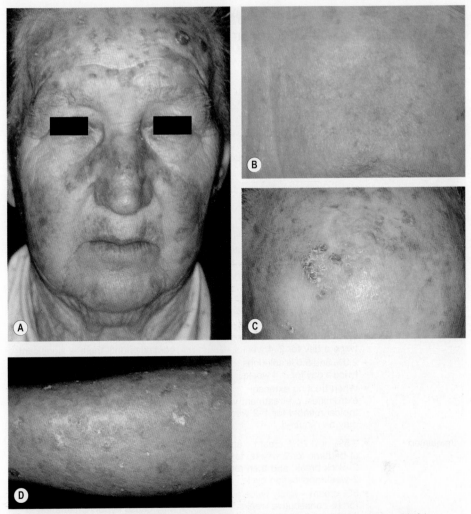

Fig. 88.2 Actinic keratoses (AKs). A Multiple AKs on the face of an elderly woman with fair complexion, blue eyes, and moderate to severe photodamage; the AKs vary in size from a few millimeters to more than 1 cm. On the left forehead, the red nodule with slight scale-crust represents a well-differentiated SCC. **B** Pink-colored atrophic AK with minimal scale on the forehead. **C** Multiple hypertrophic AKs on the bald scalp with hypopigmentation at sites of previous treatment. **D** Multiple, large hypertrophic AKs on the shin of an elderly woman; note the thick scale. *A, C, Courtesy, H. Peter Sawyer, MD; B, Courtesy, Iris Zalaudek, MD; D, Courtesy, Jean L. Bolognia, MD.*

imiquimod cream and topical 5% fluorouracil (twice daily for a longer period, e.g. 8 weeks) may be used when a surgical approach would prove difficult to perform because of location or extent.

Squamous Cell Carcinoma (SCC)

• An invasive mucocutaneous malignancy arising from keratinocytes; may develop *de novo* or from precursor AK or SCC *in situ* (see Fig. 88.1).

• More common in males than females, and incidence increases with age.

• In fair-skinned individuals, the risk factors for and the locations of invasive SCC are similar to those for AKs and SCC *in situ* (see above and Table 88.1).

• In all phototypes, invasive SCC may develop in sites of HPV infection, scars,

COMMON TREATMENT OPTIONS FOR ACTINIC KERATOSES

LOCALIZED/LESION-TARGETED TREATMENTS*

Lesion-Targeted Treatment	Helpful Hints
Liquid nitrogen cryosurgery	• No cutting or anesthesia necessary • 10- to 14-day healing period • Risk of hypopigmentation
Curettage (> curettage + electrodesiccation)	• Requires local anesthesia • Risk of hypopigmentation and scarring (less so if curettage alone)
Shave excision	• Requires local anesthesia • Risk of hypopigmentation and scarring

TOPICAL FIELD TREATMENTS**,†

Although these are the recommended FDA dosing schedules, if the patient develops significant burning with application or significant erosive erythema, the treatment should be held or discontinued.

Topical Agent	Dosing	Helpful Hints
5-Fluorouracil	• 0.5% cream – apply at bedtime × 4 weeks • 1.0% or 5.0% cream – apply twice a day for 2–4 weeks • 2.0% and 5.0% solutions – apply twice a day for 2–4 weeks • When treating extensor extremities, pretreatment with a topical retinoid for 1–2 weeks may be required	• Warn of photosensitivity, which can be severe • Optimal results occur if treatment continues until there is significant inflammation or superficial erosions • Healing usually occurs within 2 weeks of stopping treatment • Solution is best for hair-bearing areas, such as the scalp
Imiquimod	• 2.5% or 3.75% cream – apply at bedtime for 2 weeks; take a 2-week break, and then repeat 2-week application cycle • 5% cream – apply twice a week for 16 consecutive weeks • Recommended treatment area is 25 cm²	• May cause systemic flu-like symptoms • Not recommended if patient has an underlying autoimmune condition • May cause hypopigmentation at the treated site
Diclofenac	• 3% gel – apply twice a day for 90 days • A maximum amount of 8 g daily should not be exceeded	• Do not use if patient is allergic to nonsteroidal anti-inflammatory drugs (NSAIDs) • Although it may have a less severe cutaneous reaction, compliance is an issue given a longer application period
Ingenol mebutate	• 0.015% gel – apply at bedtime for 3 consecutive nights (face and scalp) • 0.05% gel – apply at bedtime for 2 consecutive nights (trunk and extremities)	• Rapid onset of action; typically within 24 hours of application, patient will experience erythema and burning • Healing occurs within 10–14 days • Supposedly does not cause hypopigmentation

Table 88.2 Common treatment options for actinic keratoses. *Continued*

Table 88.2 *Continued* **Common treatment options for actinic keratoses.**

PROCEDURAL FIELD TREATMENTS**,†	
Procedure	**Helpful Hints**
Photodynamic therapy (e.g. 5-ALA + blue light)	• Can be painful • Requires 48 hours of no outdoor exposure post-treatment • Relatively quick recovery over 1–2 weeks
Chemical peels (e.g. trichloracetic acid)	• May require local anesthesia • May cause significant irritation and temporary discoloration • Healing typically over 7 days
Ablative laser techniques (e.g. ablative fractional lasers, erbium:YAG laser)	• Requires local anesthesia • Depending on the technique, recovery period varies • Hypopigmentation a potential complication

*Most appropriate for an isolated or limited number of actinic keratoses.
**Most appropriate for numerous or larger AK lesions; there are no good comparative effectiveness studies on these topical and procedural field therapies, but the individually quoted efficacy rates are in a similar range.
†In practice, combination or sequential therapy is sometimes used (e.g. liquid nitrogen to several thicker lesions followed by imiquimod or 5-fluorouracil applied to the entire forehead).
ALA, 5-aminolevulinic acid.

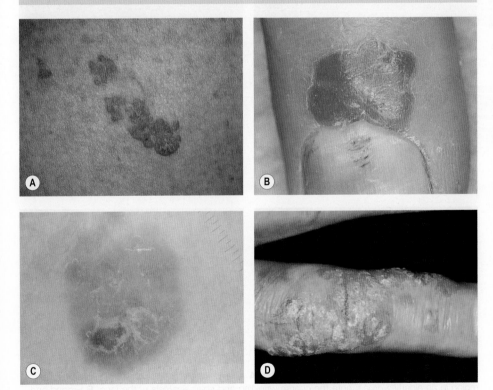

Fig. 88.3 Squamous cell carcinoma, *in situ*, Bowen's type. A Scaly red plaque on the chest with skip areas. **B** Bright-red, well-demarcated plaque on the proximal nail fold with associated horizontal nail ridging; the possibility of HPV infection needs to be considered. **C** Dermoscopic examination of a pink scaly plaque of SCC *in situ* on the chest, with tiny dotted vessels in the upper half of the lesion combined with superficial scales. **D** Extensive involvement of the finger, which is often misdiagnosed clinically as psoriasis or chronic eczema and therefore treated for years with corticosteroid creams (as was this patient). *C, Courtesy, Iris Zalaudek, MD; D, Courtesy, H. Peter Sawyer, MD.*

ACTINIC KERATOSIS, BASAL CELL CARCINOMA, AND SQUAMOUS CELL CARCINOMA

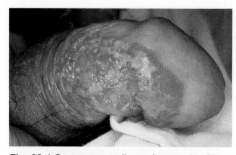

Fig. 88.4 Squamous cell carcinoma, *in situ*, of the penis, also known as penile intraepithelial neoplasia (PIN). Formerly called SCC *in situ*, erythroplasia of Queyrat type. Large eroded erythematous plaque with well-demarcated borders. The lesion began on the shaft of the penis.

chronic injury or inflammation, previous radiation therapy, or chemical exposure (e.g. polycyclic aromatic hydrocarbons; see Table 88.1).

• Common clinical presentation is an erythematous, keratotic papule or nodule that arises within a background of sun-damaged skin; tenderness common; often a history of rapid enlargement (Fig. 88.5) and sometimes a history of antecedent trauma.

• Clinical variants: keratoacanthoma (KA) (Fig. 88.6), verrucous carcinoma (Fig. 88.7), mucosal (Fig. 88.8), periungual and subungual.

• Dx: biopsy (should be deep enough to determine extent of dermal invasion); palpate regional lymph node basin.

• **DDx:**
   – *Most common*: AK, HAK, SCC *in situ*, BCC, verruca vulgaris, irritated SK.

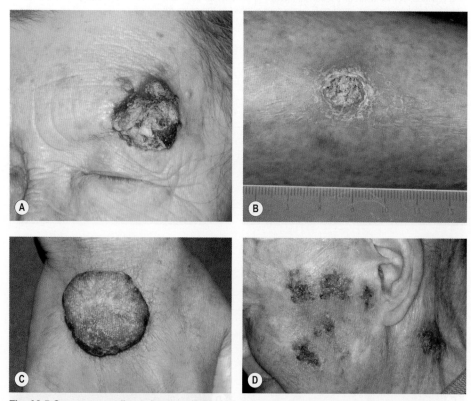

Fig. 88.5 Squamous cell carcinomas (SCCs). A A large keratotic nodule on the supraorbital region in an elderly woman; note the coarse wrinkling and solar elastosis of the face. **B** Eroded and keratotic nodule that developed rapidly at the site of trauma on the shin. **C** Large, fungating nodule on the dorsum of the hand. **D** Multiple eroded superficial SCCs in association with hypertrophic AKs on the cheek and neck of an elderly man. *A, C, D, Courtesy, H. Peter Sawyer, MD; B, Courtesy, Jean L. Bolognia, MD.* **Continued**

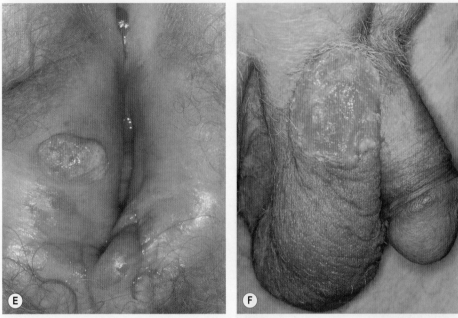

Fig. 88.5 *Continued* **E** Erosive, slightly vegetating, thick plaque arising within lichen sclerosus of the vulva. **F** Firm, eroded red plaque on the scrotum; histopathologically, the SCC was moderately differentiated. *E, F, Courtesy, H. Peter Sawyer, MD.*

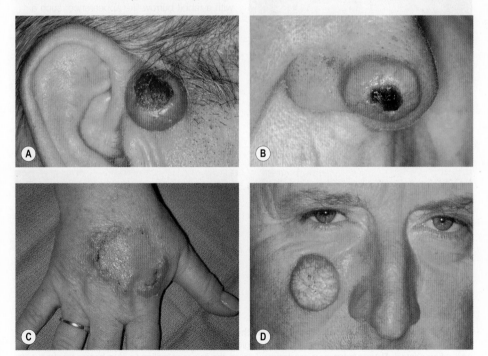

Fig. 88.6 Clinical spectrum of keratoacanthomas. A, B Rapidly growing, erythematous crateriform nodules with a rolled border and central keratotic core. **C** Progressive peripheral expansion and central involution with residual atrophy characterize keratoacanthoma centrifugum marginatum. **D** Giant keratoacanthoma with a yellow-red color and a history of rapid growth. *A, D, Courtesy, H. Peter Sawyer, MD.*

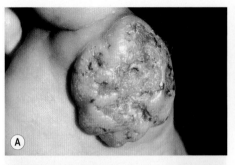

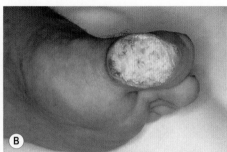

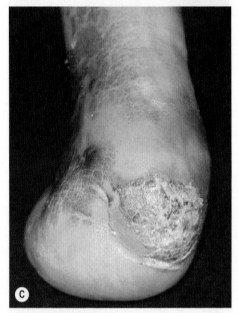

Fig. 88.7 Verrucous carcinoma. A Long-standing large nodule on the plantar surface with a rabbit burrow-like appearance; such a tumor is also referred to as an epithelioma cuniculatum. **B** Keratotic and ulcerated plaque on the ventromedial aspect of the great toe. The lesion was originally misdiagnosed as a plantar wart. **C** A classic location in an amputation stump. In general, these well-differentiated SCCs enlarge slowly. *A, C, Courtesy, H. Peter Sawyer, MD.*

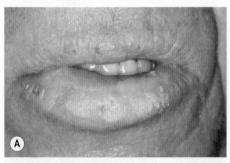

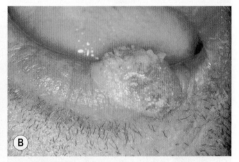

Fig. 88.8 Squamous cell carcinoma (SCC) of the lower lip. A Extensive hyperkeratosis and leukoplakia of the lower vermilion lip; histopathologically, the SCC was superficially invasive and well-differentiated. **B** Verrucous and eroded nodule on the lower vermilion lip in a heavy smoker. *A, B, Courtesy, H. Peter Sawyer, MD.*

- *Less common*: amelanotic melanoma, atypical fibroxanthoma (AFX), Merkel cell carcinoma, adnexal tumors, prurigo nodularis.

• A cutaneous SCC staging format has been proposed by the American Joint Commission on Cancer, incorporating the TNM criteria, prognostic factors (tumor thickness, ± perineural invasion, high-risk locations, ± lymph node involvement), histologic grade, and the presence or absence of lymphatic/vascular invasion on histology (Table 88.3).

• Long-term prognosis for adequately treated SCC is excellent.

• Overall, the risk of nodal metastases from invasive SCC has been estimated at 2–4%; ~20% of all skin cancer deaths are due to SCC.

• There are several risk factors for nodal metastasis: lesions on the lip, ear, and genitalia; tumor diameter ≥2 cm; poorly differentiated histology; invasion beyond the subcutaneous fat; and perineural invasion (Table 88.4).

• Significant cause of morbidity and mortality in solid organ transplant recipients, who are more likely to experience local and regional recurrences, as well as metastases.

• **Rx:** primarily excision, but based on risk factors (see Table 88.4), ranges from electrodesiccation and curettage (e.g. smaller, minimally invasive lesion in an elderly patient) to Mohs micrographic surgery (Table 88.5).

Basal Cell Carcinoma (BCC)

• Most common NMSC in humans; arises *de novo*, with no known precursor lesion.

• More common in males than females; primarily seen in middle-aged to older adults who are fair-skinned; however, the incidence is rising, especially in young women.

STAGING OF CUTANEOUS SQUAMOUS CELL CARCINOMA (SCC)	
T, N, M	
Primary tumor (T)	
TX	Primary tumor cannot be assessed
T0	No evidence of primary tumor
Tis	Carcinoma *in situ*
T1	Tumor ≤2 cm in greatest dimension with <2 high-risk features*
T2	Tumor >2 cm in greatest dimension *or* tumor any size with ≥2 high-risk features[†]
T3	Tumor with invasion of maxilla, orbit, or temporal bone
T4	Tumor with invasion of skeleton (axial or appendicular) or perineural invasion of skull base
Regional lymph nodes (N)	
NX	Regional lymph nodes cannot be assessed
N0	No regional lymph node metastasis
N1	Metastasis in a single ipsilateral lymph node, ≤3 cm in greatest dimension
N2	Metastasis in a single ipsilateral lymph node, >3 cm but <6 cm in greatest dimension (2a); or in multiple ipsilateral lymph nodes, none >6 cm in greatest dimension (2b); or in bilateral or contralateral lymph nodes, none >6 cm in greatest dimension (2c)
N3	Metastasis in a lymph node, >6 cm in greatest dimension
Distant metastasis (M)	
M0	No distant metastasis
M1	Distant metastasis

Table 88.3 Staging of cutaneous squamous cell carcinoma (SCC). *Adapted from American Joint Committee on Cancer, 2010. Continued*

Table 88.3 *Continued* **Staging of cutaneous squamous cell carcinoma (SCC).**

Stage	T	N	M
0	Tis	N0	M0
I	T1	N0	M0
II	T2	N0	M0
III	T3	N0	M0
	T1	N1	M0
	T2	N1	M0
	T3	N1	M0
IV	T1	N2	M0
	T2	N2	M0
	T3	N2	M0
	T Any	N3	M0
	T4	N Any	M0
	T Any	N Any	M1

*High-risk features for the primary tumor (T) staging:
   Depth/invasion: >2 mm thickness, Clark level ≥IV, perineural invasion.
   Anatomic location: *primary site ear, primary site hair-bearing lip.*
   Differentiation: *poorly differentiated or undifferentiated.*
†Excludes cutaneous SCC of the eyelid.

CHARACTERISTICS OF HIGH-RISK* NON-MELANOMA SKIN CANCER (NMSC)**	
Clinical Characteristics	**Histologic Characteristics**

• Area L ≥20 mm
  Area M ≥10 mm
  Area H ≥6 mm
• Poorly defined borders
• Recurrent tumor
• Immunosuppressed host
• Tumor at site of previous XRT
• Tumor at site of chronic inflammatory process (SCC only)
• Rapidly growing tumor (SCC only)
• Neurologic symptoms: pain, paresthesia, paralysis
	• Perineural involvement
	• Morpheaform (sclerosing), infiltrative, or micronodular subtypes (BCC only)
	• Poorly differentiated (SCC only)
	• Adenoid, adenosquamous, acantholytic, or desmoplastic subtypes (SCC only)
	• Arising within Bowen's disease (SCC only)
	• Depth >2 mm or Clark level IV or V (SCC only)

*High-risk of recurrence.
**Includes BCC and SCC.
Area L – low-risk anatomic sites: trunk, extremities.
Area M – middle-risk anatomic sites: cheeks, forehead, neck, scalp.
Area H – high-risk anatomic sites: 'mask areas' of face, genitalia, hands, feet.
BCC, basal cell carcinoma; SCC, squamous cell carcinoma; XRT, radiation therapy.

Table 88.4 Characteristics of high-risk non-melanoma skin cancer (NMSC).

COMMON TREATMENT OPTIONS FOR NON-MELANOMA SKIN CANCER (NMSC)*	
Squamous Cell Carcinoma	**Basal Cell Carcinoma**
Low-Risk Lesions**	**Low-Risk** Lesions**
• Tangential excision with curettage • Electrodesiccation and curettage • Standard excision with 4- to 6-mm margins • XRT† for nonsurgical candidates	• Tangential excision with curettage • Electrodesiccation and curettage • Standard excision with 4-mm margins • Topical imiquimod (superficial BCC on trunk and extremities) • XRT† for nonsurgical candidates
High-Risk Lesions**	**High-Risk** Lesions**
• Standard excision with 10+-mm margins • Mohs micrographic surgery • XRT† for nonsurgical candidates • Adjuvant XRT (if perineural involvement)	• Standard excision with 10+-mm margins • Mohs micrographic surgery • XRT† for nonsurgical candidates • Adjuvant XRT (if perineural involvement, but seen less commonly than in SCC)
Metastatic	**Inoperable or Metastatic**
• Referral to an oncologist	• Hedgehog pathway inhibitors (e.g. vismodegib)
Indications for Mohs Micrographic Surgery	

• Recurrent tumor
• High-risk** anatomic location (e.g. periorbital, perinasal, periauricular, perioral)
• Other anatomic sites where tissue preservation is imperative (e.g. fingers, toes, nail units, genitalia)
• Aggressive histologic subtype
  • Morpheaform (sclerosing), micronodular, or infiltrating BCC
  • Poorly differentiated or deeply penetrating SCC
  • Basosquamous carcinoma
• Perineural invasion
• Large size (>20 mm diameter)
• Poorly defined clinical borders
• Prior exposure to XRT
• Tumor arising within a chronic scar
• Site of positive margins on prior excision
• Immunosuppressed host
• Underlying genetic syndrome (e.g. xeroderma pigmentosum, nevoid BCC syndrome)

Includes BCC and SCC.
***High risk for recurrence; see characteristics of such lesions in Table 88.4.*
†Excluding genitalia, hands, and feet.
BCC, basal cell carcinoma; SCC, squamous cell carcinoma; XRT, radiation therapy.

Table 88.5 Common treatment options for non-melanoma skin cancer (NMSC).

ACTINIC KERATOSIS, BASAL CELL CARCINOMA, AND SQUAMOUS CELL CARCINOMA

• UV exposure is the greatest risk factor, but in contrast to AK/SCC, intense episodes of burning are more important than chronic long-term exposure; in addition, BCCs can also arise in relatively non-sun-exposed areas, e.g. retroauricular crease and inner canthus (Fig. 88.9B).
• Usually slow-growing; without adequate treatment, BCCs will gradually increase in size and they may ulcerate and cause local destruction of surrounding tissue; metastases are exceedingly rare (regional lymph nodes > lung).
• Multiple clinical variants and varied presentations.
  – *Most common*: nodular (pearly papule with telangiectasias and/or umbilica- tion; Fig. 88.9), superficial (typically an

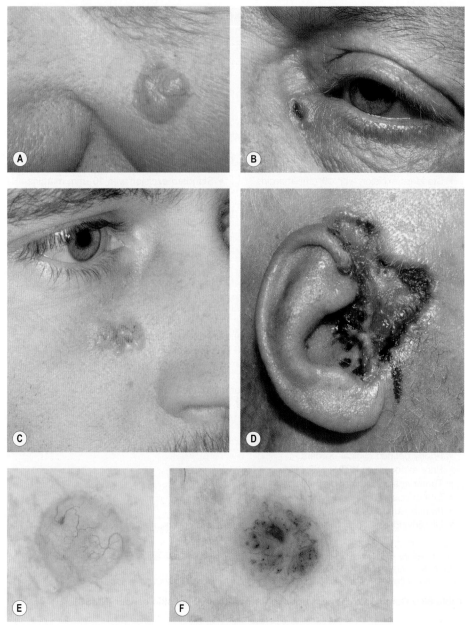

Fig. 88.9 Clinical spectrum of nodular basal cell carcinoma (BCC). A Translucent papulonodule with prominent telangiectasias on the infraorbital cheek. **B** Classic presentation with a pearly rolled border and central hemorrhagic crust. **C** Larger plaque with rolled borders and multiple telangiectasias. **D** Nodulo-ulcerative tumor of the preauricular region with translucent rolled borders, most obvious at "noon." **E** Dermoscopy of a nodular BCC with striking arborizing vessels. **F** Dermoscopy of a pigmented BCC demonstrating the classic arborizing telangiectasias and multiple blue-gray ovoid globules, pointing to the diagnosis of a small nodular BCC; the one large blue-brown structure resembles, but does not fulfill all the criteria for, a large gray-blue ovoid nest. *A, Courtesy, Stanley J. Miller, MD; C, D, Courtesy, H. Peter Sawyer, MD; E, F, Courtesy, Giuseppe Argenziano, MD.*

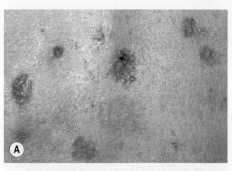

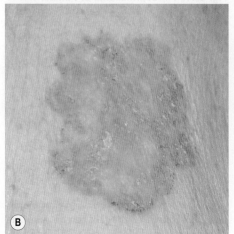

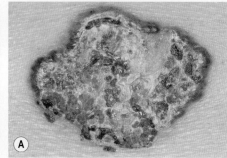

Fig. 88.10 Superficial basal cell carcinoma (BCC). **A** Numerous erythematous patches and thin plaques on the back of a man with a history of arsenic exposure decades previously. **B** A solitary large, thin, dark pink plaque. There are scattered areas of fine scaling and small foci of brown pigment within the rolled border. As a rule, these lesions are neither pruritic nor tender. *A, B, Courtesy, H. Peter Sawyer, MD.*

Fig. 88.11 Pigmented basal cell carcinoma (BCC). **A** In addition to the admixture of scale and hemorrhagic crusts centrally, there is a translucent and black rolled border superiorly. **B** The clinical differential diagnosis of this small nodular pigmented BCC includes nodular melanoma. However, the glassy translucency, in concert with characteristic dermoscopic features, will point to the diagnosis of pigmented BCC. *A, B, Courtesy, H. Peter Sawyer, MD.*

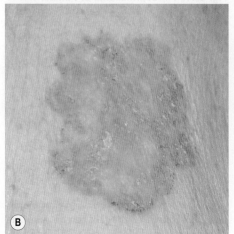

erythematous thin plaque on trunk > extremities; Fig. 88.10), pigmented (Fig. 88.11).

- *Less common*: morpheaform (scar-like; Fig. 88.12), micronodular, cystic, basosquamous, and fibroepithelioma of Pinkus (Fig. 88.13).

• Dx: biopsy; dermoscopy can assist in diagnosis (see Fig. 88.9E,F).

• **DDx:** *nodular*: intradermal melanocytic nevus, fibrous papule, sebaceous hyperplasia, invasive SCC, amelanotic melanoma; *superficial*: LPLK, AK, SCC *in situ*, isolated lesion of psoriasis, seborrheic dermatitis or num-

mular eczema, amelanotic melanoma; *morpheaform*: scar, adnexal tumors (e.g. desmoplastic trichoepithelioma, microcystic adnexal carcinoma [see Chapter 91]); *pigmented*: melanocytic nevus, seborrheic keratosis, pigmented SCC *in situ*, nodular melanoma.

• Categorize tumor into histologic subtype and whether or not meets criteria for high-risk BCC (e.g. morpheaform, micronodular, or infiltrative; see Table 88.4) or indications for Mohs micrographic surgery to determine best treatment (see Table 88.5); basosquamous lesions are treated as invasive SCCs (see above).

• Nevoid BCC syndrome: rare, autosomal dominant, caused by mutations in human

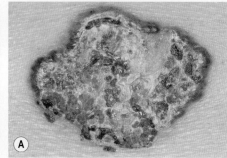

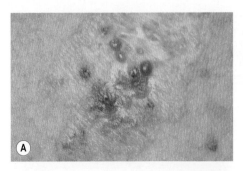

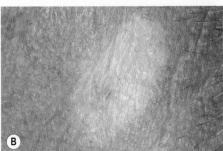

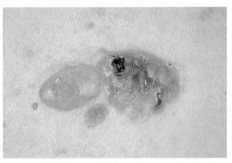

Fig. 88.13 Fibroepithelioma of Pinkus. This soft, skin-colored to light pink, broad, sessile nodule on the lower back representing a fibroepithelioma is adjacent to a classic nodular BCC. *Courtesy, H. Peter Sawyer, MD.*

Fig. 88.12 Morpheaform basal cell carcinoma (BCC). A Recurrent tumor 2 years after microscopically controlled surgery; note the scar-like appearance with superimposed glassy pink and brown papules. **B** A classic example with indistinct borders and a scar-like appearance. *A, Courtesy, Darrell S. Rigel, MD; B, Courtesy, H. Peter Sawyer, MD.*

PTCH gene; characterized by multiple BCCs, palmoplantar pits, odontogenic keratocysts of jaw, skeletal abnormalities, macrocephaly, and calcification of the falx cerebri; patients may develop medulloblastomas during childhood or ovarian fibromas.

For further information see Ch. 108. From *Dermatology, Third Edition.*

Benign Epithelial Tumors and Proliferations

89

Seborrheic Keratosis

• Begin to appear during the 4th decade of life and then gradually increase in number.

• Macular, papular, or verrucous; colors vary from white to black but most commonly brown.

• Typically has a 'stuck-on' appearance with a smooth to verrucous surface (Fig. 89.1).

• Spares the palms, soles, and mucosal surfaces.

• May resemble a melanoma clinically but has no pigment network (by dermoscopy) and has horn pseudocysts.

• Sudden appearance of multiple lesions may be associated with internal malignancy (*sign of Leser–Trélat*) or erythroderma; the former may also be associated with skin tags, irritated seborrheic keratoses, tripe palms, and acanthosis nigricans.

• Histopathology: a spectrum of different architectures, most commonly acanthotic, papillomatous and hyperkeratotic, or irritated (Fig. 89.2).

• Variants:

  – **Dermatosis papulosa nigra** (Fig. 89.3): common in dark-skinned individuals; 1- to 5-mm hyperpigmented papules on the face.

  – **Stucco keratosis** (Fig. 89.4): 1- to 4-mm gray-white papules on the lower extremities (especially dorsal feet and ankles) of older adults.

  – **Inverted follicular keratosis**: endophytic variant of seborrheic keratosis; tan to pink papule, typically on the face of adults.

Acrokeratosis Verruciformis

• Autosomal dominant disorder; sometimes associated with Darier disease.

• Multiple, skin-colored, flat-wart-like papules on dorsal aspect of hands and feet.

• Benign neoplasm of keratinocytes showing papillomatosis with overlying hyperkeratosis in 'church spires'.

• May have *ATP2A2* gene mutation.

Clear Cell Acanthoma

• Red, shiny papule or plaque, sometimes with a peripheral collarette of scale (Fig. 89.5).

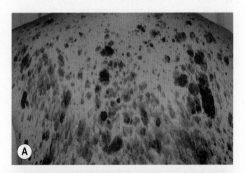

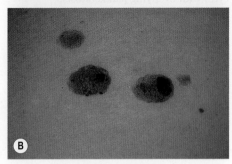

Fig. 89.1 Seborrheic keratoses. A Multiple seborrheic keratoses on the back, with some in a pattern that has been likened to raindrops. **B** Sharply demarcated pigmented papules and plaques with a papillomatous surface and horn pseudocysts. Note the 'stuck-on' appearance. *A, Courtesy, Kalman Watsky, MD.*

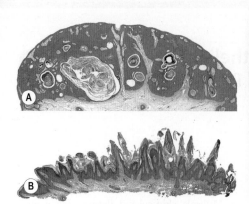

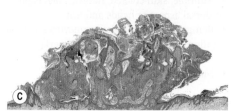

Fig. 89.2 Seborrheic keratoses – spectrum of histologic subtypes. A Acanthotic type with lobular hyperplasia with prominent horn cysts. **B** Papillomatous or hyperkeratotic type with church spires of papillomatosis and hyperkeratosis. **C** Irritated seborrheic keratosis. Exophytic lesion with papillomatosis, hyperkeratosis, hemorrhagic crust, and dermal inflammation. *A, B, Courtesy, Luis Requena, MD; C, Courtesy, Lorenzo Cerroni, MD.*

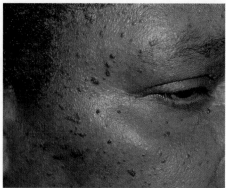

Fig. 89.3 Dermatosis papulosa nigra. Multiple hyperpigmented papules with typical location on the cheeks. *Courtesy, Luis Requena, MD.*

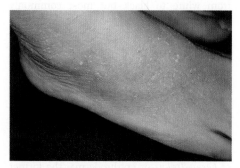

Fig. 89.4 Stucco keratoses. Multiple gray-white keratotic papules on the ankle and dorsal foot. *Courtesy, Jean L. Bolognia, MD.*

• Favors the leg.
• Histopathology: acanthosis of characteristically well-demarcated pale or clear keratinocytes with overlying parakeratosis.

Large Cell Acanthoma

• Variably colored papule or plaque in sun-exposed sites in older individuals (Fig. 89.6).
• A variant of actinic keratosis and seborrheic keratosis.
• Histopathology: orthokeratosis overlying a thin epidermis composed of enlarged keratinocytes.

Porokeratosis

• Several different types (Table 89.1; Fig. 89.7).
• All have a distinctive thread-like border of scale that corresponds histopathologically to the cornoid lamella (column of parakeratosis histologically).
• The most common form, disseminated superficial actinic porokeratosis (DSAP), is sometimes misdiagnosed as multiple actinic keratoses.

Epidermal Nevus (See Chapter 51)

• Hyperpigmented (rarely hypopigmented) papules and plaques (Fig. 89.8) along Blaschko's lines.
• Verrucous, keratotic, velvety or barely elevated.
• May have a sebaceous or other adnexal component (i.e. nevus sebaceus), especially if on the scalp or face.
• Can be caused by mosaicism for mutations in *FGFR3* (fibroblast growth factor receptor-3), *PIK3CA*, *HRAS* (also in nevus sebaceus),

TYPES OF POROKERATOSIS	
Type	**Clinical Features**
Porokeratosis of Mibelli	Plaque that arises during infancy or childhood, usually on a distal extremity; usually several cm in diameter
Disseminated superficial actinic porokeratosis	Pink to brown papules and plaques with peripheral scale; arise in sun-exposed sites, especially the forearms and shins; usually measure from a few mm to 1.5 cm; in some patients, autosomal dominant inheritance
Large-sized lesions	In immunocompromised patients, especially solid organ transplant recipients
Linear porokeratosis	Streaks along the lines of Blaschko; arise during infancy or childhood Risk of development of squamous cell carcinoma
Punctate porokeratosis	1- to 2-mm palmoplantar papules; arise during adolescence or adulthood
Porokeratosis palmaris et plantaris et disseminata	Palmoplantar papules in addition to involvement of the trunk, extremities, and even mucous membranes; onset during childhood or adolescence
Porokeratosis ptychotropica	Erythematous plaque, sometimes with smaller peripheral papules, in the gluteal cleft or folds

Table 89.1 Types of porokeratosis.

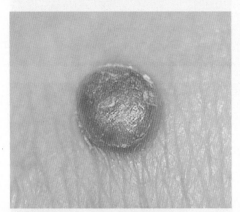

Fig. 89.5 Clear cell acanthoma. Well-demarcated, dark, red, shiny papule with a wafer-like collarette of scale. *Courtesy, Luis Requena, MD.*

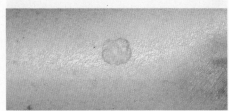

Fig. 89.6 Large cell acanthoma. Well-demarcated, thin, pink-brown plaque. *Courtesy, Luis Requena, MD.*

- 75% appear before age 5 years.
- **DDx:** primarily linear psoriasis (see Chapter 6).

Nevus Comedonicus

- Linear plaques composed of grouped comedones; may develop inflammatory acneiform lesions.
- 50% present at birth; otherwise, generally appear before age 10 years.
- May be due to mosaicism for a mutation in *FGFR2*.

Flegel's Disease (Hyperkeratosis Lenticularis Perstans)

- Rare; may have an autosomal dominant inheritance.

keratin 1 or 10 (if histologic finding of epidermolytic hyperkeratosis), and other genes.
- May be associated with extracutaneous manifestations (see Chapter 51).

Inflammatory Linear Verrucous Epidermal Nevus (See Chapter 51)

- Linear, pruritic, psoriasiform (erythematous with scale) plaques, usually on an extremity.

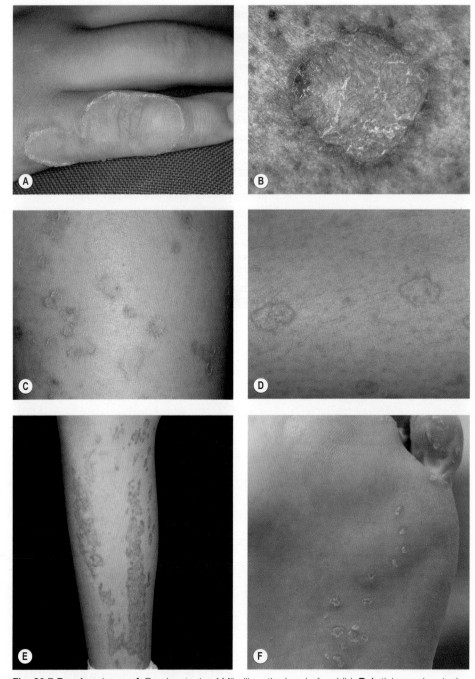

Fig. 89.7 Porokeratoses. A Porokeratosis of Mibelli on the hand of a child. **B** Actinic porokeratosis in a renal transplant patient with significant solar damage. Note the narrow, elevated rim. **C, D** Multiple lesions of disseminated superficial actinic porokeratosis (DSAP) with obvious peripheral keratotic rims; lesions can range in color from light brown to pink. **E** Several streaks of linear porokeratosis on the lower extremity. **F** Multiple keratotic papules on the plantar surface due to punctate porokeratosis. *B, C, D, Courtesy, Jean L. Bolognia, MD; F, Courtesy, Kalman Watsky, MD.*

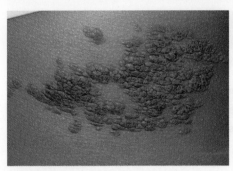

Fig. 89.8 Epidermal nevus. Verrucous hyperpigmented plaques. An individual papule, in isolation, resembles a seborrheic keratosis. *Courtesy, Kalman Watsky, MD.*

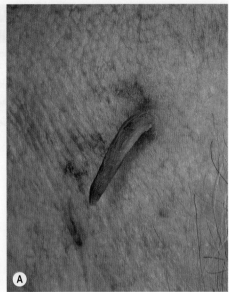

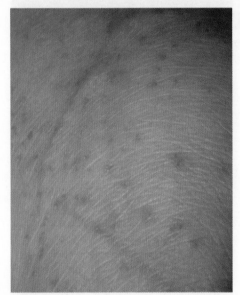

Fig. 89.9 Flegel's disease. Scaly pink to pink-brown papules on lateral foot. *Courtesy, Peter Heald, MD.*

- Onset usually during adulthood.
- Lentil-like keratotic papules on the distal lower extremities (Fig. 89.9).

Cutaneous Horn

- Clinical term for marked hyperkeratosis arising from a papule or nodule (Fig. 89.10).
- The base of the lesion most commonly represents an actinic keratosis, seborrheic keratosis, verruca, or squamous cell carcinoma.

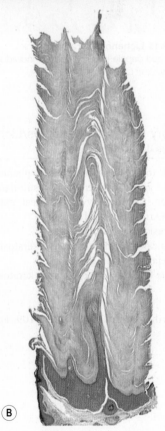

Fig. 89.10 Cutaneous horn. A This cutaneous horn arose from an actinic keratosis. **B** Striking column of hyperkeratosis with hyperplasia of the underlying epidermis. *B, Courtesy, Luis Requena, MD.*

EXAMPLES OF OTHER SOLITARY KERATOSES	
Solitary Lesion	**Histologic Features of Solitary Lesion**
Epidermolytic acanthoma	Epidermolytic hyperkeratosis (also seen in epidermolytic ichthyosis and some epidermal nevi)
Warty dyskeratoma	Resembles Darier disease
Acantholytic acanthoma	Resembles pemphigus vulgaris

Table 89.2 Examples of other solitary keratoses.

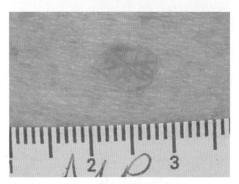

Fig. 89.11 Lichenoid keratosis. Pink, flat-topped papule in a fair-skinned individual. *Courtesy, Jean L. Bolognia, MD.*

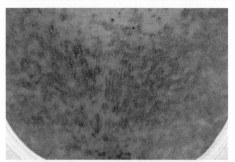

Fig. 89.12 Confluent and reticulated papillomatosis (CARP). Multiple hyperpigmented papules that are confluent centrally and assume a reticulated pattern laterally. *Courtesy, Julie V. Schaffer, MD.*

Solitary Lichenoid Keratosis/Lichen Planus-Like Keratosis

• Pink to pink-brown papule or plaque (Fig. 89.11); arises in chronically sun-damaged skin, most commonly on the chest, extensor upper extremities, and shins.
• Occasionally multiple.
• Clinically mimics an actinic keratosis and nonmelanoma skin cancer.
• Table 89.2 lists other solitary keratoses.

Confluent and Reticulated Papillomatosis (of Gougerot and Carteaud)

• Onset during puberty.
• Scaly to verrucous hyperpigmented plaques.
• Centrally confluent and reticulated at periphery (Fig. 89.12).
• Favors neck, central chest, submammary regions.
• **Rx:** oral tetracyclines (e.g. minocycline).

For further information see Ch. 109. From *Dermatology, Third Edition.*

Cysts 90

Introduction

- Variably sized papules or nodules.
- Cysts can be divided into true cysts with an epithelial lining (histologically and sometimes visible clinically) and false cysts without such a lining.
- Appreciation of the actual size of the cyst often requires palpation.
- Different types of cysts often have characteristic anatomic locations and histologic features.
- Treatment of true cysts (if symptomatic) is primarily surgical.

True Cysts – Common

Epidermoid Inclusion Cyst (EIC) (Epidermal Inclusion Cyst, 'Sebaceous Cyst')

- Most commonly on the face and the trunk; skin-colored to yellow-white unless inflamed;

size varies from several millimeters to centimeters.
- A visible comedonal-like opening or pore (resembles a blackhead) may be seen on the surface of the papule or nodule (Fig. 90.1A).
- A soft cheese-like, sometimes malodorous, material composed primarily of keratin can usually be expressed from the opening.
- Cyst contents may rupture into the dermis, eliciting an acute and chronic inflammatory reaction, leading to significant redness and pain; this inflammation is often confused with a bacterial infection (Fig. 90.1B).
- Most commonly sporadic; multiple lesions rarely associated with Gardner syndrome or Gorlin syndrome.
- **DDx:** see Fig. 95.17.
- **Rx:** *inflamed* lesions: if fluctuant, can be incised and drained ± packed with gauze (a wick); if nonfluctuant, can be injected with intralesional CS; *non-inflamed* ('cold') lesions can be excised surgically but may result in a significant scar.

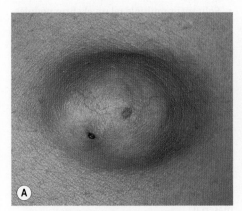 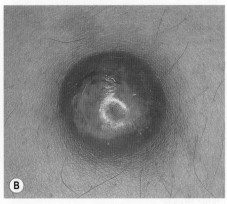

Fig. 90.1 Epidermoid inclusion cysts. A Typical clinical appearance of an epidermoid inclusion cyst with a yellowish hue. Two pores are present in this example. **B** Painful inflammatory reactions to cyst rupture are a frequent cause for presentation to a physician. Culture will often prove these lesions to be sterile, even if draining pus. Antibiotic treatment can be helpful due to their anti-inflammatory effects. *B, Courtesy, Mary S. Stone, MD.*

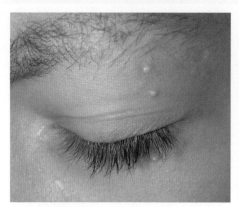

Fig. 90.2 Milia. Tiny (1–2 mm), white, dome-shaped papules on the face.

CONDITIONS ASSOCIATED WITH MULTIPLE MILIA
• Trauma, e.g. burn
• Bullous diseases Metabolic (e.g. porphyria cutanea tarda) Autoimmune (e.g. epidermolysis bullosa   acquisita >> bullous pemphigoid) Inherited (e.g. epidermolysis bullosa) Exposures (e.g. poison ivy)
• Other genodermatoses (e.g. Bazex–   Dupré–Christol syndrome)
• Follicular mycosis fungoides

Table 90.1 Conditions associated with multiple milia.

Milium (Milia – Plural)

• A small, superficial (1–2 mm), firm cyst that is white in color and is sometimes confused with a whitehead (Fig. 90.2); occasionally they are grouped.

• Occurs most frequently on the face, especially the periorbital region; seen in both children and adults.

• Commonly observed on the face in newborns; in this setting, they often resolve spontaneously.

• The majority of patients with multiple facial milia have no underlying condition; however, there may be a secondary cause (Table 90.1).

• **DDx:** whitehead (closed comedone), syringoma.

• **Rx:** because a milium lies beneath intact epidermis, the lesion must be punctured with

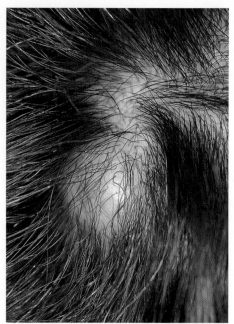

Fig. 90.3 Pilar cyst. A non-inflamed pilar cyst is skin-colored, mobile, and has a smooth surface. *Courtesy, Mary S. Stone, MD.*

a needle or sharp blade in order to express the keratin contents.

Pilar Cyst (Wen)

• Most common location is the scalp; sometimes there is associated overlying alopecia (Fig. 90.3).

• Solitary or multiple relatively firm nodules.

• May be inherited (autosomal dominant).

• Surgical removal is easier than for an EIC because less dissection from surrounding normal tissue is required; a small incision with lateral pressure may be all that is necessary.

Pilonidal Cyst

• Most common location is the upper gluteal cleft in association with a sinus tract ± fragments of hairs.

• May have a history of draining malodorous material.

• More common in men.

• May be associated with acne conglobata, hidradenitis suppurativa, and dissecting cellulitis (follicular occlusion tetrad).

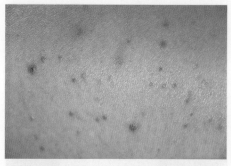

Fig. 90.4 Eruptive vellus hair cysts.
Pigmented small papules on the thigh of a young woman. *Courtesy, Mary S. Stone, MD.*

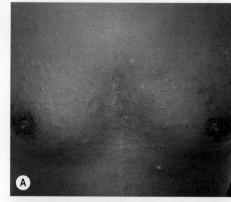

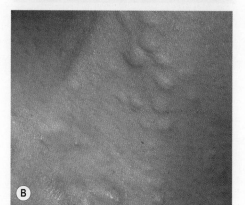

Fig. 90.5 Steatocystoma multiplex.
A, B Numerous cystic papules on the trunk and multiple cystic nodules on the neck. *A, Courtesy, Mary S. Stone, MD.*

True Cysts – Less Common

Vellus Hair Cyst

- 2- to 3-mm, skin-colored to brown-blue papule(s), commonly on the trunk (Fig. 90.4).
- Occasionally inflamed.
  - When multiple, may be inherited (autosomal dominant); can be associated with pachyonychia congenita 6b/17 > 6a/16.
  - Bedside diagnostic test: nick the cyst and examine expressed contents for vellus hairs.
- **DDx:** acne, steatocystomas (can be overlap).

Steatocystoma

- 2- to 10-mm, skin-colored to pigmented papule or nodule, usually multiple and grouped; commonly develop on the trunk or in the axillae and groin (Fig. 90.5).
- May drain oily fluid.
- Multiple lesions may be inherited as an isolated finding (autosomal dominant, *KRT17* mutation) or represent a clinical feature of pachyonychia congenita 6b/17 > 6a/16.

Hidrocystoma

APOCRINE

- Often a solitary, translucent to bluish papule on the eyelid margin (Fig. 90.6).
- Histology: the lining resembles that of an apocrine gland (decapitation secretion).
- **Rx:** if bothersome or symptomatic, excision by an experienced surgeon.

ECCRINE

- Multiple or solitary bluish, translucent papule(s) on the face (Fig. 90.7).
- Can become more prominent with sweating.
- Bedside diagnostic test: nicking the surface results in drainage of clear liquid.

'False' Cysts (No True Epithelial Lining)

Mucocele

- Compressible mucosal-colored to bluish papule or nodule, most commonly seen on the lower, inner mucosal lip (Fig. 90.8).
- Secondary to disruption of the minor salivary ducts.

881

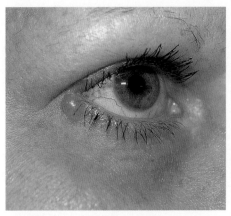

Fig. 90.6 Apocrine hidrocystoma. A single, slightly bluish, translucent papule on the lower eyelid near the lateral canthus. *Courtesy, Mary S. Stone, MD.*

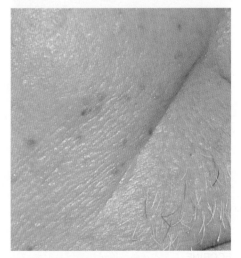

Fig. 90.7 Eccrine hidrocystomas. Numerous, tiny translucent or bluish papules on the cheek.

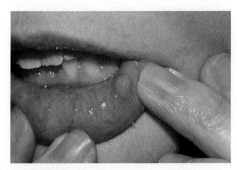

Fig. 90.8 Mucocele. A bluish translucent papule on the lower mucosal lip. *Courtesy, Mary S. Stone, MD.*

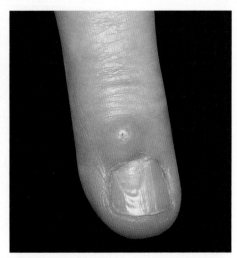

Fig. 90.9 Digital mucous cyst. A translucent papule on the dorsal distal phalanx of the finger causing a depression in the nail plate. *Courtesy, Mary S. Stone, MD.*

- May resolve spontaneously.
- **Rx:** if persistent, excision or other destructive procedure, intralesional CS.

Digital Mucous Cyst

- Translucent, skin-colored to bluish papule or nodule most commonly on digits, in particular the dorsal, distal finger near the distal interphalangeal joint (Fig. 90.9).
- There may be a connection to the joint space.
- Occurs in the setting of osteoarthritis.
- Longitudinal nail deformity may be present when the lesion compresses the nail matrix.
- Puncture can result in drainage of a gelatinous material.
- **Rx:** observation, intralesional CS, repeated incision and drainage, excision.

Ganglion Cyst

- Soft, cystic nodule most commonly on the wrist > ankle.
- Seen more often in women than in men.
- **Rx:** may spontaneously resolve but recurrence common; treatment modalities include compression, aspiration and intralesional CS, excision.

Pseudocyst of the Auricle

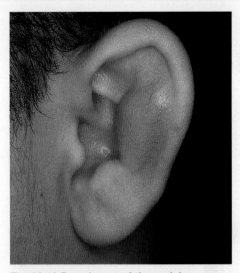

- Painless swelling, generally unilateral, of the scaphoid fossa of the ear (Fig. 90.10).
- More common in men than in women.
- **Rx:** aspiration ± intralesional CS, incision and drainage; any treatment should be followed by pressure dressings.

Fig. 90.10 Pseudocyst of the auricle.
Erythematous firm nodule on the ear.

For further information see Ch. 110. From *Dermatology, Third Edition*.

91 | Adnexal Neoplasms

- Adnexal neoplasms are tumors, more commonly benign, that show features of cutaneous adnexal structures (Fig. 91.1), e.g. hair (Table 91.1), sebaceous glands (Table 91.2), apocrine glands and eccrine glands (Table 91.3).

FOLLICULO-SEBACEOUS-APOCRINE UNIT AND ECCRINE SWEAT GLAND

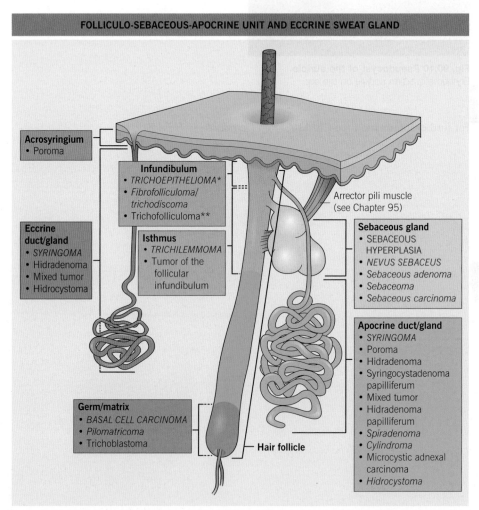

Acrosyringium
- Poroma

Infundibulum
- *TRICHOEPITHELIOMA**
- *Fibrofolliculoma/ trichodiscoma*
- Trichofolliculoma**

Arrector pili muscle
(see Chapter 95)

Eccrine duct/gland
- *SYRINGOMA*
- Hidradenoma
- Mixed tumor
- Hidrocystoma

Isthmus
- *TRICHILEMMOMA*
- Tumor of the follicular infundibulum

Sebaceous gland
- SEBACEOUS HYPERPLASIA
- *NEVUS SEBACEUS*
- *Sebaceous adenoma*
- *Sebaceoma*
- *Sebaceous carcinoma*

Apocrine duct/gland
- *SYRINGOMA*
- Poroma
- Hidradenoma
- Syringocystadenoma papilliferum
- Mixed tumor
- Hidradenoma papilliferum
- *Spiradenoma*
- *Cylindroma*
- Microcystic adnexal carcinoma
- *Hidrocystoma*

Germ/matrix
- *BASAL CELL CARCINOMA*
- *Pilomatricoma*
- Trichoblastoma

Hair follicle

Fig. 91.1 Folliculo-sebaceous-apocrine unit and eccrine sweat gland. Adnexal tumors showing differentiation toward the hair follicle, sebaceous gland, apocrine gland, and eccrine gland are listed in correspondingly colored boxes. Important entities are in capital letters; entities associated with syndromes are in italics (see Tables 91.1–91.3). *Can show germinal differentiation; **differentiation toward entire follicle.

BENIGN AND MALIGNANT TUMORS WITH FOLLICULAR DIFFERENTIATION

	Morphology	Common Site(s)	Distinctive Characteristic(s)	Association(s)*
Benign				
Pilomatricoma	Firm to hard (calcified) papule, nodule, or dermal plaque	Head > upper trunk (Fig. 91.2)	Common in children; may have a characteristic 'shelf-like' feel, possibly due to calcification; sometimes has associated anetoderma	Tumor has *CTNNB1* mutation (encodes β-catenin) Occasionally associated with myotonic dystrophy, Gardner syndrome (when cystic; *APC* mutation), Rubinstein–Taybi syndrome
Trichilemmoma	Skin-colored papule > nodule	Central face, especially nose or upper lip	May be wart-like (verrucous)	Cowden disease (PTEN hamartoma tumor syndrome) (*PTEN* mutation) (Fig. 91.15)
Desmoplastic trichoepithelioma	Skin-colored to erythematous plaque	Cheek or upper lip	Annular; more common in women	
Trichofolliculoma	Papule or nodule	Face > scalp > upper trunk	Occasionally has a tuft of white, wispy hairs protruding from center (Fig. 91.3)	
Fibrofolliculoma/ trichodiscoma	Subtle skin-colored to hypopigmented papule	Face, ears (Fig. 91.4), neck > scalp > upper trunk		Birt–Hogg–Dubé syndrome (*BHD* mutation) (Fig. 91.15)
Tumor of the follicular infundibulum	Hypopigmented, subtle macule or papule or plaque	Face (Fig. 91.5)	Sometimes atrophic	Rarely, Cowden disease (PTEN hamartoma tumor syndrome) (Fig. 91.15)
Trichoepithelioma	Pink-red to skin-colored papule or nodule	Face (especially medial cheeks, nose) > upper trunk (Fig. 91.6)		Brooke–Spiegler syndrome (*CYLD* mutation), multiple familial trichoepitheliomas
Trichoblastoma	Nodule	90% of cases on scalp		Most common tumor to develop in nevus sebaceus
Proliferating pilar tumor	Skin-colored to pink-red nodule			
Malignant†				
Basal cell carcinoma	See Chapter 88			

*Patients generally have multiple tumors when associated with a syndrome.
†Rare tumors include pilomatrical carcinoma and trichollemmal carcinoma.

Table 91.1 Benign and malignant tumors with follicular differentiation. Cysts (e.g. epidermoid and pilar) are discussed in Chapter 90. *BHD* encodes folliculin, a tumor suppressor; *CYLD* encodes a deubiquinating enzyme; *APC* encodes a protein that regulates cell adhesion/migration.

ADNEXAL NEOPLASMS

BENIGN AND MALIGNANT TUMORS WITH SEBACEOUS DIFFERENTIATION			
	Morphology	Site(s)	Distinctive Characteristic(s)	Association(s)
Benign				
Nevus sebaceus (see Chapter 51)	Yellow-orange, hairless linear plaque	Scalp > face/neck	Along lines of Blaschko, minimally raised and waxy during childhood, becoming thicker and verrucous at puberty; can develop secondary tumors, most commonly trichoblastoma	Mosaic *HRAS > KRAS* mutation; more extensive lesions may be associated with Schimmelpenning syndrome (see Chapter 51)
Sebaceous hyperplasia	Yellowish papule (Fig. 91.7)	Face (rarely other sites)	Sometimes telangiectatic, with central dell	
Sebaceous adenoma	Papule or nodule	Head and neck > upper trunk		Muir–Torre syndrome (especially in patients <50 years of age; *MSH2* or *MLH1 >> MSH6* mutation) (Fig. 91.15)**
Sebaceoma	Deep nodule or 'cyst'	Face (especially nose) > upper trunk		Muir–Torre syndrome (Fig. 91.15)
Malignant				
Sebaceous carcinoma	Occasionally yellowish nodule or plaque, sometimes ulcerated or crusted	Eyelid or other sites	Early lesions may resemble blepharitis or ocular rosacea	Muir–Torre syndrome (Fig. 91.15)

**MSH2, MLH1, *and* MSH6 *encode mismatch repair proteins.*

Table 91.2 Benign and malignant tumors with sebaceous differentiation.

ADNEXAL NEOPLASMS

BENIGN AND MALIGNANT TUMORS WITH APOCRINE/ECCRINE (GLANDULAR) DIFFERENTIATION

	Morphology	Site(s)	Distinctive Characteristic(s)	Associated Syndrome(s)*
Benign				
Syringoma	2–4 mm firm, skin-colored to yellow or pink papule	Most commonly eyelids > vulva > disseminated on trunk and upper extremities (Fig. 91.8)	More discrete than xanthelasma	Down syndrome, rarely metabolic syndrome (diabetes) with clear cell syringomas (Fig. 91.15)
Mixed tumor	Nodule	Head and neck (Fig. 91.9)		
Poroma	Red-blue papule, plaque, or nodule	Head and neck or palmoplantar	May have a vascular appearance (Fig. 91.10)	
Hidradenoma	Dermal or subcutaneous nodule (Fig. 91.11)			
Syringocystadenoma papilliferum	Papule or plaque, often crusted	Scalp (Fig. 91.12)	May arise within nevus sebaceus	
Hidradenoma papilliferum	Smooth dermal or subcutaneous nodule	Vulva		
Spiradenoma	Dermal or subcutaneous papule or nodule, may have bluish hue		Sometimes painful	Brooke–Spiegler syndrome (Fig. 91.15)
Cylindroma	Pink, single or multiple papule(s) or nodule(s)	Head and neck, especially scalp (Fig. 91.13)	May become confluent/extensive on head ('turban' tumor)	Cylindromatosis, Brooke–Spiegler syndrome (Fig. 91.15)
Malignant†				
Microcystic adnexal carcinoma	Nodule or plaque	Face (Fig. 91.14)	Young or middle-aged adults, female > male; more aggressive than basal cell carcinoma	

*Patients generally have multiple tumors when associated with a syndrome.
†Other rare tumors include porocarcinoma and adenoid cystic carcinoma.

Table 91.3 Benign and malignant tumors with apocrine/eccrine (glandular) differentiation. Cysts (e.g. hidrocystoma) are discussed in Chapter 90.

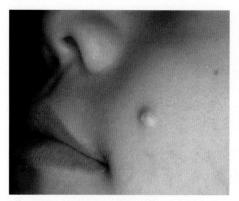

Fig. 91.2 Pilomatricoma. A nodule on the cheek of a child.

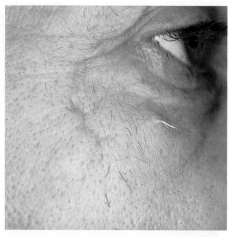

Fig. 91.3 Trichofolliculoma. Wispy vellus hairs emerge from a skin-colored papule with a dilated central pore.

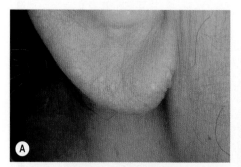

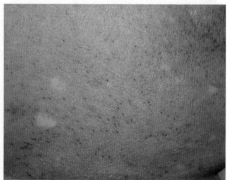

Fig. 91.5 Tumor of the follicular infundibulum. Multiple hypopigmented thin papules on the cheek.

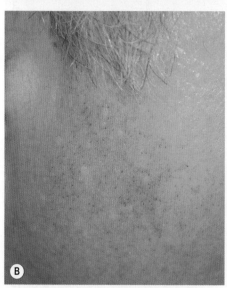

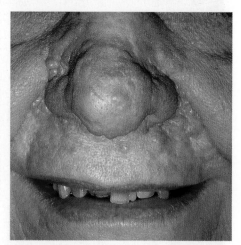

Fig. 91.4 Fibrofolliculomas in association with Birt–Hogg–Dubé syndrome. A Several skin-colored papules are present on the ear. **B** Multiple smooth papules of the lateral cheek that are relatively hypopigmented and lack the telangiectasias of the background skin.

Fig. 91.6 Multiple familial trichoepitheliomas. Numerous skin-colored papules and nodules on the mid-face.

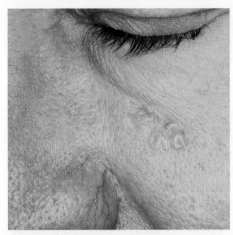

Fig. 91.7 Sebaceous hyperplasia. Skin-colored to yellowish papules with a central dell.

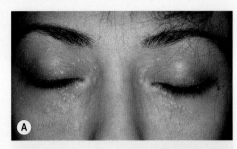

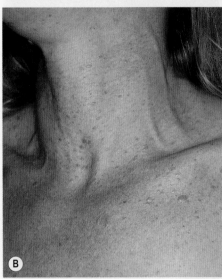

Fig. 91.8 Syringomas. A Aggregated skin-colored papules on the eyelids. **B** Multiple skin-colored to pink, smooth papules on the neck and upper chest. The lesions favor the ventral surface of the trunk, a distribution pattern referred to as *'en demicuirasse'*. *B, Courtesy, Jean L. Bolognia, MD.*

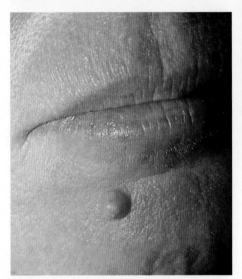

Fig. 91.9 Mixed tumor (chondroid syringoma). Nodule on the chin. *Courtesy, Ronald P. Rapini, MD.*

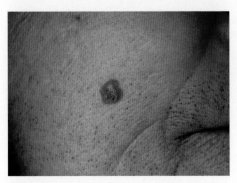

Fig. 91.10 Poroma. A biopsy specimen is necessary to establish a definitive diagnosis.

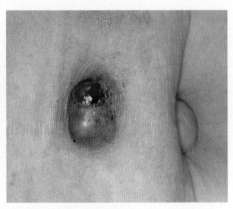

Fig. 91.11 Hidradenoma. A solitary violaceous nodule on the abdomen with serous drainage.

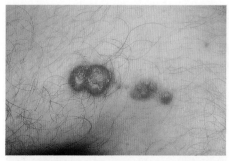

Fig. 91.12 Syringocystadenoma papilliferum. Grouped papules and nodules. The possibility of an associated nevus sebaceus needs to be considered.

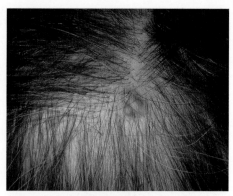

Fig. 91.13 Cylindroma. Whereas numerous tumors aggregated on the scalp are called turban tumors, solitary lesions usually present as smooth erythematous nodules.

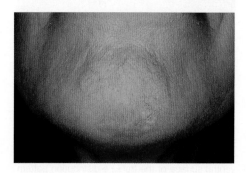

Fig. 91.14 Microcystic adnexal carcinoma. This tumor presents as a slowly expanding, firm plaque.

APPROACH TO MULTIPLE FACIAL PAPULES

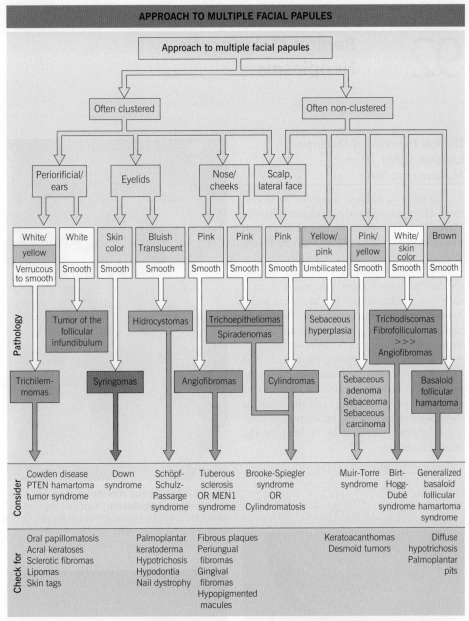

Fig. 91.15 Approach to multiple facial papules. As a general rule, multiple lesions are suggestive of a syndrome, but exceptions are syringoma and tumor of the follicular infundibulum (rarely syndromic). Other causes of multiple facial papules include BCCs, miliary osteomas, milia, verrucae, and acne. MEN, multiple endocrine neoplasia.

For further information see Ch. 111. From *Dermatology, Third Edition*.

92 | Benign Melanocytic Neoplasms

Benign Pigmented Cutaneous Lesions Other Than Melanocytic Nevi

• This group of lesions can further be divided into: (1) predominantly epidermal lesions (Table 92.1; Figs. 92.1–92.5); and (2) dermal melanocytoses (Table 92.2; Figs. 92.6 and 92.7).

• In the predominantly epidermal lesions, the tan to brown color can result from a variety of mechanisms – e.g. increased melanocyte activity (melanogenesis), increased melanin content in keratinocytes, and a mild increase in the number of melanocytes.

• In dermal melanocytoses, the skin is blue to blue-gray in color (ceruloderma) due to the presence of melanin-producing melanocytes in the mid to lower dermis and the resultant Tyndall phenomenon (the preferential scattering of shorter wavelengths of light by the dermal melanin).

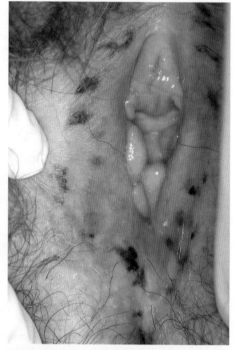

Fig. 92.2 Anogenital melanotic macules (anogenital lentiginosis). Biopsy of the darker lesion (at 7 o'clock) showed no cellular atypia. Over a period of 10 years, several of the macules faded. *Courtesy, Jean L. Bolognia, MD.*

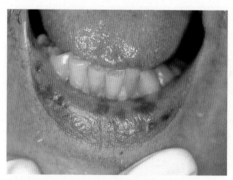

Fig. 92.1 Oral melanotic macules (labial lentigines). Multiple hyperpigmented macules on the lower lip in a patient with Laugier–Hunziker syndrome. Additional lesions are present on the tongue. Peutz–Jeghers syndrome can have a similar clinical appearance.

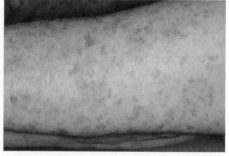

Fig. 92.3 Solar lentigines. Numerous light brown macules, some of which have an irregular border, on chronically sun-exposed skin. *Courtesy, Raymond Barnhill, MD.*

BENIGN PIGMENTED LESIONS OTHER THAN MELANOCYTIC NEVI (PREDOMINANTLY EPIDERMAL LESIONS)	
Lesion	**Major Clinical Features**
Ephelid (freckle)	• Onset in childhood (UVR-induced) and tends to fade with age and in the absence of sun exposure (e.g. winter months) • Small, well-circumscribed, usually multiple, tan to brown macules on sun-exposed areas in fair-skinned individuals
Lentigo simplex (typical type)	• Onset usually in childhood; not related to sun exposure • Small, sharply circumscribed, brown to black macules that can occur at any site, including mucosae; typically a few lesions • Multiple or generalized lentigines may be an isolated phenomenon or a marker of an underlying disorder (Table 92.3)
• Labial melanotic macule	• Onset in adulthood • Typically, an isolated to a few, brown to brown-black macule(s) on the vermilion portion of the lower lip; occasionally on the gingiva, buccal mucosa, tongue, or palate (Fig. 92.1) • Multiple lesions may be a marker of Peutz–Jeghers or Laugier–Hunziker syndromes
• Anogenital melanotic macule (Fig. 92.2)	• Onset typically in adulthood; females > males • One or more brown to black macules, sometimes with irregular or jagged borders, mottled pigmentation, and occasionally of large size (>1 cm) • In *females* favors the labia minora > labia majora, vaginal introitus, perineum; in *males* favors the glans penis and penile shaft • Multiple lesions are a feature of lichen sclerosis, Laugier–Hunziker syndrome, and Bannayan–Riley–Ruvalcaba syndrome (see Table 52.1)
• Conjunctival melanotic macule or conjunctival melanosis	• Conjunctival brown to black pigmented macules, streaks, or patches • While congenital form is typically benign, primary acquired ocular melanosis is considered a precursor lesion of conjunctival melanoma
Solar lentigo (lentigo senilis, 'liver spot' [Fig. 92.3])	• Onset in adulthood (UVR-induced); persists throughout life and may darken with sun exposure, but does not fade • Typically, multiple tan to dark brown macules, often with irregular borders, ranging from a few millimeters to >1 cm in diameter • Distribution limited to sun-exposed sites, favoring those areas of greatest cumulative exposure (e.g. face, dorsal hands and forearms, upper trunk) • Clinical variants: ink spot lentigo, PUVA lentigo, tanning bed lentigo, sunburn lentigo • If present or widespread in young children, consider: xeroderma pigmentosum, type 2 oculocutaneous albinism (lesions are unusually large and jagged)
Café-au-lait macule (CALM [Fig. 92.4])	• Onset at birth or in early childhood; not UVR-induced, but may first become noticeable following sun exposure • Uniformly colored, tan to brown macule or patch, varying in size from a few millimeters to >15 cm; grows proportionately with the child • Usually isolated but occasionally multiple; single CALM seen in ~25–35% of children; <1% of children have ≥3 CALMs • Multiple CALMs may be associated with a variety of disorders (see Table 50.3)

Table 92.1 Benign pigmented lesions other than melanocytic nevi (predominantly epidermal lesions). *Continued*

Table 92.1 *Continued* **Benign pigmented lesions other than melanocytic nevi (predominantly epidermal lesions).**

Lesion	Major Clinical Features
Becker's nevus (Fig. 92.5; see Fig. 57.3 and Table 57.1)	• May be present at birth, but the majority appear around puberty; male:female ratio ~5:1; stimulated by androgens • Classically, unilateral, tan to brown patch or thin plaque on the shoulder and/or upper trunk, but can occur elsewhere; margins typically irregular and break up into 'islands' at the periphery; hypertrichosis in ~50% • Associated smooth muscle hamartoma often present and is clinically apparent by the presence of perifollicular papules that are accentuated with rubbing • Infrequently associated with ipsilateral developmental anomalies (e.g. supernumerary nipples, breast hypoplasia, hypoplasia of the pectoralis major muscle, bony abnormalities)

PUVA, psoralens plus ultraviolet A phototherapy.

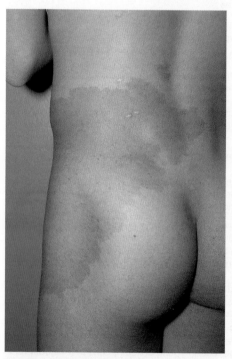

Fig. 92.4 Café-au-lait macule. Large tan patch in a geographic pattern on the lateral trunk. The patient did not have McCune–Albright syndrome.

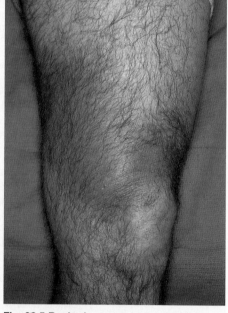

Fig. 92.5 Becker's nevus. Large patch of hyperpigmentation on the leg, which is medium brown in color. These lesions may be misdiagnosed as café-au-lait macules or congenital melanocytic nevi, especially when they do not occur on the upper trunk. *Courtesy, Jean L. Bolognia, MD.*

Acquired Melanocytic Nevi (Moles)

• Benign proliferations of a type of melanocyte called a 'nevus cell'.

• Nevus cells differ from 'ordinary' melanocytes, which typically reside as single units in the basal layer of the epidermis, in that they: (1) usually cluster as nests in the lower epidermis and/or dermis; and (2) do not have dendritic processes (except when found in a blue nevus).

• Both 'ordinary' melanocytes and nevus cells can produce melanin.

THE SPECTRUM AND CLINICAL FEATURES OF DERMAL MELANOCYTOSES	
Lesion	**Major Clinical Features**
Congenital dermal melanocytosis (Mongolian spots) (Fig. 92.6)	• Typically apparent at birth or within the first few weeks of life • Regresses in >95% of patients by age 18 years; more likely to persist in extensive or extra-sacral variants; most common in Asians and blacks • Presents as a single or multiple, uniform, blue-gray patch(es) with indefinite borders; favors the lumbosacral area and buttocks > back; varies in size from a few centimeters to >20 cm • CALM and melanocytic nevi that reside within these areas often have a 'halo' that lacks dermal melanocytes (Fig. 92.6) • DDx: ecchymosis, child abuse, patch blue nevus, venous malformation • Extensive lesions may be associated with a port-wine stain (phakomatosis pigmentovascularis; see Chapter 85), developmental abnormalities (e.g. cleft lip), or inborn errors of metabolism (e.g. Hurler syndrome)
Nevus of Ota*,** (oculodermal melanocytosis, nevus fuscocaeruleus ophthalmo-maxillaris) (Fig. 92.7)	• Bimodal age of onset, with the majority (50–60%) present at birth or in infancy (before 1 year of age), and the remainder (40–50%) appearing at or around puberty; lifelong persistence • More common in Asians and blacks; females > males • Involves those areas innervated by the first and second divisions of the trigeminal nerve, including the skin, conjunctiva, sclera, tympanic membrane, and/or oral and nasal mucosa; 10% of cases are bilateral • Lesions are characterized by speckled or mottled, grayish-brown to blue-black patches; may extend in size over time but usually stable by adulthood • Occasionally associated with neurocutaneous melanosis, glaucoma, ipsilateral sensorineural hearing loss, ocular melanoma (yearly ophthalmologic exams recommended)
Nevus of Ito* (nevus fuscocaeruleus acromiodeltoideus)	• Favored populations and clinical appearance are similar to nevus of Ota (see above) • Involves areas of skin innervated by the posterior supraclavicular and lateral brachiocutaneous nerves, namely the supraclavicular, scapular, or deltoid regions; typically unilateral
Nevus of Ota-like macules** (acquired dermal melanocytosis, acquired bilateral nevus of Ota-like macules, Hori's nevus)	• Most often seen in middle-aged Asian females • Multiple grayish-brown macules arising in a symmetric, bilateral distribution on the malar cheeks and forehead and sometimes the eyelids, temple, and nose; does not involve mucosa • Important to distinguish from melasma, as laser therapy improves nevus of Ota-like macules

*DDx for nevus of Ota or Ito: patch or plaque blue nevus, ecchymosis, venous malformation; for nevus of Ito: extra-sacral Mongolian spot.
**Rx (if desired): pulsed Q-switched lasers (e.g. Q-switched ruby, alexandrite, or Nd:YAG lasers) beneficial but often requires multiple sessions.
CALM, café-au-lait macule.

Table 92.2 The spectrum and clinical features of dermal melanocytoses.

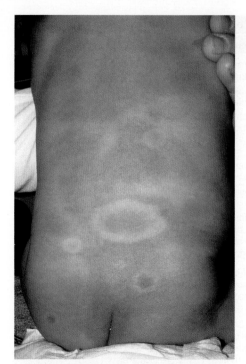

Fig. 92.6 Dermal melanocytosis (Mongolian spots) in a child with neurofibromatosis 1. Surrounding each café-au-lait macule, there is an absence of the characteristic blue discoloration.

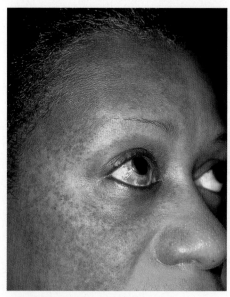

Fig. 92.7 Nevus of Ota (oculodermal melanocytosis). Unilateral blue-gray discoloration of the face, which is either mottled or confluent. There is also involvement of the sclera.

• Acquired melanocytic nevi can be categorized as **common** (banal) or **atypical** (dysplastic), and they are further named based on the histologic location of the collections of nevus cells (Fig. 92.8):
  – *Junctional* melanocytic nevus: dermal-epidermal junction.
  – *Compound* melanocytic nevus: dermal–epidermal junction plus dermis.
  – *Intradermal* melanocytic nevus: dermis.
• Variants include halo, blue, Spitz, and 'special site' nevi (Fig. 92.9).
• Risk factors for developing acquired melanocytic nevi: (1) a family history of numerous nevi; (2) a greater degree of sun exposure during childhood, especially intermittent and intense; and (3) lightly pigmented skin (individuals with phototype II have the greatest number of nevi).
• The vast majority of acquired melanocytic nevi remain as benign neoplasms throughout one's life and do not require treatment.
• Having >100 melanocytic nevi (8- to 10-fold increased relative risk) or multiple atypical nevi (>5 = 4- to 6-fold increased relative risk) are phenotypic markers for an entire skin surface at risk for developing cutaneous melanoma; such persons should have lifelong surveillance with periodic total body skin examinations (beginning around puberty) and counseling regarding home self-skin examinations and sun protective measures.
• Cutaneous melanoma may arise within a pre-existing nevus, but more than half of cutaneous melanomas arise *de novo* – i.e. in previously normal-appearing skin.
• Most patients with numerous nevi and atypical nevi will have a prominent morphologic type of nevus ('signature nevus'); by recognizing signature nevi, the 'ugly duckling' can be identified and closely examined.
• Persons with more darkly pigmented skin will typically have darker colored nevi.
• **Rx:** it is not necessary to remove clinically atypical nevi prophylactically in order to confirm the presence of histological atypia; biopsies of nevi are indicated primarily when a severely atypical nevus or cutaneous melanoma is in the **DDx** (Table 92.4); if banal nevi become irritated (e.g. by clothing or jewelry), shave removal can be done.

BENIGN MELANOCYTIC NEOPLASMS

DISORDERS ASSOCIATED WITH MULTIPLE LENTIGINES

Disorder Inheritance Gene Mutation	Comments
Generalized	
LEOPARD syndrome AD *PTPN11* gene	• Lentigines present in infancy/early childhood • Café-noir macules • ECG changes (conduction defects, hypertrophic cardiomyopathy), ocular hypertelorism, *pulmonary stenosis, abnormal genitalia, growth retardation and deafness*
Generalized lentigines AD	• Café-au-lait macules
Carney complex (NAME/LAMB syndrome) AD *PRKAR1A* gene	• Lentigines, mucocutaneous myxomas, blue nevi (including epithelioid) • Psammomatous melanotic schwannomas • Atrial myxoma • Myxoid mammary fibroadenomas • Pigmented nodular adrenocortical disease; testicular (calcifying Sertoli cell), thyroid, and pituitary tumors
Arterial dissection plus lentiginosis	• Cutaneous lentigines with onset in childhood • Dissection of aortic, internal carotid, and vertebral arteries
Localized	
Head and neck (including oral mucosa) ± acral	
Peutz–Jeghers syndrome AD *STK11* gene	• Lentigines favor perioral region,[†] oral mucosa,[‡] and hands; longitudinal melanonychia • Multiple hamartomatous GI polyps • Pancreatic carcinoma; ovarian (adenoma malignum)/testicular tumors
Laugier–Hunziker syndrome	• Similar distribution of lentigines as in Peutz–Jeghers, including lips, oral mucosa, and digits • Longitudinal melanonychia and genital melanosis
Cantú (hyperkeratosis–hyperpigmentation) syndrome AD	• Punctate palmoplantar keratoderma • Multiple small (1 mm) macules on the face, forearms, hands/feet
Cowden disease AD *PTEN* gene (See Chapter 52 and Table 52.1)	• Periorificial and acral pigmented macules

Table 92.3 Disorders associated with multiple lentigines. *Adapted from Bolognia JL. Disorders of hypopigmentation and hyperpigmentation. In Harper J, Oranje A, Prose N (eds.), Textbook of Pediatric Dermatology, 2nd edn. Oxford: Blackwell, 2006;997–1040. Continued*

Table 92.3 *Continued* **Disorders associated with multiple lentigines.**

Disorder Inheritance Gene Mutation	Comments
Centrofacial lentiginosis AD	• Lentigines in a butterfly distribution on the nose, cheeks > forehead, eyelids, upper lip • Onset in infancy; increase in number in childhood • Possibly associated with neuropsychiatric illness and osseous anomalies
Inherited patterned lentiginosis AD	• African-Americans with light brown skin • Pigmented macules appear in early childhood • Present on central face and lips > buttocks, elbows, hands/feet • Occasional oral mucosal involvement
Cronkhite–Canada syndrome	• Typically affects older men • Lentigines of buccal mucosa, face, hands/feet • Alopecia (diffuse, nonscarring), nail dystrophy, intestinal polyposis
Genital	
Bannayan–Riley–Ruvalcaba syndrome AD *PTEN* gene (see Table 52.1)	• Penile > vulvar pigmented macules
'Photodistribution'	
Xeroderma pigmentosum AR Mutations in genes encoding DNA repair proteins	• Lentigines favor, but are not limited to, chronically sun-exposed sites • Multiple skin cancers
Segmental	
Partial unilateral lentiginosis	• Multiple lentigines in a segmental distribution • Café-au-lait macules in same distribution

†May fade.
‡Persists.
AD, autosomal dominant; AR, autosomal recessive; ECG, electrocardiogram; GI, gastrointestinal; LEOPARD, lentigines/ECG abnormalities/ocular hypertelorism/pulmonary stenosis/abnormalities of genitalia/retardation of growth/deafness syndrome; NAME, nevi/atrial myxoma/myxoid neurofibroma/ephelides syndrome; LAMB, lentigines/atrial myxoma/mucocutaneous myxoma/blue nevi syndrome.

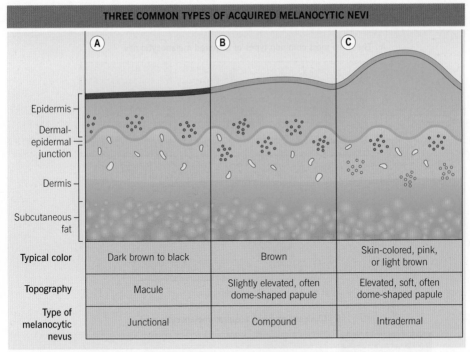

THREE COMMON TYPES OF ACQUIRED MELANOCYTIC NEVI

	A	B	C
Typical color	Dark brown to black	Brown	Skin-colored, pink, or light brown
Topography	Macule	Slightly elevated, often dome-shaped papule	Elevated, soft, often dome-shaped papule
Type of melanocytic nevus	Junctional	Compound	Intradermal

(Left labels: Epidermis, Dermal-epidermal junction, Dermis, Subcutaneous fat)

Fig. 92.8 Three common types of acquired melanocytic nevi. A Junctional, **B** compound, and **C** intradermal. The latter may also be pedunculated or papillomatous (see Chapter 1).

POTENTIAL INDICATIONS FOR BIOPSY OF MELANOCYTIC NEVI

- **Patient concern for cutaneous melanoma** (e.g. new nevus, changing nevus, anxiety-provoking nevus)
- **Symptoms** (e.g. pruritus, pain, bleeding)
- **Physician concern for cutaneous melanoma**
  - Marked asymmetry (e.g. irregular *b*orders, variegated *c*olor) – i.e. the ABCs of cutaneous melanoma*
  - Areas of regression (often seen as white or blue-gray areas)
  - Development of areas of pink or red color that are not easily explained by a benign etiology (e.g. acne or trauma)
  - Surrounding cloak of erythema ('little red riding hood sign')
  - History or photographic evidence of worrisome change in size, color, configuration
  - 'Ugly duckling' nevus (i.e. a nevus with a different phenotype than most of the other nevi in a given patient)
- **Acral nevus** – marked asymmetry, mottled pigmentation, or diameter >5 mm
- **Nail matrix-derived nevus** – single band that is dark or has an irregular color, width ≥4 mm, progressive darkening with time, or extension of pigmentation beyond the nailfold
- **Halo nevus** – the central nevus is markedly atypical or has worrisome features
- **Cellular blue nevus** – has undergone change (e.g. a new papule or nodule)
- **Spitz nevus with clinically atypical features** – see text
- **Congenital melanocytic nevus** – new papulonodule whose color can vary from red to black, new area of induration or ulceration

*D and E represent large diameter and evolution.

Table 92.4 Potential indications for biopsy of melanocytic nevi. Patients with numerous nevi can continue to develop new nevi, and banal nevi can increase in size over time.

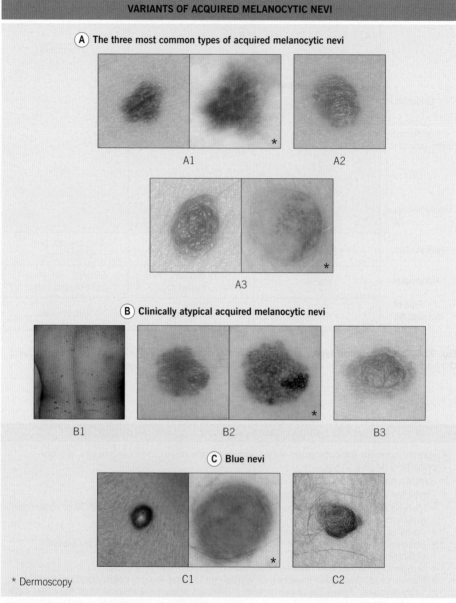

VARIANTS OF ACQUIRED MELANOCYTIC NEVI

A The three most common types of acquired melanocytic nevi

A1

A2

A3

B Clinically atypical acquired melanocytic nevi

B1

B2

B3

C Blue nevi

C1

C2

* Dermoscopy

Fig. 92.9 Variants of acquired melanocytic nevi. A The three most common types of acquired melanocytic nevi. **A1** Junctional nevus. Clinically, a brown macule with central hyperpigmentation. Dermoscopically, a uniform pigment network. **A2** Compound nevus. Light to medium brown papule. **A3** Intradermal nevus. A light tan, soft, raised papule. Dermoscopically, focal globular-like structures, whitish structureless areas, and fine comma vessels. **B** Clinically atypical acquired melanocytic nevi. **B1** Multiple pigmented macules and papules of varying sizes on the back. **B2** Close-up photo; the dermoscopy pattern is reticular-disorganized and can be seen with uncertain lesions. **B3** 'Fried egg' appearance, with a central elevated soft papule and macular rim. **C** Blue nevi. **C1** Common blue nevus. By dermoscopy, blue homogeneous color typically found in blue nevi. **C2** Cellular blue nevus. A firm blue plaque is a common presentation. *Continued*

VARIANTS OF ACQUIRED MELANOCYTIC NEVI

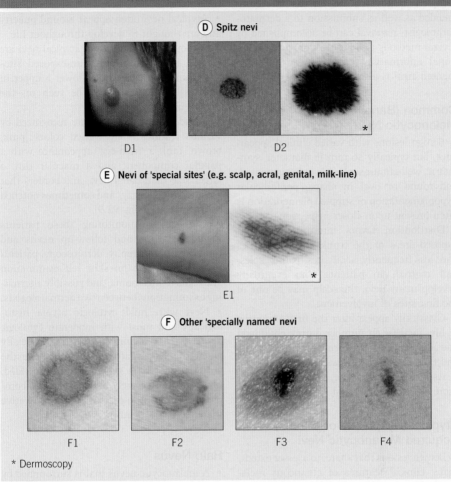

D Spitz nevi

D1   D2

E Nevi of 'special sites' (e.g. scalp, acral, genital, milk-line)

E1

F Other 'specially named' nevi

F1   F2   F3   F4

* Dermoscopy

Fig. 92.9 *Continued* **D** Spitz nevi. **D1** Classic Spitz nevus. Red dome-shaped papule on the ear of a child. **D2** Reed nevus, typified dermoscopically by the classic starburst pattern (regular streaks at the periphery of a heavily pigmented and symmetric small macule). **E** Nevi of 'special sites' (e.g. scalp, acral, genital, milk-line). **E1** Acral nevus. A brown macule on the sole of the foot. Dermoscopically, a lattice-like pattern is seen. **F** Other 'specially named' nevi. **F1** Eclipse nevus. A tan center and thinner brown rim; note the stellate appearance of the brown rim. **F2** Cockade or target nevus. Central lightly pigmented papule surrounded by a tan annulus then a brown ring. **F3** One variant of combined melanocytic nevus. Dark brown to black papule within an otherwise uniformly pigmented light brown nevus. The differential diagnosis includes the possibility of a melanoma developing in a nevus. **F4** Recurrent nevus. Dark brown pigmentation within the center of a circular scar; the pigmentation reflects the proliferation of melanocytes within the epidermis. *Courtesy, Giuseppe Argenziano, MD, Raymond L. Barnhill, MD, Jean L. Bolognia, MD, Lorenzo Cerroni, MD, Harold S. Rabinovitz, MD, Ronald P. Rapini, MD, and Iris Zalaudek, MD.*

- When cutaneous melanoma is in the **DDx**, complete removal of the nevus is recommended as well as submission to a dermatopathologist; removal can be accomplished by several methods (see Fig 1.6); providing additional information (e.g. eccentric hyperpigmented area) is also helpful.

Common (Banal) Acquired Melanocytic Nevi

- Benign lesions with varied clinical appearance, but typically ≤6 mm in diameter, symmetric, well-circumscribed, evenly pigmented, and round or oval in shape; perifollicular hypopigmentation or stippled pigmentation is often present upon closer inspection.
- Distribution favors intermittently sun-exposed areas of the trunk and extremities and, less frequently, acral sites (palms, soles, nail matrix); in patients who eventually develop many nevi, the scalp may be one of the first sites of involvement.
- Classically appear after the first 6 months of life, increase in number during childhood and adolescence, peak during the third decade, and then slowly regress with age.
- As nevi 'age' over time, they often become more elevated, softer, and less pigmented.

Atypical (Dysplastic or Clark's) Acquired Melanocytic Nevi

- Benign lesions that share, to a lesser extent, many clinical features of cutaneous melanoma (e.g. asymmetry, border irregularity, color variegation, and diameter >6 mm) but usually they 'age' in a manner similar to banal nevi and only a tiny proportion may develop melanoma within them.
- Histologically, architectural disorder is seen and cytologic atypia may be present; sometimes the latter is categorized as mild, moderate, or severe.
- The major risk factor for developing atypical nevi is genetic predisposition.
- The 'atypical mole syndrome' has been variably described in the literature, ranging from individuals with atypical nevi but no personal or family history of melanoma to the familial atypical multiple mole and melanoma syndrome (FAMMM syndrome), in which an individual with numerous nevi and ≥2 first-degree relatives with cutaneous

melanoma has a very high risk of developing melanoma.
- Atypical nevi often appear around puberty and are thought to develop throughout life.
- Although the majority of atypical nevi are located in intermittently sun-exposed sites (e.g. trunk and extremities [lower > upper in females]), often they can be seen on the breasts and buttocks.
- *Clinically*, atypical nevi are recognized by various features – e.g. varied colors (pink, brown, tan), a 'fried-egg' appearance with a papular component and a macular rim, a larger size than banal nevi, and borders that are ill-defined, 'fuzzy,' and sometimes notched or irregular (see Fig. 92.9).
- Adjuncts to monitoring these patients include baseline and follow-up nevus and total body photography; dermoscopy; patient/partner education on skin self-examination and signs of melanoma; and possibly alternating examinations between two dermatologists.
- Nevi with mild cytologic atypia histologically and most with moderate cytologic atypia do not require re-excision, especially when the biopsy attempted to remove the entire nevus; it is generally recommended, however, that severely atypical nevi be completely excised or re-excised with conservative margins (e.g. 3–5 mm).

Halo Nevus

- A melanocytic nevus that is surrounded by a round or oval, usually symmetric, halo of complete depigmentation (i.e. white color).
- The central nevus is most often a common acquired melanocytic nevus, but it can also be other nevus subtypes.
- The halo of depigmentation is believed to represent a T-cell-mediated immune response against nevus antigens, analogous to vitiligo (see Chapter 54).
- Halo nevi are seen in up to 5% of Caucasian children aged 6–15 years; they are more common in patients with an increased number of nevi and a personal or family history of vitiligo.
- The most common location is the back; multiple halo nevi are seen in ~50% of cases.
- There are four clinical stages in the life of a halo nevus, and the evolution usually occurs over years to decades (Fig. 92.10).

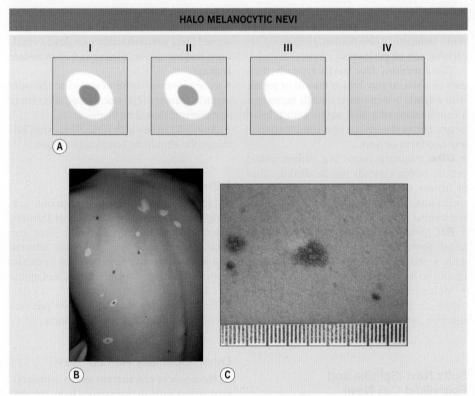

Fig. 92.10 Halo melanocytic nevi. A Four potential clinical stages in the life of a halo nevus. *Stage I*: central pigmented melanocytic nevus with a halo of depigmentation; *Stage II*: central nevus is pink with a halo of depigmentation; *Stage III*: no central nevus, just a depigmented macule; *Stage IV*: repigmentation (partial or complete). **B** Multiple halo nevi (seen here in all four of the various stages) are seen most commonly in children and young adults with numerous nevi. **C** A benign compound melanocytic nevus with an asymmetric halo. *C, Courtesy, Jean L. Bolognia, MD.*

- The central nevus should be assessed for suspicious or clinically atypical features; if none are present, then no treatment is necessary (vast majority of lesions); if present, then biopsy of just the central nevus should be performed.
- A new onset of multiple halo nevi is unusual in middle-aged and older adults; this clinical scenario should raise the possibility of the halo nevi representing an autoimmune reaction against a cutaneous or ocular melanoma.
- **DDx:** other pigmented lesions that can have halos (e.g. solar lentigo, seborrheic keratosis), halo primary cutaneous melanoma, halo melanoma metastasis.

Blue Nevi

- Benign lesions due to a proliferation of dendritic melanocytes within the dermis; blue in color because of the Tyndall effect (see above).
- Sites of predilection are those areas in which active dermal melanocytes are still present at the time of birth (e.g. head, neck, dorsal hands and feet, sacral region).
- Most blue nevi have a somatic activating mutation in *GNAQ*, which encodes the Q-class of G-protein α subunits.
- The ***common blue nevus*** typically presents as a solitary, blue to blue-black, dome-shaped papule, usually <1 cm in diameter and most often occurring on the dorsal hands or feet (see Fig. 92.9); frequently arises in adolescence; no malignant potential.
- The ***cellular blue nevus*** tends to be larger in size (i.e. more plaque-like), and it can be congenital or acquired (see Fig. 92.9); favors the head, sacral region, and buttocks; melanoma (malignant blue nevus) can develop

within cellular blue nevi (see Chapter 93); if location (e.g. scalp) or patient awareness prevents satisfactory observation, then complete excision can be performed.

• The **combined blue nevus** typically presents as a blue to gray-brown macule or papule with a subtle brown rim; it usually represents a combination of a blue nevus with a banal nevus, but in theory can be a combination of any two types of nevi.

• **DDx:** traumatic tattoo (e.g. carbon from a pencil), which typically can be distinguished by history, or a venous lake (compressible) > melanoma metastasis, primary cutaneous melanoma.

• **Rx:** none for common blue nevi and as noted above for cellular blue nevi; lesions with a history of recent growth or change should be biopsied.

• Multiple blue nevi (normal in Asians) may signify an underlying syndrome, e.g. Carney complex (see Table 92.3).

Spitz Nevi (Spindle and Epithelioid Cell Nevi)

• Benign proliferations of epithelioid and/or spindled melanocytes.

• Majority appear during childhood or young adulthood and most commonly occur on the face and lower extremities.

• Classically, a Spitz nevus is symmetric, well-circumscribed, <1 cm in diameter, uniformly pink, tan, red, or red-brown, smooth, and dome-shaped (see Fig. 92.9); occasionally, lesions are verrucous or darkly pigmented.

• **Pigmented spindle cell nevus of Reed** is a variant that typically presents in young women as a very dark brown to black minimally elevated papule, most often on the thigh; characteristic 'starburst pattern' on dermoscopy (see Fig. 92.9).

• **DDx:** *clinical:* intradermal melanocytic nevus, juvenile xanthogranuloma, molluscum contagiosum, pyogenic granuloma, verruca vulgaris, dermatofibroma, cutaneous melanoma; *histologic:* when atypical features, cutaneous melanoma.

• Molecular techniques (e.g. FISH or CGH analysis, *BRAF*^{V600E} and *H-RAS* mutational status) may help better categorize difficult lesions.

• Spitz nevi have a tendency to involute over time, and monitoring is an option for a presumed Spitz nevus that develops during childhood and has classic clinical and dermoscopic features.

• Any presumed Spitz nevus with *clinically* atypical features (e.g. size >1 cm, ulceration, asymmetry) should be biopsied.

• Any Spitz nevus with unusual features *histologically* should be completely excised.

Nevi of Special Sites

• Nevi in certain anatomic locations (e.g. scalp) may exhibit *atypical clinical* features, whereas those in several specific sites (e.g. acral, genital, auricular, milk line, flexural, and scalp nevi) may have *atypical histologic* features that simulate cutaneous melanoma (see Fig. 92.9).

• Recognition of this phenomenon prevents overdiagnosis of cutaneous melanoma.

Other 'Specially Named' Nevi

• **Meyerson or eczematous nevus**: a melanocytic nevus with an eczematous halo; eczematous reaction typically resolves spontaneously or with the application of a topical CS.

• **Eclipse nevus**: benign melanocytic nevus most often found on the scalp of children; presents as a tan, occasionally pink, central macule or papule with a brown, often stellate rim (see Fig. 92.9); ages into an intradermal nevus; when present on the scalp, may be a marker for developing numerous nevi elsewhere over time.

• **Cockade nevus**: a benign melanocytic nevus with a target configuration, namely a central pigmented papule surrounded by a concentric tan rim, which is then surrounded by another pigmented annulus (see Fig. 92.9); occurs in patients with eclipse nevi.

• **Recurrent nevus**: the reappearance of pigment within the scar of a previously biopsied or excised nevus (see Fig. 92.9); if symmetric, re-evaluation of the original histology and observation is generally all that is required; if asymmetric or continues to enlarge after its initial appearance, then biopsy is prudent.

• **Agminated nevus**: a clustering of melanocytic nevi within normal-appearing skin.

Congenital Melanocytic Nevi (CMN)

• Classically defined as a melanocytic nevus present at birth; may be subtle at birth and not readily apparent for a few months.

• Melanocytic nevi that become apparent after 3 months of age, but before 2 years of age, have been termed 'tardive CMN,' 'congenital nevus-like nevi,' or 'early onset nevi'.

• CMN are due to a proliferation of melanocytes that arise during embryogenesis; melanocytes extend deep into the dermis and subcutaneous tissues and often follow follicular and neurovascular structures; *NRAS* mutations have been detected in CMN and associated neurologic lesions (see below).

• Incidence of small CMN is estimated at 1–2%, with large CMN having an incidence of ~1 in 20 000 individuals.

• CMN are classified into four groups, based on their **final adult size**:

- *Small CMN*: <1.5 cm (Fig. 92.11A).
- *Medium CMN*: 1.5–20 cm (Fig. 92.11B–D).
- *Large CMN*: >20–40 cm (in a neonate, large CMN are >9 cm on the head or >6 cm on the body).
- *Giant CMN*: >40 cm (Fig. 92.11E).

• *Small* or *medium-sized CMN* are usually solitary, can occur anywhere on the body, range in color from tan to black, and may have increased terminal hair growth (hypertrichosis).

• *Giant CMN* are sometimes referred to as 'bathing suit' or 'garment' nevi because of their distribution pattern; multiple smaller, widely disseminated 'satellite' nevi are also commonly associated with these giant CMN.

• CMN grow proportionally with the child and over time can change from initially flat, evenly pigmented patches to elevated, mottled, pebbly or verrucous plaques; scalp CMN may lighten in color and gradually regress; papules or nodules can develop within the CMN, but signs of rapid growth, induration, or ulceration should raise suspicion for the development of melanoma and prompt a biopsy.

• CMN are a known risk factor for melanoma and neurocutaneous melanosis (NCM), with the absolute risk being associated with the severity of the cutaneous phenotype.

• The risk of developing melanoma within a small or medium-sized CMN is thought to be <1% over a lifetime; the risk for giant CMN is ~5%, with greater risk being a function of nevus size and number of satellite lesions; in giant CMN, the majority of melanomas develop in childhood (~50% in the first 5 years of life).

• Cutaneous melanomas can arise within the dermis or subcutaneous tissues of a CMN, making clinical diagnosis difficult.

• Patients with a giant CMN in a posterior axial location that is associated with multiple satellite nevi (≥20) have the greatest risk of developing melanoma; although the melanoma can develop within the CMN itself (not the satellite lesions), the CNS, or the retroperitoneum, the primary site may remain unknown.

• In **neurocutaneous melanosis (NCM)**, also referred to as leptomeningeal melanocytosis, there is a proliferation of melanocytes in the CNS (as well as the skin); individuals with multiple (≥3, but usually 10–20+), disseminated medium-sized CMN are at greatest risk of NCM, followed by those with a giant CMN in a posterior axial location with multiple satellites.

• NCM-associated signs – e.g. hydrocephalus, seizures, developmental delay, increased intracranial pressure, cranial nerve palsies, sensorimotor defects, and hypotonia – tend to manifest by 2–3 years of age.

• An approach to the management of CMN is presented in Table 92.5 and Fig. 92.12.

Speckled Lentiginous Nevus (SLN, Nevus Spilus)

• A subtype of CMN with a prevalence of ~2% in the general population.

• Often presents at or around birth as a tan patch; over time numerous macules and papules develop within the tan patch, ranging from lentigines to junctional, compound and intradermal nevi to Spitz and blue nevi (Fig. 92.13).

• The risk of developing melanoma within the SLN is thought to be similar to classic CMN of the same size range, but may be related to the type of nevi that develop within it.

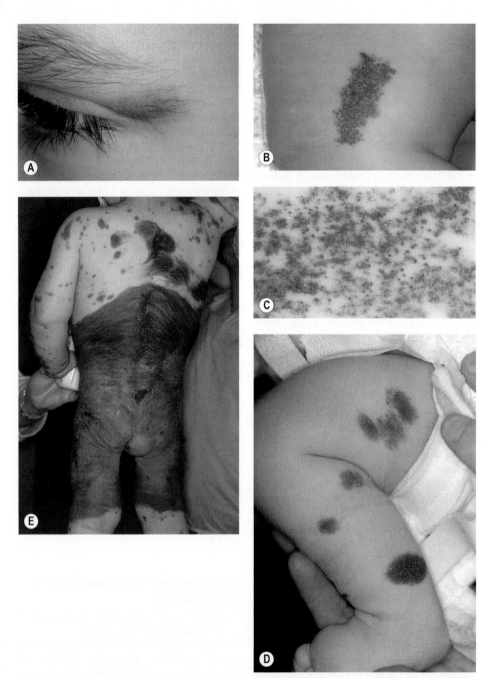

Fig. 92.11 Congenital melanocytic nevi (CMN). A Small CMN. Note the hypertrichosis and slight heterogeneity in pigmentation, reflecting its hamartomatous nature. **B** Medium-sized CMN. Note the pebbly appearance on clinical examination and the globular pattern with hyphae-like structures on dermoscopy **(C)**. **D** Multiple medium-sized CMN. This patient had 25–30 such lesions. This presentation can be associated with neurocutaneous melanosis (NCM). **E** Giant CMN, also called a 'bathing suit' nevus. It is situated in a posterior axial location with numerous satellite nevi, some of which have hypertrichosis. This patient died of intractable ascites due to the migration of benign melanocytes from the brain to the peritoneal cavity via his VP shunt. In the perianal region, the nevus was softer and somewhat 'boggy' due to neurotization. *A, Courtesy, Lorenzo Cerroni, MD; B, C, Courtesy, Raymond L. Barnhill, MD, and Harold S. Rabinovitz, MD; D, E, Courtesy, Jean L. Bologna, MD.*

APPROACH TO THE PATIENT WITH A SMALL OR MEDIUM-SIZED CONGENITAL MELANOCYTIC NEVUS (CMN)

Longitudinal Evaluation*	Excision
• No worrisome features	• Worrisome clinical or histologic features

• Observation is easy because of:
  • Location
  • Color
  • Smooth surface and uniform texture
	• Observation is difficult because of:
	  • Location (e.g. scalp)
	  • Color (e.g. black)
	  • Irregular or multinodular surface
	  • Dense hypertrichosis

• Parents/patient are:
  • Motivated and knowledgeable
  • Not anxious regarding the small chance (<1%) of melanoma
  • Not concerned regarding cosmetic appearance
	• Parents/patient are:
	  • Reluctant to observe
	  • Anxious regarding small chance (<1%) of melanoma
	  • Concerned regarding cosmetic appearance

Includes baseline photography, measurements, and periodic skin examinations.

Table 92.5 Approach to the patient with a small or medium-sized congenital melanocytic nevus (CMN).

AN APPROACH TO THE PATIENT WITH GIANT OR MULTIPLE MEDIUM-SIZED CONGENITAL MELANOCYTIC NEVI (CMN)

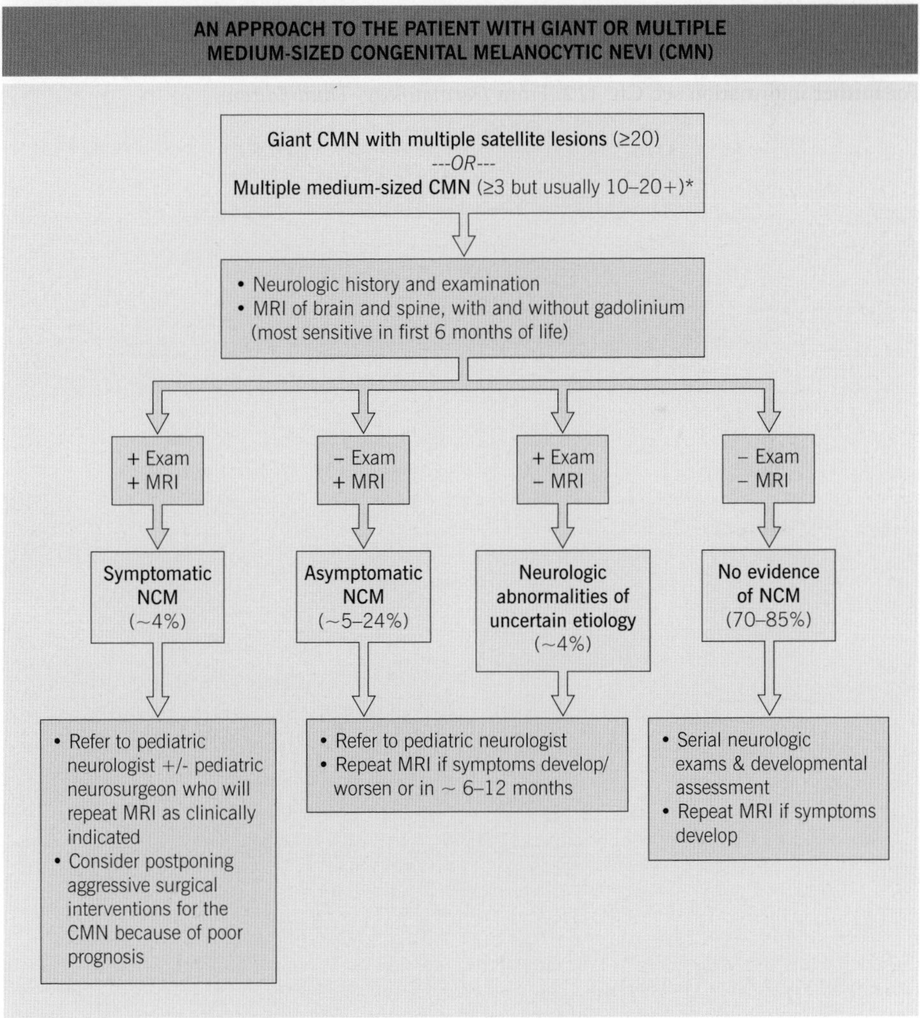

Fig. 92.12 An approach to the patient with giant or multiple medium-sized congenital melanocytic nevi (CMN). For large lesions that are on an extremity or the abdomen, with few, if any, satellite lesions, the risk of neurocutaneous melanosis (NCM) is low. *A higher proportion of these patients may have NCM compared to those with a giant CMN with multiple satellite lesions.

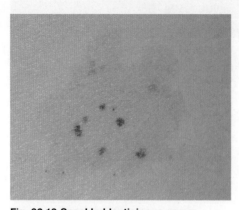

Fig. 92.13 Speckled lentiginous nevus (nevus spilus). Multiple brown macules and papules superimposed upon a tan patch.
Courtesy, Raymond L. Barnhill, MD, and Harold S. Rabinovitz, MD.

- **DDx:** agminated nevi (see above); partial unilateral lentiginosis.
- SLN should be followed with periodic examinations, photography, and biopsies as clinically indicated.

For further information see Ch. 112. From *Dermatology, Third Edition*.

Cutaneous Melanoma | 93

- A malignant tumor of melanocytes, most commonly arising from cutaneous melanocytes; can also develop from melanocytes residing elsewhere – e.g. in the uveal tract, retinal pigment epithelium, gastrointestinal mucosa, or leptomeninges.

- Some cutaneous melanomas (CMs) arise *de novo*, whereas others arise within precursor lesions (e.g. melanocytic nevi; see Chapter 92).

- Tremendous advances have been made in understanding the molecular pathways and mutations from which many CMs originate, resulting in identification of genetic markers, tools for aiding in the histologic diagnosis, and targeted treatments for CM (Figs. 93.1 and 93.2; see Table 93.11).

Epidemiology

- There has been a marked increase in the incidence of CM during the past 40–50 years, with a modest increase in mortality, especially among older males (Figs. 93.3 and 93.4).

- Death occurs at a younger age than for most other cancers.

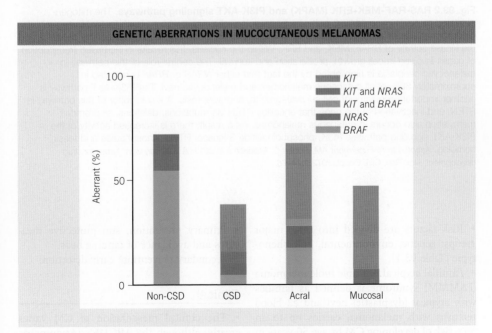

GENETIC ABERRATIONS IN MUCOCUTANEOUS MELANOMAS

Fig. 93.1 Genetic aberrations in mucocutaneous melanomas. CSD, skin with chronic sun-induced changes such as marked solar elastosis; non-CSD, skin without chronic sun-induced damage. *From Curtin JA, Busam K, Pinkel D, Bastian BC. Somatic activation of KIT in distinct subtypes of melanoma. J. Clin. Oncol. 2006;24:4340–4346.*

RAS-RAF-MEK-ERK (MAPK) AND PI3K-AKT SIGNALING PATHWAYS

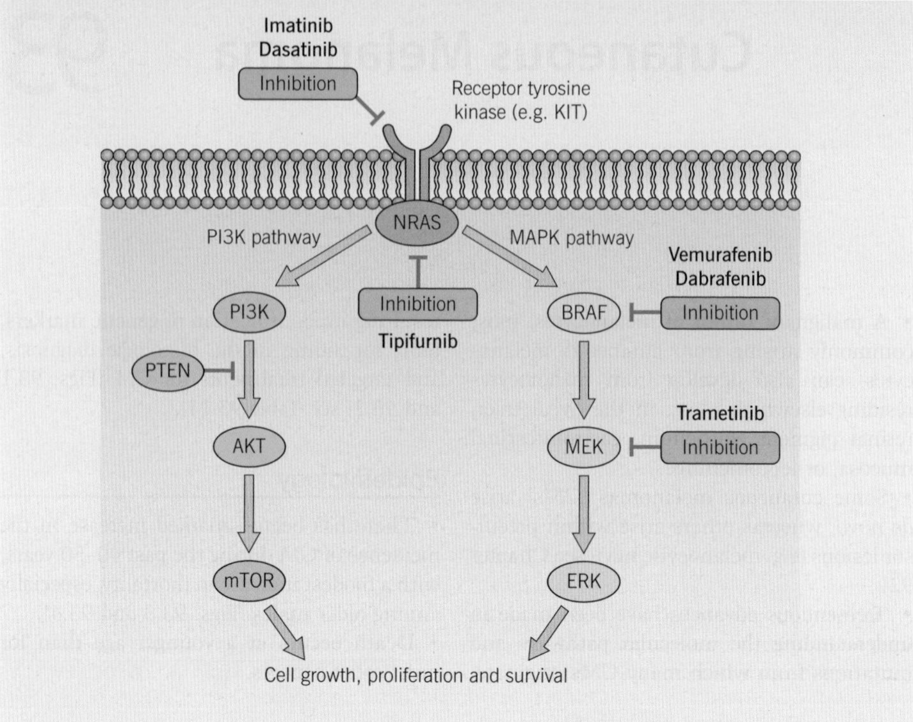

Fig. 93.2 RAS-RAF-MEK-ERK (MAPK) and PI3K-AKT signaling pathways. The mitogen-activated protein kinase (MAPK) pathway is physiologically activated by growth factor binding to receptor tyrosine kinases. The stimulus is relayed to the nucleus via the GTPase activity of NRAS and the kinase activity of BRAF, MEK, and ERK. Within the nucleus, this results in increased transcription of genes involved in cell growth, proliferation and survival. The central role of this pathway in melanocytic neoplasia is highlighted by the fact that either *NRAS* or *BRAF* is mutated in approximately 80% of all cutaneous melanomas and melanocytic nevi. The PI3K-AKT pathway is another important regulator of cell survival, growth, and apoptosis. A key inhibitor of this pathway is PTEN, and inactivation of the gene that encodes PTEN via mutations, deletions, or promoter methylation also occurs in cutaneous melanomas. As a result, there is increased activity of the PI3K-AKT signaling pathway. PI3K, phosphoinositide 3-kinase; PTEN, phosphatase and tensin homolog. *Adapted from Eggermont AM, Robert C. Melanoma in 2011: A new paradigm tumor for drug development. Nat. Rev. Clin. Oncol. 2012;9:74–76.*

- Risk factors are divided into three major groups: genetic, environmental, and phenotypic (Table 93.1).
- Familial *a*typical *m*ultiple *m*ole *m*elanoma (FAMMM) syndrome is defined as families with atypical (dysplastic) nevi and ≥2 blood relatives with melanoma; carries up to an 85% risk of developing CM by age 50 years in affected family members; some families with *CDKN2A* mutations have both melanoma and pancreatic cancer.

- Primary prevention: sun protective measures and avoidance of tanning beds.
- Secondary prevention: early detection.

Clinical

- The clinical presentation of CM varies greatly; although the **ABCDE**'s (**A**symmetry, **B**order irregularity, **C**olor variegation, **D**iameter >6 mm, **E**volution) are often used in public awareness campaigns to help promote

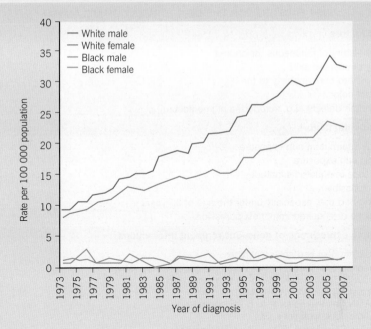

Fig. 93.3 Age-adjusted incidence rates of melanoma in the United States (1973–2007). The incidence has increased in the male and female Caucasian populations during the past three decades, and this trend has not yet stopped. The African-American population shows a constant low incidence, mostly caused by acral and mucosal melanomas. *Data from the Surveillance, Epidemiology, and End Results (SEER) program of the National Cancer Institute.*

AGE-ADJUSTED MORTALITY FROM MELANOMA IN THE US (1969–2006)

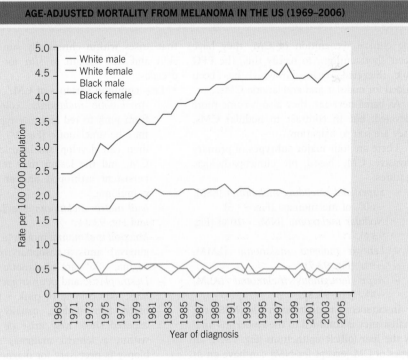

Fig. 93.4 Age-adjusted mortality from melanoma in the United States (1969–2006). The mortality has increased, especially for the male Caucasian population, during the past three decades. For females, the increase was less pronounced and has leveled off since the 1980s. *Data from the Surveillance, Epidemiology, and End Results (SEER) program of the National Cancer Institute.*

RISK FACTORS FOR THE DEVELOPMENT OF MELANOMA
Genetic factors
• Family history of cutaneous melanoma
• Lightly pigmented skin
• Tendency to burn, inability to tan
• Red hair color
• DNA repair defects (e.g. xeroderma pigmentosum)
Environmental factors
• Intense intermittent sun exposure
• Chronic sun exposure
• Residence in equatorial latitudes
• PUVA (possible)
• Tanning bed use, especially under the age of 35 years
• Iatrogenic or acquired immunosuppression
Phenotypic expressions of gene–environment interactions
• Melanocytic nevi and solar lentigines:
– Increased total number of acquired melanocytic nevi (MN)
>100 MN, relative risk ~8- to 10-fold increased
– Atypical melanocytic nevi (AMN)
>5 AMN, relative risk ~4- to 6-fold increased
– Multiple solar lentigines (SL)
Multiple SL, relative risk ~3- to 4-fold increased
Relative risks (RR) are multiplicative: e.g. a person with >100 MN + >5 AMN + multiple SL has a relative risk ~ $10 \times 5 \times 3 = 150$-fold
• Personal history of cutaneous melanoma

Table 93.1 Risk factors for the development of melanoma.

the clinical recognition of CM, they have their shortcomings; to rectify this, the **EFG** rule (**E**levated, **F**irm, **G**rowing) has been added for nodular and amelanotic CMs.

• As banal nevi age, they also become more elevated, but in contrast to nodular CMs, they are soft to palpation.

• There are four **major subtypes** of primary invasive CM, based on clinicopathologic features:

  – *Superficial spreading melanoma* (SSM; ~60% of melanomas) (Fig. 93.5).

  – *Nodular melanoma* (NM; ~20%) (Fig. 93.6).

  – *Lentigo maligna melanoma* (LMM; ~9%) (Fig. 93.7).

  – *Acral lentiginous melanoma* (ALM; ~4%) (Fig. 93.8).

• In cutaneous melanoma *in situ* (MIS), the malignancy is confined to the epidermis and/or the hair follicle epithelium (Fig. 93.9); all types of CM (except for NM) can have an *in situ* phase; *lentigo maligna* is a type of MIS

that arises within chronically sun-damaged skin and can remain *in situ* for years to decades.

• **Less common variants of CM:**

  – *Amelanotic melanoma*: color ranges from pink to red and any type of CM may be amelanotic (Fig. 93.10); children can develop amelanotic nodular CM, and the lesion may resemble a persistent arthropod bite or pyogenic granuloma.

  – *Nail matrix melanoma*: see Table 58.3 and Fig. 93.11.

  – *Mucosal melanoma*: mouth (e.g. palate, gingiva), anus > nasopharynx, larynx, vagina; ~35% are amelanotic.

  – *Desmoplastic* and *neurotropic melanomas*: skin-colored or pink > brown to black, firm nodule, usually in sun-exposed sites; may arise *de novo* or within a lentigo maligna; a deeper biopsy is necessary for diagnosis; local recurrence is a common problem.

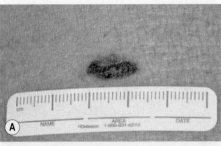

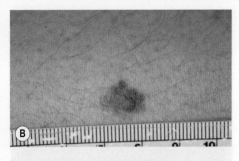

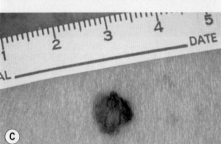

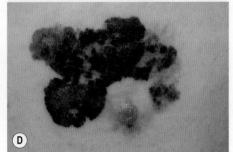

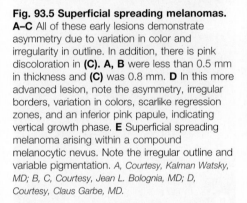

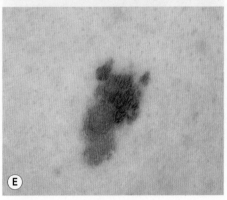

Fig. 93.5 Superficial spreading melanomas.
A–C All of these early lesions demonstrate asymmetry due to variation in color and irregularity in outline. In addition, there is pink discoloration in **(C)**. **A, B** were less than 0.5 mm in thickness and **(C)** was 0.8 mm. **D** In this more advanced lesion, note the asymmetry, irregular borders, variation in colors, scarlike regression zones, and an inferior pink papule, indicating vertical growth phase. **E** Superficial spreading melanoma arising within a compound melanocytic nevus. Note the irregular outline and variable pigmentation. *A, Courtesy, Kalman Watsky, MD; B, C, Courtesy, Jean L. Bolognia, MD; D, Courtesy, Claus Garbe, MD.*

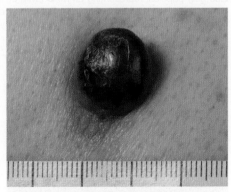

Fig. 93.6 Nodular melanoma. Rapidly growing black nodule that was >15 mm in diameter on the back of a male patient. *Courtesy, Claus Garbe, MD.*

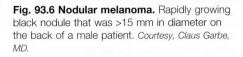

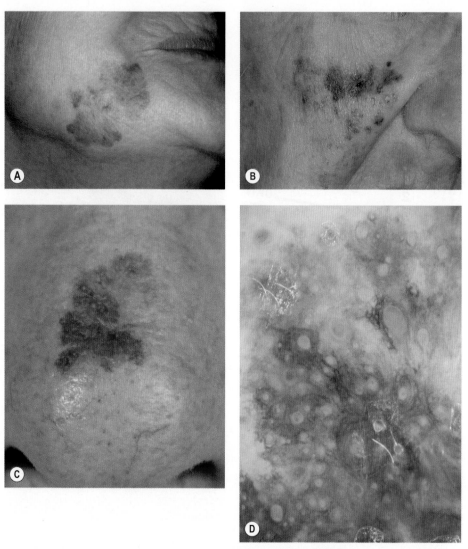

Fig. 93.7 Lentigo maligna (LM) and lentigo maligna melanoma (LMM). **A** Large-sized brown patch with some variation in color representing lentigo maligna. **B** Similarly sized lesion, but with marked variation in color and topography. There was invasion to a depth of 1.1 mm within the blue-gray papules, representing LMM. **C** LMM on the dorsal nose, with irregular borders, light to dark brown color, and marked asymmetry. **D** Dermoscopy of this lesion demonstrating annular structures corresponding to follicular openings surrounded by melanoma cells ('circle in a circle'). *B, Courtesy, Kalman Watsky, MD; C, D, Courtesy, Claus Garbe, MD.*

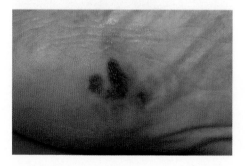

Fig. 93.8 Acral lentiginous melanoma. Irregularly pigmented lesion on the plantar surface of the foot. These tumors may become amelanotic and are then easily overlooked or misdiagnosed as verrucae or other benign lesions, often resulting in a significantly delayed diagnosis. *Courtesy, Claus Garbe, MD.*

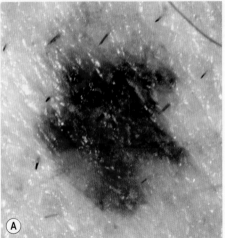
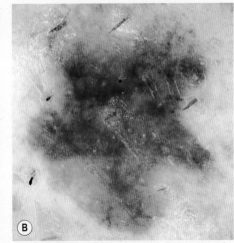
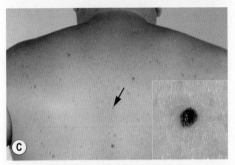

Fig. 93.9 Melanoma *in situ*. A Note the asymmetry, border irregularity, color variation, and erythema ('little red riding hood' sign). **B** The dermoscopic findings include a broadened network, dots, and some globules. **C** This melanoma *in situ* measured less than 3 mm in diameter. Small melanomas can be easily overlooked, especially if they are less heavily pigmented. This lesion was the 'ugly duckling' of all of this patient's nevi. Dermoscopy assists in making an earlier diagnosis. *Courtesy, Claus Garbe, MD.*

• Childhood CM is rare; prepubertal patients tend to have thicker lesions that can be difficult to distinguish from atypical Spitz nevi histologically, and overall the prognosis is favorable.

• Controlling for Breslow depth (in sites where the Breslow depth can be measured), all CMs have the same prognosis, including pregnancy-associated CM; however, some types of CM tend to have a deeper Breslow depth due to delayed diagnosis (e.g. amelanotic, ALM).

Diagnosis

• Early detection is key to improved survival; diagnosis is based on clinical suspicion, followed by histologic confirmation.

• The biopsy should attempt to remove the entire lesion, including a depth adequate to determine an accurate Breslow depth (Fig. 93.12); if limited by large size, representative samples should be obtained; evaluation is then performed by a dermatopathologist.

• When doing a total body skin examination (TBSE), signs such as the 'ugly duckling sign' (a pigmented lesion that stands out as atypical within the context of surrounding nevi; see Fig. 93.9C and Chapter 92) and the 'little red riding hood sign' can prove useful (see Fig. 93.9A).

• Photography and dermoscopy can aid in diagnosis (Figs. 93.13 and 93.14); for the latter, the first step is to determine if the lesion is melanocytic (Table 93.2) and then

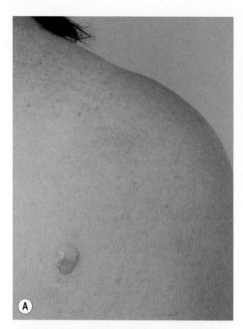

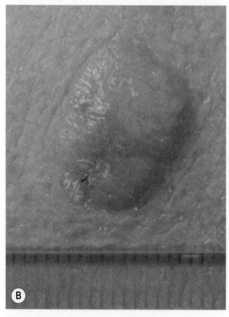

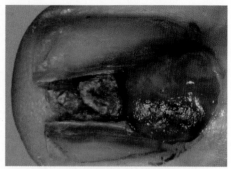

Fig. 93.11 Melanoma of the nail matrix. Ulcerated tumor destroying the nail plate. The longitudinal pigmentation of the nail plate adjacent to the nodular portion is a clue to the diagnosis of melanoma. *Courtesy, Claus Garbe, MD.*

Fig. 93.10 Amelanotic melanoma. **A, B** Skin-colored to light pink nodule on the right scapula of a female patient. Pathology revealed an amelanotic nodular melanoma with a tumor thickness of 4 mm. *Courtesy, Claus Garbe, MD.*

assess for worrisome features (Tables 93.3 and 93.4).

• **DDx:** outlined in Table 93.5.

Prognosis and Staging

• Of the histologic features of a primary invasive CM, the Breslow depth (in millimeters) is the strongest predictor of survival (see Fig. 93.12); the presence or absence of lymph node involvement is an even stronger predictor of survival.

• The American Joint Committee on Cancer's (AJCC) TNM classification and staging system for CM are outlined in Tables 93.6 and 93.7.

• As with other cancers, prognosis is dependent on the stage at the time of diagnosis (Fig. 93.15); other independent prognostic factors for survival have also been identified (Table 93.8).

Management

• Once the histologic diagnosis of CM is confirmed, evaluation includes TBSE and palpation of the surrounding skin and lymph node basins prior to re-excision (Table 93.9).

• **Sentinel lymph node biopsy (SLNB):**
  – SLNB is useful as a diagnostic and prognostic tool, but to date its usefulness as a therapeutic modality has not been established.

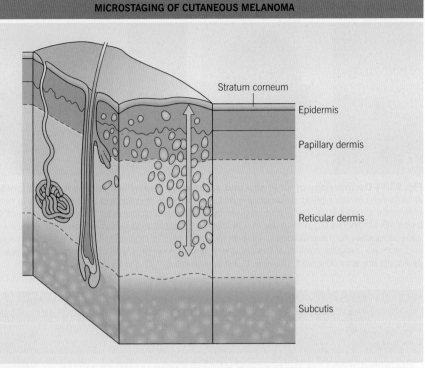

Fig. 93.12 Microstaging of cutaneous melanoma: Breslow tumor thickness. Breslow method: measure in millimeters from the top of the granular layer of the epidermis (or the base of an ulcer) to the deepest part of the tumor.

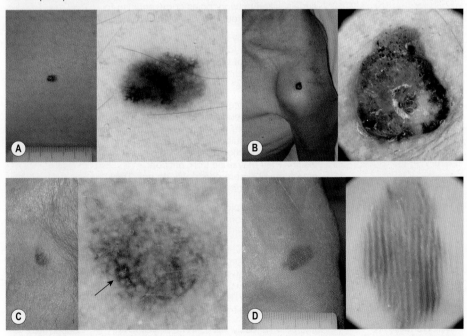

Fig. 93.13 The four most common types of cutaneous melanoma. A Small superficial melanoma typified dermoscopically by asymmetry of color and structure, atypical network, blue-white structures, and irregular streaks at the periphery. **B** Large thick nodular melanoma with predominant blue-white veil. The combination of blue color with irregular black to brown dots, globules, and blotches is highly specific for the diagnosis of thick melanoma. **C** Small facial melanoma *in situ* (lentigo maligna) typified by gray color and rhomboidal structures (arrow) by dermoscopy. **D** Acral melanoma *in situ* typified by the characteristic parallel-ridge pattern. *Courtesy, Giuseppe Argenziano, MD, and Iris Zalaudek, MD.*

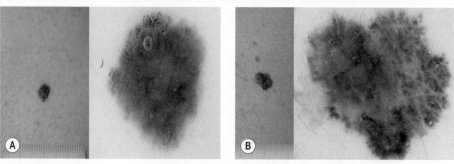

Fig. 93.14 Dermoscopy of an *in situ* and an invasive superficial cutaneous melanoma.
A Melanoma *in situ* typified dermoscopically by asymmetry of color and structure, atypical network, blue-white structures centrally, and irregular black dots and globules (at the upper portion of the lesion). **B** Melanoma 0.9 mm in depth. Clinically, a palpable area is visible, corresponding dermoscopically to the presence of blue-white veil, a sign of increased tumor thickness. Irregular dots and globules, irregular streaks at the periphery, and uneven brown to black pigmented areas (blotches) are also observed. *Courtesy, Giuseppe Argenziano, MD, and Iris Zalaudek, MD.*

DERMOSCOPIC PATTERN ANALYSIS: FIRST-STEP ALGORITHM FOR DIFFERENTIATION BETWEEN MELANOCYTIC AND NON-MELANOCYTIC LESIONS		
Dermoscopic Criterion	**Definition**	**Diagnostic Significance**
Pigment network – pseudo-network[†]	Network of brownish interconnected lines over a background of tan diffuse pigmentation. In facial skin, a peculiar pigment network, also called a pseudo-network, is typified by round, equally sized network holes corresponding to the pre-existing follicular ostia.	Melanocytic lesion
Aggregated globules	Numerous, variously sized, more or less clustered, round to oval structures with various shades of brown and gray-black. They should be differentiated from multiple blue-gray globules.	Melanocytic lesion
Streaks	These have been previously described separately as pseudopods and radial streaming, but are now combined into the one term. They are bulbous and often kinked or finger-like projections seen at the edge of a lesion. They may arise from network structures but more commonly do not. They range in color from tan to black.	Melanocytic lesion
Homogeneous blue pigmentation[‡]	Structureless blue pigmentation in the absence of pigment network or other distinctive local features	Melanocytic lesion
Parallel pattern	Seen in melanocytic lesions of palms/soles and mucosal areas. On palms/soles, the pigmentation may follow the sulci or the cristae (i.e. furrows or ridges) of the dermatoglyphics. Rarely arranged at right angles to these structures.	Melanocytic lesion
Multiple milia-like cysts	Numerous, variously sized, white or yellowish, roundish structures	Seborrheic keratosis

Table 93.2 Dermoscopic pattern analysis: first-step algorithm for differentiation between melanocytic and non-melanocytic lesions. *Adapted from Argenziano G, Soyer HP, Chimenti S, et al. Dermoscopy of pigmented skin lesions: Results of a consensus meeting via the Internet. J. Am. Acad. Dermatol. 2003;48:679–693. Continued*

Table 93.2 *Continued* **Dermoscopic pattern analysis: first-step algorithm for differentiation between melanocytic and non-melanocytic lesions.**

Dermoscopic Criterion	Definition	Diagnostic Significance
Comedo-like openings	Brown-yellowish to brown-black, round to oval, sharply circumscribed keratotic plugs in the ostia of hair follicles. When irregularly shaped, comedo-like openings are also called irregular crypts.	Seborrheic keratosis
Light brown fingerprint-like structures	Light brown, delicate, network-like structures with the pattern of a fingerprint	Seborrheic keratosis
Cerebriform pattern	Dark brown furrows between ridges typifying a brainlike appearance	Seborrheic keratosis
Arborizing vessels	Tree-like branching telangiectasias	Basal cell carcinoma*
Leaf-like structures	Brown to gray/blue discrete bulbous structures forming leaflike patterns. They are discrete pigmented nests (islands) never arising from a pigment network and usually not arising from adjacent confluent pigmented areas.	Basal cell carcinoma*
Large blue-gray ovoid nests	Well-circumscribed, confluent or near confluent, pigmented, ovoid or elongated areas, larger than globules, and not intimately connected to a pigmented tumor body	Basal cell carcinoma*
Multiple blue-gray globules	Multiple globules (not dots) that should be differentiated from multiple blue-gray dots (melanophages)	Basal cell carcinoma*
Spoke-wheel areas	Well-circumscribed radial projections, usually tan in color but sometimes blue or gray, meeting at an often darker (dark brown, black or blue) central axis	Basal cell carcinoma*
Ulceration§	Absence of the epidermis, often associated with congealed blood, not due to a well-described recent history of trauma	Basal cell carcinoma*
Red-blue lacunae	More or less sharply demarcated, roundish or oval areas with a reddish, red-bluish, or dark red to black coloration	Vascular lesion
Red-bluish to reddish-black homogeneous areas	Structureless homogeneous areas of red-bluish to red-black coloration	Vascular lesion
None of the listed criteria	Absence of the above-mentioned criteria	Melanocytic lesion

*To diagnose a basal cell carcinoma, the negative feature of pigment network must be absent and one or more of the positive features listed here must be present.
†Exception 1: Pigment network or pseudo-network is also present in solar lentigo and rarely in seborrheic keratosis and pigmented actinic keratosis. A delicate, annular pigment network is also commonly seen in dermatofibroma and accessory nipple (clue for diagnosis of dermatofibroma and accessory nipple: central white patch).
‡Exception 2: Homogeneous blue pigmentation (dermoscopic hallmark of blue nevus) is also seen (uncommonly) in some hemangiomas and basal cell carcinomas and (commonly) in intradermal melanoma metastases.
§Exception 3: Ulceration is also seen less commonly in invasive melanoma.

DERMOSCOPIC PATTERN ANALYSIS: SECOND-STEP ALGORITHM FOR DIFFERENTIATION BETWEEN MELANOCYTIC NEVI AND MELANOMA		
Dermoscopic Criterion	**Definition**	**Diagnostic Significance**
Global features		
Reticular pattern	Pigment network covering most parts of the lesion	Melanocytic nevus
Globular pattern	Numerous, variously sized, round to oval structures with various shades of brown and gray-black	Melanocytic nevus
Cobblestone pattern	Large, closely aggregated, somehow angulated globule-like structures resembling a cobblestone	Dermal nevus
Homogeneous pattern	Diffuse, brown, gray-blue to gray-black pigmentation in the absence of other distinctive local features	Melanocytic (blue) nevus
Starburst pattern	Pigmented streaks in a radial arrangement at the edge of the lesion	Spitz/Reed nevus
Parallel pattern	Pigmentation on palms/soles that follows the sulci or the cristae (furrows or ridges), rarely arranged at right angles to these structures	Acral nevus/ melanoma (see below)
Multicomponent pattern	Combination of three or more of the above patterns	Melanoma
Nonspecific pattern	Pigmented lesion lacking above patterns	Possible melanoma
Local features		
Pigment network	Typical pigment network: light to dark brown network with small, uniformly spaced network holes and thin network lines distributed more or less regularly throughout the lesion and usually thinning out at the periphery	Benign melanocytic lesion
	Atypical pigment network: black, brown, or gray network with irregular holes and thick lines	Melanoma
Dots/globules	Black, brown, round to oval, variously sized structures regularly or irregularly distributed within the lesion	If regular, benign melanocytic lesion. If irregular, melanoma
Streaks	These have been previously described separately as pseudopods and radial streaming. Streaks are bulbous and often kinked or finger-like projections seen at the edge of a lesion. They may arise from network structures but more commonly do not. They range in color from tan to black.	If regular, benign melanocytic lesion (Spitz/Reed nevus). If irregular, melanoma
Blue-whitish veil	Irregular, structureless area of confluent blue pigmentation with an overlying white 'ground-glass' film. The pigmentation cannot occupy the entire lesion and usually corresponds to a clinically elevated part of the lesion.	Melanoma

Table 93.3 Dermoscopic pattern analysis: second-step algorithm for differentiation between melanocytic nevi and melanoma. *Adapted from Argenziano G, Soyer HP, Chimenti S, et al. Dermoscopy of pigmented skin lesions: Results of a consensus meeting via the Internet. J. Am. Acad. Dermatol. 2003;48:679–693. Continued*

Table 93.3 *Continued* **Dermoscopic pattern analysis: second-step algorithm for differentiation between melanocytic nevi and melanoma.**

Dermoscopic Criterion	Definition	Diagnostic Significance
Regression structures	White scarlike depigmentation and/or blue pepper-like granules usually corresponding to a clinically flat part of the lesion	Melanoma
Hypopigmentation	Areas with less pigmentation than the overall pigmentation of the lesion	Nonspecific
Blotches	Black, brown, and/or gray structureless areas with symmetrical or asymmetrical distribution within the lesion	If symmetrical, benign melanocytic lesion If asymmetrical, melanoma
Site-related features		
Face	Typical pseudo-network (round, equally sized network holes corresponding to the pre-existing follicular ostia)	Benign melanocytic lesion
	Annular–granular structures (multiple blue-gray dots surrounding the follicular ostia with an annular–granular appearance)	Melanoma
	Gray pseudo-network (gray pigmentation surrounding the follicular ostia, formed by the confluence of annular–granular structures)	Melanoma
	Rhomboidal structures (gray-brown pigmentation surrounding the follicular ostia with a rhomboidal appearance)	Melanoma
	Asymmetric pigmented follicles (eccentric annular pigmentation around follicular ostia)	Melanoma
Palms/soles	Parallel-furrow pattern (pigmentation following the sulci)	Acral nevus
	Lattice-like pattern (pigmentation following and crossing the furrows)	Acral nevus
	Fibrillar pattern (numerous, finely pigmented filaments perpendicular to the furrows and ridges)	Acral nevus
	Parallel-ridge pattern (pigmentation aligned along the cristae)	Melanoma

DEFINITIONS OF DERMOSCOPIC CRITERIA FOR THE 3-POINT CHECKLIST

Criterion	Definition
Asymmetry	Asymmetrical distribution of colors and dermoscopic structures
Atypical network*	More than one type of network (in terms of color and thickness of the meshes) irregularly distributed within the lesion
Blue-white structures†	Presence of any type of blue and/or white color

*Usually found in early melanoma.
†Usually found in both melanoma and pigmented basal cell carcinoma.

Table 93.4 Definitions of dermoscopic criteria for the 3-point checklist. The presence of more than one criterion suggests a suspicious lesion. *Adapted from Argenziano G, Puig S, Zalaudek I, et al. Dermoscopy improves accuracy of primary care physicians to triage lesions suggestive of skin cancer. J. Clin. Oncol. 2006;24:1877–1882.*

DIFFERENTIAL DIAGNOSIS OF CUTANEOUS MELANOMA	
General	**Location-Based**
If pigmented • Atypical (dysplastic) nevus • Other nevi (e.g. black [hypermelanotic], blue, genital, acral, Spitz, recurrent) • Seborrheic keratosis • Pigmented BCC • Pigmented Bowen's disease • Thrombosed hemangioma If amelanotic (pink, red) • Pyogenic granuloma (nodular) • BCC; SCC, *in situ* or invasive • Merkel cell carcinoma • Pink intradermal nevus • Spitz nevus • Lichen planus-like keratosis (LPLK) • Isolated patch of psoriasis or eczema	Lentigo maligna (LM) • Pigmented actinic keratosis • Macular seborrheic keratosis Nail matrix melanoma • Longitudinal melanonychia (see Table 58.3) • Drug-induced nail pigmentation (see Table 58.2) • Subungual hematoma • Wart Mucosal melanoma • Melanosis of mucosal regions • Venous lake (vermilion lip) • Amalgam tattoo • Angiokeratoma (genital) • SCC, *in situ* or invasive Acral lentiginous melanoma • Black heel (*talon noir*; see Fig. 74.9) • Plantar wart

BCC, basal cell carcinoma; SCC, squamous cell carcinoma.

Table 93.5 Differential diagnosis of cutaneous melanoma.

MELANOMA TNM CLASSIFICATION		
T Classification	**Thickness**	**Ulceration Status/Mitoses**
Tis	NA	NA
T1	≤1.0 mm	a. Without ulceration and mitosis <1/mm^2 b. With ulceration or mitoses ≥1/mm^2
T2	1.01–2.0 mm	a. Without ulceration b. With ulceration
T3	2.01–4.0 mm	a. Without ulceration b. With ulceration
T4	>4.0 mm	a. Without ulceration b. With ulceration
N Classification	**No. of Metastatic Nodes**	**Nodal Metastatic Mass**
N0	0	NA
N1	1 node	a. Micrometastasis* b. Macrometastasis[†]
N2	2–3 nodes	a. Micrometastasis* b. Macrometastasis[†] c. In-transit met(s)/satellite(s)[‡] without metastatic node(s)

Table 93.6 Melanoma TNM classification. For defining T1 melanomas, Clark level of invasion is used as default criterion only if mitotic rate cannot be determined. Histologic evaluation of lymph nodes must include at least one immunohistochemical marker (e.g. HMB45, Melan-A/MART-1).
Adapted from Balch CM, Gershenwald JE, Soong SJ, et al. Final version of 2009 AJCC melanoma staging and classification. J. Clin. Oncol. 2009;27:6199–6206. Reprinted with permission from the American Society of Clinical Oncology. Continued

Table 93.6 *Continued* **Melanoma TNM classification.**

N Classification	No. of Metastatic Nodes	Nodal Metastatic Mass
N3	4 or more metastatic nodes, matted nodes, or in-transit met(s)/satellite(s)‡ with metastatic node(s)	

M Classification	Site	Serum Lactate Dehydrogenase
M0	No distant metastases	NA
M1a	Distant skin, subcutaneous or nodal metastases	Normal
M1b	Lung metastases	Normal
M1c	All other visceral metastases Any distant metastasis	Normal Elevated

Micrometastases are diagnosed after sentinel or elective lymphadenectomy.
†*Macrometastases are defined as clinically detectable nodal metastases confirmed by therapeutic lymphadenectomy or when nodal metastasis exhibits gross extracapsular extension.*
‡*In-transit metastases are >2 cm from the primary tumor but not beyond the regional lymph nodes, whereas satellite lesions are within 2 cm of the primary.*
NA, not applicable.

	Survival (%)*	Clinical Staging†			Pathologic Staging‡		
		T	N	M	T	N	M
0		Tis	N0	M0	Tis	N0	M0
IA	97	T1a	N0	M0	T1a	N0	M0
IB	93	T1b T2a	N0	M0	T1b T2a		
IIA	82 79	T2b T3a	N0	M0	T2b T3a	N0	M0
IIB	68 71	T3b T4a	N0	M0	T3b T4a	N0	M0
IIC	53	T4b	N0	M0	T4b	N0	M0
III§		Any T	N1 N2 N3	M0			
IIIA	78				T1–4a T1–4a	N1a N2a	M0
IIIB	59				T1–4b T1–4b T1–4a T1–4a T1–4a	N1a N2a N1b N2b N2c	M0

STAGE GROUPINGS FOR CUTANEOUS MELANOMA

Table 93.7 Stage groupings for cutaneous melanoma. *Adapted from Balch CM, Gershenwald JE, Soong SJ, et al. Final version of 2009 AJCC melanoma staging and classification. J. Clin. Oncol. 2009;27: 6199–6206. Reprinted with permission from the American Society of Clinical Oncology.* **Continued**

CUTANEOUS MELANOMA

Table 93.7 *Continued* **Stage groupings for cutaneous melanoma.**

	Survival (%)*	Clinical Staging†			Pathologic Staging‡		
		T	N	M	T	N	M
IIIC	40				T1–4b T1–4b T1–4b Any T	N1b N2b N2c N3	M0
IV	9–27ǁ	Any T	Any N	Any M1	Any T	Any N	Any M1

*Approximate 5-year survival (%), modified from Balch et al. (2009).
†Clinical staging includes microstaging of the primary melanoma and clinical/radiologic evaluation for metastases. By convention, it should be used after complete excision of the primary melanoma with clinical assessment for regional and distant metastases.
‡Pathologic staging includes microstaging of the primary melanoma and pathologic information about the regional lymph nodes after partial or complete lymphadenectomy. Pathologic stage 0 or stage IA patients are the exception.
§There are no stage III subgroups for clinical staging.
ǁHigher survival rate associated with normal serum LDH levels and lower rate with elevated LDH levels.

COMPARISON OF SURVIVAL CURVES IN FOUR STAGES OF MELANOMA

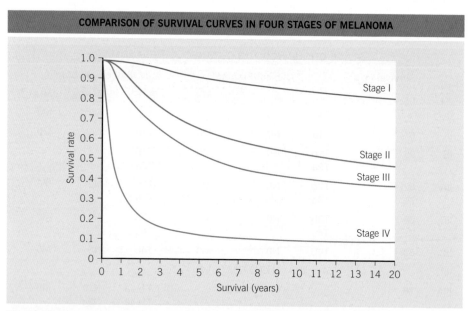

Fig. 93.15 Comparison of survival curves in four stages of melanoma. *Redrawn from Balch CM. Melanoma of the skin. In Edge SB, Byrd DR, Compton CC, et al., eds., AJCC Cancer Staging Manual, 7th edn. New York: Springer, 2009.*

- Indications for consideration of SLNB: CM with T ≥1 mm and no clinically involved regional lymph nodes or distant metastases; selected patients with T <1 mm but with ulceration and/or mitoses ≥1/mm².

- Typically performed at the time of re-excision (Fig. 93.16).
- Currently, if SLNB reveals micrometastases, then a complete lymph node dissection is performed; there are ongoing trials to determine if this is necessary.

MAJOR INDEPENDENT PROGNOSTIC FACTORS FOR SURVIVAL IN MULTIVARIATE ANALYSES	
Prognostic Factor	**Commentary**
Tumor thickness	≤1 mm, low risk; >1 mm, higher risk melanoma
Ulceration	Worse prognosis with ulceration
Mitotic rate	Worse prognosis with ≥1 mitoses/mm^2
Age	Worse prognosis with older age
Sex	Men have poorer prognosis (only for localized disease)
Anatomic site	Trunk, head, and neck associated with poorer prognosis than extremities
Number of involved lymph nodes	Cutoff points: 1, 2–3, 4 or more lymph nodes (see Table 93.6)
Regional lymph node tumor burden	Macroscopic (palpable) nodal metastases with poorer prognosis than microscopic (nonpalpable) nodal metastases
Site of distant metastases	Visceral metastases associated with poorer prognosis than nonvisceral metastases (skin, subcutaneous, distant lymph nodes)

Table 93.8 Major independent prognostic factors for survival in multivariate analyses.

SURGICAL TREATMENT OF PRIMARY CUTANEOUS MELANOMA		
Tumor Thickness	**Excision Margins (cm)**	**Comments**
In situ	0.5	Lentigo maligna of the face may be excised with 1-cm margins (especially when lesions are >1.5–2 cm in diameter) or treated by Mohs micrographic surgery or radiotherapy; postoperative topical imiquimod is often used
≤1 mm	1.0	Mohs micrographic surgery may be employed in acral and facial melanomas
1.01–2 mm	1.0–2.0	
>2 mm	2.0	

Table 93.9 Surgical treatment of primary cutaneous melanoma. Evidence from available randomized trials is insufficient to address the optimal margins for the excision of primary cutaneous melanoma, but multiple expert international committees have produced fairly consistent guidelines, as summarized here. Of note, further investigative efforts will likely alter the standards of care over time. *Adapted from Sladden MJ, et al. Surgical excision margins for primary cutaneous melanoma.* Cochrane Database Syst. Rev. 2009;(4):CD004855.

– *Advantages*: provides additional diagnostic and staging information; allows for entry into clinical trials.

– *Disadvantages*: can cause lymphedema; expensive; usually requires general anesthesia.

• Imaging studies for identification of metastases include: ultrasound of lymph node basins; CT scan of the chest, abdomen, and pelvis or PET scan in high-risk patients; and if symptoms, cranial MRI; serum LDH is measured serially as it influences prognosis (see Table 93.7).

• Additional **Rx** is outlined in Tables 93.10 and 93.11.

• A melanoma patient worksheet can help organize all of this information for both the patient and the clinician (see Appendix).

SENTINEL LYMPH NODE BIOPSY (SLNB)

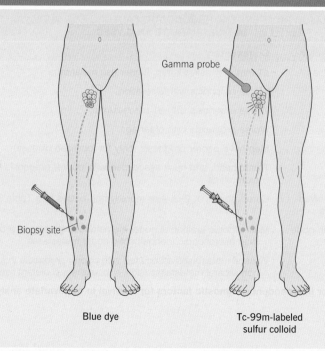

Gamma probe

Blue dye

Tc-99m-labeled
sulfur colloid

Biopsy site

Fig. 93.16 Sentinel lymph node biopsy (SLNB). Identification of the sentinel node(s) using the injection of blue dye, technetium-99m-labeled sulfur colloid, or both. Re-excision is performed after the injections. *Redrawn from Olhoffer IH and Bolognia JL. What's new in the treatment of cutaneous melanoma.* Semin. Cutan. Med. Surg. *1998;17(2):96–107.*

GENERAL GUIDELINES FOR TREATMENT OF CUTANEOUS MELANOMA (CM) BASED ON STAGE AT DIAGNOSIS, IN ADDITION TO RE-EXCISION OF THE PRIMARY CM

Stage 0 (Melanoma *In Situ*)

- Re-excision (Table 93.9)

Stages I and II

- T <1 mm (no ulceration and mitoses <1/mm^2)
  - Re-excision (Table 93.9)
- T ≥1 mm or T <1 mm but with ulceration and/or mitoses ≥1/mm^2
  - Consider SLNB before performing re-excision

Stage III

- Lymph node metastases, including micrometastases noted by SLNB
  - Consider clinical trial enrollment or interferon-α
- In-transit metastases
  - 1st: <5, surgery vs. >5, extremity perfusion*
  - 2nd: Consider topical therapy (e.g. imiquimod, miltefosine)
  - 3rd: Systemic therapy

Stage IV

- Skin or subcutaneous metastases
  - Single to a few: Surgery
  - Multiple: Surgery vs. topical (see above) vs. systemic therapy (Table 93.11)
- Solid organ metastases
  - Systemic therapy +/– surgery or radiotherapy (including stereotactic)

Should be performed as part of a controlled study.
SLNB, sentinel lymph node biopsy.

Table 93.10 General guidelines for treatment of cutaneous melanoma (CM) based on stage at diagnosis, in addition to re-excision of the primary CM.

DRUGS RECENTLY APPROVED OR IN CLINICAL DEVELOPMENT FOR UNRESECTABLE OR METASTATIC MELANOMA	
Immunotherapy	
Mechanism	*Examples*
CTLA-4 inhibition	• Ipilimumab (IV)
PD-1 inhibition	• Nivolumab (IV) • Lambrolizumab (IV)
PD-L1 inhibition	• RG-7446, MEDI-4736
Mutated Oncogene-Directed Therapy (Figs. 93.1 and 93.2)	
Mutated Oncogene	*Examples*
c-KIT	• Imatinib • Dasatinib
NRAS	• Tipifarnib
BRAF	Selective for V600E* • Vemurafenib • Dabrafenib Nonselective • Sorafenib
MEK1/2	• Trametinib

*Of melanomas with BRAF mutations, at least ~80% lead to an amino acid change at position 600, most commonly glutamic acid (E) substitutes for valine (V); can also be V600D or V600K.
IV, intravenous

Table 93.11 Drugs recently approved or in clinical development for unresectable or metastatic melanoma. With the discovery of genetic mutations that lead to dysfunction of signal transduction pathways, targeted therapies are being developed.

Follow-Up

• Primary objectives include identification of potentially curable local recurrences (~4% of patients; Fig. 93.17) or regional metastases (e.g. in transit, lymph node; Fig. 93.18) and to identify second primary CMs (up to 5% of patients).

• In addition to TBSE and lymph node examination, visits should include a review of systems that focuses on signs or symptoms of metastases to soft tissue, liver, lung, the gastrointestinal tract, and CNS.

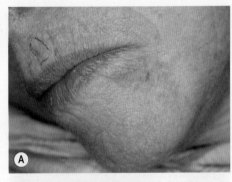

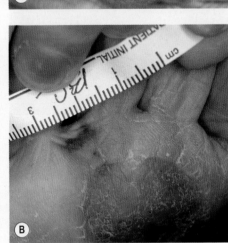

Fig. 93.17 Local recurrence of cutaneous melanoma. A Recurrent lentigo maligna along upper lateral margin of the excision on the chin; inked lesion on central upper lip is an actinic keratosis. **B** Recurrent, *in situ* acral lentiginous melanoma at the 10 o'clock position on the split-thickness skin graft. *Continued*

• Follow-up intervals during the first 3–5 years after diagnosis vary from 3 to 6 months, depending on stage, in addition to the number of primary melanomas, melanocytic nevi, and atypical nevi as well as family history of melanoma; lifelong follow-up is recommended.

• Patients should be counseled to adhere to sun protective measures; perform skin self-examinations at home; stay up-to-date on their other health maintenance and recommended cancer screenings; and take an oral vitamin D supplement if needed.

• Family members can be screened by a dermatologist, who can then determine frequency of subsequent screenings.

• Although up to 10% of patients with CM have familial melanoma, mutations have

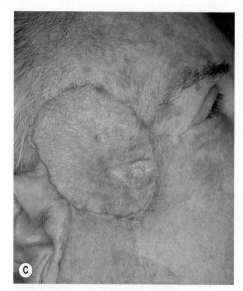

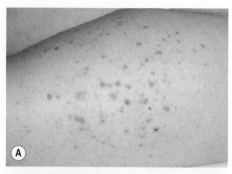

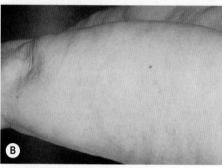

Fig. 93.17 *Continued* **C** Amelanotic nodular recurrence of a desmoplastic melanoma within the skin graft. *Courtesy, Jean L. Bolognia, MD.*

been detected in a limited number of high-penetrance genes (e.g. *CDKN2A* >> *CDK4*); when a patient with CM has multiple primaries, ≥2 family members with CM, and/or a family history of pancreatic cancer, consideration of genetic counseling should be discussed.

Fig. 93.18 In-transit metastases of melanoma. A Multiple pink papulonodules along the lymphatics were treated with intralesional low-dose IL-2 for 6 weeks. **B** Complete remission after 1 year, which persisted during the follow-up period of 7 years. *Courtesy, Claus Garbe, MD.*

For further information see Ch. 113. From *Dermatology, Third Edition.*

Vascular Neoplasms and Reactive Proliferations

94

Lesions of vascular origin are broadly, and somewhat imperfectly, classified as neoplasms (tumors), malformations, telangiectasias, or reactive proliferations. The growth of a neoplasm is largely autonomous (i.e. not reactive). Malformations, in general, are not actively proliferating (see Chapter 85). Telangiectasias represent pre-existing capillaries that are persistently dilated but lack a proliferative component (see Chapter 87). Reactive proliferations represent endothelial cell proliferation that is in response to some factor (e.g. fibrin, hypoxia, trauma).

Neoplasms/Tumors

Infantile Hemangioma and Congenital Hemangioma

• See Chapter 85.

Cherry Angioma

• Bright red, 1- to 6-mm papule, commonly on the trunk or upper extremities (Fig. 94.1); appears during adulthood; early, tiny lesions can be macular.
• Dermoscopy: red to red-blue lacunas (well-demarcated round to oval red to red-blue structures).

Glomus Tumor

• Solitary, painful papule or nodule on the extremities, or in the nail bed (beneath the nail plate) in young adults (Fig. 94.2).
• A glomus cell is a perivascular contractile cell that influences vessel diameter as a means of controlling temperature.

Tufted Angioma

• Pink to dark red patches and plaques with superimposed papules (Fig. 94.3) that slowly enlarge and occasionally regress.
• Commonly found on the neck and trunk.
• Congenital or acquired during childhood or young adulthood.
• On a spectrum with kaposiform hemangioendothelioma.
• Early-onset lesions can be associated with Kasabach–Merritt phenomenon (consumptive coagulopathy with decreased platelets).

Hobnail Hemangioma/Targetoid Hemosiderotic Hemangioma

• Uncommon red-purple papule on the trunk or extremities of children or young adults; papule may have a surrounding pale area and outer ecchymotic ring, thus creating a target lesion (Fig. 94.4).

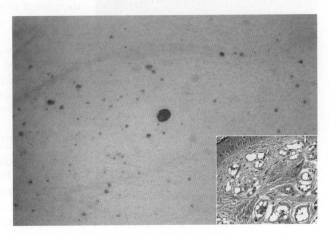

Fig. 94.1 Cherry angiomas. Multiple, slightly compressible red papules. Histologically, congested capillaries and postcapillary venules expand the papillary dermis (insert). *Courtesy, Jean L. Bolognia, MD.*

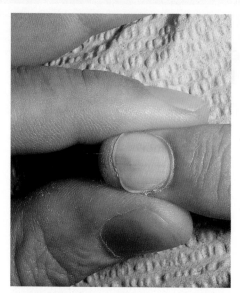

Fig. 94.2 Glomus tumor. The lesion presented with pain and ill-defined subungual erythema. *Courtesy, Ronald P. Rapini, MD.*

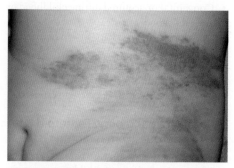

Fig. 94.3 Tufted angioma. Mottled red patches and superimposed papules are typical clinical features. *Courtesy, Julie V. Schaffer, MD.*

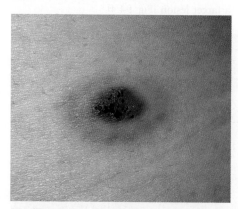

Fig. 94.4 Hobnail hemangioma (targetoid hemosiderotic hemangioma). Note the target-like appearance. *Courtesy, Ronald P. Rapini, MD.*

Kaposiform Hemangioendothelioma

• Ill-defined, pink to violaceous plaques or nodules (Fig. 94.5); sometimes deeply seated; any site.

• May be congenital and generally appears by 2 years of age.

• Locally aggressive, persistent.

• Associated with Kasabach–Merritt phenomenon (treated with rapamycin or vincristine).

Kaposi's Sarcoma

• Multifocal systemic disease; extramucocutaneous sites include gastrointestinal tract, lymph nodes, and lungs.

• Four main variants: (1) older men from the Mediterranean basin or of Ashkenazi Jewish descent with lesions on the lower extremities (Fig. 94.6); (2) African endemic; (3) iatrogenic/immunocompromised; and (4) AIDS-related epidemic (Fig. 94.7).

• Pink to dark violet patches and plaques; with time, can become nodular.

• May have mucosal involvement, e.g. oral.

• Associated with HHV-8 infection.

• Histopathology varies from a subtle increase in slit-like vessels to nodular proliferations of spindle cells; HHV-8 can be detected in endothelial cells by immunohistochemistry.

• **Rx:** observation, surgical excision, laser removal, radiotherapy, intralesional or systemic vinblastine, taxanes, liposomal anthracyclines, reduction of immunosuppression.

Angiosarcoma

• Begins as a bruise-like patch in the head and neck region of older adults with color varying from pink to dark purple (likened to the color of an eggplant).

• With time nodules and ulceration can develop.

• Associated with lymphedema (Fig. 94.8).

• 15% survival at 5 years.

• **Rx:** wide excision ± radiotherapy; consider systemic therapy with taxanes, sorafenib, or bevacizumab for larger lesions.

Malformations (See Chapter 85)

Glomuvenous Malformation (Previously Referred to as Glomangioma)

• Often multiple, bluish, partially compressible papulonodules that appear during infancy

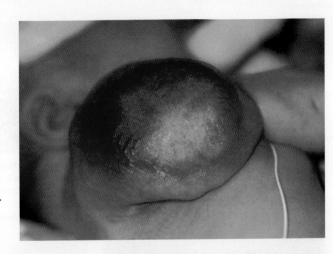

Fig. 94.5 Kaposiform hemangioendothelioma complicated by Kasabach–Merritt phenomenon. A large red-purple mass on the upper flank of an infant.

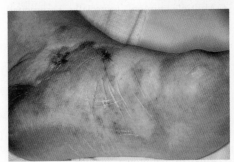

Fig. 94.6 Classic Kaposi's sarcoma. Red macules and patches on the plantar surface of the foot, with violaceous plaques on the ankle. *Courtesy, Paula North, MD.*

or childhood (Figs. 94.9 and 94.10); may be tender.
• Autosomal dominant inheritance with incomplete penetrance.
• Mutations in glomulin gene.
• **DDx:** venous malformations or blue rubber bleb nevus syndrome (see Chapter 85).

Reactive Proliferations

• Some consider pyogenic granuloma, angiolymphoid hyperplasia with eosinophilia, and glomeruloid hemangioma to be tumors.

Pyogenic Granuloma

• Rapidly growing, friable, red papulonodule that is sometimes pedunculated; often

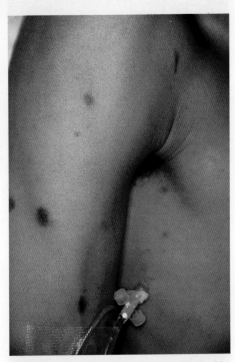

Fig. 94.7 Kaposi's sarcoma in a patient with AIDS. Violet-red papules or nodules are often oval to lance-ovate and are usually more widely distributed than in classic KS. *Courtesy, Paula North, MD.*

ulcerates and bleeds; common in children and young adults.
• Gingival and fingers > lips > face > tongue (Fig. 94.11).
• May arise on the gingiva of pregnant women (granuloma gravidarum).

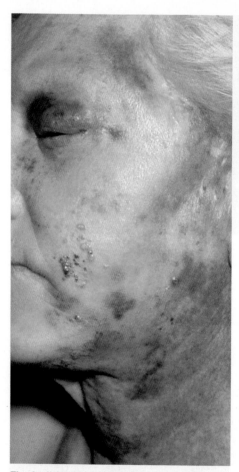

Fig. 94.8 Angiosarcoma. Erythematous and purple hemorrhagic plaques as well as grouped vesicles with clear or hemorrhagic fluid (reminiscent of microcystic lymphatic malformation) are present. There is also induration and a pink hue to the left side of the face in addition to evidence of previous excisions and radiotherapy. *Courtesy, Lorenzo Cerroni, MD.*

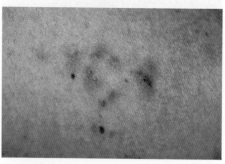

Fig. 94.9 Glomuvenous malformation ('glomangioma'). Note the cluster of slightly compressible blue papules.

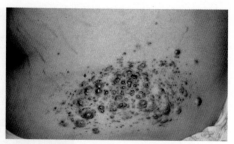

Fig. 94.10 Glomuvenous malformation ('glomangioma'). Large cluster of blue papulonodules becoming confluent centrally.

- Multiple tumors (especially periungual) may be seen in association with medications (e.g. oral retinoids, anti-retroviral protease inhibitors, EGFR inhibitors).
- **DDx:** need to distinguish from amelanotic melanoma.

Angiolymphoid Hyperplasia with Eosinophilia

- Pink to red-brown nodules or plaques, often multiple and grouped.
- Favors the head and neck region, especially around ears (Fig. 94.12).
- May be painful, pruritic, or rarely pulsatile.
- Occasionally, peripheral eosinophilia.

Glomeruloid Hemangioma

- Firm red papules or nodules on the trunk and proximal extremities.
- Associated with POEMS (polyneuropathy, organomegaly, endocrinopathy, monoclonal gammopathy, and skin findings) syndrome.

Reactive Angioendotheliomatosis

- Rare, self-limited.
- Erythematous nodules or plaques, often with petechiae or purpura.
- Associated with cryoglobulinemia (type I) or systemic disorders (e.g. renal failure).
- The form due to severe atherosclerosis leads to ulceration.

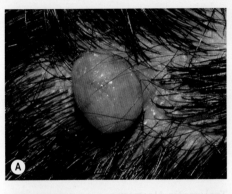

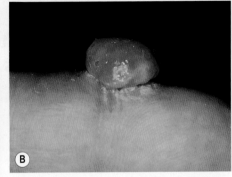

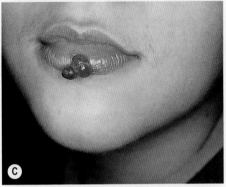

Fig. 94.11 Pyogenic granuloma. A Eroded pink-red papulonodule with a narrow base on the scalp. **B** Pedunculated papule on the finger. **C** Grouped red papules on the lip. The latter two are both common sites. By dermoscopy, red homogenous areas are intersected by white lines. *A, Courtesy, Julie V. Schaffer, MD; B, C, Courtesy, Paula North, MD.*

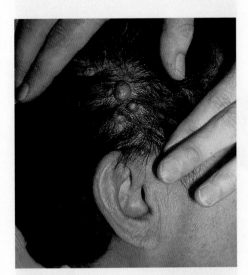

Fig. 94.12 Angiolymphoid hyperplasia with eosinophilia. Multiple pink papulonodules are often seen on the scalp.

Diffuse Dermal Angiomatosis

• Some consider this a variant of reactive angioendotheliomatosis.

• This term has been used to describe an ulcerated lesion in the setting of severe atherosclerosis or vascular compromise; these ulcers usually occur on the lower extremities and resolve with revascularization; less often occurs on the breast.

For further information see Ch. 114. From *Dermatology, Third Edition.*

95 | Common Soft Tissue Tumors/ Proliferations

Neural/Neuroendocrine

Neurofibroma

• Skin-colored to pink, soft papulonodule, often on the trunk (see Fig. 50.2).
• Compressible (the tumor often herniates inward upon palpation – this is referred to as the 'button-hole' sign); it is sometimes pedunculated.
• Usually solitary in most individuals.
• When multiple, need to distinguish linear form (segmental; mosaic) from a generalized distribution pattern (neurofibromatosis type I) (see Chapter 50).
• Histopathology: wavy, delicate spindle cells with tapered nuclei in a pink stroma.
• Plexiform type has been likened to a 'bag of worms' (Fig. 95.1); it is generally on the trunk and proximal extremities, highly associated with neurofibromatosis type I, and prone to malignant degeneration (2–13%).

Schwannoma/Neurilemmoma

• Solitary, pink-yellow, soft, smooth papulonodule; generally seen in adults.
• Often on the extremities or head (Fig. 95.2).
• Asymptomatic (rarely painful).
• Histopathology: encapsulated tumor with foci of wavy, spindled nuclei in palisades and foci of myxoid change.

Granular Cell Tumor

• Often in adults; skin-colored to brown-red, firm papulonodule; sometimes ulcerated or verrucous.
• 30% on the tongue.
• Multiple tumors in 10% of patients.
• Histopathology: polygonal cells with oval nuclei and characteristic granular cytoplasm.

Traumatic Neuroma

• Skin-colored papulonodule(s) at a site of prior trauma.
• Often painful or 'sensitive' (Fig. 95.3).
• Histopathology: haphazardly distributed fascicles of spindle cells with tapered nuclei.

Merkel Cell Carcinoma

• In older adults; solitary, rapidly growing, pink to red to violaceous nodule (Fig. 95.4).

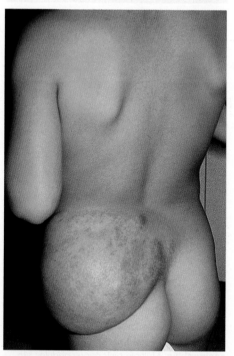

Fig. 95.1 Plexiform neurofibroma in a child with neurofibromatosis. Bag-like mass with overlying patches of hyperpigmentation. *Courtesy, Zsolt B. Argenyi, MD.*

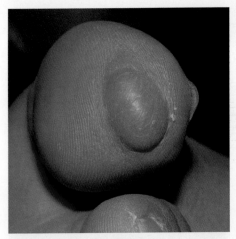

Fig. 95.2 Solitary schwannoma. Skin-colored nodule on the plantar surface of the great toe. *Courtesy, Julie V. Schaffer, MD.*

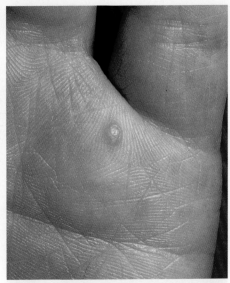

Fig. 95.3 Traumatic neuroma. A painful, firm papule that appeared after a deep puncture injury. *Courtesy, Zsolt B. Argenyi, MD.*

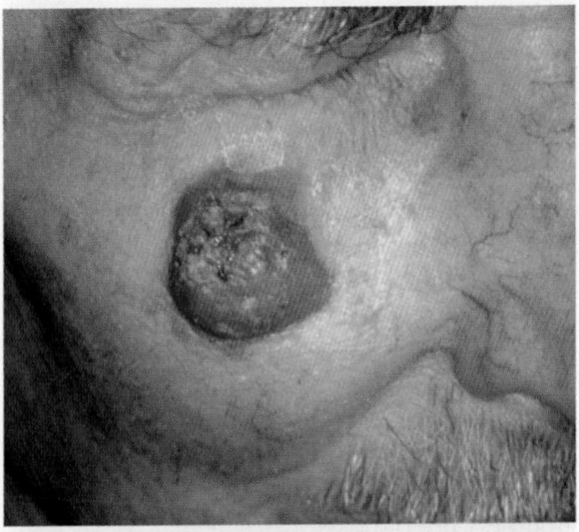

- Commonly on the head and neck.
- Aggressive behavior: distant metastases in 40%; 70% survival at 5 years if primary lesion is <2 cm in diameter; 18% survival at 5 years if distant metastatic disease.
- Histopathology: islands or trabeculae of blue cells that on high-power magnification have chromatin that appears speckled like 'salt and pepper'; characteristically cytokeratin 20 (CK20)-positive and thyroid transcription factor-1 (TTF1)-negative.
- **Rx:** optimally includes wide excision, accompanied by sentinel lymph node biopsy (SLNB); adjuvant radiation treatment recommended for most patients (exceptions: primary ≤1 cm, SLNB negative, no immunosuppression).

Fibrous/Fibrohistiocytic

Skin Tag (Acrochordon, Fibroepithelial Polyp, Soft Fibroma)

- Common; skin-colored to pink or occasionally hyperpigmented, pedunculated papule.
- Sites of predilection: neck, axilla, groin (Fig. 95.5).
- Can become irritated or infarcted.

Fig. 95.4 Merkel cell carcinoma (primary cutaneous neuroendocrine carcinoma). Eroded erythematous nodule arising within sun-damaged skin of the cheek. *Courtesy, Lorenzo Cerroni, MD.*

Angiofibroma (Fibrous Papule)

- Solitary, skin-colored to pink, shiny papule; commonly on the nose (Fig. 95.6).
- When multiple, need to consider genodermatoses (e.g. tuberous sclerosis, multiple endocrine neoplasia type I).
- Histopathology: stellate spindle cells in a hyalinized stroma with dilated vessels.
- **DDx:** basal cell carcinoma, intradermal melanocytic nevus, adnexal tumors.

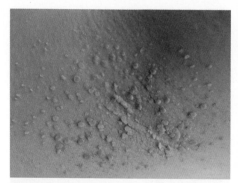

Fig. 95.5 Multiple skin tags in the axilla. The lesions are skin-colored, soft, and pedunculated.

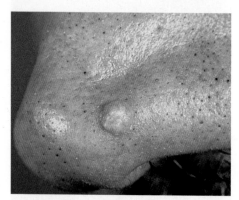

Fig. 95.6 Fibrous papule of the nose. A smooth, dome-shaped, skin-colored papule. *Courtesy, Hideko Kamino, MD.*

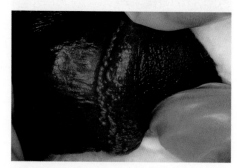

Fig. 95.7 Pearly penile papules. Multiple small white papules along the corona of the glans penis. Note the multilayered distribution. *Courtesy, Kalman Watsky, MD.*

Pearly Penile Papules

• Multiple, small, white to light pink papules along the corona of the glans penis, often with a multilayered distribution (Fig. 95.7).

• **Rx:** reassurance.

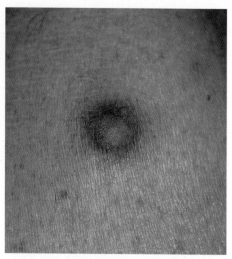

Fig. 95.8 Dermatofibroma. Hyperpigmented firm papule on the lower extremity. *Courtesy, Jean L. Bolognia, MD.*

Dermatofibroma

• 6- to 10-mm pink (especially in fair-skinned individuals), tan, or brown papule (Fig. 95.8); firm; dimples inward with lateral pressure.

• Often on the lower extremities; women > men.

• Common; multiple lesions can be seen in normal individuals but also are associated with lupus erythematosus and immunosuppresion (e.g. HIV infection).

• Histopathology: epidermal hyperplasia (sometimes with basaloid induction that resembles basal cell carcinoma) above a spindle cell proliferation that entraps collagen.

• Dermoscopic features are shown in Fig. 1.13.

Acral Fibrokeratoma

• 4- to 10-mm solitary, skin-colored to pink, cone-shaped, keratotic papule with a collarette of elevated skin (Fig. 95.9).

• Located on the fingers and sometimes the palms.

Sclerotic Fibroma

• 2- to 9-mm dome-shaped, pearly papule or nodule in adults.

• Slight predilection for the head and neck.

• Can be seen in patients with Cowden disease.

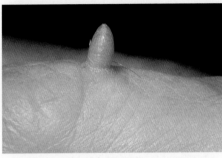

Fig. 95.9 Acral fibrokeratoma. A light pink exophytic papule arising from the dorsal surface of the finger. *Courtesy, Hideko Kamino, MD.*

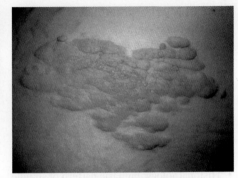

Fig. 95.11 Connective tissue nevus. Coalescence of multiple tan papules and plaques on the lower back. The lesion was firm to palpation and histologically had increased collagen.

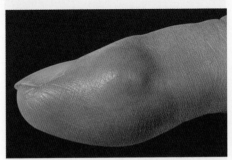

Fig. 95.10 Giant cell tumor of tendon sheath. A skin-colored nodule on the lateral aspect of the index finger. *Courtesy, Hideko Kamino, MD.*

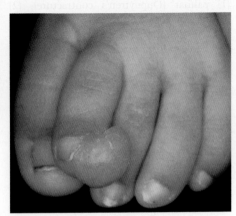

Fig. 95.12 Infantile digital fibroma. Firm skin-colored nodule on the dorsolateral aspect of the second toe in a young child.

Giant Cell Tumor of Tendon Sheath

- Firm nodule (1–2 cm), generally on the fingers or toes (Fig. 95.10).
- 30% of tumors recur locally.

Nodular Fasciitis

- Benign, reactive process in young adults.
- Rapidly growing subcutaneous nodule (1–5 cm in diameter).
- Commonly on the distal upper extremity.
- Sometimes associated with trauma.
- Histopathology: subcutaneous nodule of elongated spindle cells in a myxoid matrix.

Connective Tissue Nevus

- Skin-colored to yellow-tan (more yellow when composed predominantly of elastic tissue), firm papulonodules or plaques; solitary or multiple (often grouped) (Fig. 95.11).
- Present at birth or arise during childhood.

- May be associated with genodermatoses (e.g. tuberous sclerosis, Buschke–Ollendorf syndrome, Proteus syndrome).
- Histopathology: increased collagen (sometimes subtle) and/or elastic tissue; diagnosis may require special stains for elastic fibers and collagen.

Infantile Digital Fibroma

- Firm, skin-colored to pink papulonodule on the fingers or toes (tends to spare the thumb and great toe) (Fig. 95.12).
- Solitary or multiple; generally present before 1 year of age.
- May recur.

Infantile Myofibromatosis

- One or more skin-colored to pink to violet, firm to rubbery dermal/subcutaneous nodules.
- Most commonly on the head and neck or trunk.
- Rare; lesions present at birth or appear during the first 2 years of life.
- Can have cutaneous lesions alone or systemic involvement (bone, gastrointestinal, kidneys, lungs, heart).
- Tumors tend to self-regress.
- Histopathology: biphasic pattern of spindle cells in nodular arrangements with vessels at the periphery.

Fibromatoses

- Five subtypes, four of which are superficial: (1) palmar (Dupuytren's contracture); (2) plantar (Ledderhose disease); (3) penile (Peyronie's); and (4) knuckle pads (Fig. 95.13).
- One deep form: extra-abdominal desmoid tumor.
- Slowly growing nodules or plaques or cord-like tumors.
- Palmar fibromatosis can result in flexion contractures, especially of the 4th and/or 5th finger (see Chapter 81).
- Penile fibromatosis can result in pain and erectile dysfunction.

Muscle/Adipose

Leiomyoma

- Solitary or multiple red-brown papules or nodules, often grouped (Fig. 95.14).
- Sometimes painful.
- Generally on the trunk.

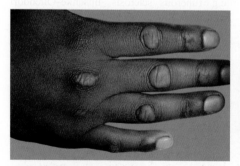

Fig. 95.13 Knuckle pads. Note the localization to the skin overlying the knuckles. *Courtesy, Ronald P. Rapini, MD.*

- When multiple, consider association with uterine leiomyomas and papillary renal cell carcinoma (Reed syndrome).
- Histopathology: fascicles of spindle cells with cigar-shaped nuclei that have perinuclear vacuoles.

Smooth Muscle Hamartoma

- Congenital or acquired, skin-colored to hyperpigmented plaque on the trunk > proximal extremities (Fig. 95.15).

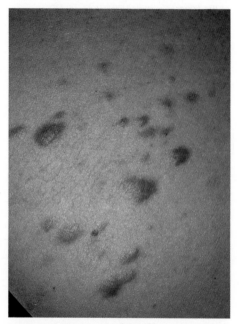

Fig. 95.14 Clustered piloleiomyomas on the back. The trunk is a common location for multiple piloleiomyomas. Patients with this clinical presentation need to be evaluated for the possibility of Reed syndrome.

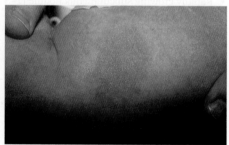

Fig. 95.15 Smooth muscle hamartoma. This infant presented with a firm plaque on the thigh. *Courtesy, Ronald P. Rapini, MD.*

• Follicular prominence and hypertrichosis may be present.
• May be confused with a congenital melanocytic nevus.
• Is on a clinicopathologic spectrum with Becker's nevus.

Lipoma

• Common tumor of mature fat; soft, mobile subcutaneous nodule.
• Generally on the trunk and extremities, but any site possible.
• Occasionally painful.
• Multiple lesions may be associated with a lipomatosis (e.g. familial type; Fig. 95.16) or a genodermatosis (e.g. Gardner syndrome, Proteus syndrome).
• **DDx:** see Fig. 95.17.

Angiolipoma

• Soft, mobile, subcutaneous nodule; often on the forearm in young adults.
• Often painful.

Nevus Lipomatosus

• Grouped, soft, yellow to skin-colored papulonodules on the hips and/or upper thighs (Fig. 95.18).
• Develops during infancy to the first two decades of life.

Soft Tissue Sarcomas
(See Table 95.1)

• Rare in comparison to benign soft tissue tumors.
• Generally presents as a nonspecific, deep-seated nodule.
• Dermatofibrosarcoma protuberans (DFSP) is characteristically multinodular (Fig. 95.19).
• Most DFSPs have a translocation t(17;22) that fuses the collagen I and platelet-derived growth factor genes; expression of this fusion gene results in high levels of platelet-derived growth factor that stimulates proliferation of fibroblasts.

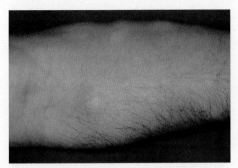

Fig. 95.16 Familial multiple lipomatosis. Several discrete lipomas are present on the forearm.

SELECTED SOFT TISSUE SARCOMAS
Angiosarcoma (can arise in setting of lymphedema and on the scalp of elderly patients) (see Chapter 94)
Dermatofibrosarcoma protuberans (often multinodular)
Pleomorphic undifferentiated sarcoma (previously referred to as malignant fibrous histiocytoma*)
Malignant peripheral nerve sheath tumor
Epithelioid sarcoma
Fibrosarcoma
Leiomyosarcoma
Liposarcoma

*Some pathologists consider atypical fibroxanthoma (AFX) to be a superficial variant of malignant fibrous histiocytoma (MFH); dermatologists see AFXs more commonly than MFHs.

Table 95.1 Selected soft tissue sarcomas.

APPROACH TO A "LUMP UNDER THE SKIN" IN ADULTS

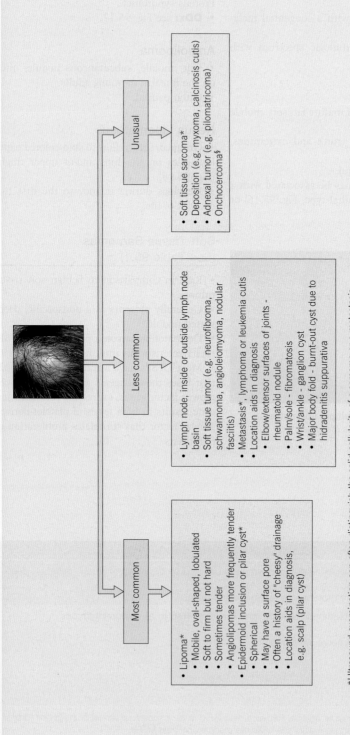

APPROACH TO A "LUMP UNDER THE SKIN" IN ADULTS

```
                    ┌──────────────┐  ┌──────────────┐  ┌──────────────┐
                    │ Most common  │  │ Less common  │  │   Unusual    │
                    └──────────────┘  └──────────────┘  └──────────────┘
```

Most common

- Lipoma*
  - Mobile, oval-shaped, lobulated
  - Soft to firm but not hard
  - Sometimes tender
  - Angiolipomas more frequently tender
- Epidermoid inclusion or pilar cyst*
  - Spherical
  - May have a surface pore
  - Often a history of "cheesy" drainage
  - Location aids in diagnosis, e.g. scalp (pilar cyst)

Less common

- Lymph node, inside or outside lymph node basin
- Soft tissue tumor (e.g. neurofibroma, schwannoma, angioleiomyoma, nodular fasciitis)
- Metastasis*, lymphoma or leukemia cutis
- Location aids in diagnosis
  - Elbow/extensor surfaces of joints - rheumatoid nodule
  - Palm/sole - fibromatosis
  - Wrist/ankle - ganglion cyst
  - Major body fold - burnt-out cyst due to hidradenitis suppurativa

Unusual

- Soft tissue sarcoma*
- Deposition (e.g. myxoma, calcinosis cutis)
- Adnexal tumor (e.g. pilomatricoma)
- Onchocercoma§

*Ultrasound examination can often distinguish the solid cellularity of a sarcoma or a metastasis from the fat of a lipoma and the cystic architecture of an epidermal inclusion cyst.

§Tropical regions of Latin America and Africa.

Fig. 95.17 Approach to a "lump under the skin" in adults. Incisional biopsy is preferred for the histopathologic evaluation of subcutaneous nodules while a punch biopsy suffices for dermal lesions. For bedside diagnosis of an epidermal inclusion cyst: after local anesthesia and superficial incision with a #11 blade, keratin is expressed.

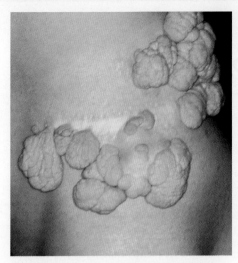

Fig. 95.18 Nevus lipomatosus superficialis.
This hamartoma is characterized by grouped,
soft, pedunculated, skin-colored tumors; a partial
resection had been performed. *With permission
from Kopf AW and Bart RS,* J. Dermatol. Surg. Oncol.
9:279–281, 1983.

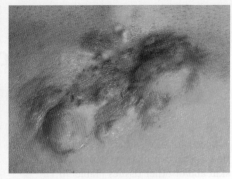

**Fig. 95.19 Dermatofibrosarcoma
protuberans.** A broad, pink-brown,
multinodular, firm plaque on the back.
Histopathologically, bland spindle cells are
arranged in storiform ('cartwheel') patterns.
Courtesy, Hideko Kamino, MD.

For further information see Chs. 115, 116 and Ch. 117. From *Dermatology, Third Edition*.

96 Mastocytosis

- Spectrum of disorders caused by proliferation and accumulation of mast cells in the skin and/or other tissues (Table 96.1).
- The onset of cutaneous mastocytosis is at birth in 25%, before 2 years of age in ~60%, and before puberty in ~70% of affected individuals; familial mastocytosis occasionally occurs.
- Childhood-onset mastocytosis generally has a benign course with spontaneous remission prior to puberty, whereas adult-onset mastocytosis typically persists and may be associated with systemic involvement (Fig. 96.1).
- The majority of pediatric and adult mastocytosis patients have a somatic activating mutation (most frequently involving codon 816) in the gene encoding the KIT tyrosine kinase receptor expressed on mast cells.

Clinical Features of Cutaneous Mastocytosis

- Patients frequently experience pruritus and may have episodic urtication (redness and swelling) of mastocytosis lesions.
- Lesions in infants and preschool-aged children can blister due to release of proteases from densely packed mast cells.
- Firmly rubbing or stroking cutaneous lesions of mastocytosis often causes urtication (Darier's sign) (Fig. 96.2); this is generally more pronounced in children.

WHO CLASSIFICATION OF MASTOCYTOSIS	
Variants	**Subvariants**
Cutaneous mastocytosis	Urticaria pigmentosa (maculopapular), diffuse, mastocytoma(s)
Indolent systemic mastocytosis*	Smoldering systemic mastocytosis, isolated bone marrow mastocytosis
Systemic mastocytosis with *associated* clonal *h*ematological *non-m*ast cell-lineage *d*isease (AHNMD)	Associated with myeloproliferative disorder, CMML, myelodysplastic disorder, AML, non-Hodgkin lymphoma, HES†
Aggressive systemic mastocytosis	Lymphadenopathic with eosinophilia**
Mast cell leukemia	Aleukemic
Mast cell sarcoma	e.g. larynx, colon, brain
Extracutaneous mastocytoma	e.g. lung

*Patients have no evidence of dysfunction of the bone marrow or other extracutaneous organs; they have a low rate of disease progression (<2% after 10 years), and overall their life expectancy is normal.
†Myeloproliferative form of HES characterized by FIP1L1/PDGFRA fusion gene (see Chapter 25).
**Some patients have FIP1L1/PDGFRA fusion gene.
AML, acute myelogenous leukemia; CMML, chronic myelomonocytic leukemia; HES, hypereosinophilic syndrome.
Adapted from Horny H-P, Akin C, Metcalfe DD, et al. Mastocytosis. In: Swerdlow SH, Campo E, Harris NL, et al. (eds.), WHO Classification of Tumours of Haematopoietic and Lymphoid Tissues. Lyon, France: IARC Press, 2008:54–63.

Table 96.1 WHO classification of mastocytosis. Patients with disorders in the bottom two rows usually do not have cutaneous lesions.

- In approximately half of patients, hiving develops after stroking clinically uninvolved skin (dermatographism).
- Several clinical patterns of cutaneous mastocytosis are recognized, but overlap between these groups can occur.

Mastocytomas (Solitary or Multiple)

- Typically present at birth or appear during infancy.
- One to several papules, nodules, or plaques with a yellow-tan to red-brown color and leathery (peau d'orange) texture (Fig. 96.3).
- Can occur anywhere on the skin surface, including acral sites.
- Smaller mastocytomas frequently go unrecognized and are likely underrepresented in series of pediatric mastocytosis patients.
- **DDx:** melanocytic nevus (e.g. congenital, Spitz), café-au-lait macule, arthropod bite, juvenile xanthogranuloma, pseudolymphoma, bullous impetigo.

Urticaria Pigmentosa (UP; Maculopapular or Plaque-Type Cutaneous Mastocytosis)

- Occurs in children and adults.
- Multiple (often numerous) pink-tan to red-brown macules, papules, and/or (particularly in infants/young children) plaques (Fig. 96.4).
- Hyperpigmentation is less prominent in patients with lightly colored skin.
- A subtle leathery texture is usually evident in larger lesions, and fine telangiectasias may be seen (especially in adults).
- Favors the trunk and proximal extremities, usually sparing the central face, palms, and soles.
- **DDx:** lentigines, melanocytic nevi.

Diffuse Cutaneous Mastocytosis

- Occurs primarily in infants, with rare reports in adults.
- Confluence of yellow-tan plaques to produce generalized, doughy thickening of the skin with a leathery texture, sometimes with deep creases.
- Flushing, blistering, and erosions are common (Fig. 96.5).

- **DDx:** epidermolysis bullosa, autoimmune bullous dermatoses.

Telangiectasia Macularis Eruptiva Perstans (TMEP)

- Rare variant that occurs primarily in adults.
- Telangiectatic macules and patches without significant hyperpigmentation (Fig. 96.6).
- Lower density of mast cells than other forms of mastocytosis, so Darier's sign may not be present.
- **DDx:** photodamage, poikiloderma, multiple spider telangiectasias (e.g. in the setting of cirrhosis) and other telangiectatic conditions (see Chapter 87).

Systemic Manifestations of Mastocytosis

- In patients with a higher mast cell burden (e.g. extensive cutaneous disease, a large mastocytoma, extracutaneous involvement), release of mast cell mediators such as histamine can lead to systemic symptoms, which range from flushing to abdominal pain and diarrhea to lightheadedness and syncope (Fig. 96.7).
- Systemic disease is extremely rare in childhood mastocytosis, with the occasional exception of severe diffuse cutaneous mastocytosis.
- Although the bone marrow is frequently involved in adult patients with cutaneous mastocytosis, hematologic sequelae are uncommon (see Table 96.1).
- Criteria for the diagnosis of systemic mastocytosis are presented in Table 96.2.
- Patients with systemic mastocytosis (primarily adults) occasionally develop osteoporosis, osteosclerosis, hepatosplenomegaly, lymphadenopathy, and infiltration of the GI tract.

Evaluation and Treatment

- An approach to the evaluation of a patient with cutaneous mastocytosis is presented in Fig. 96.8.
- Treatment of cutaneous and indolent systemic mastocytosis is directed at alleviating symptoms, if present.

DIFFERENCES IN CLINICAL PRESENTATIONS OF CHILDHOOD- AND ADULT-ONSET MASTOCYTOSIS

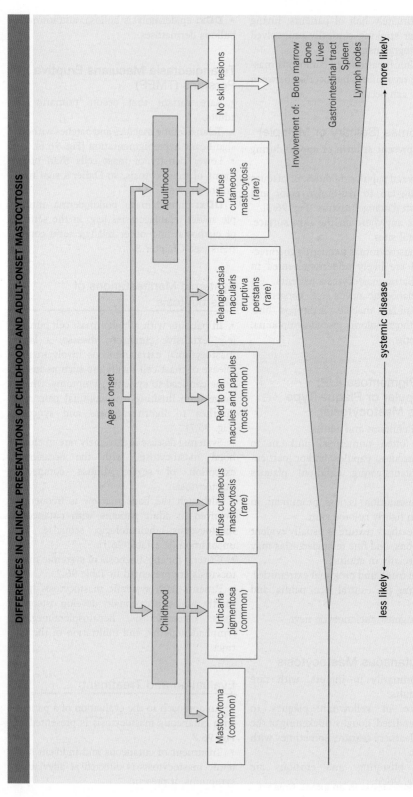

Fig. 96.1 Differences in clinical presentations of childhood- and adult-onset mastocytosis. *Courtesy, Michael Tharp, MD.*

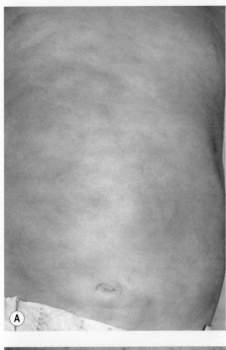

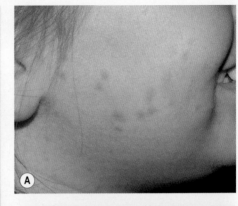

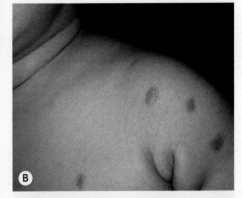

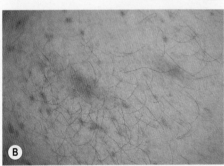

Fig. 96.2 Darier's sign in mastocytosis. An infant with extensive cutaneous involvement **(A)** and an adult with macular and papular lesions **(B).** *A, Courtesy, Julie V. Schaffer, MD; B, Courtesy, Thomas Horn, MD.*

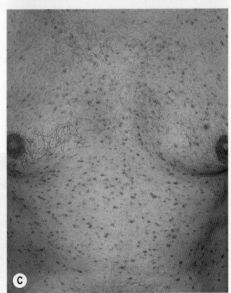

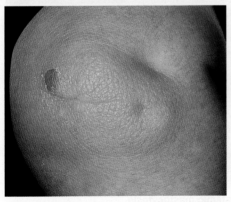

Fig. 96.3 Mastocytoma in an infant. Note the leathery appearance of the skin and the two erosions. *Courtesy, Michael Tharp, MD.*

Fig. 96.4 Urticaria pigmentosa. Papular **(A)** and papulonodular **(B)** lesions can be seen in children. The degree of associated hyperpigmentation as well as the size of the lesions varies. **C** Adult urticaria pigmentosa typically presents with small, red-brown macules and papules. *A, Courtesy Julie V. Schaffer, MD; B, C, Courtesy, Michael Tharp, MD.*

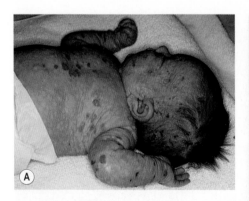

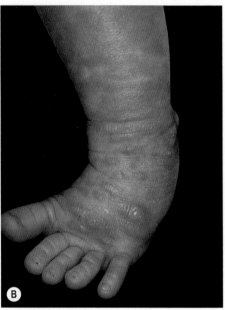

Fig. 96.5 Diffuse cutaneous mastocytosis in infants. A Diffuse infiltration with multiple erosions. **B** Spontaneous blister superimposed on a plaque; note the leathery appearance of the lesions on the shin.

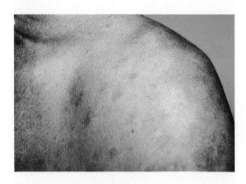

Fig. 96.6 Telangiectasia macularis eruptiva perstans. Multiple lesions composed of telangiectasias are present.

WHO CRITERIA FOR THE DIAGNOSIS OF SYSTEMIC MASTOCYTOSIS
Requires either the major criterion plus one minor criterion or three minor criteria
Major Criterion
• Multifocal dense infiltrates of mast cells (aggregates of ≥15 mast cells) in bone marrow or extracutaneous tissues
Minor Criteria
• >25% of mast cells in bone marrow samples or extracutaneous tissues are spindle-shaped or otherwise atypical
• Extracutaneous mast cells (CD117+) express CD2, CD25, or both (often bone marrow; determined via flow cytometry)
• Presence of c-*KIT* codon 816 mutation in blood, bone marrow, or extracutaneous tissues
• Serum total tryptase level is persistently >20 ng/ml (unless there is an associated clonal myeloid disorder, in which case this parameter is not valid)

Table 96.2 WHO criteria for the diagnosis of systemic mastocytosis.

MAST CELL MEDIATORS AND ASSOCIATED SYMPTOMS OF MASTOCYTOSIS

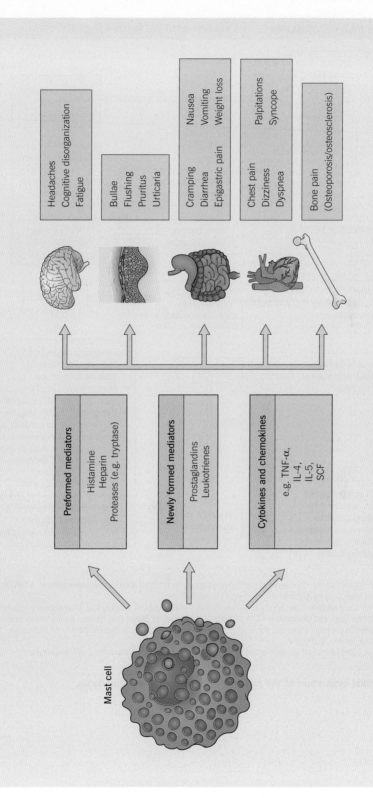

Mast cell

Preformed mediators

Histamine
Heparin
Proteases (e.g. tryptase)

Newly formed mediators

Prostaglandins
Leukotrienes

Cytokines and chemokines

e.g. TNF-α,
IL-4,
IL-5,
SCF

Headaches
Cognitive disorganization
Fatigue

Bullae
Flushing
Pruritus
Urticaria

Cramping   Nausea
Diarrhea   Vomiting
Epigastric pain Weight loss

Chest pain   Palpitations
Dizziness   Syncope
Dyspnea

Bone pain
(Osteoporosis/osteosclerosis)

Fig. 96.7 Mast cell mediators and associated symptoms of mastocytosis. SCF, stem cell factor (binds to KIT receptor).

INITIAL EVALUATION OF THE PATIENT WITH CUTANEOUS MASTOCYTOSIS

Biopsy of lesional skin demonstrating mast cell infiltrates* → Consider evaluation for c-*KIT* mutation

Inquire about constitutional (e.g. fever, malaise, weight loss) and other systemic symptoms (see Fig. 96.7)

Gastrointestinal symptoms → (+) → Further evaluation as indicated (e.g. barium study or endoscopy)

Bone pain or history of fracture → (+) → Radiographic skeletal survey or bone scan†

Examine for lymphadenopathy and hepatosplenomegaly → (+) → Ultrasonography or CT scan; liver function tests → Abnormal

Perform complete blood count (CBC) with manual differential* → Abnormal → Bone marrow biopsy†:
- Immunohistochemical staining for tryptase
- Mast cell immunophenotyping (e.g. CD2 and CD25 expression)
- Cytogenetic studies (e.g. for abnormalities indicative of an associated clonal hematological non-mast cell-lineage disease)
- Analysis of c-*KIT* for codon 816 and other mutations‡

In adults and the subset of children with evidence of systemic disease, determine serum tryptase level and follow as marker of mast cell burden

Presence of eosinophilia → (+) → Screen peripheral blood or bone marrow sample for the *FIP1L1-PDGFRA* fusion gene

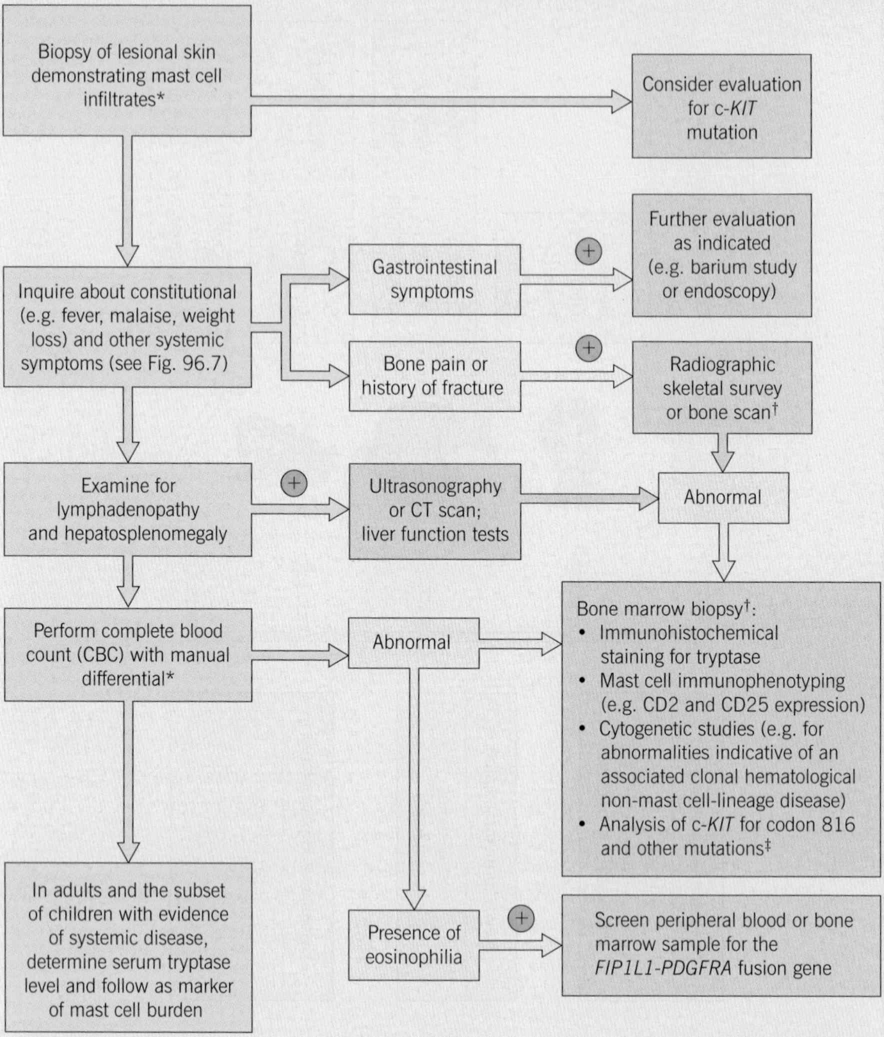

* The diagnosis can sometimes be made clinically, especially in children with classic presentations; a CBC is usually not necessary for children with a mastocytoma
† Can also be considered in other adults with evidence of a high mast cell burden, e.g. a consistently elevated serum tryptase level and extensive (>50% of body surface area) or dense skin lesions; bone marrow biopsy rarely needed in children. However, some groups recommend bone marrow examination in all individuals with tryptase level > 100ng/ml.
‡ It is also possible to analyze paraffin-embedded lesional skin biopsy specimens for c-*KIT* mutations.

Fig. 96.8 Initial evaluation of the patient with cutaneous mastocytosis.

STIMULANTS OF MAST CELL DEGRANULATION
Physical
• Friction
• Exercise
• Heat (e.g. hot bath) or cold (e.g. swimming)
Dietary
• Hot beverages
• Spicy foods
• Alcohol
Medications
• Aspirin
• Nonsteroidal anti-inflammatory drugs
• Narcotics (e.g. morphine, codeine)
• Anticholinergics (e.g. scopolamine)
• Dextromethorphan (a cough suppressant)
• Polymyxin B sulfate
• Some systemic anesthetics (e.g. lidocaine*, etomidate, thiopental, isoflurane)
• Iodine-based radiographic dyes
• Dextran (in some IV solutions)
Allergic
• Allergens causing an immediate-type hypersensitivity reaction in that patient

*Local injections are safe.

Table 96.3 Stimulants of mast cell degranulation.

• Triggers of mast cell degranulation (Table 96.3) should be avoided when possible.

• **Rx:** low-sedating H$_1$ antihistamine(s); addition of a sedating H$_1$ antihistamine at night, an H$_2$ antagonist (especially if upper GI symptoms), or cromolyn sodium (topical or oral) may be beneficial.

• An Epipen® or Epipen Jr® for emergency use can be given to patients with a high mast cell burden.

• Topical therapy with a potent CS or calcineurin inhibitor and narrowband UVB phototherapy may be helpful in patients with refractory symptoms.

• Aggressive systemic disease can be treated with agents such as cladribine or (depending on the underlying mutation) imatinib.

For further information see Ch. 118. From *Dermatology, Third Edition*.

97 | B-Cell Lymphomas of the Skin

General

• Cutaneous lymphomas can involve the skin as either the exclusive site of involvement (*primary cutaneous lymphoma*) or as the result of cutaneous involvement in association with a systemic (usually nodal) lymphoma (*secondary cutaneous lymphoma*).

• Primary cutaneous lymphomas are defined as malignant lymphomas confined to the skin at presentation only after a complete staging evaluation has been performed to exclude a systemic lymphoma.

• Primary cutaneous lymphomas differ significantly from their nodal counterparts in terms of their natural history and thus require a specialized approach to their evaluation and treatment.

• Primary cutaneous lymphomas can originate from B cells (PCBCL), T cells (CTCL), or natural killer (NK) cells.

• Unlike most extranodal lymphomas, T-cell rather than B-cell lymphomas are more prevalent in the skin.

PCBCL

• Primary cutaneous B-cell lymphomas are derived from B lymphocytes in different stages of differentiation.

• B-cell lineage is identified by the presence of CD20 and CD79a and the absence of CD3 markers.

• PCBCLs constitute approximately 20% of all primary cutaneous lymphomas, but there may be regional variation in incidence and specific types of CBCLs.

• Usually affects older adults and males > females.

• Pathogenesis unknown, but in certain areas of the world, *Borrelia* species are thought to play a role; marked immune suppression/dysregulation is also a risk factor.

• Precise classification can be achieved only after a complete synthesis of clinical, histopathologic, immunophenotypic, and molecular features.

• Once the diagnosis of a B-cell lymphoma in the skin has been made, complete staging (Table 97.1) is recommended to distinguish between primary and secondary cutaneous lymphoma.

• The new World Health Organization–European Organization for Research and Treatment of Cancer (WHO–EORTC) classification provides the basis for a consistent classification of patients and divides PCBCL into four major types (Table 97.2).

• Primary cutaneous marginal zone B-cell lymphoma (PCMZL) and primary cutaneous follicle center lymphoma (PCFCL) are indolent lymphomas with 5-year survival rates of ≥95% (Table 97.3).

• Diffuse large B-cell lymphoma, leg type (DLBCLLT) and diffuse large B-cell lymphoma, other (DLBCLO) are in a group with intermediate clinical behavior, worse 5-year survival estimates, and require more aggressive treatment (see Table 97.3).

• An approach to the patient with a suspected diagnosis of cutaneous B-cell lymphoma is shown in Fig. 97.1.

Plasma Cell Dyscrasias, Including Multiple Myeloma

• Plasma cell dyscrasias include monoclonal gammopathy of undetermined significance (MGUS), smoldering/asymptomatic myeloma and active/symptomatic myeloma, as well as light chain and heavy chain deposition diseases and amyloidosis (AL).

• While proliferations of plasma cells in the skin are unusual, cutaneous disorders associated with or thought to be related to a monoclonal gammopathy are more common (Table 97.4).

RECOMMENDED STAGING EVALUATION FOR PATIENTS WITH CONFIRMED DIAGNOSIS OF B-CELL LYMPHOMA INVOLVING THE SKIN

Staging Procedures

History and Physical Examination

- Presence/absence of 'B' symptoms, including fever, night sweats, weight loss, malaise
- Complete lymph node examination
- Palpation of abdomen for hepatosplenomegaly
- Examination of oral cavity

Laboratory Studies

- Complete blood count with differential and platelets
- Comprehensive serum chemistries
- Serum LDH
- Flow cytometry of peripheral blood mononuclear cells
- HIV testing

Imaging Studies

- CT of chest, abdomen, and pelvis with contrast, alone or with integrated whole body PET
- CT or ultrasound of neck, if clinically indicated

Additional Studies as Clinically Indicated

- Bone marrow biopsy and aspirate
- Excisional biopsy of enlarged lymph nodes or other suspicious lesions
- PCR analysis for *Borrelia* spp. DNA in patients from endemic areas (Europe)

LDH, lactate dehydrogenase; CT, computerized tomography; PET, positron emission tomography; HIV, human immunodeficiency virus; PCR, polymerase chain reaction.

Table 97.1 Recommended staging evaluation for patients with confirmed diagnosis of B-cell lymphoma involving the skin.

WHO–EORTC 2005 CLASSIFICATION OF B-CELL LYMPHOMAS WITH PRIMARY CUTANEOUS MANIFESTATIONS [CORRESPONDING ENTITY IN THE WHO 2008 CLASSIFICATION]

- Primary cutaneous follicle center lymphoma (PCFCL) [Same]
- Primary cutaneous marginal zone B-cell lymphoma (PCMZL)* [Extranodal marginal zone lymphoma of *mucosa-associated lymphoid tissue* – MALT lymphoma]
- Primary cutaneous diffuse large B-cell lymphoma, leg type (DLBCLLT) [Same]
- Primary cutaneous diffuse large B-cell lymphoma, other (DLBCLO) [Diffuse large B-cell lymphoma, NOS]
- Intravascular diffuse large B-cell lymphoma [Same]

*Includes cases previously designated as primary cutaneous immunocytoma and primary cutaneous plasmacytoma.
NOS, not otherwise specified.

Table 97.2 WHO–EORTC 2005 classification of B-cell lymphomas with primary cutaneous manifestations [corresponding entity in the WHO 2008 classification].

THE PRIMARY CUTANEOUS B-CELL LYMPHOMAS (PCBCLs): CLINICAL AND DIAGNOSTIC FEATURES AND RECOMMENDED TREATMENT OPTIONS

Primary Cutaneous B-Cell Lymphoma Subtype	Preferred Location	Clinical Features	Other Distinguishing Features	DDx	Rx	Outcome
Indolent Behavior						
Primary cutaneous marginal zone B-cell lymphoma (PCMZL)	• Extremities: upper > lower • Trunk • Occasionally generalized	• Multifocal, red to red-brown, asymptomatic papules, plaques and nodules (Fig. 97.2) • Rare ulceration; may resolve with anetoderma • Can occur in areas of acrodermatitis chronica atrophicans (Fig. 97.2B)	• Bcl-2 (+), Bcl-6 (−), CD10 (−) • Monoclonal rearrangement of *IGH* genes • Intracytoplasmic monotypic expression of Ig light chains (Fig. 97.3) • May be linked to infection with *Borrelia* species in endemic areas (e.g. Europe)	• Distinguish between the various PCBCLs • Benign reactive processes (e.g. lymphocytic infiltrate of Jessner, cutaneous lymphoid hyperplasia) • Leukemia cutis (e.g. cutaneous CLL)	Solitary or few lesions (trunk, occasionally more generalized) • Watchful waiting • Intralesional CS • RT • Surgical excision • Surgical excision plus postoperative RT • Intralesional rituximab Multiple lesions at different body sites or diffuse PCFCL with disseminated lesions or if located on legs • Intralesional CS • Subcutaneous or intralesional interferon α-2a • Systemic rituximab • Systemic chemotherapy plus rituximab	• 5-year survival ≥95% • Skin relapse common • Occasionally spontaneous resolution • Progression to systemic involvement is rare
Primary cutaneous follicle center lymphoma (PCFCL)	• Scalp, forehead, trunk (especially back), rarely legs (~5%)	• Solitary or grouped, asymptomatic, pink to plum-colored papules, plaques, or tumors (Fig. 97.4) • Surrounding skin erythema • Ulceration uncommon	• Bcl-6 (+), MUM1 (−) • Usually Bcl-2 (−), t(14;18) (−) ; if either (+) suspect systemic involvement • (−) monoclonal Ig gene rearrangement • (+) monotypic surface Ig expression	• Secondary involvement from a systemic lymphoma • Solid organ metastases		

Intermediate to Aggressive Behavior

	Clinical	Diagnostic	Immunophenotype	Differential	Treatment	Prognosis
Primary cutaneous diffuse large B-cell lymphoma, leg type (DLBCLLt)	• Distal leg • Unilateral > bilateral • May occur elsewhere (10–15%)	• Solitary or clustered, red to red-brown nodules • Often see small red papules adjacent to larger nodules (Fig. 97.5)	• Bcl-2 (+), MUM1 (+) • Usually Bcl-6 (+) • CD10 (–) • ± monoclonal rearrangement of *IGH* genes • (+) monotypic surface and/or intracytoplasmic Ig expression	• Secondary cutaneous involvement from systemic lymphoma • Cutaneous infiltrates from AML • Solid organ metastases	• Systemic rituximab • Systemic chemotherapy plus rituximab • Consider local RT for small solitary lesions	• 5-year survival ~50% • Extracutaneous involvement in ~50% • Multiple lesions on leg = poor prognosis

Other

Intravascular diffuse large B-cell lymphoma	• Indurated, red to violaceous patches and plaques • Neoplastic CD20(+) cells are located within vessels that are CD31(+) and CD34(+) • Systemic involvement is common and treatment is with systemic chemotherapy
Plasmablastic lymphoma	• Expanding oral lesion, most often arising in the setting of HIV infection • Loss of typical B-cell markers (CD20, CD79a) • Very aggressive with poor prognosis and treatment requires systemic chemotherapy

Ig, immunoglobulin; CLL, chronic lymphocytic leukemia; PCR, polymerase chain reaction; RT, radiotherapy; AML, acute myelogenous leukemia.

Table 97.3 The primary cutaneous B-cell lymphomas (PCBCLs): clinical and diagnostic features and recommended treatment options.

B-CELL LYMPHOMAS OF THE SKIN

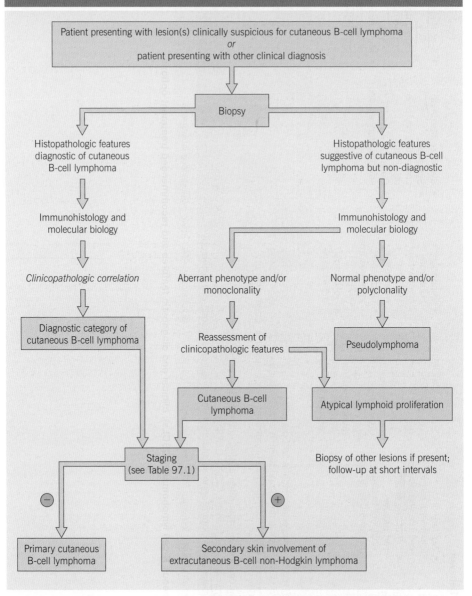

Fig. 97.1 Evaluation of the patient with a suspected diagnosis of cutaneous B-cell lymphoma. Algorithm outlining approach to the patient. *Courtesy, Lorenzo Cerroni, MD.*

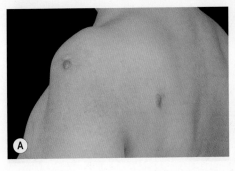

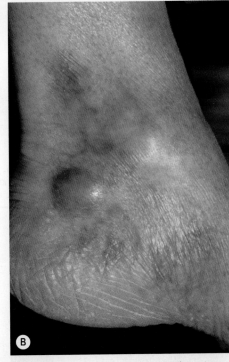

Fig. 97.2 Cutaneous marginal zone B-cell lymphoma. A Two well-circumscribed, erythematous nodules on the shoulder. **B** Dome-shaped erythematous nodule with smooth surface. The surrounding area shows features of acrodermatitis chronica atrophicans. This tumor, which demonstrated prominent lymphoplasmacytic differentiation histopathologically, was classified as a cutaneous immunocytoma in the past. *A, B, Courtesy, Lorenzo Cerroni, MD.*

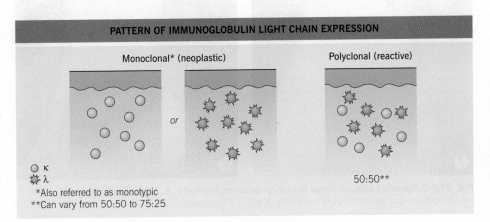

PATTERN OF IMMUNOGLOBULIN LIGHT CHAIN EXPRESSION

Monoclonal* (neoplastic)

Polyclonal (reactive)

or

○ κ

☼ λ

50:50**

*Also referred to as monotypic
**Can vary from 50:50 to 75:25

Fig. 97.3 Pattern of immunoglobulin light chain expression.

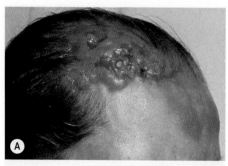
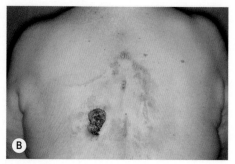

Fig. 97.4 Cutaneous follicle center lymphoma. A Large ulcerated tumors on the scalp surrounded by infiltrated erythematous nodules and plaques. **B** Large ulcerated tumor on the back. Note surrounding erythematous papules, patches, and plaques (Crosti's lymphoma). *A, B, Courtesy, Lorenzo Cerroni, MD.*

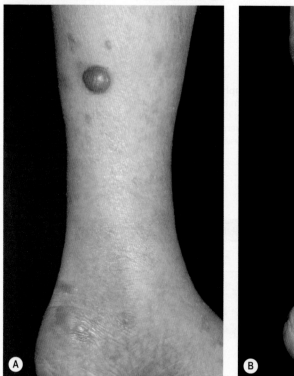
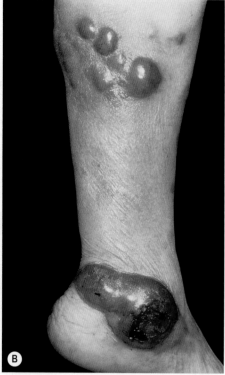

Fig. 97.5 Cutaneous diffuse large B-cell lymphoma, leg type. A, B Multiple red-brown papulonodules and tumors on the lower leg. *A, B, Courtesy, Lorenzo Cerroni, MD.*

CUTANEOUS CONDITIONS ASSOCIATED WITH A MONOCLONAL GAMMOPATHY

Proliferation of lymphoplasmacytic cells in the skin
- Extramedullary cutaneous plasmacytoma*
- Cutaneous Waldenström's macroglobulinemia (IgM)

Deposition of the monoclonal protein in the skin, by definition
- Primary systemic amyloidosis (light chains)
- Cryoglobulinemic occlusive vasculopathy (type I cryoglobulins)
- Hyperkeratotic spicules (follicular > nonfollicular)
- Crystal-storing histiocytosis
- IgM storage papules (cutaneous macroglobulinosis)
- Subepidermal bullous dermatosis associated with IgM gammopathy

Deposition of the monoclonal protein in the skin frequently observed
- Plasma cell dyscrasia-associated acquired cutis laxa, acral or generalized (amyloid and/or IgG)
- Plasma cell dyscrasia-associated reactive angioendotheliomatosis (type I cryoglobulins or amyloid)

Almost always associated with monoclonal gammopathy
- Scleromyxedema
- POEMS syndrome (polyneuropathy, organomegaly, endocrinopathy)
- AESOP syndrome – adenopathy and extensive skin patch overlying a plasmacytoma; may coexist with POEMS syndrome
- Schnitzler's syndrome (IgM)
- Necrobiotic xanthogranuloma

Frequently associated with monoclonal gammopathy
- Normolipemic plane xanthoma
- Scleredema (type 2)
- Angioedema secondary to acquired C1 esterase inhibitor deficiency
- Clarkson's syndrome (idiopathic systemic capillary leak syndrome)

Significant association with monoclonal gammopathy (at least 15% of cases)
- Erythema elevatum diutinum
- Subcorneal pustular dermatosis (SPD) and SPD-type IgA pemphigus
- Pyoderma gangrenosum

Occasionally associated with monoclonal gammopathy
- Sweet's syndrome
- Cutaneous small vessel vasculitis
- Xanthoma disseminatum
- Epidermolysis bullosa acquisita
- Paraneoplastic pemphigus

*In the current WHO–EORTC classification (see Table 97.2), primary cutaneous plasmacytoma is classified as primary cutaneous marginal zone B-cell lymphoma.

Table 97.4 Cutaneous conditions associated with a monoclonal gammopathy.

For further information see Ch. 119. From *Dermatology, Third Edition.*

98 | Cutaneous T-Cell Lymphoma

- *Primary* cutaneous lymphomas present in the skin without evidence of extracutaneous disease at the time of diagnosis.
- *Secondary* cutaneous lymphomas are skin manifestations of systemic (nodal) lymphomas and will not be discussed (see oncology texts).
- Primary cutaneous lymphomas may be of **T-**cell origin (75–80%) or **B-**cell origin (20–25%) and are termed **CTCL** and **CBCL**, respectively.
- The term CTCL will be used herein to describe the heterogeneous group of primary cutaneous lymphomas composed of neoplastic T cells or natural killer (NK) cells (Table 98.1).
- As different types of CTCLs, CBCLs, and even secondary cutaneous lymphomas may present with similar clinical and histopathological features, it is imperative to combine clinical and staging data with histologic, immunophenotypic, and genetic data before making a definitive diagnosis (classification).
- Immunophenotyping, as determined from immunohistochemical studies done on skin biopsy specimens, can help distinguish between a T-cell vs. an NK-cell vs. a B-cell lymphoma and can aid in subtyping.
- T-cell receptor (TCR) gene rearrangement analysis, either with Southern blot analysis or by more sensitive PCR-based techniques, is useful in detecting the presence or absence of a clonal T-cell population in skin biopsy specimens.
- The presence of a clonal T-cell population cannot be used as an absolute criterion of malignancy, as several benign conditions may also demonstrate clonality (e.g. pityriasis lichenoides et varioliformis acuta, lichen planus, pigmented purpuric dermatosis, lichen sclerosus, and some pseudolymphomas).

- An approach to the evaluation of a patient with suspected CTCL is presented in Fig. 98.1.
- Of the various CTCLs, approximately 65% are mycosis fungoides (MF), MF variants, or Sézary syndrome (SS) (see Table 98.1); 25% are within the spectrum of CD30+ lymphoproliferative disorders (see Table 98.1 and Fig. 98.2); and the remainder (10%) are composed of other rare entities (see Table 98.1).
- In general, the aggressive-behaving CTCLs (see Tables 98.1 and 98.2) require more extensive staging, referral to a hematologist–oncologist, and systemic chemotherapy or targeted immunotherapy (e.g. rituximab, brentuximab).

Mycosis Fungoides (MF)

- The most common subtype of CTCL, representing about 50% of all *primary* cutaneous lymphomas.
- The term MF should be restricted to the classic 'Alibert–Bazin' type, characterized by the typical evolution of patches, plaques, and tumors.
- Other clinical variants with similar behavior include hypo- and hyperpigmented MF and bullous MF.
- Three rare clinical variants of MF with distinctive clinicopathologic features are considered separately, namely pagetoid reticulosis (Fig. 98.3), folliculotropic MF (Fig. 98.4), and granulomatous slack skin (Fig. 98.5).
- Classic MF is an uncommon disease; more prevalent in males (> females), older adults, and African-Americans; pathogenesis unknown.
- Clinical presentation depends on stage at diagnosis (Tables 98.3 and 98.4), but classically patients progress from persistent patch/plaque stage to tumor stage over years to decades (Fig. 98.6).

WHO–EORTC CLASSIFICATION FOR AND FEATURES OF CUTANEOUS T-CELL LYMPHOMAS

WHO–EORTC Classification	Frequency (%)	Clinical Features	Immunophenotypic Profile	DDx
Indolent Clinical Behavior				
5-year survival rate (%)				
Mycosis Fungoides				
Overall ~88% **US Data** • Stage IA same life expectancy as age-matched controls • Stage IB/IIA median survival of 11–12 years • Stage IIB/III median survival of 3–5 years • Stage IVA/IVB median survival of 1.5–3 years	54%	• Variable progression from patch to plaque to tumor stage over years–decades (see Fig. 98.6) • **Patch stage:** variably sized red, finely scaling lesions with atrophy and poikiloderma; predilection for sun-protected sites • **Plaque stage:** infiltrated red-brown scaling plaques; often annular, polycyclic or horseshoe-shaped • **Tumor stage:** often have combination of patches, plaques, and tumors; many with ulceration	CD3⁺ CD4⁺ CD8⁻ CD7⁻ Occasionally CD4⁻, CD8⁺ Rarely CD4⁻, CD8⁻	• Eczema • Psoriasis • Superficial fungal infection • Drug reaction • Other types of epidermotropic CTCL
Mycosis Fungoides Variants				
Folliculotropic MF Overall ~80% **US Data** • Early stage (≤IIA) 5/10/15-year survival rates of 87%/82%/41% • Late stage (≥IIB) 5/10/15-year survival rates of 83%/67%/25%	6%	• Grouped follicular papules, acneiform lesions, indurated plaques (see Fig. 98.4) • Favors head and neck • Pruritus, alopecia, mucinorrhea • Pruritus often severe • Survival similar to tumor stage MF • Requires more aggressive treatment from the onset	CD3⁺ CD4⁺ CD8⁻ Occasionally CD30⁺	• Acne vulgaris • Chloracne • Alopecia mucinosa • Seborrheic dermatitis • Atopic dermatitis
Pagetoid Reticulosis 100%	1%	• Slowly progressive, solitary or localized psoriasiform or hyperkeratotic patch or plaque • Favors extremities (see Fig. 98.3) • Histologically purely intraepidermal proliferation	CD3⁺, CD4⁺, CD8⁻ —OR— CD3⁺, CD4⁻, CD8⁺ CD30⁺ in many cases	• Isolated patch of psoriasis or eczema • Other types of CTCL

Table 98.1 WHO–EORTC classification for and features of cutaneous T-cell lymphomas. *Continued*

CUTANEOUS T-CELL LYMPHOMA

Table 98.1 *Continued* **WHO–EORTC classification for and features of cutaneous T-cell lymphomas.**

WHO–EORTC Classification	Frequency (%)	Clinical Features	Immunophenotypic Profile	DDx
Granulomatous Slack Skin				
100%	<1%	• Circumscribed areas of pendulous, atrophic, lax skin (see Fig. 98.5) • Favors axillae and groin	CD3$^+$ CD4$^+$ CD8$^-$	• Acquired generalized cutis laxa • Pseudoxanthoma elasticum
Primary Cutaneous CD30$^+$ Lymphoproliferative Disorders				
Primary Cutaneous Anaplastic Large Cell Lymphoma (CALCL) 95%	10%	• Solitary or localized nodules or tumors, often with ulceration (see Fig. 98.8) • Occasionally will spontaneously regress	CD30$^+$ CD4$^+$ >> CD8$^+$ ALK$^-$ EMA$^-$ CD15$^-$ TIA-1$^+$	• CD30$^+$ large cell lymphoma secondary to MF transformation • HIV-associated or post-transplant lymphoma • Skin manifestations of systemic ALCL
Lymphomatoid Papulosis (LyP) 100%	16%	• Red-brown papules and nodules that can develop central hemorrhage, necrosis, and crusting (see Fig. 98.9) • Spontaneously disappear over 3–8 weeks • Different stages of evolution coexist • May last months to >40 years • ~20% preceded by/followed by/associated with another cutaneous lymphoma (e.g. MF, CALCL, HD)	Type B may be CD30$^-$ negative	• Pityriasis lichenoides et varioliformis acuta (PLEVA) • Pityriasis lichenoides chronica (PLC) • Folliculitis • If clustered, Majocchi's granuloma • Arthropod bites

Subcutaneous Panniculitis-Like T-Cell Lymphoma				
82%	<1%	• Subcutaneous nodules and plaques • Extremities > trunk (see Fig. 98.10) • ± Fever, fatigue, weight loss	CD3+ CD4− CD8+ CD56− βF1+ (TCR α/β+)	• Other types of panniculitis (see Chapter 83)
Primary Cutaneous CD4+ Small/Medium-Sized Pleomorphic T-Cell Lymphoma				
75%	3%	• Most often a solitary plaque or tumor on face, neck, upper trunk	CD3+ CD4+ CD8− βF1+ (TCR α/β+) CD30− CD56−	
Aggressive Clinical Behavior				
5-year survival rate (%)				
Sézary Syndrome (SS)				
24%	4%	• Exfoliative erythroderma (see Fig. 98.7) • Intense pruritus with lichenification • Lymphadenopathy • Alopecia • Palmoplantar keratoderma	CD3+ CD4+ CD8− CD7− CD26−	• Other erythrodermic syndromes (see Chapter 8) • Actinic reticuloid

Table 98.1 *Continued* **WHO–EORTC classification for and features of cutaneous T-cell lymphomas.**

WHO–EORTC Classification	Frequency (%)	Clinical Features	Immunophenotypic Profile	DDx
Adult T-Cell Leukemia/Lymphoma (ATLL)				
NDA	NDA	• Associated with HTLV-1 infection • More common in SW Japan, Caribbean islands • **Acute presentation:** leukemia, lymphadenopathy, hypercalcemia, skin lesions • **Smoldering variant:** resembles MF	CD3$^+$ CD4$^+$ CD8$^-$ CD25$^+$	Smoldering variant • MF
Extranodal NK/T-Cell Lymphoma, Nasal Type				
<5%	1%	• Almost always associated with EBV • **Nasal type:** mid-facial destructive tumor* (see Fig. 98.11) • **Skin only:** ulcerated plaques or tumors on trunk/extremities	CD2$^+$ CD3 epsilon$^+$ TIA-1$^+$ EBER-1$^+$ CD56$^+$ CD4$^-$ CD8$^{-/+}$	Nasal type • Mucormycosis • Leishmaniasis Skin only • Other cutaneous lymphomas

Primary Cutaneous Aggressive Epidermotropic CD8+ Cytotoxic T-Cell Lymphoma

18%	<1%	• Eruptive papulonodules with ulceration (see Fig. 98.12) —OR— • Keratotic patches and plaques	CD3+ CD4- CD8+ TIA-1+ βF1+ (TCR α/β+)	• Other CD8+ CTCLs (pagetoid reticulosis, MF, LyP, CALCL)

Primary Cutaneous γ/δ T-Cell Lymphoma

<5%	1%	• Disseminated plaques and/or ulceronecrotic nodules or tumors • Hemophagocytic syndrome common	CD3+ CD4- CD8- TCR γ/δ+ βF1- (TCR α/β+) TIA-1+ CD56+	• Other panniculitides (see Chapter 83)

Primary Cutaneous Peripheral T-Cell Lymphoma, Unspecified

16%	3%	• Generalized > solitary or localized nodules and tumors (see Fig. 98.13)	CD4+ CD30- CD56-	• Other cutaneous lymphomas

*Previously called lethal midline granuloma.

NDA, no data available; EBV, Epstein-Barr virus; HD, Hodgkin disease; HTLV-1, human T-lymphotrophic virus 1; TCR, T-cell receptor.

AN APPROACH TO THE PATIENT WITH A SUSPECTED CUTANEOUS T-CELL LYMPHOMA (CTCL)

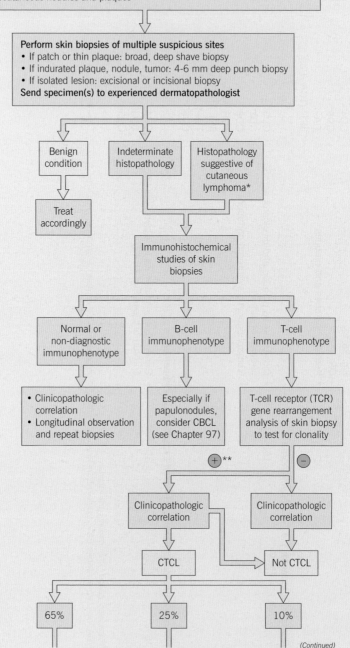

Skin lesions suspicious for CTCL
• Persistent patches and/or plaques in non-photodistributed areas
• Erythroderma
• Indurated plaques of the head and neck
• Solitary, localized, or generalized nodules or tumors, +/- ulceration and necrosis
• Subcutaneous nodules and plaques

Perform skin biopsies of multiple suspicious sites
• If patch or thin plaque: broad, deep shave biopsy
• If indurated plaque, nodule, tumor: 4-6 mm deep punch biopsy
• If isolated lesion: excisional or incisional biopsy
Send specimen(s) to experienced dermatopathologist

Benign condition

Indeterminate histopathology

Histopathology suggestive of cutaneous lymphoma*

Treat accordingly

Immunohistochemical studies of skin biopsies

Normal or non-diagnostic immunophenotype

B-cell immunophenotype

T-cell immunophenotype

• Clinicopathologic correlation
• Longitudinal observation and repeat biopsies

Especially if papulonodules, consider CBCL (see Chapter 97)

T-cell receptor (TCR) gene rearrangement analysis of skin biopsy to test for clonality

+**

−

Clinicopathologic correlation

Clinicopathologic correlation

CTCL

Not CTCL

65%

25%

10%

(Continued)

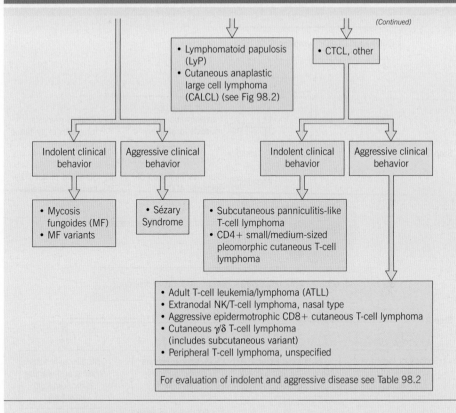

(Continued)

Fig. 98.1 An approach to the patient with a suspected cutaneous T-cell lymphoma (CTCL).

CBCL, cutaneous B-cell lymphoma
*If classic clinical and histopathological findings for MF, immunohistochemical and TCR/clonality studies may not be necessary
**The presence of a clonal T-cell population cannot be used as an absolute criterion of malignancy, as several benign conditions may also demonstrate clonality (e.g. pityriasis lichenoides et varioliformis acuta, lichen planus, pigmented purpuric dermatosis)

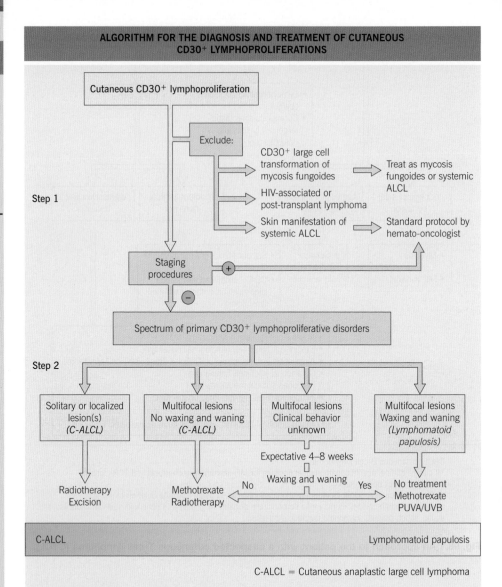

Fig. 98.2 Algorithm for the diagnosis and treatment of primary cutaneous CD30⁺ lymphoproliferations. Brentuximab targets CD30 and is used to treat systemic ALCL. *From Bekkenk M, Geelen FAMJ, van Voorst Vader PC, et al. Primary and secondary cutaneous CD30-positive lymphoproliferative disorders: long term follow-up data of 219 patients and guidelines for diagnosis and treatment. A report from the Dutch Cutaneous Lymphoma Group. Blood. 2000;95:3653–61.*

RECOMMENDED STAGING EVALUATION FOR INDOLENT- AND AGGRESSIVE-BEHAVIOR CUTANEOUS T-CELL LYMPHOMAS (CTCL)
Indolent-Behavior CTCL
• Physical examination, including lymph nodes and palpation for hepatosplenomegaly • Laboratory studies: CBC with differential, platelets, chemistry panel, calcium, LDH • Biopsy of persistently enlarged lymph node(s)
Aggressive-Behavior CTCL *In addition to that performed for indolent, also include*
• CT vs. CT/PET scan • Referral to hematology-oncology
Special Tests, If Clinically Indicated
• Detection of peripheral blood involvement (flow cytometry, TCR gene rearrangement, Sézary cell buffy coat preparation) • HTLV-1 serology, Southern blot analysis, or PCR in at-risk populations
CBC, complete blood count; LDH, lactate dehydrogenase; TCR, T-cell receptor; PCR, polymerase chain reaction; CT, computed tomography; PET, positron emission tomography.

Table 98.2 Recommended staging evaluation for indolent- and aggressive-behavior cutaneous T-cell lymphomas (CTCL).

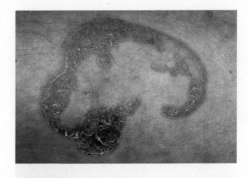

Fig. 98.3 Pagetoid reticulosis. Solitary plaque on the left upper leg. *Courtesy, Rein Willemze, MD.*

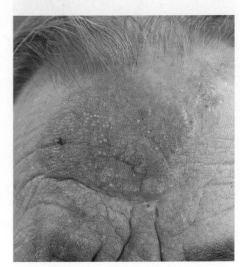

Fig. 98.4 Folliculotropic mycosis fungoides. Infiltrated erythematous plaques and acneiform lesions on the forehead and eyebrows with concurrent hair loss. The infiltration, thickening, and accentuation of the skin folds is referred to as a 'leonine facies.' *Courtesy, Rein Willemze, MD.*

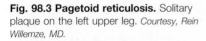

TNMB CLASSIFICATION OF MYCOSIS FUNGOIDES AND SÉZARY SYNDROME

T (skin)

T_1	Limited patch/plaque (involving <10% of total skin surface)
T_2	Generalized patch/plaque (involving ≥10% of total skin surface)
T_3	Tumor(s)
T_4	Erythroderma

N (lymph node)

N_0	No enlarged lymph nodes
N_1	Enlarged lymph nodes, histologically uninvolved
N_2	Enlarged lymph nodes, histologically involved (nodal architecture uneffaced)
N_3	Enlarged lymph nodes, histologically involved (nodal architecture [partially] effaced)

M (viscera)

M_0	No visceral involvement
M_1	Visceral involvement

B (blood)

B_0	No circulating atypical (Sézary) cells (or ≤5% of lymphocytes)
B_1	Low blood tumor burden (>5% of lymphocytes are Sézary cells, but not B_2)
B_2	High blood tumor burden (≥1000/microliter Sézary cells + positive clone)

Table 98.3 TNMB classification of mycosis fungoides and Sézary syndrome.

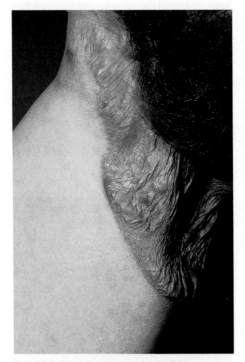

Fig. 98.5 Granulomatous slack skin.
Pendulous fold of atrophic lax skin in the right inguinal area. *Courtesy, Rein Willemze, MD.*

CLINICAL STAGING SYSTEM FOR MYCOSIS FUNGOIDES AND SÉZARY SYNDROME

Clinical Stage				
IA	T_1	N_0	M_0	B_{0-1}
IB	T_2	N_0	M_0	B_{0-1}
IIA	T_{1-2}	N_{1-2}	M_0	B_{0-1}
IIB	T_3	N_{0-1}	M_0	B_{0-1}
IIIA	T_4	N_{0-2}	M_0	B_0
IIIB	T_4	N_{0-2}	M_0	B_1
IVA$_1$	T_{1-4}	N_{0-2}	M_0	B_2
IVA$_2$	T_{1-4}	N_3	M_0	B_{0-2}
IVB	T_{1-4}	N_{0-3}	M_1	B_{0-2}

Table 98.4 Clinical staging system for mycosis fungoides and Sézary syndrome.

- Most patients have years of nonspecific eczematous or psoriasiform skin lesions and nondiagnostic biopsies before a definitive diagnosis of MF is made.
- There can be gradual progression or relapse at a similar stage of disease; advancement to a higher stage usually transpires after years and multiple treatment failures.
- Extracutaneous disease is extremely rare in patch/plaque stage, uncommon with

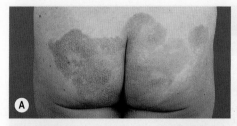
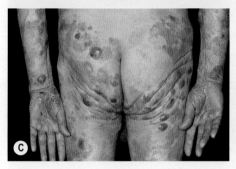
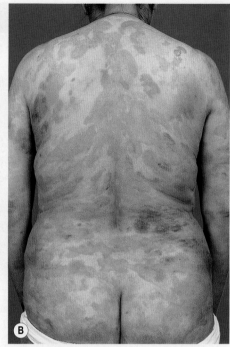

Fig. 98.6 Mycosis fungoides. A Limited patch/plaque stage disease (stage 1A). Patches on the buttocks, involving less than 10% of the skin surface. **B** Generalized patch/plaque disease (stage 1B). Extensive patches and plaques involving more than 10% of the skin surface. **C** Tumor stage. Multiple skin tumors in combination with typical patches and plaques. *Courtesy, Rein Willemze, MD.*

generalized plaques, and most likely with extensive tumors or erythroderma.

• Extracutaneous involvement almost always initially involves regional lymph nodes draining the areas of greatest skin involvement; visceral involvement can develop subsequently; bone marrow involvement is rare.

• Histopathologic examination of persistently enlarged lymph nodes can help distinguish between dermatopathic (reactive) lymphadenopathy and involvement with MF.

• Treatment is dependent on the stage at diagnosis, the host's immune status, and the general condition of the patient (Table 98.5).

• Available therapies are effective in controlling disease but usually do not prolong life.

• Three main treatment categories are available: (1) skin-directed therapies (SDT); (2) systemic biologic therapies; and (3) systemic chemotherapies; combination therapy is also utilized (Table 98.6).

• Prognosis depends on stage, the type and extent of skin lesions, and the presence of extracutaneous disease (see Table 98.3).

• An aggressive course is seen in patients with effaced lymph nodes, visceral involvement, or transformation into a large T-cell lymphoma.

• Death is usually due to systemic involvement or profound immunosuppression with resultant opportunistic infection.

Sézary Syndrome (SS)

• Leukemic variant of MF.

• Defined historically by the triad of (1) erythroderma; (2) generalized lymphadenopathy; and (3) the presence of neoplastic T cells (Sézary cells) in the skin, lymph nodes, and peripheral blood (Fig. 98.7).

• Diagnosis aided by the presence of one of the following: (1) absolute Sézary cell count of ≥1000 cells/mm³; (2) CD4:CD8 ratio ≥10 and/or an abnormal immunophenotype, including the loss of CD7 (>40%) or CD26 (>30%) by flow cytometry; and (3) evidence of T-cell clonality in the blood.

PRIMARY TREATMENT OF MYCOSIS FUNGOIDES (MF) AND SÉZARY SYNDROME (SS) BASED ON CLINICAL STAGE

STAGE IA/IIA (T1) with B_0

- SDT for limited skin disease

STAGE IB/IIA (T2) with B_0

- SDT for generalized skin disease

STAGE IA/IB/IIA with B_1

- Systemic biologic therapies

STAGE IIB (limited tumors) with B_0

- Local radiation for localized and limited tumors
- Systemic biologic therapies
- Use SDT for any patch/plaque disease

STAGE IIB (generalized tumors) with B_0 or IIB (any tumors) with B_1

- TSEBT ± adjuvant systemic biologic therapies
- Combination therapies
- Systemic chemotherapies
- ± SDT for any patch/plaque disease

STAGE III with B_0

- SDT for generalized skin disease
- And/or systemic biologic therapies

STAGE III with B_1

- Systemic biologic therapies ± SDT

STAGE IV: Sézary syndrome ± lymph node disease

- Systemic biologic therapies
- Combination therapies

STAGE IV: Visceral disease or lymph node disease (*not* SS)

- Systemic chemotherapies
- ± Radiation therapy for local control

Folliculotropic MF

- TSEBT ± adjuvant systemic biologic therapies
- Combination therapies
- Systemic chemotherapies
- ± SDT for any patch/plaque disease

Pagetoid reticulosis

- Surgical excision
- Local radiation

SDT, skin directed therapy; TSEBT, total skin electron beam therapy.

Table 98.5 Primary treatment of mycosis fungoides (MF) and Sézary syndrome (SS) based on clinical stage.

- Prognosis is generally poor and most patients die from opportunistic infections due to immunosuppression.
- Systemic treatment is required, with skin-directed therapies sometimes being used as adjuvant therapy (see Tables 98.4 and 98.5).

For further information see Ch. 120. From *Dermatology, Third Edition.*

TREATMENT OPTIONS FOR MYCOSIS FUNGOIDES (MF) AND SÉZARY SYNDROME (SS)
Skin-Directed Therapies (SDT)
<ul><li>Topical corticosteroids (high potency* and mid potency**)</li><li>Topical retinoids (tazarotene, bexarotene)*</li><li>Topical imiquimod*</li><li>Topical chemotherapy (nitrogen mustard, carmustine/BCNU)</li><li>Local radiation (for localized tumors)*</li><li>Phototherapy for patches and thin plaques (UVB, narrowband and broadband)</li><li>Phototherapy for thicker plaques (PUVA)</li><li>Total skin electron beam radiation therapy (TSEBT)**</li></ul>
Systemic Biologic Therapies
<ul><li>Interferons (IFN-α, IFN-γ)</li><li>Methotrexate</li><li>Oral retinoids (bexarotene, isotretinoin, acitretin)</li><li>Extracorporeal photopheresis (ECP)</li><li>Denileukin diftitox, brentuximab</li><li>HDAC-inhibitors (vorinostat, romidepsin)</li></ul>
Systemic Chemotherapies
<ul><li>e.g. liposomal doxorubicin, gemcitabine</li></ul>
Relapsed or Refractory Disease
<ul><li>Pralatrexate</li><li>Allogeneic hematopoietic stem-cell transplantation</li></ul>
Combination Therapies
Skin-Directed Therapy + Systemic (e.g. phototherapy + oral retinoid *or* interferon)
Systemic + Systemic (e.g. oral retinoid + interferon; ECP + interferon)

*Limited skin disease.
**Generalized skin disease.

Table 98.6 Treatment options for mycosis fungoides (MF) and Sézary syndrome (SS).

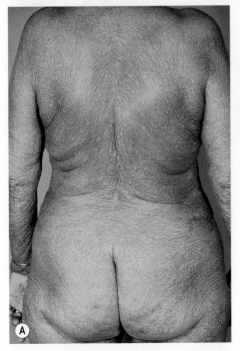

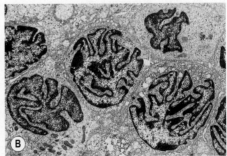

Fig. 98.7 Sézary syndrome. A Diffuse erythroderma is present. **B** Electron photomicrograph of a skin biopsy showing characteristic Sézary cells. *Courtesy, Rein Willemze, MD.*

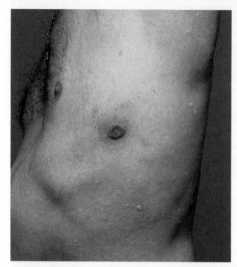

Fig. 98.8 Primary cutaneous anaplastic large cell lymphoma. Characteristic clinical presentation with a solitary ulcerating tumor. *Courtesy, Rein Willemze, MD.*

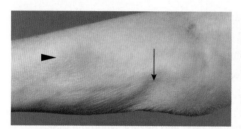

Fig. 98.10 Subcutaneous panniculitis-like T-cell lymphoma (SPTCL). Pink nodular skin lesions (arrowhead) as well as an area of lipoatrophy (arrow) at the site of a resolved nodule. *Courtesy, Rein Willemze, MD.*

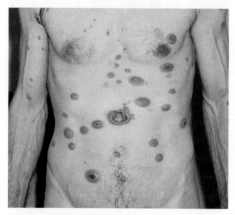

Fig. 98.12 Aggressive epidermotropic CD8⁺ cutaneous T-cell lymphoma. Generalized skin tumors with central ulceration. *Courtesy, Rein Willemze, MD.*

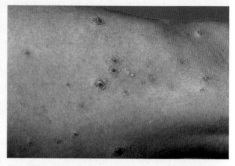

Fig. 98.9 Lymphomatoid papulosis (LyP). Clinical presentation with papulonecrotic skin lesions at different stages of evolution. *Courtesy, Rein Willemze, MD.*

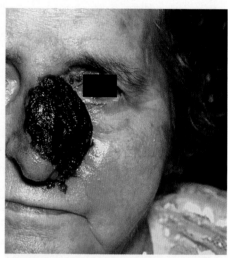

Fig. 98.11 Extranodal NK/T-cell lymphoma, nasal type. An extensive ulceronecrotic nasal mass, previously referred to as lethal midline granuloma. *Courtesy, Rein Willemze, MD.*

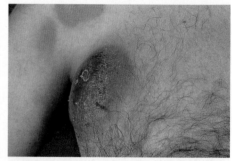

Fig. 98.13 Primary cutaneous peripheral T-cell lymphoma, unspecified. Rapidly growing nodules and tumors. Note: The skin lesions in the left upper corner do not represent patches but, rather, deep plaques present for 2 weeks. *Courtesy, Rein Willemze, MD.*

Other Lymphoproliferative and Myeloproliferative Diseases

99

Benign Lymphoctic Infiltrates

Lymphocytic Infiltrate of Jessner

- A benign skin-limited disorder that overlaps with other entities, including dermal lupus erythematosus, cutaneous lymphoid hyperplasia, and polymorphic light eruption (PMLE).
- Males = females; onset typically during middle age; very rare in children.
- Most commonly appears on the head, neck, and upper back as one or several asymptomatic, erythematous papules, plaques (often annular) > nodules (Fig. 99.1); no secondary or surface changes (such as scale or crust).
- May last several weeks to months and will typically resolve spontaneously over months to years without sequelae.
- No systemic manifestations.
- **DDx:** see Fig. 99.2.
- **Rx:** watch-and-wait approach is often acceptable; if Rx desired, consider topical (class I) or intralesional CS; less often hydroxychloroquine is used.

Cutaneous Lymphoid Hyperplasia (CLH); also known as 'Pseudolymphoma' or 'Lymphocytoma Cutis'

- A benign, reactive lymphocytic proliferation that is thought to represent an exaggerated local immunologic reaction to a trigger that is usually unidentified.
- Females > males; adults > children.
- Inciting agents that have been reported include arthropod bites, tattoos, vaccinations, medications (e.g. antihistamines, antidepressants, angiotensin II receptor blockers), and in Europe, *Borrelia burgdorferi* infection.
- Presents most often on the head, neck, and upper extremities as one or several firm, erythematous to violaceous papules, plaques, or nodules (Fig. 99.3); usually no surface changes.
- Often spontaneously resolves without scarring.
- **DDx** (see Fig. 99.2): lymphocytic infiltrate of Jessner, lymphoma cutis, leukemia cutis, solid organ metastases, and occasionally adnexal tumors.
- **Rx:** topical (class I) or intralesional CS.

Extramedullary Hematopoiesis

- Most commonly seen in neonates secondary to underlying bone marrow dysfunction; rarely in adults secondary to myelofibrosis, other myeloproliferative disorders or after splenectomy.
- Most often associated with TORCH (*t*oxoplasmosis, *o*ther [e.g. parvovirus B19], *r*ubella, *c*ytomegalovirus) infections in neonates.
- Clinically presents with erythematous to violaceous papules and nodules > plaques, ulcers, or nasal polyps (Fig. 99.4).
- When widely disseminated (typically in neonates) it leads to the classic 'blueberry muffin baby' presentation (Table 99.1).
- Diagnosis is made by histopathology (dermal infiltrates of immature erythrocytes, leukocytes, and megakaryocytes).
- **DDx:** see Table 99.1 for neonates, leukemia cutis in adults.
- **Rx:** treat underlying bone marrow dysfunction; spontaneous resolution typically occurs in cases related to viral infections.

Malignant Hematopoietic Infiltrates

Leukemia Cutis

- Cutaneous lesions associated with both acute and chronic leukemias may be either (1) *nonspecific* reactive skin lesions (Table

973

99.2) or (2) *specific* infiltrates, called 'leukemia cutis'.

• Leukemia cutis typically presents as erythematous to violaceous firm papules or nodules (Fig. 99.5); less often purpura, ulcers, and rarely bullae; lesions may be hemorrhagic due to thrombocytopenia.

• Favors head, neck, trunk, and sites of scars or trauma.

• Less common presentations of leukemia cutis: chloromas, gingival hyperplasia.

• In most patients with acute leukemia, cutaneous lesions (if present) appear at the time of diagnosis or recurrence.

• Occasionally, leukemia cutis antedates the appearance of leukemia in the peripheral smear ('aleukemic leukemia cutis'); rarely predates apparent bone marrow involvement by months.

• **DDx:** lengthy list because of the protean clinical presentations of leukemia cutis, but may include lymphoma cutis, infectious emboli, vasculitis, drug eruptions, Sweet's syndrome and other neutrophilic disorders, extramedullary hematopoiesis.

• **Rx:** treat the underlying leukemia.

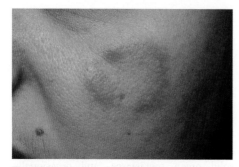

Fig. 99.1 Lymphocytic infiltrate of Jessner. Annular erythematous plaque with central clearing on the face.

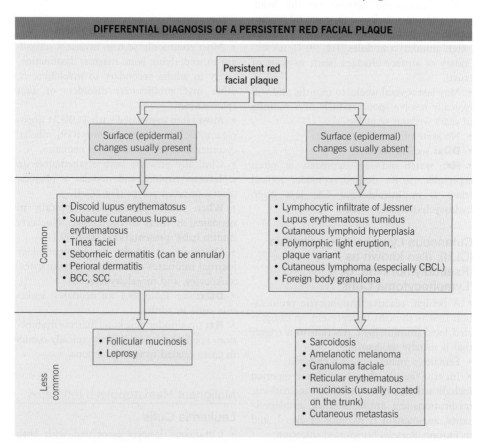

DIFFERENTIAL DIAGNOSIS OF A PERSISTENT RED FACIAL PLAQUE

Persistent red facial plaque

Surface (epidermal) changes usually present

Surface (epidermal) changes usually absent

Common

• Discoid lupus erythematosus
• Subacute cutaneous lupus erythematosus
• Tinea faciei
• Seborrheic dermatitis (can be annular)
• Perioral dermatitis
• BCC, SCC

• Lymphocytic infiltrate of Jessner
• Lupus erythematosus tumidus
• Cutaneous lymphoid hyperplasia
• Polymorphic light eruption, plaque variant
• Cutaneous lymphoma (especially CBCL)
• Foreign body granuloma

Less common

• Follicular mucinosis
• Leprosy

• Sarcoidosis
• Amelanotic melanoma
• Granuloma faciale
• Reticular erythematous mucinosis (usually located on the trunk)
• Cutaneous metastasis

Fig. 99.2 Differential diagnosis of a persistent red facial plaque. BCC, basal cell carcinoma; CBCL, cutaneous B-cell lymphoma; SCC, squamous cell carcinoma.

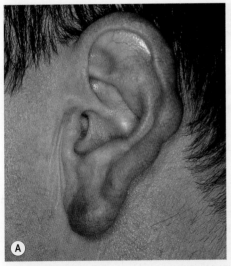

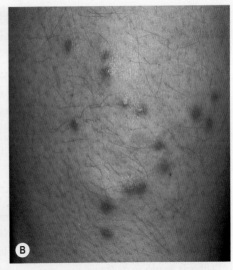

Fig. 99.3 Cutaneous lymphoid hyperplasia (lymphocytoma cutis). A Violet papulonodules on the helix and lobe of the ear (unknown etiology). **B** Multiple red-brown to violet papules at the sites of *Hirudo medicinalis* (medicinal leech) application. *B, Courtesy, Josef Smolle, MD.*

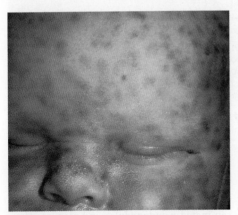

Fig. 99.4 Extramedullary hematopoiesis. 'Blueberry muffin baby' secondary to congenital rubella. *Courtesy, James Graham, MD.*

Hodgkin Disease (HD; Hodgkin Lymphoma)

• **Primary** or isolated cutaneous HD is very unusual; typically presents as one or several ulcerated nodules and usually follows a more indolent course, with prognosis similar to those patients with early stage HD.

• **Secondary** cutaneous HD, occurring in patients with advanced systemic disease, constitutes the vast majority of cutaneous HD

DIFFERENTIAL DIAGNOSIS OF 'BLUEBERRY MUFFIN BABY'

Disseminated extramedullary hematopoiesis
• Prenatal infections (e.g. TORCH)
  – Congenital rubella
  – Cytomegalovirus
  – Toxoplasmosis
  – Coxsackievirus
  – Parvovirus
• Severe and chronic prenatal anemias
  – Severe hemolytic anemias
    • Congenital spherocytosis
    • Rhesus hemolytic disease
    • ABO incompatibility
  – Twin–twin transfusion
  – Chronic fetomaternal hemorrhage
  – Severe internal bleeding (e.g. intracranial)
  – Myelodysplasia, congenital leukemia

Congenital leukemia cutis
Neonatal neuroblastoma
Congenital Langerhans cell histiocytosis
Congenital alveolar cell rhabdomyosarcoma
Hemangiomatosis, other vascular lesions (e.g. multifocal lymphangioendotheliomatosis, glomuvenous malformations)

Table 99.1 Differential diagnosis of 'blueberry muffin baby'.

'INFLAMMATORY' DISORDERS ASSOCIATED WITH ACUTE AND CHRONIC LEUKEMIAS	
Disorder	**Associated Leukemias**
Neutrophilic Dermatoses	
Sweet's syndrome	AML > CML, hairy cell leukemia, CNL > ALL, CLL
Pyoderma gangrenosum*	AML, CML, hairy cell leukemia > ALL, CLL
Neutrophilic eccrine hidradenitis	AML >> ALL, CML, CLL
Reactive Erythemas	
Exaggerated arthropod reactions (eosinophilic dermatosis associated with hematologic disorders)	CLL
Erythroderma	CLL[†]
Vasculitis	
Polyarteritis nodosa	Hairy cell leukemia >> CMML
Vasculitis (small vessel/leukocytoclastic)	Hairy cell leukemia, CLL > AMML, ALL
Erythema elevatum diutinum	Hairy cell leukemia, CLL
Panniculitis	
Erythema nodosum**	AML, CML, CMML
Other panniculitides[‡]	Hairy cell leukemia, AML, CMML
Other	
Paraneoplastic pemphigus	CLL

*Especially bullous.
[†]Many probably represent Sézary syndrome.
**Isolated case reports; may occur concomitantly with Sweet's syndrome.
[‡]Sweet's syndrome may have a subcutaneous component.
ALL, acute lymphoblastic leukemia; AML, acute myelogenous leukemia; AMML, acute myelomonocytic leukemia; CLL, chronic lymphocytic leukemia; CML, chronic myelogenous leukemia; CMML, chronic myelomonocytic leukemia; CNL, chronic neutrophilic leukemia.

Table 99.2 'Inflammatory' disorders associated with acute and chronic leukemias.

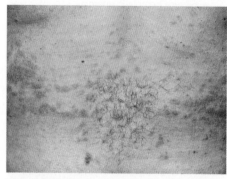

Fig. 99.5 Leukemia cutis. Multiple red-brown papules and plaques in a patient with hairy cell leukemia.

cases and as expected carries a worse prognosis.

• **Secondary** cutaneous HD usually presents with the rapid appearance of multiple, disseminated papulonodules and plaques, often on the trunk (Fig. 99.6), along with locations distal to affected lymph nodes.

Angioimmunoblastic T-Cell Lymphoma (AITL)

• Previously referred to as 'angioimmunoblastic lymphadenopathy' (AILD).

• Now known to be the second most common peripheral T-cell lymphoma with the recent identification of the follicular helper T (T_{FH}) cell as the cell of origin.

• Unique in that it characteristically presents *acutely* with widespread, non-bulky

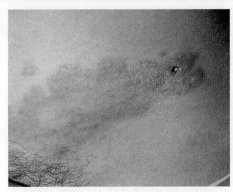

Fig. 99.6 Cutaneous Hodgkin disease (HD). A large pink plaque with central clearing is noted on the lower abdomen.

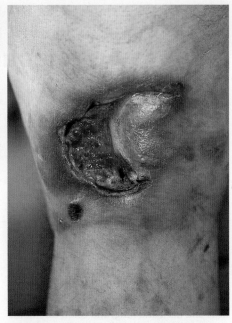

Fig. 99.7 Lymphomatoid granulomatosis. Ulcerated violaceous plaque in the popliteal fossa. *Courtesy, Jean L. Bolognia, MD.*

lymphadenopathy; fever; and a diffuse, pruritic morbilliform eruption mimicking an acute viral infection or drug eruption.

• Other systemic findings include hepatosplenomegaly, polyclonal hypergammaglobulinemia, immune dysregulation resulting in autoantibody production (e.g. ANA, rheumatoid factor, antiphospholipid antibodies, false (+) Lyme serologies), cytopenias and hypereosinophilia.

• The morbilliform eruption and lymphadenopathy typically wax and wane, making suspicion and diagnosis of this malignancy even more elusive.

• The usual course is aggressive with a poor prognosis (median survival is <3 years); up to 30% may have longer-term survival.

• **DDx:** reactive lymphadenopathy due to a viral infection; drug eruption, infectious mononucleosis, or other systemic inflammatory diseases.

• **Rx:** combination chemotherapy; high-dose chemotherapy with autologous stem cell support; allogeneic stem cell transplantation, and newer immunomodulators.

Lymphomatoid Granulomatosis (LYG)

• A rare, EBV-associated, angio-centric/destructive lymphoproliferative disorder that primarily affects the lungs, skin, and nervous system (less often the kidneys and gastrointestinal tract).

• Although previously classified as a reactive process, in most patients it represents a form of large B-cell lymphoma.

• LYG can be divided into grades 1, 2, or 3 depending on the proportion of CD20(+) large lymphoid cells.

• Most often seen in adults; males > females; can occur in the setting of immune dysfunction (e.g. Sjögren's syndrome, rheumatoid arthritis, renal transplantation, HIV infection).

• Frequently presents with cough, dyspnea, chest pain, fever, weight loss, malaise, arthralgia, and myalgia.

• Cutaneous lesions are present in ~25–50% of patients, usually ranging from nodules to ulcerated plaques (Fig. 99.7); rarely an exanthematous eruption develops.

• Typically follows an aggressive, fatal course with a 5-year mortality rate of 60–90%.

• **DDx:** other cutaneous lymphomas, infections (e.g. tuberculosis), pyoderma gangrenosum, medium vessel vasculitis, Wegener's granulomatosis, sarcoidosis.

• **Rx:** rituximab, multidrug chemotherapy, or perhaps interferon-α in earlier stage disease.

For further information see Ch. 121. From *Dermatology, Third Edition.*

100 Cutaneous Metastases

- Relatively rare with the exception of breast cancer and melanoma metastases.
- May be the presenting sign of a malignancy.
- Often associated with a poor prognosis.
- Overall, breast carcinoma most commonly metastasizes to the skin and prostate carcinoma least commonly (Table 100.1).
- Most common skin metastases: women – breast carcinoma, melanoma; men – melanoma, squamous cell carcinoma of the head and neck and lung, and colon carcinoma (Table 100.2).
- In general, nonspecific morphology: firm, mobile, painless papulonodule(s), often skin-colored to pink or red-brown and occasionally ulcerated (Fig. 100.1).
- Other clinical morphologies may be characteristic of a particular primary malignancy (Table 100.3).
- Melanoma metastases vary from pink to blue to black and they may develop along the lymphatic drainage between the primary site and regional lymph nodes (referred to as in-transit metastases; AJCC Stage III) or at distant sites (AJCC Stage IV) (Fig. 100.2).
- Location of cutaneous metastases is generally near the primary tumor, especially when secondary to intralymphatic spread (e.g. squamous cell carcinoma of the head and neck, breast carcinoma).

Metastatic Breast Carcinoma

- May have distinctive clinical morphologies (Fig. 100.3): (1) *carcinoma erysipeloides* – well-demarcated elevated erythema that resembles erysipelas or cellulitis; (2) *carcinoma telangiectoides* – telangiectasias and red papules; and (3) *carcinoma en cuirasse* – begins on the chest as induration with a *peau d'orange* appearance reminiscent of scleredema.

PERCENTAGES OF PATIENTS WITH METASTATIC CANCER WHO HAD CUTANEOUS METASTASES		
Primary Malignancy	Patients with Metastatic Disease (*n* = 4020)	Patients with Cutaneous Metastases (*n* = 420; 10%)
Melanoma	172	77 (45%)
Breast	707	212 (30%)
Squamous cell carcinoma of the head and neck (e.g. laryngeal, oral)	221	29 (13%)
Colon/rectum	413	18 (4.5%)
Lung	802	21 (2.5%)
Prostate	207	0

Adapted from Lookingbill DP, Spangler N, Helm KF. Cutaneous metastases in patients with metastatic carcinoma: A retrospective study of 4020 patients. J. Am. Acad. Dermatol. 1993;29(2 Pt 1):228–236.

Table 100.1 Percentages of patients with metastatic cancer who had cutaneous metastases.

RANKING OF UNDERLYING PRIMARY MALIGNANCIES IN PATIENTS WITH CUTANEOUS METASTASES – MEN VERSUS WOMEN			
Primary Malignancy	**Men with Cutaneous Metastases (n = 127)**	**Primary Malignancy**	**Women with Cutaneous Metastases (n = 300)**
Melanoma	41 (32%)	Breast	212 (70%)
Squamous cell carcinoma of the head and neck	21 (16.5%)	Melanoma	36 (12%)
Lung	15 (12%)		
Colon/rectum	14 (11%)		

Adapted from Lookingbill DP, Spangler N, Helm KF. Cutaneous metastases in patients with metastatic carcinoma: A retrospective study of 4020 patients. J. Am. Acad. Dermatol. 1993;29(2 Pt 1):228–236.

Table 100.2 Ranking of underlying primary malignancies in patients with cutaneous metastases – men versus women.

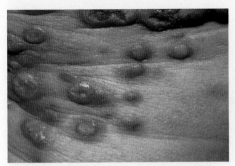

Fig. 100.1 Metastases of adenocarcinoma of the lung. Ulcerated erythematous nodules on the anterior trunk.

Alopecia Neoplastica

- Scarring alopecia of the scalp (Fig. 100.4).
- Associated with breast, lung, gastric, and renal carcinomas.

Sister Mary Joseph Nodule

- Pink to red-brown papule, umbilical or periumbilical (Fig. 100.5).
- Originally described in association with gastric carcinoma.
- May be associated with any abdominal malignancy.

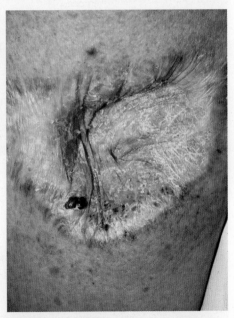

Fig. 100.2 Localized melanoma metastases. Discrete black papules are present within and at the periphery of the skin graft placed at the excision site. *Courtesy, Ronald P. Rapini, MD.*

CLINICAL PRESENTATIONS OF CUTANEOUS METASTASES AND HISTOLOGIC CORRELATES			
Type	**Clinical Description**	**Histology**	**Associated Primary Malignancy**
Dermal or subcutaneous nodules	Small miliary lesions to large tumors; single or multiple	Tumor cells infiltrating among collagen bundles or replacing dermis; Grenz zone often present	Most common presentation; any type
Inflammatory carcinoma (carcinoma erysipeloides)	Erythematous patch with spreading border; resembles erysipelas	Tumor cells within dilated lymphatic vessels	Breast >> lung, ovary, prostate, GI, others
En cuirasse	Morpheaform or sclerodermoid, depending on extent; indurated with *peau d'orange* appearance	Fibrosis with infiltrating tumor cells	Breast >> lung, GI, kidney, others
Carcinoma telangiectoides	Red-violet papules	Tumor cells within superficial blood vessels and RBC sludging	Breast
Paget's disease*	Patches extending from the nipple and areola that resemble dermatitis	Large, atypical epithelial cells with abundant pale cytoplasm arranged in solitary units and small nests within all layers of the epidermis	Breast
Alopecia neoplastica	Nodules or plaques on the scalp in association with alopecia	Cords of tumor cells between collagen bundles	Breast > lung, renal, others
Pyogenic granuloma-like	Rapidly growing nodule resembling a vascular tumor (particularly a pyogenic granuloma)	Neoplastic cells in cords and lobules admixed with prominent hemorrhage and 'pseudovascular' spaces	Renal clear cell carcinoma, hepatocellular carcinoma > others

Lesions of extramammary Paget's disease share similar histopathologic features with those of Paget's disease of the breast, but they usually represent (>75% of patients) primary cutaneous adenocarcinomas (see Table 60.6); an underlying visceral malignancy is most likely when there is perianal involvement. GI, gastrointestinal; RBC, red blood cell.

Table 100.3 Clinical presentations of cutaneous metastases and histologic correlates.
An individual patient can have an admixture of the various types. Occasionally, cutaneous metastases have a zosteriform distribution pattern and clinically they can resemble dermatoses, including eczema, vasculitis, and erythema annulare centrifugum. Obviously, they can also mimic epidermoid or pilar cysts as well as cutaneous tumors, including non-melanoma skin cancers, lipomas, granular cell tumors, or angiosarcoma.

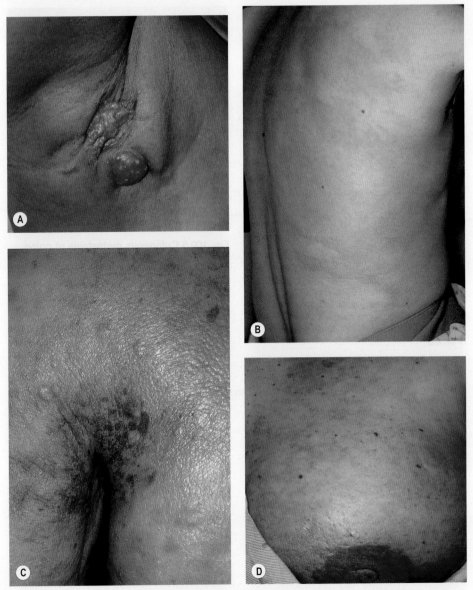

Fig. 100.3 Various presentations of cutaneous metastases of breast carcinoma. A Eroded erythematous nodules in the axilla. **B** Inflammatory form (carcinoma erysipeloides) with patches of erythema that may initially be misdiagnosed as infectious cellulitis. **C** Primarily *en cuirasse* form with obvious induration and *peau d'orange* appearance in addition to papulonodules. **D** Mixed pattern – reticulated erythema of carcinoma erysipeloides as well as *peau d'orange* appearance near the areola. *A, D, Courtesy, Matthew B. Zook, MD, and Stuart R. Lessin, MD.*

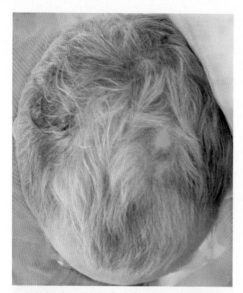

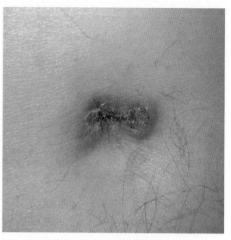

Fig. 100.5 Cutaneous metastasis of colon carcinoma. A Sister Mary Joseph nodule presenting as a pink plaque with scale-crust. *Courtesy, Matthew B. Zook, MD, and Stuart R. Lessin, MD.*

Fig. 100.4 Alopecia neoplastica secondary to metastatic breast carcinoma.
Erythematous, indurated plaques of scarring alopecia on the scalp. *Courtesy, Joslyn S. Kirby, MD.*

For further information see Ch. 122. From *Dermatology, Third Edition.*

Appendix

DETERMINATION OF THE SUN PROTECTION FACTOR (SPF)

- 10 human subjects
- Skin type I or II
- Instrumentation: light source that mimics solar spectrum
- Procedure: determine minimal erythema dose (MED) in protected* and unprotected skin

$$SPF = \frac{MED\ protected}{MED\ unprotected}$$

- To test substantivity – after application and before MED testing:

Water resistant (40): 2 × 20-min water immersions (whirlpool bath)[†]

Water resistant (80): 4 × 20-min water immersions (whirlpool bath)[†]

*Sunscreen product applied at 2 mg/cm².
[†]Air drying in between immersions.

RELATIONSHIP OF THE SUN PROTECTION FACTOR (SPF) TO BLOCKAGE OF ERYTHEMAL RADIATION

SPF	Blockage of Erythemal Radiation (%)
10	90
15	92.5
20	95
40	97.5

LABELING OF SUNSCREENS: ULTRAVIOLET B (UVB) AND ULTRAVIOLET A (UVA) PROTECTION (2011).

Ultraviolet B (UVB) Protection

- Sun protection factor (SPF)*: up to 50+

Ultraviolet A (UVA) Protection

- Either no label or BROAD SPECTRUM
- BROAD SPECTRUM can be used if the critical wavelength is ≥370 nm

Substantivity

- WATER RESISTANT (40 min) or WATER RESISTANT (80 min)
- No use of the following designations: 'WATERPROOF,' 'SUNBLOCK,' 'ALL DAY PROTECTION,' or 'SWEAT PROOF'

Additional Labeling

- If a sunscreen has an SPF ≥15 *and* is BROAD SPECTRUM, then can state that the product can help to reduce the risk of skin cancer and the risk of early skin aging, when used regularly and as directed in combination with other sun protection measures
- If the SPF of the sunscreen is <15 *or* it is not BROAD SPECTRUM, then it must have the following Skin Cancer/Skin Aging Alert: 'Spending time in the sun increases your risk of skin cancer and early skin aging. This product has been shown only to help prevent sunburn, not skin cancer or early skin aging.'

*SPF is also referred to as sunburn protection factor.
Based on the 2011 FDA Final Rule for 'Labeling and Effectiveness Testing; Sunscreen Drug Products for Over-the-Counter Human Use.'

SUNSCREEN AGENTS – MECHANISMS OF ACTION

Sunscreen agents	Inorganic	Organic
Common names	Sunblocks Physical blockers	Sunscreens Chemical absorbers
Mechanism of action	Scatter photons	Absorb photons

- ● Sunblock particle
- ⬡ Sunscreen molecules
- → UV photons
- --→ IR photons

SUNSCREEN AGENTS

	Absorption			
	UVB 290-320	UVA2 320-340	UVA1 340-400	Visible 400-800
Organic or 'chemical absorbers'				
• PABA derivatives [e.g. Padimate O (octyl dimethyl PABA)]				
• Cinnamates				
• Salicylates				
• Benzophenones				
- Oxybenzone (benzophenone-3)				
- Sulisobenzone (benzophenone-4)				
- Dioxybenzone (benzophenone-8)				
• Others				
- Octocrylene				
- Ensulizole (phenylbenzimidazole sulfonic acid)				
- Avobenzone (butyl methoxydibenzoyl methane, Parsol 1789)				
- Menthyl anthranilate (meradimate)				
- Ecamsule (Mexoryl™ SX, terephthalylidene dicamphor sulfonic acid)				
Inorganic or 'physical blockers'*				
• Titanium dioxide				
• Zinc oxide				
Other agents (not considered active screens)				
• Dihydroxyacetone				
• Iron oxide				

*Depending on particle size. Lighter colored bars represent variable efficacy.

FITZPATRICK SCALE OF SKIN PHOTOTYPES

Skin Phototype	Skin Color	Response to UV Irradiation
I	White	Always burns, does not tan
II	White	Burns easily, tans with difficulty
III	Beige	Mild burns, tans gradually
IV	Brown	Rarely burns, tans easily
V	Dark brown	Very rarely burns, tans very easily
VI	Black	Never burns, tans very easily

POTENCY RANKING OF SOME COMMONLY USED TOPICAL GLUCOCORTICOSTEROIDS

Class 1 (superpotent)

- Clobetasol propionate gel, ointment, cream, lotion, foam, spray and shampoo 0.05%
- Betamethasone dipropionate gel* and ointment* 0.05%
- Diflorasone diacetate ointment* 0.05%
- Fluocinonide cream 0.1%
- Flurandrenolide tape 4 mcg/cm^2
- Halobetasol propionate ointment and cream 0.05%

Class 2 (high potency)

- Amcinonide ointment 0.1%
- Betamethasone dipropionate cream*, lotion*, gel and ointment 0.05%
- Clobetasol propionate solution ("scalp application") 0.05%
- Desoximetasone ointment and cream 0.25% and gel 0.05%
- Diflorasone diacetate ointment and cream* 0.05%
- Fluocinonide gel, ointment, cream and solution 0.05%
- Halcinonide ointment, cream and solution 0.1%
- Mometasone furoate ointment 0.1%
- Triamcinolone acetonide ointment 0.5%

Class 3 (high potency)

- Amcinonide cream and lotion 0.1%
- Betamethasone dipropionate cream and lotion 0.05%
- Betamethasone valerate ointment 0.1%
- Diflorasone diacetate cream 0.05%
- Fluticasone propionate ointment 0.005%
- Triamcinolone acetonide ointment 0.1% and cream 0.5%

Class 4 (medium potency)

- Betamethasone valerate foam 0.12%
- Desoximetasone cream 0.05%

- Fluocinolone acetonide ointment 0.025%
- Flurandrenolide ointment 0.05%
- Hydrocortisone valerate ointment 0.2%
- Mometasone furoate cream and lotion 0.1%
- Triamcinolone acetonide ointment (Kenalog®) and cream 0.1% or spray 0.2%

Class 5 (medium potency)

- Betamethasone dipropionate lotion 0.05%
- Betamethasone valerate cream and lotion 0.1%
- Clocortolone pivalate cream 0.1%
- Fluocinolone acetonide cream 0.025% or oil and shampoo 0.01%
- Fluticasone propionate cream and lotion 0.05%
- Flurandrenolide cream and lotion 0.05%
- Hydrocortisone butyrate ointment, cream and lotion 0.1%
- Hydrocortisone probutate cream 0.1%
- Hydrocortisone valerate cream 0.2%
- Prednicarbate ointment and cream 0.1%
- Triamcinolone acetonide ointment 0.025% and lotion 0.1%

Class 6 (low potency)

- Alclometasone dipropionate ointment and cream 0.05%
- Triamcinolone acetonide cream 0.1% (Aristocort®)
- Betamethasone valerate lotion 0.1%
- Desonide gel, ointment, cream, lotion and foam 0.05%
- Fluocinolone acetonide cream and solution 0.01%
- Triamcinolone acetonide cream and lotion 0.025%

Class 7 (low potency)

- Topicals with hydrocortisone, dexamethasone and prednisolone

*Optimized vehicle.

SPECIAL CONSIDERATIONS FOR CORTICOSTEROID AND ANTIHISTAMINE USE DURING PREGNANCY

Corticosteroids

Topical	• Overuse of high-potency products can lead to systemic absorption, and halogenated corticosteroids do cross the placenta; they may also add to the already considerable risk of striae
	• Class 6 and 7 corticosteroids are safest
	• Corticosteroids that have enhanced cutaneous metabolism (e.g. mometasone furoate, prednicarbate, and methylprednisolone aceponate) can also be considered
Systemic	• Prednisolone is the systemic corticosteroid of choice for dermatologic indications because it is largely inactivated in the placenta (mother : fetus = 10 : 1)
	• During the first trimester, particularly between weeks 8 and 11, there is a possible (debated) slightly increased risk of cleft lip/cleft palate, especially if high doses prescribed and for >10 days; during this same period, a longer duration of therapy appears safe if dosages are <10–15 mg daily
	• If use is long term and extends late into gestation, fetal growth should be monitored and the risk of adrenal insufficiency in the newborn should be addressed

Antihistamines

| Systemic | • During the first trimester, the classic sedating agents (e.g. chlorpheniramine, clemastine, dimethindene) are preferred |
| | • During the second and third trimesters, if a nonsedating agent is requested, loratadine and cetirizine are considered safe |

Courtesy, Christina M. Ambros-Rudolph, MD.

CORTICOSTEROID CLASSES

Class A: Hydrocortisone and tixocortol type	Class C: Betamethasone type
Cortisone	Betamethasone
Cortisone acetate	Betamethasone disodium phosphate
Hydrocortisone	Desoximetasone
Hydrocortisone acetate	Dexamethasone
Methylprednisolone	Dexamethasone disodium phosphate
Methylprednisolone acetate	Fluocortolone
Prednisolone	**Class D: Hydrocortisone 17-butyrate and clobetasone 17-butyrate type**
Prednisolone acetate	
Tixocortol pivalate	Aclometasone dipropionate
Class B: Triamcinolone acetonide type	Betamethasone dipropionate
	Betamethasone 17-valerate
Triamcinolone acetonide	Clobetasone butyrate
Triamcinolone alcohol	Clobetasol proprionate
Halcinonide	Fluocortolone hexanoate
Flucinonide	Fluocortolone pivalate
Fluocinolone acetonide	*Hydrocortisone butyrate*
Desonide	Hydrocortisone valerate
Budesonide	Mometasone furoate
Amcinonide	Prednicarbate

Suggested patch test screening agents are in italics for when allergic contact dermatitis to topical CS is suspected; all but hydrocortisone are in the NACDG screening series.

CUTANEOUS MELANOMA PATIENT WORKSHEET

MICROSTAGING OF CUTANEOUS MELANOMA

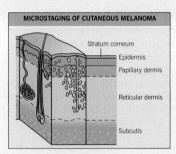

- Stratum corneum
- Epidermis
- Papillary dermis
- Reticular dermis
- Subcutis

Patient name: _____
Date of initial biopsy: _____
Location of lesion: _____
Histologic diagnosis: _____
- Breslow depth: _____
- Ulceration: _____ + or _____ −
- Mitoses/mm^2: _____
- Margins: _____
- Other: _____

MELANOMA TNM CLASSIFICATION

T classification	Thickness	Ulceration status/Mitoses
Tis	NA	NA
T1	≤1.0 mm	a: Without ulceration and mitosis <1/mm2
		b: With ulceration or mitoses ≥1/mm2
T2	1.01–2.0 mm	a: Without ulceration
		b: With ulceration
T3	2.01–4.0 mm	a: Without ulceration
		b: With ulceration
T4	>4.0 mm	a: Without ulceration
		b: With ulceration

N classification	Number of metastatic nodes	Nodal metastatic mass
N0	0	NA
N1	1 node	a: Micrometastasis
		b: Macrometastasis
N2	2–3 nodes	a: Micrometastasis
		b: Macrometastasis
		c: In-transit met(s)/satellite(s) without metastatic node(s)
N3	4 or more metastatic nodes, matted nodes, or in-transit met(s)/satellite(s) with metastatic node(s)	

M classification	Site	Serum lactate dehydrogenase
M0	No distant metastases	NA
M1a	Distant skin, subcutaneous or nodal metastases	Normal
M1b	Lung metastases	Normal
M1c	All other visceral metastases	Normal
	Any distant metastasis	Elevated

STAGE GROUPINGS FOR CUTANEOUS MELANOMA

Survival (% at ~5 years)	Clinical staging T	N	M	Pathologic staging T	N	M
0		Tis	N0	M0	Tis	N0	M0
IA	97	T1a	N0	M0	T1a	N0	M0
IB	93	T1b	N0	M0	T1b		
		T2a			T2a		
IIA	82	T2b	N0	M0	T2b	N0	M0
	79	T3a			T3a		
IIB	68	T3b	N0	M0	T3b	N0	M0
	71	T4a			T4a		
IIC	53	T4b	N0	M0	T4b	N0	M0
III		Any T	N1 N2 N3	M0			
IIIA	78				T1-4a	N1a	M0
					T1-4a	N2a	
IIIB	59				T1-4b	N1a	M0
					T1-4b	N2a	
					T1-4a	N1b	
					T1-4a	N2b	
					T1-4a	N2c	
IIIC	40				T1-4b	N1b	M0
					T1-4b	N2b	
					T1-4b	N2c	
					Any T	N3	
IV	9–27	Any T	Any N	Any M1	Any T	Any N	Any M1

COMPARISON OF SURVIVAL CURVES IN FOUR STAGES OF MELANOMA

Survival rate vs Survival (years), with curves labeled Stage I, Stage II, Stage III, Stage IV.

TNM classification: _____
Stage (clinical): _____
Stage (pathologic): _____

SURGICAL TREATMENT OF PRIMARY CUTANEOUS MELANOMA

Tumor thickness	Excision margins (cm)	Comments
In situ	0.5	Lentigo maligna of the face may be excised with 1cm margins (especially when lesions are >1.5–2 cm in diameter) or treated by Mohs micrographic surgery or radiotherapy; postoperative topical imiquimod is often used
≤1 mm	1.0	Mohs micrographic surgery may be necessary in acral and facial melanomas
1.01–2 mm	1.0–2.0	
>2 mm	2.0	

Treatment plan:
- [ ] Re-excision with _____ cm margins
- [ ] Referral for SLNB and re-excision
- [ ] Referral to oncologist
- [ ] CBC, LFTs, LDH   [ ] CT chest, abdomen, pelvis
- [ ] CXR   [ ] PET/CT
- [ ] Ultrasound: _____
- [ ] MRI: _____
- [ ] Other: _____

SLNB, sentinel lymph node biopsy; CBC, complete blood count; LFTs, liver function tests; LDH, lactate dehydrogenase; CXR, chest x-ray; CT, computed tomography; CT/PET, computed tomography/positron emission tomography; MRI, magnetic resonance imaging.

SLICC* CLASSIFICATION CRITERIA FOR SYSTEMIC LUPUS ERYTHEMATOSUS (2012)

Clinical Criteria	Immunologic Criteria
• Acute^ or subacute cutaneous lupus • Chronic cutaneous lupus^^ • Oral or nasal ulcers • Non-scarring alopecia • Arthritis (synovitis involving ≥ 2 joints) • Serositis (e.g. pleural or pericardial) • Renal (proteinuria ≥ 500mg/24 hours OR RBC casts) • Neurologic (e.g. seizures, psychosis, mononeuritis multiplex, myelitis) • Hemolytic anemia • Leukopenia (<4000/mm^3) OR lymphopenia (<1000/mm^3) • Thrombocytopenia (<100,000/mm^3)	• ANA (above lab reference range) • Anti-ds-DNA (above lab reference range) • Anti-Sm positivity • Antiphospholipid antibody positivity (e.g. positive lupus anticoagulant, false-postive rapid plasma reagin, medium- or high-titer anticardiolipin antibody level, or positive anti-β_2-glycoprotein I antibody) • Low complement (C3, C4, CH50) • Direct Coombs' test (in the absence of hemolytic anemia)

• Criteria for the classification of SLE include: ≥ **4** criteria (at least 1 clinical and 1 immunologic criteria) OR biopsy-proven lupus nephritis with either positive ANA or anti-ds-DNA

*SLICC, Systemic Lupus International Collaborating Clinics.
^Includes malar rash (but not discoid lesions), bullous lupus, toxic epidermal necrolysis variant of SLE, maculopapular lupus rash, photosensitive lupus rash (in the absence of dermatomyositis).
^^Discoid lesions (localized or generalized), hypertrophic lupus, lupus panniculitis, mucosal lupus, LE tumidus, chilblains lupus, discoid lupus/lichen planus overlap.
These revised criteria are intended to be more clinically relevant and to incorporate new immunologic information. They have not been tested for the purposes of SLE diagnosis.
Adapted from Petri M et al. Arthritis Rheum 2012;64:2677.

INSTRUCTIONS FOR OPEN WET DRESSINGS

1. Use a single thickness of thin white cotton material such as a pillowcase, handkerchief, or bed sheet. Do not use a towel or washcloth.

2. Place the material in either (depending upon what is recommended):
   • Warm tap water
   • Domeboro® solution (one packet per 16 oz of water stored in the refrigerator, then brought to room temperature).

3. Squeeze out excess water, do not wring dry.

4. Unravel material and cover red, itchy areas with the wet dressing – **apply as only one (1) layer**. Do not apply additional materials such as a blanket.

5. Allow the wet dressing to remain on the skin for 10–15 minutes.

6. Remove the wet dressing and allow skin to air dry. When the skin is dry, apply the topical corticosteroid prescribed.

7. You may feel chilled if you have covered large areas of your body. If you are treating the entire body then place dressings to one side of the body at a time.

Open wet dressings allow cooling by continuous evaporation of water. They are used to decrease redness, itching, burning and weeping of skin lesions. They will help to make you more comfortable. Apply two to three times per day.

Refer to www.expertconsult.com for a blank template of the drug eruption chart.

Index

Page numbers followed by 'f' indicate figures, 't' indicate tables, and 'b' indicate boxes.

A

B

Index

Index